D1373678

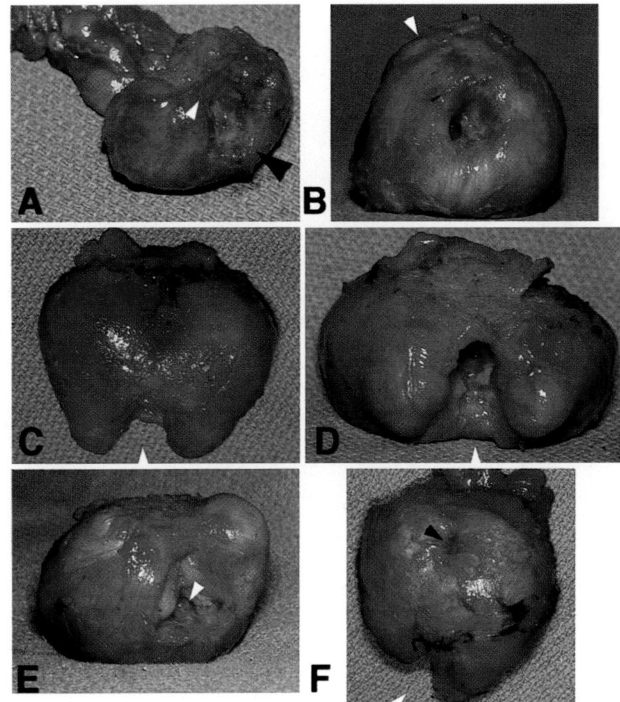

FIGURE 1-1. Variable gross (apical) morphology. **A:** Anterior apical notch with posterior lip (*black arrowhead*). Note tiny anterior commissure (*white arrowhead*). **B:** Doughnut-shaped apex with massive anterior commissure (*white arrowhead*) due to benign prostatic hyperplasia (BPH). **C:** Anterior and posterior apical notches (*white arrowhead*), view from above onto anterior surface of prostate. **D:** Same specimen as in **(C)**. Head-on apical view (*white arrowhead* points to apical urethral opening). **E:** Unusual distortion of apex by BPH nodules (*white arrowhead* points to verumontanum). **F:** Asymmetric apex (*white arrowhead*), bladder neck (*black arrowhead*).

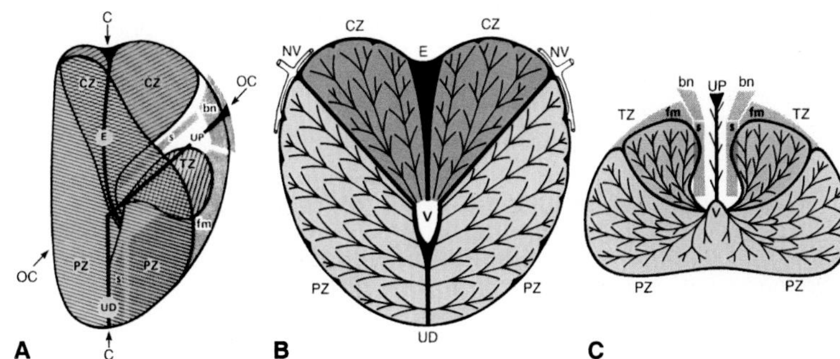

FIGURE 1-2. Zonal architecture of the prostate. **A:** Sagittal. **B:** Coronal. **C:** Oblique coronal. Note duct radiation from verumontanum (V). bn, bladder neck; C, coronal plane; CZ, central zone; E, ejaculatory duct; fm, fibromuscular stroma; NV, neurovascular tissue; OC, oblique coronal plane; PZ, peripheral zone; s, sphincter; TZ, transition zone; UD, distal prostatic urethra; UP, proximal prostatic urethra. (From McNeal JE. The prostate gland: morphology and pathobiology. *Monogr Urol* 1988;9:36–54, with permission of Thomas A. Stamey.)

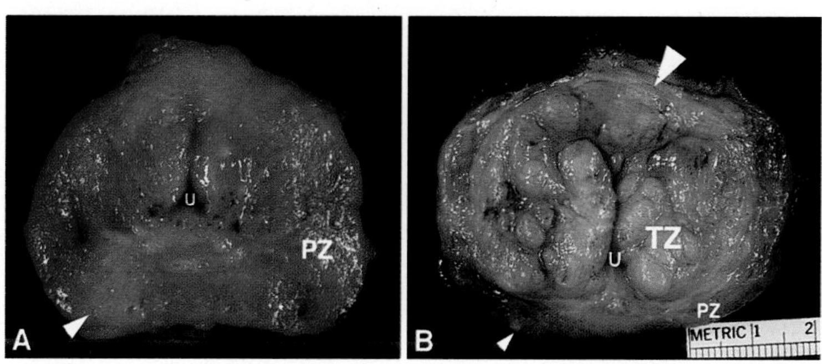

FIGURE 1-3. Prostate cancer in gross axial section. **A:** Peripheral zone (PZ) cancer (*arrowhead*). Cut surface is homogeneous with no evidence of either transition zone (TZ) or lobulation. **B:** TZ cancer (*large arrowhead*) and PZ cancer (*small arrowhead*). Prominent benign prostatic hyperplasia of TZ displaces peripheral zone outward. U, urethra. (Courtesy of Dr. David G. Bostwick.)

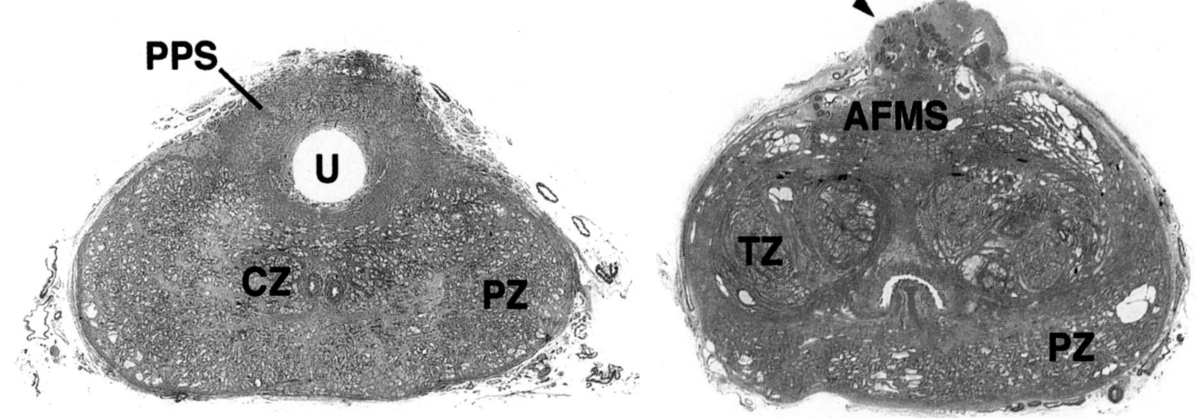

FIGURE 1-4. Axial section morphology (Masson trichrome). **A:** Section at base of prostate from 44-year-old patient without benign prostatic hyperplasia (BPH) shows relatively homogeneous acini without visible lobulation. Central zone (CZ) acini next to ejaculatory ducts seen below urethra (U) have sparse basophilic stroma compared with rich eosinophilic stroma of peripheral zone (PZ) acini. **B:** In section near apex, bilateral nodular BPH [transition zone (TZ)] distorts and compresses PZ outward. Venous plexus was bunched anteriorly before fixation. Note bundled detrusor fibers (*arrowhead*) from anterior detrusor apron. AFMS, anterior fibromuscular stroma; PPS, preprostatic sphincter.

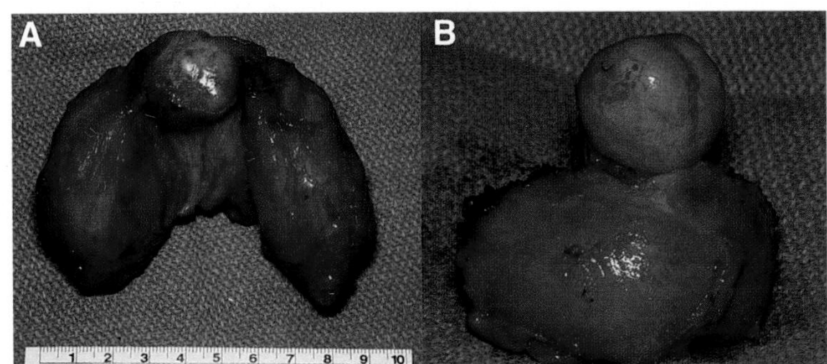

FIGURE 1-6. Lobes of benign prostatic hyperplasia (BPH). **A:** Enucleated trilobar BPH specimen weighing 105 g. **B:** Radical prostatectomy specimen with "ball valve" median lobe BPH at the bladder neck.

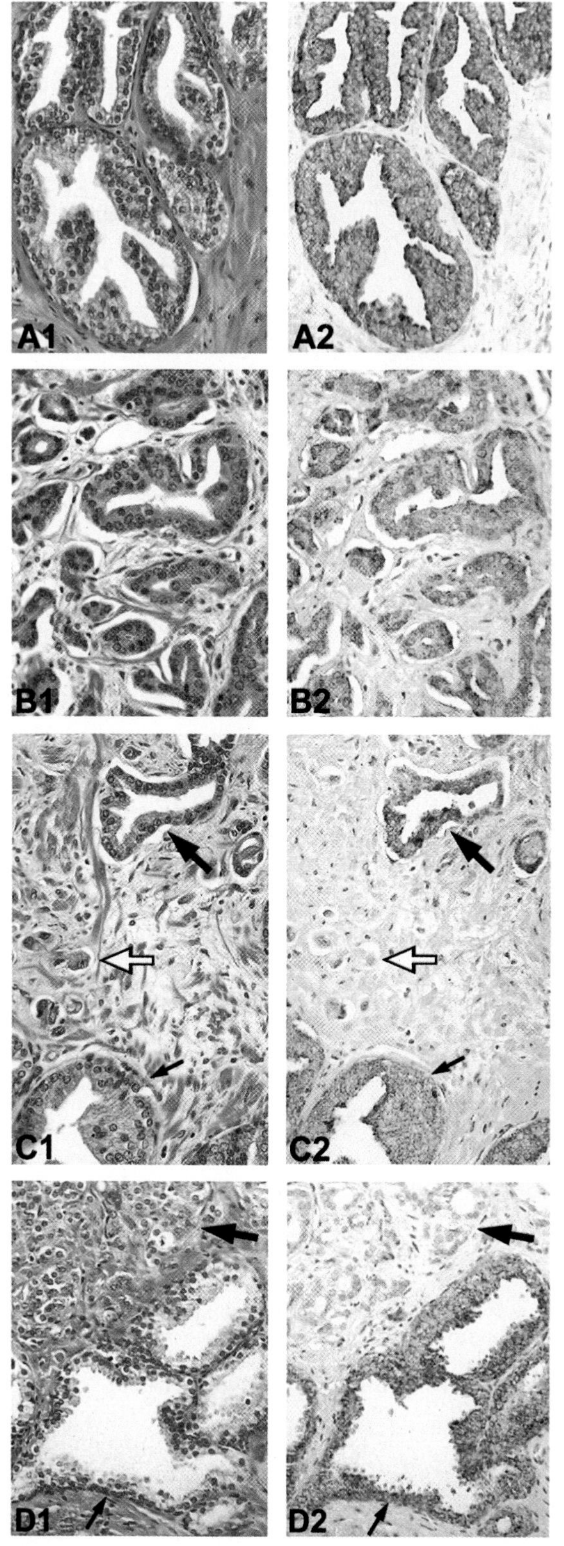

FIGURE 20-2. PTEN expression in prostate tissue. **A:** Hematoxylin-eosin (H&E) of prostatic intraepithelial neoplasia (PIN) **(A1)** and staining for PTEN **(A2)**. **B:** H&E-stained section of prostate cancer (CaP) (Gleason 6) **(B1)** and staining for PTEN **(B2)**. **C:** H&E-stained sections of CaP, Gleason grade 3 (*large black arrow*), and grade 5 cancer (*open arrow*), and PIN (*short black arrow*) **(C1)**. Gleason grade 3 CaP (*large black arrow*) and PIN (*short black arrow*) are PTEN positive, whereas Gleason grade 5 CaP is PTEN negative (*open arrow*) **(C2)**. **D:** H&E of benign prostatic acinus (*small arrow*) with surrounding Gleason 7 CaP (*large arrow*) **(D1)**. Positive staining for PTEN in benign prostate tissue and absence of staining for PTEN in CaP **(D2)**.

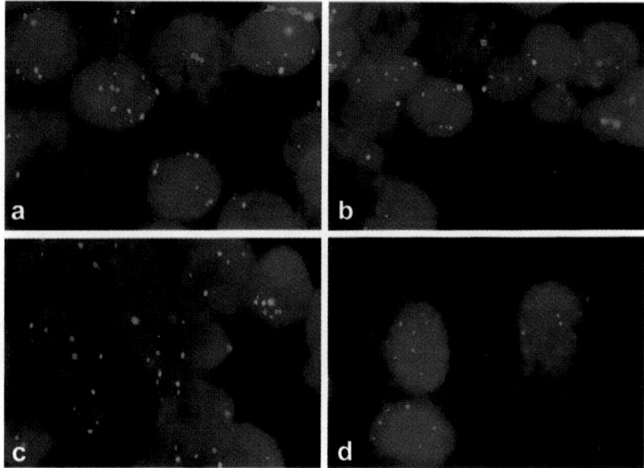

FIGURE 20-3. Fluorescent in situ hybridization analysis looking at c-myc and prostate stem cell antigen (PSCA) copy number in two patients with locally advanced prostate cancer. In **(A)** and **(C)**, for case No. 34 there is simple gain of chromosome 8 without any additional increase in c-myc or PSCA copy number. **A:** Most nuclei have three signals for both c-myc (*red*) and a probe for the centromere (*green*). A similar result is seen in **(C)**, with three signals for PSCA (*red*) and CEP-8 (green). In **(B)** and **(D)**, for case No. 75 there is additional increase in PSCA and c-myc copy number compared with the centromere, indicative of amplification of these two loci. **B:** There are, on average, five red signals (c-myc) and two green signals (CEP-8). Similarly, **(D)** there are five red signals (PSCA) and two green signals (CEP-8), again consistent with an additional increase of PSCA copy number.

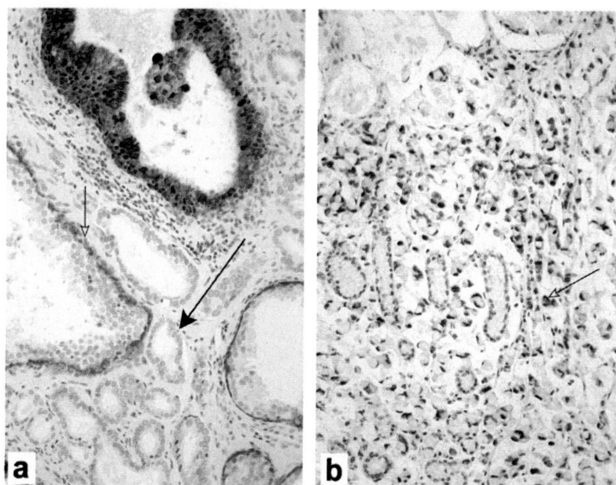

FIGURE 20-4. **A:** Positive staining for maspin localized to the basal cells (*small arrow*) and prostate intraepithelial neoplasia (*top*) and absence of staining in Gleason grade 3 tumor (*large arrow*). **B:** Positive staining for maspin in androgen-independent tumor (*small arrow*).

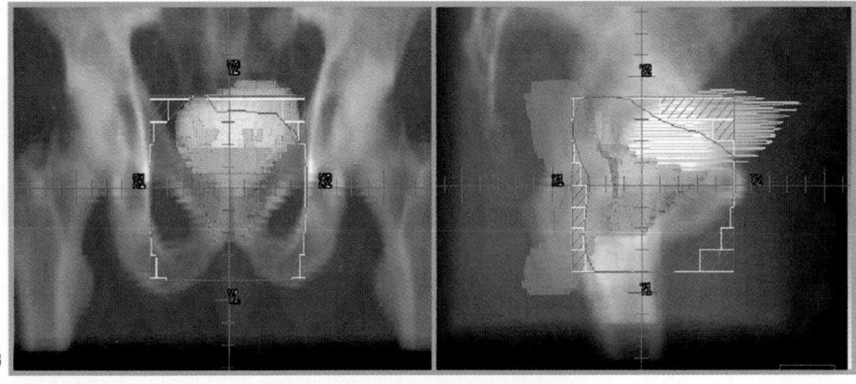

A,B

FIGURE 33-1. Example of adjuvant conformal radiation therapy fields. The prostate bed is shown in tomato, the rest of the bladder in yellow, surgical clips in blue (green when overlaying yellow), and the rectum in green. **A:** Anterior-posterior view. **B:** Right lateral view.

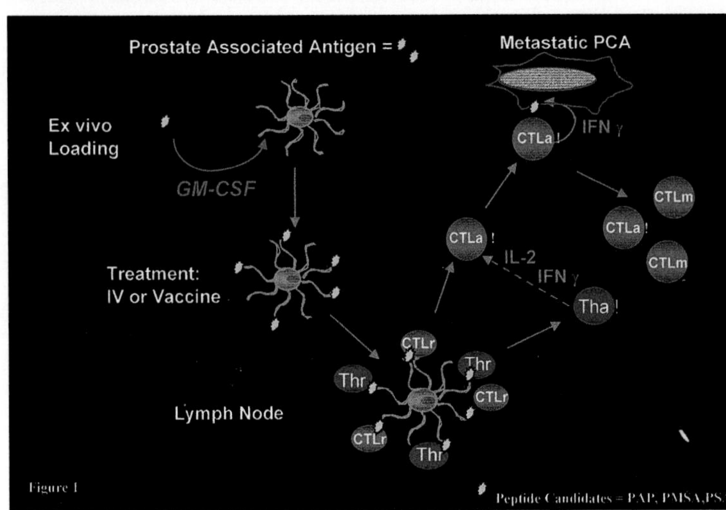

FIGURE 54-1. Prostate peptide loading of dendritic cells. CTLa, cytoxic T lymphocyte–associated antigen; CTLm, CTL memory; GM-CSF, granulocyte-macrophage colony stimulating factor; IFNγ, interferon γ; IL-2, interleukin 2; PAP, prostatic acid phosphatase antigen; PCA, prostate cancer; PSA, prostate-specific antigen; PSMA, prostate-specific membrane antigen; Tha, T-cell helper activate; Thr, threonine.

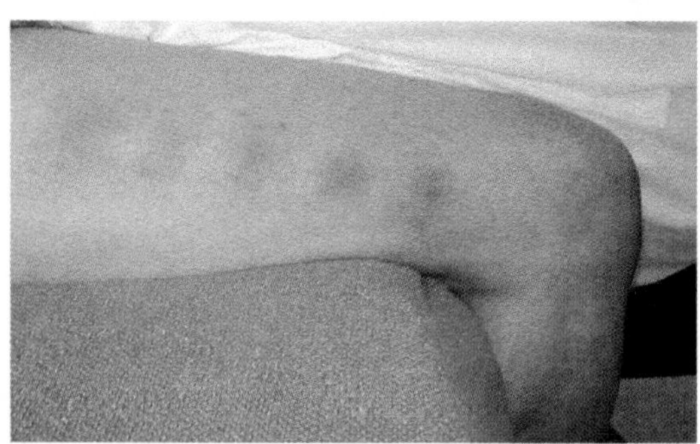

FIGURE 54-4. Outpatient safety of genetically engineered prostate cancer vaccines: activating dendritic cell antigen presentation intradermally 24 hours postvaccination. Allogeneic granulocyte-macrophage colony-stimulating factor gene–transduced irradiated prostate cancer vaccine cells.

PROSTATE CANCER: PRINCIPLES AND PRACTICE

PROSTATE CANCER: PRINCIPLES AND PRACTICE

Editors

PHILIP W. KANTOFF, M.D.

PETER R. CARROLL, M.D.

ANTHONY V. D'AMICO, M.D., PH.D.

Section Editors

RONALD K. ROSS, M.D.

JOHN T. ISAACS, PH.D.

HOWARD I. SCHER, M.D.

LIPPINCOTT WILLIAMS & WILKINS

A **Wolters Kluwer** Company

Philadelphia • Baltimore • New York • London
Buenos Aires • Hong Kong • Sydney • Tokyo

Acquisitions Editor: Jonathan Pine
Developmental Editor: Joanne Bersin and William Wiebalck
Production Editor: Erica Broennle, Silverchair Science + Communications
Manufacturing Manager: Benjamin Rivera
Cover Designer: Mark Lerner
Compositor: Silverchair Science + Communications
Printer: Edwards Brothers

530 Walnut Street
Philadelphia, PA 19106 USA
LWW.com

Printed in the USA

Library of Congress Cataloging-in-Publication Data

Prostate cancer : principles and practice / edited by Philip Kantoff, Peter Carroll, Anthony V. D'Amico ; with sections edited by John Isaacs, Ronald Ross, Howard Scher.-- 1st ed.
p. ; cm.
Includes bibliographical references and index.
ISBN 0-7817-2006-0
1. Prostate--Cancer. I. Kantoff, Philip. II. Carroll, Peter R. III. D'Amico, Anthony V.
[DNLM: 1. Prostatic Neoplasms. WJ 752 P9655352 2001]
RC280.P7598 2001
616.99'463--dc21

2001038420

---

10 9 8 7 6 5 4 3 2 1

The editors would like to dedicate this book to our patients and their families, from whom we have learned a great deal about prostate cancer and ourselves.

CONTENTS

SECTION IV: EARLY PROSTATE CANCER—SINGLE MODALITY TREATMENT

Anthony V. D'Amico and Peter R. Carroll

SECTION V: EARLY PROSTATE CANCER—MULTIMODALITY TREATMENT

Anthony V. D'Amico and Peter R. Carroll

SECTION VI: ADVANCED HORMONE-SENSITIVE DISEASE

Peter R. Carroll and Philip W. Kantoff

SECTION VII: HORMONE-REFRACTORY DISEASE

Howard I. Scher and Philip W. Kantoff

SECTION VIII: HORMONE REFRACTORY DISEASE—CURRENT STANDARDS AND FUTURE DIRECTIONS

Philip W. Kantoff and Howard I. Scher

CONTRIBUTING AUTHORS

Cory Abate-Shen, Ph.D. Associate Professor, Center for Advanced Biotechnology and Medicine, University of Medicine and Dentistry of New Jersey—Robert Wood Johnson Medical School, Piscataway, New Jersey

Peter C. Albertsen, M.D., M.S. Professor, Division of Urology, University of Connecticut School of Medicine; Chief, Division of Urology, University of Connecticut Health Center, Farmington, Connecticut

Gerald L. Andriole, M.D. Professor and Chief, Division of Urologic Surgery, Washington University School of Medicine, St. Louis, Missouri

John C. Blasko, M.D. Department of Radiation Oncology, University of Washington School of Medicine, Seattle, Washington

Elizabeth Breen, M.D. Assistant Professor of Surgery, Harvard Medical School; Attending Surgeon, Brigham and Women's Hospital, Boston, Massachusetts

David C. Brooks, M.D., F.A.C.S. Associate Professor of Surgery, Harvard Medical School; Director, Minimally Invasive Surgery, Brigham and Women's Hospital, Boston, Massachusetts

James D. Brooks, M.D. Assistant Professor of Urology, Stanford University School of Medicine, Stanford, California

Myles A. Brown, M.D. Associate Professor of Medicine, Harvard Medical School; Department of Adult Oncology, Dana-Farber Cancer Institute, Boston, Massachusetts

Glenn J. Bubley, M.D. Associate Professor of Medicine, Harvard Medical School; Department of Cancer Biology, Beth Israel Deaconess Medical Center, Boston, Massachusetts

Arnold D. Bullock, M.D. Assistant Professor of Urology, Department of Surgery, Division of Urology, Washington University School of Medicine, St. Louis, Missouri

Michael A. Carducci, M.D. Assistant Professor of Oncology, The Johns Hopkins University School of Medicine, Baltimore, Maryland

Peter R. Carroll, M.D. Professor and Chair, Department of Urology, University of California, San Francisco, School of Medicine, San Francisco, California

Barrie R. Cassileth, Ph.D. Chief, Integrative Medicine Service, Memorial Sloan-Kettering Cancer Center, New York, New York

Gerald W. Chodak, M.D. Clinical Professor of Surgery, University of Chicago Pritzker School of Medicine; Weiss Memorial Hospital, Chicago, Illinois

Gerhard A. Coetzee, Ph.D. Associate Professor of Urology, Microbiology, and Preventative Medicine, Norris Comprehensive Cancer Center, University of Southern California School of Medicine, Los Angeles, California

Gerald R. Cunha, Ph.D. Professor of Anatomy, University of California, San Francisco, School of Medicine, San Francisco, California

Anthony V. D'Amico, M.D., Ph.D. Associate Professor of Radiation Oncology, Harvard Medical School; Chief, Genitourinary Radiation Oncology, Dana-Farber Cancer Institute; Brigham and Women's Hospital, Boston, Massachusetts

Rajvir Dahiya, Ph.D. Department of Urology, University of California, San Francisco, School of Medicine, San Francisco, California

Nancy A. Dawson, M.D. Professor of Medicine, Greenebaum Cancer Center, University of Maryland School of Medicine, Baltimore, Maryland

Angelo M. De Marzo, M.D., Ph.D. Assistant Professor of Pathology, Urology, and Oncology, Department of Pathology, The Johns Hopkins University School of Medicine, Baltimore, Maryland

Samuel R. Denmeade, M.D. Assistant Professor, Department of Oncology, The Johns Hopkins University School of Medicine, Baltimore, Maryland

Theodore L. DeWeese, M.D. Assistant Professor of Radiation Oncology and Urology; Director, Radiation Biology Program, Department of Oncology, The Johns Hopkins University School of Medicine, Baltimore, Maryland

Annemarie A. Donjacour, Ph.D. Assistant Research Anatomist, Department of Anatomy, University of California, San Francisco, School of Medicine, San Francisco, California

Beverly Drucker, M.D., Ph.D. Senior Postdoctoral Fellow, Department of Oncology, The Johns Hopkins University School of Medicine, Baltimore, Maryland

Mario A. Eisenberger, M.D. Professor of Oncology and Urology, Department of Oncology, The Johns Hopkins University School of Medicine, Baltimore, Maryland

Jonathan I. Epstein, M.D. Professor of Pathology, Urology, and Oncology, The Johns Hopkins University School of Medicine, Baltimore, Maryland

Phillip G. Febbo, M.D. Instructor in Medicine, Harvard Medical School; Lank Center for Genitourinary Oncology, Department of Adult Oncology, Dana-Farber Cancer Institute, Boston, Massachusetts

Daniel J. George, M.D. Instructor in Medicine, Harvard Medical School; Lank Center for Genitourinary Oncology, Department of Adult Oncology, Dana-Farber Cancer Institute, Boston, Massachusetts

Edward L. Giovannucci, M.D., Sc.D. Associate Professor, Departments of Nutrition and Epidemiology, Harvard University School of Public Health, Harvard Medical School, Boston, Massachusetts

Peter D. Grimm, D.O. Director, Seattle Prostate Institute, Seattle, Washington

Gary D. Grossfeld, M.D. Assistant Professor of Urology, Mt. Zion Comprehensive Cancer Center, University of California, San Francisco, School of Medicine, San Francisco, California

M. Craig Hall, M.D. Associate Professor of Urology, Wake Forest University School of Medicine; Wake Forest University Baptist Medical Center, Winston-Salem, North Carolina

Simon W. Hayward, Ph.D. Assistant Professor, Department of Urology, University of California, San Francisco, School of Medicine, San Francisco, California

Brent K. Hollenbeck, M.D. Resident Physician, Department of Surgery-Urology, University of Michigan Medical School, Ann Arbor, Michigan

Hedvig Hricak, M.D., Ph.D. Professor of Radiology, Weill Medical College of Cornell University; Memorial Sloan-Kettering Cancer Center, New York, New York

John T. Isaacs, Ph.D. Professor of Oncology and Urology, Department of Oncology, The Johns Hopkins University School of Medicine, Baltimore, Maryland

William B. Isaacs, Ph.D. Professor of Urology and Oncology, Department of Urology, The Johns Hopkins University School of Medicine, Baltimore, Maryland

Philip W. Kantoff, M.D. Associate Professor of Medicine, Harvard Medical School; Director, Lank Center for Genitourinary Oncology, Dana-Farber Cancer Institute, Boston, Massachusetts

Nathaniel P. Katz, M.D. Assistant Professor of Anesthesia, Harvard Medical School, Boston, Massachusetts

Donald S. Kaufman, M.D. Clinical Professor of Medicine, Harvard Medical School; Director, Genitourinary Oncology Disease Center, Massachusetts General Hospital, Boston, Massachusetts

William K. Kelly, D.O. Assistant Professor of Medicine, Genitourinary Oncology Service, Memorial Sloan-Kettering Cancer Center; Department of Medicine, Weill Medical College of Cornell University, New York, New York

Hakan Kuyu, M.D. Staff Oncologist/Hematologist, Spokane Veterans Administration Medical Center, Spokane, Washington

Paul H. Lange, M.D. Professor and Chairman of Urology, University of Washington School of Medicine, Seattle, Washington

Menachem Laufer, M.D. Oncology Center, The Johns Hopkins University School of Medicine, Baltimore, Maryland

Daniel W. Lin, M.D. Fellow, Urologic Oncology, Department of Urology, Memorial Sloan-Kettering Cancer Center, New York, New York

Mark S. Litwin, M.D., M.P.H. Associate Professor of Urology and Health Services, University of California, Los Angeles, UCLA School of Medicine, Los Angeles, California

Massimo Loda, M.D. Associate Professor of Pathology, Harvard Medical School; Lank Center for Genitourinary Oncology, Department of Adult Oncology, Dana-Farber Cancer Institute; Department of Pathology, Brigham and Women's Hospital, Boston, Massachusetts

John P. Long, M.D. Associate Professor of Urology, Tufts University School of Medicine; New England Medical Center, Boston, Massachusetts

Paul C. Marker, Ph.D. Postdoctoral Fellow, Department of Anatomy, University of California, San Francisco, School of Medicine, San Francisco, California

Maxwell V. Meng, M.D. Clinical Instructor, Department of Urology, University of California, San Francisco, School of Medicine, San Francisco, California

Jeff M. Michalski, M.D. Assistant Professor of Radiology, Mallinckrodt Institute of Radiology, Washington University School of Medicine, St. Louis, Missouri

James E. Montie, M.D. Chairman and Valassis Professor of Urologic Oncology, Department of Urology, University of Michigan Medical School, Ann Arbor, Michigan

Michael J. Morris, M.D. Clinical Assistant Physician, Department of Medicine, Memorial Sloan-Kettering Cancer Center, New York, New York

Judd W. Moul, M.D., F.A.C.S. Colonel, Medical Corps, U.S. Army and Professor of Surgery, Uniformed Services University of the Health Sciences F. Edward Hébert School of Medicine; Director, Department of Defense Center for Prostate Disease Research; Attending Urologic Oncologist, Walter Reed Army Medical Center, Washington, District of Columbia

Robert P. Myers, M.D. Professor of Urology, Mayo Medical School, Rochester, Minnesota

William G. Nelson, M.D., Ph.D. Associate Professor of Oncology, Urology, Pharmacology, Medicine, and Pathology, Department of Medical Oncology, Division of Experimental Therapeutics, The Johns Hopkins University School of Medicine, Baltimore, Maryland

William K. Oh, M.D. Assistant Professor of Medicine, Harvard Medical School; Lank Center for Genitourinary Oncology, Department of Adult Oncology, Dana-Farber Cancer Institute, Boston, Massachusetts

Michael O'Leary, M.D. Instructor in Surgery, Division of Urology, Brigham and Women's Hospital, Boston, Massachusetts

Alan W. Partin, M.D., Ph.D. Bernard L. Schwartz Distinguished Professor of Urologic Oncology, Department of Urology and Oncology, The Johns Hopkins University School of Medicine, Baltimore, Maryland

Daniel P. Petrylak, M.D. Assistant Professor of Medicine, Columbia University College of Physicians and Surgeons, New York, New York

Roberto Pili, M.D. Assistant Professor of Oncology, Oncology Center, The Johns Hopkins University School of Medicine, Baltimore, Maryland

Elizabeth A. Platz, Sc.D., M.P.H. Assistant Professor of Epidemiology, The Johns Hopkins University School of Hygiene and Public Health, Baltimore, Maryland

Alan Pollack, M.D., Ph.D. Professor and Chairman, Department of Radiation Oncology, Fox Chase Cancer Center, Philadelphia, Pennsylvania

Brent Andrew Ponce, M.D. Resident, Combined Orthopaedic Surgery Residency Program, Harvard Medical School, Boston, Massachusetts

Steven R. Potter, M.D. Instructor of Urology, The Johns Hopkins University School of Medicine, Baltimore, Maryland

Isaac J. Powell, M.D. Professor of Urology, Wayne State University School of Medicine; Harper University Hospital, Detroit, Michigan

Joseph C. Presti, Jr., M.D. Associate Professor of Urology, Stanford University School of Medicine, Stanford, California

Derek Raghavan, M.D., Ph.D., F.R.A.C.P., F.A.C.P. Chief, Division of Medical Oncology; Professor of Medicine and Urology; Associate Director, Norris Comprehensive Cancer Center, University of Southern California School of Medicine, Los Angeles, California

John E. Ready, M.D. Instructor, Harvard Medical School; Orthopedic Surgeon, Brigham and Women's Hospital, Boston, Massachusetts

David M. Reese, M.D. Associate Clinical Professor of Medicine, University of California, San Francisco, School of Medicine, San Francisco, California

Jason Reingold Medical Student Scholar, Winship Cancer Institute, Emory University School of Medicine, Atlanta, Georgia

Jerome P. Richie, M.D. Elliott C. Cutler Professor of Surgery, Department of Urology, Harvard Medical School, Boston, Massachusetts

Brian I. Rini, M.D. Assistant Professor, Department of Medicine, University of California, San Francisco, School of Medicine, San Francisco, California

Mack Roach III, M.D. Professor of Radiation Oncology, Medical Oncology, and Urology, University of California, San Francisco, School of Medicine, San Francisco, California

Ronald K. Ross, M.D. Professor and Chair, Department of Preventative Medicine, Norris Comprehensive Cancer Center, University of Southern California, Los Angeles, California

Martin G. Sanda, M.D. Associate Professor of Urology and Oncology, University of Michigan Medical School, Ann Arbor, Michigan

Oliver Sartor, M.D. Patricia Powers Strong Professor of Oncology and Chief, Hematology/Oncology Section, Department of Medicine, Louisiana State University School of Medicine in New Orleans, New Orleans, Louisiana

Charles L. Sawyers, M.D. Professor of Medicine and Urology, Departments of Medicine and Hematology-Oncology, University of California, Los Angeles, UCLA School of Medicine, Los Angeles, California

Paul F. Schellhammer, M.D. Professor and Chairman, Department of Urology, Eastern Virginia Medical School of the Medical College of Hampton Roads; Program Director, Virginia Prostate Center of the Sentara Cancer Institute, Norfolk, Virginia

Howard I. Scher, M.D. Professor of Medicine, Weill Medical College of Cornell University, New York, New York

David Schiff, M.D. Assistant Professor of Neurological Surgery, Neurology, and Medicine, University of Pittsburgh School of Medicine, Pittsburgh, Pennsylvania

William R. Sellers, M.D. Assistant Professor of Medicine, Harvard Medical School; Lank Center for Genitourinary Oncology, Department of Adult Oncology, Dana-Farber Cancer Institute, Boston, Massachusetts

John W. Sharp, M.S.S.A. Web Administrator, Information Technology Division, Cleveland Clinic, Cleveland, Ohio

Michael M. Shen, Ph.D. Associate Professor of Pediatrics, Center for Advanced Biotechnology and Medicine and Department of Pediatrics, University of Medicine and Dentistry of New Jersey—Robert Wood Johnson Medical School, Piscataway, New Jersey

Katsuto Shinohara, M.D. Associate Professor of Urology, University of California, San Francisco, School of Medicine, San Francisco, California

William U. Shipley, M.D. Professor of Radiation Oncology, Harvard Medical School; Deputy Head for Clinical Research, Department of Radiation Oncology, Massachusetts General Hospital, Boston, Massachusetts

Jonathan W. Simons, M.D. Professor and Chair of Hematology and Oncology and Director, Winship Cancer Institute, Emory University School of Medicine, Atlanta, Georgia

Eric J. Small, M.D. Clinical Professor of Medicine and Urology, University of California, San Francisco, School of Medicine; Co-Director, Urologic Oncology Practice, Comprehensive Cancer Center, University of California Medical Center, San Francisco

Lewis G. Smith, M.D. Instructor, Department of Radiation Oncology, M. D. Anderson Cancer Center, Houston, Texas

Matthew R. Smith, M.D., Ph.D. Assistant Professor of Medicine, Harvard Medical School; Massachusetts General Hospital, Boston, Massachusetts

David B. Solit, M.D. Department of Medicine, Weill Medical College of Cornell University; Clinical Assistant Attending, Genitourinary Oncology Service, Memorial Sloan-Kettering Cancer Center, New York, New York

Mark S. Soloway, M.D. Professor and Chairman, Department of Urology, University of Miami School of Medicine, Miami, Florida

Joycelyn L. Speight, M.D., Ph.D. Clinical Instructor, Department of Radiation Oncology, University of California, San Francisco, School of Medicine, San Francisco, California

Graeme Scott Steele, M.D., F.C.S. Assistant Professor, Urological Surgery, Harvard Medical School; Brigham and Women's Hospital, Boston, Massachusetts

John E. Sylvester, M.D. Director of Education and Training, Seattle Prostate Institute; Swedish Hospital, Seattle, Washington

James A. Talcott, M.D., S.M. Assistant Professor of Medicine, Harvard Medical School; Department of Medicine, Division of Hematology-Oncology, Massachusetts General Hospital, Boston, Massachusetts

George V. Thomas, M.D., M.R.C.P.I. Research Fellow, University of California, Los Angeles, UCLA School of Medicine; Department of Pathology and Laboratory Medicine, Center for Health Sciences, University of California, Los Angeles, California

Axel A. Thomson, Ph.D. Principal Investigator, Medical Research Council, Human Reproductive Sciences Unit, Edinburgh, United Kingdom

Frank M. Torti, M.D. Professor of Medicine and Chairman, Department of Cancer Biology, Wake Forest University School of Medicine; Director, Comprehensive Cancer Center, Wake Forest University Baptist Medical Center, Winston-Salem, North Carolina

Robert L. Vessella, Ph.D. Professor of Urology, University of Washington School of Medicine, Seattle, Washington

Andrew J. Vickers, D.Phil. Assistant Attending Research Methodologist, Department of Integrative Medicine Service and Department of Biostatistics, Memorial Sloan-Kettering Cancer Center, New York, New York

Nicholas J. Vogelzang, M.D. Fred C. Buffett Professor of Medicine, Surgery (Urology), and the Ben May Institute for Cancer Research, University of Chicago Pritzker School of Medicine; Director, University of Chicago Cancer Research Center, Chicago, Illinois

Ashani T. Weeraratna, Ph.D. Postdoctoral Fellow, National Human Genome Research Institute Cancer Genetics Branch, National Institutes of Health, Bethesda, Maryland

Antje E. Wefer, M.D. Department of Radiology, Hannover Medical School, Hannover, Germany

Patrick Y. Wen, M.D. Associate Professor of Neurology, Harvard Medical School; Center for Neuro-oncology, Dana-Farber Cancer Institute, Boston, Massachusetts

Jeff A. Wieder, M.D. Fellow and Clinical Instructor, Department of Urology, University of California, Los Angeles, UCLA School of Medicine, Los Angeles, California

George Wilding, M.D. Professor of Medicine and Associate Director, Comprehensive Cancer Center, University of Wisconsin Medical School, Madison, Wisconsin

Jianfeng Xu, M.D., Dr.PH. Associate Professor of Public Health, Center for Human Genomics, Wake Forest University School of Medicine, Winston-Salem, North Carolina

Michael J. Zelefsky, M.D. Chief of Brachytherapy, Associate Professor of Radiation Oncology, Memorial Sloan-Kettering Cancer Center, New York, New York

Anthony L. Zietman, M.D. Associate Professor of Radiation Oncology, Harvard Medical School; Massachusetts General Hospital, Boston, Massachusetts

PREFACE

Prostate cancer has emerged as a major public health issue and significant cause of morbidity and mortality in the United States. This has resulted from a congruence of factors, including the introduction and widespread use of prostate-specific antigen testing, heightened public awareness, the aging of the American populace, and increasing interest in men's health issues. Although a large and expanding body of knowledge is available on the etiology, diagnosis, and treatment of this disease, much remains to be learned. There remains no consensus on the benefits, if any, of early prostate cancer detection and what constitutes the best form of treatment for most stages of disease. The editors are concerned about the apparent compartmentalization of information between basic and clinical scientists, as well as between the different disciplines involved in patient care. *Prostate Cancer: Principles and Practice* was created out of a need to improve the connection of the basic and clinical sciences, to help bridge the gaps between the different clinical disciplines, and to provide a current and comprehensive assessment of the field for all involved in research and treatment of prostate cancer. We hope that *Prostate Cancer: Principles and Practice* will be a critical reference to physicians caring for patients, as well as function as a platform for future progress. *Prostate Cancer: Principles and Practice* addresses basic cancer biology, as well as current and future treatment types. We called on a large and diverse group of authors to cover the entire spectrum of prostate cancer research and treatment. We hope our readers find this book comprehensive and useful.

Philip W. Kantoff, M.D.
Peter R. Carroll, M.D.
Anthony V. D'Amico, M.D., Ph.D.

ACKNOWLEDGMENTS

The editors would like to acknowledge the contributions of Diane Azzoto, Barbara Daly, and Kathleen Keavany, as well as the dedicated work of Stuart Freeman, Will Wiebalck, and Joanne Bersin at Lippincott Williams & Wilkins.

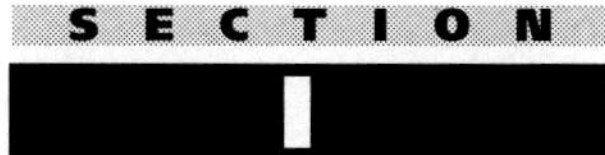

BIOLOGY

1

GROSS AND APPLIED ANATOMY OF THE PROSTATE

ROBERT P. MYERS

The prostate as an accessory reproductive organ has perhaps been the subject of more head-scratching than any other gland. "Something of a mystery" (1), "unknown physiologic function" (2), "What is the prostate and what is it for?" (3), and "*l'objet de nomenclatures différentes et contradictoires*" (4) all allude to the perplexity surrounding the only gland with wildly different forms found in all orders of mammals, even monotremes (5). There is a tremendous body of research with respect to the role of the prostate's secretory products. The secretions from the male accessory sex glands, including the prostate, function in such events as (a) semen gelation, coagulation, and liquefaction; (b) coating and decoating of spermatozoa; and (c) conditioning of the urethral surface, among others (6). However, the precise biologic contribution of the prostate, *per se*, remains to be determined.

The first description of the prostate has been attributed to Herophilus, an Alexandrian Greek anatomist in the fourth century BC (7). In *Glandular Partners*, he described more convincingly the seminal vesicles with a strict interpretation of Galen, but a clearly unambiguous reference to the prostate is lacking (8). If Herophilus described the seminal vesicles, it is inconceivable that he didn't encounter the prostate. *Prostate* literally means "that which stands before." Like the Propylaea, the impressive entryway to the ancient Acropolis, the prostate stands before the entryway or neck of the bladder. However, in a procreative sense, the prostate stands before the male external genitalia.

As a gland, the prostate is composed of many acini that empty into multiple tiny ductules streaming toward posterior urethral termination in proximity to the seminal colliculus or verumontanum (veru). (The veru, or remnant Müllerian tubercle, is a small prominence in the prostatic urethra that projects into the urethral lumen from its dorsal or posterior aspect.) The human prostate, a tubuloalveolar gland in which ducts and acini have similar secretory function, is predominantly apocrine because the apical portion of the cell is cast off with some of its secretory products, especially enzymes. Electron microscopy brilliantly shows the apocrine nature of prostatic secretion (9). In activity termed *merocrine*, other soluble secretory products, such as citrate, cross the apical membrane by an active transport process to accumulate in very high concentration in the acinar lumen (10). The acinar and ductal secretory epithelial cells produce a great number of measurable substances, which have produced more fascination and speculation than complete understanding, including acid phosphatase; lactic dehydrogenase; kallikrein proteases, such as prostate-specific antigen and HK-2; prostaglandin; spermine; fibrinogenase; aminopeptidase; zinc; citrate; cholesterol; tissue plasminogen activator; pepsinogen II; lactoferrin; and others (9,11–13).

The prostate parenchyma of the adult is supported by a smooth muscle and connective tissue stroma. At its exterior surface, the prostate has a fibrous capsule that is focally absent at its base, where it attaches to the bladder and seminal vesicles, and at its apex, where it abuts the external sphincter. There is a histologically identifiable layer of fibromuscular tissue at the posterolateral periphery. This layer is continuous with the adjacent periacinar smooth muscle (9). Grossly, the excised radical prostatectomy specimen has an apparent thick white capsular coat even if denuded of its visceral fascia.

In textbooks of anatomy and clinical urology published in the twentieth century, the human prostate is widely portrayed as Valentine heart shaped with a rounded apex in coronal section (14,15). Illustrations commonly show the most distal tip of the prostate, its apex, touching a plate of transverse muscle, usually labeled *urogenital diaphragm*, and occasionally *striated urethral sphincter*. This stylized coronal section of the prostate and immediately surrounding tissue (15) could not be further from anatomic truth. Magnetic resonance images capture a completely different anatomy (16). Because there is so much individual variation with respect to size and shape in any decade, from childhood to old age, medical illustrators have always been at a loss as to how to draw a prostate. The normal prostate has been compared to a walnut or chestnut, which suggests something small, round, and hard. It also has been described as ranging in average size and shape from small apricot to large plum (16), which speaks for (a) the age range when benign prostatic hyperplasia (BPH) is variably present, and (b) palpable fruitlike consistency.

DIGITAL RECTAL EXAMINATION

The most common method of assessing the size and consistency of the prostate involves use of the tip of an index finger to palpate digitally the posterior surface of the prostate through the anterior rectal wall. In the absence of BPH, the normal prostate as appreciated digitally is palpably smooth, mobile, and symmetric with a soft "benign" consistency, not unlike that of the thenar eminence on stretch. Prostates on examination encompass a wide range of sizes. Taking the normal prostate as the size of the surface of a table tennis ball as palpated rectally, one can assess prostate sizes in grades: 1, a golf ball; 2, a racquet ball; 3, a tennis ball; and 4, a baseball or cricket ball.

Cancer has a firm consistency, not unlike that of the knuckle of the thumb just beyond the thenar eminence (first metacarpal-phalangeal joint). Cancers often present as asymmetric nodules. To the examining index finger, cancers with extraprostatic extension are often associated with some degree of local prostate fixation. Because they blend so well into the capsule and stroma, the most malignant infiltrative cancers—for example, those having Gleason scores 8, 9, or 10—may lack any palpable induration. For local staging of prostate cancer according to the TNM (tumor-node-metastasis) classification, please see Chapter 19.

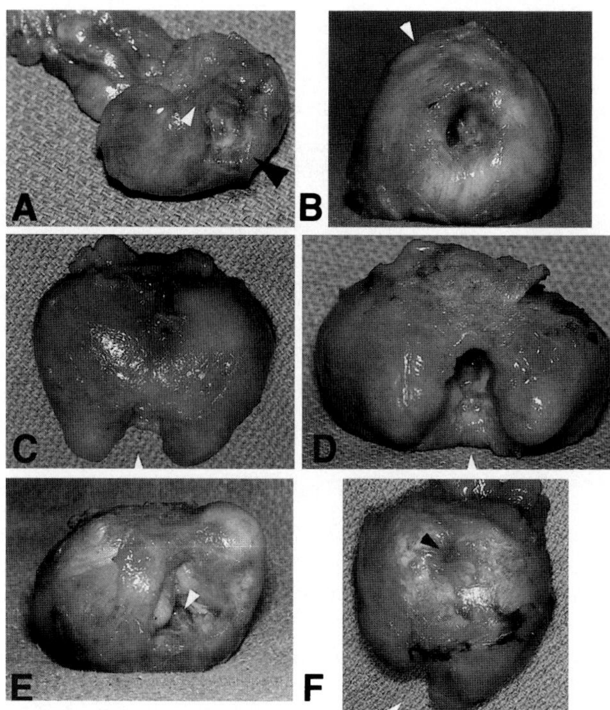

FIGURE 1-1. Variable gross (apical) morphology. **A:** Anterior apical notch with posterior lip (*black arrowhead*). Note tiny anterior commissure (*white arrowhead*). **B:** Doughnut-shaped apex with massive anterior commissure (*white arrowhead*) due to benign prostatic hyperplasia (BPH). **C:** Anterior and posterior apical notches (*white arrowhead*), view from above onto anterior surface of prostate. **D:** Same specimen as in **(C)**. Head-on apical view (*white arrowhead* points to apical urethral opening). **E:** Unusual distortion of apex by BPH nodules (*white arrowhead* points to verumontanum). **F:** Asymmetric apex (*white arrowhead*), bladder neck (*black arrowhead*). (See also color Figure 1-1.)

ADULT RELATIONS

Irrespective of variable human size and form (especially at the apex) (Fig. 1-1), the prostate has a base situated proximally against the vesical neck. Distally, at its apex, the prostate is in contact with the sphincteric [membranous (17); intermediate (18)] portion of the urethra (16) above the bulb of the corpus spongiosum of the penis. As a gland, it has anterior, posterior, and inferolateral surfaces. The bridge of fibromuscular tissue connecting the right and left halves of the prostate anterior to the urethra is known as its *commissure* or *isthmus*. The right and left halves of the prostate are often called *lobes*, despite the fact that none are demonstrable unless there is BPH (see below).

As the prostate enlarges, it raises the base of the bladder, which is attached anteriorly to the pubis by musculofascial bands that are true pubovesical [puboprostatic (17,18)] ligaments (16,19). In the anterior surgical approach in radical retropubic prostatectomy, the prostate is always obscured from view by overlying bladder and the ventrally situated, preprostatic, vascular (pudendal, Santorini's, dorsal vein) plexus derived from dorsal veins of the penis.

Posteriorly, the prostate abuts the wall of the rectum. The two seminal vesicles and the two ampullae of the vasa deferentia exit from the upper posterior surface of the prostate adjacent to the posterior prostatovesical junction.

PROSTATE DEVELOPMENT

It is useful to think about development of the prostate and the state of the male by first considering the female bladder, the urethra including external sphincter, and the neurovascular bundles in anatomic relationship to each other. Then, to the female state, add a prostate of increasing size, including progressive degrees of BPH within the prostate.

Into the urogenital sinus mesenchyme, primarily of endodermal origin, situated posterior and in juxtaposition to the Müllerian tubercle (veru) and the urethra, periurethral ductal budding begins sometime between 9 and 11 weeks of gestation as the initial event of prostate development. No evidence of budding is apparent at 9 weeks (9). Florid development from the eleventh week to the sixteenth week occurs along an ejaculatory duct axis, as shown in wax models (20). Growth is thus primarily posterolateral. Anteriorly, the upper portion of the external sphincter will come to be splayed out across the anterior surface of the prostate (21).

Embryologic studies fully support the McNeal prostate (see below). Using computer-assisted three-dimensional reconstruction of serial sections, Timms and colleagues (22) found that ductal budding and branching patterns in the developing prostate correlated to McNeal's adult regional anatomy.

In 100 newborns and infants (J. E. McNeal, *personal communication*, 1999), McNeal (23) found only stromal, but not glandular, characteristics to define what he termed *peripheral* and *central* zones with respect to the ejaculatory ducts. In the coronal section of the prostate of a 5-month-old, a relatively dense concentration of stroma in the central zone can be readily appreciated (24). All acini are responsive to some degree to androgenic and estrogenic hormonal stimulation. The periurethral mucosal and submucosal glands are particularly responsive to maternal estrogen, resulting in the squamous metaplasia that can be seen at birth. In response to hormonal influence and reciprocal stromal-epithelial interaction (25), the peripheral and central glandular zones of the adult develop within the stromal matrix. Differential response of the two zones has been suggested based on disparate origin. The central zone acini have exclusive secretory products (9).

That cytokeratin expression in prostate glandular epithelium is similar in fetal prostate and BPH supports the concept that BPH represents a "reawakening of the fetal prostate" (26). Developmental congenital anomalies of the prostate include absence, heterotopia, persistent anterior lobe (7), and unilateral absence of the central zone and seminal vesicle (27).

PROSTATE ARCHITECTURE

Discussions in the literature of prostate architecture always seem to hearken back to Lowsley (28). Lowsley described five groups of periurethral embryonic tubules: (a) middle ("prespermatic and posturethral"), (b) right lateral, (c) left lateral, (d) posterior ("postspermatic and posturethral"), and (e) ventral (anterior to the urethra). *Prespermatic* and *postspermatic* referred to location with respect to the two ejaculatory ducts. For want of a better term, he called all these groups of tubules *lobes*, thereby causing ensuing confusion among anatomists and urologists for virtually the entire twentieth century.

McNeal (29) directly challenged Lowsley's lobe concept. Currently, most urologists (following McNeal's admonition) do not adhere to a true lobar architecture, except in the context of BPH.

McNeal Prostate

The structure of the prostate as defined by McNeal became firmly established in American urology during the last quarter of the twentieth century, and his zonal anatomy is applied herein for purposes of discussion and illustration.

Microscopic Zonal Anatomy

In a series of studies of the prostate (30–33) that addressed conflicting views about the anatomy of the prostate, McNeal defined three histologically distinctive glandular zones: peripheral (70% to 75%), central (20% to 25%), and transition (5% to 10%) (Fig. 1-2). Even though the prostate without BPH is macroscopically homogeneous on cut section (Fig. 1-3A), the acini can be regionalized into specific zones histologically (Fig. 1-4A).

The *peripheral zone* was characterized by ducts radiating laterally from the distal prostatic urethra (veru to apex) and was visualized as an extension coinciding with the ejaculatory duct axis (33). The *central zone* was a proximal wedge-shaped glandular region surrounding the ejaculatory ducts, broad laterally at the base of the prostate, and funneling to duct orifices at the veru. This zone was defined in relation to the ejaculatory ducts and not the urethra. It was discovered based on a coronal section parallel to the ejaculatory ducts, and the coronal plane of section was adopted to focus on prostate morphology vis-à-vis the Wolffian duct origin of the ejaculatory ducts as opposed to the urogenital sinus origin of the prostate proper. The peripheral zone was peripheral to the central zone, with the ejaculatory ducts as a reference point. Standard sections of the prostate had always been in an axial plane and perpendicular more or less to the urethra, and the coronal plane was a new and physiologic way of looking at prostate acinar structure. In an axial section through the ejaculatory ducts, the central

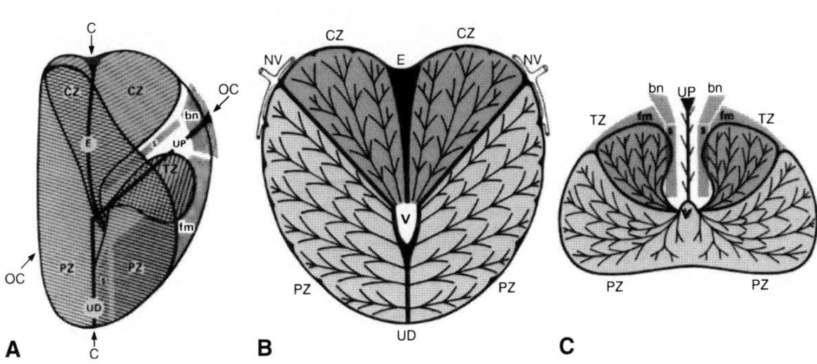

FIGURE 1-2. Zonal architecture of the prostate. **A:** Sagittal. **B:** Coronal. **C:** Oblique coronal. Note duct radiation from verumontanum (*V*). bn, bladder neck; C, coronal plane; CZ, central zone; E, ejaculatory duct; fm, fibromuscular stroma; NV, neurovascular tissue; OC, oblique coronal plane; PZ, peripheral zone; s, sphincter; TZ, transition zone; UD, distal prostatic urethra; UP, proximal prostatic urethra. (From McNeal JE. The prostate gland: morphology and pathobiology. *Monogr Urol* 1988;9:36–54, with permission of Thomas A. Stamey.) (See also color Figure 1-2.)

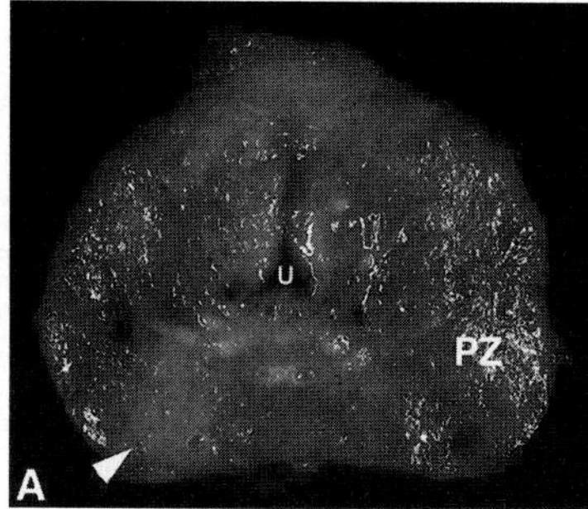

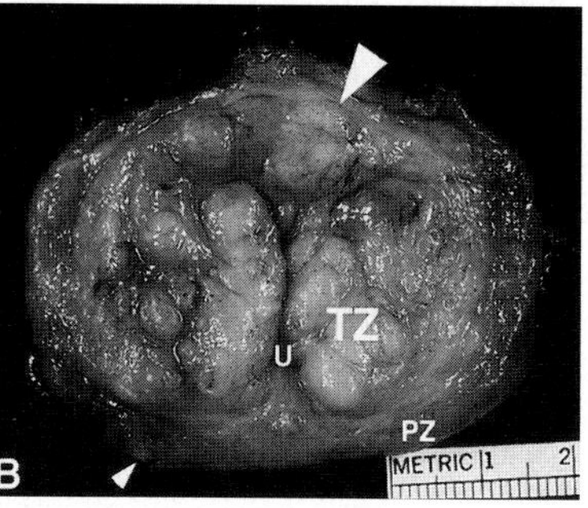

FIGURE 1-3. Prostate cancer in gross axial section. **A:** Peripheral zone (PZ) cancer (*arrowhead*). Cut surface is homogeneous with no evidence of either transition zone (TZ) or lobulation. **B:** TZ cancer (*large arrowhead*) and PZ cancer (*small arrowhead*). Prominent benign prostatic hyperplasia of TZ displaces peripheral zone outward. U, urethra. (Courtesy of Dr. David G. Bostwick.) (See also color Figure 1-3.)

zone is marked by acini with little stroma when compared with peripheral zone acini (Fig. 1-4A).

McNeal found that the peripheral zone had typically smaller acini and less complex ductal branching and sacculation than the central zone. The epithelium was histologically different between zones. The zones were distinct without transition. He suggested that the two histologically different zones must therefore be functionally different. McNeal also observed an important stromal difference: "looser" in the peripheral zone, "denser" in the central zone. Carcinoma and inflammation were found to have less predilection for the central zone than the peripheral zone. The normal central zone contained approximately 50% of the prostate epithelium, but only 5% of small cancers (J. E. McNeal, *personal communication*, 1999). It is a personal observation that isolated midline cancer nodules at the base of the prostate (central zone) on digital rectal examination are practically nonexistent.

A third zone, the *transition zone,* constituting less than 5% of the glandular prostate, was found by McNeal, when normal, to be composed of two separate gland groups bilateral to the urethra, just proximal to the veru, and entirely external to the preprostatic sphincter, which separated the transition zone from the randomly arranged periurethral glands (32). Ducts for transition zone acini were found to arise from the urethra at a single focus (bilaterally) just proximal to the veru. These ducts branched entirely anteriorly and anterolaterally in a course taking them away from the other two zones. Because their stroma mingled freely with preprostatic sphincter stroma medially and bladder neck smooth muscle proximally, the zone was designated the *transition zone*; the transition from prostate to bladder was stromal, not glandular. The term *transition* should not be taken as referring to transition from one histologic type to another or from one type of zone to another. Parenthetically, this zone is a unique zone, apart from the central and peripheral zones, that is prone to the transition of continued growth throughout life in the process of BPH.

McNeal (9) was able to determine that most clinically significant BPH represented expansion of adenomatous nodules in the transition zone. Nodules found in periurethral tissue were typically stromal without gland growth—that is, they remained very small and contributed negligibly to BPH mass (J. E. McNeal, *personal communication*, 1999).

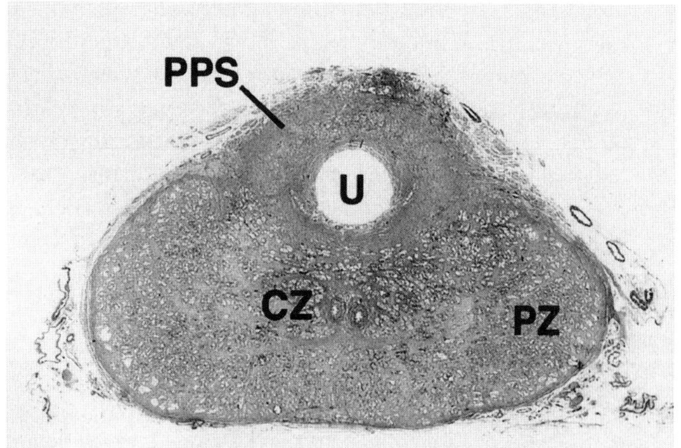

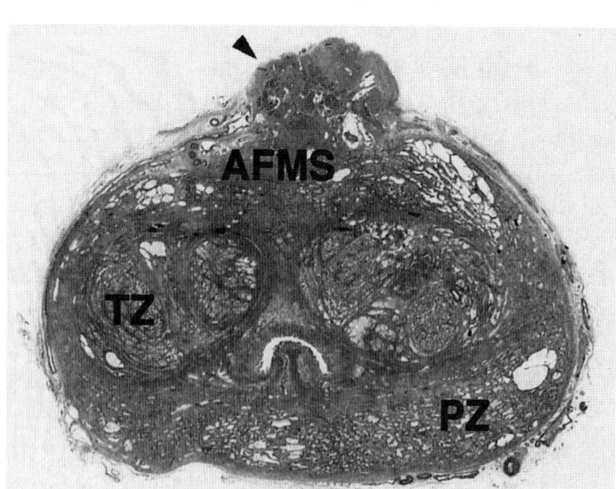

FIGURE 1-4. Axial section morphology (Masson trichrome). **A:** Section at base of prostate from 44-year-old patient without benign prostatic hyperplasia (BPH) shows relatively homogeneous acini without visible lobulation. Central zone (CZ) acini next to ejaculatory ducts seen below urethra (U) have sparse basophilic stroma compared with rich eosinophilic stroma of peripheral zone (PZ) acini. PPS, preprostatic sphincter. **B:** In section near apex, bilateral nodular BPH [transition zone (TZ)] distorts and compresses PZ outward. Venous plexus was bunched anteriorly before fixation. Note bundled detrusor fibers (*arrowhead*) from anterior detrusor apron. AFMS, anterior fibromuscular stroma. (See also color Figure 1-4.)

To define this zone accurately, McNeal cut the prostate in an oblique coronal section taken parallel to the urethra above the veru (supramontanal or supracollicular urethra) (Fig. 1-2C). In customary axial sections, any BPH of typical lateral lobe distribution is transition zone (Figs. 1-3B and 1-4B).

Transition Zone Boundary

Between the peripheral and transition zones in axial section, a transition zone boundary of stromal connective tissue is readily demonstrable with implications relative to the spread or confinement of carcinoma. Franks (34) used *ill-defined capsule* to describe this stromal interposition between outer and inner prostates. Many carcinomas of peripheral zone origin are confined to the peripheral zone (Fig. 1-3). Likewise, tumors of transition zone origin are often wholly contained within the transition zone (Fig. 1-3B). Many cancers, after increase in volume, exhibit a proclivity to invade and perforate the transition zone boundary, but usually in limited patterns.

McNeal (9) emphasized that the combined central and peripheral zone size is relatively constant throughout adult life until demonstrable atrophy appears in the 70s. It is therefore the transition zone that is subject to BPH enlargement and primarily responsible for increased gland size and weight.

Fibromuscular Stroma

The term *anterior fibromuscular stroma* was coined by McNeal (23). It includes the isthmus or commissure mentioned previously. This region is best evident in axial whole-mount histologic sections of the prostate (Fig. 1-4). In 1972, McNeal's (31) diagrammed components of the fibromuscular stroma included preprostatic sphincter, anterior detrusor muscle, internal sphincter, and a portion of the striated urethral sphincter (external sphincter). In 1988, his fibromuscular stroma was labeled simply "FM" in sagittal section without the above components (Fig. 1-2) (23). It is important to remember the components and the tissue diversity of the fibromuscular stroma. In the axial or transverse plane, the anterior fibromuscular stroma is a "thick, nonglandular apron" forming "the entire anterior surface of the prostate" (33). In some cases, that apron can be relatively sparse and histologically simple (Fig. 1-4A), but in others, relatively dense and histologically complex (Fig. 1-4B).

This anteromedial apron contains a prominent extension of outer longitudinal detrusor muscle that ends at the pubovesical (puboprostatic) ligament attachments to the pubis. The detrusor muscle fibers intermingle with prominent thick fascia and provide the scaffolding for the rich venous plexus (Santorini's, pudendal, dorsal vein, ventral vascular, with respect to prostate and urethra) (16) emanating from the penis. When sutures are used in radical retropubic prostatectomy to bunch together and secure this ventral vascular plexus, smooth muscle bundles from the detrusor are included (Fig. 1-4B). McNeal's work (31) confirmed Santorini's in showing that the bladder musculature does not end where the bladder forms a neck, but continues distally to cover a portion of the anterior surface of the prostate (35,36).

Preprostatic Sphincter

In McNeal's illustrated oblique coronal plane, the midline anterior fibromuscular stroma contains the smooth muscle of a "preprostatic" sphincter surrounding the urethral lumen (31). The *preprostatic sphincter* is composed of circularly oriented, smooth muscle fibers (Fig. 1-4A) extending distally from the circular smooth muscle of the distal trigone at the bladder neck and ending at the base of the veru. The extent of the preprostatic sphincter and its continuity with the vesical neck was captured and confirmed by Blacklock in whole-mount section (Fig. 1-5) (24,37).

It is well known that this sphincter of smooth muscle is α-adrenergically innervated and therefore responsive to relaxation by the administration of α-adrenergic blocking agents, such as tamsulosin hydrochloride. The result is decreased outflow resistance and an improved urinary stream. The prostate stroma is similarly innervated, and one of the side effects of tamsulosin hydrochloride is the inability to produce an ejaculate with the prostate stroma in a seeming state of smooth muscle paralysis.

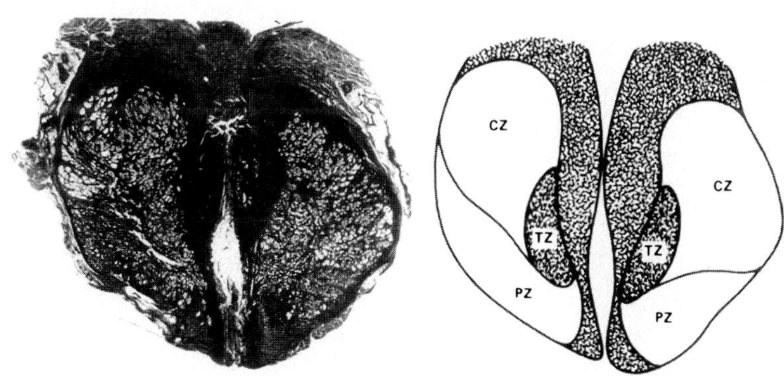

FIGURE 1-5. Coronal section morphology. Preprostatic and vesical neck sphincters are one continuous entity. CZ, central zone; PZ, peripheral zone; TZ, transition zone. (From Blacklock NJ. Surgical anatomy. In Chisholm GD, Fair WR, eds. *Scientific foundations of urology,* 3rd ed. Chicago: Heinemann Medical Books, Oxford, and Year Book Medical Publishers, 1990;340–350, with permission of Geoffrey D. Chisholm and William R. Fair.)

When BPH is absent, the presence of a cylinder of smooth muscle around the urethra distal to the vesical neck can be confirmed grossly in radical retropubic prostatectomy. With a clean plane of dissection, the prostate can be dissected away from the preprostatic sphincter, which is initially embedded within the prostate proximal to the veru. When the preprostatic sphincter has been properly dissected and transected with urethra distal to the bladder neck, the result is a bladder neck with an attached thick sphincter. This smooth muscle sphincter is found in direct continuity with the subtrigonal detrusor circular smooth muscle for 360 degrees. There is no visibly evident discontinuity to conclude that there are two sphincters, one at the bladder neck and another in the proximal prostatic urethra (38). The conclusion from looking at radical prostatectomy specimens is that the preprostatic sphincter is continuous with the vesical neck, which is immediately surrounded by a prostate that has enveloped the bladder neck by cephalad extension. The circular smooth muscle of the preprostatic sphincter and the inner subtrigonal circular layer are visibly in continuity. (The outer longitudinal detrusor layer is not in continuity.) Histologically, McNeal (9) found "no boundary" between detrusor smooth muscle and preprostatic sphincter. The gross finding of one sphincter is consistent with the fact that "the upper prostatic urethra, above the level of the colliculus seminalis at the site of the Müllerian tubercle, is derived from the vesicular portion of the primitive cloaca . . . " (7).

Benign Prostatic Hyperplasia

When BPH begins, periurethral nodules develop with concentration within and inward from the preprostatic sphincter (32). The integrity of the preprostatic sphincter and the bladder neck is disturbed. The appearance of a middle lobe makes this especially true, but involvement of the bladder neck by BPH is sometimes circumferential, or what is described as a collar-type growth of BPH at the bladder neck. The ability to find and dissect out a preprostatic sphincter at the time of radical prostatectomy disappears. When there is considerable BPH, removal of the prostate from the bladder neck during radical prostatectomy leaves a wide, gaping opening into the bladder lumen.

Normal prostates do not have BPH; thus, BPH is an abnormal condition despite its widespread prevalence to varying degrees in men beyond the age of 35. The lobar nature of BPH is captured in the enucleation specimen shown in Figure 1-6A. In suprapubic prostatectomy or adenectomy, the transition zone is effectively removed with a surgeon's index finger. What is left is the smooth inner surface of the combined and severely outwardly compressed central and peripheral zones, which subsequently reexpand.

Flocks (39) stated the lobar nature of BPH very nicely in 1937: "Masses of hyperplastic tissue present posteriorly are called median lobes; present laterally, lateral lobes; and present anteriorly, anterior lobes." The enucleated specimen shown in Figure 1-6A accounts for three of the five sites of development of BPH with respect to the veru: left lateral, right lateral, and middle, including a combined subcervical (bladder neck) and subtrigonal component. The anterior midline at the vesical neck is an uncommon fourth location. The fifth location is the peripheral zone. Very rarely, separate BPH nodules develop within the peripheral zone (40). Usually no more than 1 cm in diameter, such soft nodules can be appreciated on digital rectal examination very close to the rectal surface at the tip of the examining index finger. They do not require biopsy if sufficiently soft.

Acinar hyperplasia of the transition zone results in prostate hypertrophy of variable degrees in different individuals. The middle lobe, when present, appears in different configurations at the bladder neck. When disposed as a ball valve, pronounced obstruction to urinary outflow is possible (Fig. 1-6B). The various types of adenomatous hyperplasia have been classified as types I through VIII. The different configurations depend on which group of glands becomes hyperplastic and "the resistance to growth of the surrounding prostate and vesical neck" (41).

As BPH progresses, certain anatomic elements stay fixed with respect to each other. They include the pubis, the pubovesical (puboprostatic) ligaments, and the external sphincter. The fibromuscular stroma (including the isthmus or commissure) becomes thinner and more extensive. The urethra becomes more angulated above the veru. The examining finger on digital rectal examination encounters the prostate as an enlarged smooth, symmetric mound of benign consistency projecting into the rectal lumen,

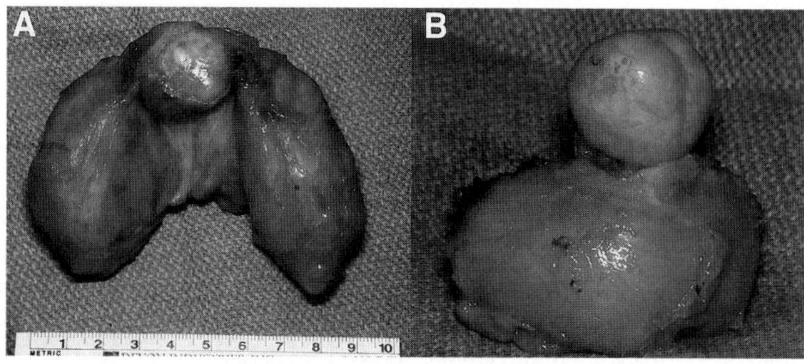

FIGURE 1-6. Lobes of benign prostatic hyperplasia (BPH). **A:** Enucleated trilobar BPH specimen weighing 105 g. **B:** Radical prostatectomy specimen with "ball valve" median lobe BPH at the bladder neck. (See also color Figure 1-6.)

whereas the nonhyperplastic prostate is expected to be small and flat against the rectum. Cephalad growth of the prostate induced by BPH elevates the bladder base. An adenomatous middle lobe situated beneath the distal trigone may be so pronounced as to obscure visualization of the ureteral orifices during endoscopy.

The process of BPH results in prostate glands of many remarkably different configurations and ultimately external shapes (Fig. 1-1) (42,43). Because there is shape variation in nonhyperplastic prostates (44), BPH is thus superimposed on nonhyperplastic prostates of variable shape to produce the final shape or configuration. This all translates into complicating the apical dissection in radical retropubic prostatectomy.

BPH results in not only increased girth of the prostate to interfere with surgery. In caudad growth, adenoma overlaps with remarkable variability the external sphincter ["BPH overlap" (45)] and sphincteric (membranous) urethra. This anatomic change brought about by BPH greatly complicates the surgeon's mission not to leave the transected residual urethra too short in radical prostatectomy and thereby sacrifice urinary control.

Alternative Architecture?

Unfortunately, while McNeal was dividing the gland into peripheral, central, and transition zones (Fig. 1-2), Tisell and Salander (46) were dissecting 3-day-old cadaveric specimens prone to artifact and identifying dorsal, lateral, and median lobes, situated in what they ultimately described as an "onion pattern." They concluded that "the anatomical relation of the lobes of the adult human prostate cannot be defined simply as dorsal, lateral, and median according to their position vis-à-vis the ejaculatory ducts." At best, their explanation is difficult to interpret, and their follow-up histologic study (47) is hardly convincing. Both of their unconfirmed gross and histologic studies appear to contain serious artifact.

Anatomists have carried lobes in their prostate nomenclature in six successive editions of the *Nomina Anatomica* (*NA*) (17) and in the *Terminologia Anatomica* (*TA*) in 1998 (18). Inspired by the unproved Tisell and Salander effort (46,47), the *TA* has introduced into current nomenclature *inferoposterior*, *inferolateral*, *superomedial*, and *anteromedial* lobules as subdivisions of right and left lobes of the prostate. Notably, in 1935, the Jena *NA* departed from *lobus* [*dexter et sinister*], preferring *partes laterales*, and discarded *lobus medius* (48). No reference to lobules as subdivisions of lobes is carried in any edition of the *NA*. But, Lich and colleagues (14) described the "outer" portion of the prostate as consisting of lobules "whose apices converge toward the posterior urethral surface." They also said, " . . . seven clinically recognizable lobes of the prostate are produced, but they are anatomically indistinguishable." Certainly, the *TA* (18) continues to promulgate uncertain ground.

Cranial gland and *caudal gland* were applied to the prostate by Gil Vernet (49). Gil Vernet's caudal zone is essentially the same as McNeal's peripheral zone, but, as noted by Villers and colleagues (50), his cranial zone appears to have included both McNeal's central and transition zones. The concept of a human cranial and caudal prostate has appeal because several species of monkey have prostates of just that configuration (3,51). Benoit and colleagues (4) also follow the cranial/caudal analogy.

Currently, the McNeal prostate, once understood, makes the most sense. However, the published literature exhibits no universal agreement with respect to prostate architecture, as is clearly apparent in the recently released *TA* (18).

Many observers conceive of the prostate as a periurethral organ because they are used to seeing, especially in illustrated coronal and axial sections, the urethra coring straight through the middle of the prostate; they have what might be termed a *urethrocentric* view of the prostate. There has been confusion in terminology, because McNeal's "central" does not refer to the urethra. Benoit and colleagues (4) see "central" as being applied logically to the urethra and the immediately surrounding parenchyma—that is, it is appropriate in their view to say that BPH is central as opposed to any portion of the prostate that is displaced peripherally. To such observers, it is a fundamental problem that McNeal's central zone is central with respect to an ejaculatory duct axis but peripheral with respect to the urethra. And, conventional pictures of the prostate do not always show the ejaculatory ducts. The urethrocentric point of view also adheres to the fact that the prostate develops as epithelial buds from the urethra and is a urethral gland as well as an accessory sex gland (6). At the prostate apex, the urethra is a common conduit for both semen and urine.

Furthermore, because BPH flanks the urethra, some radiologists refer to BPH as the *central gland*, also known as McNeal's *transition zone*. *Central gland*, of course, causes confusion with McNeal's *central zone*. With evidence that early prostate cancer is relatively rare in McNeal's *central zone* but common in the transition zone, Stamey and Hodge (52) decried the use of the term *central gland* as "dangerous."

A purely urethrocentric view, however, is not acceptable because, as demonstrated by McNeal, there is a primary ejaculatory duct axis for all of the prostatic duct orifices. The ejaculatory duct-centric view was confirmed by both Johnson in wax casts (20) and Blacklock in whole-mount histology (24,37).

The urethrocentric view mirrors Franks' (34). Franks defined the prostate as having a thick outer layer of "'external' glands—the prostate glands proper" and a small inner group of glands separated from the outer by an indefinite capsule. What he described essentially was an inner and outer prostate. His inner group contained both urethral mucosal and submucosal glands. When Lich and colleagues (14) described the prostate, they also adhered to similar external and internal "portions." Thus, for those who hold a

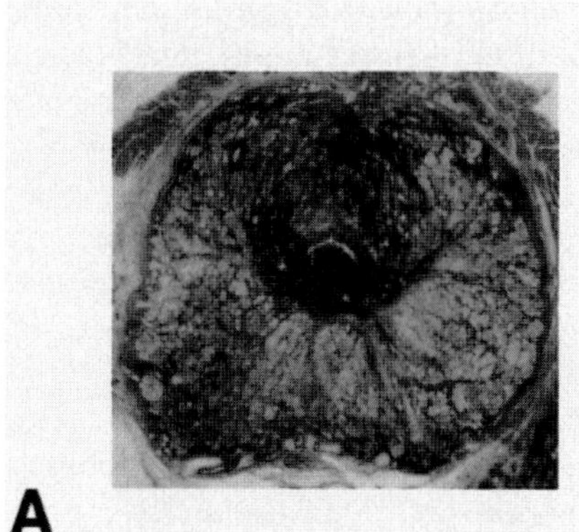

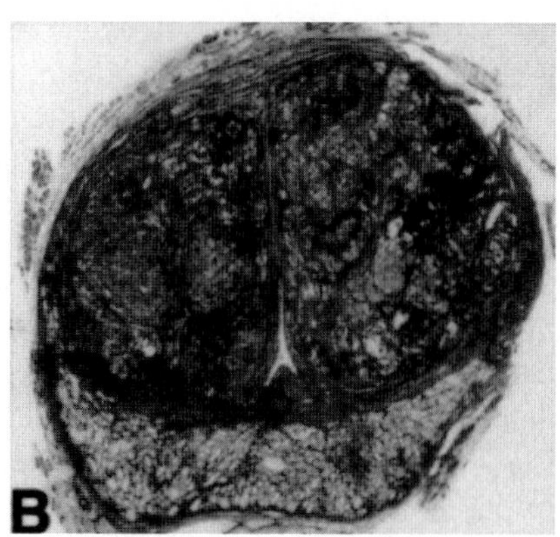

FIGURE 1-7. Axial section histology of prostate. **A:** Minimal benign prostatic hyperplasia (BPH). **B:** Advanced BPH anteriorly with marked posterior compression of peripheral zone. (From Franks LM. Benign nodular hyperplasia of the prostate: a review. *Ann R Coll Surg Engl* 1954;14:92–106, with permission of the Royal College of Surgeons of England.)

urethrocentric view of the prostate, there is considerable conceptual, but flawed, precedence for an inner and outer prostate that conflicts with the obvious embryologic development of the prostatic ducts along an ejaculatory duct axis.

Inner versus *outer* prostate fails in the context of advancing BPH. This can be confirmed by looking at Franks' own published sections (34) (Fig. 1-7). *Inner zone* or *inner prostate* may appear to work in routine whole-mount axial sections when there is minimal or no BPH (Fig. 1-7A). However, BPH expands predominantly anterolateral to the urethra with very minimal posterior extension. The peripheral and central zones become compressed into a shelf of tissue posterolateral to the urethra. Thus, from the urethra all the way to the anterior surface of the prostate, the tissue is virtually all adenoma when BPH is advanced. The transition zone becomes outer prostate anteriorly (Fig. 1-7B).

PROSTATIC URETHRA

That portion of the male urethra within the body of the prostate is known as the *prostatic urethra*, which is usually depicted in coronal views as a vertical open tube coring straight through the mid-prostate from prostate base to apex. A straight course through the prostate into the bladder is unusual. The urethra in most prostates has a curved or angled course through the prostate with concavity forward in the sagittal plane as it passes from the bladder forward, toward its entry into the dorsal surface of the penis. Because of the anterior angulation of the urethra above the veru, the urethra should never be illustrated in the coronal view as coring straight through to the bladder. Rather, only a portion of the urethra should be shown (53).

Normally, its vesicourethral junction and the internal urethral meatus at the prostate base are not situated in the axial plane, as often illustrated, but in an oblique coronal plane that is tipped forward from the feet. At first, the curve is backward and downward toward the veru. At the veru, the urethra generally takes a slight turn anteriorly as it heads toward the bulb. Because of its curved course, the complete prostatic urethra generally would not be seen in the coronal view, and magnetic resonance imaging substantiates this observation (16,53). The curved course means that flexible cystoscopy is more comfortable to patients than cystoscopy by means of a rigid, straight instrument.

McNeal (33) described the forward angulation above the veru as "roughly at a 35-degree angle" from the vertical. This should be taken as an average. (From personal experience looking at radical prostatectomy specimens, I have found that the angle appears to range from nearly 0 degrees to nearly 90 degrees.) Anecdotally, in an 18-year-old man, Glenister (54) found the supracollicular and infracollicular portions of the prostatic urethra at "right angles to one another." The observed angle relates to two features: (a) the degree of muscular development of the trigone, including its uvula [of Lieutaud (55)], and (b) the size of the commissure as it relates to the presence or absence of BPH. In the presence of BPH, the commissure may be massive. In the absence of BPH, the commissure may be but a very thin band (Fig. 1-1A). The veru usually occupies a site in the most distal prostatic urethra. Occasionally, there may be no prostatic urethra or prostate distal to the veru (45).

Situated in the posterior midline at variable distance from the prostate apex, the seminal colliculus is a prominent feature of the prostatic urethra. Urologists usually refer to the seminal colliculus as the *veru*. Anatomists prefer *seminal colliculus*. Lowsley (28) used *verum montanum*, meaning "mountainous spit or broach." Later, he fused the two words into *verumontanum* (1). [The word for *spit* or *broach* in Latin exists in two neuter-singular forms: *veru* and the variation, *verum* (56). The word *verumontanum* has been present in the English language at least since 1728, according to the *Oxford English Dictionary* (57). The metaphor would seem to be a mountainous spit of land in the sea.]

No one would disagree that the veru is a distinct promontory with a prominent dimple or tiny crater at its top marking the prostatic utricle, a Müllerian remnant. Along the posterior prostatic urethra and with considerable individual variation, orifices of the multiple prostatic and two ejaculatory ducts flank the veru.

FASCIA AND THE PROSTATE

The prostate is invested by fascia on all of its surfaces, save where it is attached to the bladder and to the striated urethral sphincter at the prostate apex. Fascia belonging to and enveloping the prostate is called *visceral.* On its anterolateral surface, the prostate is covered by fascia overlying a vascular plexus (large veins, venous spaces, and tiny arteries) embedded in a framework of thick fascia [fascia of Zuckerkandl (58)] and longitudinal bands of detrusor muscle. Its inferolateral surfaces are closely embraced by levator ani muscle, whose medial fascia (superior fascia of the pelvic diaphragm) is actually adherent to the visceral fascia of the prostate, creating multiple layers on the side of the prostate. The fascia associated with the levator ani is called *parietal,* and the lateral surfaces of the prostate are tightly bound by this fascia and the associated levator muscle. When the levator muscle is pushed off the lateral surfaces of the prostate in radical prostatectomy, the most superficial layer of fascia abandoned on and adherent to the lateral surfaces of the prostate is the parietal fascia belonging to the dislodged adjacent levator ani. The levator muscle dissected away laterally appears denuded of fascia.

When the bladder is exposed retroperitoneally, overlying fascia and detrusor muscle obscure the prostate. The initial view into the pelvis reveals retropubic adipose tissue, and beneath this lies the pelvic (endopelvic) fascia, which includes a visceral fascial component covering the bladder and a parietal fascial component covering the levator ani and obturator internus lateral to the bladder. The two fasciae, visceral of bladder and parietal of levator ani (fascia covering the superior surface of the pelvic diaphragm), converge on a thickened (white) line of fascia called the *tendinous fascial arch of the pelvis* (*arcus tendineus fasciae pelvis, NA, TA*). This thickened line of fascia sits in sulci deep on either side of the bladder and extends from the takeoff of the pubovesical (puboprostatic) ligaments in a curvilinear path to end at the ischial spine (43). The tendinous fascial arch of the pelvis defines the lateral junction of the bladder and the prostate, the latter immediately subjacent to the arch. The lateral surfaces of the prostate cannot be visualized unless the parietal fascia covering the superior surface of the pelvic diaphragm is opened. In the course of radical retropubic prostatectomy, the sides of the prostate are first exposed by (a) incising the parietal fascia just lateral and parallel to the course of the tendinous fascial arch, and (b) pushing away laterally the levator ani muscle. Only then can the prostate first be seen.

On the posterior surface of the prostate, there is a very prominent and relatively thick fascia adherent to the prostate as it sits anterior to the rectum. It is a true prostato-rectal fascia with respect to its position, but it is inherently prostatic, with midline adherence to the prostate in many cases (59). This prostato-rectal (Denonvilliers') fascia continues superiorly to cover the seminal vesicles all the way to their tips. Confusion exists as to the number of layers constituting this fascia—that is, whether it has one or two, or more, layers. From a study of embryos, Silver (60) concluded that this fascia was a single layer only. (In more than 2,000 radical retropubic prostatectomies, I have found almost consistently one layer covering the prostate, but often multiple layers covering the seminal vesicles. The fascia is smooth and unrelated to the cul-de-sac of the peritoneum.) In the course of radical retropubic prostatectomy, neurovascular bundle preservation involves incising this fascia medial to each bundle on the rectal surface. Also involved is an initial release of the neurovascular bundles from their attachment to the posterolateral prostate by incising, above each bundle, the most superficial fascia [lateral pelvic fascia (61)] on the sides of the prostate. If the incisions are not carried out properly, an important triangular layer of the prostato-rectal fascia will not be left in position on the excised prostate to cover the posterior capsule and possible breach points by carcinoma. With this technique, portions of the fascia, two strips, are left covering the neurovascular bundles. The prostate then is denuded of two strips of fascia along the course of the previously adherent bundles. This means that patients for the nerve-sparing operation must be chosen carefully for organ-confined disease in the region of each neurovascular bundle. Wide resection to sacrifice the bundle as a covering over the cancer is paramount to complete cancer excision if there is any doubt about possible extraprostatic spread.

NEUROVASCULAR BUNDLES

On its posterolateral aspects, the prostate is closely invested by neurovascular bundles. These bundles contain multiple autonomic nerves coursing from the prostatic plexuses, flanking the vesicoprostatic junction, to the cavernous plexuses en route to the corpora cavernosa and corpus spongiosum. As they pass along the lateral prostate, they give off at right angles very tiny nerve fibers in tiny pedicles that enter the capsular surface. These tiny branch points (including tiny capsular arteries and veins) require division to release the bundle properly when doing a nerve-sparing operation, and magnification is very helpful to see them properly.

In 1836, Müller (19) described major and minor cavernous nerves from the hypogastric and pelvic plexuses to the penis, but knowledge of this work was lost at a practical level. In 1982, on the basis of exquisite dissection and mapping study of those nerves in stillborn male neonates, Walsh and Donker (62) were the first, from a urologic point of view, to track the cavernous nerves in relationship to how they might be preserved in radical prostatectomy. Their effort translated into the possibility of preserving potency by very precise surgical technique. That *neurovascular bundles* were indeed identifiable as an intraoperative landmark for the cavernous nerves and could be dissected free from the posterolateral surfaces of the prostate revolutionized radical prostatectomy (63). An important localization study with respect to cavernous nerve distribution in the adult and its relationship to radical prostatectomy followed (64). Before 1982, a potent patient after radical prostatectomy was a haphazard event at best, and patients undergoing radical prostatectomy almost uniformly became impotent. This was due primarily either to ligation or to transection of the bundles located along the posterolateral aspect of the prostate. As of the year 2000, results of surgery have markedly changed, and patients who are appropriate candidates for a cavernous nerve-sparing technique can look forward to a highly successful outcome with respect to the preservation of potency (65).

When the prostate is small, the bundles in their posterolateral position are not obscured by the lateral surfaces of the prostate. Rather, the bundles may obscure the lateral surfaces. With BPH, the peripheral zone is compressed further and further posterolaterally (Figs. 1-3B and 1-4B). Coursing along the posterolateral aspect of the peripheral zone, the bundles remain in essentially the same position to each other and to the rectal surface. As the prostate fattens with transition zone expansion, its lateral surfaces bulge laterally without displacing the bundles. With pronounced BPH, the surgeon will find the bundles tucked much more underneath. Furthermore, there may be more angulation of the bundles at the prostatourethral junction. This angulation can approach 90 degrees as the bundles hug the prostate and then head distally along the urethra and into and around the striated urethral sphincter. Tethering of the bundles to produce the angulation is generated by a tiny capsular vessel and nerve branch point that flanks the prostatourethral junction.

During surgery, with suitable contrast, the largest cavernous nerves may be visible with surgical loupes but are generally obscured because fibrofatty tissue, veins, arteries, and blood hide them. Measurement of the transverse diameters of 64 nerves in a single neurovascular bundle of a 44-year-old revealed a mean diameter of 0.12 mm (range, 0.04 to 0.37 mm). There were ten major cavernous nerves with a diameter of 0.20 to 0.37 mm. A reference human hair was 0.02 mm in diameter (R. P. Myers, *previously unpublished data*).

There are multiple points of vulnerability with respect to successful neurovascular preservation. Special attention must be directed to (a) the apical dissection, (b) tension-free mobilization of the bundles laterally along the mid-prostate, (c) correct vascular pedicle ligation suitably anterior to the bundles, and (d) very careful dissection of the seminal vesicles medially away from the pelvic plexuses.

ARTERIES AND VEINS OF THE PROSTATE

The arterial supply to the prostate originates from the internal iliac arteries in a vascular pedicle or bundle shared with the inferior vesical arteries with anastomotic connections inferiorly to internal pudendal and anal canal (inferior rectal) arteries. The main pedicle is located at the posterolateral junction of the bladder and prostate in proximity to the base of each seminal vesicle. Flocks (39) defined the arterial blood supply to the prostate in 1937. The arteries enter at the prostatovesical junction and divide into urethral and capsular branches supplying the inner and outer prostate, respectively. The urethral group is found from 1 to 5 o'clock and from 7 to 11 o'clock, beginning at the bladder neck and coursing distally. During transurethral resection of the prostate for BPH, starting the resection at the bladder neck and coagulating those vessels can prevent much bleeding. In BPH, both urethral and capsular groups are more luxurious. Not only a narrow band of stroma, but also an artery, defines the boundary of the peripheral and central zone (30).

Most of the veins surrounding the prostate are associated with the plexus of veins derived from the dorsal surface of the penis, thus the name *dorsal vein complex.* However, the relationship of this plexus to the prostate is not dorsal, but anterolateral or ventrolateral. Once the dorsal veins of the penis pass posterior to the pubic arch, the penile hilus (66) is reached. From the penile hilus, major branches turn superiorly and are disposed anterolaterally to the sphincteric (membranous) portion of the urethra and prostate. The veins have many anastomoses with each other, to the point of forming tiny lakes or lacunae, as described originally by Santorini (35). This plexus is an obvious source of profound bleeding for the uninitiated surgeon. (I met one once; he was so proud to tell me that he had gone to the regular use of a cell saver, prompted by the loss of 23 units of blood during one of his cases. Little did he understand that he should not have been operating in the first place.)

A preprostatic superficial vein often exits the fascia between the pubovesical (puboprostatic) ligaments and then reenters the vesico-venous plexus (67). This vein has several variations and is absent approximately 10% of the time. The superficial vein is usually nestled in the retropubic adipose tissue and, if large, can be a source of troublesome bleeding during radical retropubic prostatectomy.

The rest of the veins associated with the prostate are found beneath fascia. The major group is anterolateral, associated with the detrusor apron on the ventral surface of the prostate. A very variable minor component accompanies the neurovascular pedicles that run along the posterolateral aspect of the prostate in the groove between the prostate and anterior rectal wall. Anastomoses between the major and minor component over the lateral surface of the prostate are also quite variable and bilaterally unequal, thus the name *plexus pubicus impar* (unequal) used by Santorini (35). It is not uncommon to see a rich plexus of veins on the lateral surface of the prostate on one side and the other side to be relatively devoid of veins (45). Many of these veins join the vesico-venous plexus and drain into the internal iliac system. Anastomoses to the internal pudendal veins through the levator ani are often present just lateral and proximal to the pubovesical (puboprostatic) ligaments.

Veins that actually drain the prostate communicate directly with this periprostatic system. When deep transurethral resection of the prostate for BPH or cancer violates the prostatic capsule opening venous sinuses, troublesome and sometimes life-threatening venous sinus bleeding can occur, as well as unrecognized fluid overload from irrigant flowing into the vascular system. The threat to life comes from (a) uncontrolled blood loss and shock, (b) hemolysis and renal failure when nonisotonic solutions are used as irrigants, and (c) hypervolemia and congestive heart failure.

FINAL COMMENT ON THE PROSTATE, PERIPROSTATIC TISSUE, AND TERMINOLOGY

With respect to the prostate and its surrounding tissues, there is a case for clarity and precision with respect to names. The prostate is situated in a milieu of contiguous structures that include urinary bladder, rectum and anal canal, urethra, penis, pubis, and all of the investing fascia and various neurovascular tissues. Language that surgeons use to describe some of the periprostatic tissues is misleading, certainly to the uninitiated. For example, the prostate has a prominent posterior fascia, but the common parlance term *Denonvilliers' fascia* provides no hint to medical students regarding its anatomic location versus using "combined prostato-rectal and seminal vesicular fascia," which characterizes it. Eponyms serve no useful purpose; it was the recommendation of the International Anatomical Nomenclature Committee in 1975 that "eponyms . . . be rejected" (68).

Lateral pelvic fascia is commonly applied to fascia that must be incised on the lateral surfaces of the prostate. The term explains its levator ani origin (superior fascia of the pelvic diaphragm), but the intimate association with the prostate, as in "most superficial layer of the lateral periprostatic fascia," is not captured in the language.

Securing the dorsal vein complex of the penis inside the pubic arch is key to successful hemostasis in radical retropubic prostatectomy, but the surgeon in that operation operates not on the penis, but on the prostate and urethra. The plexus is ventral with respect to those foci of surgical attention. Because the plexus contains arteries as well as veins, it is not just a venous plexus but a "ventral vascular plexus" (16). The issue of whether to call it dorsal or ventral could be resolved simply by referring to "the prostatourethral vascular plexus."

Urologists say "puboprostatic ligaments." However, as in women, the ligaments are fundamentally pubovesical in origin; the only difference is that, in the male, the prostate grows to encroach on the bladder and its pubovesical ligaments from underneath. It is always an illusion that they are puboprostatic. During radical retropubic prostatectomy, after the retropubic adipose tissue has been carefully excised to expose the visceral vesical fascia, the pubovesical attachment is obvious. As condensations of the vesical visceral fascia, the ligaments from their pubic termination merge straight back into the bladder proper from the distal third of the pubis as the patient is positioned supine; they do not attach to the prostate.

There is a recognized pubourethral component to the ligaments (69) but not a true puboprostatic component. Importantly, there is a thick vascular plexus interposed between the ligaments and the prostate. As illustrated by Parry and Dawson (70) in radical perineal prostatectomy, the prostate can be removed without ever encountering the ligaments or the ventral vascular plexus. There is a free plane of dissection from the prostatourethral junction along the anterior commissure to the point of attachment of the bladder. The ligaments are situated anterior to the vascular plexus, which is effectively sandwiched between the ligaments and the prostate. Illustrations (and there are many) that show a direct downward, linear connection of the ligaments to the anterior surface of the prostate without vesical continuity are simply wrong. The larger the anterior commissure of the prostate in BPH, the more the illusion that the ligaments span from pubis to prostate. Even Santorini (35,36), who coined the term *prostate ligament*, described and illustrated its vesical origin and attachment. To call these ligaments puboprostatic is to belie the fact that they contain remnant detrusor smooth muscle [*m. pubovesicalis* (17,18)] and are intrinsically pubovesical. Some authors exclaim that they can improve the chances of urinary control after radical retropubic prostatectomy if they do not "take down" the puboprostatic ligaments (71). But, for removal of the prostate retropubically, the continuity of these ligaments with the bladder must be interrupted at some point: if not at the pubis, as some have suggested, then more proximally, as others have illustrated (72).

Cited above are examples of potentially misleading terminology. In rebuttal to an argument for insisting on precise nomenclature, one reviewer for the *Journal of Urology* in 1997 replied, "The authors believe that more precise terminology that is based upon anatomic considerations is advantageous. This of course is arguable, since so many of our terms are anatomically incorrect but the surgeon knows what they refer to and what to do with the structure during an operation." Such commentary reveals that common parlance often holds pragmatic sway over common sense. When language and illustration are not precise, the confusion generated may breed not only misunderstanding, but also resultant surgical error by those who have been misled. There is no adequate rebuttal or justification for anatomically imprecise nomenclature when patient quality of life is at stake, and failure to understand pelvic floor anatomy leads to unacceptable rates of urinary incontinence and sexual impotence. The interrelationship of the prostate and contiguous structures is complex, and the anatomy must be understood clearly to obtain successful surgical results.

ACKNOWLEDGMENTS

The final form of this chapter would not have been possible without the kind input of Norman Blacklock, David Bostwick, John McNeal, Arnaud Villers, and Patrick C. Walsh.

REFERENCES

1. Lowsley OS. Embryology, anatomy and surgery of prostate gland with report of operative results. *Am J Surg* 1930; 8:526–541.
2. Coffey DS, Isaacs JT. Control of prostate growth. *Urology* 1981;17[Suppl 3]:17–24.
3. Blandy JP, Lytton B, eds. *The prostate.* London: Butterworths, 1986;1–11.
4. Benoit G, Jardin A, Gillot C. Reflections and suggestions on the nomenclature of the prostate. *Surg Radiol Anat* 1993;15:325–332.
5. Price D. Comparative aspects of development and structure in the prostate. *Natl Cancer Inst Monogr* 1963;12:1–25.
6. Aumuller G, Seitz J. Protein secretion and secretory processes in male accessory sex glands. *Int Rev Cytol* 1990;121: 127–231.
7. Skandalakis JE, Gray SW, Broecker B. The male reproductive tract. In: Skandalakis JE, Gray SW, eds. *Embryology for surgeons: the embryological basis for the treatment of congenital anomalies,* 2nd ed. Baltimore: Williams & Wilkins, 1994;773–815.
8. Von Staden H. *Herophilus: the art of medicine in early Alexandria.* Cambridge, New York: Cambridge University Press, 1989.
9. McNeal JE. Prostate. In: Sternberg SS, ed. *Histology for pathologists,* 2nd ed. Philadelphia: Lippincott–Raven Publishers, 1997;997–1017.
10. Costello LC, Franklin RB. Concepts of citrate production and secretion by prostate. 1. Metabolic relationships. *Prostate* 1991;18:25–46.
11. Kumar VL, Majumder PK. Prostate gland: structure, functions and regulation. *Int Urol Nephrol* 1995;27:231–243.
12. de Voogt HJ. Biology of the prostate. *Prog Clin Biol Res* 1991;370:207–212.
13. Young CY, Andrews PE, Tindall DJ. Expression and androgenic regulation of human prostate-specific kallikreins. *J Androl* 1995;16:97–99.
14. Lich R Jr., Howerton LW, Amin M. Anatomy and surgical approach to the urogenital tract in the male. In: Harrison JH, Gittes RF, Permutter AD, et al., eds. *Campbell's Urology,* 4th ed. Vol. 1. Philadelphia: WB Saunders, 1978;17–18.
15. Netter FH. *Atlas of human anatomy.* Summit, New Jersey: CIBA-GEIGY Corporation; Sect. 5, Plate 361, 1989.
16. Myers RP, Cahill DR, Devine RM, et al. Anatomy of radical prostatectomy as defined by magnetic resonance imaging. *J Urol* 1998;159:2148–2158.
17. International Nomenclature Committee. *Nomina anatomica,* 6th ed. Edinburgh, UK: Churchill Livingstone, 1989.
18. Federative Committee on Anatomical Terminology. *Terminologia anatomica: international anatomical terminology.* Stuttgart, Germany: Thieme, 1998.
19. Müller J. *Über die organischen Nerven der erectilen männlichen Geschlectsorgane des Menschen and der Säugethiere.* (Concerning the autonomic nerves of the male erectile genital organs of man and mammals.) Berlin: F. Dümmler, 1836.
20. Johnson FP. The later development of the urethra in the male. *J Urol* 1920;4:447–501.
21. Oelrich TM. The urethral sphincter muscle in the male. *Am J Anat* 1980;158:229–246.
22. Timms BG, Mohs TJ, Didio LJ. Ductal budding and branching patterns in the developing prostate. *J Urol* 1994;151:1427–1432.
23. McNeal JE. The prostate gland: morphology and pathobiology. *Monogr Urol* 1988;9:36–54.
24. Blacklock NJ. Surgical anatomy of the prostate. In: Williams DI, Chisholm GD, eds. *Scientific foundations of urology.* Vol. 2. Section 2. London: William Heinemann Medical Books, 1976;113–118.
25. Hayward SW, Rosen MA, Cunha GR. Stromal-epithelial interactions in the normal and neoplastic prostate. *Br J Urol* 1997;79[Suppl 2]:18–26.
26. Shapiro E, Gitlin JS, Sun T-T, Wu X-R. Expression of cytokeratin in human fetal prostate and bladder. *J Urol* 1998;159[Suppl]:108(abst).
27. Argani P, Walsh PC, Epstein JI. Analysis of the prostatic central zone in patients with unilateral absence of wolffian duct structures: further evidence of the mesodermal origin of the prostatic central zone. *J Urol* 1998;160: 2126–2129.
28. Lowsley OS. The development of the human prostate gland with reference to the development of other structures at the neck of the urinary bladder. *Am J Anat* 1912–1913;13:299–346.
29. McNeal JE. Anatomy of the prostate: an historical survey of divergent views. *Prostate* 1980;1:3–13.
30. McNeal JE. Regional morphology and pathology of the prostate. *Am J Clin Pathol* 1968;49:347–357.
31. McNeal JE. The prostate and prostatic urethra: a morphologic synthesis. *J Urol* 1972;107:1008–1016.
32. McNeal JE. Origin and evolution of benign prostatic enlargement. *Invest Urol* 1978;15:340–345.
33. McNeal JE. The zonal anatomy of the prostate. *Prostate* 1981;2:35–49.
34. Franks LM. Benign nodular hyperplasia of the prostate: a review. *Ann R Coll Surg Engl* 1954;14:92–106.
35. Santorini GD. De virorum naturalibus. (Concerning the male genitalia.) In: *Observationes anatomicae.* Venice: G Baptista Recurti, 1724;173–205.
36. Santorini GD. *Septemdecim tabulae* (seventeen tables). Girardi M, ed. Parma: Ex Regia Typographia, 1775.
37. Blacklock NJ. Surgical anatomy. In Chisholm GD, Fair WR, eds. *Scientific foundations of urology,* 3rd ed. Chicago: Heinemann Medical Books, Oxford, and Year Book Medical Publishers, 1990;340–350.
38. Dröes JT. Observations on the musculature of the urinary bladder and the urethra in the human foetus. *Br J Urol* 1974;46:179–185.
39. Flocks RH. The arterial distribution within the prostate gland: its role in transurethral prostatic resection. *J Urol* 1937;37:524–548.

40. Kerley SW, Corica FA, Qian J, et al. Peripheral zone involvement by prostatic hyperplasia. *J Urol Pathol* 1997;6:87–94.
41. Randall A, Hinman F Jr. Surgical anatomy of the prostatic lobes. In: Hinman F Jr., ed. *Benign prostatic hypertrophy.* New York: Springer Verlag, 1983;672–673.
42. Myers RP, Goellner JR, Cahill DR. Prostate shape, external striated urethral sphincter and radical prostatectomy: the apical dissection. *J Urol* 1987;138:543–550.
43. Myers RP. Practical pelvic anatomy pertinent to radical retropubic prostatectomy. *AUA Update Series* 1994;13:26–31.
44. Myers RP. An anatomic approach to the pelvis in the male. In: Crawford ED, Das S, eds. *Genitourinary cancer surgery,* 2nd ed. Baltimore: Williams & Wilkins, 1997;155–169.
45. Myers RP. Radical prostatectomy: pertinent surgical anatomy. *Atlas Urol Clin North Am* 1994;22:1–18.
46. Tisell L-E, Salander H. The lobes of the human prostate. *Scand J Urol Nephrol* 1975;9:185–191.
47. Salander H, Johansson D, Tisell L-E. The histology of the dorsal, lateral, and medial prostatic lobes in man. *Invest Urol* 1981;18:479–483.
48. Kopsch F. *Nomina anatomica; vergleichende Ubersicht der Basler, Jenaer and Pariser Nomenklatur.* Stuttgart, Germany: Georg Thieme, 1957.
49. Gil Vernet S. *Patologia urogenital: biologia y patologia de la prostata.* Book 2. Vol. 1. Madrid: Editorial Paz Montalvo, 1953.
50. Villers A, Steg A, Boccon-Gibod L. Anatomy of the prostate: review of the different models. *Eur Urol* 1991;20:261–268.
51. Blacklock NJ, Bouskill K. The zonal anatomy of the prostate in man and in the rhesus monkey (*Macaca mulatta*). *Urol Res* 1977;5:163–167.
52. Stamey TA, Hodge KK. Ultrasound visualization of prostate anatomy and pathology. *Monogr Urol* 1998;9:55–63.
53. Myers RP. Male urethral sphincteric anatomy and radical prostatectomy. *Urol Clin North Am* 1991;18:211–227.
54. Glenister TW. The development of the utricle and of the so-called “middle” or “median” lobe of the human prostate. *J Anat* 1962;96:443–455.
55. Lieutaud J. Planche 5, Fig. 2 d. *Essais anatomiques: contenant l'historie exacte de toutes les parties qui composent le Corps de l'Homme* (Nouvelle edition). Paris: D'Houry, 1766.
56. Anthon C. *A Latin-English and English-Latin Dictionary.* New York: Harper, 1868.
57. *The Oxford English dictionary,* 2nd ed. Oxford: Clarendon Press, 1989;566.
58. Haines RW. The striped compressor of the prostatic urethra. *Br J Urol* 1969;41:481–493.
59. Villers A, McNeal JE, Freiha FS, et al. Invasion of Denonvilliers' fascia in radical prostatectomy specimens. *J Urol* 1993;149:793–798.
60. Silver PHS. The role of the peritoneum in the formation of the septum rectovesicale. *J Anat* 1956;90:538–546.
61. Walsh PC. Anatomic radical prostatectomy: evolution of the surgical technique. *J Urol* 1998;160:2418–2424.
62. Walsh PC, Donker PJ. Impotence following radical prostatectomy: insight into etiology and prevention. *J Urol* 1982;128:492–497.
63. Walsh PC, Lepor H, Eggleston JC. Radical prostatectomy with preservation of sexual function: anatomical and pathological considerations. *Prostate* 1983;4:473–485.
64. Lepor H, Gregerman M, Crosby R, et al. Precise localization of the autonomic nerves from the pelvic plexus to the corpora cavernosa: a detailed anatomical study of the adult male pelvis. *J Urol* 1985;133:207–212.
65. Catalona WJ, Carvalhal GF, Mager DE, et al. Potency, continence and complication rates in 1,870 consecutive radical retropubic prostatectomies. *J Urol* 1999;162:433–438.
66. Devine CJ Jr., Angermeier KW. Anatomy of the penis and male perineum: part I. *AUA Update Series* 1994;13:9–16.
67. Myers RP. Anatomical variation of the superficial preprostatic veins with respect to radical retropubic prostatectomy. *J Urol* 1991;145:992–993.
68. Warwick R. Introduction. In: International Anatomical Nomenclature Committee. *Nomina anatomica,* 4th ed. Amsterdam: Excerpta Medica, 1977;A1–A9.
69. Steiner MS. The puboprostatic ligament and the male urethral suspensory mechanism: an anatomic study. *Urology* 1994;44:530–534.
70. Parry WL, Dawson CB. Surgery for malignant disease of the prostate. In: Glenn JF, Boyce WH, eds. *Urologic surgery.* New York: Hoeber Medical Division, 1969;342–397.
71. Poore RE, McCullough DL, Jarow JP. Puboprostatic ligament sparing improves urinary continence after radical retropubic prostatectomy. *Urology* 1998;51:67–72.
72. Myers RP. Improving the exposure of the prostate in radical retropubic prostatectomy: longitudinal bunching of the deep venous plexus. *J Urol* 1989;142:1282–1284.

2

CELLULAR AND MOLECULAR BIOLOGY OF PROSTATIC DEVELOPMENT

GERALD R. CUNHA
ANNEMARIE A. DONJACOUR
SIMON W. HAYWARD
AXEL A. THOMSON
PAUL C. MARKER
CORY ABATE-SHEN
MICHAEL M. SHEN
RAJVIR DAHIYA

The concept that neoplasia is a "caricature of differentiation" was proposed by Barry Pierce of the University of Colorado (1). This concept is based on the idea that virtually all aspects of tumor biology have a counterpart in normal embryonic development. Embryonic cells and tissues, as well as carcinoma cells, may exhibit proliferation, invasiveness, morphogenesis, and differentiation. During normal development, the process of differentiation is tightly controlled and highly orchestrated. In carcinomas, the state of differentiation is frequently diagnostic of the aggressiveness of the tumor (more differentiated tumors are usually less aggressive). Another feature of some malignant tumors is the ability of malignant cells to generate progeny that undergo normal differentiation with complete loss of malignant properties (1). The most striking example of this phenomenon is the regulation of malignant embryonal carcinoma cells by the blastocyst (2).

In the prostate, it should be noted that both prostatic carcinomas and the developing normal prostate undergo epithelial proliferation, form new ductal or acinar tissue, and undergo ductal branching morphogenesis. The process of ductal growth and branching morphogenesis in both contexts is inherently invasive. Epithelial and stromal differentiation is an important aspect of both the developing prostate and prostatic carcinomas. The biology of the developing prostate and certain carcinomas is sufficiently similar that embryonic prostatic mesenchyme can induce the Dunning prostatic carcinoma to differentiate, reduce its growth rate, and diminish its tumorigenic potential (3). For these reasons, the developing prostate serves as a particularly good model for understanding some of the biologic processes that occur in prostatic carcinomas. Moreover, the application of developmental principles to prostatic carcinomas has the potential of developing new therapeutic strategies (differentiation therapy), the goal of which is to revert carcinoma cells to a more highly differentiated nonproliferative state. This chapter reviews the cellular and molecular biology of the prostate and, where appropriate, emphasizes common themes between developing and malignant prostates of rodent and human origin. Unless specified otherwise, descriptions of specific experiments refer to animal models; however, information on rodent models is usually applicable to human prostate.

DEVELOPMENT OF THE MALE REPRODUCTIVE SYSTEM

Development of the male reproductive system begins during the ambisexual stage, when male and female embryos are indistinguishable anatomically, having a pair of undifferentiated gonads and two sets of mesodermally derived ducts, the Wolffian and Müllerian ducts. In men, the gonadal primordia differentiate into testes, which produce two hormones: testosterone and Müllerian inhibiting substance. In male embryos, testosterone or its metabolites maintain the Wolffian ducts (4), whereas Müllerian ducts regress in response to Müllerian inhibiting substance (5). Fetal testicular androgens further stimulate the Wolffian ducts to differentiate into epididymis; ductus deferens; and, in most species, the seminal vesicles (6). The mesonephric tubules attached to the cranial end of the Wolffian ducts are also maintained by androgens and differentiate into the efferent ductules, which connect the testis to the epididymis. In the absence of testosterone or functional androgen receptors, the mesonephric tubules and the Wolffian ducts degenerate (7).

The urogenital sinus, whose epithelium is endodermal in origin, is also a component of the ambisexual stage in both genders. In females, the urogenital sinus forms the urethra and the lower portion of the vagina. In males, the urogenital sinus forms the masculine urethra, the prostate, periurethral glands, and bulbourethral glands. Androgens from the fetal testis stimulate budding of the endodermally derived urogenital sinus epithelium just caudal to the bladder neck to form the prostate and even more caudally to form the bulbourethral glands. The female urogenital sinus will also form a prostate if stimulated by androgens during critical periods of development (8). Masculine development of the urogenital sinus and Wolffian duct does not occur in the absence of androgens, or functional androgen receptors, or when androgen action is blocked by administration of antiandrogens (7).

Ductal Branching Morphogenesis

The prostate is a ductal-acinar gland whose growth and development begin in fetal life and are complete at sexual maturity. Normal development of prostatic ducts requires many coordinated cellular processes, including epithelial proliferation, ductal branching morphogenesis, ductal canalization, and epithelial and mesenchymal differentiation. In many respects, ductal branching morphogenesis in the prostate resembles that of many other organs (e.g., mammary gland, lung, salivary gland, pancreas). The prostate differs from these other organs in that its development is androgen dependent and occurs mostly during the postnatal period.

Development of prostatic ducts begins when solid prostatic buds emerge from the urogenital sinus. These buds grow into the surrounding urogenital sinus mesenchyme. Prostatic buds appear on day 17 in embryonic mice, on day 19 in embryonic rats, and during the tenth week in human fetuses (9). The emergence of prostatic buds from the urogenital sinus is spatially patterned to generate the anlage of the various lobes of the rodent prostate (dorsal, ventral, lateral, and anterior) (10). In the mouse, the ventral prostate develops from two to four main ducts, while approximately 40 to 50 main ducts constitute the dorsolateral prostate. The anterior prostate develops from one or two main ducts per side, which grow cranially into the mesenchyme surrounding the seminal vesicle (11). In contrast to the rodent prostate, true lobar subdivisions are not present in the adult human prostate, which instead is organized into zones (central, peripheral, and transitional zones) (12).

Individual prostatic buds emerge from the urethra, elongate, and then branch. Eighty percent of the branching of the prostatic ducts occurs in the first 15 days of postnatal life in the mouse (11). During this time, circulating androgen levels are exceedingly low. If neonatal mice are castrated and treated with antiandrogen, prostatic ductal branching is significantly reduced (13). Re-administration of androgens in adulthood does not restore the normal number of ductal tips to animals deprived of androgen during development (13). Therefore, it appears that there is a critical period during which ductal branching morphogenesis must occur and that these early branching events are very sensitive to the low levels of circulating androgens present in the neonatal period.

Ductal branching patterns are characteristic for each lobe of the rodent prostate. The ventral prostatic buds branch dichotomously at fairly regular intervals, resulting in a pattern that resembles an elm tree, while the ducts of the dorsal prostate elongate considerably before giving rise to numerous tightly spaced ducts. Thus, the pattern of branching in the dorsal prostate resembles that of a palm tree. The primary ducts of the lateral lobe emerge from the urogenital sinus in close proximity to the dorsal ducts but wrap laterally around the periphery of the prostate and have a branching pattern similar to the ventral prostate (11).

Formation of new ductal architecture results, in part, from localized DNA synthesis at the ductal tips. Thymidine incorporation into DNA is ten- to 500-fold greater in ductal tips as compared to more proximal regions of mouse prostatic ducts (14). Based on analysis of branching morphogenesis in a variety of developing organs, differential proliferation may not, however, be the entire means by which branching morphogenesis occurs. For example, isolated lung epithelium responds to fibroblast growth factor (FGF) 1 by forming buds; however, these buds form before differential proliferation is detectable (15). FGF10 acts as a chemotactic factor for lung epithelium during development (16) but needs an associated proliferative signal to make a bud (17).

Prostatic Mesenchymal and Epithelial Differentiation

Concurrent with the process of ductal branching morphogenesis, epithelial and mesenchymal or stromal cytodifferentiation occurs in the first 2 to 3 weeks after birth in rats and mice. Prostatic development is a complex androgen-dependent process involving a coordinated set of events occurring in both the epithelial and stromal compartments of the gland. As described below androgens act upon the urogenital sinus mesenchyme to elicit a complex series of reciprocal interactions. Thus, whereas epithelial differentiation is dependent on the presence of the urogenital mesenchyme, stromal differentiation is in turn dependent on the presence and differentiation state of the developing prostatic epithelium (18). During fetal and prepubertal development, androgens act on the prostatic mesenchyme to induce ductal budding, epithelial proliferation, and growth of solid epithelial cords into the mesenchyme. When the ducts canalize, the luminal and basal epithelial cells undergo cytodifferentiation (19,20). Epithelial cells of the developing solid prostatic buds are characterized by the coexpression of cytokeratins 5, 8, 14, and 18. These solid cords elongate into the surrounding mesenchyme as a result of intense proliferative activity at their tips (14). Ductal canalization is initiated in the solid epithelial cords from the urethral terminus of the prostatic ducts and proceeds distally toward the ductal tips. As the solid epithelial cords canalize, the epithelium reorganizes into two distinct cell populations. Basal epithelial cells become localized along the basement membrane to form a discontinuous layer of cells expressing cytokeratins 5 and 14 in the rat and mouse. Concomitantly, tall columnar luminal cells, which express cytokeratins 8 and 18, differentiate and line the ductal lumina (19,21). By this process, the original homogenous epithelium of the solid epithelial buds (expressing both luminal and basal cell cytokeratins) differentiates into the distinct luminal and basal cell lineage, each expressing their characteristic subset of cytokeratins. Finally, as testosterone production increases, the production of prostatic secretory proteins is initiated in rats as early as 13 days postnatally and increases dramatically at puberty (22).

Another important differentiation marker for prostatic epithelium is the androgen receptor. Epithelial androgen receptors are not expressed in the embryonic prostatic buds, even though the surrounding urogenital sinus mesenchyme expresses high levels of androgen receptors. As the solid prostatic cords canalize in the neonatal period, the differentiating prostatic epithelium expresses low levels of androgen receptors (23). In the mouse and rat prostate, epithelial androgen receptors are detectable at approximately 2 to 6 days postnatally, even though species and strain differences in the timing of expression of epithelial androgen receptors have been noted (19,24). The number of androgen-receptor-positive epithelial cells, as well as the percentage of positive cells, increases until approximately 15 days of age, when all of the luminal cells are intensely androgen receptor positive (25). The question of whether androgen receptors are expressed in basal epithelial cells is still debated (25,26).

In all fetal male reproductive organs, androgen receptors are initially detectable in the mesenchyme during the ambisexual stage (9). Thus, androgen receptors are present in urogenital sinus mesenchyme before the initiation of prostatic budding (20,24). As mesenchymal differentiation proceeds, the smooth muscle cells remain androgen receptor positive, while interductal fibroblasts become androgen receptor negative (20,24). Therefore, many key androgen-dependent developmental processes occur in fetal life, when androgen receptor levels are high in the mesenchyme and undetectable or low in the epithelium. This suggests a paracrine mechanism of androgen action in the developing male reproductive tract.

As prostatic epithelial differentiation proceeds, starting at the prostatic urethra and extending distally toward the ductal tips, the peri-epithelial mesenchymal cells differentiate into androgen-receptor-positive smooth muscle cells. Initially, the mesenchymal cells predominantly express vimentin, although some mesenchymal cells also express smooth muscle α-actin (20). Indeed, peristaltic contractions have been reported in the urogenital sinus of the fetal mouse demonstrating that even at this early stage, some muscular activity is possible. As development progresses, the mesenchymal cells become organized into sheathes of smooth muscle expressing a range of markers, including desmin, myosin, and laminin (20).

Adult prostatic tissue in humans and rodents has an extremely low rate of cell division, even though androgen levels are high in adulthood. It is believed that in the adult prostate, androgens act on epithelial and smooth muscle cells to maintain the cytodifferentiation and function of an essentially growth-quiescent gland. Interactions between adult prostatic epithelium and smooth muscle are certainly involved in this process, even though these interactions in adulthood are fundamentally different from the morphogenetic mesenchymal-epithelial interactions occurring during development. Nemeth and Lee suggest that epithelial proliferation in the ductal tips of adult rat ventral prostate is mediated by interactions of prostatic epithelium with fibroblasts that are particularly abundant in association with ductal tips (27). Epithelial proliferation does not occur in the proximal or intermediate portions of the prostatic ducts where the epithelial cells are surrounded by smooth muscle cells. We have proposed similar ideas in relation to the control of epithelial proliferation during human prostatic carcinogenesis (18).

Role of Androgen Receptors and 5α-Reductase

Prostatic development, growth, and function are androgen dependent. While testosterone is the major androgen secreted by the testis, it is metabolized to dihydrotestosterone (DHT) by the enzyme Δ^4-3-ketosteroid-5α-reductase (5α-reductase) in the prostate (28). DHT has a tenfold greater affinity for the androgen receptor than for testosterone (29). Prostatic development is severely impaired when 5α-reductase activity is inhibited chemically or by mutation of the gene encoding this enzyme (31). This has been interpreted to indicate that DHT is the active androgen in masculinization of the embryonic urogenital sinus. 5α-Reductase is now known to consist of two isoforms, type 1 and type 2 (28). It is the type 2 enzyme that is required for normal prostatic development (32).

Mesenchymal-Epithelial Interactions in Prostatic Development

As indicated, the prostate develops from the endoderm-derived urogenital sinus, which also gives rise to the bladder and bulbourethral gland. Organogenesis of the prostate is absolutely dependent on mesenchymal-epithelial interactions, as differentiation of both the epithelium and mesenchyme is abortive if the epithelium and mesenchyme are grown by themselves. This concept applies not only to the prostate, but also to other male and female urogenital organs and other organ rudiments, which are composed of an epithelial parenchyma and mesenchyme.

Development of the prostate is dependent on inductive signals from the mesenchyme (10), and these prostatic inducing signals emanate from spatially discrete areas within the urogenital sinus mesenchyme (33,34). Regional differences in inductive activity of the urogenital sinus mesenchyme are responsible for the development of the well-defined lobar subdivisions of the prostate. The lobe-specific differences in prostatic differentiation are induced by regionally distinct subpopulations of mesenchyme within the urogenital sinus (33,34,35). For example, developing urethral epithelium is surrounded by a loose mesenchyme that is in turn partially surrounded by areas of condensed mesenchyme, the most obvious of which is the so-called ventral mesenchymal pad (34). This condensed area of mesenchyme lies ventral to the urethra and can induce the formation of the ventral prostate (34). Similarly, condensed mesenchyme overlying the dorsolateral areas of the urethra is known to induce dorsolateral prostate (36). These lobe-specific inductive activities can be experimentally identified owing to lobar differences in the secretory proteins expressed by epithelium. Surprisingly, the ventral mesenchymal pad also develops in the female embryos, and the female ventral mesenchymal pad is able to induce the formation of a prostate in the presence of androgens (34).

The outcome of epithelial-mesenchymal interactions is dependent not only on the source of the inducing mesenchyme, but also on the germ layer origin and responsiveness of the epithelium (37). Although mesenchyme induces and specifies the differentiation of the epithelium, developmental end points induced by mesenchyme are limited by the developmental repertoire of the germ layer origin of the epithelium. For example, prostatic morphogenesis and differentiation has been elicited only from endodermal epithelia derived from the urogenital sinus (vaginal, bladder, urethral, and prostatic epithelia). Attempts to induce prostatic differentiation from foregut endoderm have been unsuccessful (G. R. Cunha, *unpublished data*, 1986). Likewise, seminal vesicle differentiation has only been induced from mesodermal epithelium derived from the Wolffian duct (37). Thus, the origin of the responding epithelium plays a critical role in determining developmental outcome of experimental tissue recombinants.

While mesenchyme induces epithelial differentiation, the epithelium in turn induces smooth muscle differentiation in the mesenchyme. Indeed, both differentiation and morphologic patterning of smooth muscle in the prostate is regulated via cell-cell interactions with epithelium. For example, when urogenital sinus mesenchyme was grafted and grown for 1 month in male hosts, little if any smooth muscle differentiated in the mesenchyme. However, when urogenital sinus mesenchyme was grafted with rodent urogenital sinus–derived epithelia, actin-positive smooth muscle cells differentiated and became organized into thin sheathes, as is appropriate for the rodent prostate (38). Conversely, rat urogenital sinus mesenchyme formed thick sheets of smooth muscle surrounding the epithelial ducts in tissue recombinants composed of rat urogenital sinus mesenchyme (UGM) plus human prostatic epithelium (39). A thick smooth muscle layer is the pattern characteristic of human prostate and demonstrates that human prostatic epithelium not only induced the rat mesenchyme to undergo smooth muscle differentiation, but also to become organized into the human prostatic smooth muscle pattern. These observations suggest that prostatic smooth muscle differentiation is induced and spatially patterned by epithelium. Similar findings have been made for the uterus, urinary bladder, and intestine.

Although mesenchymal-epithelial interactions play a fundamental role in development of the prostate, the overall developmental process is elicited by androgens, which regulate prostatic development, growth, and function via androgen receptors. During fetal or neonatal periods, or both, androgens induce the appearance of prostatic epithelial buds, ductal elongation, and branching. Because prostatic development is androgen dependent and is induced by mesenchyme, androgenic effects on epithelial development have been shown to be mediated via mesenchyme. To clarify the respective roles of epithelial versus mesenchymal androgen receptors in the developing prostate, tissue recombinants were prepared with epithelium and mesenchyme from wild-type and androgen-receptor-negative testicular feminization (Tfm) mice (40). Analysis of chimeric prostates composed of wild-type mesenchyme plus Tfm epithelium has demonstrated that androgen-receptor-deficient Tfm epithelium can undergo androgen-dependent ductal morphogenesis, epithelial proliferation, and columnar cytodifferentiation (41). This suggests that certain "androgenic effects" on epithelium may be independent of androgen receptors in the epithelium. Instead, many androgenic effects on epithelium appear to be elicited by paracrine factors produced by androgen-receptor-positive mesenchyme.

If many androgenic effects on prostatic epithelium are elicited via stromal androgen receptors, then what is the function of epithelial androgen receptors? The role of epithelial androgen receptors was demonstrated by the analysis of tissue recombinants containing androgen-receptor-negative Tfm epithelium plus androgen-receptor-positive wild-type mesenchyme. In such tissue recombinants, the Tfm epithelium was induced to undergo prostatic differentiation but failed to express secretory activity (42,43). In a broader context, it is known that androgens, estrogens, and progesterone induce or inhibit epithelial proliferation in their respective target organs of male and female genital tracts. Comparable chimeric wild-type and steroid receptor–null tissue recombinants have been prepared with androgen receptor–null, estrogen receptor–α–null, or progesterone receptor–null mice. From such experiments, it has been demonstrated that, for all three classes of steroids, epithelial proliferation *in vivo* is regulated via the appropriate hormone receptors in the stromal cells (44–46). Thus, regulation of epithelial proliferation by sex steroids occurs via paracrine mechanisms in normal epithelium *in vivo*. Conversely, hormonal regulation of epithelial differentiation and function requires epithelial hormone receptors (42,43,47,48).

Homeobox Genes in Prostatic Development

Although prostatic development is clearly dependent on androgens, developmental regulatory molecules downstream of androgen action have yet to be elucidated. It is clear that mesenchymal-epithelial interactions are critical to this process, but factors intrinsic to the epithelium also play an important role. One class of regulatory molecules that might fit this role is the homeobox genes. These encode a family of transcription factors that have a highly conserved DNA-binding domain (the homeodomain) and have been shown to be important in organogenesis through control of the expression of downstream genes (49). In some systems, especially invertebrates where these genes were originally identified, homeobox genes appear to act as major developmental switches, conferring segment identity in *Drosophila* (50). In vertebrates, homeobox genes are often expressed in areas of mesenchymal-epithelial interactions (51). Two homeobox genes, *Nkx3.1* and *HoxD-13*, are of particular interest in prostatic development.

The human *NKX3.1* gene was first identified during a search for prostate-specific genes among a large expressed-sequence tag database of tissue-specific cDNA sequences (52). Human *NKX3.1* maps to the region of 8p21 that is deleted in approximately 80% of all prostate carcinomas (52). The murine *Nkx3.1* homeobox gene (53) is the earliest known marker of prostatic development, being expressed in urogenital sinus epithelium two days before the appearance of prostatic buds (54). Its restricted, "parenthesis" pattern of expression within the urogenital sinus epithelium appears to identify the prospective prostatic epithelium, such that the dorsal boundaries of *NKX3.1* expression correspond to the location of the prospective anterior prostate, the intermediate regions to the dorsolateral prostate, and the ventral boundaries of *NKX3.1* expression correspond to the ventral prostate. *Nkx3.1* expression is also observed in the endodermally derived bulbourethral gland, an androgen-dependent glandular outgrowth of the caudal urethra, but it is not observed in any of the other male secondary sex organs. *Nkx3.1* expression in the prostate continues throughout development and into adulthood. Initially, expression of this gene does not depend on direct testosterone stimulation of the epithelium, because it is expressed in androgen-receptor-negative (Tfm) epithelium that is induced to form prostate by wild-type UGM in tissue recombination experiments (54). Later expression of *Nkx3.1* does appear to require epithelial androgen receptors, as its expression decreases in Tfm epithelium once ductal morphogenesis is complete and secretory cytodifferentiation is initiated in the wild-type UGM + Tfm epithelium tissue recombinants (54). In the androgen-receptor-positive LNCap prostatic carcinoma cell line, *Nkx3.1* is induced by androgen (55).

Nkx3.1 mutant mice have been generated by targeted gene disruption (54). The prostates and derived bulbourethral glands in these mutant male mice exhibit a reduction in ductal complexity and show alterations in their secretory protein production. Moreover, both homozygous and heterozygous *Nkx3.1* mutant mice display prostatic epithelial hyperplasia and dysplasia of increasing severity with age (54).

Another class of homeobox genes expressed in the prostate is the *Hox* genes. The human and murine *Hox* genes are localized in four clusters, A, B, C, and D. The genes that occupy the same relative position within their respective clusters are thought to be functionally and structurally conserved (49). Thus, for example, *HoxD-13* has three paralogs, *HoxA-13, HoxB-13,* and *HoxC-13* (56) that are expressed in the genital region, suggesting that they may also play a role in prostatic development (57,58). *HoxD-13* is expressed in the developing and adult prostate (59), and *HoxD-13* knockout mice have prostates that are reduced in overall size and in the number of primary ducts (60). *HoxA-10* is expressed in the urogenital sinus and Wolffian duct posterior to the epididymis (61). Maximum expression of *HoxA-10* was seen at embryonic day 18, and maintenance of *HoxA-10* expression in urogenital sinus cultures was not dependent on testosterone. *HoxA-10*–null mice had decreased seminal vesicle complexity and some anterior prostate gland abnormalities (61). Seminal vesicle morphogenesis was also altered in *HoxA-13* mutant mice. This homeotic gene was broadly expressed in the urogenital tract, including the urogenital sinus, seminal vesicle, and bladder (62). Compound mutations in *HoxD-13* and *HoxA-13* result in agenesis in the male secondary sex organs (63), pointing to an overlapping function of the *Hox* genes in the prostate.

One candidate regulator of prostatic homeotic genes is *Sonic hedgehog (Shh). Shh* expression has been observed in urogenital sinus epithelium before prostatic bud formation and in prostatic ducts, mainly in the proximal regions (64). Expression of *Shh* is androgen dependent in the urogenital sinus, and its levels are highest during the early postnatal period, when branching morphogenesis is occurring. Antibodies to *Shh* appear to inhibit early prostatic morphogenesis (64). The homeotic genes and their regulatory molecules are clearly key players in prostatic development and possibly in carcinogenesis.

Growth Factors in Prostatic Development

Fibroblast Growth Factors in Prostatic Development

The FGF family presently consists of 19 structurally related proteins, some of which play an important role in prostatic development. There are four known FGF receptors (FGFR1, 2, 3, and 4), although the ligand specificity of FGFRs is known for only some FGF receptor pairs. FGFs play many different roles during embryonic development, and evidence that FGFs play a key role in directing male urogenital development is considerable.

Keratinocyte growth factor (KGF, also known as FGF7) has been shown to function as a growth regulator in the prostate (65) and seminal vesicle (66). Recombinant KGF protein directly stimulates growth of prostate and seminal vesicle epithelia when added to cultures of neonatal rat ventral prostate and mouse seminal vesicle. KGF is produced by mesenchymal cells and acts via the FGFR2 (iiib splice form), which is restricted to epithelial cells. Thus, KGF signaling is paracrine, because mesenchymal cells make KGF but do not express the receptor (FGFR2 iiib), and epithelial cells express the receptor (FGFR2 iiib) but do not make KGF. Transcripts for KGF are abundant during neonatal development of the seminal vesicle and ventral prostate and are highest during periods of active growth (67). When recombinant KGF was added to organ cultures of ventral prostate and seminal vesicle, it resulted in growth and development very similar to that induced by testosterone (65,66). Furthermore, a neutralizing monoclonal antibody to KGF inhibited testosterone-induced development of both the seminal vesicle and ventral prostate. These data supported the hypothesis that KGF functions as a mediator of androgen action, or *andromedin* (68,69). Studies on prostatic stromal cells grown *in vitro* suggested that KGF might be directly regulated by androgens (69). However, KGF messenger RNA (mRNA) was not regulated by androgens in ventral prostate or seminal vesicle organ cultures grown *in vitro*, or during development *in vivo* (67). Taken together, it is clear that KGF plays a key role as a mesenchymal factor, which regulates epithelial growth in the ventral prostate and seminal vesicle. How androgens are involved in regulating KGF activity is less clear, and it is possible that KGF is not directly regulated by androgens during prostatic or seminal vesicle development.

FGF10 has been shown to act as a paracrine regulator of development of the ventral prostate and seminal vesicle (70). FGF10 mRNA was shown to be abundant during prenatal and neonatal periods of prostatic organogenesis, but it was low or absent in adult organs (which are growth quiescent). In both the ventral prostate and seminal vesicle, FGF10 was observed in a subset of mesenchymal cells in a pattern consistent with a role as a paracrine regulator of epithelial development. In the neonatal ventral prostate, FGF10 transcripts were localized in the mesenchyme peripheral to the periurethral mesenchyme and distal to the tips of the elongating ventral prostate epithelial buds, whereas at later stages, FGF10 mRNA was observed in the mesenchyme surrounding epithelial buds undergoing branching morphogenesis. FGF10 transcripts also did not appear to be regulated by androgens when examined in organs grown *in vitro*. Although FGF10 mRNA increased fourfold after treatment with testosterone in the seminal vesicle (but not the ventral prostate), this increase could not be antagonized with an antiandrogen. Also, FGF10 transcripts were observed in embryonic female reproductive tracts in a position analogous to that of the male ventral prostate, suggesting that FGF10 expression is not dependent on androgens.

Recombinant FGF10 protein has been shown to stimulate growth of prostatic epithelial cell lines, but did not stimulate growth of either Dunning tumor stromal cells or primary seminal vesicle mesenchyme. Additionally, recombinant FGF10 stimulated the development of ventral prostate and seminal vesicle organ rudiments in serum-free organ cultures, eliciting development similar to that induced by testosterone (or KGF). When FGF10 and testosterone were added simultaneously to ventral prostate or seminal vesicle organ cultures, synergism was not observed. Furthermore, development induced by FGF10 could not be completely inhibited by the antiandrogen cyproterone acetate, demonstrating that the effects of FGF10 were not mediated by the androgen receptor. Thus, it is likely that FGF10 functions as a mesenchymal paracrine regulator of epithelial growth in the ventral prostate and seminal vesicle and that the FGF10 gene is not directly regulated by androgens (70). Despite the observations that KGF and FGF10 genes are not directly androgen regulated *in vivo*, it is possible that androgens are involved in the function of these molecules. The level at which androgens might regulate FGF10 or KGF activity is unknown, but it may be at the protein level and may involve regulation of protein distribution or other essential components of FGF signaling (e.g., heparan sulphate).

The high degree of biochemical and functional similarity between FGF10 and KGF (71) might lead to the erroneous conclusion that these molecules are interchangeable or functionally redundant, as discussed below. One of the key differences between KGF and FGF10 is in the localization of their transcripts within mesenchyme. KGF mRNA is diffusely distributed throughout mesenchyme (72), whereas FGF10 mRNA is restricted to a subset of mesenchymal cells closely associated with actively growing epithelium (16,70). This is an important difference and may account for the phenotypes observed in the KGF and FGF10-null mice. KGF knockout mice have a very mild phenotype and have no significant loss of function of organs, which normally show high levels of KGF expression (73). This may be because FGF10 can compensate for the lack of KGF. In contrast, the FGF10 knockout mouse shows a very severe phenotype and shows loss of organs known to express high levels of FGF10 (e.g., lungs, limbs, and prostate) (74,75) (A. A. Donjacour, G. R. Cunha, *unpublished data*, 2001). Clearly, KGF is not able to compensate for the lack of FGF10, and this may be due to the different expression patterns observed for KGF and FGF10 transcripts. It is possible that, because FGF10 is expressed abundantly in a spatially restricted pattern, locally high levels of FGF10 enable it to compensate for a lack of KGF, but the opposite is not true for KGF, which is diffusely expressed throughout mesenchyme.

An important difference in the mechanism of action of KGF and FGF10 is that KGF-induced growth is sensitive to antagonism by the antiandrogen cyproterone acetate (65,67), whereas FGF10-induced prostatic development is not. Thus, KGF signaling may intersect with androgen receptor signaling, whereas FGF10 signaling may not (70). These observations are in agreement with studies in the lung demonstrating different biologic effects of KGF and FGF10 (16,17). Consequently, it is possible that although KGF and FGF10 show many biochemical and functional similarities, they may have distinct as well as partially overlapping functions in development of the prostate and seminal vesicle.

Transforming Growth Factor Beta in Prostatic Development

The transforming growth factor beta (TGF-beta) superfamily represents a large group of molecules, which signal through similar cell surface receptors (76,77). This superfamily contains at least five TGF-betas, of which three (TGF-beta-1, -2 and -3) are known to be present in the prostate of humans and rodents. TGF-betas signal through a heterodimeric transmembrane receptor composed of two elements: TGF types 1 and 2 receptors (77,78). Signaling through the TGF-beta receptor heterodimer results in phosphorylation of Smad proteins (mammalian homolog of the *Drosophila Mad* gene), ultimately resulting in the activation of target genes. TGF-betas have been reported to elicit a variety of effects on cells, which reflect the target cell type and the conditions under which experiments are performed. These ligands can be either mitogenic or growth inhibitory and may also play a role in differentiation (76–78). Specific effects seem to depend on the target tissue. For example, TGF-betas are often mitogenic for fibroblasts, while acting as epithelial growth inhibitors. The growth-inhibitory effects of TGF-betas have been reported for cultures of prostatic epithelial cells (79). It is also important to note that the sites of production and action of TGF-beta do not have to be physically close. Maternal TGF-beta-1, for example, is known to cross the placenta and be active in fetal tissues (80). TGF-betas are secreted as inactive precursors, which have to be proteolytically cleaved to bind to their receptors (76). Both TGF-beta-1 and -2 have been shown to bind to extracellular matrix components, especially collagen type IV, where they are able to retain biologic activity (81). Therefore, when considering the biology of these molecules, it is important to be aware of the sites of expression, extracellular binding, and activation, as well as the location of TGF-beta receptors.

TGF-beta ligands and receptors are known to be expressed in the prostate (82,83). Ligands are differentially expressed in epithelial versus stromal compartments. For example, we have shown in tissue recombination models that TGF-beta-1 is not expressed in the epithelium of developing prostatic structures, although it is present in the stroma (39,84). In the same model system TGF-beta-3 was detected in both epithelial and stromal compartments (84).

TGF-beta is suggested to play a role in the differentiation of prostatic smooth muscle (85). It is possible that changes in either expression or activation of the ligand may affect the overall balance of cell proliferation, differentiation, and cell death. Thus, TGF-beta has been implicated as a mediator of apoptosis in both the maintenance of normal glandular architecture (86,87) and after castration (87–93). TGF-beta mRNA and protein are both repressed by androgens *in vivo* (92,93). TGF-beta-1 has recently been shown to be capable of altering the nuclear to cytoplasmic distribution of androgen receptor in rat prostatic smooth muscle cells *in vitro* (94). Although the significance of this observation for prostatic biology is at present unclear, it does emphasize the potential of this family of molecules to play a key role in the steroidal regulation of tissues.

TGF-beta-1 gene knockout mice, at least on some strain backgrounds, are viable. At 45 days of age, male mice are approximately 35% of the weight of wild-type littermates. Dissection of the male reproductive organs revealed a range of organ weights in the knockout animals, from 26% (epididymis) to 4% (seminal vesicle) of values of wild-type littermates (ventral prostate, 10%; dorsolateral prostate, 15%; testis, 17%). Dissection of the prostatic lobes showed that ductal tip number was reduced by approximately 50% (A. A. Donjacour, J. Letterio, *unpublished data*, 1997). These data illustrate that although TGF-beta-1 is not absolutely required for prostatic development, its absence leads to severe impairment of growth and development.

Epidermal Growth Factor Ligands in Prostatic Development

In its mature form, epidermal growth factor (EGF) is a 6-kDa polypeptide with potent mitogenic activity in many tissues. EGF is found in a number of exocrine secretions, including saliva, intestinal secretions, milk, seminal fluid, and urine (95). EGF-like activity has been reported in extracts of human prostate, testis, epididymis, and seminal vesicle (96). Further reports indicated that EGF was present in human prostatic fluid, with the fluid titer being significantly lower in BPH patients than in normal controls (97). A number of groups have shown that primary monolayer cultures of prostatic epithelium are responsive to the mitogenic effects of EGF (98).

Levels of immunoreactive EGF decrease markedly in the mouse ventral prostate after castration (99). Other reports demonstrate a relationship between androgen status and high-affinity EGF receptors in the rat prostate (100). Castration elicits a two- to sixfold increase in receptor expression, whereas treatment of castrated animals with DHT results in decreased expression. A similar inverse relationship between nuclear steroid receptors (androgen, estrogen, and progesterone) and EGF-receptor-binding capacity has been found in human BPH samples (101). This regulation of the EGF receptor has been interpreted as indicating a possible role for the EGF ligand family as autocrine or paracrine mediators of steroid hormone action. This idea is supported by data showing that EGF was crucial for androgen-dependent development of the Wolffian duct (102) and in estrogenic response in the uterus and vagina (103).

Work on the androgen-responsive prostatic cancer cell line, LNCaP, has shown an opposite form of regulation in that androgenic stimulus increased the expression of EGF receptor in these cells (104). Similar results have been obtained in PC3 cells transfected with the androgen receptor gene (105). These findings may represent peculiarities of these cell lines or may be related to the aberrant phenotype of these transformed cells. It is notable that other hormonally responsive cancer cell lines—for example, the human breast line MCF-7—also secrete a variety of growth factors, in some cases in an estrogen-regulated manner (106).

Transforming growth factor alpha (TGF-alpha) is a 5.6-kDa polypeptide with sequence and structural homology to EGF (107). Assays in cell culture show similar biologic activities for the two growth factors. TGF-alpha has been found in both embryonic and adult normal tissue (107). The potential role of TGF-alpha in disease processes has been underlined by studies of transgenic mice overexpressing TGF-alpha (108). Overexpression of TGF-alpha in these animals led to epithelial hyperplasia, dysplasias, and neoplasia in a number of tissues, notably the breast, liver, pancreas, and prostate. These findings clearly illustrate that control of growth factor expression is crucial to the maintenance of normal adult tissues, and that any breakdown of this control could induce the types of abnormalities described.

Four additional mammalian EGF family ligands have been described. These are heparin-binding EGF-like growth factor (HB-EGF), amphiregulin, betacellulin, and epiregulin. The receptor family has also expanded to four molecules: HER1 (EGF receptor or erbB-1), HER2 (neu or erbB-2), HER3 (erbB-3) and HER4 (erbB-4). TGF-alpha, amphiregulin, and EGF signal exclusively through HER1 (109). HB-EGF is an activating ligand for the EGF receptor (HER1 or erbB-1). HB-EGF has been detected in human prostate in interstitial and vascular smooth muscle cells and has been suggested to be an epithelial mitogen (110).

Insulinlike Growth Factors in Prostatic Development

Insulinlike growth factors 1 and 2 (IGF-1 and IGF-2) are circulating, single-chain polypeptides with significant amino acid similarity to proinsulin (111). Both polypeptides bind to and act through the type 1 IGF receptor (IGF-R1) to affect various aspects of cell function (e.g., proliferation, cell cycle progression, differentiation, apoptosis) in a wide variety of tissues (112). The IGF-R1 is a heterotetrameric transmembrane tyrosine kinase. IGF-2 can also bind to the IGF-2 or mannose 6-phosphate receptor, which also binds mannose-6-phosphate–containing extracellular proteins. This receptor is believed to be important in IGF-2 turnover (113). Both IGF-1 and IGF-2 are bound in the vasculature and in tissue by at least six different IGF-binding proteins (IGFBPs) (114). These IGFBPs modulate the activity of the IGFs. Although originally identified as circulating hormones stimulated by growth hormone secretion (115), the widespread tissue production and action of IGFs 1 and 2 imply that these are also autocrine and paracrine factors (116).

The IGFs appear to play a major role in normal prostatic growth as well as in carcinogenesis. The earliest indications of this came from *in vitro* studies. Both insulin and IGF-1 are mitogenic for human and rodent prostatic epithelial cells *in vitro* (98). Moreover, insulin (or IGF-1) has been demonstrated to be an important component of serum-free media, and, in the case of the neonatal mouse seminal vesicle, it is required to obtain maximal response to testosterone (117). IGF-1 gene expression has been reported in human and rat prostates, in the Dunning R-3327 prostatic tumor, and in some of its variants (118). Prostatic epithelial cells express IGFBPs (119). Little is known concerning the temporal and spatial pattern of expression of IGF-1, IGF-2, IGF-receptors, or IGFBPs in relation to the temporal and spatial pattern of DNA synthesis or differentiation in the growing prostate *in vivo*. An epidemiologic study in 1998 linked higher circulating IGF-1 levels with prostate cancer risk in humans (120).

IGF-1 knockout (IGF-1-KO) and type 1 IGF receptor knockout (IGF-R1-KO) mice have been created (121,122), and such mice are approximately 60% of normal size at the end of gestation. In most genetic backgrounds, IGF-1-KO and IGF-R1-KO mice usually die immediately at birth. However, even in the most severely affected strains, a small percentage (1% to 2%) of the IGF-1-KO mice survives past puberty. The prostates of these mice have been examined (123) and were found to be very small and retarded in their degree of ductal branching morphogenesis (124). Some of the parameters measured (e.g., terminal ductal tips and branch points) were proportional to the size of the animal, whereas others (e.g., gland area) were more severely reduced (124). Administration of testosterone or IGF-1 in adulthood to the homozygous null mice increased prostatic size and ductal tip number significantly. The growth-promoting effects of testosterone and IGF-1 were synergistic (124).

The authors have used an alternate method of analyzing prostates from IGF-1-KO and IGF-R1-KO mice. Prostatic rudiments were excised from IGF-R1 or IGF-1–null mouse fetuses and transplanted under the renal capsule of adult athymic nude mice. One month after transplantation, grafts of both the ligand and receptor knockout mice were significantly smaller than wild-type prostatic grafts (less than 1 mg vs. approximately 50 to 60 mg wet weight, A. A. Donjacour et al., *unpublished observations*, 1998). It is not known whether this effect on wet weight is due to changes in the rate of proliferation or of apoptosis. However, it has been shown that the cell cycle time is 2.5 times longer in IGF-R1 null fibroblasts versus normal fibroblasts (125). Despite the reduced size of transplants of prostatic rudiments from IGF-R1 or IGF-1–null donors, mature prostatic epithelial cells—which were tall, columnar, and expressed normal prostatic secretory proteins—differentiated. In both IGF-1-KO and IGF-R1-KO prostatic transplants, the stromal cells were concentrically organized around the ducts and resembled smooth muscle. Thus, IGF-1 appears to primarily affect cell number through regulation of proliferation or apoptosis, or both, and not cellular differentiation. The similarity of the results between the ligand and receptor knockout tissues suggested that local, and not circulating (in this case, from the host) IGF-1 was responsible for prostatic growth.

Many questions remain about the role of IGF-1 in prostatic development. The site of IGF-1 production must be described and its mode of action, autocrine, paracrine, or both, must be elucidated. The potential relationship of testosterone with IGF-1 deserves examination. In viable mutant strains, IGF-1-KO mice have lower testosterone levels in adulthood, owing to testicular defects that lead to infertility. In addition, in transient transfection assays, IGF-1 has been shown to stimulate androgen receptor–dependent transcription in the absence of testosterone (126). Finally, the role of the IGFBPs, which are present at least in human prostate (127), needs to be thoroughly investigated.

CONCLUSION

Secreted signaling molecules, along with their receptors and signal transduction pathways, are critical mediators of cell-cell and mesenchymal-epithelial communication that serve to regulate prostatic development and homeostasis. Other classes of molecules secreted into the extracellular space and at the cell surface are also important regulators of prostatic development and homeostasis. Examples of these molecules include (a) non-receptor proteins that bind secreted signaling molecules and modulate their activity, (b) extracellular proteases that can either activate or inactivate their target proteins, (c) extracellular matrix proteins that serve structural and other functions, (d) adhesion molecules, and (e) cell-surface enzymes that modify lipids and proteins.

In this regard, adhesive interactions between cells and tissues are also critical for controlling the movements, differentiation state, and proliferation of prostatic cells. These interactions can be mediated by cell-surface proteins, as well as by complex carbohydrate structures on the cell surface. An example is the type-2 cell surface carbohydrates implicated in cell-cell and cell-matrix adhesion interactions. The distribution of these complex carbohydrates in prostate cancer has suggested their role in regulating prostate biology (128). These carbohydrate structures can be found on proteins and lipids at the cell surface. They result from the activities of enzymes in the Golgi and at the cell surface that add, modify, and catabolize carbohydrate groups (129). Recent data from the authors' lab has shown that at least one of the enzymes, a fucosyltransferase that acts in the Golgi and at the cell surface to modify complex carbohydrates and synthesize type 2 structures, is spatially and temporally restricted during prostatic development. Furthermore, an antibody directed against this enzyme inhibits growth and branching morphogenesis of prostatic rudiments *in vitro* (130). These data suggest that control of the spatial distribution of cell-cell and cell-matrix adhesion interactions may be crucial in regulating cell movements, cell proliferation, and the spatial distribution of growth factor signaling during growth and morphogenesis of the prostate.

In summary, the extracellular space and cell surfaces within the prostate are not mere conduits for growth factors that mediate cell-cell and mesenchymal-epithelial interactions. This compartment hosts complex interactions among secreted signaling molecules, receptors, binding proteins, proteases, matrix proteins, adhesion molecules, and other enzymatic activities. The net result of these interactions is the coordinated growth, ductal branching morphogenesis, and differentiation of epithelial and stromal cells. The relative importance of secreted signaling molecules, receptors, binding proteins, proteases, matrix proteins, adhesion molecules, and other cell-surface enzymatic activities for prostatic development will ultimately be clarified as knockout mice for genes in each of these categories are made and analyzed. It seems likely that molecules in each of these categories will be found that are crucial for regulating prostatic development.

REFERENCES

1. Pierce G, Shikes R, Fink L. *Cancer: a problem of developmental biology.* Englewood Cliffs, New Jersey: Prentice Hall, 1978.
2. Mintz B. Genetic mosaicism and in vivo analyses of neoplasia and differentiation. In: Saunders G, ed. *Cell differentiation and neoplasia.* New York: Raven Press, 1978:27–56.
3. Cunha GR, Hayashi N, Wong YC. Regulation of differentiation and growth of normal adult and neoplastic epithelial by inductive mesenchyme. In: Isaacs JT, ed. *Prostate cancer: cell and molecular mechanisms in diagnosis and treatment.*

Cold Spring Harbor: Cold Spring Harbor Laboratory Press, 1991:73–90.
4. Wilson JD, Griffin JE, George FW, et al. Recent studies on the endocrine control of male phenotypic development. In: Serio M, Zanisi M, Motta M, et al., eds. *Sexual differentiation: basic and clinical aspects.* New York: Raven Press, 1984:223–232.
5. Donahoe PK, Budzik G, Trelstad R, et al. Müllerian inhibiting substance: an update. *Rec Prog Horm Res* 1982;38:279–330.
6. Jost A. Gonadal hormones in the sex differentiation of the mammalian fetus. In: Urpsrung RL, DeHaan H, eds. *Organogenesis.* New York: Holt, Rinehart and Winston, 1965:611–628.
7. Wilson JD. Syndrome of androgen resistance. *Biol Reprod* 1992;46:168–173.
8. Jost A. Problems of fetal endocrinology: the gonadal and hypophyseal hormones. *Rec Prog Horm Res* 1953;8:379–418.
9. Cunha GR, Cooke PS, Bigsby R, et al. Ontogeny of sex steroid receptors in mammals. In: Parker MG, ed. *The structure and function of nuclear hormone receptors.* New York: Academic Press, 1991:235–268.
10. Cunha GR, Donjacour AA, Cooke PS, et al. The endocrinology and developmental biology of the prostate. *Endocrine Rev* 1987;8:338–362.
11. Sugimura Y, Cunha GR, Donjacour AA. Morphogenesis of ductal networks in the mouse prostate. *Biol Reprod* 1986;34:961–971.
12. McNeal JE. The prostate gland: morphology and pathobiology. *Monogr Urology* 1983;4:3–37.
13. Donjacour AA, Cunha GR. The effect of androgen deprivation on branching morphogenesis in the mouse prostate. *Develop Biol* 1988;128:1–14.
14. Sugimura Y, Cunha GR, Donjacour AA, et al. Whole-mount autoradiography study of DNA synthetic activity during postnatal development and androgen-induced regeneration in the mouse prostate. *Biol Reprod* 1986;34: 985–995.
15. Nogawa H, Morita K, Cardoso WV. Bud formation precedes the appearance of differential cell proliferation during branching morphogenesis of mouse lung epithelium in vitro. *Dev Dyn* 1998;213:228–235.
16. Bellusci S, Grindley J, Emoto H, et al. Fibroblast growth factor 10 (FGF10) and branching morphogenesis in the embryonic mouse lung. *Development* 1997;124:4867–4878.
17. Park WY, Miranda B, Lebeche D, et al. FGF-10 is a chemotactic factor for distal epithelial buds during lung development. *Dev Biol* 1998;201:125–134.
18. Hayward SW, Grossfeld GD, Tlsty TD, et al. Genetic and epigenetic influences in prostatic carcinogenesis. *Int J Oncol* 1998;13:35–47.
19. Hayward SW, Baskin LS, Haughney PC, et al. Epithelial development in the rat ventral prostate, anterior prostate and seminal vesicle. *Acta Anatomica* 1996;155:81–93.
20. Hayward SW, Baskin LS, Haughney PC, et al. Stromal development in the ventral prostate, anterior prostate and seminal vesicle of the rat. *Acta Anatomica* 1996;155:94–103.
21. Hayward SW, Brody JR, Cunha GR. An edgewise look at basal cells: Three-dimensional views of the rat prostate, mammary gland and salivary gland. *Differentiation* 1996; 60:219–227.
22. Lopes ES, Foster BA, Donjacour AA, et al. Initiation of secretory activity of rat prostatic epithelium in organ culture. *Endocrinology* 1996;137:4225–4234.
23. Prins GS. Neonatal estrogen exposure induces lobe-specific alterations in adult rat prostate androgen receptor expression. *Endocrinology* 1992;130:2401–2412.
24. Prins GS, Birch L. The developmental pattern of androgen receptor expression in rat prostate lobes is altered after neonatal exposure to estrogen. *Endocrinology* 1995;136:1303–1314.
25. Prins G, Birch L, Greene G. Androgen receptor localization in different cell types of the adult rat prostate. *Endocrinology* 1991;129:3187–3199.
26. Soeffing WJ, Timms BG. Localization of androgen receptor and cell-specific cytokeratins in basal cells of rat ventral prostate. *J Androl* 1995;16:197–208.
27. Nemeth JA, Lee C. Prostatic ductal system in rats: regional variation in stromal organization. *Prostate* 1996;28:124–128.
28. Russell DW, Wilson JD. Steroid 5 alpha-reductase: two genes/two enzymes. *Annu Rev Biochem* 1994;63:25–61.
29. Carlson KE, Katzenellenbogen JA. A comparative study of the selectivity and efficiency of target tissue uptake of five tritium-labeled androgens in the rat. *J Steroid Biochem* 1990;36:549–561.
30. Deslypere JP, Young M, Wilson JD, et al. Testosterone and 5 alpha-dihydrotestosterone interact differently with the androgen receptor to enhance transcription of the MMTV-CAT reporter gene. *Mol Cell Endocrinol* 1992;88:15–22.
31. Imperato-McGinley J, Peterson RE, Gautier T. Primary and secondary 5α-reductase deficiency. In: Serio M, Zanisi M, Motta M, et al., eds. *Sexual differentiation: basic and clinical aspects.* New York: Raven Press, 1984:233–245.
32. Berman DM, Tian H, Russell DW. Expression and regulation of steroid 5 alpha-reductase in the urogenital tract of the fetal rat. *Mol Endocrinol* 1995;9:1561–1570.
33. Sugimura Y, Norman JT, Cunha GR, et al. Regional differences in the inductive activity of the mesenchyme of the embryonic mouse urogenital sinus. *Prostate* 1985;7:253–260.
34. Timms B, Lee C, Aumuller G, et al. Instructive induction of prostate growth and differentiation by a defined urogenital sinus mesenchyme. *Microsc Res Tech* 1995;30:319–332.
35. Takeda H, Suematsu N, Mizuno T. Transcription of prostatic steroid binding protein (PSBP) gene is induced by epithelial-mesenchymal interaction. *Development* 1990;110:273–282.
36. Hayashi N, Cunha GR, Parker M. Permissive and instructive induction of adult rodent prostatic epithelium by heterotypic urogenital sinus mesenchyme. *Epithelial Cell Biol* 1993;2:66–78.
37. Tsuji M, Shima H, Boutin G, et al. Effect of mesenchymal glandular inductors on the growth and cytodifferentiation of neonatal mouse seminal vesicle epithelium. *J Andrology* 1994;15:565–574.
38. Cunha GR, Battle E, Young P, et al. Role of epithelial-mesenchymal interactions in the differentiation and spatial organization of visceral smooth muscle. *Epithelial Cell Biol* 1992;1:76–83.
39. Hayward SW, Haughney PC, Rosen MA, et al. Interactions between adult human prostatic epithelium and rat urogenital sinus mesenchyme in a tissue recombination model. *Differentiation* 1998;63:131–140.

40. He WW, Kumar MV, Tindall DJ. A frameshift mutation in the androgen receptor gene causes complete androgen insensitivity in the testicular-feminized mouse. *Nucleic Acids Res* 1991;19:2373–2378.
41. Cunha GR, Alarid ET, Turner T, et al. Normal and abnormal development of the male urogenital tract: role of androgens, mesenchymal-epithelial interactions and growth factors. *J Androl* 1992;13:465–475.
42. Donjacour AA, Cunha GR. Assessment of prostatic protein secretion in tissue recombinants made of urogenital sinus mesenchyme and urothelium from normal or androgen-insensitive mice. *Endocrinology* 1993;131: 2342–2350.
43. Cunha GR, Young P. Inability of Tfm (testicular feminization) epithelial cells to express androgen-dependent seminal vesicle secretory proteins in chimeric tissue recombinants. *Endocrinology* 1991;128:3293–3298.
44. Sugimura Y, Cunha GR, Bigsby RM. Androgenic induction of deoxyribonucleic acid synthesis in prostatic glands induced in the urothelium of testicular feminized (Tfm/y) mice. *Prostate* 1986;9:217–225.
45. Cooke P, Buchanan D, Young P, et al. Stromal estrogen receptors (ER) mediate mitogenic effects of estradiol on uterine epithelium. *Proc Natl Acad Sci U S A* 1997;94:6535–6540.
46. Kurita T, Young P, Brody J, et al. Stromal progesterone receptors mediate the inhibitory effects of progesterone on estrogen-induced uterine epithelial cell (UtE) proliferation. *Endocrinology* 1998;139:4708–4713.
47. Buchanan DL, Setiawan T, Lubahn DL, et al. Tissue compartment-specific estrogen receptor participation in the mouse uterine epithelial secretory response. *Endocrinology* 1998;140:484–491.
48. Buchanan DL, Kurita T, Taylor JA, et al. Role of stromal and epithelial estrogen receptors in vaginal epithelial proliferation, stratification and cornification. *Endocrinology* 1998;139:4345–4352.
49. Krumlauf R. Hox genes in vertebrate development. *Cell* 1994;78:191–201.
50. Lawrence PA, Morata G. Homeobox genes: their function in *Drosophila* segmentation and pattern formation. *Cell* 1994;78:181–189.
51. Davidson D. The function and evolution of Msx genes: pointers and paradoxes. *Trends Genet* 1995;11:405–411.
52. He WW, Sciavolino PJ, Wing J, et al. A novel human prostate-specific, androgen-regulated homeobox gene (NKX3.1) that maps to 8p21, a region frequently deleted in prostate cancer. *Genomics* 1997;43:69–77.
53. Sciavolino PJ, Abrams EW, Yang L, et al. Tissue-specific expression of murine Nkx3.1 in the male urogenital system. *Dev Dyn* 1997;209:127–138.
54. Bhatia-Gaur R, Donjacour AA, Sciavolino PJ, et al. Roles for Nkx3.1 in prostate development and cancer. *Genes Dev* 1999;13:966–977.
55. Prescott JL, Blok L, Tindall DJ. Isolation and androgen regulation of the human homeobox cDNA, NKX3.1. *Prostate* 1998;35:71–80.
56. Zeltser L, Desplan C, Heintz N. Hoxb-13: a new Hox gene in a distant region of the HOXB cluster maintains colinearity. *Development* 1996;122:2475–2484.
57. Dolle P, Izpisua-Belmonte JC, Brown JM, et al. HOX-4 genes and the morphogenesis of mammalian genitalia. *Genes Dev* 1991;5:1767–1777.
58. Dolle P, Izpisua-Belmonte JC, Boncinelli E, et al. The Hox-4.8 gene is localized at the 5' extremity of the Hox-4 complex and is expressed in the most posterior parts of the body during development. *Mech Dev* 1991;36:3–13.
59. Oefelein M, Chin-Chance C, Bushman W. Expression of the homeotic gene Hox-d13 in the developing and adult mouse prostate. *J Urol* 1996;155:342–346.
60. Podlasek CA, Duboule D, Bushman W. Male accessory sex organ morphogenesis is altered by loss of function of Hoxd-13. *Dev Dyn* 1997;208:454–465.
61. Podlasek CA, Seo RM, Clemens JQ, et al. Hoxa-10 deficient male mice exhibit abnormal development of the accessory sex organs. *Dev Dyn* 1999;214:1–12.
62. Podlasek CA, Clemens JQ, Bushman W. Hoxa-13 gene mutation results in abnormal seminal vesicle and prostate development. *J Urol* 1999;161:1655–1661.
63. Warot X, Fromental-Ramain C, Fraulob V, et al. Gene dosage-dependent effects of the Hoxa-13 and Hoxd-13 mutations on morphogenesis of the terminal parts of the digestive and urogenital tracts. *Development* 1997;124: 4781–4797.
64. Podlasek CA, Barnett DH, Clemens JQ, et al. Prostate development requires Sonic hedgehog expressed by the urogenital sinus epithelium. *Dev Biol* 1999;209:28–39.
65. Sugimura Y, Foster BA, Hom YK, Rubin JS, et al. Keratinocyte growth factor (KGF) can replace testosterone in the ductal branching morphogenesis of the rat ventral prostate. *Int J Develop Biol* 1996;40:941–951.
66. Alarid ET, Rubin JS, Young P, et al. Keratinocyte growth factor functions in epithelial induction during seminal vesicle development. *Proc Natl Acad Sci USA* 1994;91:1074–1078.
67. Thomson AA, Foster BA, Cunha GR. Analysis of growth factor and receptor mRNAs during development of the rat seminal vesicle and prostate. *Development* 1997;124:2431–2439.
68. Peehl D, Rubin J. Keratinocyte growth factor: an androgen-regulated mediator of stromal-epithelial interactions in the prostate. *World J Urol* 1995;13:312–317.
69. Yan G, Fukabori Y, Nikolaropoulos S, et al. Heparin-binding keratinocyte growth factor is a candidate stromal to epithelial cell andromedin. *Molecular Endocrinology* 1992;6: 2123–2128.
70. Thomson AA, Cunha GR. Prostatic growth and development are regulated by FGF10. *Development* 1999;126: 3693–3701.
71. Igarashi M, Finch PW, Aaronson SA. Characterization of recombinant human fibroblast growth factor (FGF)-10 reveals functional similarities with keratinocyte growth factor (FGF-7). *J Biol Chem* 1998;273:13230–13235.
72. Finch PW, Cunha GR, Rubin JS, et al. Pattern of KGF and KGFR expression during mouse fetal development suggests a role in mediating morphogenetic mesenchymal-epithelial interactions. *Dev Dyn* 1995;203:223–240.
73. Guo L, Degenstein L, Fuchs E. Keratinocyte growth factor is required for hair development but not for wound healing. *Genes Dev* 1996;10:165–175.

74. Sekine K, Ohuchi H, Fujiwara M, et al. Fgf10 is essential for limb and lung formation. *Nat Genet* 1999;21:138–141.
75. Min H, Danilenko D, Scully S, et al. Fgf-10 is required for both limb and lung development and exhibits striking functional similarity to *Drosophila* branchless. *Genes Dev* 1998;20:3156–3161.
76. Sporn MB, Roberts AB. Transforming growth factor-beta: recent progress and new challenges. *J Cell Biol* 1992; 119:1017–1021.
77. Derynck R. TGF-beta-receptor-mediated signaling. *Trends Biochem Sci* 1994;19:548–553.
78. Derynck R, Feng XH. TGF-beta receptor signaling. *Biochim Biophys Acta* 1997;1333:F105–150.
79. Lucia MS, Sporn MB, Roberts AB, et al. The role of transforming growth factor-beta1, -beta2, and -beta3 in androgen-responsive growth of NRP-152 rat prostatic epithelial cells. *J Cell Physiol* 1998;175:184–192.
80. Letterio JJ, Geiser AG, Kulkarni AB, et al. Maternal rescue of transforming growth factor-beta 1 null mice. *Science* 1994;264:1936–1938.
81. Paralkar VM, Vukicevic S, Reddi AH. Transforming growth factor beta type 1 binds to collagen IV of basement membrane matrix: Implications for development. *Dev Biol* 1991;143:303–308.
82. Timme TL, Truong LD, Merz VW, et al. Mesenchymal-epithelial interactions and transforming growth factor-beta expression during mouse prostate morphogenesis. *Endocrinology* 1994;134:1039–1045.
83. Gerdes MJ, Larsen M, McBride L, et al. Localization of transforming growth factor-beta1 and type II receptor in developing normal human prostate and carcinoma tissues. *J Histochem Cytochem* 1998;46:379–388.
84. Haughney PC, Hayward SW, Dahiya R, et al. Species-specific detection of growth factor gene expression in developing prostatic tissue. *Biol Reprod* 1998;59:93–99.
85. Peehl DM, Sellers RG. Induction of smooth muscle cell phenotype in cultured human prostatic stromal cells. *Exp Cell Res* 1997;232:208–215.
86. Nemeth JA, Sensibar JA, White RR, et al. Prostatic ductal system in rats: tissue-specific expression and regional variation in stromal distribution of transforming growth factor-beta 1. *Prostate* 1997;33:64–71.
87. Lee C, Sintich SM, Mathews EP, et al. Transforming growth factor-beta in benign and malignant prostate. *Prostate* 1999;39:285–290.
88. Kim IY, Ahn HJ, Zelner DJ, et al. Expression and localization of transforming growth factor-beta receptors type I and type II in the rat ventral prostate during regression. *Mol Endocrinol* 1996;10:107–115.
89. Kyprianou N, Tu H, Jacobs SC. Apoptotic versus proliferative activities in human benign prostatic hyperplasia. *Hum Pathol* 1996;27:668–675.
90. Lindstrom P, Bergh A, Holm I, et al. Expression of transforming growth factor-beta 1 in rat ventral prostate and Dunning 83327 PAP prostate tumor after castration and estrogen treatment. *Prostate* 1996;29:209–218.
91. Saez C, Gonzalez-Baena AC, Japon MA, et al. Regressive changes in finasteride-treated human hyperplastic prostates correlate with an upregulation of TGF-beta receptor expression. *Prostate* 1998;37:84–90.
92. Kyprianou N, Isaacs JT. Expression of transforming growth factor-beta in the rat ventral prostate during castration-induced programmed cell death. *Mol Endocrinol* 1989; 3:1515–1522.
93. Kyprianou N, Isaacs JT. Identification of a cellular receptor for transforming growth factor-beta in rat ventral prostate and its negative regulation by androgens. *Endocrinology* 1988;123:2124–2131.
94. Gerdes MJ, Dang TD, Larsen M, et al. Transforming growth factor-beta1 induces nuclear to cytoplasmic distribution of androgen receptor and inhibits androgen response in prostate smooth muscle cells. *Endocrinology* 1998;139: 3569–3577.
95. Jacobs SC, Story MT. Exocrine secretion of epidermal growth factor by the rat prostate: effect of adrenergic agents, cholinergic agents and vasoactive intestinal peptide. *Prostate* 1988;13:79–87.
96. Elson SD, Browne CA, Thorburn GD. Identification of epidermal growth factor-like activity in human male reproductive tissues and fluids. *J Clin Endocrinol Metab* 1984;58:589–597.
97. Gregory H, Willshire IR, Kavanagh JP, et al. Urogastrone-epidermal growth factor concentrations in prostatic fluid of normal individuals and patients with benign prostatic hypertrophy. *Clin Sci (Colch)* 1986;70:359–363.
98. McKeehan WL, Adams PS, Rosser MP. Direct mitogenic effects of insulin, epidermal growth factor, glucocorticoid, cholera toxin, unknown pituitary factors and possibly prolactin, but not androgen, on normal rat prostate epithelial cells in serum-free, primary cell culture. *Cancer Res* 1984;44:1998–2010.
99. Hiramatsu M, Kashimata M, Minami N, et al. Androgenic regulation of epidermal growth factor in the mouse ventral prostate. *Biochem Intl* 1988;17:311–317.
100. St Arnaud R, Poyet P, Walder P, et al. Androgens modulate epidermal growth factor receptor levels in the rat ventral prostate. *Molec Cell Endocrinol* 1988;56:21–27.
101. Lubrano C, Petrangeli E, Catizone A, et al. Epidermal growth factor binding and steroid receptor content in human benign prostatic hyperplasia. *J Steroid Biochem* 1989;34:499–504.
102. Gupta C, Siegel S, Ellis D. The role of EGF in testosterone-induced reproductive tract differentiation. *Dev Biol* 1991; 146:106–116.
103. Nelson KG, Takahashi T, Bossert NL, et al. Epidermal growth factor replaces estrogen in the stimulation of female genital-tract growth and differentiation. *Proc Natl Acad Sci U S A* 1991;88:21–25.
104. Schuurmans AL, Bolt J, Veldscholte J, et al. Stimulatory effects of antiandrogens on LNCaP human prostate tumor cell growth, EGF-receptor level and acid phosphatase secretion. *J Steroid Biochem Mol Biol* 1990;37: 849–853.
105. Brass AL, Barnard J, Patai BL, et al. Androgen up-regulates epidermal growth factor receptor expression and binding affinity in PC3 cell lines expressing the human androgen receptor. *Cancer Res* 1995;55:3197–3203.
106. Lippman ME, Dickson RB, Kasid A, et al. Autocrine and paracrine growth regulation of human breast cancer. *J Steroid Biochem* 1986;24:147–154.

107. Bascom CC, Sipes NJ, Coffey RJ, et al. Regulation of epithelial cell proliferation by transforming growth factors. *J Cell Biochem* 1989;39:25–32.
108. Sandgren EP, Luetteke NC, Palmiter RD, et al. Overexpression of TGF alpha in transgenic mice: induction of epithelial hyperplasia, pancreatic metaplasia, and carcinoma of the breast. *Cell* 1990;61:1121–1135.
109. McInnes C, Sykes BD. Growth factor receptors: structure, mechanism, and drug discovery. *Biopolymers* 1997;43: 339–366.
110. Freeman MR, Paul S, Kaefer M, et al. Heparin-binding EGF-like growth factor in the human prostate: synthesis predominantly by interstitial and vascular smooth muscle cells and action as a carcinoma cell mitogen. *J Cell Biochem* 1998;68:328–338.
111. Rinderknecht E, Humbel RE. Primary structure of human insulin-like growth factor II. *FEBS Lett* 1978;89:283–286.
112. Jones JI, Clemmons DR. Insulin-like growth factors and their binding proteins: biological actions. *Endocr Rev* 1995;16:3–34.
113. Ludwig T, Eggenschwiler J, Fisher P, et al. Mouse mutants lacking the type 2 IGF receptor (IGF2R) are rescued from perinatal lethality in Igf2 and Igf1 null backgrounds. *Dev Biol* 1996;177:517–535.
114. Cohen P, Rosenfeld RG. Physiologic and clinical relevance of the insulin-like growth factor binding proteins. *Curr Opin Pediatr* 1994;6:462–467.
115. Salmon W, Daughaday W. A hormonally controlled serum factor which stimulates sulfate incorporation by cartilage in vitro. *J Lab Clin Med* 1957;49:825–836.
116. Han VK, D'Ercole AJ, Lund PK. Cellular localization of somatomedin (insulin-like growth factor) messenger RNA in the human fetus. *Science* 1987;236:193–197.
117. Tsuji M, Shima H, Cunha GR. Morphogenetic and proliferative effects of testosterone and insulin on the neonatal mouse seminal vesicle in vitro. *Endocrinology* 1991;129: 2289–2297.
118. McKeehan WL. Growth factor receptors and prostate cell growth. In: Isaacs JT, ed. *Prostate cancer: cell and molecular mechanisms in diagnosis and treatment.* Cold Spring Harbor: Cold Spring Harbor Laboratory Press, 1991:165–176.
119. Cohen P, Graves HC, Peehl DM, et al. Prostate-specific antigen (PSA) is an insulin-like growth factor binding protein-3 protease found in seminal plasma. *J Clin Endocrinol Metab* 1992;75:1046–1053.
120. Chan JM, Stampfer MJ, Giovannucci E, et al. Plasma insulin-like growth factor-I and prostate cancer risk: a prospective study. *Science* 1998;279:563–566.
121. Liu JP, Baker J, Perkins AS, et al. Mice carrying null mutations of the genes encoding insulin-like growth factor I (Igf-1) and type 1 IGF receptor (Igf1r). *Cell* 1993;75:59–72.
122. Powell-Braxton L, Hollingshead P, Warburton C, et al. IGF-I is required for normal embryonic growth in mice. *Genes Dev* 1993;7:2609–2617.
123. Baker J, Hardy MP, Zhou J, et al. Effects of an Igf1 gene null mutation on mouse reproduction. *Mol Endo* 1996;10: 903–918.
124. Ruan W, Powell-Braxton L, Kopchick JJ, et al. Evidence that insulin-like growth factor I and growth hormone are required for prostate gland development. *Endocrinology* 1999;140:1984–1989.
125. Sell C, Dumenil G, Deveaud C, et al. Effect of a null mutation of the insulin-like growth factor I receptor gene on growth and transformation of mouse embryo fibroblasts. *Mol Cell Biol* 1994;14:3604–3612.
126. Culig Z, Hobisch A, Cronauer MV, et al. Activation of the androgen receptor by polypeptide growth factors and cellular regulators. *World J Urol* 1995;13:285–289.
127. Cohen P, Peehl DM, Baker B, et al. Insulin-like growth factor axis abnormalities in prostatic cells from patients with benign prostatic hyperplasia. *J Clin Endocrinol Metab* 1994;79:1410–1415.
128. Jorgensen T, Berner A, Kaalhus O, et al. Up-regulation of the oligosaccharide sialyl LewisX: a new prognostic parameter in metastatic prostate cancer. *Cancer Res* 1995;55:1817–1819.
129. Clausen H, Hakomori S. ABH and related histo-blood group antigens; immunochemical differences in carrier isotypes and their distribution. *Vox Sang* 1989;56:1–20.
130. Marker PC, Stephan JP, Lee J, et al. Fucosyltransferase 1 and H-type complex carbohydrates modulate epithelial cell proliferation during prostatic branching morphogenesis. *Dev Biol* 2001 (*in press*).

3

NUCLEAR RECEPTORS IN NORMAL PROSTATIC GROWTH AND DISEASE

PHILLIP G. FEBBO
MYLES A. BROWN

This chapter focuses on the superfamily of proteins that are referred to as *nuclear receptors* (NRs) and their participation in normal and pathologic states of the prostate. NRs are intracellular proteins that bind lipophilic-steroid molecules. Once NRs are associated with their respective ligands, they undergo a conformational change (including dimerization for some receptors), recognize and bind to specific steroid response elements within DNA, and control transcription of specific target genes, thereby exerting control of cellular metabolism and growth.

The superfamily of NRs comprises a diverse class of proteins that most likely evolved from a common precursor (1–3). Early work comparing the highly conserved DNA-binding domains of 30 known NRs classified members of the superfamily into three major categories: (a) thyroid and retinoid hormone receptors, (b) orphan receptors, and (c) steroid receptors (3). More recent work and discovery of new members of this family have increased the number of groups to five (2), and most recently six, subfamilies (1).

Throughout the chapter, NRs are organized in two general categories: (a) steroid receptors, including the androgen receptor (AR), estrogen receptor (ER), glucocorticoid receptor (GR), progesterone receptor (PR), and mineralocorticoid receptor (MR), and (b) nonsteroid NRs that include the subfamilies thyroid hormone receptors (TRs), retinoic acid receptors (RARs), peroxisome proliferator-activated receptors (PPARs), vitamin D receptors (VDRs), ecdysone receptors, and numerous orphan receptors (1). Many of the nonsteroid NRs have not been identified in the prostate and are not discussed.

In the next sections, the general discovery, structure, and function of NRs are reviewed. The evolving understanding of transcriptional control by NRs and associated proteins is discussed, along with known modulatory and regulating effects. In the second part of this chapter, individual NRs are discussed in the context of prostate development, growth, senescence, and pathologic states, including prostate cancer (CaP).

HISTORICAL OVERVIEW

The class of NRs was first discovered with the recognition of estrogen binding within estrogen-responsive uterine cells (4,5). With the discovery of an intracellular receptor for estrogen, other binding proteins for steroid ligands were sought and found, including glucocorticoid, progesterone, and androgen-binding proteins (6–8).

Most ligand-free NRs were isolated from the cytosol and, after binding ligand, the receptor-ligand complex would be isolated in the nuclear fraction of protein. This suggested a ligand-induced translocation and a phenomenon that was referred to as the "two-step" hypothesis (4,9). With further refinement of molecular tools and intense investigation, it became clear that unbound receptors existed in both the cytoplasmic and nuclear fractions and a strict adherence to the "two-step" model did not fully explain all observations (9).

In the late 1980s, cloning of the NR genes resulted in a preliminary understanding of NR protein structure (10). Comparative analyses across known steroid receptors quickly identified the group as a family of proteins with conserved features (Table 3-1). The identification of complementary DNA (cDNA) sequence also facilitated cDNA cross-hybridization screening and identification of an unexpectedly large number of members of the growing superfamily (11). Some of the identified receptors lacked known ligands and were referred to as *orphan receptors*. The first reported examples of orphan receptors included estrogen receptor–related 1 and 2 proteins (12). Analysis of cDNA also implicated some previously described receptors, such as VDR, as being part of the NR superfamily (13).

Cloning of the specific genes and identification of orphan receptors facilitated further research investigating the tissue specific expression, intracellular location, and function of NRs. The region of greatest homology between family members was found to encode two zinc fingers that bind to DNA. This region was implicated in specific DNA

TABLE 3-1. NUCLEAR RECEPTOR CLASSES AND CHARACTERISTICS IN PROSTATE AND PROSTATE CANCER (CaP)

	Developing prostate	Adult prostate	Expression in benign prostatic hypertrophy (BPH)	Expression in CaP	Castration response	Clinical response
Steroid receptors						
Androgen receptor	First mesenchymal, then epithelial (132)	TE > EBC > SC (greater in peripheral zone) (148,151)	Increased (171)	Increased (heterogeneous) (171)	Markedly decreased (338)	Antagonists: decrease PSA, decrease symptoms, improve mortality (339,340)
Estrogen receptor alpha	Largely mesenchymal (230)	SC > TE and EBC (transitional zone) (151)	± Increased (256)	Little to no (161)	Increased (161)	Agonists: decreased CaP activity, high cardiovascular morbidity (265) Antagonists: no effect (266)
Estrogen receptor beta	Epithelium and mesenchymal (236)	TE and EBC > SC (226)	NA	Expressed in cell lines (261)	Decreased (236)	NA
Progesterone receptor	NA	SC only (271)	Increased (174)	Increased (<BPH) (174)	NA	Agonists: only modest activity (275)
Glucocorticoid receptor	NA	SC > TE and EBC (171)	Increased (171)	Increased (171)	Increased (276)	Agonists: decreased CaP activity (282)
Nonsteroid receptors						
Vitamin D receptor	NA	TE > SC (303)	Expressed (285)	Expressed (303)	NA	Agonists: may slow progression (341)
Retinoic acid receptor	Beta and gamma expressed at day 0 (311)	Alpha, beta, and gamma all expressed (312)	NA	Decreased (312)	NA	Agonists: all-*trans*-retinoic acid with no efficacy (323)
Peroxisome-proliferator activated receptor (PPAR)–gamma	NA	Low levels of PPAR-gamma (331)	NA	Increased (331)	NA	Agonists: PSA stabilization in men with metastatic disease (332)

EBC, epithelial basal cells; NA, not available; PSA, prostate-specific antigen; SC, stromal cells; TE, tubular epithelium.

binding by sophisticated work that resulted in GR-activated transcription of estrogen-responsive genes when the first of the GR zinc fingers was replaced by the DNA-binding zinc finger of the ER (14). Subsequent work (described in more detail below) identified most members of the family to contain three major functional domains: a DNA-binding domain, a ligand-binding domain, and a transactivational domain.

The development of antibodies directed against NRs in the 1990s has resulted in further description of the regulatory role of NRs and identified a host of receptor-associated proteins. Unbound NRs have been shown to associate with chaperone molecules such as heat shock protein 90, heat shock protein 70, and smaller proteins, such as immunophilins (15). The association between these chaperone molecules and steroid receptors is thought to stabilize the receptor and contribute to the receptor's ability to bind ligand and activate transcription. Once ligand is bound, however, the aggregate of receptor and chaperones is thought to disassociate as the receptor translocates into the nucleus, dimerizes, and binds specific recognition sites adjacent to regulated genes.

Although NRs bind directly to DNA, DNA binding and transcriptional activation also involves a number of directly and indirectly associated proteins. A class of NR co-stimulatory and co-inhibitory proteins have been immunoprecipitated with different receptors and demonstrated to have modulatory affect on receptor function [reviewed in (16)]. The complex interactions between NRs and modulatory proteins likely contribute to the tissue specificity of some receptors' functions.

In conclusion, the early model of a ligand-bound NR's affecting transcription of target genes to affect cellular physiology remains intact. The advances over the past thirty years have refined the model, identified NRs as a superfamily, associated structure with function, and identified a host of proteins that associate and modulate the function of NRs.

NUCLEAR RECEPTOR STRUCTURE AND FUNCTION

This section reviews what is known about the structure and function of the superfamily of nuclear hormone receptors. First, the section focuses on the structure of the family of NRs and comments on structure and function relationships. Second, the regulation and function of NRs within target cells is discussed and NR-associated cellular proteins are identified with respect to the NR superfamily.

A general overview is provided with specific examples to give the reader a general understanding of the importance and activity of each major domain of the NRs. For more exhaustive reviews of the NR superfamily, the reader is directed to previous comprehensive reviews (9,17–20) and texts (21,22).

Structure

Members of the NR superfamily share three major functional domains: (a) a central DNA-binding domain, (b) a carboxy-terminal ligand-binding domain, and (c) an amino-terminal transactivational domain (Fig. 3-1) (20).

Central and DNA-Binding Domain

Early on, a critical region of 66 amino acids was recognized as being homologous between all identified NRs and highly conserved across species (23). In the GR, insertional mutations disrupting this domain abrogated the receptor's ability to activate transcription (24). In the ER, this region is required for the receptor to achieve tight nuclear binding (25). Further work in the ER (26) and GR (27) demonstrated that this region alone was sufficient for transcriptional activation.

The amino acid sequence of this domain is rich in cysteine, lysine, and arginine and was anticipated to constitute a DNA-binding domain based on its similarity to regions within known DNA-binding proteins (e.g., TFIIa) (28,29). The amino acid sequence encodes two DNA-binding zinc fingers (30). The amino-terminus zinc finger is involved in DNA binding. The second zinc finger is more likely involved in receptor dimerization or interaction with NR coactivators. Crystallography has confirmed and expanded the understanding of NR-DNA binding (31).

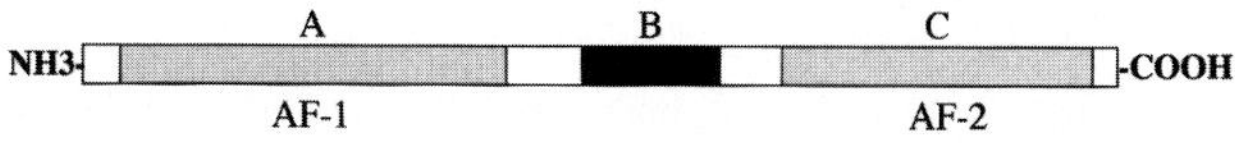

FIGURE 3-1. Generic nuclear receptor structure: schematic depiction of the primary organization of the nuclear receptor superfamily. The transactivation domain **(A)** has the greatest sequence variation between members of the superfamily and contains the activator function 1 region (AF1) with ligand-independent transcriptional activity. The DNA-binding domain **(B)** has the least sequence variation between members and contains two zinc fingers. The ligand-binding domain **(C)** is located toward the carboxy terminus and also contains an activator function (AF2) that is ligand dependent. NH3, amino terminus; COOH, carboxy terminus.

Variations within the DNA-binding domain of NRs are one method for each receptor to target specific genes. In a seminal experiment, when a chimeric receptor was created by replacing the DNA-binding domain within the ER with that of the GR, ER targets were no longer inducible, whereas glucocorticoid targets were activated (14).

Carboxy Terminus and Ligand-Binding Domain

The carboxy terminus of each NR contains the ligand-binding domain and has been implicated in many receptor functions, including nuclear localization, transcriptional regulation (ligand dependent), and receptor dimerization (11).

Ligand-Binding Domain

NRs bind ligand on the carboxy terminus. The specificity of ligand interaction is determined by the ligand-binding domain (LBD) of each receptor with some overlap in specificity, as would be predicted based on sequence homology among NR members. Relatively short carboxy-terminal truncation mutants will fail to bind to hormones, whereas mutations within the amino terminus or DNA-binding domain continue to bind ligand (24,32). A heptad repeat of hydrophobic residues exists in the carboxy region of the ER that is shared by all members of the superfamily (33). Mutations within this hydrophobic region decrease ligand binding (33).

Crystal structure of NR family members (specifically the thyroid receptor) has revealed the hydrophobic residues to form a cavity in which ligand binds (34). A comparison between the x-ray structures of ligand-free retinol X receptor-alpha, ligand-bound RAR-gamma, and TR-alpha-1 reveals a common tertiary structure called an antiparallel alpha-helical sandwich with 12 helices (35). Based on the similarities in specific regions of the LBD, it was predicted that all members of the steroid receptor superfamily would have a similar structure (36). Structural analysis of the ER-LBD has supported this hypothesis and suggested that the LBD interacts differently with agonists and antagonists, resulting in differential binding to potential coactivators (37).

Nuclear Localization Domain

Many NRs are located in the nucleus in both ligand-bound and ligand-free states (38,39). In the PR, a constitutively active nuclear localization signal, similar to that of the SV40 virus large-T antigen, has been identified (40). In the absence of ligand, receptors with mutations replacing these amino acids remain cytoplasmic. The translocation of mutated receptor to the nucleus in the presence of progesterone (40), along with research into the intracellular localization of the GR (41), implicate a second, ligand-dependent, nuclear localization signal. This second signal may act indirectly by binding chaperone proteins that result in the translocation of the receptor.

Transcriptional Regulation

Most members of the NR superfamily have two identified regions with transcriptional activating activity [termed activator function 1 and 2 (AF1 and AF2)] (19,42,43). The ligand-binding domain has ligand-dependent transcriptional regulating activity (AF2). Without ligand, this region appears to inhibit transcriptional activation. Evidence suggesting this includes the truncation of the ligand-binding domain, resulting in a constitutively active receptor (26). This regulatory role seems to be independent of protein structure, as described in the GR, where the ligand-free binding domain can suppress DNA binding and transcriptional activation when rearranged and positioned at the amino terminus, as well as when it is placed on a separate, unrelated protein such as E1A (44). Once ligand is bound, the presence of this region of the protein increases transcriptional activation.

Dimerization

As discussed below, most members of the NR superfamily undergo dimerization after ligand binding. Most studies locating the protein domain as important for dimerization have suggested that dimerization activity is contained within the ligand-binding domain (40,45). Mutation of the ligand-binding domain of the ER abrogates dimerization (33). Thyroid, vitamin D, and RAR receptors, which undergo heterodimerization with the RXR receptor, also share a similar region in the ligand-binding domain (46).

Protein Stability

This region of steroid receptors may also be involved in protein stability. The ER has a tyrosine at amino acid number 537, mutation of which has a minimal effect on ligand binding or transcriptional activation but results in a significant decrease in the stability of the ER, as measured by ligand binding over time (47). How the phosphorylation of residues within the LBD region effects protein stability and how phosphorylation effects receptor function remain largely unknown.

Amino Terminus and Transactivation Domain

The amino terminus contains the second transactivational domain of NR that is ligand independent (AF1) (24,25,32). Of the three major domains shared by NRs, this region exhibits the greatest variation between receptors (23). Many receptors contain monoacidic repeats. The AR, for example, has a polyglutamine tract, a polyglycine repeat, and multiple smaller repeats (48). The polyglutamine tract in the AR, which is highly polymorphic, has been shown to modulate AR function (49,50). The mechanistic explanation for such an affect on AR transactivation is yet to be explained.

This domain may directly interact with the transcriptional machinery for target genes or indirectly through costimulatory proteins associated with the AR. In a recent report, flanking sequences such as monoacidic repeats have been shown to affect the interaction of SRC-1 and NRs that may in part explain the effect observed on transcription (51). The monoacidic repeats may also affect transactivation by decreasing (or increasing) protein stability.

For some NRs, the amino terminus is not critical for transactivation, as complete deletion reduces but does not fully abrogate transcriptional control by NR (24,26). For the AR, deletion of two regions with activator functions (AF1a and AF1b) has been found to decrease transactivational activity by up to 90% (52).

Nuclear Receptor and Ligand Interaction

The critical roles in cellular growth and metabolism of NR are underscored by the complexity of their regulation and the growing number of proteins that are directly involved in their regulation. In this section, the cellular pathway from receptor formation and regulation to the penultimate function of control of target gene expression is discussed.

Regulation of Nuclear Receptors

NRs are regulated at many levels with frequent regulatory feedback loops to maintain homeostasis and respond to specific stimuli in the target tissue. Regulation of the specific ligand for any NR is likely the predominant regulatory feature for mammals. The reader is referred to endocrinology texts for descriptions of the hormonal regulation.

Cellular expression of NRs can be regulated through transcription, translation, and posttranslational modification. Transcriptional control of NRs has been demonstrated for the AR with testosterone's having the ability to both down-regulate (53–55) and up-regulate (56,57) the expression of AR messenger RNA (mRNA) depending on the cellular assay used. There is also a suggestion that AR mRNA expression is controlled within the prostate by Ca^{2+} regulation (58) or mRNA stabilization (59). Methylation of a CpG island within the AR promoter may represent a third method of regulating AR mRNA production in CaP (60).

There is also evidence that posttranscriptional and posttranslational regulations of NRs are important for the biology of responsive cells. Steroid receptors are phosphoproteins, and phosphorylation appears to be an important posttranslational mode of regulation for steroid and NRs (61). A few examples of kinases found to phosphorylate steroid receptors include src-kinase (62), mitogen-activated protein kinases (63), protein kinases A and C (64), and cell-cycle kinases (65).

The functional implications of receptor phosphorylation have been more difficult to define. Receptor phosphorylation has been suggested to affect ligand binding, receptor dimerization, DNA binding, transcriptional activation, protein stability, and interaction with co-regulatory proteins (61,66,67). Mutational analysis of the serine, tyrosine, and threonine residues found on NRs tend to have a modest affect on receptor function (67–70). Studies investigating the effect of forskolin-induced dephosphorylation of the AR have had conflicting results as to the effect on receptor activity but seem to favor increased transcriptional activation with dephosphorylation (64,71–73). Conversely, there are interesting examples of steroid receptor phosphorylation resulting in increased transcriptional activation as well as ligand-independent activation (63,71,74,75). A recent powerful example of AR activation by Her2/neu activation of the MAPK pathway underscores the potential importance of phosphorylation of steroids and NRs (76). Most of these studies have been performed *in vitro* and the biologic significance of phosphorylation of NRs in the prostate remains to be clearly demonstrated.

Other modalities of posttranslational modification are also used to control the activity of NRs. One example involving the AR includes an association with Ubc9. Ubc9 is a member of the E2 class of ubiquitin-conjugating enzymes that enhance AR-dependent transcription by associating with the AR in the hinge regions of the protein (77). The mechanism of this enhancement of transcription remains unknown but is not dependent on Ubc9-mediated SUMO-conjugation of the AR (77).

Location and Status of Unbound Receptor

The “two-step” hypothesis reflected the belief that unbound NRs were located in the cytoplasm (4). The development of monoclonal antibodies directed against specific receptors located most NRs within the nucleus, regardless of their association with ligand. The cellular localization of ligand-free steroid receptors (GR, ER, MR, PR, AR) is a dynamic process; receptors can shuttle in and out of the nuclear pore complex (78,79). The amount of receptors in the nucleus is due to the balance of nuclear import (energy dependent and via the nuclear pore complex) and export (default, nonspecific pathway) (80). Ligand binding to SRs shifts more receptors into the nucleus either by exposing a ligand-dependent nuclear localization signal (41), disrupting a cytoplasmic heteromeric protein complex (81), or resulting in SR’s binding to DNA, thus altering the equilibrium of SR transport across the nuclear membrane (82).

In both the cytoplasm and nucleus, ligand-free receptors are not alone; there are a growing number of associated proteins identified by coimmunoprecipitation that may modulate NR function. The first class recognized to be associated with NR proteins in the absence of ligand were the heat shock proteins, specifically heat shock protein 70 and heat shock protein 90 (83). Now included in the growing list of associated proteins are heat shock protein 70–interacting protein, heat shock protein 70– and 90–organizing protein, immunophilin, and p23, among others [reviewed in(84)]. The complexes of NR and associated proteins may not be stable but rather constitute a dynamic, energy-dependent process of constant association (requiring energy) and dissociation (spontaneous) (Fig. 3-2) (85). The concerted functions for these interacting proteins remain to be elucidated but likely include increasing SR-ligand affinity, protein stability, and transcriptional inhibition (44,83,86–88).

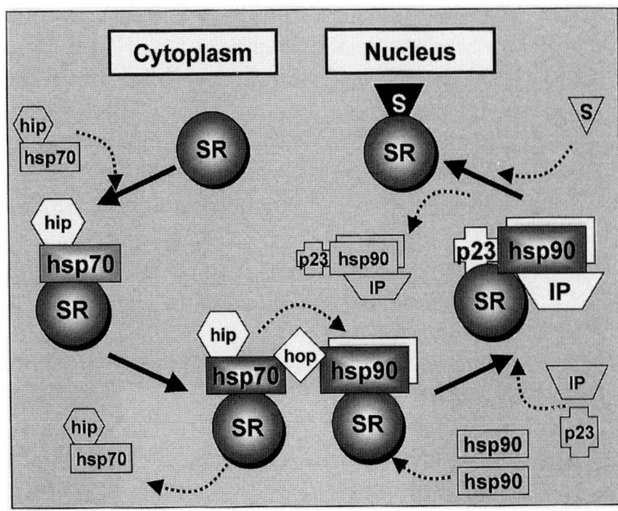

FIGURE 3-2. Steroid receptor (SR) chaperones. Before binding ligand, SRs associate with a dynamic cast of chaperone proteins. After translation, SRs bind to heat-shock protein 70 (hsp70) and hsp70 interacting protein (hip). The hsp-70 and -90 organizing protein (hop) then facilitates a switch from hsp70 to hsp90, interacting with SR. Immunophilin (IP) and p23 associate with the SR through hsp90, at which point the SRs are competent to bind to ligand (S). Once S is bound, hsp90, IP, and p23 dissociate from the SR and the ligand-bound SR translocates to the nucleus.

Interaction with Ligand

The known lipophilic ligands enter cells and bind to their cognate receptors through what appears to be a passive, nonfacilitated process. NR-ligand binding stoichiometry is 1:1 for most receptors studied (89,90). The steroid receptor subfamily generally binds to ligand while existing as monomeric receptors, whereas many NRs bind ligand when they are already dimerized and bound to DNA (91). Ligand binding initiates a cascade of activity, beginning with a conformational change in protein structure and eventually resulting in transcriptional activation or repression.

Comparing the crystal structures of the ligand-free RXR-alpha and ligand-bound RAR-gamma suggests that the structural changes result in physical trapping of the ligand within the receptor (35,92). In the SR subgroup, ligand-induced structural changes may also be responsible for a reshuffling of SR-associated proteins and exposure of a nuclear translocation signal as mentioned previously. The ER LBD has been specifically shown to undergo a different conformational change with agonists versus antagonists; most noteworthy is the observation that after binding to an antagonist, the LBD structure prevents the binding of a co-stimulator peptide, whereas the agonist-bound structure is permissive (37).

As part of the conformational change resulting from ligand binding, steroid receptors dimerize. Receptors such as GR, ER, PR, and AR homodimerize before binding to DNA. Other NRs may already exist as dimers and, in the case of RAR, VDR, and PPAR, exist as heterodimers with the RXR-NR and are already associated with DNA response elements. Along with dimerization, NRs associate with a growing list of co-stimulators and co-inhibitors. These proteins—and in one exceptional case, RNA species—have been shown either to augment ligand-dependent transcriptional activity or to diminish the NR's effect. How these co-stimulating proteins function remains unclear. It has been postulated that they may augment NR transcriptional control by stabilizing a direct association between NR and the transcription initiation complex (TIC) or by acting as a bridge between NR and the TIC (93).

Nuclear Receptor and DNA Binding

As transcription factors, NRs specifically controlling the expression of target genes is paramount to their function. NRs bind to specific hormone-response elements (HRE), thereby influencing the transcriptional initiation of target genes (94). Mutational analysis and comparative sequencing have determined consensus HRE sequences for many NRs, whereas x-ray crystallographic and nuclear magnetic resonance modeling of NR-DNA complexes have determined those amino acid residues critical for DNA binding. These studies support the current model of the interaction between members of this superfamily and DNA, but much remains to be described.

The amino-terminus zinc finger and the residues immediately adjacent to this region appear to be most important for DNA binding (95). Three clusters of residues found within this region associate with DNA and have been referred to as DNA hooks (96). In general, residues within this region bind to DNA bases; the phosphate backbone; structurally conserved, DNA-associated water molecules through hydrogen bonds and van der Waals forces; or a combination of these. Based on comparative crystal structures, as few as three amino acid residues within these DNA-binding hooks can determine DNA half-site recognition (97). However, adjacent amino acids as well as residues from the hinge region of NR, make significant contributions to HRE recognition and specificity through direct DNA binding, allosteric interference, and dimerization (96).

With the cloning of promoter regions of NR-target genes, consensus sequences were identified. There are two distinct consensus sequences that function as hexameric half-sites for many members of the NR superfamily. A consensus glucocorticoid response element of 5'AGAACA3' exists that also functions as the HRE for most of the steroid receptors (GR, PR, MR, AR) (98). The other major response element is an estrogen response element of 5'AGGTCA3' that represents a consensus sequence for many of the NRs [TR, RXR, VDR, RAR, PPAR, chicken ovalbumin upstream promoter-transcription factor (COUP-TF), and nerve growth factor–inducible-B] (99,100).

NRs most often bind to two cognate half-site response elements as dimers, and the orientation of each HRE half-site, as well as the spacing between the half sites, is important for receptor binding. Steroid receptor response elements bind to two palindromic half-sites separated by three base pairs. ERs, as well as all steroid receptors, bind to their response elements as homodimers (45,101). Most nonsteroid NRs bind DNA as heterodimers with RXR (102), although some bind as monomers (103).

Nuclear Receptor Transcriptional Activation and Repression

DNA-bound NR regulate the transcription of target genes through direct and indirect mechanisms. A simple model of transcriptional control includes an NR binding DNA and directing RNA polymerase II to initiate transcription. For many NRs, there is evidence for direct association with constituents of the TIC. For example, the steroid receptors ER, PR, and COUP-TF have been shown to directly interact with transcription factor IIB (TFIIB), an early transcription factor (104). Such a direct interaction is not unique for steroid receptors within this superfamily, as the NRs TR, VDR, and RXR each interact directly with components of the transcription initiation factor, including TFIIB, TFIID, and the multimeric TATA–binding protein (105–107).

The interactions between NR and the TIC can affect transcription in multiple ways. Ligand-dependent transcriptional activation of target genes has been reproducibly demonstrated for most known NRs. Specifically, the ligand-dependent AF2 region of multiple NRs has been demonstrated to activate transcription of target genes for the ER, PR, GR, TR, and RAR (43,108–113). Alternatively, ligand activation of NR can result in transcriptional repression of target genes with early examples identified for GR and TR (114–116) [reviewed in (117)]. Finally, ligand-activated relief of constitutive transcriptional repression or activation has also been described for NR superfamily members (118,119).

The observed phenomenon of transcriptional squelching (i.e., decreased transcription of an NR's target gene in the presence of an active, second NR) questioned the simple model of a direct and exclusive association between NR and the TIC and predicted the presence of co-regulatory proteins (120). Co-regulatory proteins were envisioned to act as bridging molecules between activation domains and basal transcription machinery (93,121).

It is now clear that many co-regulator proteins are involved in the transcriptional control of NR. A major family of proteins called the p160 coactivators includes at least three proteins in humans that have been found to directly interact with steroid receptors: SRC-1 (also known as *NcoA-1*), transcription initiation factor–2 (also known as *GRIP1* and *NcoA-2*), and AIB-1 (also known as *p/CIP*, *TRAM*, and *ACTR*) (122–124). There are also examples of co-regulatory proteins that are more specific to certain members of the nuclear and steroid receptor superfamily [e.g., ARA70 interacting with AR (125) and, recently, PPAR-gamma (126)].

Although the complete functions of this family of proteins remains to be fully understood, they do serve to physically bridge NRs with two other, highly related coactivators: CREB-binding protein and p300 (127). These two proteins contain potent histone acetyltransferase activity that is critical for their ability to mediate steroid receptor transcriptional activation (Fig. 3-3). Nuclear and steroid receptor coactivators may also serve an important integrative function through their interaction with AP-1, KfkappaB, NFAT, and STAT pathways.

Two examples of known co-repressors include the related proteins NcoR and SMRT (128,129). In 1999, an

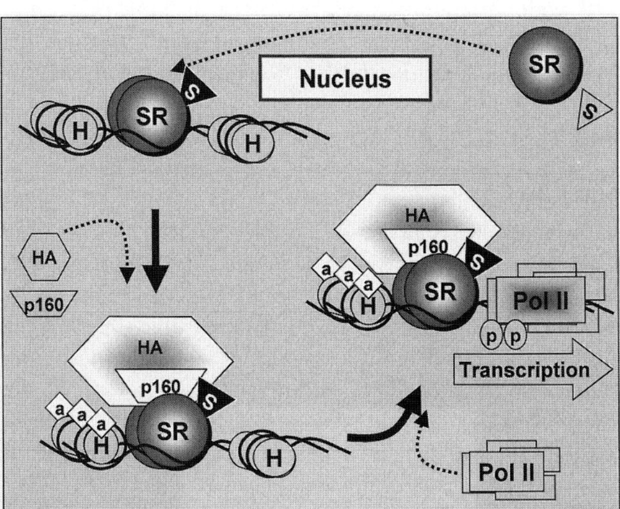

FIGURE 3-3. Steroid receptor (SR) co-regulators. Once bound to ligand, SRs bind to DNA, and the initial co-regulators recruited include members of the p160 family and proteins with histone acetylase (HA) activity. Histone acetylation occurs, and the Pol II transcription complex is approximated to the transcription start site. Phosphorylation of Pol II occurs, and transcription begins. The SR-associated complex then detaches from the DNA and repeats the cycle. The specific members of the p160 family as well as the proteins involved in histone acetylation and polymerase phosphorylation likely vary, depending on SR and cell origin. a, acetyl groups; H, histone; p, phosphate; S, ligand.

exciting observation implicated a possible new class of NR co-regulators that are functionally active as RNA transcripts (130).

There are different models to explain how these co-regulator proteins bind to NR and modulate transcription. First, there is evidence that they stabilize the interaction between NR and the TIC. Second, they may independently associate with components of the TIC and thus alter the efficiency of transcription initiation. Evidence is also growing that co-regulators affect chromatin acetylation and thereby affect DNA organization and structure. The exact mechanisms and biologic significance of the interaction between NR and coactivators is an extremely active area of current investigation.

ANDROGEN RECEPTOR IN THE GROWTH AND DEVELOPMENT OF THE PROSTATE

The development and growth of the prostate and the development of CaP are dependent on the presence of androgens and the AR (131). This section reviews the literature exploring the expression of AR in the developing and adult prostate, the presence and expression of AR in disease states of the prostate, and, finally, what is known about the function of AR in the prostate.

Embryology and Early Development

Expression of the AR during embryogenesis and early development has been described for the mouse, rat, and marsupial (132–134). The first expression of murine AR by *in situ* hybridization occurs at day 12.5 and is found in the genital tubercle, mesonephric mesenchyme, mammary mesenchyme, and other less strongly staining regions, such as the glandular part of the pituitary, the adrenal gland, and the levator ani muscle (132). The epithelial buds from which the prostate develops (135) are negative for AR staining in the developing embryo, but the surrounding mesenchyme stains strongly (132). As the mesonephric (Wolffian) ducts develop, there is a shift from AR expression in the mesenchyme to the ductal epithelium (132). Shortly after birth, there is an increase in the AR content of the ventral prostate epithelium in the immediate neonatal period of the rat (136).

Marsupials offer a good model to study the development of the genitourinary system because of their immature state at the time of birth and neonatal maturation (134). AR protein expression is not detected until postnatal day 5, when it is expressed in the scrotum, genital tubercle, and mesenchyme of the Cowper's gland and less intensely in the mesenchyme of the prostate. Like the development in the mouse, with increasing postnatal age, there is an increased expression in the prostatic mesenchyme and a late switch (at or after postnatal day 80) to expression in the epithelium of the prostate, as seen in the adult (137).

When human tissue, preserved in paraffin blocks, is examined by *in situ* hybridization and immunohistochemical staining, expression of AR mRNA is found in the prostatic epithelium from early fetuses, but no protein is seen (138). Later fetal specimens and infantile specimens did have immunohistochemical reactivity for AR, but in a largely cytoplasmic pattern. In pubertal and adult tissues, the level of mRNA expression appears to be decreased compared to that of the fetal prostate, but AR protein, now with a nuclear staining pattern, is readily detected (138). The mechanisms regulating or causing a slow sequential development of mRNA expression, cytoplasmic AR expression, and, finally, nuclear AR expression remain unknown.

AR knockout models occur naturally and underscore the importance of the AR in the development of the prostate. In the mouse, cat, and dog, the lack of a functional AR results in the formation of only a very rudimentary prostate (139–141). Mice with a syndrome of complete androgen insensitivity, referred to as *testicular feminization* (Tfm), have a frame shift mutation in the AR gene, causing early protein truncation (142). The use of chimeric recombinations of wild-type stromal cells and bladder epithelial cells from Tfm mice have demonstrated that AR activity within the stroma of the developing prostate is sufficient for prostatic gland bud formation, even though the epithelial cells remain AR negative (143–145). In androgenized heterozygote female mice (Tfm/wt), AR-positive and -negative cells formed small patches throughout the urogenital mesenchyme, and, on exposure to androgens, only those stromal cells positive for AR were found adjacent to forming prostatic buds (146).

Together, these observations suggest that prostate gland formation is dependent on stromal expression of AR, and, as the prostate matures, AR expression shifts from the stroma to the epithelium. It remains an active area of investigation to determine the downstream targets of AR activity that result in the formation and maturity of the prostate.

Expression of the Androgen Receptor in the Adult Prostate

The AR was initially shown to be present in the prostate in 1971 (147). In the adult prostate, there is also a suggestion that AR expression is higher in the peripheral zone [location of the majority of CaP tumors] than in the periurethral (internal) zone (148,149) although there is a report suggesting the opposite (150). The AR is expressed in the differentiated epithelium, basal cells, stromal cells, and vascular smooth muscle cells within the prostate (138). The relative expression levels vary with cell type; tubular epithelial cells have more intense and consistent staining than either basal epithelial cells or stromal cells (151,152).

Immunohistochemistry and hormone-binding studies suggest that most AR in prostatic epithelium is nuclear (48,153). In androgen-depleted states, increased AR is within the cytoplasm (154,155). In elderly men, with lower circulating levels of androgens, increased cytoplasmic AR is also observed (149). Cytoplasmic AR will shift into the nucleus, with replacement of androgens supporting the presence of a ligand-dependent nuclear localization signal (156,157).

Androgen ablation results in prostatic atrophy with a decrease in the number, size, and secretory function of luminal epithelial cells (158–160). There is often basal cell predominance that replaces the well-differentiated luminal epithelium and, at times, frank basal cell hyperplasia (161). On castration, AR mRNA content within prostatic epithelial cells initially increases (151,162) but eventually declines (54,163,164). Along with the total cellular content of AR decreasing, castration also results in a shift of AR into the cytoplasm (163).

Expression of the Androgen Receptor in Benign Prostatic Hypertrophy, Prostatic Intraepithelial Neoplasm, and Prostate Cancer

Much work has focused on the expression pattern of AR in the normal adult prostate compared to that of disease states such as benign prostatic hypertrophy (BPH), prostatic intraepithelial neoplasm (PIN), and CaP. In general, the staining pattern of AR within normal prostates is homogeneous within cell nuclei (Fig. 3-4A). In BPH, PIN, and CaP, AR expression becomes increasingly heterogeneous, with wide variation between regions of the same prostate or tumor (Fig. 3-4B) (165–169). Although androgen-binding studies have identified both cytoplasmic and nuclear AR (170), immunohistochemical analysis generally detects nuclear AR (171). Quantitative studies have focused on the association between AR content and disease states as well as CaP behavior.

In general, AR expression is higher in BPH, PIN, and CaP than in normal prostatic tissue (165,166,171–174), although exceptions are found in the literature (175). Within the epithelial cells, it appears that the differences in AR content (as measured by androgen binding) are not found within the cytoplasm but rather the nucleus (170). The differences among BPH and CaP with respect to AR content are less clear, and studies have suggested that AR content in BPH is greater than (165,168,171,176), equal to (170,173), or less than (149) in CaP. Similarly conflicting results were found with PIN epithelial cells and CaP or BPH (169,177,178). When AR expression in lymph node metastases was compared to primary tumor expression, no difference was detected (175). Thus, there is little additional information provided by AR status with respect to the type of prostate pathology or to the stage of tumor.

It is still possible, however, that AR content may help to better CaP prognosis or response to treatment. Early observations suggested that CaP of a higher Gleason grade had

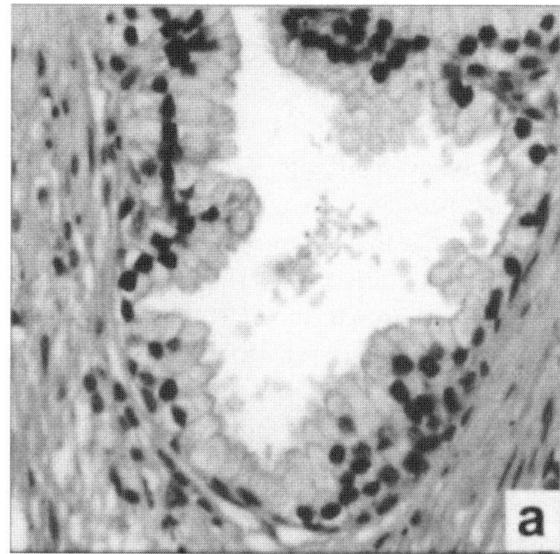

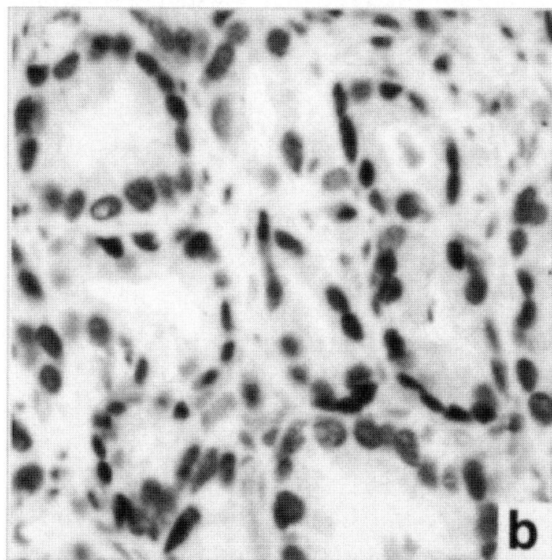

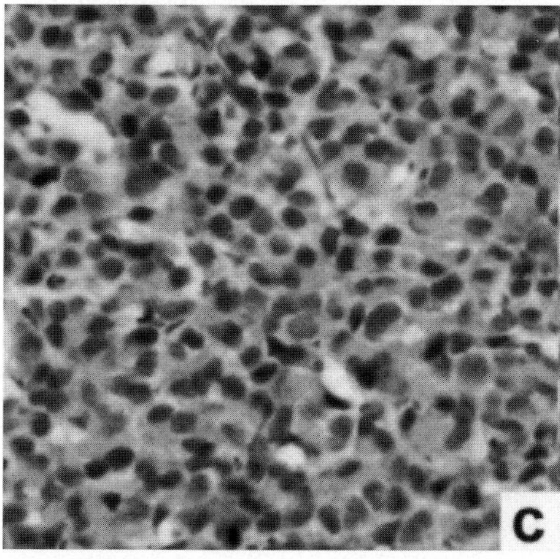

FIGURE 3-4. Androgen receptor (AR) staining in the prostate. AR staining is mainly nuclear for tubular epithelial cells within normal prostate glands, and staining is relatively homogeneous **(A)**. With prostatic intraepithelial neoplasm (not shown) and prostate cancer (CaP) **(B)**, AR staining becomes less homogeneous and can vary widely from cell to cell. AR expression is largely maintained at relatively high levels in both androgen-dependent **(C)** and androgen-independent metastatic CaP. (Photomicrographs of formalin-fixed tissue stained with hematoxylin before immunohistochemistry with an anti-AR antibody provided courtesy of M. Loda, Dana-Farber Cancer Institute, Boston.)

decreased nuclear AR expression (166). However, other studies have failed to support this association (173) or demonstrate the opposite (169). Such inconsistent results are likely due to variability in tissue acquisition, differences in AR assays, and the heterogeneity of AR expression within the same tumor. It does appear that with increasing Gleason grade, AR staining becomes more heterogeneous (169). It is also noteworthy that patients with CaP tumors with marked AR heterogeneity have poorer survival regardless of the amount of AR (179). Whether this suggests a change in the functional role of AR with more aggressive CaP or is merely the result of an unrelated process remains to be demonstrated.

Investigators have addressed whether AR content or staining pattern predicts an individual's response to androgen withdrawal. Two early studies found that increased nuclear androgen binding capacity was statistically correlated with a longer response to hormonal therapy (180,181). Although an initial immunohistochemical study (182) with a small number of patients failed to support this observation, larger, more recent immunohistochemical studies have suggested that increased AR staining is associated with a higher response rate to hormonal therapy and increased duration of response (183,184).

Outside of the clinical response to hormonal withdrawal, it is less clear that AR content or staining predicts disease behavior. One study has demonstrated that patients with paraffin-embedded tumors that stain negatively for AR have a poorer survival than those that stain positively for AR (185). However, a large retrospective study from the Mayo Clinic found no association between mean number of AR immunoreactive nuclei as a univariate or multivariate variable and clinical progression, biochemical progression, or overall survival (178). Also, when newer automated immunohistochemical techniques are used, all of 40 advanced cancers evaluated expressed AR, with 85% of tumors having more than half of all cells positive (169).

One final area of investigation involves AR expression in androgen-independent tumors. Based on initial observations from androgen-independent tumors in the Dunning rat model (186) and the *in vitro* cell lines PC3 and DU145, loss of AR expression was thought to be important in androgen-independent growth of CaP. However, the vast majority of androgen-independent tumors in men continue to have high levels of AR staining (187–190). In a subset of androgen-independent tumors, continued AR expression may be increased owing to selection for clones that have undergone amplification of the AR gene (190,191). Mutations within the AR ligand-binding domain have also been identified in hormone-independent CaP and may maintain AR transcriptional activity in androgen-depleted states (187,192,193). It seems to be clear, that even with the development of androgen-independent CaP, the AR continues to be involved in cell growth.

Thus, AR is expressed within the prostate, BPH, and CaP. BPH tends to have the highest expression of AR when compared to normal or malignant prostatic tissue, whereas CaP has the most heterogeneous staining. Decreased staining of AR within CaP is associated with a decreased response to androgen withdrawal therapy, but few other definitive conclusions can be made. Understanding the true significance of these observations lies in describing the function of the AR within the prostate epithelium and how this functional role changes with malignant transformation.

Function of the Androgen Receptor within the Prostate and Prostate Cancer

A functional AR is necessary for the development of the prostate and CaP (131,194). As discussed earlier, the AR is clearly expressed during prostate organogenesis, in the mature prostate epithelium, and during all stages of prostate cancer. Animal models of CaP demonstrate that increased rates of CaP carcinogenesis are dramatically facilitated by androgens (195,196). However, the mechanisms behind AR's critical role and the important AR target genes in the developing prostate, the adult prostate, and the diseased prostate, have yet to be comprehensively described.

AR clearly acts as a transcription factor in the prostate. Prostate-specific antigen (PSA) is regulated by the AR; two androgen response elements are located within the promoter of PSA, and transcription of this gene is up-regulated by ligand-bound AR (197–200). Other androgen-responsive genes in prostatic cells include prostatic acid phosphatase (201), kallikrein (202,203), clathrin heavy and light chains (204), steroid-conjugating uridine diphosphate–glucuronosyltransferase enzymes (205,206), cyclin-dependent kinases 2 and 4 (CDK2 and CDK4) (207), p21 (208), and the homeobox gene NKX3.1 (209), among many others. However, it is not clear that all of these genes are under direct control of AR, nor has it been sufficiently demonstrated that AR regulation of these genes is necessary for the growth and development of the prostate or CaP.

The necessity for AR to act as a transcriptional factor in normal prostate development is demonstrated by androgen insensitivity syndromes. The most complete androgen insensitivity syndromes (with no or only a rudimentary prostate present) are caused by mutations that severely limit DNA or ligand binding (210–212). Although the AR target genes required for prostate development have not been identified, AR expression is only required in the developing prostatic stroma, suggesting that important genes may be involved in paracrine functions.

One example of an AR-regulated gene with paracrine activity potentially important in prostate development is the fibroblast growth factor 7 (FGF7 or keratinocyte growth factor) (213,214). FGF7 is expressed in the developing stroma, and early prostatic epithelial cells contain receptors for FGF7 (215). *In vitro*, exogenous FGF7 (and androgen-free media) can stimulate early prostate glandular formation, mimicking the effects of androgens (216). Although a good example of an AR-regulated gene that has paracrine activity potentially important to prostatic development, the knockout of FGF7 has a normal prostate; thus, this gene, and regulation of this gene by AR, are not necessary for prostate development (217). Other AR-regulated genes that may be important paracrine factors for stromal-epithelial interaction in the developing prostate include insulinlike growth factor II, basic FGF, transforming growth factor alpha (TGF-alpha), TGF-beta, and nerve growth factor (218).

For CaP, there is a clear example that a functional AR within the neoplastic epithelial cells is sufficient for androgen-dependent growth. An AR-positive human CaP cell line, PC-82, was placed into an AR-negative murine host to abrogate any potential AR-regulated stromal paracrine effects (219). On castration, these tumors had decreased proliferation and increased apoptosis (219). Again, although this model provides clear evidence that the AR, most likely via transcriptional regulation, controls the expression of genes required for cell proliferation and survival, the important genes remain unknown.

Attempting to comprehensively describe which genes are regulated by the AR in the prostate and CaP and their importance in cellular survival and growth remains a difficult task. In a comprehensive review of the genes known to be regulated by the prostate, one author refers to the complex group of genes as the Janus Face of androgen action (220). In this review, AR's regulation of CDKs (CDK1, CDK2, and CDK4), cyclins (D3 and A), PSA, FGF7, TGF-beta, vascular endothelial growth factor (VEGF), and maspin is advantageous to cell growth but the regulation of insulinlike growth factor binding protein 5, neutral endopeptidase 24.11, and Bcl-2 is disadvantageous to prostatic cell growth (220). It will take exquisite molecular experiments with precise gene knockout or knockin models before we are able to definitively know what the most important AR-regulated genes are for the prostate and CaP.

Androgens may also have other functions within prostate cells unrelated to the AR or transcriptional control, or both. Some steroids have very rapid actions that are too rapid to be explained by their traditional role in transcriptional regulation (221). Such potential mechanisms include cell-signaling pathways involving protein kinase C, phospholipase C, or induction of Ca^{2+} mobilization and Ca^{2+} channels (222). Androgens have been found to rapidly alter cytoplasmic Ca^{2+} levels of macrophages and lymphocytes (223,224). Using the CaP model ALVA-41, androgens have been shown to provide a proliferative stimulus in the presence of sex hormone–binding globulin and not in its absence (225). The role that nontranscriptional effects of androgens and the coordinated association with AR have in prostate development or CaP has yet to be explored.

OTHER NUCLEAR RECEPTORS IN PROSTATE DEVELOPMENT AND DISEASE STATES

Although the role of AR in the development of the prostate and CaP has received the most attention by investigators, it has long been recognized that other NRs play an important role in the biology of the prostate and CaP. Of the other NRs, members of the steroid receptor subgroup have received most of the attention. However, with recent discovery of the importance of previously identified orphan receptors in the metabolism and biology of epithelial cells, there are more studies addressing the expression and functional role of such receptors in the prostate and CaP. These studies are reviewed below.

Other Steroid Receptors

Estrogen Receptor

An NR that binds estrogens was one of the first steroid receptors identified (4,5). Although initially investigated as a single receptor, a second NR with homology to the initial ER has been identified with specific estrogen avidity, and multiple variants are now known to exist (226–229). The two major receptors are now identified as ER-alpha (the initial receptor cloned) and ER-beta (cloned in 1996). ER-beta was cloned from a prostate cDNA library and has resulted in renewed interest in the distribution of both receptors in the developing and normal prostate, and changes that are associated with BPH and CaP. Work before the identification of ER-beta, using antibodies and *in situ* probes, was most likely specifically looking at ER-alpha expression. However, ER-beta probably contributed to the estrogen-binding activity in early experiments and may have contributed to inconsistent findings.

Estrogen Receptors in the Developing and Normal Prostate

ER-alpha is present within the prostatic mesenchyme of newborn mice and not in the epithelium (230). As the mesenchyme differentiates into mature stroma, ER staining remains positive and much stronger than does the epithelium of the prostate (151,231). The relative ER expression between fibroblasts and smooth muscle cells of the prostate remains unclear (230,232). *In vitro* prostatic smooth muscle cells retain ER staining and proliferate with estrogenic stimulation (233), whereas prostatic fibroblasts have been found to be ER negative and unresponsive to estrogens (234). Whether this difference is reflective of the cell's *in situ* biology or an artifact from cell isolation and culture is unclear. With aging, and most rapidly during puberty, ER expression decreases in the stroma of the prostate (235).

ER-beta is expressed at low levels at the time of birth within the mesenchyme and the epithelial cells of the prostate (236). From day 1 of life on, there is a trend for decreasing stromal expression (eventually to no greater than background on *in situ* stains) and increasing epithelial staining (236). The adult prostate clearly has expression of ER-beta in the epithelium of the prostate and not in the smooth muscle cells or fibroblasts of the stroma (226). Although ER-beta expression in men is high in the prostatic epithelium, other tissues expressing ER-beta include the lung, kidney, adrenals, bladder, heart, hypothalamus, testes, and the epididymis (226,237–240), although there is some discrepancy between studies.

Prostatic expression of ER-alpha and ER-beta changes on androgen withdrawal. Many studies have followed ER-alpha expression within the stromal cells of the prostate after androgen deprivation, with mixed results. Although two studies report the ER-alpha expression to be decreased after castration (151,241), the majority appears to implicate increased ER-alpha expression after castration (161,231,242–244). ER expression is also increased in the prostate with exogenous estrogen neonatally or in the adult (151,245). The single paper reporting ER-beta expression after castration found decreased expression (236).

The functional role of ER in the development of the prostate has been explored using neonatal estrogen exposure and knockout models for both ER-alpha and ER-beta. Neonatal estrogen exposure causes a lasting influence on the prostate's growth and response to androgens (246–248). Although the mechanisms remain unclear, estrogen exposure delays prostatic epithelial maturation, as determined by expression of luminal proteins, AR, prostate-binding protein, and the development of a mature basal and luminal epithelial cell layer (247). Perhaps most interesting, in the adult prostates of mice exposed to neonatal estrogens, preneoplastic lesions have been observed (249,250). The mechanism for such alterations remains unclear. There is decreased AR content in the adult prostates of mice exposed to neonatal estrogens (251,252) and alterations in the periductal fibroblasts and extracellular matrix within treated prostates (253), but these observations have not been shown to have a causal role in the subsequent prostatic dysplasia.

ER-alpha male knockout mice have normal-appearing prostates but are infertile, owing to disruption of spermatogenesis and degeneration of the seminiferous tubules (254). ER-beta knockout mice, both male and female, retain fertility, with slight compromise in female mice owing to decreased ovarian efficiency (255). The ER-beta knockout male mice, while mostly without phenotype, have hyperplasia noted within the prostate and bladder (255). This specific phenotype in an otherwise normal-appearing mouse has the potential to result in further clarification of the role of ER in prostate development and adult growth. However, in more recent work, the finding of hyperplasia in ER-beta knockout mice was not confirmed, leaving the true role for ER-beta in the development of the prostate unclear.

Estrogen Receptors in Disease States of the Prostate

Estrogens, and ER, have been implicated in the development of BPH. Exogenous estrogens act synergistically with androgens to induce BPH in dogs but not in rats (256). In general, ER expression has been found to be higher in prostates with BPH as compared to normal prostates (256,257), although a few studies fail to detect a difference (258). Regionally, within the prostate, ER has been demonstrated to have slightly higher expression in the transitional zone, which is more prone to BPH (148). ER mRNA is specifically expressed in fibromyoadenomatous hyperplasia and myoadenomatous hyperplasia, but not adenomatous hyperplasia, continuing to emphasize the stromal bias in its expression (243). Although work describing ER-beta expression in BPH has not been published, the hyperplasia seen with ER-beta knockout mice suggests a possible preventive role for this form of ER. The functional implications of ER in BPH are unclear, and a review of the literature suggested that estrogens act to induce AR expression, alter the metabolism of androgens to increase the cellular levels of dihydrotestosterone, and decrease the rate of cell death within the prostate (256).

CaP, in agreement with the expression pattern of epithelial cells from which the cancer is derived, tends to have little or no expression of ER-alpha (161,174,259). Although some reports find CaP specimens to have estrogen-binding capacity and thus are assumed to be ER-positive, these reports have used homogenized tissue likely with a significant amount of ER positive stromal cells (258,260). When *in situ* hybridization is combined with immunohistochemistry, ER mRNA and protein staining tends to be positive in the nonmalignant stromal cells and not in the epithelial cells (243). With androgen deprivation during the treatment of CaP, ER expression was observed to increase in the stromal cells adjacent to the epithelial cancer cells, along with an associated hyperplasia of basal cells (243). The mechanism of repression for ER-alpha and ER-beta is not clear, but it may be related to promoter methylation (261,262), a frequent mechanism in CaP to decrease gene expression.

The consistent lack of ER-alpha staining in the epithelial cells of primary prostatic tumors makes the observations of ER expression in the CaP cell lines LNCaP, DU145, and PC3 of unclear biologic significance (261,263,264). LNCaP cells have been documented to express ER and, on stimulation with physiologic concentrations of estrogens, demonstrate growth stimulation (263), although this may be partially mediated through the mutated AR in LNCaP cells. DU145 and PC3 cells, both effectively AR-negative, experience growth inhibition when treated with estrogens (PC3) or antiestrogens (PC3 and DU145) (261).

Clinically, as discussed in Chapter 40, estrogens have been used to effectively palliate symptomatic CaP in men, although cardiovascular morbidity has limited its current use (265). Antiestrogens such as tamoxifen (266,267) or similar compounds have had minimal activity on CaP. Recently, PC-SPES, an herbal-based therapy with estrogenic activity (268) has demonstrated impressive clinical activity in patients with CaP (269). However, it remains to be seen if the clinical activity of PC-SPES is mediated through the ER (alpha or beta).

Progesterone Receptor

The PR, similar to the ER, is expressed in the prostate (270) and has higher expression in stromal cells than epithelial cells (271). Similar binding activity is found throughout the prostate without a bias toward any specific region (148). PR binding within prostatic stromal cells is predominantly localized to the cytosol. This is unusual for steroid receptors and suggests that other progestin-binding proteins may exist within the prostate (272). Immunohistochemical studies have found strong PR staining within the nuclei of stromal cells, rather than the cytoplasm, and rare staining of epithelial nuclei (174). Although of unclear significance, PR expression does seem to be up-regulated by estrogen stimulation in the prostate (231,273).

PR (as detected by progesterone binding) is detected in BPH and CaP specimens (260,273). Compared to normal prostatic stroma, increased PR staining within the stromal cell nuclei of BPH samples has been observed (174). When high-grade (273) or metastatic (274) CaP lesions are compared with primary tumors, there is a tendency toward decreased PR staining. However, it is possible that this decrease represents an artifact from less positively staining, nonmalignant stromal cells and is not of biologic significance.

Medroxyprogesterone acetate has been used to treat men with metastatic and hormone-refractory CaP. However, the efficacy of treatments acting through the PR appear to be very inferior to those targeting the androgen and less effective than estrogen therapy (275).

Glucocorticoid Receptor

The GR is another steroid receptor expressed in the prostate. After castration, GR levels have been found to increase and may occupy similar DNA-binding sites as the AR (276).

In specimens of BPH and CaP, GR stains intensely in the stromal cells but had low (CaP) or intermediate (BPH) staining in epithelial cells (171). In the same study, no relationship between GR staining and Gleason score, clinical stage, or pathologic stage was found (171).

The GR in prostatic cell lines has been shown to induce expression of the androgen-responsive gene PSA but to have no or inhibitory growth effects. Expression of wild-type GR in the LNCaP tumor line (normally GR negative) has been shown to induce the activity of a transfected PSA-promoter-luciferase construct as well as the endogenous PSA gene (277). Although GR activation with dexamethasone increased PSA expression, no increased proliferation of LNCaP was seen (277). In fact, three different GR-expressing prostate cell lines exhibited growth inhibition on exposure to corticosteroids (278–280). In the AR-negative, rat PA-111 prostate carcinoma cell line, GR stimulation results in decreased proliferation (281). This decreased proliferation may be due to reduced protein kinase C cellular concentrations, coupled with sphinganine antagonism of protein kinase C activation (280). GR stimulation also results in decreased proliferation of androgen-independent PC3 cells, possibly through up-regulating TGF-beta (279). Thus, it appears that GR can bind to and initiate transcription for genes that are responsive also to AR (e.g., PSA), but a difference exists in that GR is unable to stimulate increased proliferation.

Clinically, high doses of corticosteroids palliate symptoms from CaP and have been incorporated into palliative regimens, including chemotherapy (282,283). However, whether steroids work directly on CaP through the GR or through GR-mediated effects on the expression of local growth factors remains unclear (284).

Nonsteroid Nuclear Receptors

Vitamin D Receptor

VDRs are expressed by epithelial and stromal cells of the prostate and CaP cells (285–287). Interest in the functional role of vitamin D metabolism and VDRs stems from epidemiologic studies that suggest a link between CaP and calcium metabolism, vitamin D levels, and genetic polymorphisms within the VDR (288–302). Although inconsistent, these studies suggest that vitamin D and its metabolites may have a protective effect against CaP.

Primary cultures of prostatic epithelial cells and stromal cells expressed VDR and were growth inhibited by vitamin D metabolites (285). With antibodies directed against the VDR, receptors were found within the nuclei of prostatic epithelial cells as well as a few stromal cells (303).

In CaP cell lines, activation of the VDR has been shown to induce the transcription of PSA and prostate-specific acid phosphatase, which suggests that this receptor may play a role in differentiation (304,305). Along with a more differentiated phenotype, *in vitro* CaP cell lines tend to be growth arrested by VDR activation (287,306,307). LNCaP and Alva-31 cell lines express relatively high levels of VDR and are sensitive to growth inhibition by vitamin D metabolites, whereas the insensitive cell lines of PC3 and DU145 have low levels of VDR expression (308).

Although not well described, growth regulation by VDR is thought to involve such mechanisms as decreased retinoblastoma protein phosphorylation, repressed E2F transcriptional activity, increased levels of the CDK inhibitor p21 (WAF1, CIP-1), and decreased CDK2 activity (287,306). Another potential mechanism for VDR-mediated inhibition of CaP cell growth is through up-regulation of AR (309,310).

These observations suggest that there may be a role for agents that bind to and activate VDR in chemoprevention or treatment of CaP, although this remains untested.

Retinoic Acid Receptor

RAR is another NR expressed and functioning within the prostate. Both RAR-beta and RAR-gamma are expressed in the day 0 prostate of rats and treatment with 13-*cis*-retinoic acid and all-*trans*-retinoic acid during prostatic development inhibited epithelial budding (311). RAR-alpha, RAR-beta, and RAR-gamma are all expressed in the adult prostate and in prostate tumors (312).

In general, exposure to different forms of retinoic acid inhibits *in vitro* growth of CaP cell lines (313–316). In LNCaP cells, exposure to 13-*cis*-retinoic acid decreased expression of PSA, decreased growth and soft agar colony formation, and resulted in smaller xenographic tumors (313). Other studies have not found significant effects on PSA expression (317), but there is a general agreement that growth inhibition occurs. A specific example is the expression of RAR-beta in PC3 cells (normally RAR-beta negative), resulting in growth inhibition on exposure to ligands for RAR-beta (318).

It is unclear the mechanisms by which RARs exert their growth arrest in CaP, but one mechanism, similar to VDR, is possibly through regulation of the AR (310,319,320). It is also becoming clearer that the three subtypes of RAR (alpha, beta, and gamma), as well as the three subtypes of RXR (alpha, beta, and gamma), may have distinct roles, as evidenced by the diverse responses to different specific ligands (315,318,321,322).

A phase II study looking at the response of hormone-refractory CaP patients to all-*trans*-retinoic acid failed to demonstrate any antitumor, although the negative finding may have been contributed to by inadequate tissue levels of the agent (323). However, with the growing knowledge that synthetic retinoids can target specific subtypes of RAR and RXR, there remains the possibility that a potent, antitumor retinoid exists and can play a role in the treatment of CaP.

Peroxisome Proliferator–Activated Gamma Receptors

The PPARs were identified after the observation that transcriptional control of genes involved in fatty acid metabolism was induced by agents that increased the size and number of hepatic peroxisomes (324,325). Three PPAR subtypes exist, PPAR-alpha, PPAR-gamma, and PPAR-delta. Specific ligands for PPAR-alpha and PPAR-gamma have been shown to have cytostatic and prodifferentiating activities, respectively (326–328). PPAR-gamma selective agents have resulted in increased differentiation of lipoblasts in tumors of patients with liposarcoma (329,330).

The prostate epithelium expresses relatively low levels of PPAR-gamma, whereas the PC3 cell line has higher levels of expression (331). Exposure of PC3 cells to a PPAR-gamma selective agent, troglitazone, reduced growth in immunodeficient mice and perhaps resulted in a more differentiated phenotype of cells grown in culture (331). The cell line DU145 is similarly growth inhibited when exposed to PPAR-gamma ligands (332). These initial findings have translated into some observed clinical activity of troglitazone in metastatic CaP where an unexpectedly high percentage of patients had stabilization of their serum PSA levels (332). Although troglitazone has been removed from the market owing to concerns with hepatotoxicity, other PPAR-gamma ligands are available and under investigation.

Other Nuclear Receptors

There are many other NRs, the roles of which, in the prostate and CaP, have yet to be explored. In the developing prostate, mRNA for the COUP-TF has been found to be present (333). Another example of orphan receptors pulled from prostatic cDNA libraries includes the subfamily including TR2 (334), TR3, and TR4 (335). Although the role of these receptors in the prostate remains unknown, there have been two published reports exploring possible functions. The orphan receptor TR3 has been found to be up-regulated by androgens in LNCaP and may be involved in drug metabolism (336). When a chimeric receptor is made between TR3 and AR, there is evidence of constitutive activity, although the significance of this observation remains unclear (337).

As more NRs are identified and the reagents created to rapidly assay for their expression, undoubtedly the profile of NRs within the prostate and CaP will become more complex. The profound clinical effect of the AR in the development of the prostate and CaP suggests that other NRs may provide avenues for profound clinical interventions.

CONCLUSIONS AND THE FUTURE

NRs represent a superfamily of transcription factors with major importance in the development of the prostate and CaP. The AR remains the most important target for CaP therapy and the only receptor whose inhibition has been demonstrated to prolong the life of men diagnosed with metastatic disease (339,340). However, most men will eventually have tumors that progress to androgen independence, and men with androgen-independent CaP generally succumb to their disease within a year. Our growing understanding of the cellular biology involved in AR-mediated transcription, the identification and characterization of co-regulatory proteins, and the coexpression of other members of the NR superfamily in CaP collectively create increased opportunities to design rational treatments and improve the survival of men with metastatic disease.

Although it is clear that the major function of NRs is mediated through transcriptional regulation, it remains a major challenge to identify those genes whose regulation by NRs is critical to observed cellular phenotype. Even in tumors that are refractory to hormonal therapy, there is evidence that AR-mediated transcriptional activation continues. The sequencing of the human genome and growing expertise in global expression analysis will aid in the identification and characterization of the most important regulated genes. These downstream genes offer great potential for further development of targeted therapies in CaP.

The discovery of the complex cascade of proteins that interact with NRs, from translation to ligand binding and to eventual transcriptional activation, is also an area with incredible opportunity. As the implications of each protein's interaction with the AR and other NRs important in CaP are better characterized, the interactions most important for receptor function can be targeted for disruption.

ER (alpha and beta), PR, GR, and many of the non-steroid NRs that are expressed in prostatic tissue and therapies targeting these receptors have also demonstrated some activity in CaP. The discovery of ER-beta has opened up the possibility that preferentially stimulating one variant of a receptor over another may offer biologic and clinical opportunities. The initial clinical effectiveness of PC-SPES, representing a complex pharmacologic mix containing some estrogenic compound(s), suggests that combinatorial approaches to NR stimulation or inhibition, or both, may prove to be more effective than therapies targeting any single receptor.

Over the next decade, the NRs most important to the prostate and CaP will be better characterized, the proteins associated with these receptors as chaperones or co-regulators will be identified and described, and the genes whose regulation is critical to the effects of receptor activation will be determined. It is very possible that these fundamental discoveries will rapidly improve therapy for CaP so that there will be a dramatic decrease in the number of men dying of this disease.

REFERENCES

1. Laudet V. Evolution of the nuclear receptor superfamily: early diversification from an ancestral orphan receptor. *J Mol Endocrinol* 1997;19:207–226.
2. Detera-Wadleigh SD, Fanning TG. Phylogeny of the steroid receptor superfamily. *Mol Phylogenet Evol* 1994;3:192–205.
3. Laudet V, Hanni C, Coll J, et al. Evolution of the nuclear receptor gene superfamily. *Embo J* 1992;11:1003–1013.
4. Jensen E, Sujuki T, Kawashima T, et al. A two-step mechanism for the interaction of estradiol with rat uterus. *Proc Natl Acad Sci U S A* 1968;59:632–638.

5. Toft D, Gorsky J. A receptor molecule for estrogens: isolation from the rat uterus and preliminary characterization. *Proc Natl Acad Sci U S A* 1966;5:1574–1581.
6. Baxter J, Tomkins G. Specific cytoplasmic glucocorticoid hormone receptors in hepatoma tissue culture cells. *Proc Natl Acad Sci U S A* 1971;68:932–937.
7. Corvol P, Falk R, Freifeld M, et al. In vitro studies of progesterone binding protein in guinea pig uterus. *Endocrinology* 1972;90:1464–1469.
8. Bauulieu EE, Jung I, Blondeau J, et al. Androgen receptors in rat ventral prostate. *Adv Biosci* 1971;7:179-191.
9. Gorski J, Gannon F. Current models of steroid hormone action: a critique. *Ann Rev Physiol* 1976;38:425-450.
10. Jensen, E. Overview of the nuclear receptor family, In: Parker M, ed. *Nuclear hormone receptors: molecular mechanisms, cellular functions, and clinical abnormalities.* London: Academic Press 1991;1–14.
11. O'Malley B. The steroid receptor superfamily: more excitement predicted for the future. *Mol Endocrinol* 1990;4:363–369.
12. Giguere V, Yang N, Segui P, et al. Identification of a new class of steroid hormone receptors. *Nature* 1988;331:91–94.
13. McDonnell DP, Pike JW, O'Malley BW. The vitamin D receptor: a primitive steroid receptor related to thyroid hormone receptor. *J Steroid Biochem* 1988;30:41–46.
14. Green S, Chambon P. Oestradiol induction of a glucocorticoid-responsive gene by a chimeric receptor. *Nature* 1987;325:75–78.
15. Silverstein A, Galigniana M, Kanelakis K, et al. Different regions of the immunophilin FKBP52 determine its association with the glucocorticoid receptor, hsp90, and cytoplasmic dynein. *J Biol Chem* 1999;274:36980-36986.
16. Glass C, Rosenfeld M. The coregulator exchange in transcriptional functions of nuclear receptors. *Genes Dev* 2000;14:121–141.
17. Parker MG. Structure and function of nuclear hormone receptors. *Semin Cancer Biol* 1990;1:81–87.
18. Lazar MA. Steroid and thyroid hormone receptors. *Endocrinol Metab Clin North Am* 1991;20:681–695.
19. Carson-Jurica MA, Schrader WT, O'Malley BW. Steroid receptor family: structure and functions. *Endocr Rev* 1990;11:201–220.
20. Tsai S, Tsai M, O'Malley B. The steroid receptor superfamily: transactivators of gene expression. In: Parker M, ed. *Nuclear hormone receptors: molecular mechanisms, cellular functions, clinical abnormalities.* London: Academic Press, 1991;103–124.
21. Parker M. *Nuclear hormone receptors: molecular mechanisms, cellular functions, clinical abnormalities.* London: Academic Press, 1991.
22. Freedman L. *Molecular biology of steroid and nuclear hormone receptors.* Boston: Birkhauser, 1998;319.
23. Green S, Chambon P. A superfamily of potentially oncogenic hormone receptors. *Nature* 1986;324:615–617.
24. Giguére V, Hollenberg S, Rosenfeld M, et al. Functional domains of the human glucocorticoid receptor. *Cell* 1986;46:645–652.
25. Kumar V, Green S, Stack G, et al. Functional domains of the human estrogen receptor. *Cell* 1987;51:941–951.
26. Waterman M, Adler S, Nelson C, et al. A single domain of the estrogen receptor confers deoxyribonucleic acid binding and transcriptional activation of the rat prolactin gene. *Mol Endocrinol* 1988;2:14–21.
27. Miesfeld R, Godowski P, Maler B, et al. Glucocorticoid receptor mutants that define a small region sufficient for enhancer activation. *Science* 1987;236:423–427.
28. Weinberger C, Hollenberg S, Ong E, et al. Identification of human glucocorticoid receptor complementary DNA clones by epitope selection. *Science* 1985;228:740–742.
29. Weinberger C, Hollenberg S, Rosenfeld M, et al. Domain structure of human glucocorticoid receptor and its relationship to the v-erbA oncogene product. *Nature* 1985;318: 670–672.
30. Freedman L, Luisi B, Korszun Z, et al. The function and structure of the metal coordination sites within the glucocorticoid receptor DNA binding domain. *Nature* 1988;334: 543–546.
31. Schwabe JW, Chapman L, Finch JT, et al. The crystal structure of the estrogen receptor DNA-binding domain bound to DNA: how receptors discriminate between their response elements. *Cell* 1993;75:567–578.
32. Lees J, Fawell S, Parker M. Identification of two transactivation domains in the mouse oestrogen receptor. *Nucleic Acids Res* 1989;17:5477–5488.
33. Fawell SE, Lees JA, White R, et al. Characterization and colocalization of steroid binding and dimerization activities in the mouse estrogen receptor. *Cell* 1990;60:953–962.
34. Wagner RL, Apriletti JW, McGrath ME, et al. A structural role for hormone in the thyroid hormone receptor. *Nature* 1995;378:690–697.
35. Bourguet W, Ruff M, Chambon P, et al. Crystal structure of the ligand-binding domain of the human nuclear receptor RXR-alpha. *Nature* 1995;375:377–382.
36. Wurtz J-M, Bourguet W, Renaud J-P, et al. A canonical structure for the ligand-binding domain of nuclear receptors. *Nat Struct Biol* 1996;3:87–94.
37. Shiau AK, Barstad D, Loria M, et al. The structural basis of estrogen receptor/coactivator recognition and the antagonism of this interaction by tamoxifen. *Cell* 1998;95:927–937.
38. Husmann DA, Wilson CM, McPhaul MJ, et al. Antipeptide antibodies to two distinct regions of the androgen receptor localize the receptor protein to the nuclei of target cells in the rat and human prostate. *Endocrinology* 1990; 126:2359–2368.
39. Hiroi H, Inoue S, Watanabe T, et al. Differential immunolocalization of estrogen receptor alpha and beta in rat ovary and uterus. *J Mol Endocrinol* 1999;22:37–44.
40. Guiochon-Mantel A, Loosfelt H, Lescop P, et al. Mechanisms of nuclear localization of the progesterone receptor: evidence for interaction between monomers. *Cell* 1989;57: 1147–1154.
41. Picard D, Yamamoto K. Two signals mediate hormone-dependent nuclear localization of the glucocorticoid receptor. *EMBO J* 1987;6:3333–3340.
42. Jensen EV. Steroid hormone receptors. *Curr Top Pathol* 1991;83:365–431.
43. Tora L, White J, Brou C, et al. The human estrogen receptor has two independent nonacidic transcriptional activation functions. *Cell* 1989;59:477–487.

44. Picard D, Salser SJ, Yamamoto KR. A movable and regulable inactivation function within the steroid binding domain of the glucocorticoid receptor. *Cell* 1988;54:1073–1080.
45. Kumar V, Chambon P. The estrogen receptor binds tightly to its responsive element as a ligand-induced homodimer. *Cell* 1988;55:145–156.
46. Kurokawa R, Yu VC, Naar A, et al. Differential orientations of the DNA-binding domain and carboxy-terminal dimerization interface regulate binding site selection by nuclear receptor heterodimers. *Genes Dev* 1993;7:1423–1435.
47. Yudt M, Vorojeikina D, Zhong L, et al. Function of estrogen receptor tyrosine 537 in hormone binding, DNA binding, and transactivation. *Biochemistry* 1999;38:14146–14156.
48. Lubahn DB, Joseph DR, Sar M, et al. The human androgen receptor: complementary deoxyribonucleic acid cloning, sequence analysis and gene expression in prostate. *Mol Endocrinol* 1988;2:1265–1275.
49. Kazemi-Esfarjani P, Trifiro MA, Pinsky L. Evidence for a repressive function of the long polyglutamine tract in the human androgen receptor: possible pathogenetic relevance for the (CAG)n-expanded neuronopathies. *Hum Mol Genet* 1995;4:523–527.
50. Chamberlain NL, Driver ED, Miesfeld RL. The length and location of CAG trinucleotide repeats in the androgen receptor N-terminal domain affect transactivation function. *Nucleic Acids Res* 1994;22:3181–3186.
51. Needham M, Raines S, McPheat J, et al. Differential interaction of steroid hormone receptors with LXXLL motifs in SRC-1a depends on residues flanking the motif. *J Steroid Biochem Mol Bio* 2000;72:35–46.
52. Chamberlain NL, Whitacre DC, Miesfeld RL. Delineation of two distinct type 1 activation functions in the androgen receptor amino-terminal domain. *J Biol Chem* 1996;271: 26772–26778.
53. Wolf DA, Herzinger T, Hermeking H, et al. Transcriptional and posttranscriptional regulation of human androgen receptor expression by androgen. *Mol Endocrinol* 1993;7: 924–936.
54. Mora GR, Prins GS, Mahesh VB. Autoregulation of androgen receptor protein and messenger RNA in rat ventral prostate is protein synthesis dependent. *J Steroid Biochem Mol Biol* 1996;58:539–549.
55. Lin MC, Rajfer J, Swerdloff RS, et al. Testosterone downregulates the levels of androgen receptor mRNA in smooth muscle cells from the rat corpora cavernosa via aromatization to estrogens. *J Steroid Biochem Mol Biol* 1993;45:333–343.
56. Dai JL, Burnstein KL. Two androgen response elements in the androgen receptor coding region are required for cell-specific up-regulation of receptor messenger RNA. *Mol Endocrinol* 1996;10:1582–1594.
57. Wiren KM, Zhang X, Chang C, et al. Transcriptional upregulation of the human androgen receptor by androgen in bone cells. *Endocrinology* 1997;138:2291–2300.
58. Gong Y, Blok LJ, Perry JE, et al. Calcium regulation of androgen receptor expression in the human prostate cancer cell line LNCaP. *Endocrinology* 1995;136:2172–2178.
59. Yeap BB, Krueger RG, Leedman J. Differential posttranscriptional regulation of androgen receptor gene expression by androgen in prostate and breast cancer cells. *Endocrinology* 1999;140:3282–3291.
60. Jarrard DF, Kinoshita H, Shi Y, et al. Methylation of the androgen receptor promoter CpG island is associated with loss of androgen receptor expression in prostate cancer cells. *Cancer Res* 1998;58:5310–5314.
61. Blok LJ, de Ruiter E, Brinkmann AO. Androgen receptor phosphorylation. *Endocr Res* 1996;22:197–219.
62. Arnold S, Notides A. An antiestrogen: a phosphotyrosyl peptide that blocks dimerization of the human estrogen receptor. *Proc Natl Acad Sci U S A* 1995;92:7475–7479.
63. Kato S, Endoh H, Masuhiro Y, et al. Activation of the estrogen receptor through phosphorylation by mitogen-activated protein kinase. *Science* 1995;270:1491–1494.
64. Blok LJ, de Ruiter E, Brinkmann AO. Forskolin-induced dephosphorylation of the androgen receptor impairs ligand binding. *Biochemistry* 1998;37:3850–3857.
65. Hu J, Bodwell J, Munck A. Cell cycle-dependent glucocorticoid receptor phosphorylation and activity. *Mol Endocrinol* 1994;8:1709–1713.
66. Karin M, Hunter T. Transcriptional control by protein phosphorylation: signal transmission from the cell surface to the nucleus. *Curr Biol* 1995;5:747–757.
67. Garabedian M, Rogatzky I, Hittelman A, et al. Regulation of glucocorticoid and estrogen receptor activity by phosphorylation. In: Freedman L, ed. *Molecular biology of steroid and nuclear hormone receptors*. Boston: Birkhauser, 1998.
68. Kuiper GG, de Ruiter E, Trapman J, et al. Localization and hormonal stimulation of phosphorylation sites in the LNCaP-cell androgen receptor. *Biochem J* 1993;291:95–101.
69. Bai W, Tullos S, Weigel N. Phosphorylation of ser530 facilitates hormone-dependent transcriptional activation of the chicken progesterone receptor. *Mol Endocrinol* 1994;8: 1465–1473.
70. LeGoff P, Montano M, Schodin D, et al. Phosphorylation of the human estrogen receptor. *J Biol Chem* 1994;269: 4458–4466.
71. Nazareth LV, Weigel NL. Activation of the human androgen receptor through a protein kinase A signaling pathway. *J Biol Chem* 1996;271:19900–19907.
72. Sadar MD. Androgen-independent induction of prostate-specific antigen gene expression via cross-talk between the androgen receptor and protein kinase A signal transduction pathways. *J Biol Chem* 1999;274:7777–7783.
73. Rana S, Bisht D, Chakraborti K. Synergistic activation of yeast-expressed rat androgen receptor by modulators of protein kinase-A. *J Mol Biol* 1999;286:669–681.
74. Power R, Mani S, Codina J, et al. Dopaminergic and ligand-independent activation of steroid hormone receptors. *Science* 1991;254:1636–1639.
75. Bunone G, Briand P, Miksicek R, et al. Activation of the unliganded estrogen receptor by EGF involves the MAP kinase pathway and direct phosphorylation. *EMBO J* 1996;15:2174–2183.
76. Yeh S, Lin HK, Kang HY, et al. From HER2/Neu signal cascade to androgen receptor and its coactivators: a novel pathway by induction of androgen target genes through MAP kinase in prostate cancer cells. *Proc Natl Acad Sci U S A* 1999;96:5458–5463.
77. Poukka H, Aarnisalo P, Karvonen U, et al. Ubc9 interacts with the androgen receptor and activates receptor-dependent transcription. *J Biol Chem* 1999;274:19441–19446.

78. Guiochon-Mantel A, Lescop P, Chrisin-Maitre S, et al. Nucleocytoplasmic shuttling of the progesterone receptor. *EMBO J* 1991;10:3851–3859.
79. Madan A, DeFranco D. Bidirectional transport of glucocorticoid receptors across the nuclear envelope. *Proc Natl Acad Sci U S A* 1993;90:3588–3592.
80. DeFranco D. Subcellular and subnuclear trafficking of steroid receptors. In: Freedman L, ed. *Molecular biology of steroid and nuclear receptors*. Boston: Birkhauser, 1998;19–34.
81. Yang J, DeFranco D. Assessment of glucocorticoid receptor-heat shock protein 90 interactions in vivo during nucleocytoplasmic trafficking. *Mol Endocrinol* 1996;10:3–13.
82. Sackey F, Hache R, Reich T, et al. Determinants of subcellular distribution of the glucocorticoid receptor. *Mol Endocrinol* 1996;10:1191–1205.
83. Pratt W. The role of heat shock proteins in regulating the function, folding, and trafficking of the glucocorticoid receptor. *J Biol Chem* 1993;268:21455–21458.
84. Pratt W, Toft D. Steroid receptor interactions with heat shock protein and immunophilin chaperones. *Endocr Rev* 1997;18:306–360.
85. Smith D. Dynamics of heat shock protein 90-progesterone receptor binding and the disactivation loop model for steroid receptor complexes. *Mol Endocrinol* 1993;7:1418–1429.
86. Bresnick E, Dalman F, Sanchez E, et al. Evidence that the 90-kDa heat shock protein is necessary for the steroid binding conformation of the L cell glucocorticoid receptor. *J Bio Chem* 1989;264:4992–4997.
87. Rafestin-Oblin M-E, Couette B, Radanyi C, et al. Mineralocorticosteroid receptor of the chick intestine. *J Bio Chem* 1989;264:9304–9309.
88. Yamamoto K, Godowski PJ, Picard D. Ligand regulated nonspecific inactivation of receptor function: a versatile mechanism for signal transduction. *Cold Spring Harb Symp Quant Biol* 1988;53:803–811.
89. Estes P, Suba E, Lawler-Heavner J, et al. Immunologic analysis of human breast cancer progesterone receptors. 1. Immunoaffinity purification of transformed receptors and production of monoclonal antibodies. *Biochemistry* 1987; 26:6250–6262.
90. Seielstad D, Carlson K, Katzenellenbogen J, et al. Molecular characterization by mass spectrometry of the human estrogen receptor ligand binding domain expressed in *Escherichia coli*. *Mol Endo* 1995;9:647–658.
91. Simons S. Structure and function of the steroid and nuclear receptor ligand binding domain. In: Freedman L, ed. *Molecular biology of steroid and nuclear hormone receptors*. Boston: Birkhauser, 1998;35–104.
92. Renaud J, Rochel N, Ruff M, et al. Crystal structure of the RAR-gamma ligand-binding domain bound to all-*trans* retinoic acid. *Nature* 1995;378:681–689.
93. Bagchi L. Molecular mechanisms of nuclear receptor-mediated transcriptional activation and basal repression. In: Freedman L, ed. *Molecular biology of steroid and nuclear hormone receptors*. Boston: Birkhauser, 1998;159–189.
94. Tora L, Gronemeyer H, Tucotte B, et al. The N-terminal region of the chicken progesterone receptor specifies target gene activation. *Nature* 1988;333:185–188.
95. Green S, Kumar V, Theulaz I, et al. The N-terminal DNA binding zinc finger of oestrogen and glucocorticoid receptors determines target gene specificity. *EMBO J* 1988;7: 3037–3044.
96. Rastinejad F. Structure and function of the steroid and nuclear receptor DNA binding domain. In: Freedman LP, ed. *Molecular biology of steroid and nuclear hormone receptors*. Boston: Birkhauser, 1998;105–131.
97. Mader S, Kumar V, deVerneui H, et al. Three amino acids of the oestrogen receptor are essential to its ability to distinguish an oestrogen from a glucocorticoid-responsive element. *Nature* 1989;338:271–274.
98. Scheidereit C, Westphal H, Carlson C, et al. Molecular model of the interaction between the glucocorticoid receptor and the regulatory elements of inducible genes. *DNA* 1986;5:383–391.
99. Ryffel G, Klein-Hitpass L, Druege P, et al. The estrogen-responsive DNA element: structure and interaction with the estrogen receptor. *J Cell Biochem* 1988;35:219–227.
100. Klock G, Strahle U, Schutz, G. Oestrogen and glucocorticoid responsive elements are closely related but distinct. *Nature* 1987;375:734–736.
101. Tsai S, Carlstedt-Duke J, Weigel N, et al. Molecular interactions of steroid hormone receptor with its enhancer element: evidence for receptor dimer formation. *Cell* 1988;55: 361–369.
102. Cheskis B, Freedman L. Modulation of steroid/nuclear receptor dimerization and DNA binding by ligands. In: Freedman L, ed. *Molecular biology of steroid and nuclear hormone receptors*. Boston: Birkhauser, 1998;133–158.
103. Lazar M, Harding H. Monomeric nuclear receptors. In: Freedman L, ed. *Molecular biology of steroid and nuclear hormone receptors*. Boston: Birkhauser, 1998.
104. Ing N, Beekman J, Tsai S, et al. Members of the steroid receptor superfamily interact with TFIIB (S300-II). *J Biol Chem* 1992;267:17617–17623.
105. Baniahmad A, Ha I, Reinberg D, et al. Interaction of human thyroid hormone receptor beta with transcription factor TFIIB may mediate target gene derepression and activation by thyroid hormone. *Proc Natl Acad Sci U S A* 1993;90:8832–8836.
106. Hadzic E, Desai-Yajnik V, Helmer E, et al. A 10-amino acid sequence in the N-terminal A/B domain of thyroid hormone receptor alpha is essential for transcriptional activation and interaction with the general transcription factor TFIIB. *Mol Cell Biol* 1995;15:4507–4517.
107. Schulman I, Chrakravarti D, Juguilon H, et al. Interactions between the retinoid X receptor and a conserved region of the TATA-binding protein mediate hormone-dependent transactivation. *Proc Natl Acad Sci U S A* 1995;92:8288–8292.
108. Hollenberg S, Evans R. Multiple and cooperative transactivation domains of the human glucocorticoid receptor. *Cell* 1988;55:899–906.
109. Webster N, Green S, Jin JR, et al. The hormone-binding domains of the estrogen and glucocorticoid receptors contain an inducible transcription activation function. *Cell* 1988;54:199–207.
110. Meyer M, Pornon A, Ji J, et al. Agonistic and antagonistic activities of RU486 on the functions of the human progesterone receptor. *EMBO J* 1989;9:3923–3932.
111. Danielian P, White R, Lees J, et al. Identification of a conserved region required for hormone dependent transcrip-

tional activation by steroid hormone receptors. *EMBO J* 1992;11:1025–1033.

112. Saatcioglu F, Bartunek P, Dent T, et al. A conserved C-terminal sequence that is deleted in v-ErbA is essential for the biological activities of c-ErbA (the thyroid hormone receptor). *Mol Cell Biol* 1993;13:3675–3685.
113. Nagpal S, Saunders M, Kastner P, et al. Promoter context- and response element-dependent specificity of the transcriptional activation and modulating functions of retinoic acid receptors. *Cell* 1992;70:1007–1019.
114. Shupnik M, Chin W, Habener J, et al. Transcriptional regulation of the thyrotropin subunit genes by thyroid hormone. *J Biol Chem* 1985;260:2900–2903.
115. Charron J, Drouin H. Glucocorticoid inhibition of transcription from episomal proopiomelanocortin gene promoter. *Proc Natl Acad Sci U S A* 1986;83:8903–8907.
116. Drouin J, Trifiro M, Plante R, et al. Glucocorticoid receptor binding to a specific DNA sequence is required for hormone-dependent repression of proopiomelanocortin gene transcription. *Mol Cell Biol* 1989;9:5305–5314.
117. Akerblom I, Mellon P. Repression of gene expression by steroid and thyroid hormones, In: Parker M, ed. *Nuclear hormone receptors: molecular mechanisms, cellular functions, clinical abnormalities*. San Diego: Academic Press, 1991:175–196.
118. Baniahmad A, Kohne A, Renkawitz R. A transferable silencing domain is present in the thyroid hormone receptor, in the v-erbA oncogene product and in the retinoic acid receptor. *EMBO J* 1992;11:1015–1023.
119. Damm K, Thompson C, Evans R. Protein encoded by v-erbA functions as a thyroid hormone receptor antagonist. *Nature* 1989;339:593–597.
120. Meyer M, Gronemeyer H, Turcotte B, et al. Steroid hormone receptors compete for factors that mediate their enhancer function. *Cell* 1989;57:433–442.
121. Ptashne M. How do eukaryotic transcriptional activators work? *Nature* 1988;335:683–689.
122. Onate S, Tsai S, Tsai M, et al. Sequence and characterization of a coactivator for the steroid hormone receptor superfamily. *Science* 1995;270:1354–1357.
123. LeDuoarin B, Nielsen A, Garnier J, et al. A possible involvement of TIF1-alpha and TIF1-beta in the epigenetic control of transcription by nuclear receptors. *EMBO J* 1996;15: 6701–6715.
124. Voegel J, Heine M, Zechel C, et al. TIF2, a 160kDa transcriptional mediator for the ligand-dependent activation function AF-2 of nuclear receptors. *EMBO J* 1996;15: 3667–3675.
125. Yeh S, Chang C. Cloning and characterization of a specific coactivator, ARA70, for the androgen receptor in human prostate cells. *Proc Natl Acad Sci U S A* 1996;93:5517–5521.
126. Heinlein CA, Ting HJ, Yeh S, et al. Identification of ARA70 as a ligand-enhanced coactivator for the peroxisome proliferator-activated receptor gamma. *J Biol Chem* 1999;274: 16147–16152.
127. Kwok R, Lundblad J, Chrivia J, et al. Nuclear protein CBPO is a coactivator for the transcription factor CREB. *Nature* 1994;370:223–226.
128. Chen J, Evans R. A transcriptional co-repressor that interacts with nuclear hormone receptors. *Nature* 1995;377: 3741–3751.
129. Horlein A, Naar A, Heinzel T, et al. Ligand-independent repression by the thyroid hormone receptor mediated by a nuclear receptor co-repressor. *Nature* 1995;377:397–403.
130. Lanz RB, McKenna NJ, Onate SA, et al. A steroid receptor coactivator, SRA, functions as an RNA and is present in an SRC-1 complex. *Cell* 1999;97:17–27.
131. Coffey D. The molecular biology, endocrinology, and physiology of the prostate and the seminal vesicles. In: Walsh PC, Retik AB, Starney TA, eds. *Campbell's urology*, 6th ed. Philadelphia: WB Saunders, 1992;221–266.
132. Crocoll A, Zhu CC, Cato AC, et al. Expression of androgen receptor mRNA during mouse embryogenesis. *Mech Dev* 1998;72:175–178.
133. Bentvelsen F, Brinkmann A, VanderSchoot P, et al. Developmental pattern and regulation by androgens of androgen receptor expression in the urogenital tract of the rat. *Mol Cell Endocrinol* 1995;113:245–253.
134. Tyndale-Biscoe H, Renfree M. *Reproductive physiology of marsupials*. Cambridge: Cambridge University Press. 1987; 3–28.
135. Cunha G. Role of mesenchymal-epithelial interactions in normal and abnormal development of the mammary gland and prostate. *Cancer* 1994;74:1030–1044.
136. Zhang YL, Zhou ZX, Zhang YD, et al. Expression of androgen receptors and prostatic steroid-binding protein during development of the rat ventral prostate. *J Endocrinol* 1988;117:361–366.
137. Sonea IM, Iqbal J, Prins GS, et al. Ontogeny of androgen receptor-like immunoreactivity in the reproductive tract of male Monodelphis domestica. *Biol Reprod* 1997;56:852–860.
138. Aumuller G, Holterhus M, Konrad L, et al. Immunohistochemistry and in situ hybridization of the androgen receptor in the developing human prostate. *Anat Embryol (Berl)* 1998;197:199–208.
139. Meyers-Wallen VN. Genetics of sexual differentiation and anomalies in dogs and cats. *J Reprod Fertil Suppl* 1993;47:441–452.
140. McPhaul MJ. Molecular defects of the androgen receptor. *J Steroid Biochem Mol Biol* 1999;69:315–322.
141. Wieacker F, Knoke I, Jakubiczka, S. Clinical and molecular aspects of androgen receptor defects. *Exp Clin Endocrinol Diabetes* 1998;106:446–453.
142. Gaspar ML, Meo T, Bourgarel P, et al. A single base deletion in the Tfm androgen receptor gene creates a short-lived messenger RNA that directs internal translation initiation. *Proc Natl Acad Sci U S A* 1991;88:8606–8610.
143. Cunha GR, Donjacour AA, Sugimura Y. Stromal-epithelial interactions and heterogeneity of proliferative activity within the prostate. *Biochem Cell Biol* 1986;64:608–614.
144. Shannon JM, Cunha GR. Characterization of androgen binding and deoxyribonucleic acid synthesis in prostate-like structures induced in the urothelium of testicular feminized (Tfm/Y) mice. *Biol Reprod* 1984;31:175–183.
145. Lasnitzki I, Mizuno T. Prostatic induction: interaction of epithelium and mesenchyme from normal wild-type mice and androgen-insensitive mice with testicular feminization. *J Endocrinol* 1980;85:423–428.
146. Takeda H, Lasnitzki I, Mizuno T. Change of mosaic pattern by androgens during prostatic bud formation in XTfm/X+ heterozygous female mice. *J Endocrinol* 1987;114:131–137.

147. Hansson V, Tveter K, Attramadal A, et al. Androgenic receptors in human benign nodular prostatic hyperplasia. *Acta Endocrinol* 1971;68:79.
148. Feneley MR, Puddefoot JR, Xia S, et al. Zonal biochemical and morphological characteristics in BPH. *Br J Urol* 1995;75:608–613.
149. Sanchez-Visconti G, Herrero L, Rabadan M, et al. Ageing and prostate: age-related changes in androgen receptors of epithelial cells from benign hypertrophic glands compared with cancer. *Mech Ageing Dev* 1995;82:19–29.
150. Monti S, Di Silverio F, Toscano V, et al. Androgen concentrations and their receptors in the periurethral region are higher than those of the subcapsular zone in benign prostatic hyperplasia (BPH). *J Androl* 1998;19:428–433.
151. Bacher M, Rausch U, Goebel HW, et al. Stromal and epithelial cells from rat ventral prostate during androgen deprivation and estrogen treatment—regulation of transcription. *Exp Clin Endocrinol* 1993;101:78–86.
152. Bonkhoff H, Remberger K. Widespread distribution of nuclear androgen receptors in the basal cell layer of the normal and hyperplastic human prostate. *Virchows Arch* 1993;422:35–38.
153. Takeda H, Chodak G, Mutchnik S, et al. Immunohistochemical localization of androgen receptors with mono- and polyclonal antibodies to the androgen receptor. *J Endocrinology* 1989;126:17–25.
154. Callaway TW, Bruchovsky N, Rennie S, et al. Mechanisms of action of androgens and antiandrogens: effects of antiandrogens on translocation of cytoplasmic androgen receptor and nuclear abundance of dihydrotestosterone. *Prostate* 1982;3:599–610.
155. Brinkmann AO, Lindh LM, Breedveld DI, et al. Cyproterone acetate prevents translocation of the androgen receptor in the rat prostate. *Mol Cell Endocrinol* 1983;32:117–129.
156. Blondeau, JP, Baulieu EE, Robel P. Androgen-dependent regulation of androgen nuclear receptor in the rat ventral prostate. *Endocrinology* 1982;110:1926–1932.
157. Paris F, Weinbauer GF, Blum V, et al. The effect of androgens and antiandrogens on the immunohistochemical localization of the androgen receptor in accessory reproductive organs of male rats. *J Steroid Biochem Mol Biol* 1994;48: 129–137.
158. deVoogt H, Rau B, Geldof A, et al. Androgen action blockade does not result in reduction in size but changes the histology of the normal human prostate. *Prostate* 1987;11:305–313.
159. Aumuller G. Functional anatomy of the prostate. In: Vahlensieck W, Rutishauer G, eds. *Benign prostatic diseases*. New York: Georg Thieme Verlag, 1992;4–16.
160. Kiplesund K, Halgunset J, Fjosne H, et al. Light microscopic morphometric analysis of castration effects in the different lobes of the rat prostate. *Prostate* 1988;13:221–232.
161. Kruithof-Dekker IG, Tetu B, Janssen J, et al. Elevated estrogen receptor expression in human prostatic stromal cells by androgen ablation therapy. *J Urol* 1996;156:1194–1197.
162. Blok LJ, Bartlett JM, Bolt-De Vries J, et al. Effect of testosterone deprivation on expression of the androgen receptor in rat prostate, epididymis and testis. *Int J Androl* 1992;15: 182–198.
163. Mobbs BG, Johnson IE, Connolly JG, et al. Concentration and cellular distribution of androgen receptor in human prostatic neoplasia: Can estrogen treatment increase androgen receptor content? *J Steroid Biochem* 1983;19:1279–1290.
164. Prins GS, Birch L. Immunocytochemical analysis of androgen receptor along the ducts of the separate rat prostate lobes after androgen withdrawal and replacement. *Endocrinology* 1993;132:169–178.
165. van Aubel OG, Bolt-de Vries J, Blankenstein MA, et al. Nuclear androgen receptor content in biopsy specimens from histologically normal, hyperplastic, and cancerous human prostatic tissue. *Prostate* 1985;6:185–194.
166. Chodak GW, Kranc DM, Puy LA, et al. Nuclear localization of androgen receptor in heterogeneous samples of normal, hyperplastic and neoplastic human prostate. *J Urol* 1992;147:798–803.
167. Brolin J, Lowhagen T, Skoog L. Immunocytochemical detection of the androgen receptor in fine needle aspirates from benign and malignant human prostate. *Cytopathology* 1992;3:351–357.
168. Miyamoto KK, McSherry SA, Dent GA, et al. Immunohistochemistry of the androgen receptor in human benign and malignant prostate tissue. *J Urol* 1993;149:1015–1019.
169. Magi-Galluzzi C, Xu X, Hlatky L, et al. Heterogeneity of androgen receptor content in advanced prostate cancer. *Mod Pathol* 1997;10:839–845.
170. Barrack ER, Bujnovszky P, Walsh C. Subcellular distribution of androgen receptors in human normal, benign hyperplastic, and malignant prostatic tissues: characterization of nuclear salt-resistant receptors. *Cancer Res* 1983;43:1107–1116.
171. Mohler JL, Chen Y, Hamil K, et al. Androgen and glucocorticoid receptors in the stroma and epithelium of prostatic hyperplasia and carcinoma. *Clin Cancer Res* 1996;2:889–895.
172. Donnelly BJ, Lakey WH, McBlain WA. Androgen binding sites on nuclear matrix of normal and hyperplastic human prostate. *J Urol* 1984;131:806–811.
173. Elhilali M, Lehoux JG, Carmel M, et al. Nuclear androgen receptors of human prostatic tissue—a quantitative histological study. *Arch Androl* 1983;10:21–27.
174. Brolin J, Skoog L, Ekman P. Immunohistochemistry and biochemistry in detection of androgen, progesterone, and estrogen receptors in benign and malignant human prostatic tissue. *Prostate* 1992;20:281–295.
175. Sweat SD, Pacelli A, Bergstralh EJ, et al. Androgen receptor expression in prostate cancer lymph node metastases is predictive of outcome after surgery. *J Urol* 1999;161:1233–1237.
176. Grimaldo JI, Meikle AW. Increased levels of nuclear androgen receptors in hyperplastic prostate of aging men. *J Steroid Biochem* 1984;21:147–150.
177. Harper ME, Glynne-Jones E, Goddard L, et al. Expression of androgen receptor and growth factors in premalignant lesions of the prostate. *J Pathol* 1998;186:169–177.
178. Sweat SD, Pacelli A, Bergstralh EJ, et al. Androgen receptor expression in prostatic intraepithelial neoplasia and cancer. *J Urol* 1999;161:1229–1232.
179. Sadi MV, Barrack ER. Image analysis of androgen receptor immunostaining in metastatic prostate cancer. Heterogeneity as a predictor of response to hormonal therapy. *Cancer* 1993;71:2574–2580.

180. Fentie DD, Lakey WH, McBlain WA. Applicability of nuclear androgen receptor quantification to human prostatic adenocarcinoma. *J Urol* 1986;135:167–173.
181. Benson RC Jr., Gorman A, O'Brien C, et al. Relationship between androgen receptor binding activity in human prostate cancer and clinical response to endocrine therapy. *Cancer* 1987;59:1599–1606.
182. Sadi MV, Walsh C, Barrack ER. Immunohistochemical study of androgen receptors in metastatic prostate cancer. Comparison of receptor content and response to hormonal therapy. *Cancer* 1991;67:3057–3064.
183. Takeda H, Akakura K, Masai M, et al. Androgen receptor content of prostate carcinoma cells estimated by immunohistochemistry is related to prognosis of patients with stage D2 prostate carcinoma. *Cancer* 1996;77:934–940.
184. Pertschuk LP, Macchia RJ, Feldman JG, et al. Immunocytochemical assay for androgen receptors in prostate cancer: a prospective study of 63 cases with long-term follow-up. *Ann Surg Oncol* 1994;1:495–503.
185. Pertschuk LP, Schaeffer H, Feldman JG, et al. Immunostaining for prostate cancer androgen receptor in paraffin identifies a subset of men with a poor prognosis. *Lab Invest* 1995;73:302–305.
186. Quarmby VE, Beckman WC Jr., Cooke DB, et al. Expression and localization of androgen receptor in the R-3327 Dunning rat prostatic adenocarcinoma. *Cancer Res* 1990;50:735–739.
187. Taplin ME, Bubley GJ, Shuster TD, et al. Mutation of the androgen-receptor gene in metastatic androgen-independent prostate cancer [see comments]. *N Engl J Med* 1995;332:1393–1398.
188. Hobisch A, Culig Z, Radmayer C, et al. Distant metastases from prostate carcinoma express androgen receptor protein. *Cancer Res* 1995;55:3068–3072.
189. Hobisch A, Culig Z, Radmayr C, et al. Androgen receptor status of lymph node metastases from prostate cancer. *Prostate* 1996;28:129–135.
190. Koivisto P, Kononen J, Palmberg C, et al. Androgen receptor gene amplification: a possible molecular mechanism for androgen deprivation therapy failure in prostate cancer. *Cancer Res* 1997;57:314–319.
191. Visakorpi T, Hyytinen E, Koivisto P, et al. In vivo amplification of the androgen receptor gene and progression of human prostate cancer. *Nat Genet* 1995;9:401–406.
192. Veldscholte J, Berrevoets CA, Ris-Stalpers C, et al. The androgen receptor in LNCaP cells contains a mutation in the ligand binding domain which affects steroid binding characteristics and response to antiandrogens. *J Steroid Biochem Mol Biol* 1992;41:665–669.
193. Veldscholte J, Ris-Stalpers C, Kuiper GG, et al. A mutation in the ligand binding domain of the androgen receptor of human LNCaP cells affects steroid binding characteristics and response to anti-androgens. *Biochem Biophys Res Commun* 1990;173:534–540.
194. Wilding G. The importance of steroid hormones in prostate cancer. *Cancer Surv* 1992;14:113–130.
195. Bosland M. The etiopathogenesis of prostate cancer with special reference to environmental factors. *Adv Cancer Res* 1988;51:1–106.
196. Noble RL. The development of prostatic adenocarcinoma in Nb rats following prolonged sex hormone administration. *Cancer Res* 1977;37:1929–1933.
197. Riegman H, Vlietstra RJ, van der Korput JA, et al. The promoter of the prostate-specific antigen gene contains a functional androgen responsive element. *Mol Endocrinol* 1991;5:1921–1930.
198. Wolf DA, Schulz P, and Fittler F. Transcriptional regulation of prostate kallikrein-like genes by androgen. *Mol Endocrinol* 1992;6:753–762.
199. Henttu P, Liao SS, Vihko P. Androgens up-regulate the human prostate-specific antigen messenger ribonucleic acid (mRNA), but down-regulate the prostatic acid phosphatase mRNA in the LNCaP cell line. *Endocrinology* 1992;130:766–772.
200. Young CY, Montgomery BT, Andrews E, et al. Hormonal regulation of prostate-specific antigen messenger RNA in human prostatic adenocarcinoma cell line LNCaP. *Cancer Res* 1991;51:3748–3752.
201. Henttu P, Vihko P. Steroids inversely affect the biosynthesis and secretion of human prostatic acid phosphatase and prostate-specific antigen in the LNCaP cell line. *J Steroid Biochem Mol Biol* 1992;41:349–360.
202. Shan JD, Porvari K, Ruokonen M, et al. Steroid-involved transcriptional regulation of human genes encoding prostatic acid phosphatase, prostate-specific antigen, and prostate-specific glandular kallikrein. *Endocrinology* 1997;138:3764–3770.
203. Yu DC, Sakamoto GT, Henderson DR. Identification of the transcriptional regulatory sequences of human kallikrein 2 and their use in the construction of calydon virus 764, an attenuated replication competent adenovirus for prostate cancer therapy. *Cancer Res* 1999;59:1498–1504.
204. Prescott JL, Tindall DJ. Clathrin gene expression is androgen regulated in the prostate. *Endocrinology* 1998;139:2111–2119.
205. Belanger G, Beaulieu M, Marcotte B, et al. Expression of transcripts encoding steroid UDP-glucuronosyltransferases in human prostate hyperplastic tissue and the LNCaP cell line. *Mol Cell Endocrinol* 1995;113:165–173.
206. Guillemette C, Levesque E, Beaulieu M, et al. Differential regulation of two uridine diphospho-glucuronosyltransferases, UGT2B15 and UGT2B17, in human prostate LNCaP cells. *Endocrinology* 1997;138:2998–3005.
207. Lu S, Tsai SY, Tsai MJ. Regulation of androgen-dependent prostatic cancer cell growth: androgen regulation of CDK2, CDK4, and CKI p16 genes. *Cancer Res* 1997;57:4511–4516.
208. Lu S, Liu M, Epner DE, et al. Androgen regulation of the cyclin-dependent kinase inhibitor p21 gene through an androgen response element in the proximal promoter. *Mol Endocrinol* 1999;13:376–384.
209. Prescott JL, Blok L, Tindall DJ. Isolation and androgen regulation of the human homeobox cDNA, NKX3.1. *Prostate* 1998;35:71–80.
210. Brinkmann AO, Trapman J. Androgen receptor mutants that affect normal growth and development. *Cancer Surv* 1992;14:95–111.
211. Brinkmann AO, Jenster G, Ris-Stalpers C, et al. Androgen receptor mutations. *J Steroid Biochem Mol Biol* 1995;53:443–448.

212. MacLean HE, Warne GL, Zajac JD. Defects of androgen receptor function: from sex reversal to motor neurone disease. *Mol Cell Endocrinol* 1995;112:133–141.
213. Peehl D, Rubin J. Keratinocyte growth factor: an androgen-regulated mediator of stromal-epithelial interactions in the prostate. *World J Urol* 1995;13:312–317.
214. Trapman J, Cleutjens KB. Androgen-regulated gene expression in prostate cancer. *Semin Cancer Biol* 1997;8:29–36.
215. Yan G, Fukabori Y, Nikolaropoulos S, et al. Heparin-binding keratinocyte growth factor is a candidate stromal-to-epithelial-cell andromedin. *Mol Endocrinol* 1992;6:2123–2128.
216. Sugimura Y, Foster B, Hom Y, et al. Keratinocyte growth factor can replace testosterone in the ductal branching morphogenesis of the rat ventral prostate. *Int J Dev Biol* 1996;40:941–951.
217. Guo L, Degenstein L, Fuchs E. Keratinocyte growth factor is required for hair development but not for wound healing. *Genes Dev* 1996;10:165–175.
218. Russell J, Bennett S, Stricker P. Growth factor involvement in progression of prostate cancer. *Clin Chem* 1998;44:705–723.
219. Gao J, Isaacs JT. Development of an androgen receptor-null model for identifying the initiation site for androgen stimulation of proliferation and suppression of programmed (apoptotic) death of PC-82 human prostate cancer cells. *Cancer Res* 1998;58:3299–3306.
220. Jenster G. The role of the androgen receptor in the development and progression of prostate cancer. *Semin Oncol* 1999;26:407–421.
221. Wehling M. Specific, nongenomic actions of steroid hormones. *Annu Rev Physiol* 1997;59:365–393.
222. Wiebe J. Nongenomic actions of steroids on gonadotropin release. *Recent Prog Horm Res* 1997;52:71–99.
223. Benten WP, Lieberherr M, Stamm O, et al. Testosterone signaling through internalizable surface receptors in androgen receptor-free macrophages. *Mol Biol Cell* 1999;10:3113–3123.
224. Benten WP, Lieberherr M, Giese G, et al. Functional testosterone receptors in plasma membranes of T cells. *Faseb J* 1999;13:123–133.
225. Nakhla AM, Rosner W. Stimulation of prostate cancer growth by androgens and estrogens through the intermediacy of sex hormone-binding globulin. *Endocrinology* 1996;137:4126–4129.
226. Kuiper GG, Enmark E, Pelto-Huikko M, et al. Cloning of a novel receptor expressed in rat prostate and ovary. *Proc Natl Acad Sci U S A* 1996;93:5925–5930.
227. Tremblay GB, Tremblay A, Copeland NG, et al. Cloning, chromosomal localization, and functional analysis of the murine estrogen receptor beta. *Mol Endocrinol* 1997;11: 353–365.
228. Ogawa S, Inoue S, Watanabe T, et al. Molecular cloning and characterization of human estrogen receptor betacx: a potential inhibitor of estrogen action in human. *Nucleic Acids Res* 1998;26:3505–3512.
229. Hanstein B, Liu H, Yancisin MC, et al. Functional analysis of a novel estrogen receptor-beta isoform. *Mol Endocrinol* 1999;13:129–137.
230. Cooke P, Young P, Hess R, et al. Estrogen receptor expression in developing epididymis, efferent ductules, and other male reproductive organs. *Endocrinology* 1991;128:2874–2879.
231. West NB, Roselli CE, Resko JA, et al. Estrogen and progestin receptors and aromatase activity in rhesus monkey prostate. *Endocrinology* 1988;123:2312–2322.
232. Tilley WD, Horsfall DJ, Skinner JM, et al. Effect of pubertal development on estrogen receptor levels and stromal morphology in the guinea pig prostate. *Prostate* 1989;15: 195–210.
233. Ricciardelli C, Horsfall DJ, Sykes J, et al. Effects of oestradiol-17 beta and 5 alpha-dihydrotestosterone on guinea-pig prostate smooth muscle cell proliferation and steroid receptor expression in vitro. *J Endocrinol* 1994;140:373–383.
234. Levine AC, Ren M, Huber GK, et al. The effect of androgen, estrogen, and growth factors on the proliferation of cultured fibroblasts derived from human fetal and adult prostates. *Endocrinology* 1992;130:2413–2419.
235. Tilley WD, Horsfall DJ, McGee MA, et al. Effects of ageing and hormonal manipulations on the level of oestrogen receptors in the guinea-pig prostate. *J Endocrinol* 1987;112: 139–144.
236. Prins GS, Marmer M, Woodham C, et al. Estrogen receptor-beta messenger ribonucleic acid ontogeny in the prostate of normal and neonatally estrogenized rats. *Endocrinology* 1998;139:874–883.
237. Saunders T, Maguire SM, Gaughan J, et al. Expression of oestrogen receptor beta (ER beta) in multiple rat tissues visualized by immunohistochemistry. *J Endocrinol* 1997; 154:R13–R16.
238. Couse JF, Lindzey J, Grandien K, et al. Tissue distribution and quantitative analysis of estrogen receptor-alpha (ERalpha) and estrogen receptor-beta (ERbeta) messenger ribonucleic acid in the wild-type and ERalpha-knockout mouse. *Endocrinology* 1997;138:4613–4621.
239. Kuiper GG, Shughrue J, Merchenthaler I, et al. The estrogen receptor beta subtype: a novel mediator of estrogen action in neuroendocrine systems. *Front Neuroendocrinol* 1998;19:253–286.
240. Taylor AH, Al-Azzawi F. Immunolocalisation of oestrogen receptor beta in human tissues. *J Mol Endocrinol* 2000; 24:145–155.
241. Suzuki K, Ito K, Suzuki T, Honma S, et al. Synergistic effects of estrogen and androgen on the prostate: effects of estrogen on androgen- and estrogen-receptors, BrdU uptake, immunohistochemical study of AR, and responses to antiandrogens. *Prostate* 1995;26:151–163.
242. Bodker A, Andersson KE, Batra S, et al. The estrogen receptor expression in the male rabbit urethra and prostate following castration. *Scand J Urol Nephrol* 1994;28:113–118.
243. Ehara H, Koji T, Deguchi T, et al. Expression of estrogen receptor in diseased human prostate assessed by non-radioactive in situ hybridization and immunohistochemistry. *Prostate* 1995;27:304–313.
244. Kirschenbaum A, Ren M, Erenburg I, et al. Estrogen receptor messenger RNA expression in human benign prostatic hyperplasia: detection, localization, and modulation with a long-acting gonadotropin-releasing hormone agonist. *J Androl* 1994;15:528–533.
245. Prins GS, Birch L. Neonatal estrogen exposure up-regulates estrogen receptor expression in the developing and adult rat prostate lobes. *Endocrinology* 1997;138:1801–1809.

246. Prins GS. Neonatal estrogen exposure induces lobe-specific alterations in adult rat prostate androgen receptor expression. *Endocrinology* 1992;130:3703–3714.
247. Prins GS, Woodham C, Lepinske M, et al. Effects of neonatal estrogen exposure on prostatic secretory genes and their correlation with androgen receptor expression in the separate prostate lobes of the adult rat. *Endocrinology* 1993; 132:2387–2398.
248. vom Saal F, Timms B, Montano M, et al. Prostate enlargement in mice due to fetal exposure to low doses of estradiol or diethylstilbestrol, and opposite effects at high doses. *Proc Natl Acad Sci U S A* 1997;94:2056–2061.
249. McLachlan J, Newbold R, Bullock B. Reproductive tract lesions in male mice exposed prenatally to diethylstilbestrol. *Science* 1975;190:991–992.
250. Pylkkanen L, Makela S, Valve, E, et al. Prostatic dysplasia associated with increased expression of C-MYC in neonatally estrogenized mice. *J Urol* 1993;149:1593–1601.
251. Turner T, Edery M, Mills KT, et al. Influence of neonatal diethylstilbestrol treatment on androgen and estrogen receptor levels in the mouse anterior prostate, ventral prostate and seminal vesicle. *J Steroid Biochem* 1989;32:559–564.
252. Prins GS, Birch L. The developmental pattern of androgen receptor expression in rat prostate lobes is altered after neonatal exposure to estrogen. *Endocrinology* 1995;136:1303–1314.
253. Chang WY, Wilson MJ, Birch L, et al. Neonatal estrogen stimulates proliferation of periductal fibroblasts and alters the extracellular matrix composition in the rat prostate. *Endocrinology* 1999;140:405–415.
254. Eddy EM, Washburn TF, Bunch DO, et al. Targeted disruption of the estrogen receptor gene in male mice causes alteration of spermatogenesis and infertility. *Endocrinology* 1996;137:4796–4805.
255. Krege JH, Hodgin JB, Couse JF, et al. Generation and reproductive phenotypes of mice lacking estrogen receptor beta. *Proc Natl Acad Sci U S A* 1998;95:15677–15682.
256. Coffey DS, Walsh C. Clinical and experimental studies of benign prostatic hyperplasia. *Urol Clin North Am* 1990;17:461–475.
257. Konishi N, Nakaoka S, Hiasa Y, et al. Immunohistochemical evaluation of estrogen receptor status in benign prostatic hypertrophy and in prostate carcinoma and the relationship to efficacy of endocrine therapy. *Oncology* 1993;50:259–263.
258. Emtage LA, Dunn J, Rowse AD. Androgen and oestrogen receptor status in benign and neoplastic prostate disease. Study of prevalence and influence on time to progression and survival in prostate cancer treated by hormone manipulation. *Br J Urol* 1989;63:627–633.
259. Seitz G, Wernert N. Immunohistochemical estrogen receptor demonstration in the prostate and prostate cancer. *Pathol Res Pract* 1987;182:792–796.
260. Kumar VL, Wadhwa SN, Kumar V, et al. Androgen, estrogen, and progesterone receptor contents and serum hormone profiles in patients with benign hypertrophy and carcinoma of the prostate. *J Surg Oncol* 1990;44:122–128.
261. Lau KM, LaSpina M, Long J, et al. Expression of estrogen receptor (ER)-alpha and ER-beta in normal and malignant prostatic epithelial cells: regulation by methylation and involvement in growth regulation. *Cancer Res* 2000;60: 3175–3182.
262. Li LC, Chui R, Nakajima K, et al. Frequent methylation of estrogen receptor in prostate cancer: correlation with tumor progression. *Cancer Res* 2000;60:702–706.
263. Castagnetta LA, Miceli MD, Sorci CM, et al. Growth of LNCaP human prostate cancer cells is stimulated by estradiol via its own receptor. *Endocrinology* 1995;136:2309–2319.
264. Carruba G, Pfeffer U, Fecarotta E, et al. Estradiol inhibits growth of hormone-nonresponsive PC3 human prostate cancer cells. *Cancer Res* 1994;54:1190–1193.
265. Robinson MR, Smith H, Richards B, et al. The final analysis of the EORTC Genito-Urinary Tract Cancer Co-Operative Group phase III clinical trial (protocol 30805) comparing orchidectomy, orchidectomy plus cyproterone acetate and low dose stilboestrol in the management of metastatic carcinoma of the prostate. *Eur Urol* 1995;28:273–283.
266. Glick JH, Wein A, Padavic K, et al. Phase II trial of tamoxifen in metastatic carcinoma of the prostate. *Cancer* 1982;49:1367–1372.
267. Spremulli E, DeSimone P, Durant J. A phase II study Nolvadex: tamoxifen citrate in the treatment of advanced prostatic adenocarcinoma. *Am J Clin Oncol* 1982;5:149–153.
268. DiPaola RS, Zhang H, Lambert GH, et al. Clinical and biologic activity of an estrogenic herbal combination (PC-SPES) in prostate cancer [see comments]. *N Engl J Med* 1998;339:785–791.
269. Small EJ, Frohlich MW, Bok R, et al. Prospective trial of the herbal supplement PC-SPES in patients with progressive prostate cancer. *J Clin Oncol* 2000;18:3595–3603.
270. Heikinheimo O, Mahony MC, Gordon K, et al. Estrogen and progesterone receptor mRNA are expressed in distinct pattern in male primate reproductive organs. *J Assist Reprod Genet* 1995;12:198–204.
271. Sirett DA, Grant JK. Effect of sodium molybdate on the interaction of androgens and progestins with binding proteins in human hyperplastic prostatic tissue. *J Endocrinol* 1982;92:95–102.
272. Akimoto S, Sato R, Kodama T, et al. Properties of progestin-binding protein in benign hypertrophic human prostate. *Endocrinol Jpn* 1986;33:423–432.
273. Mobbs BG, Johnson IE, Liu Y. Quantitation of cytosolic and nuclear estrogen and progesterone receptor in benign, untreated, and treated malignant human prostatic tissue by radioligand binding and enzyme-immunoassays. *Prostate* 1990;16:235–244.
274. Ekman P, Brolin J. Steroid receptor profile in human prostate cancer metastases as compared with primary prostatic carcinoma. *Prostate* 1991;18:147–153.
275. Pavone-Macaluso M, de Voogt HJ, Viggiano G, et al. Comparison of diethylstilbestrol, cyproterone acetate and medroxyprogesterone acetate in the treatment of advanced prostatic cancer: final analysis of a randomized phase III trial of the European Organization for Research on Treatment of Cancer Urological Group. *J Urol* 1986;136:624–631.
276. Davies P, Rushmere NK. Association of glucocorticoid receptors with prostate nuclear sites for androgen receptors and with androgen response elements. *J Mol Endocrinol* 1990;5:117–127.
277. Cleutjens C, Steketee K, Eekelen CC, et al. Both androgen receptor and glucocorticoid receptor are able to induce

prostate-specific antigen expression, but differ in their growth stimulating properties of LNCaP cells. *Endocrinology* 1997;138:5293–5300.

278. Smith RG, Syms AJ, Nag A, et al. Mechanism of the glucocorticoid regulation of growth of the androgen-sensitive prostate-derived R3327H-G8-A1 tumor cell line. *J Biol Chem* 1985;260:12454–12463.
279. Reyes-Moreno C, Frenette G, Boulanger J, et al. Mediation of glucocorticoid receptor function by transforming growth factor beta I expression in human PC-3 prostate cancer cells. *Prostate* 1995;26:260–269.
280. Sosnowski J, Stetter-Neel C, Cole D, et al. Protein kinase C mediated anti-proliferative glucocorticoid-sphinganine synergism in cultured Pollard III prostate tumor cells. *J Urol* 1997;158:269–274.
281. Koutsilieris M, Grondin F, Lehoux JG. The expression of mRNA for glucocorticoid receptor gene and functional glucocorticoid receptors detected in PA-III rat prostate adenocarcinoma cells. *Anticancer Res* 1992;12:899–904.
282. Tannock I, Osoba D, Stockler M, et al. Chemotherapy with mitoxantrone plus prednisone or prednisone alone for symptomatic hormone-resistant prostate cancer: a Canadian randomized trial with palliative end points. *J Clin Oncology* 1996;14:1756–1764.
283. Kantoff W, Halabi S, Conaway M, et al. Hydrocortisone with or without mitoxantrone in men with hormone-refractory prostate cancer: results of the cancer and leukemia group B 9182 study [see comments]. *J Clin Oncol* 1999;17:2506–2513.
284. Koutsilieris M, Reyes-Moreno C, Sourla A, et al. Growth factors mediate glucocorticoid receptor function and dexamethasone-induced regression of osteoblastic lesions in hormone refractory prostate cancer. *Anticancer Res* 1997;17:1461–1465.
285. Peehl DM, Skowronski RJ, Leung GK, et al. Antiproliferative effects of 1,25-dihydroxyvitamin D3 on primary cultures of human prostatic cells. *Cancer Res* 1994;54:805–810.
286. Miller GJ, Stapleton GE, Hedlund TE, et al. Vitamin D receptor expression, 24-hydroxylase activity, and inhibition of growth by 1 alpha,25-dihydroxyvitamin D3 in seven human prostatic carcinoma cell lines. *Clin Cancer Res* 1995;1:997–1003.
287. Hedlund TE, Moffatt KA, Miller GJ. Vitamin D receptor expression is required for growth modulation by 1 alpha,25-dihydroxyvitamin D3 in the human prostatic carcinoma cell line ALVA-31. *J Steroid Biochem Mol Biol* 1996;58:277–288.
288. Chan JM, Giovannucci E, Andersson SO, et al. Dairy products, calcium, phosphorous, vitamin D, and risk of prostate cancer (Sweden). *Cancer Causes Control* 1998;9:559–566.
289. Giovannucci E. Dietary influences of 1,25(OH)2 vitamin D in relation to prostate cancer: a hypothesis. *Cancer Causes Control* 1998;9:567–582.
290. Ingles SA, Ross RK, Yu MC, et al. Association of prostate cancer risk with genetic polymorphisms in vitamin D receptor and androgen receptor [see comments]. *J Natl Cancer Inst* 1997;89:166–170.
291. Xue L, Lipkin M, Newmark H, et al. Influence of dietary calcium and vitamin D on diet-induced epithelial cell hyperproliferation in mice. *J Natl Cancer Inst* 1999;91:176–181.
292. Nomura AM, Stemmermann GN, Lee J, et al. Serum vitamin D metabolite levels and the subsequent development of prostate cancer (Hawaii, United States). *Cancer Causes Control* 1998;9:425–432.
293. Kibel AS, Isaacs SD, Isaacs WB, et al. Vitamin D receptor polymorphisms and lethal prostate cancer. *J Urol* 1998; 160:1405–1409.
294. Ma J, Stampfer MJ, Gann H, et al. Vitamin D receptor polymorphisms, circulating vitamin D metabolites, and risk of prostate cancer in United States physicians. *Cancer Epidemiol Biomarkers Prev* 1998;7:385–390.
295. Ingles SA, Coetzee GA, Ross RK, et al. Association of prostate cancer with vitamin D receptor haplotypes in African-Americans. *Cancer Res* 1998;58:1620–1623.
296. Gross C, Musiol IM, Eccleshall TR, et al. Vitamin D receptor gene polymorphisms: analysis of ligand binding and hormone responsiveness in cultured skin fibroblasts. *Biochem Biophys Res Commun* 1998;242:467–473.
297. Giovannucci E, Rimm EB, Wolk A, et al. Calcium and fructose intake in relation to risk of prostate cancer. *Cancer Res* 1998;58:442–447.
298. Giles G, Ireland P. Diet, nutrition and prostate cancer. *Int J Cancer* 1997;[suppl 10]:13-17.
299. Taylor JA, Hirvonen A, Watson M, et al. Association of prostate cancer with vitamin D receptor gene polymorphism. *Cancer Res* 1996;56:4108–4110.
300. Gann H, Ma J, Hennekens CH, et al. Circulating vitamin D metabolites in relation to subsequent development of prostate cancer. *Cancer Epidemiol Biomarkers Prev* 1996;5:121–126.
301. Braun MM, Helzlsouer KJ, Hollis BW, et al. Prostate cancer and prediagnostic levels of serum vitamin D metabolites (Maryland, United States). *Cancer Causes Control* 1995;6:235–239.
302. Feldman D, Skowronski RJ, Peehl DM. Vitamin D and prostate cancer. *Adv Exp Med Biol* 1995;375:53–63.
303. Kivineva M, Blauer M, Syvala H, et al. Localization of 1,25-dihydroxyvitamin D3 receptor (VDR) expression in human prostate. *J Steroid Biochem Mol Biol* 1998;66:121–127.
304. Hsieh TY, Ng CY, Mallouh C, et al. Regulation of growth, PSA/PAP and androgen receptor expression by 1 alpha,25-dihydroxyvitamin D3 in the androgen-dependent LNCaP cells. *Biochem Biophys Res Commun* 1996;223:141–146.
305. Hedlund TE, Moffatt KA, Uskokovic MR, et al. Three synthetic vitamin D analogues induce prostate-specific acid phosphatase and prostate-specific antigen while inhibiting the growth of human prostate cancer cells in a vitamin D receptor-dependent fashion. *Clin Cancer Res* 1997;3:1331–1338.
306. Zhuang, SH, Burnstein KL. Antiproliferative effect of 1alpha,25-dihydroxyvitamin D3 in human prostate cancer cell line LNCaP involves reduction of cyclin-dependent kinase 2 activity and persistent G1 accumulation. *Endocrinology* 1998;139:1197–1207.
307. Ly LH, Zhao XY, Holloway L, et al. Liarozole acts synergistically with 1alpha,25-dihydroxyvitamin D3 to inhibit growth of DU 145 human prostate cancer cells by blocking 24-hydroxylase activity. *Endocrinology* 1999;140:2071–2076.
308. Zhuang SH, Schwartz GG, Cameron D, et al. Vitamin D receptor content and transcriptional activity do not fully predict antiproliferative effects of vitamin D in human prostate cancer cell lines. *Mol Cell Endocrinol* 1997;126:83–90.
309. Hsieh T, Wu JM. Induction of apoptosis and altered nuclear/cytoplasmic distribution of the androgen receptor and prostate-specific antigen by 1alpha,25-dihydroxyvita-

min D3 in androgen-responsive LNCaP cells. *Biochem Biophys Res Commun* 1997;235:539–544.
310. Zhao XY, Ly LH, Peehl DM, et al. Induction of androgen receptor by 1alpha,25-dihydroxyvitamin D3 and 9-cis retinoic acid in LNCaP human prostate cancer cells. *Endocrinology* 1999;140:1205–1212.
311. Aboseif SR, Dahiya R, Narayan P, et al. Effect of retinoic acid on prostatic development. *Prostate* 1997;31:161–167.
312. Pasquali D, Thaller C, Eichele G. Abnormal level of retinoic acid in prostate cancer tissues. *J Clin Endocrinol Metab* 1996;81:2186–2191.
313. Dahiya R, Park HD, Cusick J, et al. Inhibition of tumorigenic potential and prostate-specific antigen expression in LNCaP human prostate cancer cell line by 13-cis-retinoic acid. *Int J Cancer* 1994;59:126–132.
314. Danielpour D, Kadomatsu K, Anzano MA, et al. Development and characterization of nontumorigenic and tumorigenic epithelial cell lines from rat dorsal-lateral prostate. *Cancer Res* 1994;54:3413–3421.
315. Lu XP, Fanjul A, Picard N, et al. A selective retinoid with high activity against an androgen-resistant prostate cancer cell type. *Int J Cancer* 1999;80:272–278.
316. Sun SY, Yue P, Lotan R. Induction of apoptosis by N-(4-hydroxyphenyl)retinamide and its association with reactive oxygen species, nuclear retinoic acid receptors, and apoptosis-related genes in human prostate carcinoma cells. *Mol Pharmacol* 1999;55:403–410.
317. Esquenet M, Swinnen JV, Heyns W, et al. LNCaP prostatic adenocarcinoma cells derived from low and high passage numbers display divergent responses not only to androgens but also to retinoids. *J Steroid Biochem Mol Biol* 1997;62: 391–399.
318. Campbell MJ, Park S, Uskokovic MR, et al. Expression of retinoic acid receptor-beta sensitizes prostate cancer cells to growth inhibition mediated by combinations of retinoids and a 19-nor hexafluoride vitamin D3 analog. *Endocrinology* 1998;139:1972–1980.
319. Young CY, Murtha E, Andrews E, et al. Antagonism of androgen action in prostate tumor cells by retinoic acid. *Prostate* 1994;25:39–45.
320. Gao M, Ossowski L, Ferrari AC. Activation of Rb and decline in androgen receptor protein precede retinoic acid-induced apoptosis in androgen-dependent LNCaP cells and their androgen-independent derivative. *J Cell Physiol* 1999;179:336–346.
321. de Vos S, Dawson MI, Holden S, et al. Effects of retinoid X receptor-selective ligands on proliferation of prostate cancer cells. *Prostate* 1997;32:115–121.
322. Liang JY, Fontana JA, Rao JN, et al. Synthetic retinoid CD437 induces S-phase arrest and apoptosis in human prostate cancer cells LNCaP and PC-3. *Prostate* 1999; 38:228–236.
323. Trump DL, Smith DC, Stiff D, et al. A phase II trial of all-trans-retinoic acid in hormone-refractory prostate cancer: a clinical trial with detailed pharmacokinetic analysis. *Cancer Chemother Pharmacol* 1997;39:349–356.
324. Issemann I, Green S. Activation of a member of the steroid hormone receptor superfamily by peroxisome proliferators. *Nature* 1990;347:645–650.
325. Forman B. Orphan nuclear receptors and their ligands. In: Freedman L, ed. *Molecular biology of steroid and nuclear hormone receptors.* Boston: Birkhauser, 1998;281–305.
326. Pineau T, Hudgins WR, Liu L, et al. Activation of a human peroxisome proliferator-activated receptor by the antitumor agent phenylacetate and its analogs. *Biochem Pharmacol* 1996;52:659–667.
327. Tontonoz P, Hu E, Spiedelman B. Stimulation of adipogenesis in fibroblasts by PPAR gamma 2, a lipid-activated transcription factor. *Cell* 1994;79:1147–1156.
328. Kliewer SA, Lenhard JM, Willson TM, et al. A prostaglandin J2 metabolite binds peroxisome proliferator-activated receptor gamma and promotes adipocyte differentiation. *Cell* 1995;83:813–819.
329. Demetri GD, Fletcher CD, Mueller E, et al. Induction of solid tumor differentiation by the peroxisome proliferator-activated receptor-gamma ligand troglitazone in patients with liposarcoma. *Proc Natl Acad Sci U S A* 1999;96:3951–3956.
330. Tontonoz P, Singer S, Forman BM, et al. Terminal differentiation of human liposarcoma cells induced by ligands for peroxisome proliferator-activated receptor gamma and the retinoid X receptor. *Proc Natl Acad Sci U S A* 1997;94:237–241.
331. Kubota T, Koshizuka K, Williamson EA, et al. Ligand for peroxisome proliferator-activated receptor gamma (troglitazone) has potent antitumor effect against human prostate cancer both in vitro and in vivo. *Cancer Res* 1998;58:3344–3352.
332. Mueller E, Smith M, Sarraf P, et al. Effects of ligand activation of peroxisome proliferator-activated receptor gamma in human prostate cancer. *Proc Natl Acad Sci U S A* 2000;97: 10990–10995.
333. Pereira FA, Qiu Y, Tsai MJ, et al. Chicken ovalbumin upstream promoter transcription factor (COUP-TF): expression during mouse embryogenesis. *J Steroid Biochem Mol Biol* 1995;53:503–508.
334. Lin DL, Wu SQ, Chang C. The genomic structure and chromosomal location of the human TR2 orphan receptor, a member of the steroid receptor superfamily. *Endocrine* 1998;8:123–134.
335. Chang C, Da Silva SL, Ideta R, et al. Human and rat TR4 orphan receptors specify a subclass of the steroid receptor superfamily. *Proc Natl Acad Sci U S A* 1994;91:6040–6044.
336. Uemura H, Chang C. Antisense TR3 orphan receptor can increase prostate cancer cell viability with etoposide treatment. *Endocrinology* 1998;139:2329–2334.
337. Kokontis J, Liao S, Chang C. Transcriptional activation by TR3 receptor, a member of the steroid receptor superfamily. *Receptor* 1991;1:261–270.
338. Huggins C. Endocrine-induced regression of cancers. *Science* 1967;156:1050–1054.
339. Crawford E, Eisenberger M, McLeod D, et al. A controlled trial of leuprolide with and without flutamide in prostatic carcinoma. *N Engl J Med* 1989;321:419–424.

4

SOMATIC GENETICS OF PROSTATE CANCER: ONCOGENES AND TUMOR SUPPRESSORS

WILLIAM R. SELLERS
CHARLES L. SAWYERS

Recently, there has been a shift from the empiric development of therapeutic agents to the development of small molecule inhibitors of specific cellular proteins or "targets." This new approach is predicated on the notion that the certain molecular alterations found in cancer cells will render these cells exquisitely sensitive (more so than normal cells) to treatment with drugs designed to exploit these molecular changes. One rate-limiting step, to what is hopefully the ultimate success of this strategy, is to define each cancer on the basis of the accumulated genetic and molecular changes. This information, coupled with a functional understanding of the consequence of such changes, is required to select appropriate drug targets.

Progress in obtaining a molecular or genetic definition of prostate cancer has been hampered by the heterogeneity of prostate tumors, by the difficulty in obtaining high-quality clinical samples, and by the paucity of mutations in common oncogenes and tumor suppressors examined to date. The sequencing of the human genome, the application of genome-wide analytical approaches to the classification of prostate tumors, the development of tissue microarrays, the use of laser capture microdissection, and other developing technologies promise to allow us to overcome these barriers and to dramatically expand the existing prostate somatic-genetic database.

Here, it is important to realize that, like leukemia, prostate cancer seems to represent a diverse set of tumor types. It is likely that specific subtypes of prostate cancer, as yet undefined, will have a characteristic set of genetic lesions. For example, leukemias can often be subtyped based on the presence of specific chromosomal translocations. In this view, it may be unreasonable to expect that mutations in specific genes will be present in all or even a majority of prostate tumors. Rather, we will need to understand each prostate cancer subtype and how specific molecular defects influence prognosis with respect to the requirement for local therapy, with respect to the progression to hormone-insensitive disease, and with respect to the tailoring of novel therapeutic interventions toward specific subsets. This latter concept is best illustrated by the expanding, targeted molecular-based pharmacopoeia, which includes tamoxifen [estrogen receptor (ER) alpha]; trastuzumab [Herceptin (Her2/neu)]; all-*trans*-retinoic acid (retinoic acid receptor–APML fusion); the STI571 kinase inhibitor (BCR-ABL fusion); and, most notably, in prostate cancer, flutamide and casodex (androgen receptor). In each case, except for the androgen receptor, the presence of a particular molecular lesion is associated with the response to a specific drug. Thus, the molecular marker becomes a "predictive factor"—that is, a factor that guides and is predictive of response to particular therapies.

Another corollary of this viewpoint is that there may not be a single pathway of progression that applies to all prostate tumors. Furthermore, in our opinion, there is insufficient data in the published literature to accurately describe a sequence of events likely to be ascribed to the initiation and progression of prostate cancer. On the other hand, the function of the protein products of many oncogenes and tumor suppressor genes is now understood in great detail. More importantly, such proteins typically function within specific pathways regulating cell survival, cell proliferation, cell motility and adhesion, and genetic stability. Therefore, in trying to put genetic lesions into context, especially with a view toward the selection of drug targets, it seems reasonable to discuss genetic lesions within a given gene in the larger context of the pathway altered by such lesions. Based on these considerations, and in a departure from many previous discussions of this subject, in this chapter, the somatic-genetic alterations found in prostate cancer are presented in a pathway-specific organization. For each section, a brief description of the pathway is followed by a summary of the genetic lesions found in each pathway in prostate cancer. This *pathway* view of somatic genetics is an appropriate format for understanding how a tumor can achieve the same biologic end point through different genetic alterations, and for understanding how therapeutic interventions directed at specific pathways might, or might not, be efficacious in the setting of specific mutations.

ALTERATIONS IN SIGNALING PATHWAYS IN PROSTATE CANCER

To begin, we explore the alterations found in the major growth regulatory pathways, implicated in common epithelial cancers: the epidermal growth factor receptor (EGFR)–mitogen-activated protein kinase cascade, the insulinlike growth factor (IGF)–phosphoinositide 3-kinase (PI3K) pathway, the transforming growth factor beta (TGF-beta) cascade, and the Wnt/β-catenin pathway. In each of these pathways, extracellular soluble ligands bind to transmembrane receptors and trigger a signaling cascade that ultimately results, at least in part, in changes in nuclear transcription factor activity. There can be many cross-pathway connections in which one pathway can influence or activate another. However, for the sake of simplicity, these complexities largely are ignored.

Epidermal Growth Factor Receptor and Her2-Ras–Mitogen-Activated Protein Kinase Pathways

The Pathway

Work from numerous laboratories focused on signal transduction in normal and malignant cells has established the central importance of a signaling pathway connecting the receptor tyrosine kinases on the cell surface to the Ras G protein and its downstream effector kinases Raf, MEK, and Erk. Briefly, when a receptor tyrosine kinase such as EGFR or Her2/neu is activated by ligand, the cytoplasmic domain is capable of recruiting a complex of proteins that ultimately leads to the generation of activated Ras. Ras proteins are small enzymes that hydrolyze guanine nucleotide triphosphate (GTPases) and act as signaling intermediaries that couple the activation of the growth factor receptors to downstream signals. Specifically, when Ras is bound to GTP it is "on," and this form of Ras, in turn, activates a cascade of kinases from Raf to MEK to MAPK (the so-called Map kinase pathway). Ras then hydrolyzes the GTP back to guanine nucleotide diphosphate, and the signal is turned off (Fig. 4-1).

Abnormalities in this pathway are present in multiple cancer types and can occur at multiple levels in the pathway, from the receptor, to Ras itself, to downstream effector molecules. For example, activation can occur through amplification of the genes encoding the receptors or through oncogenic point mutations in Ras proteins. Such mutations render Ras constitutively active by keeping it in the GTP-bound state. Most research using clinical prostate cancer material has focused on identifying mutations in the receptor tyrosine kinases, or in the Ras protein; therefore, we review only these members of the pathway. It is formally possible, however, that mutation at any point in the pathway can lead to constitutive activation of Ras signaling.

Epidermal Growth Factor Receptor and Her2 Receptor Tyrosine Kinases

Her2/neu, a member of the EGF family of receptor tyrosine kinases, is best known for its role in breast cancer. Her2/neu

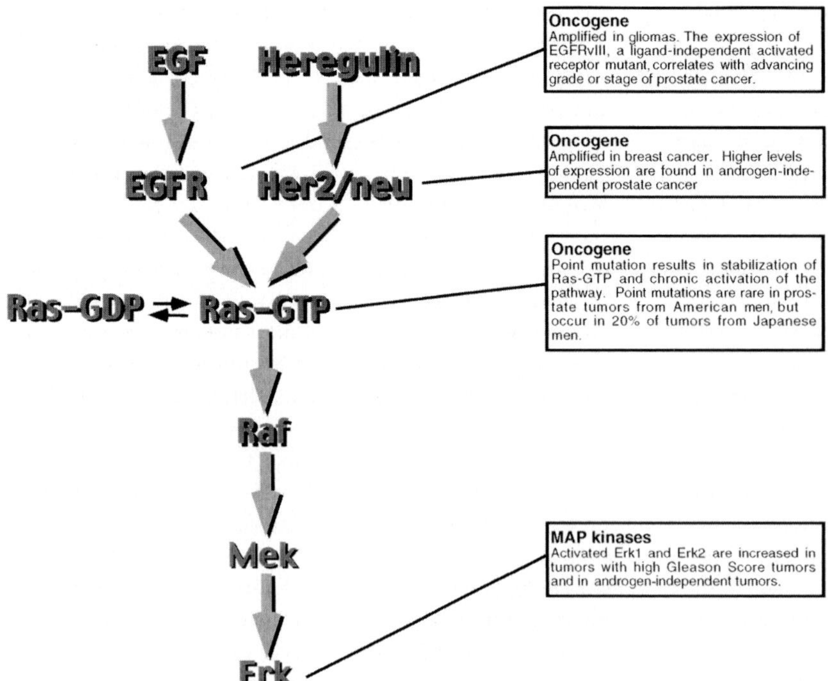

FIGURE 4-1. The Her2/neu and epidermal growth factor receptor (EGFR) signaling pathway. Secreted ligands such as EGF or heregulin bind to and activate their respective transmembrane receptors (EGFR) and Her2/neu. Activation of the receptor triggers the conversion of Ras from the inactive guanosine nucleotide diphosphate (GDP)–bound state to the active guanine nucleotide triphosphate (GTP)–bound state. In the active state, Ras triggers the activation of the mitogen-activated protein (MAP) kinase cascade, inducing Raf activation, which in turn activates MEK and then Erk kinases. Note: Recent studies indicate that Her2/neu functions primarily as a co-receptor and binds ligand only in the context of heterodimer formation with another kinase family member, such as Her1 or Her3.

is amplified, and overexpressed, in 20% to 30% of human breast and ovarian cancers, and patients whose breast tumors express high levels of Her2/neu protein have a poorer prognosis (1,2). In rodent fibroblast cells, Her2/neu functions as a classic receptor tyrosine kinase oncogene (3,4), and in murine transgenic models, mammary-specific overexpression of Her2/neu is sufficient to induce breast cancer (5,6). At the biochemical level, Her2/neu appears to function primarily by activating the Ras and MAP kinase pathways (7,8).

A number of groups have examined Her2/neu expression in prostate cancer and have reported conflicting results about the frequency of overexpression. Her2/neu is clearly normally expressed in prostate epithelial cells, particularly in the basal cell compartment (9,10). The putative ligand (neu differentiation factor or heregulin) is expressed in the stroma of the normal prostate gland (11) and is thought to play a role in the differentiation of secretory epithelial cells. Unlike breast cancer, most studies report that Her2 gene amplification does not occur in prostate cancer (12–15), although there are some exceptions (16,17). Rather, it appears that Her2 protein is overexpressed in the absence of gene amplification in a fraction of early-stage prostate cancers. The protein levels tend to be lower than those found in Her2 amplified, Herceptin-responsive (also called *3+ Her2-positive*) breast cancers. Recently, three groups have performed studies of metastatic and androgen-independent prostate cancers and have found that up to two-thirds of cases express elevated levels of Her2 protein (18) (R. Cote, C. Cardon-Cardo, *personal communication*, 2000). These results are consistent with the notion that Her2/neu protein levels increase as prostate cancers progress to advanced hormone-refractory states, but the mechanism for this increase is clearly distinct from the genomic alteration mechanism found in breast cancers and remains to be elucidated.

A growing body of literature suggests that activation of the EGFR/Her2-signaling pathway can also occur through aberrant expression of other receptors in the family, such as EGFR, and through overproduction of the ligands that activate the receptors (19,20). For example, TGF-alpha ligand and EGFR are frequently coexpressed in androgen-independent prostate cancers, raising the possibility of an autocrine loop causing pathway activation (20). Most compelling, however, is a recent report showing expression of a variant EGFRvIII receptor in a large fraction of advanced prostate cancers (19). EGFRvIII is a mutant allele, originally described in human gliomas, that lacks much of the extracellular domain (due to deletion of exons 2 to 7) and, as a result, has ligand-independent activity (21–23).

What advantage do prostate cancer cells gain from activation of the EGFR/Her2-Ras–MAP kinase pathway? One exciting possibility is based on experimental evidence demonstrating cross-talk between Her2/neu and androgen receptor (AR) signaling. Overexpression of Her2/neu in xenograft models is sufficient to activate the AR in the absence of ligand and superactivate the AR in the presence of low levels of androgen, as might be seen in men treated by medical castration with luteinizing hormone–releasing hormone agonists. Therefore, activation of the EGFR/Her2-Ras–MAP kinase pathway could rescue prostate cancer cells from the growth arrest imposed by hormone ablation therapy. Compelling evidence for this hypothesis comes from the demonstration that overexpression of Her2/neu is sufficient to convert androgen-dependent cells to androgen-independent growth (24). The mechanism for cross-talk between Her2 and AR remains to be defined, but recent work in the estrogen receptor field indicates that hormone receptors and their coactivators, such as SRC-1 or AIB-1, are targets of regulatory phosphorylation by serine and threonine kinases, such as Erk, which function downstream of Her2/neu and EGFR (25–28). Indeed, constitutive Erk activation in clinical androgen-independent prostate cancers has been reported by one group who compared signaling pathway activation in patient specimens obtained at the time of diagnosis versus progression to the hormone refractory phase (29).

Observations of EGFR/Her2 pathway abnormalities in prostate cancer raise the possibility that novel agents directed against this pathway may have utility in prostate cancer. Recent success in developing monoclonal antibodies or small molecule inhibitors targeted against EGFR or HER2/neu has already led to a series of newly initiated clinical trials that will test this concept in patients. One prediction from the AR cross-talk studies is that EGFR/Her2 pathway inhibition may convert androgen-independent prostate cancer back to a hormone-sensitive state.

Ras Mutations in Prostate Cancer

The H-ras of the ras family of genes was the first described human oncogene (30), and the introduction of Ras into a number of rodent cells results in cellular transformation (31,32). Three genes are included in this family, K-, N-, and H-ras. As mentioned earlier, Ras proteins are activated by oncogenic point mutations. Typically, these mutations are found in codons 12, 13, and 61. These mutations are common in a number of cancers, including those of the lung, pancreas, and colon. Rare activating mutations of ras in prostate cancer were first described in 1987 (33), and as detailed in Table 4-1, Ras mutations have been examined in primary prostate tumors by a number of groups. Here, results obtained by multiple investigators are quite consistent and demonstrate infrequent detection (0% to 5%) of ras mutations in primary prostate cancer samples isolated from American men. On the other hand, the rate of Ras mutations is significantly higher in prostate cancer samples isolated from Japanese men (13% to 27%). These data indicate that there may be a considerable difference in both the etiology and progression of tumors from different ethnic backgrounds. In addition, there might be a considerable difference in remaining genetic lesions detectable in tumors from American versus Japanese men.

TABLE 4-1. RAS MUTATIONS

Author	Ras genes examined	Codons examined	Mutations	Tumor type	Ethnicity
Carter (216)	H, N, and K	12, 13, 61	1/24 (4%)	P	American[a]
Anwar (217)	H, N, and K	12, 61	16/68 (24%)	Mixed[b]	Japanese
Gumerlock (218)	H, N, and K	12, 13, 61[c]	1/19 (5%)	Mixed	American[a]
Konishi (219)	H and K	12 (H,K),13(K)	6/22 (27%)	Latent[d]	Japanese
Konishi (220)	H, N, and K	12, 13, 61	9/70 (13%)	P	Japanese
			1/31 (3%)	P	American
Moul (221)	H, N and K	12, 13, 61	0/24	P	American
Moyret-Lalle (222)	H, N and K	Exons 1, 2	0/22[e]	P	European[a]
Shiraishi (223)	H, N and K	12, 13, 61	20/81 (24%)	P	Japanese

P, primary.
[a]Ethnicity not defined.
[b]Included latent, primary, and metastatic tumors.
[c]Not codon 13 of H-Ras or K-Ras.
[d]Autopsy cancers.
[e]Analyzed 27 tumors; however, 5 tumors found to have no tumor cells.

Insulinlike Growth Factor, Phosphoinositide 3-Kinase, and Phosphatase and Tensin Homologue Pathway

The Pathway

This signaling pathway begins with the binding of IGF-I to the IGF-I receptor (IGF-IR) (Fig. 4-2). Ligand binding results in receptor activation and recruitment of the PI3K complex to the plasma membrane. Next, PI3K phosphorylates a specific type of lipid found in the plasma membrane, generating a lipid product known as *phosphoinositide-3,4,5-trisphosphate* or, for short, PI-3,4,5-P3 [reviewed in (34)]. This lipid, normally absent in quiescent cells, is induced on growth factor stimulation. When present, this lipid serves to recruit and activate a second kinase, known as Akt. There are three Akt kinases (Akt-1, -2, and -3). Akt, in turn, phosphorylates a number of downstream targets, and in so doing is sufficient to block apoptosis and can promote cell proliferation [reviewed in (35)]. In addition, activation of this pathway has been linked to regulation of cell adhesion and cell motility.

The protein product of the *PTEN* tumor suppressor gene (designated as PTEN hereafter) is an enzyme that can remove phosphate moieties from other macromolecules (a phosphatase). PTEN is unique in that it specifically dephosphorylates the phosphorylated lipids (PI-3,4,5-P3) produced by PI3K (36) and dampens or blocks activation of this pathway (37–43). Tumor cells lacking PTEN protein contain elevated levels of the lipid PI-3,4,5-P3 and

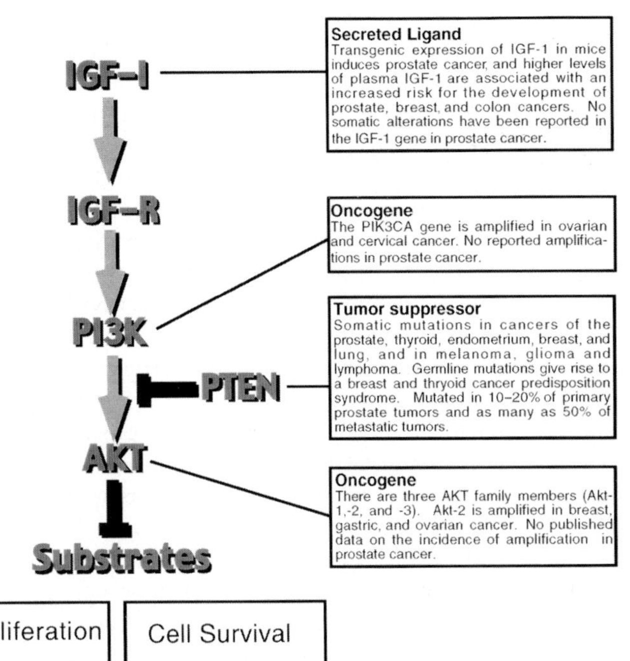

FIGURE 4-2. The insulinlike growth factor (IGF), phosphoinsotide-3 kinase, and PTEN pathway. Secreted ligands such as IGF-1 bind to and activate their transmembrane receptors (IGF-R). Receptor activation results in the recruitment of phosphoinositide 3-kinase (PI3K) to the receptor. Here, PI3K can phosphorylate membrane lipids that serve to recruit and activate kinases such as Akt. Akt activation results in the phosphorylation of a number of downstream target substrates. These substrates are typically, though not always, inactivated by Akt phosphorylation. Substrates of Akt are involved in the regulation of both cell proliferation and cell death.

consequently have constitutively activated Akt and constitutive phosphorylation of downstream Akt targets (37,41–45). In this manner, loss of PTEN leads to increased proliferation and decreased apoptosis.

Insulinlike Growth Factor I Plasma Levels Are Associated with an Increased Risk of Prostate Cancer

A number of studies have shown that increasing levels of plasma IGF-I are associated with the diagnosis of prostate cancer. For example, in case-control studies, increased IGF-I levels were found to be associated with an increased risk of having prostate cancer (46,47). Furthermore, in the prospective Physicians' Health Study, IGF-I was also a strong risk factor for the development of prostate cancer. Here, men in the highest quartile of plasma IGF-I levels (drawn on entry into the study) were found to have a relative risk of prostate cancer of 4.3 when compared to men in the lowest quartile. Furthermore, in this study, there was a linear relationship with increasing IGF-I levels and prostate cancer risk (48). In addition, such men have an elevated risk of death from prostate cancer, suggesting that IGF-I specifically contributes to the development of lethal tumors (E. Giovannucci, *personal communication*, 2000). Recent data have demonstrated an association between IGF-I plasma levels and the development of breast cancer in premenopausal women and of colorectal carcinoma in women [reviewed in (49)].

In keeping with the idea that IGF-I contributes to the development of cancer, transgenic mice that express IGF-I in prostate epithelial cells are prone to develop prostate cancer (50). To date, there have been no reported genetic lesions in prostate tumors that would result in elevated tumor secretion by IGF-I, nor has amplification of the gene been reported.

Insulinlike Growth Factor I Receptor and Prostate Cancer

As elevated levels of IGF-I increase prostate cancer risk, it would be reasonable to think that overexpression, or constitutive activation, of the IGF-I receptor could contribute to tumor induction or progression. To date, however, there is little evidence for direct overexpression, or amplification, of the IGF-IR receptor in prostate cancers. Rather, it would appear that as tumors progress, the level of the IGF-IR receptor declines (51). How can we reconcile the seemingly paradoxical results that higher levels of plasma IGF-I, but lower levels of IGF-IR, are found in association with prostate cancer? First, down-regulation of IGF-IR could occur as a result of excessive stimulation of the receptor. Specifically, receptor activation results in internalization of the receptor, and thus overactivation in fact might result in lower IGF-IR protein levels. Second, there is emerging data that the signaling "dose" that is required for tumor progression might be quite narrow and that overstimulation could, in fact, trigger cell death rather than proliferation (52) (T. Roberts, *personal communication*, 2000). There is, in fact, experimental evidence supporting this duality. For example, in murine fibroblasts, transformation by simian virus (SV)40 large-T antigen requires an intact IGF-I receptor (53). Conversely, human prostate epithelial cells transformed by SV40 large-T antigen, down-regulate IGF-R and undergo apoptosis when IGF-R is reexpressed in these cells (54–56). As described earlier, the protein product of the PTEN tumor suppressor gene is a negative regulator of PI3K signaling. Thus, it is possible, once a tumor has lost PTEN and as a result acquires constitutive activation of PI3K signaling, that IGF-R receptor activation is not required, or indeed might induce cell death. Therefore, an important area of future investigation will be to determine the state of the IGF-R receptor (activated or not) in PTEN-plus and PTEN-null tumors, and in early versus late tumors.

PTEN Loss in Prostate Cancer

The *PTEN* tumor suppressor gene, also known as MMAC1 or TEP1, localizes to the 10q23 chromosomal band (57–59). Germline mutations of PTEN give rise to a hereditary cancer predisposition syndrome, known as *Cowden disease*, in which affected individuals are predisposed to develop breast and thyroid cancers (60,61). The 10q23 region is often altered in primary prostate cancer and, more frequently, in metastatic prostate tumors. In these settings, between 20% and 60% of tumors exhibit loss of heterozygosity (LOH) in this region (62–68). Intragenic markers have demonstrated that PTEN is contained within the region most commonly targeted for loss, although there is occasional loss of 10q that excludes PTEN. Mutations and inactivation of the second allele of PTEN have been demonstrated in xenografts and in prostate tumor tissue (Table 4-2). In keeping with the results of LOH analysis at 10q23, PTEN deletion or mutation is also more frequent in higher-grade tumors and in metastatic foci (64,69). Study of the PTEN protein by immunohistochemistry (IHC) has revealed that 20% of primary tumors have lost PTEN protein staining. In keeping with the mutation data, loss of PTEN staining is associated with higher-grade and higher-stage tumors (70). Thus, loss of PTEN appears to be associated with the development of particularly aggressive tumors.

It is of interest to note that the rate of LOH at 10q23 in prostate cancer samples is considerably higher than the frequency at which one can convincingly demonstrate inactivation of the retained PTEN allele. This is similar to, although not as profound as, the data in breast cancer where 10q23 LOH is found in 40% of invasive tumors, whereas mutation of the second PTEN allele is rarely seen

TABLE 4-2. PTEN ALTERATIONS

Author	Loss of heterozygosity (LOH)	Mutation	Deletion	mRNA	Immunohistochemical (IHC) (neg)	No. of tumors	Source
Orikasa (224)	2/18 (11%)	0/18 (0%)	—	—	—	45	P
Gray (225)	24/37 (64%)	5/37[a] (14%)	—	—	—	37	P
Dong (226)	7/40[b]	1/40 (2.5%)	—	—	—	40	P[b]
Pesche (227)	12/22 (55%)[c]	1/10 (10%)	—	—	—	22	P
Vlietstra (228)[d]	—	3/11 (27%)	4/11 (36%)	—	—	11	X
Whang (76)	—	0/10 (0%)	1/10 (10%)	5/10[e]	—	10	X
Feilotter (229)	30/51 (58%)	1/51 (2%)	—	—	—	51	P[f]
Wang (230), Giri (231)	10/60 (17%)	0/2 (0%)	8/60 (13%)	—	—	60	P[f]
Teng (232)	10/24 (42%)	0/6 (0%)	—	—	—	24	P
McMenamin (70)	—	—	—	—	22 (20%)[g]	109	P
Suzuki (69)	10/18 (55%)	4/18 (22%)	2/18 (11%)	—	—	19 (50)[h]	M
Cairns (233)	23/80[i] (28%)	4/23 (17%)	6/23 (26%)	—	—	80	P, LN[j]

LN, lymph node; M, metastatic sites; mRNA, messenger RNA; P, primary; X, xenograft.
[a]Four of five mutations were identified in primary tumors associated with metastases.
[b]No markers within PTEN had loss. Tumors were typically low grade.
[c]Six of 12 had LOH of intragenic markers.
[d]Xenografts, no normal tissue available for LOH analysis.
[e]Four of ten xenografts with no mRNA, and one of ten with reduced mRNA.
[f]Primary tumors with no associated LN mets.
[g]Correlated with advanced Gleason score and advanced T stage.
[h]Fifty tumor samples from 19 different patients.
[i]Three tumors had LOH excluding PTEN.
[j]Seven of ten tumors with either deletions or mutations were nodal metastasis.

(2% to 3%) (71–73). Lack of somatic PTEN mutation is particularly puzzling, as germline mutation of PTEN is associated with an inherited predisposition to breast cancer (Cowden disease), and PTEN+/– mice develop breast cancer (74). The "two-hit" model for tumor suppressor genes argues that tumor suppressor genes are typically inactivated at two loci and, experimentally, this appears to often equate with mutations of both copies of the same gene (75). How then can we explain the discordance between the rate of LOH and the rate of PTEN mutations in prostate and breast cancers, as well as in other tumors? First, it is likely that the rate of detection of inactivating mutations understates the actual rate. In other words, methods for mutation detection are insensitive. Lack of sensitivity can arise as a result of studies that restrict the analysis to point mutations, or look at only a few of the coding exons, and do not search for deletions or mutations that affect splicing or promoter function. A second possibility is that there might be another tumor suppressor gene in this locus. Indeed Mxi-1 (see below) maps telomeric to PTEN at 10q24. In addition, the PTEN protein can be downregulated in the absence of known DNA mutation, suggesting the possibility of epigenetic regulation of PTEN (76–78). Finally, the two-hit model does not preclude the possibility that two hits can occur at separate genes. More specifically, haploinsufficiency at more than one locus might contribute to tumor formation or progression. In addition, with respect to PTEN, there is evidence to suggest that loss of one allele of PTEN is, by itself, pathologic and could contribute to tumor progression. For example, in murine fibroblasts genetically engineered to contain either two, one, or no copies of the PTEN gene, there is a gene-dosage effect with respect to activation of the downstream kinase Akt (38). Similarly, PTEN heterozygous mice develop a diffuse hyperplasia of the prostate, and eventually go on to develop prostate cancers (79). Of note, prostate cancer increases significantly when these mice are crossed to p27 heterozygous mice (P. Pandolfi, *personal communication*, 2000).

Other Mechanisms for Activation of the Phosphoinositide 3-Kinase Pathway in Cancer

There are a number of alternate mechanisms for activating the IGF/PI3K pathway (Fig. 4-2). PI3K is both the product of an avian retroviral oncogene and is a target of amplification in ovarian and cervical cancer (80–83). Likewise, an oncogenic form of the regulatory subunit p85 has been identified in transformed cells (84). Moreover, constitutive PI3K expression leads to the transformation of rodent cells (52) (T. Roberts, *personal communication*, 2000). Like PI3K, Akt-1 is found as a retroviral oncogene, and Akt-2 is the target of gene amplification in ovarian, breast, pancreatic, and gastric cancer (85–92). Thus, in the absence of PTEN mutations, amplification of these genes might serve as an alternative pathway activation mechanism. To date, however, such amplifications have not been described in prostate cancer.

Transforming Growth Factor Beta Pathway in Prostate Cancer

The Pathway

The TGF-beta superfamily is a large related group of secreted polypeptides that includes TGF-beta, bone morphogen proteins, and activin. These proteins regulate diverse processes including embryogenesis, bone development, and the regulation of epithelial cell proliferation. The signaling cascade begins at the cell surface, where TGF-beta ligand binding acts to bring together two receptors, the type I and II TGF-beta receptors [reviewed in (93)]. The type II receptor activates the type I receptor, which in turn phosphorylates and activates a group of transcription factors known as Smads. Simplistically, this phosphorylation event allows translocation of Smad proteins to the nucleus, where they induce the transcription of target genes. Signaling by TGF-beta itself is complex, and the phenotypic output of the pathway can be cell-type dependent; however, loss of the antiproliferative effects of TGF-beta is a common finding in certain common epithelial malignancies.

Alterations in Prostate Cancer

The role for TGF-beta pathway mutations in cancer is best documented in colon and pancreatic cancers. In colon cancer, mutations in the mismatch repair proteins MLH1 and MLH2 are associated with the development of a form of genetic instability characterized by defects in DNA mismatch repair. As a consequence of this mismatch repair defect, the TGF-beta II receptor is targeted for inactivating mutations (94). Downstream of TGF-beta, mutations or deletions in the Smad proteins occur at high frequency in both colon and pancreatic cancer (95–97).

In experimental systems, induced disruption of TGF-beta signaling can induce hallmarks of transformation (98). In LNCaP cells harboring a deletion of the TGF-beta-1 gene, restoration of signaling suppresses tumorigenesis (99,100). Despite the biology that links TGF-beta signaling to the regulation of the growth of prostate epithelial cells, definitive evidence for a role for inactivation of this pathway in prostate tumors is lacking. In some studies, the TGF-beta type I or II receptors appear to be lost or down-regulated in prostate cancer, when measured by IHC, and such loss may be correlated with poorer outcome (101,102). On the other hand, in some studies, TGF-beta levels measured again by IHC were higher in prostate cancer (103–105). At the genetic level, deletion or mutations of the TGF-I or -II receptors have not been reported, and mutations in Smad2 were not found in the only published report (106). Thus, whether the alterations in the protein levels represent phenomena linked casually to the progression of prostate cancer, as opposed to merely associated with the progression of prostate cancer, remains unclear. Further work is clearly needed in this area.

Wnt Signaling Pathways in Prostate Cancer

The Pathway

The first Wnt family member was discovered as a protooncogene (int-1) in virally induced murine mammary epithelial cell tumors (107). The Wnt proteins, like the TGF-beta proteins, now encompass a large family of secreted polypeptides (Wnts), which signal through the adenomatous polyposis coli (APC)/β-catenin pathway [reviewed in (108,109)]. In the absence of a Wnt signal, β-catenin is found in the cytoplasm, where it is constantly targeted for degradation by the action of a protein complex consisting of APC, axin, and the glycogen synthetase kinase (GSK)-3β. In response to Wnt, signaling the degradation function of the APC/axin/GSK-3β complex is turned off, resulting in the stabilization and accumulation of β-catenin. Under these conditions, β-catenin translocates to the nucleus, where it forms a complex with a set of transcription factors known as *lymphoid enhancer factor-1/T-cell transcription factor-1* (LEF/TCF). This trimeric complex binds to DNA and activates gene transcription.

Inappropriate activation of this pathway is linked to cellular transformation. In the colonic mucosa, it is thought that the LEF/TCF transcription complex may be required for maintenance of a crypt proliferating cell compartment. Transcriptional target genes of LEF/TCF include those that regulate proliferation, such as Myc and cyclin D1. In this view, inappropriate activation of the pathway would result in the expansion of this population of cells and the formation of a polyp. Tumors can activate the Wnt pathway through deletion or mutation of APC (which occurs in 85% of hereditary and sporadic colon cancer), through activating mutations in β-catenin (which occurs in 15% of colorectal tumors), and through overexpression of Wnt ligands [reviewed in (109)].

Alteration in Prostate Cancer

In prostate cancer, there are limited published data pertaining to the incidence of mutations in this pathway. Overexpression of the Wnt-5A messenger RNA (mRNA), a member of the Wnt ligand family, was found in one set of prostate tumors (110). LOH was found in the APC locus in 15% of prostate tumors (111), or in three of seven informative tumors (112). In studies of tumors from Japanese men, APC gene mutation was found in none of 18 tumors and 1 of 36 tumors (113,114). Finally, activating β-catenin mutations in exon 3 were found in 5 of 104 tumors (115). It is of interest to note that APC gene mutations give rise to very early premalignant lesions in the intestinal tract, and to date, the detection of reproducible genetic lesions in the earliest stages of prostate cancer (prostatic intraepithelial neoplasia) are rare. Further study of this pathway, particularly in the setting of prostatic intraepithelial neoplasia, appears warranted.

Sonic Hedgehog Pathway

The Pathway

The role of hedgehog signaling in pattern formation in the developing embryo has been studied extensively. However, recent data suggest that deregulation of this pathway can play a role in the genesis of both basal cell carcinoma and medulloblastoma [reviewed in (116)]. Hedgehog family members are secreted factors that bind to a cell surface transmembrane receptor complex of two proteins: Smoothened, which transmits the signal, and Patched (PTCH), which antagonizes signaling. As is in many signaling pathways, activation of the receptor leads to the activation of a family of transcription factors, in this case known as Gli. This family of transcription factors is opposed by the repressor activities of the so-called suppressor of fused [Su(fu)] proteins. There are three hedgehog proteins in mammalian cells, and there is an absolute requirement for one of these genes: sonic hedgehog (Shh) in prostate development in mice (117), suggesting that this pathway is active in prostate cells particularly during development. These data raise the possibility that reactivation of this pathway in adult prostate epithelial cells could contribute to the development and progression of prostate cancer.

Alterations in Prostate Cancer

Mutation of PTCH, the receptor for Shh, gives rise to medulloblastoma in mice. Interestingly, mutation, or loss of the second allele, is not seen, suggesting that haploinsufficiency is oncogenic (118). In keeping with these data, inactivating mutations in PTCH are found in 10% of human medulloblastomas (119,120). In addition, germline mutation of PTCH in humans is associated with the development of a basal cell cancer syndrome known as *Gorlin's syndrome*, and sporadic basal cell carcinomas have activating mutations in both the Smoothened receptor and in the PTCH gene (121). In keeping with these data, transgenic expression of the ligand Shh gives rise to basal cell carcinomas (122,123). Because data implicating this pathway in cancer are relatively recent, it is too early to know if alterations occur in prostate cancer. To date, there are no such reports in the prostate cancer literature. Of note, the human Su(fu) [huSu(fu)] gene product, a repressor of Gli activity, maps to the 10q24 locus, and thus could be targeted for deletion or codeletion along with *PTEN* (located at 10q23) in a number of prostate cancers (124).

P53 AND PRB TUMOR SUPPRESSOR PATHWAYS

p53 Pathway

The Pathway

p53 is a tumor suppressor gene that, in response to genotoxic stress or in response to inappropriate proliferative signals delivered by certain oncogenes, can induce either a cell-cycle arrest or apoptosis. p53 is subjected to frequent somatic mutation in a wide variety of tumors (as many as 50% of all tumors), and germline mutation of p53 results in the acquisition of a rare hereditary cancer predisposition syndrome known as *Li-Fraumani syndrome* (125–127). Patients afflicted with this illness develop breast carcinomas, sarcomas, brain tumors, and other cancers at a significantly higher rate than the general population (128).

p53 is present in low to undetectable levels in normal cells. When cells are exposed to DNA-damaging agents such as ultraviolet or gamma irradiation, p53 is stabilized and forms a homotetrameric complex that binds to promoter elements in p53 target genes and activates these genes (Fig. 4-3). These target genes include the cyclin-dependent kinase inhibitor p21, a mediator of p53-induced cell-cycle arrest, and a number of genes thought to participate in the induction of apoptosis.

p53 is regulated by a number of inputs (Fig. 4-3). First, it is thought that DNA damage is "sensed" by the gene product of the ataxia-telangiectasia gene. The Ataxia-telangiectasia gene, in turn, regulates the activity of two kinases, Chk1 and Chk2, that can phosphorylate and activate p53 in the damage response pathway (129,130). Of particular interest here is that certain Li-Fraumeni families do not harbor p53 mutations, but rather have mutations in Chk2, strongly suggesting that Chk2 is both a critical regulator of p53 and a tumor suppressor gene (131). Second, the oncogene MDM2 binds to the C-terminus of p53 and targets p53 for ubiquitin-mediated degradation (132,133). In turn, p53 can induce the MDM2 gene, creating a negative feedback loop to shut itself off. Finally, as discussed below, the gene encoding for the cell-cycle regulator $p16^{INK4a}$ also encodes a second protein, $p14^{ARF}$ in humans, or $p19^{ARF}$ in mice (referred to as *ARF*, for *alternative reading frame*, here forward) (134). The study of mice lacking an intact ARF coding sequence, but capable of making a p16 protein, revealed that the ARF loss is associated with the formation of tumors, raising the possibility that this gene, and not $p16^{INK4a}$, is the major tumor suppressor in this locus (135). Biochemically, ARF appears to function by interacting with Mdm2 to block degradation of p53 (136–139). ARF is particularly important, as it appears to act as a sensor for the inappropriate activation of certain oncogenic proteins, such as Myc or E1A (140,141). In cells expressing wild-type p53, induction of ARF by such stimuli leads to the inhibition of Mdm2, stabilization of p53, and activation of p53-dependent apoptosis. Thus, loss of ARF would provide a critical advantage to a cell that then acquires activating oncogenic mutations.

p53 Alterations in Prostate Cancer

Mutation of p53 and changes in p53 expression as detected by IHC have been extensively studied in prostate cancer. Because of space constraints, Table 4-3 presents a partial accounting of the studies of p53 in prostate cancer, primarily focusing on those investigations in which there was a

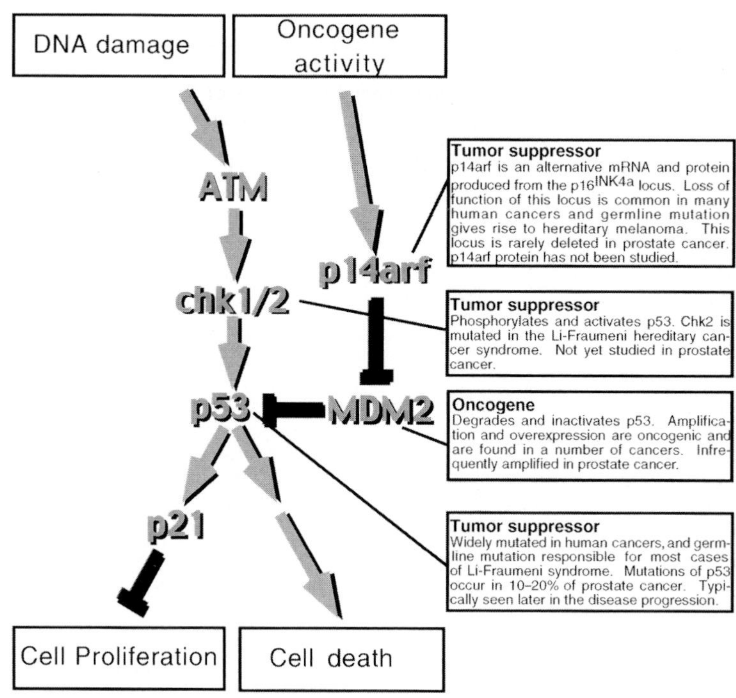

FIGURE 4-3. The p53 pathway. The p53 pathway is a damage control pathway that can respond to both genotoxic stress, such as radiation, and the inappropriate activation of oncogenes. DNA damage is thought to be "sensed" by the protein product of the ataxia-telangiectasia gene (ATM). Activation of ATM triggers the activation of the chk1 and chk2 serine-threonine kinases. Chk1 and Chk2 are kinases that can phosphorylate and activate p53. p53 is a transcription factor that can induce the production of p21 and a resulting cell-cycle arrest as a consequence of inhibition of cyclin-dependent kinase activity. In addition, p53 can induce programmed cell death through both transcriptional and nontranscriptional means. p53 is in turn negatively regulated by MDM2, which targets p53 for protein degradation. This pathway can also be triggered by the induction of ARF. ARF is a protein produced from the same genetic locus as p16^{INK4a}, using, however, an alternative reading frame for translation of the protein. ARF protein is induced by a number of oncogenic signals and blocks the ability of MDM2 to degrade p53. In this manner, induction of ARF induces p53.

direct examination of p53 mutations (typically by single-strand conformational polymorphism analysis or by direct sequencing). IHC studies were included when the IHC staining results were confirmed by limited mutation detection. Immunohistochemistry, by its very nature, is subjective and less precise. In the case of p53, enhanced IHC staining is thought to be equivalent to mutation as a result of stabilization of mutant p53 protein. In the studies listed in Table 4-3, there is a high concordance between the rate of mutation detection and the rate of IHC-positive cells. The reader should note that this is not the case with the entire body of literature, which shows a wide range in the reported frequency of p53 alterations in prostate cancer. Among studies that look directly at p53 mutations in all the tumors (not just in tumors that are positive by IHC+ in Table 4-3), the rate of mutation detection in primary prostate tumors is 10% to 20%. Another consistent finding is that the rate of p53 mutations increases in androgen-independent metastatic disease, where the rate of p53 loss can approach 30% to 40%. Clearly, p53 is inactivated in a significant fraction of prostate cancers, and biallelic inactivation appears later in tumor progression; such is the case for PTEN. In addition, the lack of p53 mutations in a substantial fraction of tumors raises the possibility that this pathway may be inactivated through an alternative mechanism in some tumors.

MDM2 Amplification in Prostate Cancer

As mentioned previously, p53 function is inhibited by binding of MDM2 to the p53 C-terminus. Inactivation of p53, by amplification of MDM2, occurs frequently in soft-tissue and bone sarcomas, but also in glioblastoma and breast, lung, and ovarian cancers (142). In one xenograft model of prostate cancer, the emergence of an androgen-independent phenotype is associated with increased levels of MDM2 protein (143), suggesting a possible role for this mechanism in human tumors. In primary and metastatic prostate tumors, MDM2 amplification has not been extensively studied. In 28 stage B tumors, Ittmann et al. found no amplification of MDM2 (144). Others have found that higher levels of MDM2 protein, as detected by IHC detection of MDM2 protein, are associated with more advanced-stage disease (145).

p14^{ARF} Alterations in Prostate Cancer

ARF is encoded by the same gene that encodes the p16^{INK4a} protein. The major method for inactivation of ARF in tumors is the simultaneous inactivation of p16^{INK4a}, along with ARF by gene deletion (typically deletion of exon 2), or by promoter methylation. Mutations in the p16^{INK4a} are presented in detail under the retinoblastoma (RB) pathway (below), although alterations in this gene are rare in prostate cancer. In families with hereditary melanoma and in sporadic breast cancers, mutation of p16^{INK4a} appears to be more tightly linked to the cancer phenotype (146–148). On the other hand, in leukemia and in some melanoma cell lines, specific mutations involving ARF and sparing p16^{INK4a}, have been found (149,150). Thus, reexamining prostate tumors for selective mutation of ARF is an important task that remains to be done.

Mutation of p21 and Waf1

p21-Mediated inhibition of cyclin-dependent kinase activity is the primary mechanism through which p53 enacts a

TABLE 4-3. P53 ALTERATIONS

Author	Loss of heterozygosity (LOH)	Mutation	Deletion	Immunohistochemistry (IHC) (pos)	No. of tumors	Source
Navone (234)	—	0/4 IHC–[a]	—	0/36 (0%)	36	P, LN, M
		8/8 IHC+[a]		21/44 (48%)[i]	44	M (AI)
Uchida (235)	—	2/21 (9.5%)	—	—	21	P[b]
Effert (236)	—	1/10 (10%)	—	—	10	P
	—	1/2 (50%)	—	—	2	LN ,M
Dinjens (237)	—	2/20[c] (10%)	—	2/20[a] (10%)	20	P[d]
		2/15[c] (13%)			17	LN
Watanabe (238,239)	—	11/90 (12%)	—	—	90	P
		1/4 (25%)			4	LN, M
Voeller (240)	—	2/34 (6%)	—	2/85[e] (2%)	85	P
Chi (241)	—	12/44 (27%)	3/44 (7%)	—	44	P
		2/4 (50%)	0/4 (0%)		4	LN
Massenkeil (242)	18/30	3/38 (8%)	—	—	39	P[b]
Kubota (243)	—	4/21 (19%)	—	—	21	P
Heidenberg (244)	—	9/11 IHC+	—	6/27 (22%)	27	P (no rx)
				4/8 (50%)	8	LN (no rx)
				20/26 (76%)	26	P (AI)
Moyret-Lalle (222)	—	2/19 (11%)	—	—	19	P
Konishi (245)	—	5/32 (16%)	—	5/32 (16%)[f]	32	P
		0/15 (0%)		0/15 (0%)	15	Latent
Mirchandani (246)	—	5/65 (8%)	—	—	65	P
Kunimi (247)	—	1/18 (6%)	—	—	18	P
Suzuki (248)	—	0/29 (0%)	—	—	29	P
		7/22 (32%)			22	P, LN, M (autopsy)
Prendergast (249)	—	3/5 IHC+	—	5/25 (20%)	25	P (no rx)
		0/5 IHC–		13/18 (17%)	18	P (rec. post-XRT)
Dahiya (250)	—	2/25 (8%)	—	2/25[g] (8%)	25	P[b]
		4/20 (20%)		4/20 (20%)	20	LN
Brooks (251)	10/55	1/55 (2%)	—	2/38 (5%)	67	P
				26/42 (62%)	42	M
Schlechte (252), Schlechte (253)	—	6/24 (25%)	—	—	24	P
Mottaz (254)	—	5/5 IHC+	—	5/100 (5%)	100	P and BPH
Salem (255)	—	2/3 IHC+	—	10/96 (10%)	96	P (stage C)
		0/3 IHC–				
Stapleton (256), Eastham (257)	—	1/6 IHC–	—	6/60 (10%)	60	P
		9/20 IHC+		20/60 (33%)	60	LN (56), M[h]
Facher (258)	—	3/57 (5%)	—	—	57	P

AI, androgen independent; BPH, benign prostate hyperplasia; LN, lymph node; M, metastatic site; P, primary.
[a]Concordance between IHC and mutation detection.
[b]Included transurethral prostatectomy (TURP) specimens.
[c]One mutation was the same in both the primary tumor and metastasis.
[d]All primary tumors obtained by TURP.
[e]One sample was positive by both mutation analysis and IHC.
[f]Three samples were positive by both mutation analysis and IHC.
[g]All six samples with mutations had >40% nuclear staining. Data are not otherwise described.
[h]Paired primary and metastatic tumors.
[i]High rate of p53 staining in AI tumors, the majority of which were bone mets. Only one androgen-dependent bone met available.

cell-cycle block. Mutation of p21 would render inactive the p53 cell-cycle-arrest function of p53 and thus could be one mechanism by which tumors evade p53 growth suppression. To date, one group has reported on the p21 mutations in prostate cancer, finding two such mutations in 18 primary tumors (151).

Retinoblastoma Pathway

The Pathway

The *RB-1* gene encodes a nuclear growth regulatory protein—pRB. The pRB protein is part of a pathway that regulates cell-cycle entry and coordinates the execution of

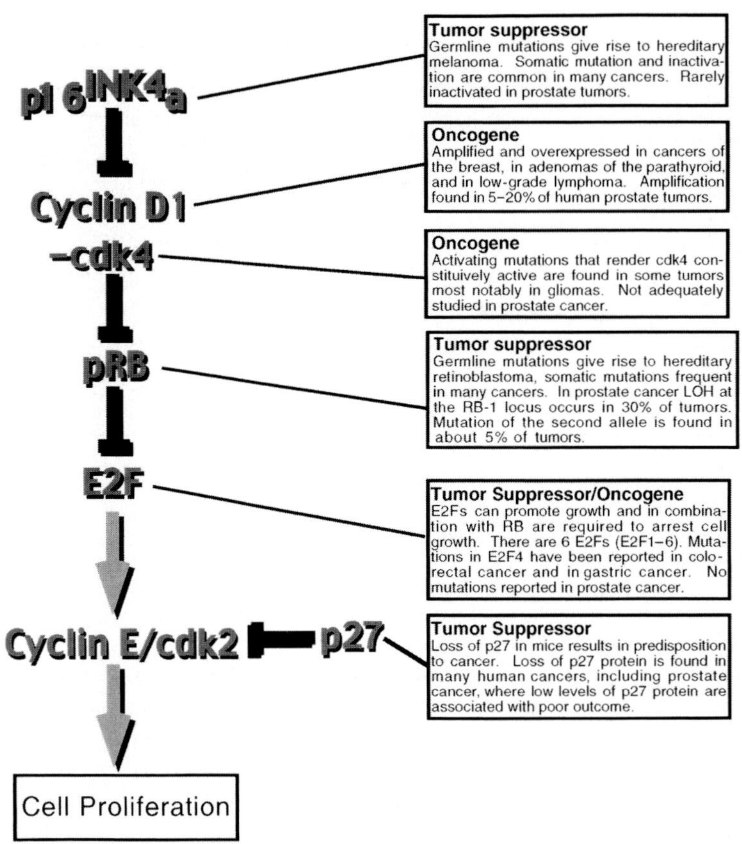

FIGURE 4-4. The retinoblastoma (RB) pathway. The RB pathway acts primarily to regulate the progression of cells from the G1 phase of the cell cycle to the initiation of DNA replication (S phase). The pathway is centered on the regulation of protein product of the retinoblastoma gene (RB) and the E2F transcription factor family. The E2F family is a critical regulator of the transcription of genes involved in cell proliferation and cell cycle progression. These genes include the cyclin E gene, DNA polymerase α, and others. When activated, for example, cyclin E can itself induce cells to enter S phase. The RB protein can bind to E2F and the RB-E2F complex acts to repress or turn off transcription of the aforementioned E2F target genes. This complex can be inactivated by phosphorylation of RB by the cyclin D1 cyclin-dependent kinase (cdk4) complex. Cyclin D1 and cdk4 itself are subjected to inhibitory regulation of the cyclin-dependent kinase inhibitor (cdki) p16^{INK4a}. LOH, loss of heterozygosity.

certain differentiation events with appropriate withdrawal from the cell cycle [for review see (152)]. The RB protein forms a complex with a transcription factor family known as E2F. The RB-E2F complex, when bound to the E2F sites in a promoter region of a gene, acts to repress transcription of the particular gene (153–155). E2F sites are found in the promoters of genes involved in DNA synthesis, such as dihydrofolate reductase and thymidylate synthetase, and in the promoters of genes that also regulate the cell cycle, such as cyclin E and the E2F genes themselves. By blocking the transcription of these genes, pRB can arrest cells in G1 (Fig. 4-4). Although E2F is a transcription factor that can turn on S-phase-specific genes and induce cell-cycle entry, it is also necessary for the recruitment of pRB to promoter elements where it represses transcription. In keeping with these two roles, forced overexpression of E2F is associated with transformation and is required for tumors that form in the absence of pRB, whereas loss of E2F can also lead to tumors (156–161). Indeed, mutations in the E2F-4 gene, one of six members of the E2F family, have been reported in colorectal and gastric cancers (162–164).

The formation and action of the RB-E2F complex is opposed by the activity of two cyclin-dependent kinase activities: D-type cyclins (cyclin D1, D2, and D3) complexed to either cdk4 or cdk6, and E-type cyclins (cyclin E1 and cyclin E2) complexed to cdk2 (Fig. 4-4). These kinase complexes can phosphorylate and inactivate pRB, leading to the activation of E2F transcription, the induction of E2F target genes, and the induction of S-phase entry. Thus, increased cyclin kinase activity is associated with an increase in cellular proliferation. Cyclin D1 is notable, as it is a cellular oncogene targeted by gene amplification events in breast cancer, parathyroid adenomas, and lymphoma (Bcl-1).

The activity of cyclin D/cdk complexes is blocked by a cyclin-dependent kinase inhibitor known as p16^{INK4a}. This inhibitor is produced by the p16/INK4A/MTS-1 gene and binds to and inhibits the association between cyclin D and cdk4, or cdk6. p16^{INK4a} is a tumor suppressor gene, and undergoes frequent somatic mutation in a number of cancers. In addition, germline mutations are associated with the development of hereditary melanoma. This same gene leads to the production of a second protein product known as p19^{ARF} (ARF) (134). As described previously, ARF is a regulator of the p53 pathway. Mutations in this gene can knock out both proteins, thereby altering both the RB and p53 pathways.

In addition to phosphorylating pRB, cyclin E is also an important transcriptional target of the RB/E2F complex. Therefore, cyclin E/cdk2 most likely acts downstream of pRB and regulates a number of proteins whose functions are connected to the regulation of the cell cycle and DNA synthesis. For example, cyclin E/cdk2 can phosphorylate NPAT, a protein that regulates the biosynthesis of histones, a critical component of chromatin (165–167).

TABLE 4-4. RETINOBLASTOMA ALTERATIONS

Author	Loss of heterozygosity (LOH)	Mutation	Deletion	Immunohistochemical (IHC) (neg)	No. of tumors	Source
Ittmann (259)	7/19 (36%)[a]	ND	0/16	4/24	26	P
Brooks (260)	11/41(27%)	—	—	—	46	P, LN (4)
Vesalainen (261)	—	—	—	1/118	118	P
Kubota (262)	—	4/25	—	—	25	P
Phillips (263)	24/40 (60%)[b]	—	—	7/9	43	P[c]
Bookstein (264)	—	1/6	—	1/6[d]	6	P, LN, M
Geradts (265)	—	—	—	2/19	19	P
Latil (266)	33/60 (55%)	—	—	—	60	—
Melamed (267)	24/80 (30%)	—	—	—	80	P, LN, M
Tricoli (268)	—	1/83	3/68[e]	—	83	P, LN (4)
Cooney (269)	13/40 (33%)	—	—	8/37[f]	40	P

LN, lymph node; M, metastatic site; P, primary.
[a]Exon 20 polymorphism screened.
[b]Twelve with LOH with one marker only.
[c]Tumors found on transurethral prostatectomy.
[d]Immunoblot detection of pRB.
[e]Deletion or rearrangement.
[f]No correlation between negative IHC and LOH.

Cyclin E/cdk2 activity is held in check by the action of another cyclin-dependent kinase inhibitor, p27.

Retinoblastoma 1 Alterations in Prostate Cancer

The pRB protein can be inactivated by the viral oncoprotein large-T antigen from SV40. This oncoprotein inactivates both pRB and p53 and is sufficient to induce prostate neoplasia when expressed in the murine prostate epithelium (168). In the renal capsule recombination model, biallelic inactivation of *RB* in murine prostate epithelial cells is also associated with the development of prostate carcinoma caused by hormonal stimulation, suggesting that loss of pRB can predispose to prostate epithelial neoplasia (169). Surprisingly little work has been done to detail the extent of biallelic loss of *RB-1* in human prostate cancer (Table 4-4). It is likely that the large size of the gene (27 exons spanning 200 kb of genomic DNA) and the lack of consistent mutational hot spots discourages investigators from vigorously pursuing the comprehensive detection of mutations. Studies looking at loss of chromosomal markers have found that loss of the *RB-1* locus on chromosome 13q is frequent (33% to 60%). However, it has been difficult to demonstrate loss or mutation of the second *RB-1* allele. To date, the best estimates are that perhaps 10% of prostate tumors harbor biallelic-inactivating mutations in *RB-1*. Loss of RB protein, as defined by IHC, has varied from less than 1% to 77%, showing the wide variation in this technique. It is likely that mutations in *RB-1* are more common and are underestimated by current technologies. In addition, the pRB pathway can be inactivated through alternative means.

Cyclin D1 Amplification in Prostate Cancer

Overexpression of cyclin D1 inactivates pRB through phosphorylation via the cdk4/6-cyclin D complex. Cyclin D1 is frequently amplified or overexpressed in breast cancer. In murine models, overexpression of D1 in the mammary gland results in breast carcinomas with a prolonged latency (170). In prostate cancer, cyclin D1 has not been studied extensively. The published data generally show low levels of amplification (0% to 5%) and a modest incidence of overexpression (4% to 24%) in primary and metastatic foci (12,171,172). Although others have reported a higher incidence of both amplification and overexpression (17,173), these discrepancies most likely result from differences in detection and scoring techniques. These data are summarized in Table 4-5.

$p16^{INK4a}$ Alterations in Prostate Cancer

Unlike the RB-1 gene, the $p16^{INK4a}$ gene is quite small, including only three exons. Furthermore, the majority of the coding sequence is contained within exon 2. Therefore, rapid sequencing of the entire gene from human tumors is possible. To date, point mutations and deletions have been found in only 2.5% and 3%, respectively, of all prostate tumors surveyed. In addition to mutational loss, $p16^{INK4a}$ is commonly inactivated by promoter methylation. Herman found frequent methylation of prostate cancer cell lines (60%) (174); however, in primary tumors, methylation was found in 7% of tumors (Table 4-6). Thus, it would appear that loss of function of $p16^{INK4a}$ occurs in less than 10% of prostate tumors.

p27 Alterations in Prostate Cancer

The paucity of pRB, $p16^{INK4a}$, and cyclin D1 alterations raises the possibility that alternative mechanisms for deregulating the G1 check point may be operational in prostate cancer. The cyclin-dependent kinase inhibitor p27 is a critical regulator of cyclin E/cdk2 activity and is a critical regulator of the G1 checkpoint downstream of

TABLE 4-5. CYCLIN D1 ALTERATIONS

Author	Amplified	Increased mRNA	Increased protein	No. of tumors	Tumor type
Bubendorf (12)	0/172 (0%)	—	—	172	P
	3/38 (7.9%)			38	LR
	2/43 (5%)			43	M (AI)
Kaltz-Wittmer (17)	2/16 (12%)[a]	—	—	22	P
	8/57 (14%)[a]			63	M (AI)
Drobnjak (270)	—	—	10 (11%)	86	P
			15 (68%)	22	M (AI)
Gumbiner (171)	—	4/93 (4%)	—	93	P
Han (172)	—	—	12 (24%)[b]	50	P
Kallakury (271)	—	—	31 (22%)	140	P
Shiraishi (272)	—	—	20 (30%)	66	P
Aaltomaa (173)	—	—	133/187 (71%)	213	P

AI, androgen independent; LR, local recurrence; M, metastatic site; P, primary.
[a]Using the authors, cut off of 30% of nuclei positive.
[b]Twelve percent of normal prostate had increased staining as well. Vast majority of both tumor and normal had no staining.

pRB. p27 heterozygous– and homozygous–null mice develop hyperplasia in multiple organs, as well as tumors, when challenged with radiation (175,176). Finally, when crossed with the PTEN+/–, mice loss of p27 results in prostate tumors (P. Pandolfi, *personal communication*, 2000). Thus, p27 appears to be a critical regulator of prostate epithelial cell proliferation. In human prostate tumors, p27 loss is associated with advanced stage and a poorer prognosis (reviewed in Chapter 20). Thus, one possibility is that loss of p27 is the major mechanism for inactivation of the pRB pathway in prostate tumors. p27 can be regulated through ubiquitin-mediated degradation, and enhanced degradation has been described in gliomas; colorectal tumors (177,178); and, more recently, in prostate tumors (M. Loda, *personal communication*, 2000).

TRANSCRIPTION FACTORS

Androgen Receptor

The AR is a critical regulator of growth and differentiation of prostate epithelial cells, both normal and transformed. In the setting of clinical administration of the AR antagonist flutamide, somatic mutations of the receptor that confers flutamide activation to the receptor can occur (179–183). However, patients with these tumors account for only a minority of those tumors that become androgen independent. Instead, direct amplification of the AR is being recognized at greater frequency in this setting (12,184,185). Clearly, this may imply a continued important role for the receptor, even in the androgen-independent state. This topic is covered in greater detail in Chapters 3 and 6.

TABLE 4-6. P16^{INK4a} ALTERATIONS

Author	Loss of heterozygosity (LOH)	Mutation	Deletion	Aberrant methylation	Immunohistochemical (IHC) (neg)	No. of tumors	Source
Chi (273)	—	1/32 (3%)	2/7[a] (29%)	—	26/60	116	P
Komiya (274)	—	1/51 (2%)	—	—	—	51	P, M (AI)
Chen (275)	—	1/18 (5%)	0/18[b] (0%)	—	—	18	P
Gaddipati (276)	—	0/18 (0%)	—	—	—	18	P
Gu (277)	—	0/30 (0%)	—	1/21	—	30	P
Jarrard (278)	12/60	0/3 (0%)	—	3/24	—	60	P
	13/28	0/7 (0%)	—	1/12	—	28	LN, M
Mangold (279)	—	—	2/63 (3%)	—	—	63	P
Park[c] (280)	—	1/32 (3%)	0/25 (0%)	—	—	32	P
Tamimi (281)	—	1/20 (5%)	0/20[a] (0%)	—	—	20	P[d]
Nguyen (282)	—	—	—	8/11[e]	—	11	P

AI, androgen independent; LN, lymph node; M, metastatic; P, primary.
[a]Judged by ability to polymerase chain reaction (PCR) amplify p16 exons.
[b]By semiquantitative PCR compared to glyceraldehyde-3-phosphate dehydrogenase.
[c]Also found no deletions or mutations in p15, p18, or p19.
[d]Primary samples obtained by transurethral prostatectomy.
[e]Methylation in exon 2 that *did not* result in loss of expression.

Myc Family

Myc is one of the first members of the large helix-loop-helix leucine zipper family of transcription factors. These members share a common three-dimensional protein structure, and the ability to recognize a DNA-binding element known as an E-box. Myc binds to DNA in partnership with Max (forming Myc:Max heterodimers) [reviewed in (186)]. The Myc:Max complex is capable of activating transcription from the E-box promoter elements. However, the Myc:Max complex is either absent or low in most quiescent cells. In these cells, Max is primarily complexed with another protein known as Mad or the Mad-related family member, Mxi-1 (forming Mad:Max or Mxi-1:Max heterodimers). This complex sits on a promotor element and turns off transcription. Thus, there are two opposing forces: one active (Myc:Max), and one repressive (Mad:Max or Mxi-1:Max). Amplification, or overexpression, of Myc results in a shift in this equilibrium from the repressive complex to the active complex, with subsequent inappropriate, or untimely, activation of Myc-responsive genes and the unregulated induction of cell-cycle entry.

Mxi-1 can bind to Mad and act to negatively regulate Myc target genes. Thus, loss of Mxi-1 due to deletion or inactivating point mutation would, like Myc amplification, shift the balance of transcription toward Myc-dependent transcriptional activation. Consistent with this notion, Mxi-1 overexpression can block Myc-dependent transformation (187), and Mxi-1 knockout mice develop hyperproliferation of the prostate epithelium, as well as multiple tumor types when either crossed to $p16^{INK4a}$-null background or exposed to carcinogens (188).

Myc Amplification or Overexpression in Prostate Cancer

Myc amplification can be identified by Southern blot, or by fluorescent *in situ* hybridization, to detect gene copy number. In the latter, one can distinguish chromosome amplification (aneuploidy) from gene-specific amplification by comparing the gene-specific signal to that obtained with a centromeric probe. For example, Bubendorf et al. required a threefold increase in the fluorescence *in situ* hybridization signal, obtained with Myc, over the chromosome 8 centromeric probe in their definition of myc amplification. In a survey of tumors studied on a tumor microarray, they found that Myc amplification occurred in 10% of metastatic tumors and 4% of locally recurrent tumors, but in none of the 168 primary tumors examined (12). In other reports, Myc amplification has been found in primary tumors, ranging from 0% to 44% (Table 4-7). Here, a significant problem is that the threshold for calling amplification, and the use of a centromeric probe for correcting for chromosomal amplification, varies from study to study. Nonetheless, Myc amplification occurs in a definitive group of prostate tumors and, in one recent study, was an independent predictor of systemic progression (189).

Mxi-1 Loss of Function in Prostate Cancer

Mxi-1 maps to the chromosomal region 10q24-25 telomeric to PTEN, located at 10q23. As mentioned earlier, this region is a frequent target of LOH; therefore, *Mxi-1* would be expected to undergo at least monoallelic loss quite frequently in prostate cancer. Mutation of the second

TABLE 4-7. MYC AMPLIFICATION AND OVEREXPRESSION

Author	Amplified	Increased mRNA	No. of tumors	Tumor type
Bubendorf (12)	0	—	168	P
	2 (4%)[a]	—	47	LR
	5 (10%)	—	47	M
Buttyan (283)	—	6/9	62	M
Latil (15)	0/21	—	—	P
Latil (284)	—	19/33	—	P
Nupponen (285)	5/17 (29%)[b]	—	—	P (AI)
Qian (286)	44%[c]	—	25	P
Kaltz-Wittmer (17)	3/15 (20%)	—	—	P
	29/62 (47%)	—	—	M (AI)
Reiter (287)	7/20 (35%)[d]	—	—	P
Sato (189)	28/144 (19%)[e]	—	157	P
Mark (288)	11/33	—	—	P

AI, androgen independent; LR, locally recurrent; M, metastatic site; P, primary.
[a]Both were also amplified in the metastatic lesion and are counted again below.
[b]Threefold Myc amplification.
[c]Percentage of tumor foci (multiple foci per patients examined) with amplification of Myc >1.1 times chromosome 8 signal.
[d]A ratio of Myc staining to chromosome 8 staining greater than 1.3 was used to define amplification. An additional 5 of 20 tumors had gain of chromosome 8.
[e]An additional 50 tumors had gain of chromosome 8 and an equivalent gain of c-Myc. Myc amplification was an independent predictor of systemic progression.

TABLE 4-8. MXI-1 ALTERATIONS

Authors	Loss of heterozygosity (LOH)	Mutation	No. of tumors	Tumor type
Gray (62)	23/37[a]	0/23	37	—
Kawamata (289)	—	0/32	32	P
Eagle (290)	—	4/10[b]	10[c]	P
Kucsyk (291)	—	0/32	32	P

P, primary.
[a]Twenty-three of 37 tumors had LOH at 10q23-25. Specific loss of Mxi-1 (as opposed to other regions or entire region) found in 1 of 23.
[b]Detected by sequencing cloned polymerase chain reaction (PCR) products. The PCR products containing the mutant alleles (repeated in 3 to 4 experiments) represented 1.6%, 2.4%, 2.1%, and 19% of all clones.
[c]All ten samples selected on the basis of LOH at 10q24-25.

allele remains controversial (Table 4-8). One group reported inactivating point mutations in four of ten tumors preselected for LOH at the 10q24 locus, although others, who have not preselected their tumors, have failed to find any mutations. For example, Gray et al. found LOH at 10q23-25 in 23 of 37 tumors, but only one had specific loss at 10q24. In the group of 23 tumors with 10q23-25 LOH, no mutations of Mxi-1 were found (62).

In addition to the open question regarding the extent of biallelic loss of Mxi-1, there are a number of questions that arise. First, could monoallelic loss of *PTEN* and monoallelic loss of *Mxi-1* cooperate to induce pathologic growth of prostate epithelial cells? Genetic experiments in mice have demonstrated that haploinsufficiency of PTEN results in a prostate hyperplasia. It is possible that the additional loss of one copy of *Mxi-1* could serve to exacerbate PTEN loss. Second, is it possible the haploinsufficiency of *Mxi-1* might cooperate with amplification of Myc to produce a more profound deregulation of this growth-control pathway? Further studies are needed to document whether these scenarios are likely.

NKX3.1

NKX3.1 is a member of a large family of homeodomain transcription factors (190,191). NKX3.1 is highly expressed in the prostate, as well as in salivary glands, the kidney, and portions of the central nervous system (192,193), and is expressed in an androgen-dependent manner (191). Genetically altered mice that lack one or both alleles of NKX3.1 develop a prostate gland; thus, NKX3.1 is not essential for prostate development but may be important for regulating production of certain secretory proteins (194). However, both the heterozygous- and homozygous-null mice develop prostate hyperplasia (194). Thus, loss of function of NKX3.1 might be associated with the development of prostate cancer. In keeping with these data, NKX3.1 is localized to chromosome 8p21 (195). LOH at this locus occurs in prostate cancer and is associated with more aggressive or invasive tumors, suggesting the presence of a tumor suppressor gene in the 8p21–8p22 interval (196–199). Mutations of the remaining NKX3.1 gene have not been identified. Thus, it is unclear whether this protein is a bona fide tumor suppressor gene in human prostate cancer (195). However, the fact that mice demonstrate a phenotypic consequence of loss of one allele of NKX3.1 raises the possibility that haploinsufficiency of this gene in human tumors results in a propensity to tumor formation or progression (194).

ADHESION FACTORS

E-Cadherin

Cadherins are a family of transmembrane proteins with a long extracellular domain composed of repetitive domains required for cell-cell adhesion. E-cadherin is the major Ca^{2+}-dependent adhesion receptor found in the adherens junctions between epithelial cells. The intracellular portion of the receptor binds to α-catenin, β-catenin, and γ-catenin, which serve to connect E-cadherin to the actin cytoskeleton [reviewed in (200)]. Functionally, E-cadherin is altered in cancer through a number of mechanisms, including germline mutation, found in familial sporadic gastric cancer; somatic mutation, found in breast cancer; and epigenetic modulation. In mice, loss of E-cadherin appears to contribute to tumor progression, but loss of E-cadherin itself is not sufficient to render a tumor invasive through basement membrane (201). Conversely, restoration of E-cadherin to tumor cell lines can suppress their neoplastic properties.

A role for loss of E-cadherin in prostate cancer was first proposed after observations that invasive Dunning rat tumors lost both E-cadherin protein and mRNA (202). Furthermore, in this model, restoration of E-cadherin expression was associated with a decrease in the invasiveness of the Dunning tumors, suggesting that loss of E-cadherin is causally associated with invasive behavior (203). In human tumors, loss of E-cadherin protein, as detected by IHC, has been observed by a number of groups. Although normal prostate epithelial cells express E-cadherin, 50% or more of prostate tumors appear to lose E-cadherin protein (204–207). Loss of

E-cadherin has been correlated with Gleason score, and, in some studies, loss of E-cadherin is prognostic for survival (208,209). E-cadherin loss, however, does not appear to add additional discrimination when combined with standard prognostic features (210).

Genetic alteration and mutation of E-cadherin is found in other tumors, but to date no evidence of allelic loss has been found for the E-cadherin locus in prostate cancer (211). Rather, loss of E-cadherin appears to occur as a result of loss, or down-regulation, of transcription (212), and this appears to result as a consequence of methylation of the E-cadherin promoter (213). Of note, a single genetic lesion in this pathway has been noted in PC3 cells, where deletion of the α-catenin gene has been described (214).

In summary, the data for E-cadherin are quite consistent from study to study and suggest that epigenetic loss of this protein is an important step in the progression of prostate cancer.

CONCLUSION

The heterogeneity of prostate cancer remains a formidable hurdle to dissecting the genetic alterations that trigger and drive prostate epithelial cell transformation. Unfortunately, at this point it does not appear that we have detailed understanding of these genetic alterations, and much work is needed in this area. There are three future goals to this ongoing work. First, we need to determine whether there exist separable molecular classes of prostate cancer. Such molecular subsets exist in breast cancer and can be defined based on known molecules, such as estrogen receptor and Her2/neu, or, more recently, based on complimentary DNA microarray analysis (215). Clearly, the definition of breast tumors, based on ER or Her2/neu status, carries therapeutic implications. The second goal is to elucidate the combination of distinct genetic and epigenetic events occurring within each molecular subset. For example, are p53 pathways and pRB pathways inactivation co-incident? Does mutation, or loss, of one allele of PTEN cooperate with loss of p27 protein? Finally, we need to determine whether there exists a specific sequence in which genetic alterations are obtained. What are the earliest lesions in prostate cancer? Can the identification of such events direct us toward preventive strategies in prostate cancer? The postgenome era brings the promise of answering these questions and leading us to the development of robust novel therapeutic agents.

REFERENCES

1. Slamon DJ, Godolphin W, Jones LA, et al. Studies of the HER-2/neu proto-oncogene in human breast and ovarian cancer. *Science* 1989;244:707–712.
2. Venter DJ, Tuzi NL, Kumar S, et al. Overexpression of the c-erbB-2 oncoprotein in human breast carcinomas: immunohistological assessment correlates with gene amplification. *Lancet* 1987;2:69–72.
3. Hudziak RM, Schlessinger J, Ullrich A. Increased expression of the putative growth factor receptor p185HER2 causes transformation and tumorigenesis of NIH 3T3 cells. *Proc Natl Acad Sci U S A* 1987;84:7159–7163.
4. Kokai Y, Myers JN, Wada T, et al. Synergistic interaction of p185c-neu and the EGF receptor leads to transformation of rodent fibroblasts. *Cell* 1989;58:287–292.
5. Muller WJ, Sinn E, Pattengale PK, et al. Single-step induction of mammary adenocarcinoma in transgenic mice bearing the activated c-neu oncogene. *Cell* 1988;54:105–115.
6. Bouchard L, Lamarre L, Tremblay PJ, et al. Stochastic appearance of mammary tumors in transgenic mice carrying the MMTV/c-neu oncogene. *Cell* 1989;57:931–936.
7. Ben-Levy R, Paterson HF, Marshall CJ, et al. A single autophosphorylation site confers oncogenicity to the Neu/ErbB-2 receptor and enables coupling to the MAP kinase pathway. *Embo J* 1994;13:3302–3311.
8. Dankort DL, Wang Z, Blackmore V, et al. Distinct tyrosine autophosphorylation sites negatively and positively modulate neu-mediated transformation. *Mol Cell Biol* 1997;17:5410–5425.
9. Ware JL, Maygarden SJ, Koontz WW Jr, et al. Immunohistochemical detection of c-erbB-2 protein in human benign and neoplastic prostate. *Hum Pathol* 1991;22:254–258.
10. Robinson D, He F, Pretlow T, et al. A tyrosine kinase profile of prostate carcinoma. *Proc Natl Acad Sci U S A* 1996;93:5958–5962.
11. Lyne JC, Melhem MF, Finley GG, et al. Tissue expression of neu differentiation factor/heregulin and its receptor complex in prostate cancer and its biologic effects on prostate cancer cells in vitro. *Cancer J Sci Am* 1997;3:21–30.
12. Bubendorf L, Kononen J, Koivisto P, et al. Survey of gene amplifications during prostate cancer progression by high-throughout fluorescence in situ hybridization on tissue microarrays [published erratum appears in *Cancer Res* 1999;59:1388]. *Cancer Res* 1999;59:803–806.
13. Mark HF, Feldman D, Das S, et al. Fluorescence in situ hybridization study of HER-2/neu oncogene amplification in prostate cancer. *Exp Mol Pathol* 1999;66:170–178.
14. Fournier G, Latil A, Amet Y, et al. Gene amplifications in advanced-stage human prostate cancer. *Urol Res* 1995;22:343–347.
15. Latil A, Baron JC, Cussenot O, et al. Oncogene amplifications in early-stage human prostate carcinomas. *Int J Cancer* 1994;59:637–638.
16. Ross JS, Sheehan C, Hayner-Buchan AM, et al. HER-2/neu gene amplification status in prostate cancer by fluorescence in situ hybridization. *Hum Pathol* 1997;28:827–833.
17. Kaltz-Wittmer C, Klenk U, Glaessgen A, et al. FISH analysis of gene aberrations (MYC, CCND1, ERBB2, RB, and AR) in advanced prostatic carcinomas before and after androgen deprivation therapy. *Lab Invest* 2000;80:1455–1464.
18. Signoretti S, Montironi R, Manola J, et al. Her-2-neu expression and progression toward androgen independence in prostate cancer. *J Natl Cancer Inst* 2000;92:1918–1925.
19. Olapade-Olaopa EO, Moscatello DK, MacKay EH, et al. Evidence for the differential expression of a variant EGF

receptor protein in human prostate cancer. *Br J Cancer* 2000;82:186–194.

20. Leav I, McNeal JE, Ziar J, et al. The localization of transforming growth factor alpha and epidermal growth factor receptor in stromal and epithelial compartments of developing human prostate and hyperplastic, dysplastic, and carcinomatous lesions. *Hum Pathol* 1998;29:668–675.
21. Malden LT, Novak U, Kaye AH, et al. Selective amplification of the cytoplasmic domain of the epidermal growth factor receptor gene in glioblastoma multiforme. *Cancer Res* 1988;48:2711–2714.
22. Steck PA, Lee P, Hung MC, et al. Expression of an altered epidermal growth factor receptor by human glioblastoma cells. *Cancer Res* 1988;48:5433–5439.
23. Sugawa N, Ekstrand AJ, James CD, et al. Identical splicing of aberrant epidermal growth factor receptor transcripts from amplified rearranged genes in human glioblastomas. *Proc Natl Acad Sci U S A* 1990;87:8602–8606.
24. Craft N, Shostak Y, Carey M, et al. A mechanism for hormone-independent prostate cancer through modulation of androgen receptor signaling by the HER-2/neu tyrosine kinase [see comments]. *Nat Med* 1999;5:280–285.
25. Kato S, Endoh H, Masuhiro Y, et al. Activation of the estrogen receptor through phosphorylation by mitogen-activated protein kinase. *Science* 1995;270:1491–1494.
26. Tremblay A, Tremblay GB, Labrie F, et al. Ligand-independent recruitment of SRC-1 to estrogen receptor beta through phosphorylation of activation function AF-1. *Mol Cell* 1999;3:513–519.
27. Font de Mora J, Brown M. AIB1 is a conduit for kinase-mediated growth factor signaling to the estrogen receptor. *Mol Cell Biol* 2000;20:5041–5047.
28. Bunone G, Briand PA, Miksicek RJ, et al. Activation of the unliganded estrogen receptor by EGF involves the MAP kinase pathway and direct phosphorylation. *Embo J* 1996;15:2174-2183.
29. Gioeli D, Mandell JW, Petroni GR, et al. Activation of mitogen-activated protein kinase associated with prostate cancer progression. *Cancer Res* 1999;59:279–284.
30. Parada LF, Tabin CJ, Shih C, et al. Human EJ bladder carcinoma oncogene is homologue of Harvey sarcoma virus ras gene. *Nature* 1982;297:474-478.
31. Parada LF, Land H, Weinberg RA, et al. Cooperation between gene encoding p53 tumour antigen and ras in cellular transformation. *Nature* 1984;312:649–651.
32. Newbold RF, Overell RW. Fibroblast immortality is a prerequisite for transformation by EJ c-Ha-ras oncogene. *Nature* 1983;304:648–651.
33. Peehl DM, Wehner N, Stamey TA. Activated Ki-ras oncogene in human prostatic adenocarcinoma. *Prostate* 1987;10: 281–289.
34. Vazquez F, Sellers WR. The PTEN tumor suppressor protein: an antagonist of phosphoinositide 3-kinase signaling. *Biochim Biophys Acta* 2000;1470:M21–M35.
35. Datta SR, Brunet A, Greenberg ME. Cellular survival: a play in three Akts. *Genes Dev* 1999;13:2905–2927.
36. Maehama T, Dixon JE. The tumor suppressor, PTEN/MMAC1, dephosphorylates the lipid second messenger, phosphatidylinositol 3,4,5-trisphosphate. *J Biol Chem* 1998;273:13375–13378.
37. Ramaswamy S, Nakamura N, Vazquez F, et al. Regulation of G1 progression by the PTEN tumor suppressor protein is linked to inhibition of the phosphatidylinositol 3-kinase/Akt pathway. *Proc Natl Acad Sci U S A* 1999;96:2110–2115.
38. Stambolic V, Suzuki A, de la Pompa JL, et al. Negative regulation of PKB/Akt-dependent cell survival by the tumor suppressor PTEN. *Cell* 1998;95:29–39.
39. Li D, Sun H. PTEN/MMAC1/TEP1 suppresses the tumorigenicity and induces G1 cell cycle arrest in human glioblastoma cells. *Proc Natl Acad Sci U S A* 1998;95:15406–15411.
40. Myers MP, Pass I, Batty IH, et al. The lipid phosphatase activity of PTEN is critical for its tumor suppressor function. *Proc Natl Acad Sci U S A* 1998;95:13513–13518.
41. Wu X, Senechal K, Neshat MS, et al. The PTEN/MMAC1 tumor suppressor phosphatase functions as a negative regulator of the phosphoinositide 3-kinase/Akt pathway. *Proc Natl Acad Sci U S A* 1998;95:15587–15591.
42. Dahia PLM, Aguiar RCT, Alberta J, et al. PTEN is inversely correlated with the cell survival factor Akt/PKB and is inactivated via multiple mechanisms in haematological malignancies. *Hum Mol Genet* 1999;8:185–193.
43. Davies MA, Koul D, Dhesi H, et al. Regulation of Akt/PKB activity, cellular growth, and apoptosis in prostate carcinoma cells by MMAC/PTEN. *Cancer Res* 1999;59:2551–2556.
44. Haas-Kogan D, Shalev N, Wong M, et al. Protein kinase B (PKB/Akt) activity is elevated in glioblastoma cells due to mutation of the tumor suppressor PTEN/MMAC. *Curr Biol* 1998;8:1195–1198.
45. Nakamura N, Ramaswamy S, Vazquez F, et al. Forkhead transcription factors are critical effectors of cell death and cell cycle arrest downstream of PTEN. *Mol Cell Biol* 2000; 20:8969–8982.
46. Mantzoros CS, Tzonou A, Signorello LB, et al. Insulin-like growth factor 1 in relation to prostate cancer and benign prostatic hyperplasia [see comments]. *Br J Cancer* 1997;76: 1115–1118.
47. Wolk A, Mantzoros CS, Andersson SO, et al. Insulin-like growth factor 1 and prostate cancer risk: a population-based case-control study [see comments]. *J Natl Cancer Inst* 1998;90:911–915.
48. Chan JM, Stampfer MJ, Giovannucci E, et al. Plasma insulin-like growth factor-I and prostate cancer risk: a prospective study [see comments]. *Science* 1998;279:563–566.
49. Giovannucci E. Insulin-like growth factor-I and binding protein-3 and risk of cancer. *Horm Res* 1999;51:34–41.
50. DiGiovanni J, Kiguchi K, Frijhoff A, et al. Deregulated expression of insulin-like growth factor 1 in prostate epithelium leads to neoplasia in transgenic mice. *Proc Natl Acad Sci U S A* 2000;97:3455–3460.
51. Chott A, Sun Z, Morganstern D, et al. Tyrosine kinases expressed in vivo by human prostate cancer bone marrow metastases and loss of the type 1 insulin-like growth factor receptor. *Am J Pathol* 1999;155:1271–1279.
52. Klippel A, Escobedo MA, Wachowicz MS, et al. Activation of phosphatidylinositol 3-kinase is sufficient for cell cycle entry and promotes cellular changes characteristic of oncogenic transformation. *Mol Cell Biol* 1998;18:5699–5711.
53. Sell C, Rubini M, Rubin R, et al. Simian virus 40 large tumor antigen is unable to transform mouse embryonic

fibroblasts lacking type 1 insulin-like growth factor receptor. *Proc Natl Acad Sci U S A* 1993;90:11217–11221.

54. Plymate SR, Tennant M, Birnbaum RS, et al. The effect on the insulin-like growth factor system in human prostate epithelial cells of immortalization and transformation by simian virus-40 T antigen. *J Clin Endocrinol Metab* 1996;81: 3709–3716.
55. Plymate SR, Bae VL, Maddison L, et al. Reexpression of the type 1 insulin-like growth factor receptor inhibits the malignant phenotype of simian virus 40 T antigen immortalized human prostate epithelial cells. *Endocrinology* 1997;138: 1728–1735.
56. Plymate SS, Bae VL, Maddison L, et al. Type-1 insulin-like growth factor receptor reexpression in the malignant phenotype of SV40-T-immortalized human prostate epithelial cells enhances apoptosis. *Endocrine* 1997;7:119–124.
57. Li J, Yen C, Liaw D, et al. PTEN, a putative protein tyrosine phosphatase gene mutated in human brain, breast, and prostate cancer. *Science* 1997;275:1943–1947.
58. Li DM, Sun H. TEP1, encoded by a candidate tumor suppressor locus, is a novel protein tyrosine phosphatase regulated by transforming growth factor beta. *Cancer Res* 1997;57:2124–2129.
59. Steck PA, Pershouse MA, Jasser SA, et al. Identification of a candidate tumour suppressor gene, MMAC1, at chromosome 10q23.3 that is mutated in multiple advanced cancers. *Nat Genet* 1997;15:356–362.
60. Liaw D, Marsh DJ, Li J, et al. Germline mutations of the PTEN gene in Cowden disease, an inherited breast and thyroid cancer syndrome. *Nat Genet* 1997;16:64–67.
61. Marsh DJ, Dahia PL, Zheng Z, et al. Germline mutations in PTEN are present in Bannayan-Zonana syndrome. *Nat Genet* 1997;16:333–334.
62. Gray IC, Phillips SM, Lee SJ, et al. Loss of the chromosomal region 10q23-25 in prostate cancer. *Cancer Res* 1995;55:4800–4803.
63. Carter BS, Ewing CM, Ward WS, et al. Allelic loss of chromosomes 16q and 10q in human prostate cancer. *Proc Natl Acad Sci U S A* 1990;87:8751–8755.
64. Rubin MA, Gerstein A, Reid K, et al. 10q23.3 loss of heterozygosity is higher in lymph node-positive (pT2-3,N+) versus lymph node-negative (pT2-3,N0) prostate cancer. *Hum Pathol* 2000;31:504–508.
65. Latil A, Baron JC, Cussenot O, et al. Genetic alterations in localized prostate cancer: identification of a common region of deletion on chromosome arm 18q. *Genes Chromosomes Cancer* 1994;11:119–125.
66. Lacombe L, Orlow I, Reuter VE, et al. Microsatellite instability and deletion analysis of chromosome 10 in human prostate cancer. *Int J Cancer* 1996;69:110–113.
67. Trybus TM, Burgess AC, Wojno KJ, et al. Distinct areas of allelic loss on chromosomal regions 10p and 10q in human prostate cancer. *Cancer Res* 1996;56:2263–2267.
68. Komiya A, Suzuki H, Ueda T, et al. Allelic losses at loci on chromosome 10 are associated with metastasis and progression of human prostate cancer. *Genes Chromosomes Cancer* 1996;17:245–253.
69. Suzuki H, Freije D, Nusskern DR, et al. Interfocal heterogeneity of PTEN/MMAC1 gene alterations in multiple metastatic prostate cancer tissues. *Cancer Res* 1998;58:204–209.
70. McMenamin ME, Soung P, Perera S, et al. Loss of PTEN expression in paraffin-embedded primary prostate cancer correlates with high Gleason score and advanced stage. *Cancer Res* 1999;59:4291–4296.
71. Rhei E, Kang L, Bogomolniy F, et al. Mutation analysis of the putative tumor suppressor gene PTEN/MMAC1 in primary breast carcinomas. *Cancer Res* 1997;57:3657–3659.
72. Feilotter HE, Coulon V, McVeigh JL, et al. Analysis of the 10q23 chromosomal region and the PTEN gene in human sporadic breast carcinoma. *Br J Cancer* 1999;79:718–723.
73. Freihoff D, Kempe A, Beste B, et al. Exclusion of a major role for the PTEN tumour-suppressor gene in breast carcinomas. *Br J Cancer* 1999;79:754–758.
74. Stambolic V, Tsao MS, Macpherson D, et al. High incidence of breast and endometrial neoplasia resembling human Cowden syndrome in pten+/– mice. *Cancer Res* 2000;60:3605–3611.
75. Knudson AG Jr., Hethcote HW, Brown BW. Mutation and childhood cancer: a probabilistic model for the incidence of retinoblastoma. *Proc Natl Acad Sci U S A* 1975;72:5116–5120.
76. Whang YE, Wu X, Suzuki H, et al. Inactivation of the tumor suppressor PTEN/MMAC1 in advanced human prostate cancer through loss of expression. *Proc Natl Acad Sci U S A* 1998;95:5246–5250.
77. Zhou XP, Gimm O, Hampel H, et al. Epigenetic PTEN silencing in malignant melanomas without PTEN mutation. *Am J Pathol* 2000;157:1123–1128.
78. Perren A, Weng LP, Boag AH, et al. Immunohistochemical evidence of loss of PTEN expression in primary ductal adenocarcinomas of the breast. *Am J Pathol* 1999;155:1253–1260.
79. Di Cristofano A, Pesce B, Cordon-Cardo C, et al. Pten is essential for embryonic development and tumour suppression. *Nat Genet* 1998;19:348–355.
80. Chang HW, Aoki M, Fruman D, et al. Transformation of chicken cells by the gene encoding the catalytic subunit of PI 3-kinase. *Science* 1997;276:1848–1850.
81. Shayesteh L, Lu Y, Kuo WL, et al. PIK3CA is implicated as an oncogene in ovarian cancer. *Nat Genet* 1999;21:99–102.
82. Ma YY, Wei SJ, Lin YC, et al. PIK3CA as an oncogene in cervical cancer. *Oncogene* 2000;19:2739–2744.
83. Racz A, Brass N, Heckel D, et al. Expression analysis of genes at 3q26-q27 involved in frequent amplification in squamous cell lung carcinoma. *Eur J Cancer* 1999;35:641–646.
84. Jimenez C, Jones DR, Rodriguez-Viciana P, et al. Identification and characterization of a new oncogene derived from the regulatory subunit of phosphoinositide 3-kinase. *Embo J* 1998;17:743–753.
85. Staal SP. Molecular cloning of the akt oncogene and its human homologues AKT1 and AKT2: amplification of AKT1 in a primary human gastric adenocarcinoma. *Proc Natl Acad Sci U S A* 1987;84:5034–5037.
86. Staal SP, Hartley JW. Thymic lymphoma induction by the AKT8 murine retrovirus. *J Exp Med* 1988;167:1259–1264.
87. Cheng JQ, Godwin AK, Bellacosa A, et al. AKT2, a putative oncogene encoding a member of a subfamily of protein-serine/threonine kinases, is amplified in human ovarian carcinomas. *Proc Natl Acad Sci U S A* 1992;89:9267–9271.
88. Bellacosa A, de Feo D, Godwin AK, et al. Molecular alterations of the AKT2 oncogene in ovarian and breast carcinomas. *Int J Cancer* 1995;64:280–285.

89. Thompson FH, Nelson MA, Trent JM, et al. Amplification of 19q13.1-q13.2 sequences in ovarian cancer. G-band, FISH, and molecular studies. *Cancer Genet Cytogenet* 1996;87:55–62.
90. Cheng JQ, Ruggeri B, Klein WM, et al. Amplification of AKT2 in human pancreatic cells and inhibition of AKT2 expression and tumorigenicity by antisense RNA. *Proc Natl Acad Sci U S A* 1996;93:3636–3641.
91. Miwa W, Yasuda J, Murakami Y, et al. Isolation of DNA sequences amplified at chromosome 19q13.1-q13.2 including the AKT2 locus in human pancreatic cancer. *Biochem Biophys Res Commun* 1996;225:968–974.
92. Ruggeri BA, Huang L, Wood M, et al. Amplification and overexpression of the AKT2 oncogene in a subset of human pancreatic ductal adenocarcinomas. *Mol Carcinog* 1998;21: 81–86.
93. Massague J, Chen YG. Controlling TGF-beta signaling. *Genes Dev* 2000;14:627–644.
94. Markowitz S, Wang J, Myeroff L, et al. Inactivation of the type II TGF-beta receptor in colon cancer cells with microsatellite instability. *Science* 1995;268:1336–1338.
95. Eppert K, Scherer SW, Ozcelik H, et al. MADR2 maps to 18q21 and encodes a TGFbeta-regulated MAD-related protein that is functionally mutated in colorectal carcinoma. *Cell* 1996;86:543–552.
96. Riggins GJ, Thiagalingam S, Rozenblum E, et al. Mad-related genes in the human. *Nat Genet* 1996;13:347–349.
97. Hahn SA, Schutte M, Hoque AT, et al. DPC4, a candidate tumor suppressor gene at human chromosome 18q21.1. *Science* 1996;271:350–353.
98. Tang B, de Castro K, Barnes HE, et al. Loss of responsiveness to transforming growth factor beta induces malignant transformation of nontumorigenic rat prostate epithelial cells. *Cancer Res* 1999;59:4834–4842.
99. Kim IY, Ahn HJ, Zelner DJ, et al. Loss of expression of transforming growth factor beta type I and type II receptors correlates with tumor grade in human prostate cancer tissues. *Clin Cancer Res* 1996;2:1255–1261.
100. Guo Y, Kyprianou N. Restoration of transforming growth factor beta signaling pathway in human prostate cancer cells suppresses tumorigenicity via induction of caspase-1-mediated apoptosis. *Cancer Res* 1999;59:1366–1371.
101. Guo Y, Jacobs SC, Kyprianou N. Down-regulation of protein and mRNA expression for transforming growth factor-beta (TGF-betal) type I and type II receptors in human prostate cancer. *Int J Cancer* 1997;71:573–579.
102. Kim IY, Ahn HJ, Lang S, et al. Loss of expression of transforming growth factor-beta receptors is associated with poor prognosis in prostate cancer patients. *Clin Cancer Res* 1998;4:1625–1630.
103. Truong LD, Kadmon D, McCune BK, et al. Association of transforming growth factor-beta 1 with prostate cancer: an immunohistochemical study. *Hum Pathol* 1993;24:4–9.
104. Steiner MS, Zhou ZZ, Tonb DC, et al. Expression of transforming growth factor-beta 1 in prostate cancer. *Endocrinology* 1994;135:2240–2247.
105. Eastham JA, Truong LD, Rogers E, et al. Transforming growth factor-beta 1: comparative immunohistochemical localization in human primary and metastatic prostate cancer. *Lab Invest* 1995;73:628–635.
106. Latil A, Pesche S, Valeri A, et al. Expression and mutational analysis of the MADR2/Smad2 gene in human prostate cancer. *Prostate* 1999;40:225–231.
107. Nusse R, van Ooyen A, Cox D, et al. Mode of proviral activation of a putative mammary oncogene (int-1) on mouse chromosome 15. *Nature* 1984;307:131–136.
108. Polakis P. Wnt signaling and cancer. *Genes Dev* 2000;14: 1837–1851.
109. Bienz M, Clevers H. Linking colorectal cancer to Wnt signaling. *Cell* 2000;103:311–320.
110. Iozzo RV, Eichstetter I, Danielson KG. Aberrant expression of the growth factor Wnt-5A in human malignancy. *Cancer Res* 1995;55:3495–3499.
111. Brewster SF, Browne S, Brown KW. Somatic allelic loss at the DCC, APC, nm23-H1 and p53 tumor suppressor gene loci in human prostatic carcinoma. *J Urol* 1994;151:1073–1077.
112. Phillips SM, Morton DG, Lee SJ, et al. Loss of heterozygosity of the retinoblastoma and adenomatous polyposis susceptibility gene loci and in chromosomes 10p, 10q and 16q in human prostate cancer. *Br J Urol* 1994;73:390–395.
113. Watanabe M, Kakiuchi H, Kato H, et al. APC gene mutations in human prostate cancer. *Jpn J Clin Oncol* 1996;26: 77–81.
114. Suzuki H, Aida S, Akimoto S, et al. State of adenomatous polyposis coli gene and ras oncogenes in Japanese prostate cancer. *Jpn J Cancer Res* 1994;85:847–852.
115. Voeller HJ, Truica CI, Gelmann EP. Beta-catenin mutations in human prostate cancer. *Cancer Res* 1998;58:2520–2523.
116. McMahon AP. More surprises in the Hedgehog signaling pathway. *Cell* 2000;100:185–188.
117. Podlasek CA, Barnett DH, Clemens JQ, et al. Prostate development requires Sonic hedgehog expressed by the urogenital sinus epithelium. *Dev Biol* 1999;209:28–39.
118. Wetmore C, Eberhart DE, Curran T. The normal patched allele is expressed in medulloblastomas from mice with heterozygous germ-line mutation of patched. *Cancer Res* 2000;60:2239–2246.
119. Zurawel RH, Allen C, Chiappa S, et al. Analysis of PTCH/SMO/SHH pathway genes in medulloblastoma. *Genes Chromosomes Cancer* 2000;27:44–51.
120. Dong J, Gailani MR, Pomeroy SL, et al. Identification of PATCHED mutations in medulloblastomas by direct sequencing. *Hum Mutat* 2000;16:89–90.
121. Xie J, Murone M, Luoh SM, et al. Activating Smoothened mutations in sporadic basal-cell carcinoma. *Nature* 1998; 391:90–92.
122. Fan H, Oro AE, Scott MP, et al. Induction of basal cell carcinoma features in transgenic human skin expressing Sonic Hedgehog. *Nat Med* 1997;3:788–792.
123. Oro AE, Higgins KM, Hu Z, et al. Basal cell carcinomas in mice overexpressing sonic hedgehog. *Science* 1997;276:817–821.
124. Stone DM, Murone M, Luoh, S, et al. Characterization of the human suppressor of fused, a negative regulator of the zinc-finger transcription factor Gli. *J Cell Sci* 1999;112: 4437–4448.
125. Li FP, Fraumeni JF Jr. Soft-tissue sarcomas, breast cancer, and other neoplasms. A familial syndrome? *Ann Intern Med* 1969;71:747–752.

126. Malkin D, Li FP, Strong LC, et al. Germ line p53 mutations in a familial syndrome of breast cancer, sarcomas, and other neoplasms. *Science* 1990;250:1233–1238.
127. Srivastava S, Zou ZQ, Pirollo K, et al. Germ-line transmission of a mutated p53 gene in a cancer-prone family with Li-Fraumeni syndrome. *Nature* 1990;348:747–749.
128. Li FP, Fraumeni JF Jr., Mulvihill JJ, et al. A cancer family syndrome in twenty-four kindreds. *Cancer Res* 1988;48: 5358–5362.
129. Shieh SY, Ahn J, Tamai K, et al. The human homologs of checkpoint kinases Chk1 and Cds1 (Chk2) phosphorylate p53 at multiple DNA damage-inducible sites [published erratum appears in *Genes Dev* 2000;14:750]. *Genes Dev* 2000;14:289–300.
130. Flaggs G, Plug AW, Dunks KM, et al. Atm-dependent interactions of a mammalian chk1 homolog with meiotic chromosomes. *Curr Biol* 1997;7:977–986.
131. Bell DW, Varley JM, Szydlo TE, et al. Heterozygous germ line hCHK2 mutations in Li-Fraumeni syndrome. *Science* 1999;286:2528–2531.
132. Honda R, Tanaka H, Yasuda H. Oncoprotein MDM2 is a ubiquitin ligase E3 for tumor suppressor p53. *FEBS Lett* 1997;420:25–27.
133. Fuchs SY, Adler V, Buschmann T, et al. Mdm2 association with p53 targets its ubiquitination. *Oncogene* 1998;17: 2543–2547.
134. Quelle DE, Zindy F, Ashmun RA, et al. Alternative reading frames of the INK4a tumor suppressor gene encode two unrelated proteins capable of inducing cell cycle arrest. *Cell* 1995;83:993–1000.
135. Kamijo T, Zindy F, Roussel MF, et al. Tumor suppression at the mouse INK4a locus mediated by the alternative reading frame product p19ARF. *Cell* 1997;91:649–659.
136. Pomerantz J, Schreiber-Agus N, Liegeois, NJ, et al. The Ink4a tumor suppressor gene product, p19Arf, interacts with MDM2 and neutralizes MDM2's inhibition of p53. *Cell* 1998;92:713–723.
137. Kamijo T, Weber JD, Zambetti G, et al. Functional and physical interactions of the ARF tumor suppressor with p53 and Mdm2. *Proc Natl Acad Sci U S A* 1998;95:8292–8297.
138. Tao W, Levine AJ. P19(ARF) stabilizes p53 by blocking nucleo-cytoplasmic shuttling of Mdm2. *Proc Natl Acad Sci U S A* 1999;96:6937–6941.
139. Zhang Y, Xiong Y, Yarbrough WG. ARF promotes MDM2 degradation and stabilizes p53: ARF-INK4a locus deletion impairs both the Rb and p53 tumor suppression pathways. *Cell* 1998;92:725–734.
140. de Stanchina E, McCurrach ME, Zindy F, et al. E1A signaling to p53 involves the p19(ARF) tumor suppressor. *Genes Dev* 1998;12:2434–2442.
141. Zindy F, Eischen CM, Randle DH, et al. Myc signaling via the ARF tumor suppressor regulates p53-dependent apoptosis and immortalization. *Genes Dev* 1998;12:2424–2433.
142. Momand J, Jung D, Wilczynski S, et al. The MDM2 gene amplification database. *Nucleic Acids Res* 1998;26:3453–3459.
143. Agus DB, Cardon-Cardo C, Fox W, et al. Prostate cancer cell cycle regulators: response to androgen withdrawal and development of androgen independence. *J Natl Cancer Inst* 1999;91:1869–1876.
144. Ittmann M, Wieczorek R, Heller P, et al. Alterations in the p53 and MDM-2 genes are infrequent in clinically localized, stage B prostate adenocarcinomas. *Am J Pathol* 1994;145:287–293.
145. Osman I, Drobnjak M, Fazzari M, et al. Inactivation of the p53 pathway in prostate cancer: impact on tumor progression. *Clin Cancer Res* 1999;5:2082–2088.
146. Liu L, Goldstein AM, Tucker MA, et al. Affected members of melanoma-prone families with linkage to 9p21 but lacking mutations in CDKN2A do not harbor mutations in the coding regions of either CDKN2B or p19ARF. *Genes Chromosomes Cancer* 1997;19:52–54.
147. Fargnoli MC, Chimenti S, Keller G, et al. CDKN2a/p16INK4a mutations and lack of p19ARF involvement in familial melanoma kindreds. *J Invest Dermatol* 1998;111: 1202–1206.
148. Brenner AJ, Paladugu A, Wang H, et al. Preferential loss of expression of p16(INK4a) rather than p19(ARF) in breast cancer. *Clin Cancer Res* 1996;2:1993–1998.
149. Kumar R, Sauroja I, Punnonen K, et al. Selective deletion of exon 1 beta of the p19ARF gene in metastatic melanoma cell lines. *Genes Chromosomes Cancer* 1998;23:273–277.
150. Gardie B, Cayuela JM, Martini S, et al. Genomic alterations of the p19ARF encoding exons in T-cell acute lymphoblastic leukemia. *Blood* 1998;91:1016–1020.
151. Gao X, Porter AT, Honn KV. Involvement of the multiple tumor suppressor genes and 12-lipoxygenase in human prostate cancer. Therapeutic implications. *Adv Exp Med Biol* 1997;407:41–53.
152. Sellers WR, Kaelin WG Jr. Role of the retinoblastoma protein in the pathogenesis of human cancer. *J Clin Oncol* 1997;15:3301–3312.
153. Weintraub SJ, Prater CA, Dean DC. Retinoblastoma protein switches the E2F site from positive to negative element. *Nature* 1992;358:259–261.
154. Weintraub SJ, Chow KN, Luo RX, et al. Mechanism of active transcriptional repression by the retinoblastoma protein. *Nature* 1995;375:812–815.
155. Sellers WR, Rodgers JW, Kaelin WG Jr. A potent transrepression domain in the retinoblastoma protein induces a cell cycle arrest when bound to E2F sites. *Proc Natl Acad Sci U S A* 1995;92:11544–11548.
156. Yamasaki L, Bronson R, Williams BO, et al. Loss of E2F-1 reduces tumorigenesis and extends the lifespan of Rb1(+/–) mice. *Nat Genet* 1998;18:360–364.
157. Yamasaki L, Jacks T, Bronson R, et al. Tumor induction and tissue atrophy in mice lacking E2F-1. *Cell* 1996;85:537–548.
158. Xu G, Livingston DM, Krek W. Multiple members of the E2F transcription factor family are the products of oncogenes. *Proc Natl Acad Sci U S A* 1995;92:1357–1361.
159. Yang XH, Sladek TL. Overexpression of the E2F-1 transcription factor gene mediates cell transformation. *Gene Expr* 1995;4:195–204.
160. Singh P, Wong SH, Hong W. Overexpression of E2F-1 in rat embryo fibroblasts leads to neoplastic transformation. *Embo J* 1994;13:3329–3338.
161. Beijersbergen RL, Kerkhoven RM, Zhu L, et al. E2F-4, a new member of the E2F gene family, has oncogenic activity and associates with p107 in vivo. *Genes Dev* 1994;8:2680–2690.

162. Souza RF, Yin J, Smolinski KN, et al. Frequent mutation of the E2F-4 cell cycle gene in primary human gastrointestinal tumors. *Cancer Res* 1997;57:2350–2353.
163. Kim JJ, Baek MJ, Kim L, et al. Accumulated frameshift mutations at coding nucleotide repeats during the progression of gastric carcinoma with microsatellite instability. *Lab Invest* 1999;79:1113–1120.
164. Yoshitaka T, Matsubara N, Ikeda M, et al. Mutations of E2F-4 trinucleotide repeats in colorectal cancer with microsatellite instability. *Biochem Biophys Res Commun* 1996;227: 553–557.
165. Zhao J, Dynlacht B, Imai T, et al. Expression of NPAT, a novel substrate of cyclin E-CDK2, promotes S-phase entry. *Genes Dev* 1998;12:456–461.
166. Zhao J, Kennedy BK, Lawrence BD, et al. NPAT links cyclin E-Cdk2 to the regulation of replication-dependent histone gene transcription. *Genes Dev* 2000;14:2283–2297.
167. Ma T, Van Tine BA, Wei Y, et al. Cell cycle-regulated phosphorylation of p220 (NPAT) by cyclin E/Cdk2 in Cajal bodies promotes histone gene transcription. *Genes Dev* 2000;14:2298–2313.
168. Greenberg NM, DeMayo F, Finegold MJ, et al. Prostate cancer in a transgenic mouse. *Proc Natl Acad Sci U S A* 1995;92:3439–3443.
169. Wang Y, Hayward S, Donjacour A, et al. Sex hormone-induced prostatic carcinogenesis in Rb-deficient prostate tissue. *Cancer Res* 2000;60:6008–6017.
170. Wang TC, Cardiff RD, Zukerberg L, et al. Mammary hyperplasia and carcinoma in MMTV-cyclin D1 transgenic mice. *Nature* 1994;369:669–671.
171. Gumbiner LM, Gumerlock PH, Mack PC, et al. Overexpression of cyclin D1 is rare in human prostate carcinoma. *Prostate* 1999;38:40–45.
172. Han EK, Lim JT, Arber N, et al. Cyclin D1 expression in human prostate carcinoma cell lines and primary tumors. *Prostate* 1998;35:95–101.
173. Aaltomaa S, Eskelinen M, Lipponen P. Expression of cyclin A and D proteins in prostate cancer and their relation to clinopathological variables and patient survival. *Prostate* 1999;38:175–182.
174. Herman JG, Merlo A, Mao L, et al. Inactivation of the CDKN2/p16/MTS1 gene is frequently associated with aberrant DNA methylation in all common human cancers. *Cancer Res* 1995;55:4525–4530.
175. Fero ML, Randel E, Gurley KE, et al. The murine gene p27Kip1 is haplo-insufficient for tumour suppression. *Nature* 1998;396:177–180.
176. Fero ML, Rivkin M, Tasch M, et al. A syndrome of multiorgan hyperplasia with features of gigantism, tumorigenesis, and female sterility in p27(Kip1)-deficient mice. *Cell* 1996;85:733–744.
177. Loda M, Cukor B, Tam SW, et al. Increased proteasome-dependent degradation of the cyclin-dependent kinase inhibitor p27 in aggressive colorectal carcinomas. *Nat Med* 1997;3:231–234.
178. Piva R, Cancelli I, Cavalla P, et al. Proteasome-dependent degradation of p27/kip1 in gliomas. *J Neuropathol Exp Neurol* 1999;58:691–696.
179. Taplin ME, Bubley GJ, Shuster TD, et al. Mutation of the androgen-receptor gene in metastatic androgen-independent prostate cancer [see comments]. *N Engl J Med* 1995;332:1393–1398.
180. Taplin ME, Bubley GJ, Ko YJ, et al. Selection for androgen receptor mutations in prostate cancers treated with androgen antagonist. *Cancer Res* 1999;59:2511–2515.
181. Newmark JR, Hardy DO, Tonb DC, et al. Androgen receptor gene mutations in human prostate cancer. *Proc Natl Acad Sci U S A* 1992;89:6319–6323.
182. Suzuki H, Sato N, Watabe Y, et al. Androgen receptor gene mutations in human prostate cancer. *J Steroid Biochem Mol Biol* 1993;46:759–765.
183. Gaddipati JP, McLeod DG, Heidenberg HB, et al. Frequent detection of codon 877 mutation in the androgen receptor gene in advanced prostate cancers. *Cancer Res* 1994; 54:2861–2864.
184. Koivisto P, Visakorpi T, Kallioniemi OP. Androgen receptor gene amplification: a novel molecular mechanism for endocrine therapy resistance in human prostate cancer. *Scand J Clin Lab Invest Suppl* 1996;226:57–63.
185. Palmberg C, Koivisto P, Hyytinen E, et al. Androgen receptor gene amplification in a recurrent prostate cancer after monotherapy with the nonsteroidal potent antiandrogen Casodex (bicalutamide) with a subsequent favorable response to maximal androgen blockade. *Eur Urol* 1997; 31:216–219.
186. Foley KP, Eisenman RN. Two MAD tails: what the recent knockouts of Mad1 and Mxi1 tell us about the MYC/MAX/MAD network. *Biochim Biophys Acta* 1999;1423:M37–M47.
187. Lahoz EG, Xu L, Schreiber-Agus N, et al. Suppression of Myc, but not E1a, transformation activity by Max-associated proteins, Mad and Mxi1. *Proc Natl Acad Sci U S A* 1994;91:5503–5507.
188. Schreiber-Agus N, Meng Y, Hoang T, et al. Role of Mxi1 in ageing organ systems and the regulation of normal and neoplastic growth. *Nature* 1998;393:483–487.
189. Sato K, Qian J, Slezak JM, et al. Clinical significance of alterations of chromosome 8 in high-grade, advanced, nonmetastatic prostate carcinoma. *J Natl Cancer Inst* 1999;91: 1574–1580.
190. He WW, Sciavolino PJ, Wing J, et al. A novel human prostate-specific, androgen-regulated homeobox gene (NKX3.1) that maps to 8p21, a region frequently deleted in prostate cancer. *Genomics* 1997;43:69–77.
191. Prescott JL, Blok L, Tindall DJ. Isolation and androgen regulation of the human homeobox cDNA, NKX3.1. *Prostate* 1998;35:71–80.
192. Tanaka M, Komuro I, Inagaki H, et al. Nkx3.1, a murine homolog of drosophila bagpipe, regulates epithelial ductal branching and proliferation of the prostate and palatine glands. *Dev Dyn* 2000;219:248–260.
193. Sciavolino PJ, Abrams EW, Yang L, et al. Tissue-specific expression of murine Nkx3.1 in the male urogenital system. *Dev Dyn* 1997;209:127–138.
194. Bhatia-Gaur R, Donjacour AA, Sciavolino PJ, et al. Roles for Nkx3.1 in prostate development and cancer. *Genes Dev* 1999;13:966–977.
195. Voeller HJ, Augustus M, Madike V, et al. Coding region of NKX3.1, a prostate-specific homeobox gene on 8p21, is not mutated in human prostate cancers. *Cancer Res* 1997;57: 4455–4459.

196. Kagan J, Stein J, Babaian RJ, et al. Homozygous deletions at 8p22 and 8p21 in prostate cancer implicate these regions as the sites for candidate tumor suppressor genes. *Oncogene* 1995;11:2121–2126.
197. Suzuki H, Emi M, Komiya A, et al. Localization of a tumor suppressor gene associated with progression of human prostate cancer within a 1.2 Mb region of 8p22-p21.3. *Genes Chromosomes Cancer* 1995;13:168–174.
198. MacGrogan D, Levy A, Bostwick D, et al. Loss of chromosome arm 8p loci in prostate cancer: mapping by quantitative allelic imbalance. *Genes Chromosomes Cancer* 1994; 10:151–159.
199. Bova GS, Carter BS, Bussemakers MJ, et al. Homozygous deletion and frequent allelic loss of chromosome 8p22 loci in human prostate cancer. *Cancer Res* 1993;53:3869–3873.
200. Semb H, Christofori G. The tumor-suppressor function of E-cadherin. *Am J Hum Genet* 1998;63:1588–1593.
201. Perl AK, Wilgenbus P, Dahl U, et al. A causal role for E-cadherin in the transition from adenoma to carcinoma. *Nature* 1998;392:190–193.
202. Bussemakers MJ, van Moorselaar RJ, Giroldi LA, et al. Decreased expression of E-cadherin in the progression of rat prostatic cancer. *Cancer Res* 1992;52:2916–2922.
203. Luo J, Lubaroff DM, Hendrix, MJ. Suppression of prostate cancer invasive potential and matrix metalloproteinase activity by E-cadherin transfection. *Cancer Res* 1999;59: 3552–3556.
204. Umbas R, Schalken JA, Aalders TW, et al. Expression of the cellular adhesion molecule E-cadherin is reduced or absent in high-grade prostate cancer. *Cancer Res* 1992;52:5104–5109.
205. Otto T, Rembrink K, Goepel M, et al. E-cadherin: a marker for differentiation and invasiveness in prostatic carcinoma. *Urol Res* 1993;21:359–362.
206. Ross JS, Figge HL, Bui HX, et al. E-cadherin expression in prostatic carcinoma biopsies: correlation with tumor grade, DNA content, pathologic stage, and clinical outcome. *Mod Pathol* 1994;7:835–841.
207. Cheng L, Nagabhushan M, Pretlow TP, et al. Expression of E-cadherin in primary and metastatic prostate cancer. *Am J Pathol* 1996;148:1375–1380.
208. Richmond PJ, Karayiannakis AJ, Nagafuchi A, et al. Aberrant E-cadherin and alpha-catenin expression in prostate cancer: correlation with patient survival. *Cancer Res* 1997;57:3189–3193.
209. Umbas R, Isaacs WB, Bringuier PP, et al. Decreased E-cadherin expression is associated with poor prognosis in patients with prostate cancer. *Cancer Res* 1994;54:3929–3933.
210. Kuczyk M, Serth J, Machtens S, et al. Expression of E-cadherin in primary prostate cancer: correlation with clinical features. *Br J Urol* 1998;81:406–412.
211. Murant SJ, Rolley N, Phillips SM, et al. Allelic imbalance within the E-cadherin gene is an infrequent event in prostate carcinogenesis. *Genes Chromosomes Cancer* 2000;27:104–109.
212. Bussemakers MJ, Giroldi LA, van Bokhoven A, et al. Transcriptional regulation of the human E-cadherin gene in human prostate cancer cell lines: characterization of the human E-cadherin gene promoter. *Biochem Biophys Res Commun* 1994;203:1284–1290.
213. Graff JR, Herman JG, Lapidus RG, et al. E-cadherin expression is silenced by DNA hypermethylation in human breast and prostate carcinomas. *Cancer Res* 1995;55:5195–5199.
214. Morton RA, Ewing CM, Nagafuchi A, et al. Reduction of E-cadherin levels and deletion of the alpha-catenin gene in human prostate cancer cells. *Cancer Res* 1993;53:3585–3590.
215. Perou CM, Sorlie T, Eisen MB, et al. Molecular portraits of human breast tumours. *Nature* 2000;406:747–752.
216. Carter BS, Epstein JI, Isaacs WB. ras gene mutations in human prostate cancer. *Cancer Res* 1990;50:6830–6832.
217. Anwar K, Nakakuki K, Shiraishi T, et al. Presence of ras oncogene mutations and human papillomavirus DNA in human prostate carcinomas. *Cancer Res* 1992;52:5991–5996.
218. Gumerlock PH, Poonamallee UR, Meyers FJ, et al. Activated ras alleles in human carcinoma of the prostate are rare. *Cancer Res* 1991;51:1632–1637.
219. Konishi N, Enomoto T, Buzard G, et al. K-ras activation and ras p21 expression in latent prostatic carcinoma in Japanese men. *Cancer* 1992;69:2293–2299.
220. Konishi N, Hiasa Y, Tsuzuki T, et al. Comparison of ras activation in prostate carcinoma in Japanese and American men. *Prostate* 1997;30:53–57.
221. Moul JW, Friedrichs PA, Lance RS, et al. Infrequent RAS oncogene mutations in human prostate cancer. *Prostate* 1992;20:327–338.
222. Moyret-Lalle C, Marcais C, Jacquemier J, et al. ras, p53 and HPV status in benign and malignant prostate tumors. *Int J Cancer* 1995;64:124–129.
223. Shiraishi T, Muneyuki T, Fukutome K, et al. Mutations of ras genes are relatively frequent in Japanese prostate cancers: pointing to genetic differences between populations. *Anticancer Res* 1998;18:2789–2792.
224. Orikasa K, Fukushige S, Hoshi S, et al. Infrequent genetic alterations of the PTEN gene in Japanese patients with sporadic prostate cancer. *J Hum Genet* 1998;43:228–230.
225. Gray IC, Stewart LM, Phillips SM, et al. Mutation and expression analysis of the putative prostate tumour-suppressor gene PTEN. *Br J Cancer* 1998;78:1296–1300.
226. Dong JT, Sipe TW, Hyytinen ER, et al. PTEN/MMAC1 is infrequently mutated in pT2 and pT3 carcinomas of the prostate. *Oncogene* 1998;17:1979–1982.
227. Pesche S, Latil A, Muzeau F, et al. PTEN/MMAC1/TEP1 involvement in primary prostate cancers. *Oncogene* 1998; 16:2879–2883.
228. Vlietstra RJ, van Alewijk DC, Hermans KG, et al. Frequent inactivation of PTEN in prostate cancer cell lines and xenografts. *Cancer Res* 1998;58:2720–2723.
229. Feilotter HE, Nagai MA, Boag AH, et al. Analysis of PTEN and the 10q23 region in primary prostate carcinomas. *Oncogene* 1998;16:1743–1748.
230. Wang SI, Parsons R, Ittmann M. Homozygous deletion of the PTEN tumor suppressor gene in a subset of prostate adenocarcinomas. *Clin Cancer Res* 1998;4:811–815.
231. Giri D, Ittmann M. Inactivation of the PTEN tumor suppressor gene is associated with increased angiogenesis in clinically localized prostate carcinoma. *Hum Pathol* 1999; 30:419–424.

232. Teng DH, Hu R, Lin H, et al. MMAC1/PTEN mutations in primary tumor specimens and tumor cell lines. *Cancer Res* 1997;57:5221–5225.
233. Cairns P, Okami K, Halachmi S, et al. Frequent inactivation of PTEN/MMAC1 in primary prostate cancer. *Cancer Res* 1997;57:4997–5000.
234. Navone NM, Troncoso P, Pisters LL, et al. p53 protein accumulation and gene mutation in the progression of human prostate carcinoma. *J Natl Cancer Inst* 1993;85: 1657–1669.
235. Uchida T, Wada C, Shitara T, et al. Infrequent involvement of p53 gene mutations in the tumourigenesis of Japanese prostate cancer. *Br J Cancer* 1993;68:751–755.
236. Effert PJ, McCoy RH, Walther PJ, et al. p53 gene alterations in human prostate carcinoma. *J Urol* 1993;150:257–261.
237. Dinjens WN, van der Weiden MM, Schroeder FH, et al. Frequency and characterization of p53 mutations in primary and metastatic human prostate cancer. *Int J Cancer* 1994;56:630–633.
238. Watanabe M, Ushijima T, Kakiuchi H, et al. p53 gene mutations in human prostate cancers in Japan: different mutation spectra between Japan and western countries. *Jpn J Cancer Res* 1994;85:904–910.
239. Watanabe M, Fukutome K, Shiraishi T, et al. Differences in the p53 gene mutational spectra of prostate cancers between Japan and Western countries. *Carcinogenesis* 1997;18:1355–1358.
240. Voeller HJ, Sugars LY, Pretlow T, et al. p53 oncogene mutations in human prostate cancer specimens. *J Urol* 1994;151:492–495.
241. Chi SG, deVere White RW, Meyers FJ, et al. p53 in prostate cancer: frequent expressed transition mutations. *J Natl Cancer Inst* 1994;86:926–933.
242. Massenkeil G, Oberhuber H, Hailemariam S, et al. P53 mutations and loss of heterozygosity on chromosomes 8p, 16q, 17p, and 18q are confined to advanced prostate cancer. *Anticancer Res* 1994;14:2785–2790.
243. Kubota Y, Shuin T, Uemura H, et al. Tumor suppressor gene p53 mutations in human prostate cancer. *Prostate* 1995;27:18–24.
244. Heidenberg HB, Sesterhenn IA, Gaddipati JP, et al. Alteration of the tumor suppressor gene p53 in a high fraction of hormone refractory prostate cancer. *J Urol* 1995;154:414–421.
245. Konishi N, Hiasa Y, Hayashi I, et al. p53 mutations occur in clinical, but not latent, human prostate carcinoma. *Jpn J Cancer Res* 1995;86:57–63.
246. Mirchandani D, Zheng J, Miller GJ, et al. Heterogeneity in intratumor distribution of p53 mutations in human prostate cancer. *Am J Pathol* 1995;147:92–101.
247. Kunimi K, Amano T, Uchibayashi T. Point mutation of the p53 gene is an infrequent event in untreated prostate cancer. *Cancer Detect Prev* 1996;20:218–222.
248. Suzuki H, Komiya A, Aida S, et al. Detection of human papillomavirus DNA and p53 gene mutations in human prostate cancer. *Prostate* 1996;28:318–324.
249. Prendergast NJ, Atkins MR, Schatte EC, et al. p53 immunohistochemical and genetic alterations are associated at high incidence with post-irradiated locally persistent prostate carcinoma. *J Urol* 1996;155:1685–1692.
250. Dahiya R, Deng G, Chen KM, et al. P53 tumour-suppressor gene mutations are mainly localised on exon 7 in human primary and metastatic prostate cancer. *Br J Cancer* 1996; 74:264–268.
251. Brooks JD, Bova GS, Ewing CM, et al. An uncertain role for p53 gene alterations in human prostate cancers. *Cancer Res* 1996;56:3814–3822.
252. Schlechte HH, Schnorr D, Loning T, et al. Mutation of the tumor suppressor gene p53 in human prostate and bladder cancers—investigation by temperature gradient gel electrophoresis (TGGE). *J Urol* 1997;157:1049–1053.
253. Schlechte H, Lenk SV, Loning T, et al. p53 tumour suppressor gene mutations in benign prostatic hyperplasia and prostate cancer. *Eur Urol* 1998;34:433–440.
254. Mottaz AE, Markwalder R, Fey MF, et al. Abnormal p53 expression is rare in clinically localized human prostate cancer: comparison between immunohistochemical and molecular detection of p53 mutations. *Prostate* 1997;31:209–215.
255. Salem CE, Tomasic NA, Elmajian DA, et al. p53 protein and gene alterations in pathological stage C prostate carcinoma [see comments]. *J Urol* 1997;158:510–514.
256. Stapleton AM, Timme TL, Gousse AE, et al. Primary human prostate cancer cells harboring p53 mutations are clonally expanded in metastases. *Clin Cancer Res* 1997;3:1389–1397.
257. Eastham JA, Stapleton AM, Gousse AE, et al. Association of p53 mutations with metastatic prostate cancer. *Clin Cancer Res* 1995;1:1111–1118.
258. Facher EA, Becich MJ, Deka A, et al. Association between human cancer and two polymorphisms occurring together in the p21Waf1/Cip1 cyclin-dependent kinase inhibitor gene. *Cancer* 1997;79:2424–2429.
259. Ittmann MM, Wieczorek R. Alterations of the retinoblastoma gene in clinically localized, stage B prostate adenocarcinomas. *Hum Pathol* 1996;27:28–34.
260. Brooks JD, Bova GS, Isaacs WB. Allelic loss of the retinoblastoma gene in primary human prostatic adenocarcinomas. *Prostate* 1995;26:35–39.
261. Vesalainen S, Lipponen P. Expression of retinoblastoma gene (Rb) protein in T12M0 prostatic adenocarcinoma. *J Cancer Res Clin Oncol* 1995;121:429–433.
262. Kubota Y, Fujinami K, Uemura H, et al. Retinoblastoma gene mutations in primary human prostate cancer. *Prostate* 1995;27:314–320.
263. Phillips SM, Barton CM, Lee SJ, et al. Loss of the retinoblastoma susceptibility gene (RB1) is a frequent and early event in prostatic tumorigenesis. *Br J Cancer* 1994;70:1252–1257.
264. Bookstein R, Rio P, Madreperla SA, et al. Promoter deletion and loss of retinoblastoma gene expression in human prostate carcinoma. *Proc Natl Acad Sci U S A* 1990;87:7762–7766.
265. Geradts J, Hu SX, Lincoln CE, et al. Aberrant RB gene expression in routinely processed, archival tumor tissues determined by three different anti-RB antibodies. *Int J Cancer* 1994;58:161–167.
266. Latil A, Bieche I, Pesche S, et al. Loss of heterozygosity at chromosome arm 13q and RB1 status in human prostate cancer. *Hum Pathol* 1999;30:809–815.
267. Melamed J, Einhorn JM, Ittmann MM. Allelic loss on chromosome 13q in human prostate carcinoma. *Clin Cancer Res* 1997;3:1867–1872.

268. Tricoli JV, Gumerlock PH, Yao JL, et al. Alterations of the retinoblastoma gene in human prostate adenocarcinoma. *Genes Chromosomes Cancer* 1996;15:108–114.
269. Cooney KA, Wetzel JC, Merajver SD, et al. Distinct regions of allelic loss on 13q in prostate cancer. *Cancer Res* 1996;56:1142–1145.
270. Drobnjak M, Osman I, Scher HI, et al. Overexpression of cyclin D1 is associated with metastatic prostate cancer to bone. *Clin Cancer Res* 2000;6:1891–1895.
271. Kallakury BV, Sheehan CE, Ambros RA, et al. The prognostic significance of p34cdc2 and cyclin D1 protein expression in prostate adenocarcinoma. *Cancer* 1997;80:753–763.
272. Shiraishi T, Watanabe M, Muneyuki T, et al. A clinicopathological study of p53, p21 (WAF1/CIP1) and cyclin D1 expression in human prostate cancers. *Urol Int* 1998;61: 90–94.
273. Chi SG, deVere White RW, Muenzer JT, et al. Frequent alteration of CDKN2 (p16(INK4A)/MTS1) expression in human primary prostate carcinomas. *Clin Cancer Res* 1997; 3:1889–1897.
274. Komiya A, Suzuki H, Aida S, et al. Mutational analysis of CDKN2 (CDK4I/MTS1) gene in tissues and cell lines of human prostate cancer. *Jpn J Cancer Res* 1995;86:622–625.
275. Chen W, Weghorst CM, Sabourin CL, et al. Absence of p16/MTS1 gene mutations in human prostate cancer. *Carcinogenesis* 1996;17:2603–2607.
276. Gaddipati JP, McLeod DG, Sesterhenn IA, et al. Mutations of the p16 gene product are rare in prostate cancer. *Prostate* 1997;30:188–194.
277. Gu K, Mes-Masson AM, Gauthier J, et al. Analysis of the p16 tumor suppressor gene in early-stage prostate cancer. *Mol Carcinog* 1998;21:164–170.
278. Jarrard DF, Bova GS, Ewing, CM, et al. Deletional, mutational, and methylation analyses of CDKN2 (p16/MTS1) in primary and metastatic prostate cancer. *Genes Chromosomes Cancer* 1997;19:90–96.
279. Mangold KA, Takahashi H; Brandigi C, et al. p16 (CDKN2/MTS1) gene deletions are rare in prostatic carcinomas in the United States and Japan. *J Urol* 1997;157:1117–1120.
280. Park DJ, Wilczynski SP, Pham EY, et al. Molecular analysis of the INK4 family of genes in prostate carcinomas. *J Urol* 1997;157:1995–1999.
281. Tamimi Y, Bringuier PP, Smit F, et al. p16 mutations/deletions are not frequent events in prostate cancer. *Br J Cancer* 1996;74:120–122.
282. Nguyen TT, Nguyen CT, Gonzales FA, et al. Analysis of cyclin-dependent kinase inhibitor expression and methylation patterns in human prostate cancers. *Prostate* 2000;43: 233–242.
283. Buttyan R, Sawczuk IS, Benson MC, et al. Enhanced expression of the c-myc protooncogene in high-grade human prostate cancers. *Prostate* 1987;11:327–337.
284. Latil A, Vidaud D, Valeri A, et al. htert expression correlates with MYC over-expression in human prostate cancer. *Int J Cancer* 2000;89:172–176.
285. Nupponen NN, Kakkola L, Koivisto P, et al. Genetic alterations in hormone-refractory recurrent prostate carcinomas. *Am J Pathol* 1998;153:141–148.
286. Qian J, Jenkins RB, Bostwick DG. Detection of chromosomal anomalies and c-myc gene amplification in the cribriform pattern of prostatic intraepithelial neoplasia and carcinoma by fluorescence in situ hybridization. *Mod Pathol* 1997;10:1113–1119.
287. Reiter RE, Sato I, Thomas G, et al. Coamplification of prostate stem cell antigen (PSCA) and MYC in locally advanced prostate cancer. *Genes Chromosomes Cancer* 2000;27:95–103.
288. Mark HF, Samy M, Santoro K, et al. Fluorescent in situ hybridization study of c-myc oncogene copy number in prostate cancer. *Exp Mol Pathol* 2000;68:65–69.
289. Kawamata N, Park D, Wilczynski S, et al. Point mutations of the Mxil gene are rare in prostate cancers. *Prostate* 1996;29:191–193.
290. Eagle LR, Yin X, Brothman AR, et al. Mutation of the MXI1 gene in prostate cancer. *Nat Genet* 1995;9:249–255.
291. Kuczyk MA, Serth J, Bokemeyer C, et al. The MXI1 tumor suppressor gene is not mutated in primary prostate cancer. *Oncol Rep* 1998;5:213–216.

5

ANTISURVIVAL THERAPY FOR METASTATIC PROSTATE CANCER

ASHANI T. WEERARATNA
JOHN T. ISAACS

In normal bone marrow, approximately 25% of the hematopoietic cells are proliferating per day to replace approximately 25% of these cells dying daily (1). Likewise, approximately 10% of the epithelium in the skin (2) and gut (3) are proliferating per day to balance the 10% daily death rate of these cells. These percentages translate into the human reality that there will be sufficient cell proliferation in a 180-lb man to produce 180 lb of new blood, skin, and gut cells per year to balance the death of 180 lb of these cells, which normally occurs annually. Because the daily rate of cell proliferation equals that of death, neither involution nor overgrowth of these tissues normally occurs. The most remarkable fact about prostate cancer is that 39,000 American men will die of this devastating disease this year (4), even though less than 5% of the metastatic prostate cancer cells proliferate per day (5). Thus, although highly lethal, metastatic prostate cancer cells are proliferating at a daily rate that is two- to fivefold lower than a variety of normal host cells. In contrast to these normal cells, however, metastatic prostate cancer cells characteristically have a remarkably low rate of death (i.e., less than 2% of these cells die per day) (5). Because more prostate cancer cells proliferate daily than die (i.e., 5% – 2% = 3% net gain in malignant prostate cells per day), prostate cancer grows continuously. Thus, the major reason for the ability of prostate cancer cells to metastasize and kill the patient is not related to their high rate of proliferation, but to their high rate of survival once they have disseminated to a distant site (5).

Presently, there is a large variety of cytotoxic chemotherapeutic agents available. Unfortunately, essentially all of the agents require the target cell to be proliferating to be killed. Because metastatic prostate cancer cells have such a low rate of cell proliferation, there is essentially no therapeutic index between these cancer cells and rapidly proliferating normal gut, skin, and blood cells when the patient is exposed to the presently available cytotoxic chemotherapeutic agents. This lack of tumor-cell specificity leads to host toxicity that limits both the dose and total length of treatment with such nontargeted cytotoxic agents. Therefore, what is needed is a method for targeting the death of prostate cancer cells without inducing such death in host normal cells.

Based on this realization, identifying the molecular pathways responsible for the high level of survivability of prostate cancer cells has become a major research focus. These studies have focused on the knowledge that androgen is the major survival factor for the androgen-responsive prostate cancer cells present within the patient. This is because sufficient levels of androgen are chronically required to antagonize the activation of the programmed (i.e., apoptotic) death of these androgen-responsive cancer cells (6). It is on this basis that androgen ablation has been used as standard systemic therapy for metastatic prostate cancer.

PROBLEM WITH ANDROGEN ABLATION THERAPY

During this year, 39,000 men will die of prostate cancer in the United States (4). Essentially, all of these patients will have received treatment with a variety of androgen ablation techniques. There is a multitude of excellent means of ablating serum androgens, including chronic treatment with luteinizing hormone–releasing hormone analogs alone and in combination with antiandrogens or surgical orchiectomy, or both. A recent, large, randomized, prospective clinical trial compared the effectiveness of gold standard androgen ablation (i.e., surgical orchiectomy) as monotherapy to a combination approach of orchiectomy plus concomitant antiandrogen treatment in patients with metastatic prostate cancer. The data demonstrated that there is no additional advantage of combination approaches when compared with orchiectomy alone, in terms of the time of progression or overall survival (7). None of the patients with definitive metastatic disease was cured by such androgen ablation therapy, regardless of how aggressively it was given (7). To understand why such androgen ablation is not curative, an understanding of the cellular basis for androgen responsiveness is necessary.

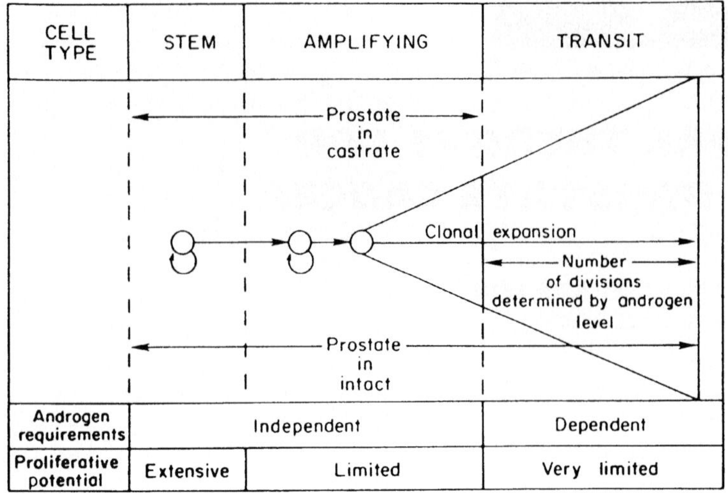

FIGURE 5-1. Heterogeneous composition of the normal prostate. The prostate is composed of a limited number of androgen-independent stem cells that can differentiate into androgen-independent, but -sensitive, amplifying cells. In the presence of physiologic androgen, the normal prostate is in a steady-state, self-renewing, maintenance condition, heterogeneously composed of androgen-independent, -sensitive, and -dependent epithelial cells. Because of the clonally expansive nature of this hierarchical stem cell organization, the vast majority of the epithelial compartment is composed of androgen-dependent glandular cells, with lower numbers of androgen-sensitive basal cells, and a limited number of androgen-independent basal stem cells.

ANDROGEN RESPONSIVENESS ON A CELLULAR BASIS

Whether normal or malignant, the growth of any cell type is dependent on the relationship between its rate of cell proliferation and death. If these rates are equivalent, no net growth occurs, even though cellular turnover (i.e., steady-state replacement) occurs continuously. In contrast, if the rate of cell proliferation is greater than death, then continuous net growth occurs; if the proliferation rate is lower than death, then cellular elimination occurs. Androgens are the major regulators of proliferation and death for the normal prostate (8–10). Androgens regulate the total prostate epithelial cell number by chronically stimulating the rate of cell proliferation (i.e., agonistic ability of androgen) while simultaneously inhibiting the rate of cell death (i.e., antagonistic ability of androgen) of specific subsets of androgen-sensitive and -dependent epithelial cells, and endothelial cells, within the prostate (8–12). The normal prostate is heterogeneously composed of a limited number of androgen-independent stem cells (i.e., a subset of basal epithelial cells) that, beside maintaining their own limited numbers, give rise to a larger subset of progeny that differentiates into androgen-independent, but -sensitive, amplifying cells (i.e., also located in the basal layer of prostate epithelial cells) (13). When sufficient androgen is not present (i.e., after androgen ablation), the amplifying cells are maintained (i.e., rate of proliferation equals rate of cell death), but do not expand into transit (e.g., luminal epithelial) cells (13–16). In contrast, when physiologically normal levels of androgen are exogenously replaced in a previously castrated host, the majority of these basally located androgen-sensitive amplifying cells differentiate into luminally located androgen-dependent transit (glandular) epithelial cells (Fig. 5-1). Once the normal number of these androgen-dependent transit (glandular) cells is reached, their rate of cell proliferation balances their rate of cell death, such that neither prostatic regression nor continuous glandular overgrowth occurs (13–16). Thus, in the presence of physiologic androgen, the normal prostate is in a steady-state, self-renewing maintenance condition, heterogenously composed of androgen-independent, -sensitive, and -dependent epithelial cells. Because of the clonally expansive nature of this hierarchical stem-cell organization, the vast majority of the epithelial compartment is composed of androgen-dependent glandular cells, with lower numbers of androgen-sensitive basal cells and a limited number of androgen-independent basal stem cells (Fig. 5-1).

CELL SURVIVAL PATHWAYS VERSUS APOPTOTIC CASCADE

If a sufficient systemic androgen level is not chronically maintained (e.g., after androgen ablation), then the entire subset of androgen-dependent prostatic glandular and epithelial cells, as well as a subset of prostatic endothelial cells, dies rapidly via the activation of an energy-dependent cascade of biochemical and morphologic changes, collectively referred to as *programmed cell death* (8–12). Normally, this programmed death is actively suppressed, owing to androgen-dependent production of cell survival signals. These include the production of secreted peptide survival factors, such as insulinlike growth factors I and II (IGF-I and -II), platelet-derived growth factor (PDGF), and vascular-endothelial growth factor (VEGF). These survival factors initiate their effect by binding to their cell-surface cognate receptor and inducing receptor dimerization. Once dimerized, each monomer transphosphorylates the opposing monomer on specific tyrosine residues. This tyrosine transautophosphorylation functions to recruit intracellular signaling proteins to bind via their src homology 2 domains to specific phosphorylated tyrosines in the ligand-occupied dimeric receptor complex (17). This autophosphorylation initiates three major kinase-dependent signaling cascades. These include: (a) the ras/raf/Mek/srk cascade, (b) the phospholipase Cγ/diacylglycerol/inositol triphosphate (IP_3)/protein kinase C cascade, and (c) the phosphotidyl-inositol 3-kinase (PI3K)/protein kinase B kinase (PKBK)/protein kinase B (PKB also called Akt)/Bcl-2 antagonist of cell death (BAD)/procaspase 9 cascade (17–24). PI3K is a heterodimer composed of an 85-kD regulatory subunit and a catalytic 110-kD subunit. The mechanism, by which growth factors activate PI3K, involves the binding of the 85-kD subunit to specific phosphotyrosines on either the cytoplasmic domain of the plasma membrane growth factor–occupied dimeric receptor or to phosphotyrosines on adapter proteins, which are themselves bound via their src homology 2 domain to the phosphorylated receptor. This binding anchors not only the 85-kD regulatory subunit but also the catalytic 110-kD subunit of PI3K to the plasma membrane. This binding allows the tyrosine kinase of the receptor to phosphorylate the 85-kD subunit of the PI3K to which it is bound. This activates the PI3K, allowing it to phosphorylate the three positions of phosphatidylinositol-4,5-bisphosphate (PI-4,5-P_2) attached to the plasma membrane to form membrane-bound phosphatidylinositol-3,4,5-trisphosphate (PI-3,4,5-P_3). An inositol 5' polyphosphatase converts PI-3,4,5-P_2 to PI-3,4-P_2 (18). Once formed, the PI-3,4-P_2 can bind to the N-terminal, pleckstrin homology (PH) domain of the serine/threonine protein kinase termed *PKB*. PH binding to PI-3,4-P_2 not only anchors the Akt protein to plasma membrane, but also causes it to undergo a conformational change, allowing it to expose its c-terminal regulatory domain, which can then be phosphorylated at threonine 308 and serine 473 (20). The phosphorylation of threonine at position 308 of Akt is catalyzed by a specific PKBK associated with the plasma membrane. This PKBK is also known as *3-phosphoinositide-dependent protein kinase 1*, because it is activated by binding PI-3,4,-P_3, but not PI-4,5-P_2 (21). The identity of the enzyme responsible for phosphorylation of the serine at 473 has not been resolved. This dual phosphorylation synergistically activates the serine/threonine kinase of Akt. IP_3, generated from PI-4,5-P_2 by phospholipase-Cγ, releases Akt from the plasma membrane to phosphorylate downstream cytoplasmic and nuclear targets (Fig. 5-2A) until inactivated by dephosphorylation by protein phosphatase 2A (18). Several downstream targets are known and include the apoptotic-inducing proteins, procaspase 9 (22), and the proapoptotic Bcl-2 family member, BAD (23). Akt phosphorylation of procaspase 9 inhibits the activation of this proapoptotic enzyme, whereas phosphorylation of the proapoptotic BAD allows it to form a complex with 14-3-3 protease, retaining the complex within the cytoplasm (23,24).

An increase in $[Ca^{2+}]_i$ results in increased Ca^{2+} binding to calmodulin, allowing the Ca^{2+}-loaded calmodulin to bind to calcineurin, activating its phosphatase activity (25). Activated calcineurin dephosphorylates the proapoptotic protein BAD (25). This active dephosphorylation of phospho-BAD is coupled to a decrease in BAD phosphorylation, due to a decrease in the activity of Akt, secondary to decreased occupancy of the survival factor receptors and PI3K signaling (Fig. 5-2B). This dephosphorylation of BAD results in its translocation from the cytosol to the mitochondrial outer membrane (25). This causes the dissociation of the apoptotic inhibitors Bc1-2 or Bcl-X_L, or both, from their dimeric complex with the proapoptotic protein BAX, allowing BAX to induce a permeability transition event via interaction with porin molecule in the inner mitochondrial membrane and translocation proteins in the outer mitochondrial membrane (25–27). This results in the release of cytochrome c from mitochondria (Fig. 5-2C). Once liberated, cytochrome c interacts with apoptotic-protease activating factor 1 to cause the processing of a series of procysteine–aspartic acid–specific proteases (e.g., procaspases 9 and 3) into enzymatically active caspases (28–31). Once activated, these caspases degrade specific intracellular proteins, including the 45-kD DNase inhibitor of the DNA fragmentation factor (DFF) complex (32,33). Once the 45-kD DNase inhibitor is inactivated, the 40-kD DNase subunit of the DFF complex is enzymatically activated and begins to fragment the cell's genomic DNA (32,33).

Increases in $[Ca^{2+}]_i$ can be caused when androgen levels are insufficient—for example, after castration, the androgen-dependent prostate glandular cells undergo an epigenetic reprogramming, involving the increased synthesis of a series of protein, including calmodulin, DNase, clusterin, γ-prochymosin, and others, coupled with decreased synthesis of survival protein, such as IGF-I and -II; PDGF; and the DNA-binding, highly charged, low-molecular-weight polyamines (i.e., spermidine and spermine) (9,34–39). Because of this reprogramming, a plasma-membrane channel for calcium is opened, allowing the high extracellular calcium (i.e., 1 to 3 μm) to influx into these cells, raising the intracellular free Ca^{2+} $[Ca^{2+}]_i$ from 20 to 40 nm to greater than 1 μm (36,38). This increase in $[Ca^{2+}]_i$ results, as previously mentioned, in the increased activity of calmodulin-dependent calcineurin. Having undergone the apoptotic cascade triggered by the calcineurin-dependent dephosphorylation of BAD, culminating in the activation of DFF, the genomic DNA is initially fragmented into high-molecular-weight sizes (i.e., 50 to 300 kb), which are subsequently degraded further into nucleosomal oligomers (i.e., multiples of a 180-base pair subunit) that lack intranucleosomal breaks in the DNA (9,35). This DNA fragmentation is subsequently followed by irreversible, morphologic changes, termed *apoptosis*, that characteristically involve chromatic condensation; nuclear disintegration; cell surface blebbing; and, eventually, cellular fragmentation into a cluster of membrane-bound apoptotic bodies within the prostate (Fig. 5-3). Comparisons

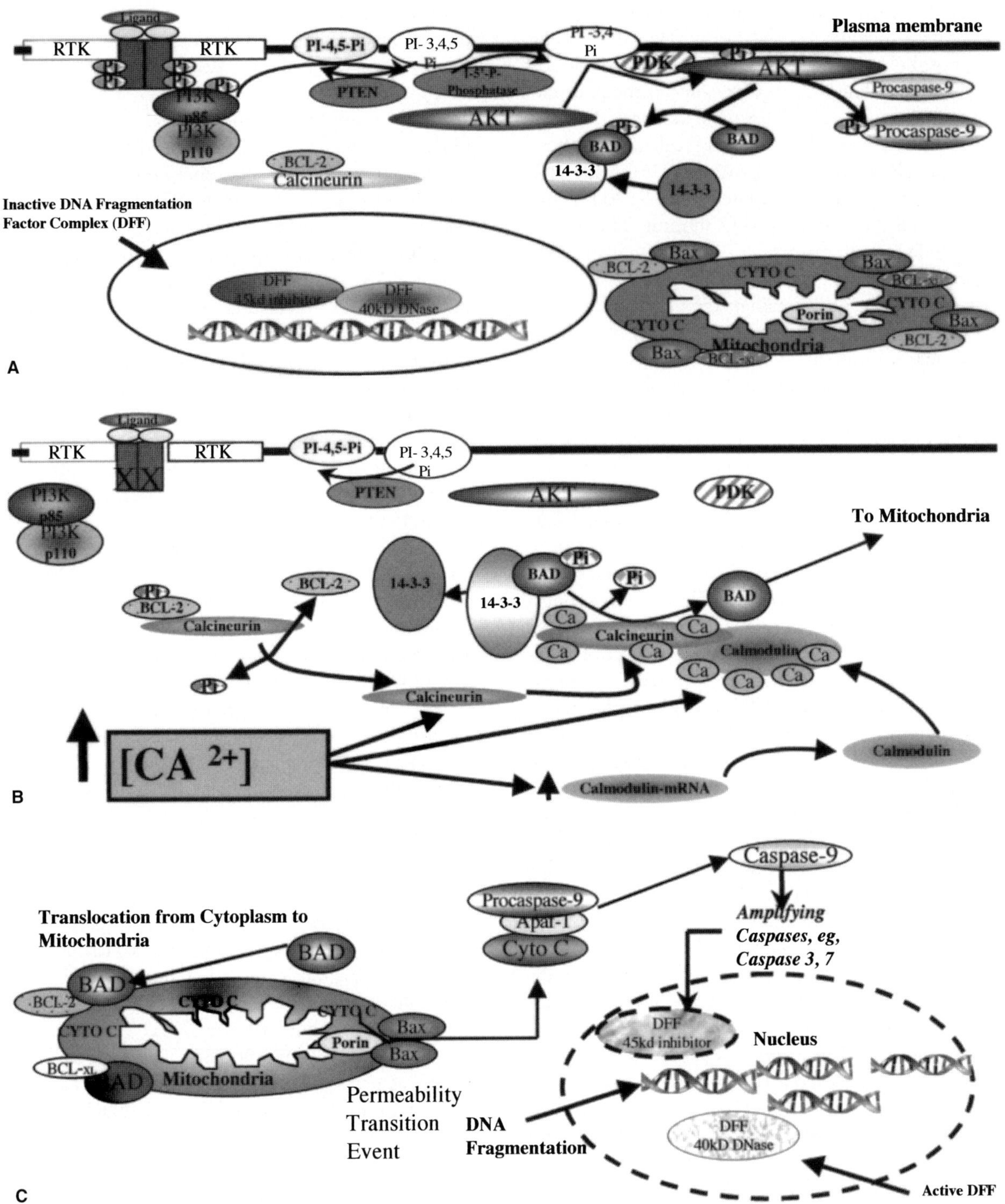

FIGURE 5-2. **A:** When activated by ligand binding, receptor autophosphorylation results in the activation of a downstream signaling cascade involving the phosphotidyl-inositol 3-kinase (PI3K)/ protein kinase B (PKB) pathway. **B:** If inactivated, either by inhibition of ligand binding or targeted deactivation of the receptor, the lack of phosphorylation of the receptor results in the dephosphorylation of PI3K and AKT. In addition, any rises in [Ca] activate the phosphatase calcineurin via its interaction with calmodulin. These two events work in tandem to dephosphorylate Bcl-2 antagonist of cell death (BAD), causing its translocation to the mitochondria. **C:** Once in the mitochondria, BAD dimerizes with Bcl-2 and Bcl-X_L, causing BAX to homodimerize and form complexes, which results in permeability transition events in the mitochondria. Cytochrome c is released and complexes with apoptotic-protease activating factor (Apaf)-1, resulting in the conversion of procaspase 9 to its active form and the subsequent activation of caspases that degrade the DNA fragmentation factor (DFF) inhibitor, resulting in the release of active DFF and subsequent DNA degradation. See text for details. mRNA, messenger RNA; RTK, receptor tyrosine kinase.

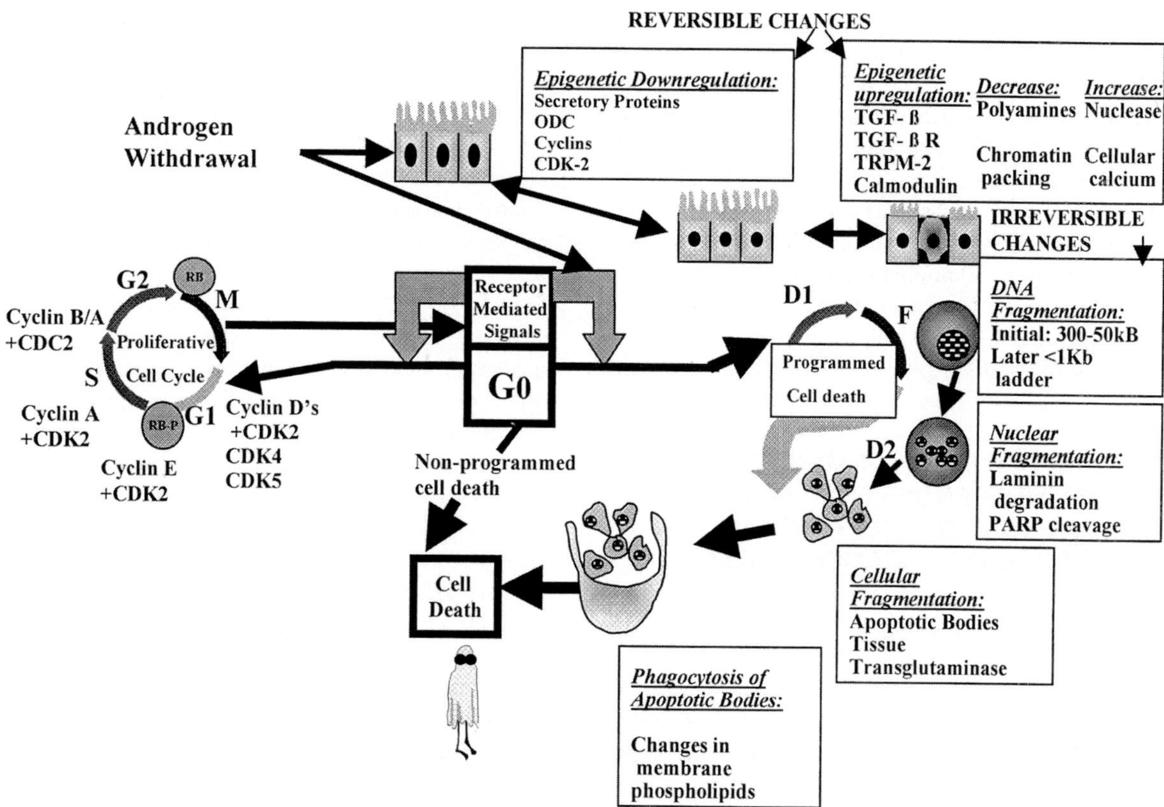

FIGURE 5-3. Schematic representation of the prostate cell cycle during proliferation, resting phase (G0) and programmed cell death. The period during which new gene and protein expression are required for the induction of DNA fragmentation (F) is termed *D1*, and the time during which the cell fragments into apoptotic bodies is termed *D2*. The biochemical and morphologic details are outlined here and further discussed in the text. CDK, cyclin-dependent kinase; ODC, orinthine decarboxylase; PARP, poly-adenosine-di-phosphate-ribose polymerase; TGF-β, transforming growth factor beta; TRPM-2, testosterone repressed prostate message 2.

of the kinetics of induction of DNA fragmentation, the appearance of apoptotic bodies, and the loss of prostatic glandular cell number after castration have demonstrated that the fragmentation of genomic DNA is the irreversible commitment step in the death of the androgen-dependent prostate cells and does not occur as a result of the cells already being dead (9,35,36).

RELATIONSHIP BETWEEN CELL OF ORIGIN FOR PROSTATE CANCER AND ANDROGEN RESPONSIVENESS

Based on the stem cell organization of the normal prostate epithelium, there are three distinct cells of origin possible for prostate cancer (40). The first alternative is that the prostate cancer is monoclonally derived from an androgen-independent stem cell. Even if the cell of origin is an androgen-independent stem cell, it is still possible for the resulting cancer to be responsive to androgen ablation. The malignant stem cell could retain the ability to progress down the hierarchical pathway described previously, giving rise to larger subsets of androgen-sensitive amplifying, and even larger numbers of androgen-dependent transit, malignant cells. Such a heterogenous cancer, composed of these three cell types, would respond to androgen ablation with the elimination of the largest subset of cancer cells (i.e., the androgen-dependent malignant transit cells) and a reduction in the growth rate of the next largest subset of cancer cells (i.e., the androgen-sensitive malignant amplifying cells). Such a response would not be curative, because neither the malignant androgen-independent stem cell nor the androgen-sensitive malignant amplifying cells would be eliminated.

A second alternative is that the original prostate cancer can be monoclonally derived from an androgen-sensitive amplifying basal cell. If this occurred, then the cancer would again be androgen responsive, because it is composed of androgen-sensitive malignant amplifying cells that retain the ability of differentiating into androgen-dependent transit cell progeny. Again, owing to clonal expansion, the major type of cancer cell present would be the androgen-dependent malignant transit cell. Such a heterogenous cancer would be responsive to androgen ablation, owing to the elimination of the major subset of malignant transit cells; however, the cancer would not be cured by such therapy, because the androgen-sensitive amplifying cells would not be eliminated.

A third alternative is that the original cancer is monoclonally derived from an androgen-dependent transit (glandular) cell. If this occurs, then the cancer would initially be highly androgen-responsive to androgen ablation. If no further malignant progression occurred, the cancer, theoretically, could be cured by such therapy; however, as will be discussed, even if this third possibility occurs, and the initial prostate cancer is homogeneously composed of androgen-dependent cancer cells, as these cells undergo sufficient cellular proliferation to produce clinically detectable prostate cancer (i.e., more than 30 population doublings), a series of mechanisms eventually leads to the heterogenous development of malignant clones of androgen-sensitive or androgen-independent prostate cancer cells, or both.

MECHANISM FOR DEVELOPMENT OF ANDROGEN-INDEPENDENT OR -SENSITIVE PHENOTYPE FROM INITIALLY ANDROGEN-DEPENDENT PROSTATE CANCER CELLS

The exact mechanism responsible for the basic alteration of the cancer cell phenotype has not been completely resolved but involves changes in the structure or regulation, or both, of the cancer cell genome. Regardless of the detailed mechanism, such a change in phenotype is inheritable. This requires that some type of basic genetic change occur in these cells. *Genetic change* is defined here as a heritable alteration of phenotype, whether resulting from gene mutations, chromosomal alterations, or alterations in gene regulation. The ability of cancer cells to undergo such genetic changes demonstrates that these tumor cells are genetically unstable (i.e., genetically changeable). This genetic instability can lead to the addition of a series of genetically altered clones of cancer cells, each with a distinct phenotype. Only such newly developed clones, in which the new phenotype allows these cells to proliferate without the requirement for androgenic stimulation (i.e., androgen-independent or -sensitive cells), are important in the development of resistance to androgen ablation therapy. Once these androgen-independent or -sensitive clones develop, they have a growth advantage after androgen ablation over all the other newly developed tumor clones that still retain androgen dependence, in addition to any original androgen-dependent cells still present in the tumor. Eventually, such a growth advantage leads, via clonal selection, to the development of resistance of androgen ablation therapy (e.g., hormonal refractory disease) (41).

The basic question becomes What causes the development of genetic instability of initially androgen-dependent prostate cancer cells? One possibility is that changes in the tumor microenvironment are critically involved in inducing the development of this genetic instability. Exactly how this could occur is not completely understood. Exposure of tissue culture cells to medium deficients in single essential amino acids results in a decrease in cellular proliferation with a specific inhibition of the cell cycle during the S phase (42). This inhibition has also been shown to induce the development of genetic instability, such that eventually, demonstrable chromosomal aberrations occur (42). The net result of this environmentally induced genetic instability is that genetically distinct androgen-independent or -sensitive cells can be added to the tumor even before any androgen ablation therapy is given.

Besides androgen ablation–independent changes in the tumor microenvironment, such change also can be directly induced by androgen ablation. For example, the continuous growth and survival of any cancer critically requires an adequate tumor blood supply. Because a critical tumor blood supply is continuously expanding (i.e., angiogenesis) with the net growth of the cancer, anything that inhibits tumor angiogenesis produces local (i.e., microenvironmental) hypoxia, acidosis, and toxic metabolic waste build-up. These microenvironmental changes could induce such instability of the cancer cells. Adequate tumor angiogenesis requires the continuous production of a series of angiogenesis factors, one of the most important of which is VEGF. VEGF induces the migration, proliferation, and survival of endothelial cells and is also produced by prostate cancer cells themselves. Recent studies have demonstrated that VEGF secretion by androgen-responsive and -dependent prostate cancer cells is under androgen regulation (11,12,43–45). Thus, androgen ablation induces a significant decrease in VEGF levels within prostate cancers, by which inhibiting tumor angiogenesis could produce significant microenvironment stress on the prostate cancer cells, inducing their genetic instability.

An alternative explanation is that changes in the host microenvironment, whether dependent or independent of androgen ablation, do not have a direct inductive role in the development of genetic instability of the initially androgen-dependent prostate cancer cells. Instead, it is possible that the development of genetic instability of the androgen-dependent prostate cancer cells occurs as a stochastic event related to the basic nature of the cancer cells (41). How such genetic instability could develop independent of microenvironmental factors is not entirely known. One possibility is that one of the earliest events in malignant transformation of prostate epithelial cells could involve deactivation of a gene locus, which increases the likelihood of subsequent genetic errors.

In prostate cancer, the gene encoding for the phase II detoxification enzyme, the π isozyme of glutathione S-transferase, has also been found to be extensively methylated in its promoter region in a completely cancer-specific fashion, with concomitant absence of expression (46). This methylation event, found in over 90% of all prostate cancers, is the earliest and most common genomic alteration yet observed in sporadic prostate cancer (46). The mechanism by which this region becomes specifically methylated in prostate cancer and the basis for its apparent selection in the carcinogenic pathway are unclear. Because this enzyme has a key part in an important cellular pathway to prevent damage from a wide range of carcinogens, inactivation of its activity may result in increased susceptibility of prostate tissue to both tumor initiation and progression, resulting from an increased rate of accumulated DNA damage (i.e., increasing its genetic instability).

Additional genetic changes may explain the progression to an androgen-independent phenotype. Bcl-2 is an oncogene located on chromosome 18q21, encoding a membrane-bound 26-kD protein that prolongs cell survival by inhibiting apoptosis (47). Bcl-2 expression is localized to the basal epithelial cells in the normal human prostate (48). Normal human prostatic secretory epithelial cells do not express the Bcl-2 protein; however, a fraction of primary untreated prostate adenocarcinoma cells do express this apoptosis-suppressing oncoprotein at significant levels (48–51). With the use of immunohistochemical examination for Bcl-2 expression in androgen-dependent and androgen-independent prostate carcinoma, Bcl-2 is undetectable in approximately 60% of androgen-dependent cancers. In contrast, androgen-independent cancers displayed diffuse high levels of Bcl-2 expression in 30% to 40% of cases (49,51). These findings suggest that enhanced Bcl-2 expression is correlated with the progression of prostate cancer androgen dependence to androgen independence. The frequency of Bcl-2 expression during the progression of human and rat prostate cancers from an androgen-sensitive nonmetastatic phenotype to an androgen-independent metastatic phenotype is statistically and significantly correlated (51). Such Bcl-2 expression is not absolutely required for either androgen-independent or metastatic ability by human prostate cancer cells (51). Experimentally, overexpressing of Bcl-2 in human prostate cancer cells protects these cells from apoptotic stimuli *in vitro* and confers resistance to androgen depletion *in vivo,* and such protection correlates with the ability to form hormone-refractory prostate tumors *in vivo* (50,51).

The androgen receptor is a key mediator of androgen function within normal and malignant prostate cells. The androgen receptor is nearly universally expressed in primary and metastatic sites in untreated patients and in patients undergoing androgen ablation but with recurrent disease, suggesting that the androgen receptor is required for the progression of prostate cancer to the androgen-unresponsive metastatic stage (52,53). Molecular analysis has demonstrated that amplification of the Xq11-q13 region, where the androgen receptor gene is located, is common in prostate cancer, recurring during androgen ablation therapy (54,55). Androgen receptor amplification has been detected in approximately 30% of recurrent prostate cancers, but not in specimens taken from the same patients before therapy (54,55). Combining these results suggests that in approximately one-third of patients, failure of androgen ablation therapy may be caused by clonal outgrowth of prostate cancer cells with increased androgen receptor expression. In addition to amplification, mutations in the gene can cause androgen receptor dysfunction, including alterations of androgen receptor specificity, binding affinity, and expression (56). Androgen receptor mutations occur in low frequency in primary prostate cancer (56,57). In contrast, the cells in the distant metastases and recurrent prostate cancer after androgen ablation often contain androgen receptor mutations (57).

Recently, a series of experimental studies demonstrated that there is "cross-talk," between the androgen receptor and the signaling pathway, induced by peptide growth factors (58). These studies have demonstrated that when the androgen receptor is not expressed, certain peptide growth factors [e.g., nerve growth factor (NGF), keratinocyte growth factor, epidermal growth factor (EGF), and IGF-1] are unable to stimulate the transcription of androgen-responsive genes by androgen-independent prostate cancer cells. In contrast, when the androgen receptor is expressed experimentally in these same androgen-independent cancer cells, these same peptide growth factors can now induce the expression of these androgen-responsive genes in an androgen ligand–independent manner. Ligand-independent androgen receptor activation of transcription of specific genes can be induced by co-stimulation of pathways involving protein kinase A or peptide growth factors (58,59). These results suggest that the androgen-regulated transcriptional pathways for growth and survival may be activated in an androgen ligand–independent manner by cross-talk with the nuclear transcriptional machinery induced by peptide growth factors. This raises the interesting possibility that, although certain prostate cancer cells can progress to become independent of androgen for growth and survival, these same cells may retain an androgen receptor dependence, independent of binding of the androgen ligand to this receptor. Thus, therapies targeted at decreasing androgen receptor expression within prostate cancer cells, independent of lower serum androgen levels, are a new approach (60). An additional new approach is to disrupt the ability of the androgen receptor to interact with a series of coactivator proteins (e.g., SRC-1) needed for efficient transcription of androgen responsive genes (61).

NEW APPROACHES FOR ANDROGEN-INDEPENDENT PROSTATE CANCER

For androgen-dependent prostate cancer cells to progress to a non-androgen-dependent phenotype, these non-androgen-dependent cancer cells must substitute alternative (i.e., non-androgen-dependent) mechanisms for activation of their survival pathway (62–67). There is a variety of growth factors and cytokines that could potentially provide activation of such survival pathways. Growth factors and cytokines vary in their ability to induce proliferation and survival, but they all function by binding to and, thereby, activating their cognate receptors, which in turn activates signal transduction pathways. These receptors can be of several types being either (a) tyrosine kinase coupled, (b) G protein coupled, or (c) adapter coupled. The ability of certain growth factors to induce proliferation is not necessarily correlated with their ability to promote survival, and indeed some growth factors and cytokines promote survival of postmitotic cells (68). For example, apoptotic cell death can often be induced *in vitro* by simply a removal of serum from the media. This is because serum contains a variety of survival factors including insulin, IGF-I and -II, PDGF, and neurotrophins, such as NGF. In contrast, when cells are grown in restricted levels of serum-containing media, they often can survive, but not proliferate. Exposure of such serum-restricted cells to exogenously added EGF or fibroblast growth factors (FGF), but not to insulin, IGF, PDGF, or NGF, often induces these cells to enter the cell cycle and proliferate [i.e., EGF and FGF are mitogenic factors, whereas insulin, IGF, PDGF, and NGF are survival factors (69)].

Regardless of the final response, each of these previously discussed factors is known to initiate its effect by binding to its cell surface cognate receptor and inducing receptor dimerization. Once dimerized, each monomer transphosphorylates the opposing monomer on specific tyrosine residues and thus generates various signaling pathways, outlined in Figure 5-2.

Recent studies have demonstrated that a gene termed PTEN, which is located on the long arm of human chromosome 10, is often physically deleted at one allele and mutated at the other in a large variety of human cancers, including prostate cancer (70). This PTEN gene normally encodes a phospholipid that can hydrolyze PI-3,4,5-P_3 at its 3 position to produce PI-4,5-P_2. Because the PH domain of Akt only binds PI-3,4-P_2 and not PI-4,5-P_2, such PTEN-catalyzed hydrolyzing inhibits the activation of Akt. The level of PI-3,4-P_2 is directly related to the level of PI-3,4,5-P_3, which itself is regulated by the relationship between the competing activity of PI3K versus PTEN. Thus, the tonic level of Akt activity effecting cell survival is determined by the relationship between PI3K versus PTEN activity (71). The importance of this PI3K/Akt pathway for survival has been demonstrated repeatedly by the observation that treatment with the PI3K inhibitors wortmannin or LY293002 can induce the apoptotic death of certain cells, and that in normal cells this death cannot be overcome by adding additional amounts of survival factors (72). In contrast, transgenetically expressing a mutated Akt gene encoding constitutively active Akt (i.e., which does not need to be activated by PI3K) allows such transfected cells to be completely resistant to the apoptosis induced by wortmannin or LY294002 treatment (73).

Although each of the ligands for tyrosine receptor kinases (i.e., EGF, FGF, IGF, VEGF, PDGF, NGF, and others) can activate both the proliferation and survival cascades, the relative magnitude of the activation to the two cascades varies between ligands. For example, EGF or FGF predominately stimulates the proliferative cascades (i.e., ras/raf/Mek/erk), whereas IGF, PDGF, and NGF predominately stimulate the survival pathway (72–76). Because in serum all of these factors are present, growing cells in serum containing media optimally stimulate both cascades, owing to the sum of the input from all of the growth factors. Although a large series of studies have demonstrated that both normal and malignant prostate cells respond to these growth factors, recent studies have identified some significant differences between normal and malignant prostate cells. The differences relate to the role of NGFs. Western blotting, immunocytochemistry, and enzyme-linked immunoabsorbent assay, demonstrate that NGF is located in the prostate epithelium and that the concentration of NGF is slightly higher in prostate cancer (i.e., 3.1 ± 1.5 ng/g) versus benign prostatic hyperplasia (BPH) tissue (i.e., 2.0 ± 0.7 ng/g), and both tissues express NGF messenger RNA (mRNA) (77). Using immunocytochemical staining of a series of normal (i.e., N = 67), BPH (N = 15), and primary prostate cancers (N = 27), NGF is present within all of these tissues (77a). NGF and its respective 140-kD high-affinity tyrosine kinase (i.e., trkA) receptors have been implicated in both normal and malignant prostate growth. Using Scatchard binding analysis, normal human prostatic glandular cells express high affinity (K_d = ~1 × 10^{-11}M) trkA receptors (78). Using immunocytochemical analysis, trkA is expressed in epithelial cells in normal human prostates (N = 67) and is homogeneously expressed (i.e., expressed in greater than or equal to 80% of the cancer cells examined) by 60% of the primary tumors (N = 59) and 80% of the metastases (N = 10) (79) (77a). In approximately one-third of these lesions, expression is actually higher than in normal prostate. Like the situation in humans, normal rat prostate and various members of the Dunning system of rat prostate cancers express measurable amounts of NGF (80). Using immunocytochemical analysis, trkA is expressed in the normal rat prostate epithelium and in all of the Dunning rat cancer sublines (79).

Reverse transcriptase-polymerase chain reaction (RT-PCR) confirmed these immunocytochemical analyses in a series of four human (i.e., LNCaP, DU145, PC3, and TSU-Pr1) and five rat (i.e., Dunning G, MatLyLu, AT-2, AT-3.1, and AT-6.1) prostate cancer cell lines, maintained as pure populations of malignant cells in tissue culture. Trk expression was also examined in a human xenograft (PC82) and a syngeneic rat tumor (Dunning H) grown *in vivo*. Each of these prostate cancer lines or tissues expressed trkA transcripts (79). These data indicate that trk expression is maintained in all established tumors and cell lines derived from spontaneous human and rodent prostate cancers. RT-PCR analysis for trkA expression was also performed on prostate tissue obtained directly from 18 patients undergoing radical prostatectomy for localized prostate cancer. These results demonstrated that 67% (12 of 18) of primary prostate cancer tissue expresses trkA mRNA (77a). In additional studies, no mutations were detected in the trkA gene within these cancers (81).

Besides high-affinity trkA receptors, NGF can also bind to a 75-kD lower-affinity plasma membrane receptor termed p75 (75,82). The function of the p75 receptor is not clear, but it is a member of the tumor necrosis factor α kD family of plasma membrane receptor proteins. Expression of the p75 low-affinity receptor is not required for signaling via the 140-kD high-affinity trkA receptor, but coexpression does enhance such signaling (75). Using a monoclonal antibody to p75, expression of p75 protein immunocytochemically in both the basal and luminal epithelial cells in all normal human prostate (N = 67) and in BPH tissue (N = 15) was determined. The level of expression is higher in the basal than the luminal epithelial cell. In direct contrast, only 4 of 27 (15%) primary prostate cancers expressed comparable levels of p75 staining, whereas in this series, 16 of 27 (60%) of the cancers had equivalent or higher levels of trkA protein expression (77a). Using RT-PCR, Western blotting, and immunocytochemical staining, none of the established human prostate cancer cell lines available (e.g., DU145, PC3, LNCaP, and TSU) expressed p75, even though all of these lines expressed trkA (82–85).

Combining these results demonstrates that, whereas both normal and malignant prostate cells produce NGF, there are differences between these cells based on their pattern of trkA versus p75 receptor expression. Using a combination of RT-PCR and Western blotting analysis, TSU and DU145 human prostate cancer cell lines produce significant amounts of NGF and in all prostate cancer lines (i.e., TSU, DU145, LNCaP, and PC3), NGF binding to trkA receptors leads to receptor dimerization and activation of both the ras/raf/Mek/erk and PI3K/PKBK/Akt cascades. Because both normal and malignant prostate cells express both NGF and trkA, the issue is raised of what would happen to these prostate cells if they were treated with an inhibitor of the tyrosine kinase activity of the NGF occupied trkA receptor. For these studies, the trk tyrosine kinase inhibitor CEP-751 was selected from a library of K-252a indolocarbazole derivatives, because it inhibits neurotrophin/trk signaling at low nanomolar concentrations *in vitro* and at low mg per kg doses *in vivo* (86).

Initial studies demonstrated that at maximally tolerated subcutaneous doses of CEP-751 inhibition of tyrosine kinase activity of trk receptors had no discernable effect on the normal rat prostate. This is not unreasonable, because inhibiting the tyrosine kinase activity of the NGF/trk receptor should not inhibit the activation of either the ras/raf/Mek/erk or PI3K/PKBK/Art cascades by the binding of the other growth factors present (i.e., IGF, FGF, and others) to their cognate receptors. What was highly unexpected was the observation that when using the same subcutaneous *in vivo* dosing regimens in nine different models of human (LNCaP, DU145, PC3, TSU, and PC82) and rodent (Dunning G, MatLyLu, AT-2, and H) prostate cancer, CEP-751 inhibited the *in vivo* growth by 40% to 80% in all of the prostatic cancer sublines tested, independent of their state of differentiation, androgen sensitivity, metastatic ability, or growth rate (79,87). Using terminal transferase end-labeling to quantitate the percentage of tumor cells dying, and bromodeoxyuridine incorporation to determine the percentage of cells in cycle, the major effect of CEP-751 treatment was documented to enhance death, not to inhibit the proliferation of these cancer cells (i.e., its major effect is cytotoxic, not antiproliferative) (79,87).

These results demonstrated that inhibiting the signaling ability of the NGF/trkA receptor complex in malignant, but not normal prostate epithelial cells, induces apoptosis. Another difference between normal and malignant prostate cells is their response to PI3K inhibition. Within 48 hours of treatment with the PI3K inhibitor, LY293002, more than 90% of normal human prostate epithelial cells in early passage, maintained in serum-free defined media containing insulin, IGF-II, EGF, basic FGF (bFGF), and NGF, underwent apoptosis (77a). In contrast, when a series of rodent (i.e., AT-3) and human (i.e., TSU, PC3, and DU145) prostate cancer cells were similarly exposed for 48 hours to PI3K inhibitors, at most only 30% of the cancer cells underwent apoptosis (A. Weeraratna, J. Issacs, *unpublished data*, 2001). These results demonstrate that, in malignant prostate cancer cells, changes have occurred, as compared to normal prostate epithelial cells, such that now the tyrosine kinase activity of the NGF/trkA receptor complex is chronically required to suppress the activation of apoptosis via stimulation of more than just PI3K.

In additional studies, exposure of human prostate cancer cells to 100-nm CEP-751 demonstrated a delayed (i.e., greater than 18 hours post initial exposure) rise in the intracellular free calcium concentration (i.e., Ca_i^{2+}) from 20 to 40 nm to 10 to 20 μm (88). This delayed rise in $[Ca^{2+}]_i$ is associated with cytochrome-c release from the mitochondria and activation of genomic DNA fragmentation, and thus apoptotic death of the cancer cells. Using a variety of methods to block this delayed rise in $[Ca^{2+}]_i$, without inhibiting the decrease in the PI3K/Akt phosphorylation pathway induced by CEP-751, documented that inhibition of the latter survival pathway, although necessary, was not sufficient for induction of apoptosis by these prostate cancer cells (88). Such apoptosis additionally requires the delayed μm $[Ca^{2+}]_i$ rise also induced by CEP-751 treatment.

There are additional therapeutic methods for producing a delayed $[Ca^{2+}]_i$ rise in prostate cancer cells, which efficiently induced this apoptotic death (89). For example, thapsigargin is a sesquiterpene lactone that selectively inhibits the sarcoplasmic and the endoplasmic reticulum Ca^{2+}-ATPases (SERCA) (90). Inhibition of the SERCA causes depletion of intracellular Ca^{2+} stores, resulting in an initial transient (i.e., less than 6 hours) rise in cytoplasmic Ca^{2+} concentration, which is followed by a delayed (i.e., greater than 18 hours) influx of extracellular Ca^{2+}, producing a secondary sustained elevation of cytoplasmic Ca^{2+} to a value greater than 10 μm (90,91). This delayed μm elevation of the cytosolic Ca^{2+} concentration activates the proliferation-independent programmed death of susceptible cells, including androgen-independent prostate cancer cells, by the calcineurin/BAD/cytochrome-c pathway outlined in Figure 5-2 (90–93). Because the SERCA is present in all cells, thapsigargin (TG) also induces apoptosis in many normal host cells. Consequently, a method of targeting the proliferation-independent cytotoxicity of TG selectively to prostate cancer cells is needed. To target TG, advantage can be taken of the secretion of prostate-specific antigen (PSA) by prostate cancer cells. PSA is a serine protease with an unusual specificity. Thus, PSA can efficiently liberate toxic compounds covalently linked via an interval amino group to the c-terminal carboxylic acid group of glutamine of a PSA-specific six–amino acid peptide, N-histidine-serine-serine-lysine-leucine-glutamine–COOH (94,95). In contrast, this covalently linked prodrug is a very poor substrate for other purified proteases and proteases present in sera (94,96). The specificity of such a prodrug has further been illustrated by incubating cancer cells with a prodrug, in which the amino group of doxorubicin is coupled to the c-terminal of glutamine in this six–amino acid peptide. Only PSA-producing cells are killed, validating that doxorubicin is only liberated in the vicinity of such cells (94). A fast inactivation of PSA outside the prostate ductal system means that the hydrolytic activity only will be of significance in the close vicinity of prostate cells and prostate cancer cells (95). The aim is to develop a prodrug consisting of a primary amine containing TG analog, which, via the amine group, is coupled to a PSA-cleavable peptide. Presently, such TG analogs have been synthesized (97) and are being coupled to the PSA-specific peptide for testing in preclinical animal models.

SUMMARY

Androgen ablation therapy has been an important modality for the treatment of disseminating prostatic cancer for nearly 60 years. Unfortunately, such therapy, when given alone, is rarely curative. The failure of this therapy to cure such tumors, even though it can induce an initially positive response, is not due to a change in the systemic effectiveness of such a treatment. Instead, the development of resistance to such therapy is related to changes in the tumor itself. Experiments by a large number of investigators have identified several of the important tumor cell and host factors involved in these tumor changes. Through the identification of these factors, a concept has evolved that there may be multiple pathways for the development of resistance to hormonal therapy based on a stem-cell model for the normal prostate (40). Although such pathways can be described in phenomenologic terms, the detailed molecular biology of such a process is still unknown. It is clear, however, that the essential feature of the development of androgen resistance is the emergence of androgen-independent or -sensitive cancer cells, or both. The critical question for future studies is, therefore, Exactly how do androgen-independent cells develop? If this question can be answered, it might be possible to design therapies that prevent the development of these independent tumor cells.

Only under such conditions would androgen ablation therapy, used as a single modality, become potentially curative. However, even if therapeutic means can be developed to prevent the emergence of androgen-independent or -sensitive tumor cells, or both, this type of blocking therapy would have to be performed before such development had already occurred to be effective. Therefore, before such therapy was begun, some type of clinical test to determine that the tumor did not already have some androgen-independent or -sensitive tumor cells, or both, present (i.e., the tumor was not already heterogeneous androgen–sensitive), would additionally be required. Because at present, neither a method for determining the homogeneous versus heterogeneous nature of the androgen requirements of a particular tumor, nor a method for prevention of the development of androgen-independent or -sensitive tumor cells, or both, from dependent prostate cancer cells is available, these should be critical areas for extensive future study. Any advancement in either of these important areas would have profound consequences on the more effective issue of androgen ablation therapy.

Until these advancements are made, it would appear appropriate that androgen ablation therapy be used in combination with other modalities of treatment (e.g., radiation or other chemotherapy, or both, and others), which are specifically targeted at the androgen-independent or -sensitive cells, or both, either initially present or developing during androgen ablation therapy. Standard antiproliferative chemotherapeutic agents may be ineffective against such androgen-independent or -sensitive prostatic cancers, or both, because these cancers have a low proliferative rate (i.e., the median daily proliferative rate of prostate cancer cells within lymph node or bone metastases was less than 5% per day). Newer agents are needed that target the greater than 95% of prostate cancer cells within a given metastatic site that are not immediately proliferating. Several approaches have been proposed that are targeted at decreasing survival signals while elevating the Ca_i^{2+} to activate the apoptotic death cascade in prostate cancer cells. Such approaches can be combined with standard androgen ablation to increase their efficiency. In such combination approaches, it will be critical to evaluate the importance of both the timing (early vs. late) and the order (sequential or simultaneous) of androgen therapy in relation to these other modalities.

REFERENCES

1. Budke H, Orazi A, Neiman RS, et al. Assessment of cell proliferation in paraffin sections of normal bone marrow by the monoclonal antibodies KI-67 and PCNA. *Mod Pathol* 1994;7:860–866.
2. Knaggs HE, Holland DB, Morris C, et al. Quantification of cellular proliferation in acne using the monoclonal antibody Ki-67. *J Invest Dermatol* 1994;102:89–92.
3. Johnston PG, O'Brien MJ, Dervan PA, et al. Immunohistochemical analysis of cell kinetic parameters in colonic adenocarcinomas, adenomas, and normal mucosa. *Hum Pathol* 1989;20:696–700.
4. Landis SH, Murray T, Bolden S, et al. Cancer statistics, 1998. *CA Cancer J Clin* 1998;48:6–29.
5. Berges RR, Vukanovic J, Epstein JI, et al. Implication of the cell kinetic changes during the progression of human prostatic cancer. *Clin Cancer Res* 1995;1:473–480.
6. Kyprianou N, English H, Isaacs JT. Programmed cell death during regression of the PC-82 human prostate cancer following androgen ablation. *Cancer Res* 1990;50:3748–3752.
7. Eisenberger MA, Blumenstein BA, Crawford ED, et al. Bilateral orchiectomy with or without flutamide for metastatic prostate cancer. *N Engl J Med* 1998;339:1036–1042.
8. Isaacs JT. Antagonistic effect of androgen on prostatic cell death. *Prostate* 1984;5:545–559.
9. Kyprianou N, Isaacs JT. Activation of programmed cell death in the rat ventral prostate following castration. *Endocrinology* 1988;122:552–562.
10. Denmeade SR, Lin XS, Isaacs JT. Role of programmed (apoptotic) cell death during the progression and therapy of prostate cancer. *Prostate* 1996;28:251–265.
11. Joseph IBJK, Isaacs JT. Potentiation of the antiangiogenic ability of Linomide by androgen ablation involves down-regulation of vascular endothelial growth factor in human androgen responsive prostatic cancer. *Cancer Res* 1997;57: 1054–1057.
12. Joseph IBJK, Nelson JB, Denmeade SR, Isaacs JT. Androgens regulate vascular endothelial growth factor content in normal and malignant prostatic tissue. *Clinical Cancer Res* 1997;3:2507–2511.
13. Isaacs JT, Coffey DS. Etiology of BPH. *Prostate Suppl* 1998;2:33.
14. Bonkhoff H, Remberger K. Differentiation pathways and histogenetic aspects of normal and abnormal prostatic growth: a stem cell model. *Prostate* 1996;28:98–106.
15. DeMarzo AM, Nelson WG, Meeker AK, et al. Stem cell features of benign and malignant prostate epithelial cells. *J Urol* 1998;160:2381–2392.
16. DeMarzo AM, Meeker AK, Epstein JI, et al. Prostate stem cell compartments: expression of the cell cycle inhibitor p27Kip1 in normal, hyperplastic, and neoplastic cells. *Am J Pathol* 1998;153:911–919.
17. Porter AC, Vaillancourt RR. Tyrosine kinase receptor-activated signal transduction pathway which lead to oncogenesis. *Oncogene* 1998;16:1343–1352.
18. Hemmings BA. Akt signaling: linking membrane events of life and death decisions. *Science* 1997;275:628–630.
19. Kaplan DR, Stephens RM. Neurotrophin signal transduction by the trk receptor. *J Neurobiol* 1994;25:1404–1417.
20. Stephens L, Anderson K, Stokoe D, et al. Protein kinase B kinases that mediate phosphatidylinositol 3,4,5-trisphosphate-dependent activation of protein kinase B. *Science* 1998;279:710–714.
21. Walker KS, Deak M, Paterson A, et al. Activation of protein kinase B β and γ isoforms by insulin in vivo and by 3-phosphoinositide-dependent protein kinase-1 in vitro: comparison with protein kinase Bα. *Biochem J* 1998;331:299–308.
22. Cardone MH, Roy N, Stennicke HR, et al. Regulation of cell death protease caspase-9 by phosphorylation. *Science* 1998;282:1318–1321.
23. Datta SR, Dudek H, Tao X, et al. Atk phosphorylation of BAD couples survival signals to the cell-intrinsic death machinery. *Cell* 1997;91:231–241.
24. Zha J, Harada H, Yang E, et al. Serine phosphorylation of death agonist BAD in response to survival factor results in binding to 14-3-3 not BCL-XL. *Cell* 1996;87:619–628.
25. Wang H-G, Pathan N, Ethell IM, et al. Ca2+-induced apoptosis through calcineurin dephosphorylation of BAD. *Science* 1999;284:339–343.
26. Narita M, Shimizu S, Ito T, et al. Bax interacts with the permeability transition pore to induce permeability transition and cytochrome c release in isolated mitochondria. *Proc Natl Acad Sci U S A* 1998;95:14681–14686.
27. Green DR, Reed JC. Mitochondria and apoptosis. *Science* 1998;281:1309–1312.
28. Zou H, Henzel WJ, Liu X, et al. Apaf-1, a human protein homologous to *C. elegans* CED-4, participates in cytochrome c-dependent activation of caspase-3. *Cell* 1997; 90:405–413.
29. Li P, Jijhawan D, Budihardjo I, et al. Cytochrome c and dATP-dependent formation of Apaf-1/caspase-9 complex initiates an apoptotic protease cascade. *Cell* 1997;91:479–489.
30. Qin H, Srinivasula SM, Wu G, et al. Structural basis of procaspase-9 recruitment by the apoptotic protease-activating factor 1. *Nature* 1999;399:549–557.
31. Cain K, Brown DG, Langlais C, et al. Caspase activation involves the formation of the aposome, a large (approximately 700 kD) caspase-activating complex. *J Biol Chem* 1999;274:22686–22692.
32. Liu X, Li P, Widlak P, et al. The 40-kDa subunit of DNA fragmentation factor induces DNA fragmentation and chromatin condensation during apoptosis. *Proc Natl Acad Sci U S A* 1998;95:8461–8466.
33. Lui X, Zou H, Widlak P, et al. Activation of the apoptotic endonuclease DFF40 (caspase-activated DNase or nuclease). Oligomerization and direct interaction with histone H1. *J Biol Chem* 1999;274:13835–13840.
34. Furuya Y, Isaacs JT. Proliferation dependent versus independent programmed cell death of prostatic cancer cells involving distinct gene regulation. *Prostate* 1994;26:301–309.
35. Kyprianou N, English H, Isaacs JT. Activation of Ca2+-Mg2+-dependent endonuclease as an early event in castra-

tion induced prostatic cell death. *Prostate* 1988;13:103–117.
36. English H, Kyprianou N, Isaacs JT. Relationship between DNA fragmentation and apoptosis in the programmed cell death in the rat prostate following castration. *Prostate* 1989;15:233–250.
37. Kyprianou N, Isaacs JT. Expression of transforming growth factor β in the rat ventral prostate during castration-induced programmed cell death. *Mol Endocrinol* 1989;3:1515–1522.
38. Martikainen P, Isaacs JT. The role of calcium in the programmed death of rat prostatic glandular cells. *Prostate* 1990;17:175–188.
39. Martikainen P, Kyprianou N, Isaacs JT. Effect of transforming growth factor-β1 on proliferation and death of rat prostatic cells. *Endocrinology* 1990;127:2963–2968.
40. Isaacs JT. The biology of hormone refractory prostate cancer. *Urol Clin North Am* 1999;26:263–273.
41. Isaacs JT, Wake N, Coffey DS, et al. Genetic instability coupled to clonal selection as a mechanism for tumor progression in the Dunning R-3327 rat prostatic adenocarcinoma system. *Cancer Res* 1982;42:2353–2361.
42. Freed JJ, Schatz SA. Chromosomal aberrations in cultured cells deprived of single essential amino acids. *Exp Cell Res* 1969;55:393–409.
43. Franck-Lissbrant I, Haggstrom S, Damber JE, et al. Testosterone stimulates angiogenesis and vascular regrowth in the ventral prostate in castrated rats. *Endocrinology* 1998;139: 451–456.
44. Jain RK, Safabakhsh N, Sckell A, et al. Endothelial cell death, angiogenesis and microvascular function following castration in an androgen-dependent tumor: role of VEGF. *Proc Natl Acad Sci U S A* 1998;95:10820–10825.
45. Benjamin LE, Golijanin D, Itin A, et al. Selective ablation of immature blood vessels in established human tumors follows vascular endothelial growth factor withdrawal. *J Clin Inves* 1999;103:159–165.
46. Lee WH, Morton RA, Epstein JI, et al. Cytidine methylation of regulatory sequences near the p-class glutathione-S-transferase gene accompanies human prostate cancer carcinogenesis. *Proc Natl Acad Sci U S A* 1994;91:11733–11737.
47. Hockenbery DM. The bcl-2 oncogene and apoptosis. *Semin Immunol* 1992;4:413–420.
48. McDonnell TJ, Troncoso P, Brisbay SM, et al. Expression of the protooncogene bcl-2 in the prostate and its association with emergence of androgen-independent prostate cancer. *Cancer Res* 1992;52:6940–6944.
49. Colombel M, Symmans F, Gil S, et al. Detection of the apoptosis-suppressing oncoprotein bcl-2 in hormone-refractory human prostate cancers. *Am J Pathol* 1993;143:390–400.
50. Raffo AJ, Perlman H, Chen MW, et al. Overexpression of bcl-2 protects prostate cancer cells from apoptosis in vitro and confers resistance to androgen depletion *in vivo. Cancer Res* 1995;55:4438–4445.
51. Furuya Y, Krajewski S, Septein JI, et al. Expression of bcl-2 and the progression of human and rodent prostatic cancers. *Clin Cancer Res* 1996;2:389–398.
52. Hobisch A, Culig Z, Radmayr C, et al. Distant metastases from prostate carcinoma express androgen receptor protein. *Cancer Res* 1995;55:3068–3072.
53. Hobisch A, Culig Z, Radmayr C, et al. Androgen receptor status of lymph node metastases from prostate cancer. *Prostate* 1996;28:129–133.
54. Viskorpi T, Hyytinen E, Koivisto P, et al. *In vivo* amplification of the androgen receptor gene and progression of human prostate cancer. *Nat Genet* 1995;9:401–406.
55. Koivisto P, Kononen J, Palmberg C, et al. Androgen receptor gene amplification: a possible molecular mechanism for androgen deprivation therapy failure in prostate cancer. *Cancer Res* 1997;57:314–319.
56. Culig Z, Hobisch A, Cronauer MV, et al. Mutant androgen receptor detected in an advanced-stage prostatic carcinoma is activated by adrenal androgens and progesterone. *Mol Endocrinol* 1993;7:1541–1550.
57. Tilley WD, Buchanan G, Hickey TT, et al. Mutations in the androgen receptor gene are associated with progression of human prostate cancer to androgen independent. *Clin Cancer Res* 1996;2:277–285.
58. Culig Z, Hobisch A, Cronauer MV, et al. Androgen receptor activation in prostatic tumor cell lines by insulin-like growth factor-I, keratinocyte growth factor and epidermal growth factor. *Cancer Res* 1994;54:5474–5478.
59. Nazareth LV, Weigel NL. Activation of the human androgen receptor through a protein kinase A signaling pathway. *J Biol Chem* 1996;271:19900–19907.
60. Chen S, Song CS, Larvorsky Y, et al. Catalytic cleavage of the androgen receptor messenger RNA and functional inhibition of androgen receptor activity by a hammerhead ribozyme. *Mol Endocrinol* 1998;12:1558–1566.
61. Xu J, Qin Y, DeMayo FJ, et al. Partial hormone resistance in mice with disruption of the steroid receptor coactivator-1 (SRC-1) gene. *Science* 1998;279:1922–1925.
62. Matuo Y, Nishi N, Matsui S, et al. Heparin binding affinity of rat prostatic growth factor in normal and cancerous prostates: partial purification and characterization of rat prostatic growth factor in the Dunning tumor. *Cancer Res* 1987;47:188–192.
63. Matuo Y, Nishi N, Tanaka H, Sasaki I, et al. Production of IGF-II-related peptide by an anaplastic cell line (AT-3) established from the Dunning prostatic carcinoma of rats. *In Vitro Cell Dev Biology* 1988;24:1053–1056.
64. Sitaras NM, Sariban E, Bravo M, et al. Constitutive production of platelet-derived growth factor-like proteins by human prostate carcinoma cell lines. *Cancer Res* 1988;48:1930–1935.
65. Fowler JE, James LT, Lau LG, et al. Epidermal growth factor and prostatic carcinoma: an immunohistochemical study. *J Urol* 1988;139:857–861.
66. Mansson P-E, Adams P, Kan M, et al. Heparin-binding growth factor gene expression and receptor characteristics in normal rat prostate and two transplantable rat prostate tumors. *Cancer Res* 1989;49:2485–2494.
67. Jarrad DF, Bussemakers MJG, Bova GS, et al. Regional loss of imprinting of the insulin-like growth factor II gene occurs in human prostate tissues. *Clin Cancer Res* 1995;1:1471–1478.
68. Raff MC, Barres BA, Burne JF, et al. Programmed cell death and the control of cell survival: lessons from the nervous system. *Science* 1993;262:695–700.
69. Harrington EA, Bennett MR, Fanidi A, Evan GI. C-Myc–induced apoptosis in fibroblasts is inhibited by specific cytokines. *EMBO J* 1994;13:3286–3295.

70. Whang YE, Wu X, Suzuki H, et al. Inactivation of the tumor suppressor PTEN/MMAC 1 in advanced human prostate cancer through loss of expression. *Proc Natl Acad Sci U S A* 1998;95:5246–5250.
71. Stambolic B, Suzuki A, de la Pompa JL, et al. Negative regulation of PKB/Akt-dependent cell survival by the tumor suppressor PTEN. *Cell* 1998;95:29–39.
72. Kenney SG, Wagner AJ, Conzen DS, et al. The PI 3-kinase/Akt signaling pathway delivers an anti-apoptotic signal. *Genes Dev* 1997;11:701–713.
73. Alessi DR, Andjelkovic M, Caudwell B, et al. Mechanism of activation of protein kinase B by insulin and IGF-1. *EMBO J* 1996;15:6541–6551.
74. Xia Z, Dickens M, Raingeaud J, et al. Opposing effects of ERK and JNK-p38 MAP kinases on apoptosis. *Science* 1995;270:1326–1331.
75. Aloyz RS, Bamji SX, Pazniak CD, et al. P53 is essential for developmental neuron death as regulated by the trkA and p75 neurotrophin receptor. *J Cell Biol* 1998;143:1691–1703.
76. Franke TF, Yang S-II, Chan TO, et al. The protein kinase encoded by the Akt proto-oncogene is a target of the PDGF-activated phosphatidylinositol 3-kinase. *Cell* 1995; 81:727–736.
77. Paul AB, Grant ES, Habib FK. The expression and localisation of β-nerve growth factor (β-NGF) in benign and malignant human prostate tissue: relationship to neuroendocrine differentiation. *Br J Cancer* 1996;74:1990–1996.

77a. Weeraratna AT, Arnold JT, George DJ, et al. Rational basis for TrK inhibition therapy for prostate cancer. *Prostate* 2000;45:140–148.

78. Pflug BR, Dionne CA, Kaplan DR, et al. Expression of the Trk high affinity nerve growth factor receptor in the human prostate. *Endocrinology* 1995;136:262–268.
79. Dionne CA, Camoratto AM, Jani JP, et al. Cell cycle-independent death of prostate adenocarcinoma is induced by the trk tyrosine kinase inhibitor CEP-751 (KT6587). *Clin Cancer Res* 1998;4:1887–1898.
80. Geldof AA, De Kleijn MAT, Rao BR, et al. Nerve growth factor stimulates *in vitro* invasive capacity of DU145 human prostatic cancer cells. *J Cancer Res Clin Oncol* 1997;123:107–112.
81. George DA, Suski H, Bova GS, et al. Mutational analysis of the trkA gene in prostate cancer. *Prostate* 1998;36:172–180.
82. Graham CW, Lynch JH, Djakiew D. Distribution of nerve growth factor-like protein and nerve growth factor receptor in human prostatic hyperplasia and prostatic carcinoma. *J Urol* 1992;147:1444–1447.
83. Pflug BR, Onoda M, Lynch JH, et al. Reduced expression of the low affinity nerve growth factor receptor in benign and malignant human prostate tissue and loss of expression in four human metastatic prostate tumor cell lines. *Cancer Res* 1992;52:5403–5406.
84. Djakiew D, Delsite R, Dalal R, et al. The role of the low affinity nerve growth factor receptor and the high affinity Trk receptor in human prostate carcinogenesis. *Radiat Oncol Investg* 1996;3:333–339.
85. Perez M, Regan T, Pflug B, et al. Loss of the low affinity nerve growth factor receptor during malignant transformation of the human prostate. *Prostate* 1997;30:274–279.
86. Camoratto AM, Jani JP, Angeles TS, et al. CEP-751 inhibits trk receptor tyrosine kinase activity in vitro and exhibits anti-tumor activity. *Int J Cancer* 1997;72:673–679.
87. George DJ, Dionne CA, Jani J, et al. Sustained in vivo regression of Dunning H rat prostate cancers treated with combinations of androgen ablation and trk tryosine kinase inhibitors CEP-751 (KT-6587) or CEP-701 (KT-5555). *Cancer Res* 1999;59:2395–2401.
88. Weeraratna AT, Tombal BT, Isaacs JT. The tyrosine kinase inhibitors CEP-751 (KT-6587) and CEP-701 (KT-5555) lead to apoptosis in prostate cancer cells via the elevation of intracellular free calcium and inhibition of the PI-3Kinase/PKB pathway. In Submission.
89. Martikainen P, Kyprianou N, Tucker RW, et al. Programmed death of nonproliferating androgen-independent prostatic cancer cells. *Cancer Res* 1991;51:4693–4700.
90. Furuya Y, Lundmo P, Short AD, et al. The role of calcium, pH and cell proliferation in the programmed (apoptotic) death of androgen-independent prostatic cancer cells induced by thapsigargin. *Cancer Res* 1994;54:6167–6175.
91. Tombal B, Denmeade SR, Isaacs JT. Assessment and validation of a microinjection method for kinetic analysis of [Ca2+]i in individual cells undergoing apoptosis. *Cell Calcium* 1999;25:19–28.
92. Furuya Y, Isaacs JT. Proliferation dependent versus independent programmed cell death of prostatic cancer cells involving distinct gene regulation. *Prostate* 1994;26:301–309.
93. Lin XS, Denmeade SR, Cisek L, et al. Mechanism and role of growth arrest in programmed (apoptotic) death of prostatic cancer cells induced by thapsigargin. *Prostate* 1997;33: 201–207.
94. Denmeade SR, Nagy A, Gao J, et al. Enzymatic activation of a doxorubicin-peptide prodrug by prostate-specific antigen. *Cancer Res* 1998;58:2537–2540.
95. Denmeade SR, Isaacs JT. Enzymatic activation of prodrugs by prostate specific antigen: targeted therapy for metastatic prostate cancer. *Cancer J Sci Am* 1998;4:15–21.
96. Denmeade SR, Lou W, Maim J, et al. Specific and efficient peptide substrates for assaying the proteolytic activity of prostate specific antigen. *Cancer Res* 1997;57:4924–4930.
97. Christensen SB, Andersen A, Kromann H, et al. Thapsigargin analogues for targeting programmed death of androgen-independent prostate cancer cells. *Bioorg Med Chem* 1999;7:1273–1280.

6

EVOLUTION OF HORMONE-REFRACTORY PROSTATE CANCER

GLENN J. BUBLEY

DIMENSIONS OF THE PROBLEM

Despite increased awareness and the use of prostate-specific antigen (PSA) screening over the past several years, more than 37,000 men still die yearly from prostate cancer (1). Almost all of these men will have had hormone-refractory prostate cancer (HRPC) or progressive disease after androgen deprivation (AD). Efforts at screening and prevention may yet reduce the number of men who progress to this stage of disease, but for the foreseeable future, at least, HRPC will be a major problem in the management of prostate cancer.

The pathogenesis of HRPC is still not understood. It has been known for more than 50 years that 80% to 90% of patients with bone metastasis will respond initially to AD. But the duration of response is almost always finite, averaging 12 to 18 months (2). AD administered earlier in the disease, for instance before the onset of bone disease, has a longer duration of response, but most men are still likely to become resistant to this form of therapy. For this reason, a better understanding of the evolution of HRPC is extremely important. Recurrence after AD carries with it, initially, the emotional burden of observing rising PSA levels and, subsequently, bone pain and other symptoms associated with the hormone-refractory state.

What has perplexed physicians for more than 50 years is the mechanism of resistance to androgen ablation. What is not understood is why this disease, which has so robust a response to AD, should inevitably recur. If it were possible to understand how cancer cells are able to thrive after extreme modification of their normal hormonal environment, then insights into therapeutic strategies might follow. In other words, if the underlying mechanisms behind resistance to AD could be elucidated, then it might be possible to at least delay the onset of this stage of disease by treating it more effectively or preventing it entirely.

In this chapter, we discuss what is currently understood about the evolution of HRPC. We define this state as progressive biochemical or clinical disease during the course of AD therapy, either luteinizing hormone releasing hormone (LHRH) analogs or orchiectomy. Therefore, we do not mean to infer that HRPC, as defined in this manner, is not sometimes responsive to additional hormonal maneuvers, such as antiandrogens or ketoconazole, as addressed in Chapter 43.

The focus in this chapter is on several critical issues. First, it is critically important to determine whether hormone-refractory cells are present at initial diagnosis or arise during the course of hormonal therapy. This question, often phrased as *adaption versus selection*, is fundamental for efforts currently under way for treatment of the disease in the adjuvant setting. Subsequent sections address the role of the androgen receptor. As will be discussed, there is evidence to suggest that androgen receptor (AR)–mediated signaling remains critical to the development of HRPC. As part of our discussion on the AR pathway, we address the possible role of a family of proteins that interact with the AR and affect its function, called *coactivators*. Other possible mechanisms through which the AR might have augmented function, including cross-talk to other signal transduction pathways, are also addressed. In addition, there may well be mechanisms of prostate cell growth independent of AR signaling. In other words, are there mechanisms of androgen-independent disease that are totally independent of the AR? Finally, we review what might be gleaned about the evolution of the hormonally refractive state from the clinical literature and suggest other possible clinical investigations that might be informative.

EFFECT OF ANDROGEN DEPLETION IN HORMONALLY SENSITIVE CELLS

The first step in attempting to understand the pathogenesis of HRPC is to appreciate how reducing androgen levels leads to the regression of prostate cancer. After androgen ablation, most normal prostate epithelial cells and most cancerous prostate cells undergo a multigene-encoded suicide pathway called *programmed cell death* or *apoptosis* (3). There is also likely to be a population of cells that do not undergo apoptosis but instead enter into a resting state in which they do not replicate. These cells may be able to survive without cycling in the G0 state (4). Because the clinical response to androgen ablation is always finite, these cells may represent the precursors that repopulate the bone marrow or other metastatic sites during relapse. Although the biologic properties of these androgen-independent cells are not known, an important issue is to understand to what degree prostate cancer, at any stage of disease, is dependent on androgen-mediated signaling for survival. Prostate cancer animal models suggest that prostate cancer, fairly early in its evolution, is heterogenous and is composed of androgen-independent and androgen-dependent cells, despite the significant apoptosis observed after androgen withdrawal (5,6). What is harder to discern in humans is to what degree prostate cancer cells can survive the withdrawal of the androgenic stimulus. Understanding this dynamic may have important implications for therapy, but we lack a full range of informative cell models to better investigate the HRPC phenotype. LNCaP cells are an androgen-responsive cell line that will stop cycling after androgen removal (4). However, for the most part, these cells do not die and are amenable to restimulation with subsequent androgen exposure. In fact, after long-term culture in minimal androgen media, this cell line is paradoxically inhibited by subsequent androgen exposure (4). The underlying mechanism behind this adaption is not known. However, cells that survive AD by any means are theoretically available to repopulate metastatic, or even the prostate at later stages in the illness. Are there cells that are androgen-independent even before the initiation of androgen deprivation therapy? Or are there cells that are able to adapt over time to the androgen-depleted environment by as-yet-not-understood mechanisms? This issue has important implications for therapy. If androgen-independent cells exist within a tumor mass from the beginning of androgen-depleting therapy, one might expect more complete, and perhaps more durable, responses by combining androgen depletion with therapies directed at androgen-independent cells, such as chemotherapy. Clearly, a better understanding of the basic biologic processes wherein cells can escape androgen-induced inhibition would enhance our capacity to investigate this problem during various stages of the illness.

ANDROGEN RECEPTOR

Much attention has focused on the AR as a possible key mediator in the evolution to HRPC. It has been suggested that AR signaling continues to be important in HRPC, because patients at this stage of the disease continue to display increased PSA serum levels with progressive disease (7). Although there may be other mechanisms regulating PSA expression, as is discussed below, a functional AR seems necessary to activate PSA expression by binding to identified androgen-responsive elements (AREs) within the PSA promoter (8). In addition, there is evidence that the AR is consistently expressed and, as is discussed below, even amplified, in many cases of HRPC.

How might the AR continue to activate androgen-inducible genes in the setting of reduced levels of serum androgen? One possible mechanism is altered AR function. The role of AR mutations in HRPC will be discussed in detail, as interesting gain of function mutations have been isolated from clinical samples obtained from men with HRPC. However, it is likely that AR mutations do not contribute to the pathogenesis of a majority of cases of HRPC. Therefore, other possibilities for modulation of AR function in HRPC will be addressed, although in most cases there is not yet firm evidence for their importance in the clinical setting.

As discussed in Chapter 3, the AR is a member of the superfamily of receptors called *steroid receptors*, which includes the estrogen, progesterone, and glucocorticoid receptors (9,10). Included in this family are also receptors that bind vitamin D, retinoic acid, and thyroid hormone. Because this family of receptors is active in the nucleus, and because of their similarity of structure, they are also called the *nuclear receptors*. In this chapter, we refer to this family as both steroid and nuclear receptors.

Like its relatives, the AR has three distinct domains: a carboxy-terminal hormone-binding domain (HBD), an amino-terminal transactivation domain, and a DNA-binding domain located between these regions (9,11). Genes whose expression is stimulated by androgen are flanked by specific DNA sequences, called AREs, which are recognized by the DNA-binding domain of the AR (11). After binding of testosterone or dihydrotestosterone (DHT) to the HBD, the receptor becomes phosphorylated and binds to AREs as dimers, stimulating transcription of *androgen-inducible* genes (8,11). A number of inducible genes have been identified, including the PSA gene. Importantly, recent observations suggest that this set of genes is reexpressed in the hormone-refractory state in at least some of the existing cell lines. Current investigation, using gene-chip technology, is focusing on the array of genes expressed at different stages of disease. If it is shown that the set of genes expressed in progressing hormonally naïve patients is very similar to the set of genes expressed in hormone-refractory patients, then it would support the hypothesis that AR-mediated signaling is important in the progression to HRPC. At this point, however, it is better to consider HRPC both as AR and non-AR mediated, although this distinction may prove to be arbitrary.

MUTATIONS OF THE ANDROGEN RECEPTOR IN HORMONE-REFRACTORY PROSTATE CANCER

If AR expression acts to maintain the cell in an androgen-dependent state, then one possible mechanism of HRPC might be down-regulation, or loss of AR expression. Although some prostate cancer cell lines, such as PC3 and DU145, do not express the AR, the weight of clinical evidence suggests that the AR, although more heterogeneous than in hormonally naïve patients, is consistently expressed, and even overexpressed, in HRPC. As early as 1991, studies by van der Kwast et al. demonstrated that more than 80% of HRPC specimens demonstrated expression of the AR as detected by a monoclonal antibody to the N-terminal region (12). Hobisch et al. confirmed this in a study published in 1995, in which they demonstrated AR staining in 21 of 22 distant metastases from HRPC patients (13). Because of the inherent genetic instability of late-stage cancer, persistent expression of the AR protein suggests that it may serve a critical function in the cell. This leads to the possibility that there are structural changes of the AR in HRPC.

The functional importance of structural change in the AR is underscored by patients with the androgen insensitivity syndrome (AIS). In this syndrome, affected individuals fail to develop normal genitalia, including prostates (14), even in the presence of normal levels of androgenic hormones. Studies performed over the past several years have shown that most of these patients have mutations in the AR (14,15). Moreover, in all AIS cases studied to date, the mutation's effects have been to inactivate or destabilize the protein (14,15).

In contrast to the inactivating mutations detected in AIS, is it possible that the AR is altered in HRPC by activating mutations? Because the AR has been mapped to the X chromosome, the effect of a mutation should be immediately evident and dominant, as there is no allele on a sister chromosome to alter its phenotype. The LNCaP mutation (codon 877, threonine to alanine) is particularly interesting in that it alters AR function in such a way that it can respond to steroid hormones other than androgen present in castrated men (17). Therefore, treatment of this cell line with relatively low levels of estrogen and progesterone results in enhanced growth, even in the absence of androgen (17). With the recognition of an AR mutation in the prostate cancer cell line, LNCaP (16,17), it became important to search for mutations in the AR that might enhance or alter its function.

One of the first systematic investigations of AR structure was performed by Newmark et al. In their study of 24 primary prostate specimens obtained before hormonal therapy, a point mutation in a tumor from one patient was detected (18). This mutation in codon 730 (GTG to ATG, valine to methionine), was detected in a minority of the cells, and the possible functional significance of this mutation was not determined. In contrast, Ruizeveld de Winter et al. did not detect any AR mutations in their study of 18 HRPC specimens, most of which were obtained from the prostate gland (19). These data suggested that AR mutations in prostate cancer are uncommon, at least before hormonal therapy or from the prostate, compared to metastases.

Supporting the hypothesis that AR mutations might be selected for by the hormone-refractory state or in metastatic sites, the first mutation with possible clinical and functional significance was isolated from a metastatic specimen from a patient with HRPC. This mutation, at codon 715 in the hormone-binding domain (GTG to ATG, valine to methionine), enhanced the sensitivity of the AR to androstenedione, an adrenal androgen, and progesterone *in vitro* (20). Taplin, working with our group, detected AR mutations in five of ten HRPC patients, focusing exclusively on tissue obtained from metastatic sites (primarily bone marrow) (21). One of these mutations was in the same codon as the LNCaP mutation but resulted in a different amino acid change (threonine to serine). The other mutations detected were located at codon 874 (histidine to tyrosine), 902 (glutamine to arginine), and 721 (alanine to tyrosine). Another patient had four separate mutations (21). All of these mutations were within the hormone-binding domain of the receptor. Two of these mutations (at codons 874 and 877) displayed an altered sensitivity to other steroid hormones, such as estrogen, progesterone, or androstenedione (Fig. 6-1) (21,22). One of the mutations, at codon 874, was later detected in a prostate cancer human xenograft propagated in immunodeficient mice (CWR22) (23). Suzuki et al. searched for AR mutations in both hormonally sensitive and resistant patients. They did not detect mutations in seven cases of hormonally sensitive disease but did detect AR mutations from patients with HRPC. In one case, disease from the primary site contained a mutation at codon 701 (threonine to alanine), and a mutation from a metastatic site in the same patient contained the LNCaP mutation (24). In fact, the LNCaP mutation was also detected in metastatic sites in two of the other 22 patients with HRPC investigated (24). Importantly, two of these three patients demonstrated a flutamide withdrawal response. As is discussed below, the clinical observation regarding the effects of discontinuing flutamide are of great interest, because some of the AR mutations, like the LNCaP mutation, can be activated by flutamide *in vitro*.

It should be noted that the functional effect of mutations, such as the one described at codon 715, have been investigated predominantly in nonprostate cancer cell lines using transient transfection assays. In this assay, expression plasmids containing mutant ARs are cotransfected cells with a reporter gene under the control of an androgen-responsive element (20–22). After transfection into cells that do not express an endogenous AR, AR-mediated signaling is assayed immediately as a readout from the reporter gene (20–22). Although the experiments are well controlled, the effects of other factors that may be specific to prostate cancer cells are not assessable.

The detection of mutations in metastases from HRPC patients, as well as their gain of function phenotype, would seem to present an organized picture regarding their pathogenesis and clinical importance. But Tilley

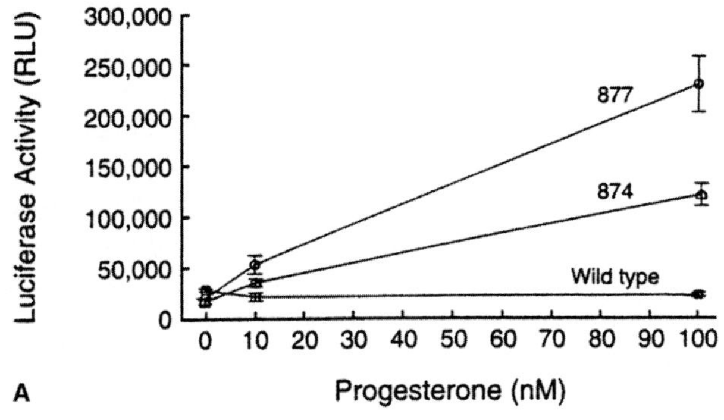

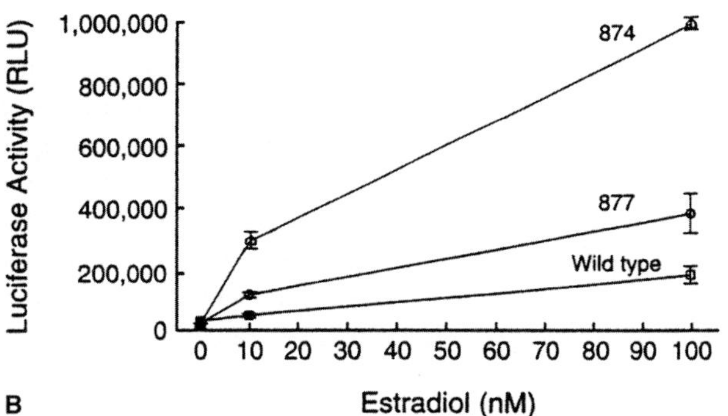

FIGURE 6-1. Functional analysis of androgen receptor mutations. Wild-type or mutant androgen receptors were transiently expressed in CV-1 cells with a luciferase reporter gene and various concentrations of progesterone **(A)** or estradiol **(B)**. The luciferase activity [expressed in relative light units (RLU)] was normalized for beta galactosidase activity to yield a standardized RLU. The maximal responses to androgen (5-alpha-dihydrotestosterone) for each androgen receptor averaged approximately 2,200,000 RLU for the wild-type androgen receptor, 1,500,000 RLU for the 874 mutant receptor, and 800,000 for the 877 mutant in three experiments. Determinations were performed in triplicate, and the mean (± standard error) results of a representative experiment are shown. (From Taplin ME, Bubley GJ, Shuster TD, et al. Mutation of the androgen-receptor gene in metastatic androgen-independent prostate cancer. *N Engl J Med* 1995;332:1393–1398, with permission.)

and his colleagues detected AR mutations in 11 of 25 cases of prostate cancer from untreated patients, suggesting that AR mutations are not as obviously important in the evolution of HRPC (25). Interestingly, the mutations they detected were not confined to the HBD of the AR. Although data regarding their activation *in vitro* was not provided, one mutation, at codon 794, is almost certainly inactivating, as it was also reported in a patient with complete AIS (25).

The importance of AR mutations to the evolution of HRPC might also differ in patients from different populations. Takahashi et al. investigated AR mutations in Japanese and American men. The incidence of clinical prostate cancer is much less prevalent in Japan, although the incidence of latent disease seems to be roughly equivalent (26). This group, therefore, analyzed disease samples obtained from both latent and clinically evident prostate cancer in both populations. They detected AR mutations only in Japanese men. Importantly, many of these AR mutations exhibited premature stop codons consistent with an inactivated receptor. These data suggested that one reason that latent disease might not progress to clinical disease in Japanese men is inactivating AR mutations, instead of the gain of function mutations that are sometimes demonstrated in HRPC.

The prevalence and potential clinical significance of AR mutations in the pathogenesis of HRPC are not immediately obvious. As discussed earlier, the frequency and kind of AR mutations may differ as a function of sampling the primary site versus metastasis, from sampling hormone-sensitive versus hormone-refractory disease, or even from sampling latent versus clinically apparent prostate cancer. Another factor that needs to be taken into consideration is the method used to detect these mutations. For instance, our group used reverse transcriptase polymerase chain reaction (RT-PCR) to amplify the AR, and then sequenced individual clones (21,22). Mutations were only confirmed as authentic, and not as a polymerase chain reaction (PCR) artifact, when a separate amplification was performed and the same mutation was detected. Furthermore, that these represented somatic and not germ line mutations was confirmed by analyzing the white cell DNA from the patient in question. Many other investigators used different techniques, such as single-stranded conformational polymorphism analysis. Tilley and colleagues carefully selected areas of analysis that demonstrated differential staining for AR expression between N- and c-terminal antibodies. They reasoned that these regions might more likely demonstrate structural changes in the AR. This very careful analysis, and careful selection of tissue sites, may have resulted in the higher mutation rate they found relative to other studies. Our group determined that a critical factor as to whether AR mutations could be detected from clinical samples is the hormonal environment of the patient at the time the sample is obtained. For instance, studies from our group suggest that AR mutations are detected most frequently from patients treated with long-term flutamide (27). This suggests that specific AR mutations can be selected among a population of prostate cancer cells. It makes sense that these cells might have a growth advantage, as flutamide is a strong agonist for cells harboring these mutations (22,27). This observation underscores the importance of attempting to understand the phenotype of the AR mutation. Given the paradigm for HRPC discussed so far in this chapter, AR mutations with a gain of function phenotype would be expected to be more critical to the acquisition of HRPC than inactivating mutations.

Chapter 3 in this book explores altered structure of the transactivation domain of the AR, particularly with respect to glutamine or glycine repeats in exon one of this gene. An alteration in the number of these repeat amino acids has an effect of AR function (28). Differences in repeat length have been demonstrated only in the germ line, and not in the affected tissue. Therefore, because this is thought to be a stable germ line mutation present in all the patient's prostate cancer cells, it is less likely to be a factor, *per se*, in the pathogenesis of HRPC. However, as shorter transactivating domains may make cells more sensitive to androgen signaling, it might affect the aggressiveness of the disease.

In summary, the significance of AR mutations to the pathogenesis of HRPC is not yet fully understood. However, the weight of evidence to date suggests that AR mutations play a role in only a minority of cases of HRPC, many of which might be the result of long-term flutamide administration.

Increased Expression of the Androgen Receptor in Hormone-Refractory Prostate Cancer

An intriguing clue regarding the evolution of HRPC is the consistent expression, and frequently apparent overexpression, of the AR observed in prostate cancer specimens obtained after AD therapy. Although AR expression can sometimes be heterogenous within the tumor tissue, immunohistochemical analysis has often demonstrated bright staining consistent with overexpression (12,13,29). One mechanism of increased protein expression is *gene amplification*, or an increase in gene copy number. Amplification is a well-known mechanism of resistance to chemotherapeutic agents in cancer therapy. For instance, cells treated *in vitro* with methotrexate over repeated passages often demonstrate a manyfold increase in copies of dihydrofolate reductase (DHFR) gene, the protein product of which can reverse methotrexate resistance. In cells, DHFR amplification can be visualized as expanded region within the chromosome in the location of the DHFR gene or as small fragments of DNA called *double minutes* (30).

Could AR amplification contribute to the evolution of HRPC? In other words, can the prostate cancer cell compensate for decreased levels of AR ligand by increasing AR expression? Using fluorescent *in situ* hybridization and other techniques, two groups have separately demonstrated AR amplification in approximately 30% of samples obtained from patients with HRPC (31,32). In contrast, AR amplification is only rarely observed in prostate cancer before hormonal therapy (31,32). Furthermore, amplification is more likely to occur in patients who have responded to androgen ablation for more than 12 months, suggesting that AR amplification is selected for over a relatively longer period of time in a setting of low levels of androgen. These observations may be important clues to the pathogenesis of HRPC. Furthermore, although amplification is observed only in a minority of HRPC cases, it should be noted that this mechanism is only one of a number of methods of increased gene expression. Therefore, it is quite possible that the frequency of AR amplification actually underestimates the degree of increased AR expression.

How might increased AR expression mediate disease progression after AD? There are a number of possibilities for investigation. For instance, increased AR expression might alter its association with other proteins that regulate the AR's localization and function within the cell (as below). Increased AR expression might also result in sufficient ligand binding, even in the setting of low levels of androgenic hormones, as is expected in the serum of men treated with AD therapy. Although there are many theoretical possibilities, an obvious explanation of how increased AR expression might result in the evolution of hormone refractory disease is not immediately obvious. In *in vitro* cell transfection experiments, hormonal independence is not established by simply increasing the amount of AR protein within the transfected cell. Also, targeting the AR in HRPC patients, using even high doses of existing antiandrogens such as bicalutamide, has not been associated with a very high response rate.

Androgen Receptor Interaction with Chaperone Proteins

It is generally believed that under normal conditions the AR undergoes a conformational alteration after binding to testosterone or DHT. This conformational change may have multiple effects in making the AR more available to affect downstream gene regulation (11). For instance, this conformational change may permit the release of AR from proteins that sequester it in a nonactive state. This group of proteins, called *heat shock proteins* (hsps), are known to bind to other steroid hormone receptors such as the glucocorticoid receptor (GR) (32–34). In the unbound state, GR is complexed to hsps in the cytoplasm. After binding glucocorticoid, the receptor undergoes a conformational change, permitting an alteration in its interaction with hsps such that it can translocate to the nucleus and bind to DNA response elements (32–35).

Is it possible that an alteration in the interaction between the AR and the hsp complex might be important in the progression to HRPC? Interesting *in vitro* experiments demonstrate that a deletion of a portion of the HBD of the AR results in a receptor that is constitutively active—that is, active in the absence of any steroid hormone or known ligands (11). The molecular basis for this is not known with certainty, although this deletion in the HBD results in an altered association with the hsp complex. Lack of a normal interaction with hsps might permit the AR to be free of the chaperoning effects of the hsps, possibly permitting translocation to the nucleus, and binding to DNA in the absence of ligand. However, large deletions have not been observed in clinical specimens from patients with HRPC. It is also possible that critical mutations in specific hsps could be selected during the evolution of HRPC, although these have also not been detected in clinical samples obtained from patients with HRPC. Increased AR expression, perhaps resulting from gene amplification, might also lead to an alteration in the AR's association with the hsp complex. These possibilities provide intriguing avenues for further investigation.

Coactivators and Corepressors of the Androgen Receptors in Hormone-Refractory Prostate Cancer

Nuclear or steroid receptors, such as the AR, interact with a number of other proteins that alter their function, often termed *coactivators* or *corepressors*. This group of proteins has the capacity to alter nuclear receptor activity, either enhancing (coactivator) or diminishing (corepressor) the function of the receptor (36–38).

Nuclear receptor modifying proteins have been identified through multiple methods. One of the more productive techniques is termed *yeast two-hybrid screening* (39). In this technique, a portion of a steroid receptor, such as the AR hormone-binding domain, is used as bait to search for proteins that interact with it in yeast. Although several AR-interacting proteins have been identified by this methodology, the challenge arises in attempting to understand the role these proteins may play in the development of prostate cancer or HRPC.

An important feature of many of the coactivators that have been identified thus far is that they can directly or indirectly trigger histone acetyl transferase activity (37,40). This activity alters chromatin formation, making it more amenable to transcription factors. Many coactivators, such as SRC-1 (steroid receptor coactivator) (41), also have the capacity to interact with a key cellular protein termed CBP/p300, which also remodels chromatin and recruits other transcription factors (40,41). As is often the case in biology, there is a class of steroid modifying proteins that have an opposite effect on transcription (38,42). This class, called *corepressors*, has been best studied for its interaction with the thyroid hormone receptor, another member of the steroid and nuclear receptor family.

A study of how coactivators interact with steroid receptors has yielded interesting insights into their function, particularly for the estrogen receptor (ER). Many coactivators interact with specific amino acid sequences in the hormone-binding domain of steroid receptors. For the ER, this is called the *activator function* (AF) 2 domain (36). Moreover, some of the family members of coactivators share a common amino acid motif (LLXXL) important for interaction with the steroid receptors, where the *Ls* stand for leucine and the *X* is any amino acid. This region of the modifying protein seems critical for direct binding to the nuclear receptor. Estrogen antagonists, such as tamoxifen, alter the position of critical protein residues in the AF2 region, which thereby alter the interaction with coactivators (36).

Is it possible that increased expression of a coactivator (or decreased expression of a corepressor) could play a role in the evolution of prostate cancer to HRPC? The steroid receptor–coactivator interaction certainly provides a possible mechanism for HRPC. However, firm evidence of their importance to the progression of HRPC does not yet exist. It would be important to determine whether coactivators exist that are relatively specific for the AR. It would also be important to ascertain whether a specific coactivator or corepressor altered AR substrate specificity or affinity. Finally, it would be interesting to detect an alteration in structure, function, or expression of the coactivator or corepressor during the evolution of HRPC.

Although most of the coactivators identified thus far are not specific for any nuclear receptor, Yeh and colleagues have identified coactivators that may be relatively specific to the AR. One, called ARA70, has some of the properties of a coactivator that may be involved in the evolution to HRPC (43,44). First, expression of ARA70 *in vitro* can enhance AR activity. Also, a number of antiandrogens, such as hydroxyflutamide and bicalutamide, seem to promote the interaction of ARA70 and AR, perhaps accounting for the partial agonist properties these antiandrogens exhibit *in vitro*. Also *in vitro*, in the setting of ARA70 overexpression, estradiol can act as a potent ligand for the AR (43,44). Although these data make it very important to determine whether during the progression to HRPC, ARA70 or a similar coactivator is altered or overexpressed, altered expression or function of coactivators or corepressors has not been detected in prostate cancer samples obtained from HRPC patients. However, this is a difficult problem to investigate in patient samples because of a lack of available antibodies or other methods to assess expression and function in sampled tumor. Currently, the role of coactivators or corepressors to the evolution of HRPC deserves to be actively investigated, but its significance is not known.

GROWTH FACTORS AND PROSTATE CANCER PROGRESSION

Growth factors, such as epidermal growth factors (EGFs) and platelet-derived growth factors, are small molecules that have been shown to be important for the growth and development of cancer. In the case of prostate cancer, epidemiologic evidence has shown that increases in one growth factor, insulinlike growth factor 1 (IGF-1), are associated with an increased risk of prostate cancer (45). Growth factors bind to specific growth factor receptors on the cell membrane. After binding to their cognate growth factor, the growth factor receptor is activated through phosphorylation in its tyrosine kinase domain and initiates a signaling cascade critical to cell growth, death, or differentiation. The biology of the large family of growth factor receptors, often called *receptor protein tyrosine kinases* (RPTKs), is of great interest for those interested in cancer treatment because of the recent availability of many highly specific, high-affinity antagonists of this family of receptors.

In general, there are two types of growth factor signaling pathways. The autocrine stimulatory pattern is one in which the cell makes both the growth factor and the ligand. The paracrine model is one in which surrounding cells provide crucial growth factors to the cancer cell. Both models are likely to contribute to the progression of prostate cancer. For instance, one group demonstrated that prostate cancer cells express both the EGF receptor and its cognate ligand, transforming growth factor alpha (46). This autocrine loop is not detected in normal prostatic epithelium. On the other hand, it is believed that the paracrine model of growth factor stimulation is also likely to be important for the progression of prostate cancer. Evidence of possible paracrine stimulation in prostate cancer progression comes from the observation that prostate cancer is very often admixed with stroma, both in the gland and at metastatic sites. It is possible that adjacent stroma produces necessary growth factors critical for the survival of the tumor. For instance, an important growth factor for prostate development is keratinocyte growth factor (KGF). KGF is produced in the stroma in response to androgen stimulation, and normal prostatic epithelial cells express the KGF receptor (47). Transforming growth factor beta normally has a negative effect on cell growth. However, one group discovered that this growth factor might paradoxically promote prostate cancer tumorigenicity (48). These basic observations, coupled with the known propensity for prostate cancer growth to be dependent on surrounding cell stroma, suggest mechanisms through which growth factor and receptor alterations might affect the progression of HRPC.

There have been some important experiments that suggest a role for growth factor signaling in the progression of prostate cancer. A critical observation is that activation of specific growth factor pathways *in vitro* can enhance AR activity, even in the absence of androgens. These observations connect pathways known to be important for cancer progression to AR function. For instance, it has been demonstrated that stimulation of LNCaP cells with KGF, EGF, or IGF-1 results in enhanced cell growth and PSA secretion independent of androgen (49). Importantly, in the LNCaP example, this effect is blocked by the antiandrogen bicalutamide, suggesting that the interaction must occur through the AR (49). Physiologic coupling between nuclear, steroid, and growth factor receptor families is also demonstrated by the example of mice in which the ER has been eradicated (ER knockout mice) (50). The normal effects of EGF stimulation in these animals, such as induction of the progesterone receptor, are not observed in animals lacking ER expression (50). Cross-talk between steroid receptors and the RPTK-induced pathways has also been demonstrated by experiments in which DHT treatment of AR-transfected PC3 cells results in enhanced EGF receptor expression (51).

The effect of tyrosine kinase growth factor stimulation and the progression of advanced prostate cancer has been investigated by Sawyers and his colleagues (52). This group demonstrated that increased expression of the Her2/neu growth factor receptor, a member of the EGF receptor family, resulted in enhanced activity of the AR, even in the absence of androgen stimulation (52). In this case, a direct physical interaction between the AR and the Her2/neu receptor appeared to activate the AR. This, of course, leads to the question of whether inhibition of the Her2/neu receptor with herceptin, an antibody directed against Her2/neu, would be effective therapy in prostate cancer therapy. Furthermore, hormone refractory disease may overexpress the Her2/neu receptor. These observations provide interesting hypotheses for the evolution of HRPC that are readily testable in the clinical setting.

Cross-talk between other signaling pathways and AR activation has also been demonstrated for other protein kinases. For instance, both the protein kinase A and protein kinase C pathways have been shown to alter AR signaling *in vitro* (53,54).

It is not known with certainty how alterations in specific signal transduction pathways affect AR function. Proteins that are kinases cause phosphorylation at specific sites in target proteins. Mitogen-activated protein (MAP) kinase, a key protein in signal transduction in the mitogen-activated pathway, is known to be activated by several growth factors. Abreu-Martin and colleagues have also shown that one of the signal-transduction proteins in the MAP kinase cascade, called *mitogen-activated protein kinase kinase kinase 1*, when activated, stimulates transcriptional activity of the AR (55). Importantly, MAP kinases have been shown to also phosphorylate the ER and stimulate transcription. In the case of ER-beta, phosphorylation of specific residues within the AF1 domain leads to an enhancement of coactivator recruitment (56). Although there are some conflicting data regarding the role receptor phosphorylation plays in AR function, one report has demonstrated a role for AR phosphorylation in agonist and antagonist activity (57).

These data are very intriguing in that there is at least the conceptual possibility that alterations in growth factor signaling can directly or indirectly affect AR function. If it is demonstrated that altered expression of a specific growth factor receptor occurs during the evolution of HRPC, it will also provide a rationale for antigrowth factor strategies.

OTHER STEROID AND NUCLEAR RECEPTORS IN HORMONE-REFRACTORY PROSTATE CANCER

Although much of the discussion in this chapter has been on the AR and other proteins that affect AR function, it is entirely possible that other steroid and nuclear receptors might play a role in mediating progression to the hormone-refractory state. There are a host of other nuclear and steroid receptors that are expressed in prostate cancer epithelium. In fact, the full spectrum of nuclear and steroid receptors in either normal prostate epithelium or prostate cancer is not known. Although there is no data showing consistent activation of a specific nuclear receptor with the progression of prostate cancer, both laboratory and clinical data have demonstrated that treatment with ligands specific for a number of nuclear receptors can affect prostate cancer biology. In this section of this chapter, we describe some of the examples of how targeting these receptors has led to a therapeutic advantage in the treatment of a minority of cases of HRPC. These clinical observations, however few, provide the beginning of an insight into the role other specific nuclear and steroid hormone receptors might play in the evolution of HRPC.

Targeting specific nuclear and steroid receptors other than AR and ER has been useful in the treatment of other solid tumors and leukemias. In the treatment of acute promyelocytic leukemia, targeting the retinoic acid receptor alpha with a specific ligand, all-*trans*-retinoic acid, a retinoid, has been demonstrated to be an integral component of therapy (58). Treatment with retinoids has also been useful in the treatment of head and neck cancer (59). In many cases, this type of therapy is thought to induce cell differentiation rather than a cytotoxic response.

Retinoids have also been used in the treatment of prostate cancer. For instance, treatment with a retinoid analog, called *fenretinide*, has been shown to result in apoptosis of prostate cancer cells *in vitro* (60). Other nuclear receptors have been targeted as well. For instance, investigators demonstrated that the peroxisome proliferator–induced receptor gamma is expressed not only in fat cells, where it is known to play a critical role in differentiation, but also in prostate cancer (61,62). Thiazolidinedione is a ligand specific for peroxisome proliferator–induced receptor gamma that is in clinical use as an antidiabetic agent. Treatment of prostate cancer cells *in vitro* led to a reduction in PSA expression by LNCaP cells and a reduction in growth for both this cell line and another prostate cancer cell line, PC3 (62). Current clinical trials using analogs of vitamin D, a ligand for the vitamin D nuclear receptor, have already shown that these agents may be active in HRPC (63).

The fact that there is some activity for these agents in the context of HRPC does not, of course, implicate these receptor pathways in the pathogenesis of HRPC. Can receptors other than the AR promulgate consistent PSA expression in prostate cancer cells? Is it possible that another nuclear receptor can bind and activate upstream regions that are normally bound and activated by AR, thus explaining the consistent secretion of PSA in HRPC? In general, the known nuclear receptors have relatively specific DNA-binding consensus regions, so that it is unlikely that other receptors would have potential binding capacity at AREs. For instance, although the AR consensus DNA-binding sequence is very similar to that of the glucocorticoid receptor, it is not known whether GR can bind *in vivo*. Because of its potential for clinical translation, this area of prostate cancer biology is under intense investigation by several laboratories.

The receptors for the ligands discussed are associated with a complex biology. In some cases, such as for retinoid and vitamin D, the receptors can bind as heterodimers with other specific members of the nuclear receptor family (9,10). In some cases, nuclear receptors in the retinoid family can bind as heterodimers to nuclear receptors without known ligands, called *orphan receptors* (64). Like other solid tumors, prostate cancer expresses a number of orphan receptors. An impediment to understanding the role of nuclear receptors in prostate cancer progression is the complexity of the system. Investigators into this field are faced with a great number of nuclear receptors, many of which function as heterodimers and many of which do not have specific ligands.

ANDROGEN RECEPTOR–INDEPENDENT PROGRESSION TO HORMONE-REFRACTORY PROSTATE CANCER AND CELL-CYCLE PROTEIN ALTERATIONS

Prostate cancer is similar to other solid tumor malignancies in that, with the progression of disease, there are multiple genetic alterations, including the acquisition of oncogenes and loss of tumor suppressor genes. In theory, any of these changes might mediate the progression to HRPC, completely independent of AR signaling or function. The challenge in prostate and other cancers is first to determine whether genetic alterations are specific to a stage in the illness, and then, even more important, to understand its biologic consequences. What are the genetic alterations observed with the progression to HRPC? Is it possible that some of these mediate progression independent of the AR or other nuclear and steroid receptors? Does the genetic database provide any clues for the alteration in expression of specific genes?

One approach to determining the spectrum of genes expressed with the progression to HRPC is to assess which genes are amplified. In one study, the myc oncogene was amplified in approximately 10% of cases in refractory stages, but only rarely in hormone-sensitive disease (32). This is of interest, as this gene product is involved in cell growth and cell division. Myc acts in the nucleus, and its overexpression is a possible method of altered gene expression, independent of signal transduction enzymes involved in amplifying signals from the cell surface or cytoplasm.

Another approach to assessing which gene products might be important in mediating the progression to HRPC is to determine whether any are capable of converting an androgen-dependent line to an androgen-independent cell line. Androgen-dependent LNCaP cells can be made androgen-independent cells by transfection of the oncogene-activated Ras (65). In the case of Ras, it is possible that the effects are through pathways similar to those involved with expression through RPTKs. Activation of Ras can induce signal transduction through pathways similar to those induced by RPTK stimulation, including possible activation of a key signal transduction intermediate, phosphatidylinositol 3'-kinase (PI3K). Activation of PI3K is pivotal to critical pathways involving cell growth, differentiation, and apoptosis. This is of great interest in prostate cancer in that, in later stages, a tumor suppressor called PTEN is frequently lost (66). The PTEN gene product encodes a phosphatidylinositol phosphatase that antagonizes activation of PI3K (67). Loss of PTEN function in a cell may, therefore, lead to maintenance of PI3K in a chronically activated state.

Progression to HRPC may also involve alterations in critical cell-cycle regulatory proteins. Detection of alterations in this group of proteins would be very interesting, as control of cell cycle is critical to cancer in general and would be expected to be important in the pathogenesis of HRPC. Therefore, there has been much investigation into alterations of some of these proteins, such as the cyclin-dependent kinase inhibitor $p27^{kip1}$ (68,69). Although there are many studies focusing on expression of some of these proteins increasing Gleason grade, there has been a paucity of studies analyzing expression with the progression of disease into HRPC. This is partly because it is very difficult to obtain and analyze metastatic deposits from patients with HRPC. Also, quite interestingly, some key cell-cycle regulatory proteins are directly or indirectly altered by androgens in prostate cancer cells. For instance, D-type cyclins (cyclins D1, D2, and D3) may complex with the AR and inhibit its transcriptional ability (70). This is something of a surprise because, when cyclin D1 binds the ER, it may activate its transcriptional capacity, even in the absence of estrogen.

There may be other alterations involving the evolution of prostate cancer to the hormone refractory state that are related to loss of the normal control for cell death. Very interestingly, increased expression of the antiapoptotic gene, Bcl-2, leads to androgen independence on LNCaP cells (71). Here again, however, rather than being totally independent of the AR pathway, there is an inverse relationship between Bcl-2 and AR expression in normal prostate epithelium.

Undoubtedly, changes in cell-cycle and cell-survival proteins are important for cell growth and survival in HRPC. The challenge is to determine, if possible, which change is integral, and which change precedes others in these pathways. Beyond investigation of human tissue and the few established cell lines, there are important insights to be learned from animal models of HRPC.

ANIMAL MODELS OF HORMONE-REFRACTORY PROSTATE CANCER

The development of cell culture and animal models is critically important to advancing our understanding of HRPC. The appropriate animal model would mimic progression in human disease. Metastases would be primarily to bone, express the AR, respond initially to androgen ablation, and recur at some later time point. Furthermore, the best HRPC models would be relatively refractory to antiandrogens, such as bicalutamide, as is typical of the human disease after androgen ablation.

Although an optimal animal model is not yet available, the TRAMP model of Greenberg, in which the SV40 T antigen is expressed in specific regions of the mouse prostate, possesses some very useful properties (72,73). The tumor can metastasize. It also often regresses after castration, only to recur eventually in castrate animals. However, because the gene responsible for inducing the SV40 T antigen is androgen regulated, regression with castration may be less significant. Still, the model may impart important biologic insights into HRPC. For instance, the IGF-1 receptor is expressed in the hormone-dependent primary disease in these animals, but not in the androgen-independent recurrence (73). Our group has also observed this phenomenon in metastatic samples derived from HRPC patients (74). Another animal model that shows promise has been developed by Klein and colleagues, in which they have had propagated samples from patients with HRPC in immune-deficient mice (75).

The propagation of cell lines under androgen-depleted conditions is another approach to understanding the evolution of prostate cancer. As discussed earlier, the LNCaP cell line after long-term growth in the absence of androgens is paradoxically inhibited by androgen reexposure. Wainstein and colleagues developed a line called CWR22 that can be propagated in an androgen-dependent fashion in animals and as an androgen-independent line *in vitro* (76). This cell line may yield insights into the problem of progression after androgen ablation. The Dunning rat model has also been of use in this regard. Androgen-dependent and -independent lines have been derived, but it is not known how closely they mimic the human disease. In contrast, the study of human prostate cancer cell lines, such as DU145 and PC3, is less useful. These lines do not permit us to study the evolution to HRPC, as they do not express the AR.

INSIGHT FROM CLINICAL STUDIES ON THE MECHANISM OF HORMONE-REFRACTORY PROSTATE CANCER

The persistence of AR and PSA expression in HRPC would suggest that this disease is still potentially dependent on AR stimulation. Yet second-line hormonal therapies are, in general, much less effective in prostate cancer when compared to breast cancer, leading to the designation of the disease as hormone refractory after primary androgen ablative therapy. A discussion of secondary hormonal therapies is provided in Chapter 43. In this chapter we will examine what might be learned regarding the evolution of HRPC from some of the clinical trials performed at this stage of the illness.

The flutamide-withdrawal response is defined as a PSA decline, and often as a clinical benefit, after the discontinuation of flutamide in HRPC patients (77). This response occurs in 40% to 50% of patients on long-term flutamide. Much of the evidence suggests that this is the result of AR mutations, for which flutamide functions paradoxically as an agonist. For instance, our group has shown that AR mutations are more likely to be detected from patients on long-term flutamide, suggesting that there is a long-term drug therapy resulting in positive selection pressure. Also, we and others have shown that these mutants are often paradoxically stimulated by flutamide *in vitro*, but not by bicalutamide. These data suggested that high-dose bicalutamide might be effective for patients with HRPC. In fact, two separate clinical trials, one performed by the author's group and another by Scher and his colleagues, demonstrated very similar outcomes (78,79). In both studies, bicalutamide responses were predominantly restricted to HRPC patients who previously had been treated with long-term flutamide as part of their androgen-ablative regimens. HRPC patients who had not been treated with flutamide had a very low response rate (79). These data indicated that prior hormone therapy changed the response rate to subsequent hormonal agents. One method of explaining this phenotype is that patients treated with flutamide developed AR mutations that could be inhibited by bicalutamide. Experiments performed by Taplin et al. seemed to confirm this, in that many of the patients responding to bicalutamide had AR mutations, for which flutamide is an agonist (27). In contrast, only rare AR mutations were detected from patients treated with LHRH analogs or orchiectomy alone, and these could not be stimulated by flutamide.

Hormone withdrawal responses have also been observed after discontinuing other antiandrogens, such as bicalutamide, but to date mutations for which this antiandrogen is an agonist have not been detected. In fact, withdrawal responses have been observed even after discontinuation of other agents that are not even antiandrogens, such as megestrol acetate (megace). Understanding the molecular basis of withdrawal responses, even though of limited duration clinically, may improve our knowledge of the evolution of HRPC. Are these responses the result of AR mutations, and if so, what does it teach us about the structure-function relationship for this receptor? Alternatively, are these responses mediated by other mechanisms? For instance, is it possible that withdrawal responses, in some cases, are the result of interaction of an antiandrogen with the AR and a coactivator, as might be expected from the phenotype induced by overexpression of ARA70?

AR amplification and mutation suggest that androgens synthesized by the adrenal gland are a potential source of ligand in HRPC. Might these hormones become a source for stimulating prostate cancer cells having these phenotypes? The hypothalamic-pituitary-adrenal axis, predominantly under the influence of ACTH, is largely intact in orchiectomized patients and in patients treated with LHRH analogs. Therefore, adrenal androgens such as dehydroepiandrosterone, dehydroepiandrosterone sulfate, and androstenedione may provide a direct source of stimulation or become converted to testosterone or dihydrotestosterone. To test this hypothesis, agents that effectively reduce adrenal cortex hormonal production have been used. But, as reviewed by Dawson in Chapter 43, only occasional responses to a "medical adrenalectomy" with aminoglutethimide have been observed (80). This suggests that, for most patients, these hormones are not sufficient alone to propagate HRPC. Even for the responders to adrenal hormone inhibition, the picture is not clear. Agents that reduce adrenal hormone synthesis, such as aminoglutethimide and ketoconazole, require the coadministration of glucocorticoids, and these alone induce responses in a minority of HRPC patients. The molecular basis of response to glucocorticoids in HRPC is not known, but this might be mediated by feedback inhibition, causing a lowering of adrenal cortical hormone production. In one study, 8 of 15 patients had PSA reductions by greater than 50% on only replacement doses of hydrocortisone (81).

CONCLUSION

Obviously, one of the more important problems facing prostate cancer patients is the progression of the disease to the hormone-refractory state. This chapter raises more questions than it answers, but hopefully provides some meaningful directions. It is the bias of the author that AR signaling will prove to be an important feature of HRPC. This might be the result of altered structure or expression of the AR, altered interaction with coactivating or co-repressing proteins, or of cross-talk with other signal transduction pathways, such as those involved from growth factor receptors. However, it is also quite possible that there are other pathways involved with progression to the hormone-refractory state that are totally independent of the AR.

It is clear that this area of prostate cancer biology is fruitful for investigation. It would be useful to inactivate the AR by a dominant-negative or antisense approach. But, to do these experiments, we need better preclinical models of HRPC. Finally, it will be important to confirm findings and find leads from clinical specimens. As frequently as possible, we need to obtain tissue specimens from patients at different stages of prostate cancer. This will permit an evaluation of molecular pathways important for progression.

Finally, students of prostate cancer biology might be at first glance quite surprised by the lack of basic understanding we currently have on mechanisms of HRPC. However, in this we are not alone. We can closely observe the progress made by our colleagues investigating the molecular basis of tamoxifen resistance in breast cancer. In fact, there may be important insights into the pathogenesis of HRPC as a result of discoveries made in hormone-refractory breast cancer. Overall, these two cancer problems, both critical to relieving suffering for so many cancer patients, are at relatively the same stage of understanding of hormonal progression.

REFERENCES

1. Landis SH, Murray T, Bolden S, et al. Cancer statistics. *CA Cancer J Clin* 1998;48:6–30.
2. Catalona WJ. Management of cancer of the prostate. *N Engl J Med* 1994; 331:996–1004.
3. English HF, Kyprianou N, Isaacs JT. Relationship between DNA fragmentation and apoptosis in the programmed cell death in the rat prostate following castration. *Prostate* 1989;15:233–250.
4. Lim DJ, Liu X-L, Sutkowski DM, et al. Growth of an androgen-sensitive human prostate cancer cell line, LNCaP, in nude mice. *Prostate* 1993;22:109–118.
5. Isaacs JT, Kyprianou N. Development of androgen-independent tumor cells and their implication for the treatment of prostatic cancer. *Urol Res* 1997;15:133–138.
6. Kokontis J, Hay N, Liao S. Progression of LNCaP prostate tumor cells during androgen deprivation: hormone-independent growth, regression of proliferation by androgen, and role of p27Kip1 in androgen-induced cell cycle arrest. *Mol Endocrinol* 1998;12:941–953.
7. Nagabhushan M, Miller CM, Pretlow TP, et al. CWR22: the first human prostate cancer with strongly androgen-independent and relapse strains both in vivo and in soft agar. *Cancer Res* 1996;56:3042–3046.
8. Riegman PH, Vliestra RJ, van der Korput JA, et al. The promoter of the prostate specific antigen gene contains a functional androgen responsive element. *Mol Endocrinol* 1991;5:1921–1930.
9. Beato M. Gene regulation by steroid hormones. *Cell* 1989;56:335–344.
10. Evans RM. The steroid and thyroid hormone receptor superfamily. *Science* 1988;240:889–895.
11. Jenster G, van der Korput HA, van Vroonhoven C, et al. Domains of the human androgen receptor involved in steroid binding, transcriptional activation, and subcellular localization. *Mol Endocrinol* 1991;5:1396–1404.
12. van der Kwast TH, Schalken J, Ruizeveld de Winter JA, et al. Androgen receptors in endocrine therapy resistant human prostate cancer. *Int J Cancer* 1991;48:189–193.
13. Hobisch A, Culig Z, Radmayr C, et al. Distant metastases from prostatic carcinoma express androgen receptor protein. *Cancer Res* 1995;55:3068–3072.
14. Marcelli M, Tilley WD, Wilson CM, et al. A single nucleotide substitution introduces a premature termination codon into the androgen receptor gene of a patient with receptor negative androgen resistance. *J Clin Invest* 1990;85:1522–1528.
15. De Bellis A, Quigley CA, Cariello NF, et al. Single base mutations in the human androgen receptor gene causing complete androgen insensitivity: rapid detection by a modified denaturing gradient gel electrophoresis technique. *Mol Endocrinol* 1992;6:1909–1920.
16. Horoszewisz JS, Leong SS, Kawanski E, et al. LNCaP model of prostatic carcinoma. *Cancer Res* 1983;43:1809–1818.
17. Olea N, Sakabe K, Soto AM, et al. The proliferative effect of "anti-androgens" on the androgen-sensitive human prostate tumor cell line LNCaP. *Endocrinology* 1990;126:1457–1463.
18. Newmark JR, Hardy DO, Tonb DC, et al. Androgen receptor gene mutations in human prostate cancer. *Proc Natl Acad Sci* 1992;89:6319–6323.
19. Ruizeveld de Winter JA, Janssen PJ, Sleddens HM, et al. Androgen receptor status in localized and locally progressive hormone refractory human prostate cancer. *Am J Pathol* 1994;144:735–746.
20. Culig Z, Hobisch A, Cronauer MV, et al. Mutant androgen receptor detected in an advanced-stage prostatic carcinoma is activated by adrenal androgens and progesterone. *Mol Endocrinol* 1993;7:1541–1550.
21. Taplin ME, Bubley GJ, Shuster TD, et al. Mutation of the androgen-receptor gene in metastatic androgen-independent prostate cancer. *N Engl J Med* 1995;332:1393–1398.
22. Fenton MA, Shuster TD, Fertig A, et al. Functional characterization of mutant androgen receptors from androgen-independent prostate cancer. *Clin Cancer Res* 1997;3:1383–1388.
23. Myers R, Oelschlager D, Coan P, et al. Changes in cyclin-dependent kinase inhibitors p21 and p27 during the castration induced regression of the CWR22 model of prostatic carcinoma. *J Urol* 1999;161:945–949.
24. Suzuki H, Sato N, Watabe Y, et al. Androgen receptor gene mutations in human prostate cancer. *J Steroid Biochem Mol Biol* 1993;46:759–765.
25. Tilley WD, Wilson CM, Marcelli M, et al. Androgen receptor gene expression in human prostate carcinoma cell lines. *Cancer Res* 1990;50:5382–5386.
26. Takahashi H, Furusato M, Allsbrook WC Jr., et al. Prevalence of androgen receptor gene mutations in latent prostatic carcinomas from Japanese men. *Cancer Res* 1995;55:1621–1624.
27. Taplin ME, Bubley GJ, Ko YJ, et al. Selection for androgen receptor mutations in prostate cancers treated with androgen antagonist. *Cancer Res* 1999;59:2511–2515.

28. Giovannucci E, Stampfer MJ, Krithivas K, et al. The CAG repeat within the androgen receptor gene and its relationship to prostate cancer. *Proc Natl Acad Sci* 1997;94:3320–3323.
29. Ruizeveld de Winter JA, Trapman J, Vermey M, et al. Androgen receptor expression in human tissues: an immunohistochemical study. *J Histochem Cytochem* 1991;39:927–936.
30. Lengauer C, Kinzler K, Vogelstein B. Genetic instabilities in human cancers. *Nature* 1998;396:643–649.
31. Visakorpi T, Hyytinen E, Kovivisto P, et al. In vivo amplification of the androgen receptor gene and progression of human prostate cancer. *Nat Genet* 1995;9:401–406.
32. Bubendorf L, Kononen J, Kiovisto P, et al. Survey of gene amplifications during prostate cancer progression by high throughput fluorescence in situ hybridization on tissue microarrays. *Cancer Res* 1999;59:803–806.
33. Knoblauch R, Garabedian MJ. Role for hsp90-associated cochaperone p23 in estrogen receptor signal transduction. *Mol Cell Biol* 1999;19:3748–3759.
34. Miyata Y, Yahara I. Cytoplasmic 8 S glucocorticoid receptor binds to actin filaments through the 90-kDa heat shock protein moiety. *Jour Biol Chem* 1996;296:8779–8783.
35. Nathan DF, Lindquist S. Mutational analysis of hsp90 function: interactions with a steroid receptor and a protein kinase. *Mol Cell Biol* 1995;15:3917–3925.
36. Mak HY, Hoare S, Henttu MA, et al. Molecular determinants of the estrogen receptor-coactivator interface. *Mol Cell Biol* 1999;19:3895–3903.
37. Torchia J, Rose DW, Inostroza J, et al. The transcriptional co-activator p/CIP binds CBP and mediates nuclear-receptor function. *Nature* 1997;387:677–684.
38. Alland L, Muhle R, Hou H Jr., et al. Role for N-Cor and histone deacetylase in Sin3-mediated transcriptional repression. *Nature* 1999;387:49–55.
39. Wang H, Peters GA, Zeng X, et al. Yeast two-hybrid demonstrates that estrogen receptor dimerization is ligand dependent in vivo. *J Biol Chem* 1995;270:23322–23329.
40. Korzus E, Torchia J, Rose DW, et al. Transcription factor-specific requirements for coactivators and their acetyltransferase functions. *Science* 1998;279:703–707.
41. Yao T-P, Ku G, Zhou N, et al. The nuclear hormone receptor coactivator src-1 is a specific target of p300. *Proc Natl Acad Sci* 1996;93:10626–10631.
42. Olson DP, Sun B, Koenig RJ. Thyroid hormone response element architecture affects corepressor release from thyroid hormone receptor dimers. *J Biol Chem* 1998;273:3375–3380.
43. Yeh S, Miyamato H, Shima H, et al. From estrogen to androgen receptor: a new pathway for sex hormones in prostate. *Proc Natl Acad Sci* 1998;95:5527–5532.
44. Miyamoto H, Yeh S, Wilding G, et al. Promotion of agonist activity of antiandrogens by the androgen receptor coactivator, ARA 70, in human prostate cancer DU145 cells. *Proc Natl Acad Sci* 1998;95:7379–7384.
45. Russell PJ, Bennett S, Stricker P. Growth factor involvement in the progression of prostate cancer. *Clin Chem* 1998; 44:705–723.
46. Scher HI, Sarkis A, Reuter V, et al. Changing pattern of expression of the epidermal growth factor receptor and transforming growth factor alpha in the progression of prostatic neoplasms. *Clin Can Res* 1995;1:545–560.
47. Planz B, Wang Q, Kirley SD, et al. Androgen responsiveness of stromal cells of the human prostate: regulation of cell proliferation and keratinocyte growth factor by androgen. *J Urol* 1998;160:1850–1855.
48. Barrack ER. TGF beta in prostate cancer: a growth inhibitor that can enhance tumorigenicity. *Prostate* 1997;31:61–70.
49. Putz T, Culig Z, Eder IE, et al. Epidermal growth factor receptor blockade inhibits the action of EGF, insulin like growth factor I, and a protein kinase activator in prostate cancer cell lines. *Cancer Res* 1999;59:227–233.
50. Curtis SW, Washburn T, Sewall C, et al. Physiologic coupling of growth factor and steroid receptor signaling pathways: estrogen receptor knockout mice lack estrogen-like response to epidermal growth factor. *Proc Natl Acad Sci* 1996;93:12626–12630.
51. Brass AL, Barnard J, Pastal BL. Androgen up-regulates epidermal growth factor binding affinity in PC3 cell lines expressing the human androgen receptor. *Cancer Res* 1995; 55:3197–3203.
52. Craft N, Shostak Y, Carey M, et al. A mechanism for hormone-independent prostate cancer through modulation of androgen receptor signaling by the HER-2/neu tyrosine kinase. *Nat Med* 1999;5:280–285.
53. Sadar MD. Androgen-independent induction of PSA expression via cross-talk between the androgen receptor and protein kinase A signal transduction pathways. *J Biol Chem* 1999;274:7777–7783.
54. De Ruiter PE, Teuwen R, Trapman J, et al. Synergism between androgens and protein kinase-C on androgen regulated gene expression. *Mol Cell Endocrinol* 1995;110:1–6.
55. Abreu-Martin M, Chari A, Palladino AA. Mitogen-activated protein kinase kinase kinase 1 activates androgen-receptor-dependent transcription and apoptosis in prostate cancer. *Mol Cell Biol* 1999;19:5143–5154.
56. Moraitis AN, Giguere V. Transition from monomeric to homodimeric DNA binding by nuclear receptors: identification of RevErbAalpha determinants required for RORalpha homodimer complex formation. *Mol Endocrin* 1999; 13:431–439.
57. Wang LG, Liu XM, Kreis W, et al. Phosphorylation/dephosphorylation of androgen receptor as a determinant of androgen agonistic and antagonistic activity. *Biochem Biophys Res Commun* 1999;259:21–28.
58. Nason-Burchenal K, Allopenna J, Begue A, et al. Targeting of PML/RARalpha is lethal to retinoic acid-resistant promyelocytic leukemia cells. *Blood* 1998;98:1758–1767.
59. Wan H, Oridinate N, Lotan D, et al. Overexpressioon of retinoic acid receptor beta in head and neck squamous cell carcinoma cells increases their sensitivity to retinoid-induced suppression of squamous differentiation by retinoids. *Cancer Res* 1999;59:3518–3526.
60. Sun SY, Yue P, Lotan R. Induction of apoptosis by N-(4-hydroxyphenyl)retinamide and its association with reactive oxygen species, nuclear retinoic acid receptors, and apoptosis-related genes in human prostate carcinoma cells. *Mol Pharmacol* 1999; 55:403–410.
61. Tontonoz P, Hu E, Spielgelman BM. Stimulation of adipogenesis in fibroblasts by PPAR gamma 2, a lipid-activated transcription factor. *Cell* 1994;79:1147–1156.

62. Kubota T, Koshizuka K, Williamson EA, et al. Ligand for peroxisome proliferator-activated receptor gamma (troglitazone) has potent antitumor effect against human prostate cancer in vitro and in vivo. *Cancer Res* 1998;58:3344–3352.
63. Blutt SE, Allegretto EA, Pike JW, et al. 1,25-dihydroxyvitamin D3 and 9 cis-retinoic acid act synergistically to inhibit the growth of LNCaP prostate cells and cause accumulation of cells in G1. *Endocrinology* 1997;138:1491–1497.
64. Kastner P, Mark M, Chambon P. Nonsteroid nuclear receptors: What are genetic studies telling us about their role in real life? *Cell* 1995;83:859–869.
65. Voeller HJ, WIlding G, Gelmann EP. v-rasH expression confers hormone-independent in vitro growth in LNCaP prostate carcinoma cells. *Mol Endocrinol* 1991;5:209–216.
66. Wu X, Senechal K, Neshat MS, et al. The PTEN/MMAC1 tumor suppressor functions as a negative regulator of the phosphoinositide 3-kinase/Akt pathway. *Proc Natl Acad Sci* 1998;95:15587–15591.
67. Whang Y, Xu X, Suzuki H, et al. Inactivation of the tumor suppressor PTEN/MMAC1 advanced prostate cancer through loss of expression. *Proc Natl Acad Sci* 1998;95:5246–5250.
68. Yang RM, Naitoh J, Murphy M, et al. Low p27 expression predicts poor disease-free survival in patients with prostate cancer. *J Urol* 1998;159:941–945.
69. Forgaro M, Tallini G, Zheng DQ, et al. p27(kip1) acts as a downstream effector of and is coexpressed with the beta 1X integrin in prostatic adenocarcinoma. *J Clin Invest* 1999; 103:321–329.
70. Knudsen KE, Cavenee WK, Arden KC. D-type cyclins complex with the androgen receptor and inhibit its transcriptional transactivation ability. *Cancer Res* 1999;59:2297–2301.
71. McDonnell TJ, Troncoso P, Brisbay SM, et al. Expression of the protooncogene bcl-2 in the prostate and its association with emergence of androgen-independent prostate cancer. *Cancer Res* 1992;52:6940–6944.
72. Gingrich J, Barrios R, Kattan M, et al. Androgen-independent prostate cancer progression in the TRAMP model. *Cancer Res* 1997;57:4687–4691.
73. Kaplan PJ, Mohan S, Cohen P, et al. The insulin-like growth factor axis and prostate cancer: lessons from the transgenic adenocarcinoma of mouse prostate (TRAMP) model. *Cancer Res* 1999;59:2203–2209.
74. Chott A, Sun Z, Morganstern D, et al. Tyrosine kinase expressed in vivo by human prostate cancer bone marrow metastases and loss of the type 1 insulin-like growth factor receptor. *Am J Pathol* 1999;155:1271–1279.
75. Klein KA, Reiter RE, Redula J, et al. Progression of metastatic human prostate cancer to androgen independence in immunodeficient SCID mice. *Nat Med* 1997;3:402–408.
76. Wainstein M, He F, Robinson D, et al. CWR22: an androgen-dependent xenograft model derived from a primary human prostatic carcinoma. *Cancer Res* 1994;54:6049–6052.
77. Scher HI, Kelly WK. Flutamide withdrawal syndrome: its impact on clinical trials in hormone-refractory prostate cancer. *J Clin Oncol* 1993;11:1566–1572.
78. Scher HI, Liebertz C, Kelly WK, et al. Bicalutamide for advanced prostate cancer: the natural versus treated history of disease. *J Clin Oncol* 1997;15:2928–2938.
79. Joyce R, Fenton MA, Rode P, et al. High dose bicalutamide for androgen-independent prostate cancer: effect of prior treatment. *J Urol* 1998;159:149–153.
80. Chang AY, Bennett JM, Pandya KJ, et al. A study of aminoglutethimide and hydrocortisone in patients with advanced and refractory prostate carcinoma. *Am J Clin Oncol* 1998;12:358–360.
81. Kelley WK, Curley T, Leibretz C, et al. Prospective evaluation of hydrocortisone and suramin in patients with androgen independent prostate cancer. *J Clin Oncol* 1995; 13:2208–2213.

7

PROSTATE CANCER PREVENTION

WILLIAM G. NELSON
THEODORE L. DEWEESE
ANGELO M. DE MARZO
JAMES D. BROOKS

Prostate cancer has become one of the leading cancers diagnosed in men in the United States and a major cause of cancer mortality (1). Fortunately, over the past two decades, new strategies for early detection of prostate cancer, featuring blood testing for prostate-specific antigen (PSA) and systematic prostate biopsies, have increased the fraction of prostate cancer cases that can be approached with curative intent using surgery or radiation therapy (2–5). Unfortunately, although systemic treatment for advanced prostate cancer has also improved, men with prostate cancer metastases at the time of prostate cancer diagnosis, or with prostate cancer metastases at the time of recurrence after surgery or radiation therapy, currently cannot be cured with systemic therapy (6–9). Most of these men die with progressive prostate cancer. Also, even though many men with localized prostate cancer enjoy long-term cancer-free survival after surgery or radiation therapy, side effects of such curative treatment frequently include erectile dysfunction and urinary incontinence (10–12). For these reasons, new strategies for prostate cancer prevention are needed.

EPIDEMIOLOGY OF PROSTATE CANCER

Prostate cancer incidence and mortality vary greatly in different geographic regions, with generally high risks of prostate cancer development characteristic of the United States and Western Europe and generally low risks of prostate cancer development characteristic of Asia (13–17). Although genetic factors likely play a significant role in the pathogenesis of life-threatening prostate cancer, environmental factors are probably the dominant influence that account for geographic differences in prostate cancer incidence and mortality. Migrants from low-risk regions to high-risk regions typically adopt a higher prostate cancer risk within one generation. For example, although Asian immigrants to the United States display a prostate cancer risk approximately one-half that of white men in the United States, prostate cancer risk among ethnic Asian men appears to increase with duration of exposure to a Western lifestyle: Asian immigrants to North America have a higher risk of prostate cancer after living in North America for more than 25 years than after living in North America for less than 10 years (18). Asian men born in the United States have a risk for life-threatening prostate cancer development similar to white men. These ecologic epidemiology observations underscore the critical role for environmental factors in fostering the epidemic of prostate cancer afflicting men in the United States.

The major environmental exposure modulating prostate cancer risk is likely diet. Clearly, stereotypical Asian diets are quite different from stereotypical Western diets. In addition, case-control epidemiology studies have implicated dietary components, such as animal fats, charred meats, and others, as candidate factors increasing prostate cancer risk, and vitamins, fruits and vegetables, and others as candidate factors decreasing prostate cancer risk (18–21). Unfortunately, whether the stereotypical Western diet makes an error of *commission* (i.e., overconsumption of saturated fats), an error of *omission* (i.e., underconsumption of fruits and vegetables), or both has not been rigorously established. Animal model studies of prostate cancer development and progression have provided support for the contention that dietary components likely influence prostate cancer development. Male rats fed the heterocyclic aromatic amine carcinogen 2-amino-1-methyl-6-phenylimidazo[4,5-β]pyridine (PhIP), rich in "charred" or "well-done" meats, specifically develop mutations in prostate cells and neoplastic prostate lesions (22,23). Human prostatic carcinoma xenografts in immunodeficient mice display attenuated growth when the mice are fed diets low in fat or supplemented with vitamin E (24,25). Thus far, the mechanisms by which such dietary components affect normal and neoplastic prostate cell behavior have yet to be fully elucidated.

Genetic factors also influence prostate cancer risks. Prostate cancer cases are often clustered in families. Statistical modeling has suggested that many such prostate cancer family case clusters reflect inheritance of a high-risk prostate cancer gene [or genes (26)]. Inherited prostate cancer often appears at a younger age, and at a more advanced stage, than sporadic prostate cancer (27). Intensive analyses of families with multiple men affected by prostate cancer have, thus far, revealed genetic linkage to candidate high-risk prostate cancer genes located at various sites on chromosomes 1p, 1q, and X (28–31). The identities of these candidate high-risk prostate cancer genes have not yet been reported. Case-control genetic epidemiology studies have tested the contribution of polymorphic variants of a number of known genes as prostate cancer risk modifiers. The gene encoding the androgen receptor *hAR* displays polymorphic variations in the lengths of a polyglutamate repeat sequence and of a polyglycine repeat sequence. In several studies, men carrying *hAR* genes encoding receptors with shorter polyglutamate repeat sequences appear to be at higher risk for prostate cancer development or for more advanced prostate cancer stage, or both, at diagnosis (32–37). Provocatively, African-American men, who characteristically have *hAR* genes encoding receptors with shorter polyglutamate repeat sequences, also appear at higher risk for prostate cancer development and for more advanced prostate cancer stage at diagnosis. Similar case-control epidemiology studies examining prostate cancer risks associated with polymorphic variants of genes encoding 5α-reductase, the vitamin D receptor, glutathione S-transferases (GSTs), and other metabolic enzymes have yielded mixed results (38–45).

MOLECULAR PATHOGENESIS OF PROSTATE CANCER

Human prostatic carcinoma cells contain a myriad of somatic genome alterations, including gene mutations, gene amplifications, gene deletions, chromosomal rearrangements, and changes in DNA methylation. In some genome changes, such as loss of DNA sequences on chromosome 8p, gain of DNA sequences on chromosome 8q, and abnormal methylation of "CpG island" sequences encompassing *GSTP1*, the gene encoding the π-class GST, appear in most prostate cancer cases (46–62). Other somatic genome alterations appear in only a fraction of cases. Whether the striking case-to-case heterogeneity of genome changes characteristic of prostatic cancers reflects chronic exposure to genome damaging stresses, defective maintenance of genome integrity, or a combination of both processes, has not been established. What is more clear is that genomic instability is likely responsible for the most malignant prostate cancer cell behaviors, including metastasis and progression to androgen independence after attempts at hormonal therapy. Autopsy studies suggest that prostatic carcinogenesis may begin at quite a young age and proceed over many years: Although the median age of prostate cancer diagnosis in the United States approaches 65 to 70 years, prostate cancer lesions have been seen in as many as 29% of men aged 30 to 40 years (63). A major goal for preventing life-threatening prostate cancer may be to reduce the rate at which neoplastic prostate cells acquire somatic genome alterations.

An emerging body of evidence supports a new hypothesis that *GSTP1* gene inactivation, via "CpG island" DNA methylation, may serve as an initiating genome lesion for prostatic carcinogenesis (59–62) (Fig. 7-1). *GSTP1* "CpG island" DNA methylation, accompanied by lack of GSTP1 expression, constitutes the most common somatic genome change recognized in prostatic carcinoma cells and in cells comprising prostatic intraepithelial neoplasia (PIN) lesions. GSTP1, like other GSTs, can inactivate electrophile or oxidant carcinogens via enzymatic conjugation with glutathione. Thus, loss of GSTP1 function may not affect prostate cell growth or survival as much as it affects prostate cell vulnerability to carcinogen damage. Compared to mice with normal *Gstp* genes, mice carrying disrupted *Gstp* genes display increased skin tumors after treatment with the carcinogen 7,12 dimethylbenzanthracene (64). Humans homozygous for null *GSTM1* gene alleles (as many as 40% of white individuals) manifest an increased risk for cancer, particularly if exposed to carcinogens, such as those present in cigarette smoke (65–67). Polymorphic *GSTP1* alleles, thought to encode low-activity GSTP1 enzymes, may confer an increased risk in women for breast cancer (68,69). During prostate carcinogenesis, somatic loss of *GSTP1* function may render normal prostate cells vulnerable to neoplastic transformation, and it may render neoplastic cells vulnerable to malignant progression, mediated by electrophile or oxidant carcinogens that inflict genome damage. In support of this mechanism, new data suggest that prostate cancer cells carrying defective *GSTP1* genes may be particularly sensitive to genome damage mediated by the dietary heterocyclic aromatic amine carcinogen PhIP (69a).

GSTs stereotypically function as inducible enzymatic defenses against oxidant and electrophile stresses. In most cell types, GST induction can be attributed to increased transcription of *GST* genes triggered by carcinogen exposure (70). The most complete analyses of GST regulation during cancer development have been obtained from studies of the pathogenesis of hepatocellular carcinoma in a variety of different species. For example, when rats are treated with various hepatocarcinogens, hyperplastic liver nodules composed of cells containing very high levels of the rat π-class GST, GST-P, typically appear (71–76). Although the majority of these hyperplastic liver nodules regress over time, perhaps as a result of increased protection against further cell and genome afforded by high-level GST-P expression, a few of the lesions progress to hepatocellular carcinoma, indicating

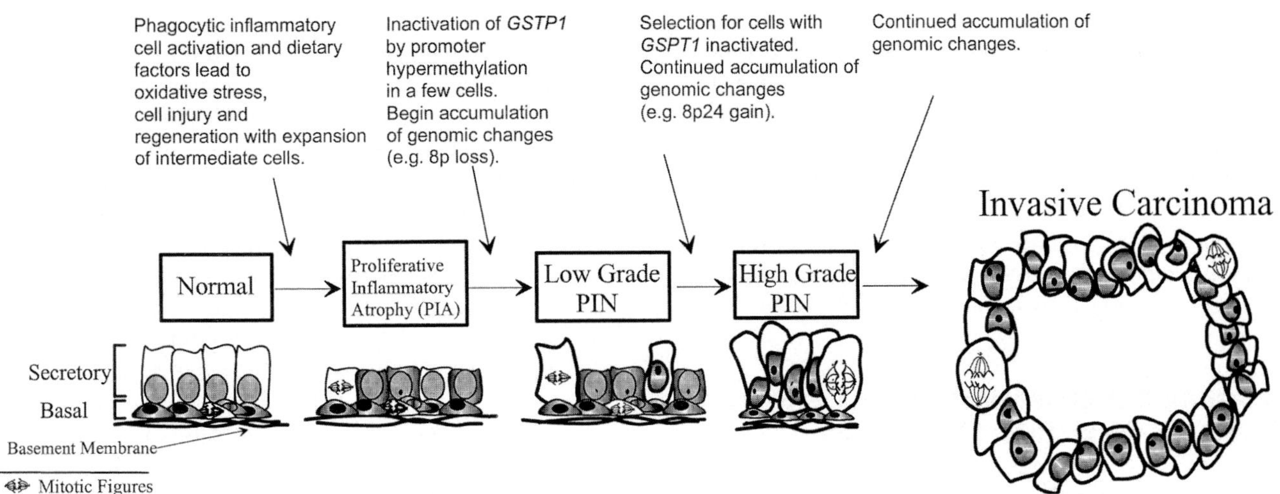

FIGURE 7-1. The pathogenesis of prostate cancer: loss of *GSTP1* function in the face of chronic genome-damaging stress. In normal prostatic epithelium, basal prostate cells express GSTP1 (shown as cytoplasmic shading), whereas columnar secretory cells do not. Chronic inflammation drives the appearance of PIA lesions in which GSTP1 expression is induced throughout the prostate epithelium. However, cells with inactivated *GSTP1* alleles incapable of GSTP1 expression appear and begin to accumulate somatic genome abnormalities (e.g., 8p loss and 8q gain) that lead to the development of prostatic intraepithelial neoplasia (PIN; shown as columnar cells devoid of GSTP1 that contain nuclei with prominent nucleoli). Further genome injury leads to the development of invasive prostatic carcinoma.

that the high GST-P–expressing hyperplastic liver nodules are cancer precursor lesions. In rainbow trout (*Onchorhynchus mykiss*), liver cells fail to readily increase GST expression on exposure to aflatoxin B_1 or 1,2-dimethylbenzanthracene (77). Instead, the carcinogen-treated fish develop both high GST-expressing hyperplastic liver nodules and low GST-expressing hyperplastic liver nodules, with the low GST-expressing hyperplastic nodules appearing more likely to progress to hepatocellular carcinoma (77). These data suggest that loss of GST expression in liver cancer precursor lesions likely increases the risk of progression to cancer (77,78). The pathogenesis of human hepatocellular carcinoma, reminiscent of the pathogenesis of human prostate cancer, has been reported to proceed via loss of GSTP1 expression, accompanying somatic *GSTP1* inactivation by "CpG island" methylation (79). *GSTP1* "CpG island" methylation changes were also reported in human livers with cirrhosis and hepatitis, characterized by proliferative hepatocytes adjacent to inflammatory cells, known to be at high risk for hepatocellular carcinoma development (79). All of these observations suggest that in the liver, carcinogen exposure triggers the appearance of cells containing high GST levels that can be considered early cancer precursors and that loss of GST expression by these cancer precursor cells likely accelerates the progression to cancer.

Immunohistochemical staining studies of human prostate tissues have revealed that increased *GSTP1* expression may be characteristic of a lesion termed *proliferative-inflammatory atrophy* (PIA) (80). PIA lesions, unlike the diffuse atrophic changes seen in prostate tissues after androgen withdrawal, are characterized by proliferation of atrophic-appearing prostate epithelial cells often adjacent to inflammatory cells (80–86). Provocatively, like the hyperplastic liver nodules seen in rats treated with carcinogens, PIA lesions may be early prostate cancer precursors. PIA lesions are commonly seen in radical prostatectomy specimens containing prostate cancer and have been observed in direct contiguity with PIN lesions (87). Inflammatory lesions in other organ sites, including the liver, stomach, and colon, are known cancer precursors. In the prostate, PIA lesion cells, which express high GSTP1 levels, may be protected, somewhat, against genome damage from inflammatory oxidants and electrophiles. However, PIA cells that acquire *GSTP1* defects may become vulnerable to progress to PIN cells, or to prostate cancer cells, when subjected to the same genome-damaging threats. The mechanism by which PIA cells acquire *GSTP1* "CpG island" DNA hypermethylation changes and become PIN cells or prostate cancer cells has not been established.

The convergence of insights from prostate cancer epidemiology, which indicate a significant role for environmental factors in life-threatening prostate cancer development, and from the molecular pathogenesis of prostate cancer, which suggest that neoplastic prostate cells may possess a phenotype of increased vulnerability to carcinogen damage, provide a framework for considering many new prostate cancer prevention strategies. Clearly, chronic damage to prostate cell genomes from oxidants and electrophiles needs to be reduced. Antioxidant micronutrients, including vitamin E, selenium, and carotenoids, such as lycopene, might be expected to reduce oxidant damage to prostate cell DNA if used for prostate cancer prevention. Also, because endogenous oxidant production in prostate cancer cells may be increased in the presence of androgens, antiandrogen treatment might also reduce oxidant genome damage and attenuate progression to life-threatening prostate cancer (88,89). Antiinflammatory agents might reduce inflammation-associated oxidant production in the prostate. Consumption of cruciferous fruits and vegetables, which contain the isothiocyanate compound sulforaphane, an inducer of GSTs and other carcinogen-detoxification enzymes, might compensate for the crippling of *GSTP1* gene function in neoplastic prostate cells (90–92).

CLINICAL DEVELOPMENT OF NEW PROSTATE CANCER PREVENTION STRATEGIES

The development and assessment of new prostate cancer prevention strategies will present considerable challenges in clinical trial design. Clinical trials have played critical roles in the development of chemoprevention for head and neck cancer, breast cancer, and colorectal cancer (93–97). Data from controlled clinical trials are needed by the U.S. Food and Drug Administration (FDA) to permit approval and labeling of all drugs, including cancer prevention agents. The FDA also monitors the safety and labeling of nutrient supplements and food products. Large-scale, randomized, placebo-controlled, investigator-blinded, clinical trials that recruit heterogeneous subject cohorts drawn from the general population and monitor subjects for end points, such as cancer development or cancer survival, have historically been the preferred tool for assessing treatment efficacy versus treatment safety. However, for cancer prevention drugs, such clinical trials are often very large, very costly, and very slow to yield useful data. For prostate cancer, several new and exciting prevention approaches have been proffered. Unfortunately, the current clinical trial capacity is inadequate to test each of these new approaches using randomized trials involving study subjects from the general population. To accelerate prostate cancer prevention drug development and approval in the future, these clinical trial deficiencies need to be addressed. One reason that cancer prevention trials have needed so many subjects and have taken so long is that the cohorts targeted for study, if drawn from the general population, display generally low rates of cancer development and mortality. Because the goals of randomized clinical trials for cancer prevention are to estimate differences in rates of cancer development or death attributable to treatment, cancer prevention trials featuring small treatment groups often require long follow-up times, whereas trials featuring short follow-up times often need large treatment groups. A second reason that cancer prevention trials typically take so long to complete is that the study end points, usually cancer development or death, may take many years to appear.

In addition to providing new opportunities for prostate cancer prevention drug discovery, the progressive understanding of the molecular pathogenesis of prostate cancer may also offer new opportunities to improve the efficiency of prostate cancer prevention drug development. Recent insights have the potential both to identify high-risk study subjects for clinical trial participation, prone to display high rates of cancer development or mortality, and to define new clinical trial end points as surrogates for cancer development. For example, as high-risk gene alleles for prostate cancer development are discovered and characterized, genotyping for such alleles can be used to identify otherwise healthy high-risk men as candidates for participation in prostate cancer prevention clinical trials. Known biomarkers, such as serum PSA levels, serum IGF-1 levels, or serum selenium levels may prove useful for risk stratification in clinical trial recruitment (98–100). New candidate biomarkers, arising from intensive efforts to fully characterize the vast array of messenger RNA and polypeptide species present in normal and neoplastic prostate cells, may also find use as predictors of prostate cancer risk. Known biomarkers, such as the presence of PIN on prostate biopsy, and new biomarkers, such as the presence of PIA on prostate biopsy; markers of oxidative damage; somatic genome alterations; and others, may serve, not only to identify men at risk for prostate cancer development, but also to provide candidate surrogate end points for prostate cancer prevention clinical trials.

PROSTATE CANCER PREVENTION AGENTS UNDER CURRENT DEVELOPMENT

5α-Reductase Inhibitors and Antiandrogens

Androgen signaling pathways have been targeted by a number of drugs, including FDA-approved drugs, for the treatment of benign prostatic hyperplasia (BPH), advanced prostate cancer, and other conditions, such as male pattern baldness. Finasteride, which has been marketed as Proscar for BPH and as Propecia for alopecia, is a selective inhibitor of type II 5α-reductase, is the enzyme responsible for converting testosterone to dihydrotestosterone in the prostate. Because finasteride has few worrisome side effects and may reduce the serum PSA in men with prostate cancer (101,102), the drug has been subjected to study in prostate cancer chemoprevention as part of the Prostate Cancer Prevention Trial (103,104). The Prostate Cancer Prevention Trial, which targeted men in the general population above age 55, has enrolled 18,882 subjects. As part of the clinical trial design, after 7 years of treatment with finasteride or placebo, all of the men in the trial are to undergo prostate biopsy. Results of the trial, expected by 2004, should reveal whether finasteride treatment reduces the period prevalence of prostate cancer. Other clinical trial data featuring finasteride treatment have not been very encouraging. In one prospective, randomized, placebo-controlled trial of finasteride for BPH (n = 3,040), 4.7% of men treated with finasteride and 5.1% of men treated with placebo were ultimately diagnosed with prostate cancer ($p = .7$) (105). In another smaller randomized trial (n = 52), men with an elevated serum PSA but no cancer on prostate biopsies received finasteride or no treatment for 12 months (106). Prostate biopsies obtained at study end were remarkable for the detection of cancer in 30% of men treated with finasteride versus 4% of men left untreated ($p = .25$). For men in the trial with PIN detected on the original biopsy, finasteride treatment did not appear to affect the PIN lesions. Furthermore, prostate cancer was evident after 12 months in six of eight of the men with PIN who were treated with finasteride versus zero of five of the men with PIN who were left untreated (106).

Antiandrogens, such as bicalutamide (Casodex) and flutamide (Eulexin), and androgen-lowering drugs, such as leuprolide acetate (Lupron), and goserelin acetate (Zoladex), have established roles in the treatment of advanced prostate cancer. As androgens are required for human prostate cancer development, these types of drugs, particularly if used at an early enough age, may well attenuate prostatic carcinogenesis. However, the prolonged and sustained use of such antiandrogenic drugs will carry a high risk of side effects, including loss of bone and muscle mass, loss of libido, and breast pain or gynecomastia, that will almost certainly restrict the broad application of such drugs to prostate cancer prevention. In a recent prospective, randomized, placebo-controlled clinical trial, the antiestrogenic drug tamoxifen citrate (Nolvadex) provided women protection against breast cancer development at the expense of increasing the risk of uterine cancer development (93). However, by targeting a group of women at particularly high risk for breast cancer, identified using a predictive tool (the Gail model) (107), the benefits of breast cancer risk reduction were found to outweigh the risks of treatment-associated side effects. For antiandrogenic drugs, if men at extremely high risk for prostate cancer development could be identified, perhaps via the use of genetic testing or new molecular biomarkers, or both, and if antiandrogen treatment reduced prostate cancer risks in such men, then it is conceivable that the risk-benefit ratio of drug treatment might be found to be favorable. Another intriguing approach might be to consider the use of antiandrogens for brief treatment periods, or with intermittent dosing schedules, for prostate cancer prevention. When administered in these ways, antiandrogenic drugs might reduce prostate cancer risks with significantly fewer side effects.

Antioxidant Micronutrients and Antiinflammatory Agents

Epidemiologic studies have provided substantial evidence that increased consumption of selenium, vitamin E, and the carotenoid lycopene decrease prostate cancer risks (108–118). These data are supported by the results of two well-publicized clinical trials (119,120). In one of the studies, 1,312 men and women with a history of nonmelanoma skin cancer were treated with 200 µg selenized brewer's yeast, or a placebo each day in an effort to reduce the risk of further skin cancer development (121). Although selenium supplementation failed to reduce skin cancer appearance in this trial, men receiving selenium supplements displayed a lower incidence of prostate cancer (121,122). In the other trial, α-tocopherol, β-carotene, a combination of α-tocopherol and β-carotene, or placebo was administered to 29,133 male Finnish smokers in an attempt to prevent lung cancer (119). Again, although neither α-tocopherol nor β-carotene supplementation reduced lung cancer development in the trial, men receiving α-tocopherol displayed a lower incidence of prostate cancer and lower prostate cancer mortality (119–122). To confirm these results, a prospective, randomized, placebo-controlled clinical trial of selenium and vitamin E (Selenium and Vitamin E Cancer Prevention Trial; n >30,000) has been planned. The results of this trial, not likely to be available for at least a decade, may provide definitive evidence for protective effects of these antioxidant micronutrients against prostatic carcinogenesis. Until the Selenium and Vitamin E Cancer Prevention Trial results become available, how can men be counseled concerning reducing prostate cancer risks by the consumption of over-the-counter antioxidants? Careful scrutiny of the epidemiology data available reveals that the highest prostate cancer risks tend to be associated with the lowest, or most inadequate, blood or tissue levels of antioxidant micronutrients (111,113,117). Micronutrient supplementation in doses sufficient to correct antioxidant deficiencies, rather than in "megadoses," will likely be safe and may be effective at reducing prostate cancer risks. Micronutrient antioxidants are often available in a variety of forms. For example, vitamin E supplementation may be accomplished using α-tocopherol or γ-tocopherol, whereas selenium supplementation may be accomplished using selenomethionine, methylselenocysteine, sodium selenite, or others (123). Each of the different compounds has different pharmacologic properties. To best determine which of these compounds may be most useful for prostate cancer prevention, in which formulation, at what dose, and at which schedule of administration, small clinical trials featuring new biomarkers, particularly markers of oxidative stress, as trial end points will be needed.

Arachidonic acid signaling pathways, the targets of widely used nonsteroidal antiinflammatory drugs, may be a critical determinant not only of inflammation, but also of carcinogenesis. Nonselective cyclooxygenase inhibitors, which have long been used as antiinflammatory and analgesic drugs, have also demonstrated provocative clinical activity against colorectal polyps, thought to represent colorectal cancer precursor lesions (96). Recently, new selective inhibitors of cyclooxygenase-2 (COX-2), celecoxib (Celebrex), and rofecoxib (Vioxx), have become available. These drugs appear to retain the antiinflammatory and analgesic properties of the nonselective cyclooxygenase inhibitors and to have substantially fewer side effects of gastroduodenal irritation and ulceration. Most intriguingly, mice prone to develop intestinal polyps that carry disrupted genes encoding COX-2 form significantly fewer polyps (124). COX-2, which is expressed at high levels in human colorectal neoplasms (125), may be a good target for human colorectal cancer prevention. In a recent clinical trial, celecoxib demonstrated significant efficacy in the treatment of colorectal polyps (97). Unfortunately, no consensus exists yet for whether COX-2 is expressed at high levels in normal prostate cells or in cells comprising PIA lesions, PIN lesions, or prostatic carcinomas (126–129). Nonetheless, celecoxib will be assessed in the near future for clinical activity against prostate cancers. R-flurbiprofen, an antiinflammatory agent that does not inhibit cyclooxygenases but may alter COX-2 messenger RNA levels (130), has demonstrated preclinical efficacy in the transgenic adenocarcinoma mouse prostate cancer model and has entered phase I/II human clinical testing against established prostate cancer. Sulindac sulfone (Exisulind), a nonsteroidal antiinflammatory agent that may target cyclic guanine monophosphate phosphodiesterase, has also entered clinical trials against established prostate cancer presenting as a rising serum PSA after primary prostate cancer treatment (131,132). 5-Lipoxygenases appear to modulate prostate cancer cell survival *in vitro* (133–139). Inhibitors of 5-lipoxygenases may be promising new drugs for prostate cancer treatment and for prostate cancer prevention.

Retinoids and Vitamin D Analogs

Differentiation agents, drugs that promote prostate cell differentiation at the expense of cell proliferation, may be attractive drugs for prostate cancer treatment and for prostate cancer prevention. Both retinoid compounds and vitamin D analogs have been reported to affect prostate cell behavior. Retinoids have also shown some ability to prevent aerodigestive cancers in clinical trials (94,95). Tretinoin (all-*trans*-retinoic acid, Vesanoid), 4-hydroxyphenylretinimide, and isotretinoin (13-*cis*-retinoic acid, Accutane), given alone or in combination with vitamin D analogs, manifest preclinical activity against prostate cancer cells *in vitro* (140–147). New retinoid compounds, such as alitretinoin (9-*cis*-retinoic acid, Panretin), an agonist against retinoic acid receptors and retinoid X receptors, and bexarotene (4-[1-(5,6,7,8-tetrahydro-3,5,5,8,8-pentamethyl-2-naphtalenyl) propenyl] benzoic acid, Targretin), a selective retinoid X receptor agonist, have also demonstrated preclinical activity against prostate cancer cells (148–150). In the near future, several of these retinoid compounds will likely be tested in men with established prostate cancer, alone and in various combinations with other drugs. If the side effects are limited and the clinical activity is encouraging for any of these retinoids, further assessment as prostate cancer chemoprevention drugs will be undertaken. Deficiencies in vitamin D intake or activation, or both, have been proposed to increase prostate cancer risks (151,152). Furthermore, vitamin D and its analogs have been shown to modulate prostate cancer cell growth and differentiation *in vitro* (140,141,143,153–165). Although analogs that bind the vitamin D receptor but cause little hypercalcemia at the doses and dosing schedules used appear the most promising in early clinical trials against established prostate cancer, vitamin D itself may find some use as a prostate cancer prevention agent.

Soy Products, Antiangiogenesis Agents, Matrix Metalloproteinase Inhibitors, and Others

Soy products are consumed in great quantities in Asia, where prostate cancer risks are low. Soy isoflavones, including genistein, have been proposed to inhibit protein kinases (166–169), topoisomerases (170,171), and 5α-reductases (172). Two new isoflavone compounds, PTI-G2535 and PTI-G4660 (Protein Technologies International), have entered phase I/II clinical trial testing against established prostate cancers. The Bowman-Birk inhibitor concentrate, an orally bioavailable protease inhibitor from soy (173–175), has entered phase I/II clinical trials against oral leukoplakia (176) and BPH. A large number of antiangiogenesis drugs and matrix metalloproteinase inhibitors that have the potential to arrest the progression of small prostate cancers, as well as other solid organ cancers (177–184), are currently under preclinical and early clinical development. Which of these agents will emerge as the most effective for established prostate cancer and have the fewest worrisome side effects is not clear. Insulinlike growth factor 1 (IGF-1) may modulate prostatic carcinogenesis (98,185–191). Drugs that decrease IGF-1 levels, increase IGF-binding protein levels, prevent PSA-mediated cleavage of IGF-binding proteins, or interfere with IGF receptor tyrosine kinases may find use in prostate cancer treatment or in prostate cancer prevention (187,188). Difluoromethylornithine (Eflornithine), an inhibitor of ornithine decarboxylase used to treat African sleeping sickness, is also under preclinical and clinical development as a prostate cancer chemoprevention drug (192).

CONCLUSIONS AND FUTURE DIRECTIONS

Of the many new candidate prostate cancer chemoprevention drugs under preclinical and early clinical development, most target various phenotypic features of prostate cancer cells, including sex-steroid hormone signaling, arachidonic acid signaling, growth factor signaling, and the regulation of differentiation. The majority of these drugs will be assessed for efficacy against established prostate cancer before being tested as prostate cancer chemoprevention drugs. Although more effective, and less toxic, treatments for established prostate cancer are needed, restriction of the prostate cancer chemoprevention pipeline to drugs useful for established prostate cancer may miss a great rational drug development opportunity. For prevention of strokes and heart attacks, treatments are directed at the "disease" atherosclerosis. For prostate cancer chemoprevention, the "disease" best treated may be prostatic carcinogenesis, not prostate cancer itself. The most compelling argument for the promise of prostate cancer prevention remains the fact that environmental factors, especially the diet, may play a dominant role in the prostate cancer epidemic in the United States. The molecular basis for these environmental effects may be that *GSTP1*, the gene encoding the π-class GST, serves a "caretaker" function for prostatic cells that is lost early during human prostatic carcinogenesis. Loss of *GSTP1* function appears to render PIN and prostate cancer cells vulnerable to genome damage inflicted by oxidants and electrophiles, including dietary components, that promote genomic instability and malignant behavior. Thus, this mechanism of prostatic carcinogenesis, featuring ongoing threats to genome integrity associated with high-risk dietary practices, may be the most critical rational "disease" target for prostate cancer prevention. To this end, the most promising prostate cancer prevention strategies under current consideration may be interventions aimed at reducing genome-damaging stresses in prostate cells, such as the use of antioxidants and anti-inflammatory agents, rather than drugs aimed at established prostate cancer cells.

Ultimately, the greatest challenge for any candidate prostate cancer prevention drug will be the daunting clinical development pathway necessary to prove efficacy for patient benefit to permit approval by the FDA. For the near future, dietary modifications and nutritional supplements that target the "disease" of prostatic carcinogenesis, not subject to the same regulatory requirements as drugs, may offer men concerned about prostate cancer the best prospect for reducing prostate cancer risks. Hopefully, such dietary interventions will be directed not only by epidemiology observations, but also by a growing body of clinical trial data.

REFERENCES

1. Landis SH, Murray T, Bolden S, et al. Cancer statistics [see comments]. *CA Cancer J Clin* 1999;49:8–31.
2. Polascik TJ, Oesterling JE, Partin AW. Prostate specific antigen: a decade of discovery—what we have learned and where we are going [see comments]. *J Urol* 1999;162:293–306.
3. Partin AW, Pound CR, Clemens JQ, et al. Serum PSA after anatomic radical prostatectomy. The Johns Hopkins experience after 10 years. *Urol Clin North Am* 1993;20:713–725.
4. Shipley WU, Thames HD, Sandler HM, et al. Radiation therapy for clinically localized prostate cancer: a multi-institutional pooled analysis. *JAMA* 1999;281:1598–1604.
5. Scher HI, Fossa S. Prostate cancer in the era of prostate-specific antigen. *Curr Opin Oncol* 1995;7:281–291.
6. Prostate Cancer Trialists' Collaborative Group. Maximum androgen blockade in advanced prostate cancer: an overview of the randomised trials [see comments]. *Lancet* 2000;355: 1491–1498.
7. Smith DC, Esper P, Strawderman M, et al. Phase II trial of oral estramustine, oral etoposide, and intravenous paclitaxel in hormone-refractory prostate cancer. *J Clin Oncol* 1999; 17:1664–1671.
8. Petrylak DP, Macarthur RB, O'Connor J, et al. Phase I trial of docetaxel with estramustine in androgen-independent prostate cancer. *J Clin Oncol* 1999;17:958–967.
9. Tannock IF, Osoba D, Stockler MR, et al. Chemotherapy with mitoxantrone plus prednisone or prednisone alone for symptomatic hormone-resistant prostate cancer: a Canadian randomized trial with palliative end points [see comments]. *J Clin Oncol* 1996;14:1756–1764.
10. Walsh PC, Marschke P, Ricker D, et al. Patient-reported urinary continence and sexual function after anatomic radical prostatectomy. *Urology* 2000;55:58–61.
11. Walsh PC, Lepor H, Eggleston JC. Radical prostatectomy with preservation of sexual function: anatomical and pathological considerations. *Prostate* 1983;4:473–485.
12. Horwitz EM, Hanlon AL, Hanks GE. Update on the treatment of prostate cancer with external beam irradiation. *Prostate* 1998;37:195–206.
13. Brawley OW, Knopf K, Thompson I. The epidemiology of prostate cancer part II: the risk factors. *Semin Urol Oncol* 1998;16:193–201.
14. Carter HB, Piantadosi S, Isaacs JT. Clinical evidence for and implications of the multistep development of prostate cancer. *J Urol* 1990;143:742–746.
15. Danley KL, Richardson JL, Bernstein L, et al. Prostate cancer: trends in mortality and stage-specific incidence rates by racial/ethnic group in Los Angeles County, California (United States). *Cancer Causes Control* 1995;6:492–498.
16. Haenszel W, Kurihara M. Studies of Japanese migrants. I. Mortality from cancer and other diseases among Japanese in the United States. *J Natl Cancer Inst* 1968;40:43–68.
17. Shimizu H, Ross RK, Bernstein L, et al. Cancers of the prostate and breast among Japanese and white immigrants in Los Angeles County. *Br J Cancer* 1991;63:963–966.
18. Whittemore AS, Kolonel LN, Wu AH, et al. Prostate cancer in relation to diet, physical activity, and body size in blacks, whites, and Asians in the United States and Canada [see comments]. *J Natl Cancer Inst* 1995;87:652–661.
19. Ross RK, Shimizu H, Paganini-Hill A, et al. Case-control studies of prostate cancer in blacks and whites in southern California. *J Natl Cancer Inst* 1987;78:869–874.
20. Kolonel LN, Yoshizawa CN, Hankin JH. Diet and prostatic cancer: a case-control study in Hawaii. *Am J Epidemiol* 1988;127:999–1012.
21. Giovannucci E, Rimm EB, Colditz GA, et al. A prospective study of dietary fat and risk of prostate cancer [see comments]. *J Natl Cancer Inst* 1993;85:1571–1579.
22. Stuart GR, Holcroft J, de Boer JG, et al. Prostate mutations in rats induced by the suspected human carcinogen 2-amino-1-methyl-6-phenylimidazo[4,5-b]pyridine. *Cancer Res* 2000; 60:266–268.

23. Shirai T, Sano M, Tamano S, et al. The prostate: a target for carcinogenicity of 2-amino-1-methyl-6-phenylimidazo[4,5-b]pyridine (PhIP) derived from cooked foods. *Cancer Res* 1997;57:195–198.
24. Fleshner N, Fair WR, Huryk R, et al. Vitamin E inhibits the high-fat diet promoted growth of established human prostate LNCaP tumors in nude mice. *J Urol* 1999;161:1651–1654.
25. Wang Y, Corr JG, Thaler HT, et al. Decreased growth of established human prostate LNCaP tumors in nude mice fed a low-fat diet [see comments]. *J Natl Cancer Inst* 1995;87:1456–1462.
26. Carter BS, Beaty TH, Steinberg GD, et al. Mendelian inheritance of familial prostate cancer. *Proc Natl Acad Sci U S A* 1992;89:3367–3371.
27. Gronberg H, Isaacs SD, Smith JR, et al. Characteristics of prostate cancer in families potentially linked to the hereditary prostate cancer 1 (HPC1) locus [see comments]. *JAMA* 1997;278:1251–1255.
28. Smith JR, Freije D, Carpten JD, et al. Major susceptibility locus for prostate cancer on chromosome 1 suggested by a genome-wide search [see comments]. *Science* 1996;274:1371–1374.
29. Gibbs M, Chakrabarti L, Stanford JL, et al. Analysis of chromosome 1q42.2-43 in 152 families with high risk of prostate cancer. *Am J Hum Genet* 1999;64:1087–1095.
30. Gibbs M, Stanford JL, McIndoe RA, et al. Evidence for a rare prostate cancer-susceptibility locus at chromosome 1p36. *Am J Hum Genet* 1999;64:776–787.
31. Xu J, Meyers D, Freije D, et al. Evidence for a prostate cancer susceptibility locus on the X chromosome. *Nat Genet* 1998;20:175–179.
32. Hsing AW, Gao YT, Wu G, et al. Polymorphic CAG and GGN repeat lengths in the androgen receptor gene and prostate cancer risk: a population-based case-control study in China. *Cancer Res* 2000;60:5111–5116.
33. Nam RK, Elhaji Y, Krahn MD, et al. Significance of the CAG repeat polymorphism of the androgen receptor gene in prostate cancer progression. *J Urol* 2000;164:567–572.
34. Edwards SM, Badzioch MD, Minter R, et al. Androgen receptor polymorphisms: association with prostate cancer risk, relapse and overall survival. *Int J Cancer* 1999;84:458–465.
35. Giovannucci E, Stampfer MJ, Krithivas K, et al. The CAG repeat within the androgen receptor gene and its relationship to prostate cancer [published erratum appears in *Proc Natl Acad Sci U S A* 1997;94:8272]. *Proc Natl Acad Sci U S A* 1997;94:3320–3323.
36. Stanford JL, Just JJ, Gibbs M, et al. Polymorphic repeats in the androgen receptor gene: molecular markers of prostate cancer risk [see comments]. *Cancer Res* 1997;57:1194–1198.
37. Ingles SA, Ross RK, Yu MC, et al. Association of prostate cancer risk with genetic polymorphisms in vitamin D receptor and androgen receptor [see comments]. *J Natl Cancer Inst* 1997;89:166–170.
38. Taylor JA, Hirvonen A, Watson M, et al. Association of prostate cancer with vitamin D receptor gene polymorphism. *Cancer Res* 1996;56:4108–4110.
39. Autrup JL, Thomassen LH, Olsen JH, et al. Glutathione S-transferases as risk factors in prostate cancer. *Eur J Cancer Prev* 1999;8:525–532.
40. Wadelius M, Autrup JL, Stubbins MJ, et al. Polymorphisms in NAT2, CYP2D6, CYP2C19 and GSTP1 and their association with prostate cancer. *Pharmacogenetics* 1999;9:333–340.
41. Harries LW, Stubbins MJ, Forman D, et al. Identification of genetic polymorphisms at the glutathione S-transferase Pi locus and association with susceptibility to bladder, testicular and prostate cancer. *Carcinogenesis* 1997;18:641–644.
42. Jaffe JM, Malkowicz SB, Walker AH, et al. Association of SRD5A2 genotype and pathological characteristics of prostate tumors. *Cancer Res* 2000;60:1626–1630.
43. Febbo PG, Kantoff PW, Platz EA, et al. The V89L polymorphism in the 5alpha-reductase type 2 gene and risk of prostate cancer. *Cancer Res* 1999;59:5878–5881.
44. Lunn RM, Bell DA, Mohler JL, et al. Prostate cancer risk and polymorphism in 17 hydroxylase (CYP17) and steroid reductase (SRD5A2). *Carcinogenesis* 1999;20:1727–1731.
45. Kantoff PW, Febbo PG, Giovannucci E, et al. A polymorphism of the 5 alpha-reductase gene and its association with prostate cancer: a case-control analysis. *Cancer Epidemiol Biomarkers Prev* 1997;6:189–192.
46. Perinchery G, Bukurov N, Nakajima K, et al. Loss of two new loci on chromosome 8 (8p23 and 8q12-13) in human prostate cancer. *Int J Oncol* 1999;14:495–500.
47. Cheng L, Song SY, Pretlow TG, et al. Evidence of independent origin of multiple tumors from patients with prostate cancer. *J Natl Cancer Inst* 1998;90:233–237.
48. Cunningham JM, Shan A, Wick MJ, et al. Allelic imbalance and microsatellite instability in prostatic adenocarcinoma. *Cancer Res* 1996;56:4475–4482.
49. Crundwell MC, Chughtai S, Knowles M, et al. Allelic loss on chromosomes 8p, 22q and 18q (DCC) in human prostate cancer. *Int J Cancer* 1996;69:295–300.
50. Vocke CD, Pozzatti RO, Bostwick DG, et al. Analysis of 99 microdissected prostate carcinomas reveals a high frequency of allelic loss on chromosome 8p12-21. *Cancer Res* 1996;56:2411–2416.
51. Macoska JA, Trybus TM, Benson PD, et al. Evidence for three tumor suppressor gene loci on chromosome 8p in human prostate cancer. *Cancer Res* 1995;55:5390–5395.
52. Emmert-Buck MR, Vocke CD, Pozzatti RO, et al. Allelic loss on chromosome 8p12-21 in microdissected prostatic intraepithelial neoplasia. *Cancer Res* 1995;55:2959–2962.
53. Suzuki H, Emi M, Komiya A, et al. Localization of a tumor suppressor gene associated with progression of human prostate cancer within a 1.2 Mb region of 8p22-p21.3. *Genes Chromosomes Cancer* 1995;13:168–174.
54. Trapman J, Sleddens HF, van der Weiden MM, et al. Loss of heterozygosity of chromosome 8 microsatellite loci implicates a candidate tumor suppressor gene between the loci D8S87 and D8S133 in human prostate cancer. *Cancer Res* 1994;54:6061–6064.
55. Cher ML, MacGrogan D, Bookstein R, et al. Comparative genomic hybridization, allelic imbalance, and fluorescence in situ hybridization on chromosome 8 in prostate cancer. *Genes Chromosomes Cancer* 1994;11:153–162.
56. Macoska JA, Trybus TM, Sakr WA, et al. Fluorescence in situ hybridization analysis of 8p allelic loss and chromosome 8 instability in human prostate cancer. *Cancer Res* 1994;54:3824–3830.

57. MacGrogan D, Levy A, Bostwick D, et al. Loss of chromosome arm 8p loci in prostate cancer: mapping by quantitative allelic imbalance. *Genes Chromosomes Cancer* 1994; 10:151–159.
58. Bova GS, Carter BS, Bussemakers MJ, et al. Homozygous deletion and frequent allelic loss of chromosome 8p22 loci in human prostate cancer. *Cancer Res* 1993;53:3869–3873.
59. Millar DS, Ow KK, Paul CL, et al. Detailed methylation analysis of the glutathione S-transferase pi (GSTP1) gene in prostate cancer. *Oncogene* 1999;18:1313–1324.
60. Lee WH, Morton RA, Epstein JI, et al. Cytidine methylation of regulatory sequences near the pi-class glutathione S-transferase gene accompanies human prostatic carcinogenesis. *Proc Natl Acad Sci U S A* 1994;91:11733–11737.
61. Lee WH, Isaacs WB, Bova GS, et al. CG island methylation changes near the GSTP1 gene in prostatic carcinoma cells detected using the polymerase chain reaction: a new prostate cancer biomarker. *Cancer Epidemiol Biomarkers Prev* 1997;6:443–450.
62. Brooks JD, Weinstein M, Lin X, et al. CG island methylation changes near the GSTP1 gene in prostatic intraepithelial neoplasia. *Cancer Epidemiol Biomarkers Prev* 1998;7:531–536.
63. Sakr WA, Grignon DJ, Crissman JD, et al. High grade prostatic intraepithelial neoplasia (HGPIN) and prostatic adenocarcinoma between the ages of 20–69: an autopsy study of 249 cases. *In Vivo* 1994;8:439–443.
64. Henderson CJ, Smith AG, Ure J, et al. Increased skin tumorigenesis in mice lacking pi class glutathione S-transferases. *Proc Natl Acad Sci U S A* 1998;95:5275–5280.
65. McWilliams JE, Sanderson BJ, Harris EL, et al. Glutathione S-transferase M1 (GSTM1) deficiency and lung cancer risk. *Cancer Epidemiol Biomarkers Prev* 1995;4:589–594.
66. Nazar-Stewart V, Vaughan TL, Burt RD, et al. Glutathione S-transferase M1 and susceptibility to nasopharyngeal carcinoma. *Cancer Epidemiol Biomarkers Prev* 1999;8:547–551.
67. Brockmoller J, Cascorbi I, Kerb R, et al. Combined analysis of inherited polymorphisms in arylamine N-acetyltransferase 2, glutathione S-transferases M1 and T1, microsomal epoxide hydrolase, and cytochrome P450 enzymes as modulators of bladder cancer risk. *Cancer Res* 1996;56:3915–3925.
68. Helzlsouer KJ, Selmin O, Huang HY, et al. Association between glutathione S-transferase M1, P1, and T1 genetic polymorphisms and development of breast cancer [see comments]. *J Natl Cancer Inst* 1998;90:512–518.
69. Lavigne JA, Helzlsouer KJ, Huang HY, et al. An association between the allele coding for a low activity variant of catechol-O-methyltransferase and the risk for breast cancer. *Cancer Res* 1997;57:5493–5497.
69a. Nelson CP, Kidd LR, Sauvgeot J, et al. Protection against 2-hydroxyamino-1-methyl-6-phenylimidazo[4,5-β]pyridine (*N*-OH-PhIP) cytotoxicity and DNA adduct formation in human prostate by glutathione *S*-transferase P1. *Cancer Res* 2001;61:103–109.
70. Hayes JD, Pulford DJ. The glutathione S-transferase supergene family: regulation of GST and the contribution of the isoenzymes to cancer chemoprotection and drug resistance. *Crit Rev Biochem Mol Biol* 1995;30:445–600.
71. Farber E, Cameron R. The sequential analysis of cancer development. *Adv Cancer Res* 1980;31:125–226.
72. Farber E, Sarma DS. Hepatocarcinogenesis: a dynamic cellular perspective. *Lab Invest* 1987;56:4–22.
73. Roomi MW, Ho RK, Sarma DS, et al. A common biochemical pattern in preneoplastic hepatocyte nodules generated in four different models in the rat. *Cancer Res* 1985;45:564–571.
74. Satoh K, Kitahara A, Soma Y, et al. Purification, induction, and distribution of placental glutathione transferase: a new marker enzyme for preneoplastic cells in the rat chemical hepatocarcinogenesis. *Proc Natl Acad Sci U S A* 1985; 82:3964–3968.
75. Sato K, Kitahara A, Satoh K, et al. The placental form of glutathione S-transferase as a new marker protein for preneoplasia in rat chemical hepatocarcinogenesis. *Gann* 1984;75:199–202.
76. Bannasch P. Preneoplastic lesions as end points in carcinogenicity testing. I. Hepatic preneoplasia. *Carcinogenesis* 1986;7: 689–695.
77. Kirby GM, Stalker M, Metcalfe C, et al. Expression of immunoreactive glutathione S-transferases in hepatic neoplasms induced by aflatoxin B1 or 1,2-dimethylbenzanthracene in rainbow trout (*Oncorhynchus mykiss*). *Carcinogenesis* 1990;11:2255–2257.
78. Hayes MA, Smith IR, Rushmore TH, et al. Pathogenesis of skin and liver neoplasms in white suckers from industrially polluted areas in Lake Ontario. *Sci Total Environ* 1990;94:105–123.
79. Tchou JC, Lin X, Freije D, et al. GSTP1 CpG island DNA hypermethylation in hepatocellular carcinomas. *Int J Oncol* 2000;16:663–676.
80. De Marzo AM, Marchi VL, Epstein JI, et al. Proliferative inflammatory atrophy of the prostate: implications for prostatic carcinogenesis. *Am J Pathol* 1999;155:1985–1992.
81. Feneley MR, Young MP, Chinyama C, et al. Ki-67 expression in early prostate cancer and associated pathological lesions. *J Clin Pathol* 1996;49:741–748.
82. Liavag I. Mitotic activity of prostatic epithelium. A study by means of Colcemid. *Acta Pathol Microbiol Scand* 1968;73: 19–28.
83. Franks LM. Atrophy and hyperplasia in the prostate proper. *J Pathology and Bacteriology* 1954;68:617–621.
84. Reese JH, McNeal JE, Goldenberg SL, et al. Distribution of lactoferrin in the normal and inflamed human prostate: an immunohistochemical study. *Prostate* 1992;20:73–85.
85. McNeal JE. Normal histology of the prostate. *Am J Surg Pathol* 1988;12:619–633.
86. Ruska KM, Sauvageot J, Epstein JI. Histology and cellular kinetics of prostatic atrophy. *Am J Surg Pathol* 1998;22: 1073–1077.
87. Putzi MJ, De Marzo AM. Morphologic transitions between proliferative inflammatory atrophy and high-grade prostatic intraepithelial neoplasia. *Urology* 2000;56:828–832.
88. Ripple MO, Henry WF, Rago RP, et al. Prooxidant-antioxidant shift induced by androgen treatment of human prostate carcinoma cells [see comments]. *J Natl Cancer Inst* 1997;89:40–48.
89. Ripple MO, Henry WF, Schwarze SR, et al. Effect of antioxidants on androgen-induced AP-1 and NF-kappaB DNA-binding activity in prostate carcinoma cells. *J Natl Cancer Inst* 1999;91:1227–1232.
90. Zhang Y, Talalay P, Cho CG, et al. A major inducer of anticarcinogenic protective enzymes from broccoli: isolation and elucidation of structure. *Proc Natl Acad Sci U S A* 1992;89:2399–2403.

91. Zhang Y, Kensler TW, Cho CG, et al. Anticarcinogenic activities of sulforaphane and structurally related synthetic norbornyl isothiocyanates. *Proc Natl Acad Sci U S A* 1994;91:3147–3150.
92. Fahey JW, Zhang Y, Talalay P. Broccoli sprouts: an exceptionally rich source of inducers of enzymes that protect against chemical carcinogens. *Proc Natl Acad Sci U S A* 1997;94:10367–10372.
93. Fisher B, Costantino JP, Wickerham DL, et al. Tamoxifen for prevention of breast cancer: report of the National Surgical Adjuvant Breast and Bowel Project P-1 Study. *J Natl Cancer Inst* 1998;90:1371–1388.
94. Hong WK, Endicott J, Itri LM, et al. 13-cis-retinoic acid in the treatment of oral leukoplakia. *N Engl J Med* 1986;315:1501–1505.
95. Hong WK, Lippman SM, Itri LM, et al. Prevention of second primary tumors with isotretinoin in squamous-cell carcinoma of the head and neck [see comments]. *N Engl J Med* 1990;323:795–801.
96. Giardiello FM, Hamilton SR, Krush AJ, et al. Treatment of colonic and rectal adenomas with sulindac in familial adenomatous polyposis. *N Engl J Med* 1993;328:1313–1316.
97. Steinbach G, Lynch PM, Phillips RK, et al. The effect of celecoxib, a cyclooxygenase-2 inhibitor, in familial adenomatous polyposis. *N Engl J Med* 2000;342:1946–1952.
98. Chan JM, Stampfer MJ, Giovannucci E, et al. Plasma insulin-like growth factor-I and prostate cancer risk: a prospective study [see comments]. *Science* 1998;279:563–566.
99. Gann PH, Hennekens CH, Stampfer MJ. A prospective evaluation of plasma prostate-specific antigen for detection of prostatic cancer [see comments]. *JAMA* 1995;273:289–294.
100. Ross KS, Carter HB, Pearson JD, et al. Comparative efficiency of prostate-specific antigen screening strategies for prostate cancer detection. *JAMA* 2000;284:1399–1405.
101. Andriole G, Lieber M, Smith J, et al. Treatment with finasteride following radical prostatectomy for prostate cancer. *Urology* 1995;45:491–497.
102. Presti JC Jr., Fair WR, Andriole G, et al. Multicenter, randomized, double-blind, placebo controlled study to investigate the effect of finasteride (MK-906) on stage D prostate cancer. *J Urol* 1992;148:1201–1204.
103. Coltman CA Jr., Thompson IM Jr., Feigl P. Prostate Cancer Prevention Trial (PCPT) update. *Eur Urol* 1999;35:544–547.
104. Feigl P, Blumenstein B, Thompson I, et al. Design of the Prostate Cancer Prevention Trial (PCPT). *Control Clin Trials* 1995;16:150–163.
105. Andriole GL, Guess HA, Epstein JI, et al. Treatment with finasteride preserves usefulness of prostate-specific antigen in the detection of prostate cancer: results of a randomized, double-blind, placebo-controlled clinical trial. PLESS Study Group. Proscar Long-Term Efficacy and Safety Study. *Urology* 1998;52:195–201; discussion 201–202.
106. Cote RJ, Skinner EC, Salem CE, et al. The effect of finasteride on the prostate gland in men with elevated serum prostate-specific antigen levels [see comments]. *Br J Cancer* 1998;78:413–418.
107. Gail MH, Brinton LA, Byar DP, et al. Projecting individualized probabilities of developing breast cancer for white females who are being examined annually [see comments]. *J Natl Cancer Inst* 1989;81:1879–1886.
108. Gann PH, Ma J, Giovannucci E, et al. Lower prostate cancer risk in men with elevated plasma lycopene levels: results of a prospective analysis. *Cancer Res* 1999;59:1225–1230.
109. Giovannucci E, Ascherio A, Rimm EB, et al. Intake of carotenoids and retinol in relation to risk of prostate cancer. *J Natl Cancer Inst* 1995;87:1767–1776.
110. Giovannucci E. Tomatoes, tomato-based products, lycopene, and cancer: review of the epidemiologic literature [see comments]. *J Natl Cancer Inst* 1999;91:317–331.
111. Hardell L, Degerman A, Tomic R, et al. Levels of selenium in plasma and glutathione peroxidase in erythrocytes in patients with prostate cancer or benign hyperplasia. *Eur J Cancer Prev* 1995;4:91–95.
112. Rao AV, Fleshner N, Agarwal S. Serum and tissue lycopene and biomarkers of oxidation in prostate cancer patients: a case-control study. *Nutr Cancer* 1999;33:159–164.
113. Yoshizawa K, Willett WC, Morris SJ, et al. Study of prediagnostic selenium level in toenails and the risk of advanced prostate cancer [see comments]. *J Natl Cancer Inst* 1998; 90:1219–1224.
114. Tzonou A, Signorello LB, Lagiou P, et al. Diet and cancer of the prostate: a case-control study in Greece. *Int J Cancer* 1999;80:704–708.
115. Deneo-Pellegrini H, De Stefani E, Ronco A, et al. Foods, nutrients and prostate cancer: a case-control study in Uruguay. *Br J Cancer* 1999;80:591–597.
116. Kristal AR, Stanford JL, Cohen JH, et al. Vitamin and mineral supplement use is associated with reduced risk of prostate cancer. *Cancer Epidemiol Biomarkers Prev* 1999;8:887–892.
117. Nomura AM, Lee J, Stemmermann GN, et al. Serum selenium and subsequent risk of prostate cancer. *Cancer Epidemiol Biomarkers Prev* 2000;9:883–887.
118. Chan JM, Stampfer MJ, Ma J, et al. Supplemental vitamin E intake and prostate cancer risk in a large cohort of men in the United States. *Cancer Epidemiol Biomarkers Prev* 1999; 8:893–899.
119. The Alpha-Tocopherol, Beta Carotene Cancer Prevention Study Group. The effect of vitamin E and beta carotene on the incidence of lung cancer and other cancers in male smokers [see comments]. *N Engl J Med* 1994;330:1029–1035.
120. Heinonen OP, Albanes D, Virtamo J, et al. Prostate cancer and supplementation with alpha-tocopherol and beta-carotene: incidence and mortality in a controlled trial [see comments]. *J Natl Cancer Inst* 1998;90:440–446.
121. Clark LC, Combs GF Jr., Turnbull BW, et al. Effects of selenium supplementation for cancer prevention in patients with carcinoma of the skin. A randomized controlled trial. Nutritional Prevention of Cancer Study Group [see comments] [published erratum appears in *JAMA* 1997;277:1520]. *JAMA* 1996;276:1957–1963.
122. Clark LC, Dalkin B, Krongrad A, et al. Decreased incidence of prostate cancer with selenium supplementation: results of a double-blind cancer prevention trial. *Br J Urol* 1998; 81:730–734.
123. Patterson BH, Levander OA. Naturally occurring selenium compounds in cancer chemoprevention trials: a workshop summary. *Cancer Epidemiol Biomarkers Prev* 1997;6:63–69.
124. Oshima M, Dinchuk JE, Kargman SL, et al. Suppression of intestinal polyposis in Apc delta716 knockout mice by inhibition of cyclooxygenase 2 (COX-2). *Cell* 1996;87:803–809.

125. Sano H, Kawahito Y, Wilder RL, et al. Expression of cyclooxygenase-1 and -2 in human colorectal cancer. *Cancer Res* 1995;55:3785–3789.
126. Gupta S, Srivastava M, Ahmad N, et al. Over-expression of cyclooxygenase-2 in human prostate adenocarcinoma. *Prostate* 2000;42:73–78.
127. Yoshimura R, Sano H, Masuda C, et al. Expression of cyclooxygenase-2 in prostate carcinoma. *Cancer* 2000;89:589–596.
128. Tanji N, Kikugawa T, Yokoyama M. Immunohistochemical study of cyclooxygenases in prostatic adenocarcinoma; relationship to apoptosis and Bcl-2 protein expression. *Anticancer Res* 2000;20:2313–2319.
129. Kirschenbaum A, Klausner AP, Lee R, et al. Expression of cyclooxygenase-1 and cyclooxygenase-2 in the human prostate. *Urology* 2000;56:671–676.
130. Tjandrawinata RR, Dahiya R, Hughes-Fulford M. Induction of cyclo-oxygenase-2 mRNA by prostaglandin E2 in human prostatic carcinoma cells. *Br J Cancer* 1997;75:1111–1118.
131. Soh JW, Mao Y, Kim MG, et al. Cyclic GMP mediates apoptosis induced by sulindac derivatives via activation of c-Jun NH2-terminal kinase 1. *Clin Cancer Res* 2000;6:4136–4141.
132. Thompson WJ, Piazza GA, Li H, et al. Exisulind induction of apoptosis involves guanosine 3',5'-cyclic monophosphate phosphodiesterase inhibition, protein kinase G activation, and attenuated beta-catenin. *Cancer Res* 2000;60:3338–3342.
133. Myers CE, Ghosh J. Lipoxygenase inhibition in prostate cancer. *Eur Urol* 1999;35:395–398.
134. Hong SH, Avis I, Vos MD, et al. Relationship of arachidonic acid metabolizing enzyme expression in epithelial cancer cell lines to the growth effect of selective biochemical inhibitors. *Cancer Res* 1999;59:2223–2228.
135. Ghosh J, Myers CE. Inhibition of arachidonate 5-lipoxygenase triggers massive apoptosis in human prostate cancer cells. *Proc Natl Acad Sci U S A* 1998;95:13182–13187.
136. Ghosh J, Myers CE. Arachidonic acid stimulates prostate cancer cell growth: critical role of 5-lipoxygenase. *Biochem Biophys Res Commun* 1997;235:418–423.
137. Anderson KM, Seed T, Vos M, et al. 5-Lipoxygenase inhibitors reduce PC-3 cell proliferation and initiate nonnecrotic cell death. *Prostate* 1998;37:161–173.
138. Anderson KM, Seed T, Ondrey F, et al. The selective 5-lipoxygenase inhibitor A63162 reduces PC3 proliferation and initiates morphologic changes consistent with secretion. *Anticancer Res* 1994;14:1951–1960.
139. Anderson KM, Harris JE. 5,8,11,14-eicosatetraynoic acid inhibits PC3 DNA synthesis and cellular proliferation, in part due to its 5'-lipoxygenase activity. *Clin Physiol Biochem* 1990;8:308–313.
140. Elstner E, Campbell MJ, Munker R, et al. Novel 20-epi-vitamin D_3 analog combined with 9-cis-retinoic acid markedly inhibits colony growth of prostate cancer cells. *Prostate* 1999;40:141–149.
141. Campbell MJ, Park S, Uskokovic MR, et al. Synergistic inhibition of prostate cancer cell lines by a 19-nor hexafluoride vitamin D_3 analogue and anti-activator protein 1 retinoid. *Br J Cancer* 1999;79:101–107.
142. Igawa M, Tanabe T, Chodak GW, et al. N-(4-hydroxyphenyl) retinamide induces cell cycle specific growth inhibition in PC3 cells. *Prostate* 1994;24:299–305.
143. Esquenet M, Swinnen JV, Heyns W, et al. Control of LNCaP proliferation and differentiation: actions and interactions of androgens, 1alpha,25-dihydroxycholecalciferol, all-trans retinoic acid, 9-cis retinoic acid, and phenylacetate. *Prostate* 1996;28:182–194.
144. Roberson KM, Penland SN, Padilla GM, et al. Fenretinide: induction of apoptosis and endogenous transforming growth factor beta in PC-3 prostate cancer cells. *Cell Growth Differ* 1997;8:101–111.
145. Hsu JY, Pfahl M. ET-1 expression and growth inhibition of prostate cancer cells: a retinoid target with novel specificity. *Cancer Res* 1998;58:4817–4822.
146. Sun SY, Yue P, Lotan R. Induction of apoptosis by N-(4-hydroxyphenyl)retinamide and its association with reactive oxygen species, nuclear retinoic acid receptors, and apoptosis-related genes in human prostate carcinoma cells. *Mol Pharmacol* 1999;55:403–410.
147. Shen JC, Wang TT, Chang S, et al. Mechanistic studies of the effects of the retinoid N-(4-hydroxyphenyl) retinamide on prostate cancer cell growth and apoptosis. *Mol Carcinog* 1999;24:160–168.
148. de Vos S, Dawson MI, Holden S, et al. Effects of retinoid X receptor-selective ligands on proliferation of prostate cancer cells. *Prostate* 1997;32:115–121.
149. Blutt SE, Allegretto EA, Pike JW, et al. 1,25-dihydroxyvitamin D_3 and 9-cis-retinoic acid act synergistically to inhibit the growth of LNCaP prostate cells and cause accumulation of cells in G1. *Endocrinology* 1997;138:1491–1497.
150. Zhao XY, Ly LH, Peehl DM, et al. Induction of androgen receptor by 1alpha,25-dihydroxyvitamin D_3 and 9-cis retinoic acid in LNCaP human prostate cancer cells. *Endocrinology* 1999;140:1205–1212.
151. Hanchette CL, Schwartz GG. Geographic patterns of prostate cancer mortality. Evidence for a protective effect of ultraviolet radiation. *Cancer* 1992;70:2861–2869.
152. Schwartz GG, Hulka BS. Is vitamin D deficiency a risk factor for prostate cancer? (Hypothesis). *Anticancer Res* 1990;10:1307–1311.
153. Barreto AM, Schwartz GG, Woodruff R, et al. 25-Hydroxyvitamin D_3, the prohormone of 1,25-dihydroxyvitamin D_3, inhibits the proliferation of primary prostatic epithelial cells. *Cancer Epidemiol Biomarkers Prev* 2000;9:265–270.
154. Chen TC, Schwartz GG, Burnstein KL, et al. The in vitro evaluation of 25-hydroxyvitamin D_3 and 19-nor-1alpha,25-dihydroxyvitamin D_2 as therapeutic agents for prostate cancer. *Clin Cancer Res* 2000;6:901–908.
155. Lokeshwar BL, Schwartz GG, Selzer MG, et al. Inhibition of prostate cancer metastasis in vivo: a comparison of 1,23-dihydroxyvitamin D (calcitriol) and EB1089. *Cancer Epidemiol Biomarkers Prev* 1999;8:241–248.
156. Schwartz GG, Whitlatch LW, Chen TC, et al. Human prostate cells synthesize 1,25-dihydroxyvitamin D_3 from 25-hydroxyvitamin D_3. *Cancer Epidemiol Biomarkers Prev* 1998;7:391–395.
157. Schwartz GG, Wang MH, Zang M, et al. 1 alpha,25-Dihydroxyvitamin D (calcitriol) inhibits the invasiveness of human prostate cancer cells. *Cancer Epidemiol Biomarkers Prev* 1997;6:727–732.
158. Konety BR, Schwartz GG, Acierno JS Jr., et al. The role of vitamin D in normal prostate growth and differentiation. *Cell Growth Differ* 1996;7:1563–1570.

159. Schwartz GG, Hill CC, Oeler TA, et al. 1,25-Dihydroxy-16-ene-23-yne-vitamin D_3 and prostate cancer cell proliferation in vivo. *Urology* 1995;46:365–369.
160. Miller GJ. Vitamin D and prostate cancer: biologic interactions and clinical potentials. *Cancer Metastasis Rev* 1998;17:353–360.
161. Hedlund TE, Moffatt KA, Uskokovic MR, et al. Three synthetic vitamin D analogues induce prostate-specific acid phosphatase and prostate-specific antigen while inhibiting the growth of human prostate cancer cells in a vitamin D receptor-dependent fashion. *Clin Cancer Res* 1997;3:1331–1338.
162. Wang X, Chen X, Akhter J, et al. The in vitro effect of vitamin D_3 analogue EB-1089 on a human prostate cancer cell line (PC-3). *Br J Urol* 1997;80:260–262.
163. Campbell MJ, Elstner E, Holden S, et al. Inhibition of proliferation of prostate cancer cells by a 19-nor-hexafluoride vitamin D_3 analogue involves the induction of p21waf1, p27kip1 and E-cadherin. *J Mol Endocrinol* 1997;19:15–27.
164. Skowronski RJ, Peehl DM, Feldman D. Vitamin D and prostate cancer: 1,25 dihydroxyvitamin D_3 receptors and actions in human prostate cancer cell lines. *Endocrinology* 1993;132:1952–1960.
165. Skowronski RJ, Peehl DM, Feldman D. Actions of vitamin D_3, analogs on human prostate cancer cell lines: comparison with 1,25-dihydroxyvitamin D_3. *Endocrinology* 1995;136:20–26.
166. Kyle E, Neckers L, Takimoto C, et al. Genistein-induced apoptosis of prostate cancer cells is preceded by a specific decrease in focal adhesion kinase activity. *Mol Pharmacol* 1997;51:193–200.
167. Agarwal R. Cell signaling and regulators of cell cycle as molecular targets for prostate cancer prevention by dietary agents. *Biochem Pharmacol* 2000;60:1051–1059.
168. Shen JC, Klein RD, Wei Q, et al. Low-dose genistein induces cyclin-dependent kinase inhibitors and G(1) cell-cycle arrest in human prostate cancer cells. *Mol Carcinog* 2000;29:92–102.
169. Akiyama T, Ishida J, Nakagawa S, et al. Genistein, a specific inhibitor of tyrosine-specific protein kinases. *J Biol Chem* 1987;262:5592–5595.
170. Okura A, Arakawa H, Oka H, et al. Effect of genistein on topoisomerase activity and on the growth of [Val 12]Ha-ras-transformed NIH 3T3 cells. *Biochem Biophys Res Commun* 1988;157:183–189.
171. Markovits J, Linassier C, Fosse P, et al. Inhibitory effects of the tyrosine kinase inhibitor genistein on mammalian DNA topoisomerase II. *Cancer Res* 1989;49:5111–5117.
172. Evans BA, Griffiths K, Morton MS. Inhibition of 5 alpha-reductase in genital skin fibroblasts and prostate tissue by dietary lignans and isoflavonoids. *J Endocrinol* 1995;147: 295–302.
173. Wan XS, Ware JH, Zhang L, et al. Treatment with soybean-derived Bowman Birk inhibitor increases serum prostate-specific antigen concentration while suppressing growth of human prostate cancer xenografts in nude mice. *Prostate* 1999;41:243–252.
174. Kennedy AR. Prevention of carcinogenesis by protease inhibitors. *Cancer Res* 1994;54:1999s–2005s.
175. Kennedy AR. The evidence for soybean products as cancer preventive agents [see comments]. *J Nutr* 1995;125:733S–743S.
176. Wan XS, Meyskens FL Jr., Armstrong WB, et al. Relationship between protease activity and neu oncogene expression in patients with oral leukoplakia treated with the Bowman Birk Inhibitor [in-process citation]. *Cancer Epidemiol Biomarkers Prev* 1999;8:601–608.
177. Heath EI, Grochow LB. Clinical potential of matrix metalloprotease inhibitors in cancer therapy. *Drugs* 2000;59: 1043–1055.
178. Gradishar WJ. An overview of clinical trials involving inhibitors of angiogenesis and their mechanism of action. *Invest New Drugs* 1997;15:49–59.
179. Bergers G, Javaherian K, Lo KM, et al. Effects of angiogenesis inhibitors on multistage carcinogenesis in mice. *Science* 1999;284:808–812.
180. O'Reilly MS, Boehm T, Shing Y, et al. Endostatin: an endogenous inhibitor of angiogenesis and tumor growth. *Cell* 1997;88:277–285.
181. Parangi S, O'Reilly M, Christofori G, et al. Antiangiogenic therapy of transgenic mice impairs de novo tumor growth. *Proc Natl Acad Sci U S A* 1996;93:2002–2007.
182. O'Reilly MS, Holmgren L, Shing Y, et al. Angiostatin: a novel angiogenesis inhibitor that mediates the suppression of metastases by a Lewis lung carcinoma [see comments]. *Cell* 1994;79:315–328.
183. Ingber D, Fujita T, Kishimoto S, et al. Synthetic analogues of fumagillin that inhibit angiogenesis and suppress tumour growth. *Nature* 1990;348:555–557.
184. Conway JG, Trexler SJ, Wakefield JA, et al. Effect of matrix metalloproteinase inhibitors on tumor growth and spontaneous metastasis. *Clin Exp Metastasis* 1996;14:115–124.
185. Mantzoros CS, Tzonou A, Signorello LB, et al. Insulin-like growth factor 1 in relation to prostate cancer and benign prostatic hyperplasia [see comments]. *Br J Cancer* 1997;76: 1115–1118.
186. Iwamura M, Sluss PM, Casamento JB, et al. Insulin-like growth factor I: action and receptor characterization in human prostate cancer cell lines. *Prostate* 1993;22:243–252.
187. Cohen P, Peehl DM, Graves HC, et al. Biological effects of prostate specific antigen as an insulin-like growth factor binding protein-3 protease. *J Endocrinol* 1994;142:407–415.
188. Cohen P, Graves HC, Peehl DM, et al. Prostate-specific antigen (PSA) is an insulin-like growth factor binding protein-3 protease found in seminal plasma. *J Clin Endocrinol Metab* 1992;75:1046–1053.
189. Wolk A, Mantzoros CS, Andersson SO, et al. Insulin-like growth factor 1 and prostate cancer risk: a population-based, case-control study [see comments]. *J Natl Cancer Inst* 1998;90:911–915.
190. Culig Z, Hobisch A, Cronauer MV, et al. Androgen receptor activation in prostatic tumor cell lines by insulin-like growth factor-I, keratinocyte growth factor and epidermal growth factor. *Eur Urol* 1995;27:45–47.
191. Pietrzkowski Z, Mulholland G, Gomella L, et al. Inhibition of growth of prostatic cancer cell lines by peptide analogues of insulin-like growth factor 1. *Cancer Res* 1993;53:1102–1106.
192. Meyskens FL Jr., Gerner EW. Development of difluoromethylornithine (DFMO) as a chemoprevention agent. *Clin Cancer Res* 1999;5:945–951.

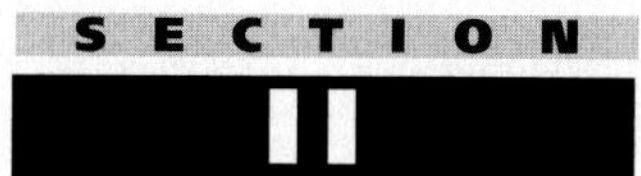

EPIDEMIOLOGY

8

NUTRITIONAL AND ENVIRONMENTAL EPIDEMIOLOGY OF PROSTATE CANCER

EDWARD L. GIOVANNUCCI
ELIZABETH A. PLATZ

In U.S. men, prostate cancer (CaP) is the second leading cause of cancer death and accounts for 30% of all cancers diagnosed. During the 1990s, the CaP incidence rate rapidly increased, mainly attributable to screening using prostate-specific antigen (PSA). Our understanding of the etiology of CaP remains far from complete. Established nonmodifiable risk factors for CaP include older age, a family history of CaP, and race. Risk is greatest among African-Americans, followed by white individuals and Asians. Few modifiable risk factors are universally accepted as established. Nonetheless, several lines of evidence indicate that nutritional or other environmental factors profoundly influence the occurrence or progression of CaP.

The first clue that exogenous factors influence prostate carcinogenesis is that CaP incidence rates display substantial variability across countries around the world. An almost 70-fold differential in CaP risk has been observed between the populations with the lowest and highest rate (1). CaP rates are lowest in the Far East and on the Indian subcontinent and highest in Western Europe, Australia, and North America. Standardizing CaP rates to a common age standard, the incidence rate was approximately 1 of 100,000 men annually in China compared to 62 of 100,000 for U.S. whites and 82 of 100,000 for African-Americans in the late 1980s (1). Mortality rates vary greatly between nations as well; in Japan, 4 of 100,000 men die of CaP per year, whereas in Canada, France, Germany, the United Kingdom, and the United States, the mortality rate ranges from 16 to 18 of 100,000 men annually (2).

Differences in medical practice leading to differential rates of detection of subclinical tumors, as well as differences in genetic susceptibility, contribute to these differences, but these differences are likely to result largely from exogenous factors, because the incidence of CaP increases in populations that have migrated from countries in which the rates are low to those where rates are high. For example, men of Asian heritage living in the United States are at lower risk for CaP than are white Americans, but they are at greater risk of the disease than are men of similar ancestries living in Asia (3–5). These rate differences do not appear to result entirely from differences in detection of early-stage tumors between the United States and Asian countries (6).

A final indication that nutritional or related factors influence risk of CaP is that high correlations are observed between *per capita* consumption of fat, animal fat, red meat, and dairy products and national CaP incidence and mortality rates (7). Among the strongest correlations are those observed for dairy products. For example, Figure 8-1 illustrates the relationship between *per capita* consumption of milk products and CaP mortality rates in different countries. It is not possible to draw firm conclusions based on such correlational data; in this case, other factors that co-vary with milk consumption could account for this association. Nonetheless, the variation in international CaP incidence rates, the increasing rates in immigrants coming to countries with higher rates of the disease, and the strong correlations between various nutritional factors and CaP incidence and mortality strongly suggest that some aspects of diet and lifestyle influence risk of CaP.

This chapter reviews the epidemiologic evidence for specific modifiable determinants for CaP. First, the natural history of CaP is discussed, because it is critical to understand when risk factors act during carcinogenesis so that interventions may be appropriately timed. After this discussion is a summary of the hormonal influences on CaP risk, including androgens, insulinlike growth factor (IGF)-1, and vitamin D. These are crucial to consider, because many nutritional and environmental components may influence CaP risk by modulating these hormonal systems. Finally, this chapter concludes with a discussion of specific modifiable risk factors, focusing especially on diet.

RISK FACTORS IN RELATION TO THE NATURAL HISTORY OF PROSTATE CANCER

Like many adult cancers, CaP likely represents the accumulation of various genetic insults that develop over the

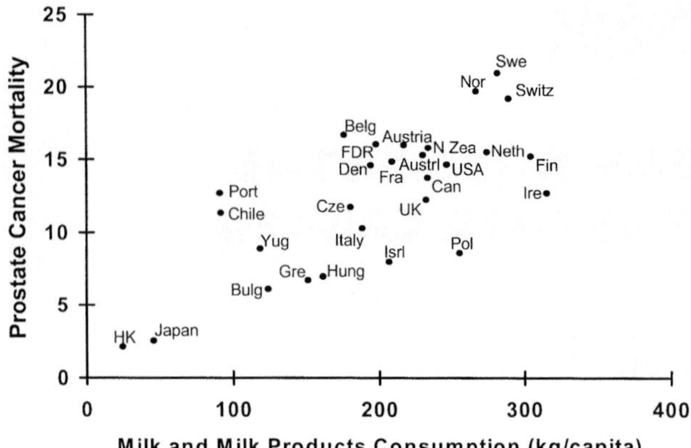

FIGURE 8-1. Age-standardized prostate cancer mortality rates (circa 1975 per 100,000 population) and milk and milk products consumption from 1970. FDR, Germany; HK, Hong Kong. (Reproduced from World Health Organization Regional Office for Europe: Copenhagen, 1993, with permission.)

course of decades. Because CaP is diagnosed on average at an older age than any other malignancy, most CaP is probably initiated quite early in life. Thus, nutritional and other environmental risk factors may influence CaP development and progression throughout most of the male life cycle. To better understand the potential role of exogenous factors in prostate carcinogenesis, it is important to consider critical periods in the development and growth of the prostate gland.

The development of the prostate gland, controlled largely by sex hormones, is initiated at approximately week 12 of fetal development, when the secretion of testosterone (T) from the embryonic testis stimulates prostate morphogenesis. The initial genetic insults for prostate carcinogenesis could occur *in utero*, but this hypothesis is difficult to study directly. Birth weight may be an indicator of *in utero* exposure to nutrients, steroid hormones, and fetal growth factors (8) and has been hypothesized to be associated with CaP risk. A small cohort study (21 cases among 366 men) found that CaP incidence was more than four times higher among those whose birth weight was in the upper quartile compared to the lower quartile (9). However, subsequent larger studies have shown little evidence for an important contribution of birth weight to risk of CaP (10,11). How strongly birth weight correlates with *in utero* hormonal exposure is unclear. One study found that preeclampsia and prematurity, which are likely correlates of pregnancy hormones and other growth factors, are inversely associated with CaP incidence and mortality (10).

In the male infant, the prostate gland weighs approximately 1 g. The prostate grows slowly during childhood and achieves a weight of approximately 4 g before the onset of puberty. The surge of androgens and other growth factors at puberty causes a rapid acceleration in the growth of the prostate, culminating in the final adult mass of approximately 25 g. Further (noncancerous) growth later in adulthood is abnormal and is usually described histologically as benign prostatic hyperplasia or hypertrophy.

Some data suggest that events around the time of puberty and adolescence influence subsequent risks of CaP. Prostatic intraepithelial neoplasia, a putative precancerous lesion, is already present in a substantial proportion of men by the third and fourth decades of life (12). Examining the correlation between hormonal patterns during adolescence and subsequent CaP development is difficult because CaP occurs decades later. However, indirect markers, such as attained height, may provide some insight. Although the available data regarding risk factors early in life are limited, they tend to support the hypothesis that early life events can influence risk of prostate carcinogenesis (see sections Height and Body Mass and Composition below), particularly at times of rapid growth of the prostate. Perhaps prostatic epithelia is most prone to the initial genetic lesions during these growth periods, as attested to by the high prevalence of prostatic intraepithelial neoplasia in young men.

The appearance of clinically relevant CaP and metastatic disease typically requires additional decades. At least some risk factors are probably involved during later periods of life, perhaps even during progression of CaP. Over time, "autonomous" clones that are less likely to be externally influenced develop. It is unknown at what point exogenous factors are no longer influential. Because men diagnosed with CaP are motivated to alter dietary and lifestyle behaviors, the potential role of modifiable risk factors in the post-diagnostic period could be critically important for survival.

HORMONAL MILIEU AND PROSTATE CANCER

Sex steroids and the IGF and vitamin D axes appear to influence the occurrence and progression of CaP. Individual CaP risk may be determined by normal variation in the blood levels of the relevant hormones, or their binding proteins, and by genetic variation in their receptors. Because this variation is influenced both by external factors and by heredity, hormonally related factors are likely to be at a critical interface between many of the nutritional and other environmental factors, and CaP risk and nutritional or genetic interactions are likely to be important. Many of the nutritional and other exogenous factors suspected to influence CaP risk are hypothesized to act through a hormonal mechanism. The roles of androgens, IGFs, and vitamin D in prostate carcinogenesis are discussed in the following sections.

Androgens

The development and progression of prostate tumors depend on androgens, including T and dihydrotestosterone (DHT) (13). The evidence that very low levels of androgens inhibit prostate carcinogenesis is substantial. CaP occurrence may be low among men with liver cirrhosis, which is associated with hyperestrogenicity and hypoandrogenicity (14). Long-term diabetic men, many of whom may have abnormally low levels of T, also appear to be at decreased risk of CaP (15). Androgen inhibition or ablation causes the regression of CaP before attainment of hormone-independent growth (16). Also, human prostate tumors implanted in castrated animals do not grow (17), and prostate tumors developed in rats administered subcutaneously T (18,19).

Whether normal between-person variation in androgen levels influences prostate carcinogenesis is less certain. Studies evaluating the relationship of CaP with plasma levels of steroid hormones and sex hormone–binding globulin (SHBG) have not yielded consistent results (20–36). Many of these studies have serious limitations, including the determination of steroid levels after the diagnosis of CaP, small sample size, failure to account for age differences between the case and comparison groups, and failure to adjust simultaneously for other hormones and SHBG. Measuring and controlling for SHBG levels are particularly critical, because this protein is thought to modulate the bioavailability of steroid hormones. Prospective studies (29–34,36) have found that a higher T to DHT ratio and higher levels of androstanediol glucuronide, a metabolite of DHT often used as an indicator of prostatic production of DHT, are related to increased CaP risk (29,31,33).

The largest and most comprehensive study of this issue to date was a nested case-control evaluation in the Physicians' Health Study (PHS) (33). This study was based on 222 cases and mutually adjusted for each hormone measured and SHBG. CaP cases had an average of more than 6 years elapsed between blood donation and diagnosis. This study showed relative risks (RRs) for CaP of 2.6 for T, 0.46 for SHBG, and 0.56 for estradiol when comparing the top quartile of the distribution of concentrations to the bottom for each hormone. These results indicate that risk of CaP can be influenced within the normal range of androgenicity.

The concept that variation in androgenicity influences CaP risk extends to studies of polymorphisms in androgen-related genes. The most consistent results have been for the androgen receptor (AR), which mediates the effect of T and DHT in androgen-responsive tissues (37). The first exon, which encodes the region of the AR responsible for transactivational control (38), contains a polymorphic region of CAG repeats encoding polyglutamine. The mean repeat number of CAGs has been reported to be approximately 22 in whites and 20 in African-Americans, and the normal range is from approximately 6 to 39 over several racial or ethnic groups (39,40). Shorter length of the CAG repeat linearly correlates with enhanced transcriptional transactivation in experimental gene constructs (38,41), and, clinically, greater CAG repeat lengths are associated with androgen insensitivity (42–44). Epidemiologic studies of AR gene CAG repeat length and CaP have reported moderately increased risks of CaP or advanced CaP when comparing shorter to longer repeat lengths (40,45,46).

Insulinlike Growth Factors

Accumulating evidence supports an important role for the IGF axis in prostate carcinogenesis. The IGF axis is organized into IGFs, IGF-binding proteins (IGFBPs), IGF proteases, and membrane-associated receptors. IGF-1, the major circulating IGF, is required by cells to progress through the cell cycle (47). IGFBPs can oppose actions of IGF-1, in part by binding and sequestering IGF-1, but perhaps also through direct effects mediated by specific IGFBP-3 membrane-associated receptors (48,49). IGFBP-3 is the major circulating IGFBP. IGF-1, several of its binding proteins, and IGF proteases (including PSA) are produced by normal prostate cells and CaP cells, and evidence from *in vitro* studies and animal models supports an important role for IGF-1, IGFBPs, and proteases for cell growth and apoptosis for both normal and neoplastic prostate tissue (50,51).

Several recent studies have linked the IGF axis directly to CaP. The first report of IGF in relation to CaP risk was from a Greek case-control study (52) that compared circulating IGF-1 levels in 52 incident CaP cases to age-matched controls. IGFBPs were not assayed in this study. High levels of IGF-1 were associated with an increased risk of CaP. These results were intriguing, but, because blood samples for cases were collected after the diagnosis of CaP, the potential impact of the tumor on IGF-1 levels could not be excluded. Shortly after this report, results from a prospective study of IGF-1 and IGFBP-3 and CaP risk were published from the PHS. In 1982, 14,916 male U.S. physicians aged 40 to 82 each provided a blood sample, which was then frozen and archived (53). Among 152 cases diagnosed through 1992, IGF-1 was found to be associated with approximately a two-and-a-half–fold increased risk, and when IGF-1 and IGFBP-3 were adjusted for each other, stronger associations emerged. Comparing top to bottom quartiles, IGF-1 was associated with a RR of 4.3 of CaP and IGFBP-3 with a RR of 0.4. Analyses limited to cases diagnosed at least 5 years from the time of blood draw yielded similar results, arguing against the impact of IGF levels by large undiagnosed tumors. Another case-control study from Sweden (54) found that high IGF-1 levels were associated with an increased risk of CaP.

Vitamin D Metabolites

Vitamin D is part of a complex hormonal axis. 1,25-dihydroxyvitamin D [$1,25(OH)_2D$], the most active metabolite of vitamin D, is a steroid hormone that activates gene transcription via binding to the cytoplasmic vitamin D receptor (VDR) (55). Circulating $1,25(OH)_2D$ levels are under tight homeostatic regulation. The prostate epithelium expresses VDRs, and physiologic levels of $1,25(OH)_2D$

bind to the VDR in established CaP cell lines and in primary cultures of human prostatic epithelial cells derived from malignant tissue (56–59). 1,25$(OH)_2$D has been shown to inhibit proliferation and induce differentiation in prostatic epithelial cells (56,60–63). A role of 1,25$(OH)_2$D or its analogs in prostate carcinogenesis is supported by a limited body of animal data (64,65).

Several lines of epidemiologic evidence also suggest that high levels of circulating vitamin D protect against risk of CaP. Supportive data include the evidence that the vitamin D endocrine system regulates prostate growth and differentiation and that black race and residence in northern latitudes, risk factors for CaP, are potentially associated with low circulating levels of vitamin D (66). Men with high circulating prediagnostic 1,25$(OH)_2$D may be at reduced risk of CaP (67). However, a more recent study did not find a strong association between 1,25$(OH)_2$D and CaP risk (68), although the lowest risk of CaP was observed in men with high 1,25$(OH)_2$D and low 25$(OH)_2$D, the parent vitamin D compound.

Further support for a role of the vitamin D axis in CaP comes from studies of the relationship between several VDR gene polymorphisms and CaP risk. These include a poly-A microsatellite in the 3'-untranslated region of the VDR gene, and the following restriction-length polymorphisms: *Bsm*I in intron 8 (denoted *b*); *Apa*I in intron 8 (denoted *a*); and *Taq*I in exon 9, which results in a base, but not amino acid change (denoted *t*). All of these polymorphisms are in strong linkage disequilibrium, but none affects the amino acid–coding sequence of the VDR. However, the *BAt* haplotype is associated with greater VDR transcription or enhanced messenger RNA stability in artificial gene constructs than is the *baT* haplotype, and individuals with the *BB* genotype have higher circulating 1,25$(OH)_2$D levels than do those with *Bb* or *bb* genotypes (69). Evidence for a relationship between these polymorphisms and CaP risk has been inconclusive (70–73), but even the least supportive data (73) have suggested complex interactions between circulating 1,25$(OH)_2$D levels and VDR gene polymorphisms. Further work in identifying physiologically relevant VDR polymorphisms may enhance our understanding of the relationship between the vitamin D axis and CaP.

NONNUTRITIONAL MODIFIABLE RISK FACTORS

Cigarette Smoking

Cigarettes are the leading cause of death from cancer, but the relationship between smoking and CaP mortality is still unclear. Some studies have indicated no connection between tobacco use and CaP (74–78), whereas others suggest an elevated risk among smokers (79–83). In general, because of the inconsistencies, smoking is not likely to be a major contributor to CaP risk.

However, an increased risk of CaP mortality with tobacco use is more consistently observed than with CaP incidence. This paradox could be explained if smokers delay diagnosis and treatment of CaP, which could result in poorer survival. The studies that found smokers to be at higher risk for CaP mortality (84–87) could not distinguish whether this association was caused by delayed diagnosis and treatment among smokers or directly from effects of tobacco. Direct effects of tobacco could be related to carcinogens, which may theoretically induce CaP to develop a more aggressive phenotype by causing mutations in genes associated with tumor progression. Alternatively, tobacco use may alter host factors, such as levels of hormones, which promote tumor growth or progression. Smoking is associated with higher plasma T levels in men (88,89). Two studies (90,91) have found smokers more likely to be diagnosed with CaPs diagnosed at an advanced stage or that have a poor histologic grade.

A recent analysis based on the Health Professionals Follow-Up Study cohort found recent smoking history to be strongly related to the subset of CaPs that are rapidly progressive and highly fatal (92). This association did not appear to result from delayed detection of cancers among smokers. Although differences in diagnosis seeking and treatment between smokers and nonsmokers cannot be entirely ruled out based on available data, the studies suggest that carcinogens in cigarette smoke enhance tumor progression by effects directly on the tumor or on the host. Although the mechanism remains unknown, smokers appear to suffer a higher mortality rate from CaP.

Alcohol Consumption

A plausible link between alcohol intake and CaP risk is suggested by effects of alcohol consumption on various hormone levels. Acute alcohol intake transiently reduces circulating T (93–95), and alcoholic cirrhosis is associated with reduced T levels in men (96). Alcohol also is associated with increases in circulating estrogen concentrations in pre- (97) and postmenopausal (98) women; a similar effect is likely in men (99; A. E. Field, *personal communication*, 1998). Despite the plausible influences of alcohol on CaP, prospective studies generally have not found these to be related (100–105). A case-control study conducted in Sweden found a statistically nonsignificant direct association between CaP risk and total grams of alcohol consumed weekly (106). Another case-control study conducted in the United States supported an association in both African-Americans and whites, and in particular for higher-grade CaP (107). However, other case-control studies have not supported this relationship (75,108,109). A recent review (110) concluded that there is little evidence for a positive or inverse association between CaP and moderate alcohol consumption, but that few studies have examined extremely high alcohol intake, which is most likely to influence hormones. Overall, alcohol consumption is unlikely to be a major determinant of CaP risk, at least below levels sufficient to induce cirrhosis.

Vasectomy

Vasectomy, used in many parts of the world for contraception, has had few documented acute or long-term adverse health effects associated with it (111–113). However, in the past decade, some studies have suggested a link between vasectomy and increased CaP risk (80,114–121). This relation is controversial, because almost an equal number of studies have found no association (122–127). Detection bias resulting from heightened detection among men who have had a vasectomy or, less likely, confounding by uncontrolled factors, has not been excluded as a possible explanation for the positive results (128,129). Moreover, the biologic basis underlying any vasectomy-CaP relation remains speculative. Elevations in antispermatozoa antibodies, decreased seminal vesicle hormone concentrations, and decreased prostatic secretions have been reported in men who underwent vasectomy and in animal models (117), but how these changes could influence prostate carcinogenesis remains unknown. Future studies should examine whether more consistent associations are observed in specific subgroups of men who have had a vasectomy. For example, one study found that an increased risk of CaP was limited to men who had their vasectomies at a relatively early age (younger than age 35) (116). Consistent patterns in subgroups, however, have not emerged.

Diabetes Mellitus

Several prospective studies have examined the relationship between type II diabetes mellitus and risk of CaP and have found an approximately 30% to 70% reduction in CaP risk among diabetic men (15,130,131). However, no clear evidence of an inverse association could be detected in another prospective study (86) or in two case-control studies (132,133). Men with severe type II diabetes have lower androgen levels, probably resulting from a toxic effect of hyperglycemia on the T-producing Leydig cells of the testis (134). The hypoandrogenism induced by chronic hyperglycemia may underlie the relationship between diabetes and CaP. Consistent with this notion, hyperglycemia tends to increase over time, and the risk of CaP appears to decrease with increasing time since the diagnosis of diabetes (15).

Sexual and Reproductive Factors

Sexual activity and reproductive history plausibly may be related to CaP through a variety of mechanisms, some causal and some indirect. Sexual hyperactivity may theoretically be secondary to higher androgenicity or may enhance exposure to sexually transmitted agents. Age at first sexual activity is likely correlated with younger age of puberty. At older ages, shortly before a diagnosis of CaP, undiagnosed CaPs may impact sexual function. These complexities may explain why the literature on sexual activity and CaP risk is inconsistent, with some studies suggesting higher activity as protective, whereas some indicate indices of sexual activity as risk factors (135). Most data are based on retrospective assessments of sexual history in CaP cases and controls. Biased reporting may add to the inconsistencies, particularly because sexual activity in CaP cases is likely to have changed from the disease and may influence reporting of past activity. Future study in this area should emphasize prospective assessments of self-reported sexual history.

Other Potential Modifiable Risk Factors

There are scattered reports of additional nondietary, potentially modifiable risk factors for CaP. Occupationally related exposures have received some study, but the data have not generated firm associations. Areas that have received the most attention to date have been farming-related exposures to pesticides and herbicides, rubber manufacturing, and occupational exposure to cadmium (136). Each of these areas has yielded some suggestive findings, but the data are far from conclusive. Although it may be prudent to prevent excessive exposures to these factors, they could account for only a small fraction of CaP, even if they are true risk factors. A recent study has indicated that nonsteroidal-antiinflammatory drugs may reduce the risk of advanced CaP (137). Such a potentially important finding requires confirmation in other studies.

DIET AND NUTRITION

The substantial variability in CaP incidence and mortality rates around the world is believed by many to result from specific dietary and nutritional patterns (1). CaP rates are lowest in Asia and highest in Western Europe, Australia, and North America. These regions differ in dietary patterns, overall nutritional status, and other lifestyle factors. National *per capita* consumption of various nutritional variables correlates strongly with national CaP mortality rates (7). A correlation with milk and dairy product consumption with CaP mortality is particularly strong (Fig. 8-1). Although the importance of nutrition is generally accepted, the specific dietary factors involved remain unclear. Total fat, saturated fat, and animal fat are hypothesized to be among the most consistently observed risk factors, but these may actually be correlates of the real dietary factors involved in prostate carcinogenesis.

Studies comparing national *per capita* consumption and cancer rates are limited by lack of individual, specific exposure data and by the inability to sufficiently control for potential confounding factors. Case-control and prospective cohort studies have provided the most important data on diet and CaP risk and are emphasized here. This section first considers the influence of total energy intake and energy balance. Then, specific hypotheses regarding saturated and unsaturated fats are considered, followed by a discussion of nonlipid components in dairy products. Finally, the potential preventive role of some micronutrients and phytochemicals is considered. Although numerous potentially protective agents have been hypothesized, this section emphasizes those compounds for which the human data, from epidemiologic studies or intervention trials, are the strongest.

Total Energy Intake and Energy Balance

Energy balance is a critical factor for cancer development, including CaP, in numerous animal models. In rodent models of transplantable prostate tumors (androgen-sensitive Dunning R3337-H adenocarcinoma), in which energy balance can be carefully controlled, a 20% to 30% energy restriction reduces tumor size (138). The tumors in the energy-restricted rats exhibit increased stroma, more homogenous and smaller glands, and reduced angiogenesis. Importantly, these changes do not differ whether the restriction is induced by lipid or carbohydrate restriction.

Unlike animal models, for which energy intake can be closely controlled, the examination of total energy intake as a risk factor for CaP in free-living human populations is fraught with difficulties. Energy balance in adults is achieved when total energy intake equals energy expenditure and there is no net weight loss or gain. The determinants of total energy expenditure are body size, particularly lean body mass, which has a greater energy requirement than adipose tissue, physical activity, and overall "metabolic efficiency." Because each of these variables is measured with some degree of error, it is not feasible to directly calculate energy balance in epidemiologic studies. However, weight change over a specific time provides an estimate of energy balance over that period. For example, an individual who has gained substantial weight over some time period is in positive energy balance, at least on average, over that time span. Body mass index (BMI) or a measure of adiposity can provide an estimate of cumulative lifetime energy balance. Metabolic efficiency, which is related to a complex interplay of multiple factors, may be related to CaP risk (139–141).

Height

Attained height reflects factors that determine growth during adolescence, including marked changes in circulating concentrations of steroid hormones, growth hormone, and IGF-1. During puberty, the prostate gland, which is responsive to the changing balance of these factors, develops and enlarges. Possibly acting as a marker for hormonal and growth factor levels, height is positively associated with risk of CaP in some populations (76,104,106,142–146) but not all (75,105,108,147–151). Height may not be a consistent risk factor in all populations, because the relative importance of nutritional and genetic factors may vary across populations.

Because tallness is a risk factor for CaP in many studies, higher energy intake is likely to be a risk factor for CaP, owing to the fact that taller men have greater lean body mass on average and, hence, greater energy requirements. The public health relevance of energy intake is dubious, because much of the variation in energy requirement is not modifiable. For example, taller men with more lean body mass would have a higher energy requirement and could not feasibly lower their energy intake to the level of men with a less lean body mass.

Body Mass and Body Composition

In men, obesity is associated with higher plasma estrogen and lower T levels (88,89,152–155), a balance of steroid hormones possibly related to lower CaP risk (33). In most epidemiologic studies, BMI is used as an indicator of obesity. BMI is defined as weight in kilograms divided by the square of height in meters. Although BMI serves as a useful indicator for adiposity, it is additionally a correlate of lean body mass, including the muscle compartment (156). This characteristic of BMI complicates studies of CaP, as endocrinologic factors, such as IGFs and sex hormones that may underlie CaP risk, also may be related to adiposity and lean body mass. Perhaps because of these complexities, studies that have examined BMI in relation to CaP have been inconsistent. BMI has not been related to CaP risk in case-control studies (75,106,108,109,147,151,157–159), with one exception (149). In prospective studies, some have found a positive relation with BMI or body weight (105,150,160–163), but as many others have not (100,104,144,148,164,165). One prospective study (166) that found a positive association between BMI and CaP showed that the elevated CaP risk was probably due to muscle, rather than fat, mass. Also, a positive association observed between BMI and fatal CaP in a large Swedish retrospective, cohort study of construction workers might possibly reflect the higher average muscle mass in construction workers (143). Measures of obesity based on waist and hip circumference measures in one study (144) were related to a slightly lower risk of advanced CaP.

The prostate gland undergoes maturation during puberty. The role of obesity during earlier life has not been extensively examined. No association between CaP and weight at puberty in comparison to classmates or weight and BMI at age 20 was observed in a Swedish case-control study (142). Conversely, in a large cohort study, higher BMI at age 21 was strongly associated with a lower risk of advanced CaP (144). In that same cohort, measures of adiposity based on body shape pictograms indicated that obesity at ages 10 to 20 years strongly predicted lower risk of advanced CaP in adulthood. The finding that tallness was a positive risk factor in the same cohort appears paradoxic in that both taller height and higher BMI would seem to relate to higher energy intake. The explanation may be that taller height signifies high energy intake complementary to a hormonal milieu related to linear growth (e.g., high IGF-1, growth hormone, androgen levels), whereas obesity in adolescence, and presumably less muscle mass, signifies low levels of androgens and growth-stimulating hormones. Although further study relying on more direct measures of lean body mass and adiposity is required, the emerging picture appears to be that adiposity may be associated with decreased risk and lean body mass with elevated risk.

Physical Activity

Relatively few studies have examined the impact of physical activity on CaP risk, and results have been mixed. Most studies have found a slight or moderate inverse relation between risk of CaP and occupational or leisure-time physical activity (109,150,167–171) or cardiorespiratory fitness (172). However, others have found no association (108,173) or, in one case, an increased risk among the most physically active (105). Most of these studies have focused on activity level in adulthood within a relatively short time period before diagnosis. However, a few have examined physical activity earlier in life. Three studies found direct positive associations between physical activity in young adulthood and subsequent risk for CaP (164,174,175), one showed an inverse association for physical activity during puberty (142), and one found an association with physical activity during youth, as well as during middle and older ages (108).

Several recent large prospective cohort studies, the Harvard Alumni cohort and the Health Professionals' Follow-Up Study, have found no overall association between physical activity and CaP risk (176,177). However, more detailed analyses revealed an interesting pattern in both studies. In the Harvard Alumni cohort (176), a lower risk among older men who had extremely high energy expenditures was observed. This pattern was essentially replicated in the Health Professionals' Follow-Up Study (177), except that this inverse association was limited to metastatic CaP. Part of this difference could be related to the fact that the Harvard Alumni Study was conducted before widespread PSA screening; thus, the CaPs diagnosed tended to be more aggressive than those diagnosed in the Health Professionals' Follow-Up Study, in which a clear relationship was only with metastatic cancer. In contrast to an inverse association with CaP suggested only with very high activity levels, both cohorts demonstrated that moderate activity levels are associated with a lower risk of colon cancer, as well as other conditions. Perhaps relevant to the CaP findings, reductions in serum T have only been observed with very high levels of physical training but not in men participating in recreational exercise (178,179).

Overall, these results suggest that exercise in adulthood is unlikely to either increase or lower risk appreciably, except perhaps for a benefit at very high levels of activity. The level of activity required for a benefit, as observed in recent cohort studies, may be too high for everyone to adopt. The tendency for studies to demonstrate a positive association between exercise earlier in life and subsequent risk of CaP is worrisome but hardly conclusive. It is possible that higher activity levels during adolescence may be secondary to other factors (greater muscle mass or higher androgen levels), and, thus, the association, if confirmed, may not be causal in nature.

Animal and Saturated Fat

International *per capita* fat consumption correlates with international CaP incidence and mortality rates (7). Animal sources of fat, primarily from red meat and dairy sources, appear most strongly related to risk based on this indirect measurement. Animal fat and saturated fat intake derived from diet histories of samples of men representing five ethnic groups residing in Hawaii correlates highly (r = 0.9) with CaP incidence rates in these five groups (180). Tables 8-1 and 8-2 summarize the extensive data available on the relationship between dietary fat, meats, and dairy products and risk of CaP from epidemiologic case-control and cohort studies. In general, a positive association between CaP and intake of dietary fat, higher-fat foods, meat, and dairy foods has been observed in most (75,108,149,157–159,181–186), but not all, (76,132,187–190) case-control studies (Table 8-1). These studies have been conducted in diverse populations, and the results have often been adjusted for potential confounding factors. In a multiethnic case-control study, positive associations between saturated fat and CaP risk, particularly for advanced cancers, have been observed separately for African-Americans, whites, Chinese-Americans, and Japanese-Americans (108). Most of these studies examined diet as recalled relatively recently before the diagnosis in cases. In a Swedish case-control study, no association was found between total dietary fat or specific fatty foods consumed during adolescence (142). However, it is unclear how well adolescent diet was recalled by middle-aged and elderly men.

Prospective cohort studies are generally less prone to recall bias than case-control studies (Table 8-2). Findings for dietary fat and CaP from early prospective cohort studies did not support the hypothesis that high intake of saturated fat increases risk of CaP (101,173). However, these studies tended to use relatively crude dietary assessment instruments, and the span between diet assessment and diagnosis may have been too long if diets changed substantially over time. These factors would tend to attenuate any

TABLE 8-1. SUMMARY OF CASE-CONTROL STUDIES OF INTAKE OF FATTY ANIMAL FOODS AND PROSTATE CANCER RISK

Reference	Year	Location(s)	Cases (no.)	Findings: Fat intake	Findings: Dairy intake	Findings: Meat intake
Rotkin et al. (253)	1977	Illinois, California	111	—	Cases ate more cheese (p = .09), margarine (p = .04), butter (p = .09), and milk (NS)	Cases ate more beef and pork (NS)
Schuman et al. (183)	1982	Minnesota	223	—	Cases ate more ice cream (NS)	No association with meat
Graham et al. (254)	1983	New York	262	Animal fat (RR, 3.0; p <.01) Total fat (RR, 2.0; p <.05)	—	Meats and fish (RR, 2.2; p <.05) (only significant for men >70 yr)
Heshmat et al. (184)	1985	Washington, DC	180	Positive association with total fat (p = .9), saturated fat (p = .08), and monounsaturated fat (p = .09) for consumption at ages 30–49, no association with consumption at >50 yr	—	—
Talamini et al. (255)	1986	Italy	166	—	Milk or dairy (RR, 2.5; p = .05)	Meat (RR,1.7; p = .05)
Ross et al. (75)	1987	California	142 black, 142 white	Black: total fat (RR,1.9; p <.05) White: total fat (RR, 1.6; NS)	—	Black: pork (RR, 2.3; p <.05) White: pork (RR,1.3; NS)
Ohno et al. (256)	1988	Japan	100	Fat intake (RR, 0.8; NS)	—	—
Kolonel et al. (157)	1988	Hawaii	452	Among men ≥70 yr: total fat (RR, 1.5; NS), saturated fat (RR, 1.7; p = .05), cholesterol (RR,1.6; p = .05)	—	—
Mettlin et al. (257)	1989	New York	371	Animal fat (RR, 1.3; NS)	Whole milk (RR, 2.5; p <.05)	—
Kaul et al. (189)	1987	Washington, DC	55	No association with total fat or saturated fat	—	—
West et al. (258)	1991	Utah	358	Risk for aggressive tumors among men >67 yr of age, total fat (RR, 2.9), saturated fat (RR, 2.2; NS), monounsaturated fat (RR,1.7), and cholesterol (RR, 1.5; NS)	—	—
LaVecchia et al. (194)	1991	Italy	96	No association with fat	Milk (RR,5.0; p <.05)	No association with meat
Talamini et al. (182)	1992	Italy	271	No association with oils	Milk (RR,1.6; p <.03); no association with cheese or butter; among ≥70 yr: milk (RR, 1.9; p = .03) and butter (RR, 1.7; p = .14)	Meat (RR, 1.4; p = .07)
Whittemore et al. (108)	1995	United States	1655	Positive association with total and saturated fat for advanced cancers in African-Americans, whites, Chinese-Americans, and Japanese-Americans	Saturated fat from dairy-positive association	Saturated fat from meat-positive association

(*continued*)

TABLE 8-1. (*continued*)

Reference	Year	Location(s)	Cases (no.)	Findings		
				Fat intake	Dairy intake	Meat intake
Ewings and Bowie (185)	1996	Great Britain	159	—	No association with milk consumption	Positive association with meat consumption (RR, 2.67; p = .005)
Andersson et al. (259)	1996	Sweden	526 total	No association with fat independent of total energy	Dairy Total: (RR, 1.49; p <.05)	Meat Total: (RR, 1.39; p = .06)
Chan et al. (260)	1998	—	296 advanced	—	(RR, 1.64; p <.05)	(RR, 1.60; p <.05)
Key et al. (235)	1997	Great Britain	328	No association with total fat, saturated or monounsaturated fat	—	No association with meat of any type, or roasted or grilled meat
Tzonou (236)	1999	Greece	320	—	Nonsignificant positive association with milk and dairy products (RR, 1.59; p = .1)	No association with meats, fish, and eggs
Hayes et al. (186)	1999	United States	449 black, 483 white	Positive association for total fat and animal fat for blacks and whites	Significantly positive risk factor for whites, but not blacks	Significantly positive risk factor for blacks, but not whites
Walker et al. (190)	1992	South Africa	166	Positive association with fat (RR, 2.6; p <.01)	—	Positive association with meat (RR, 2.0; p <.05)

NS, association not statistically significant; RR, relative risk.

associations. In two cohort studies of Seventh-Day Adventists (100,161), men with relatively high consumption of animal products had a greater CaP risk. Two cohort studies, in which diet was assessed at most 5 years before diagnosis, found that men with higher consumption of red meat, total animal fat, and fatty animal foods had double the risk of CaP (104,191). In a cohort of relatively young Norwegians (163), no association was observed for overall fat consumption, but a positive relation with CaP for consumption of certain high-fat meats (e.g., hamburger and meatballs) was seen.

In some studies, associations with fat were stronger for advanced CaP than for total CaP occurrence (108,159,161,191). These findings suggest that dietary fat influences late stages of carcinogenesis or that fat primarily or solely influences lesions that have the capacity to progress.

Dairy Products and Calcium

National *per capita* milk consumption correlates highly with national CaP mortality rates (Fig. 8-1). In fact, the magnitude of the correlation between CaP mortality and milk (r = 0.69) is greater than it is for other foods high in animal fat (e.g., meats, r = 0.39) (192,193). Relative to nondrinkers, or men who rarely drink milk, men consuming substantial milk, as well as other dairy products, are at increased risk for CaP in case-control (149,181–183,188,194,195) and prospective cohort (104,161,196) studies (Tables 8-1 and 8-2). The results based on inter- and intranational studies, as well as case-control and cohort studies, indicate that milk and dairy products increase CaP occurrence or progression. Although this association may be related to the fat content of these products, in some cases skim or low-fat milk appears to be a risk factor (185,196,197), suggesting that milk imparts an excess risk beyond that of fat alone.

A positive association between calcium intake and CaP risk has been postulated (196). This relation may be indirectly inferred by the observed association with skim or low-fat milk and dairy consumption, the primary sources of calcium in most countries. A U.S. prospective cohort study (196) and a Swedish case-control study (195) found a positive association between calcium intake and CaP risk. In the cohort study (196), both dietary and supplemental sources of calcium were independently associated with increased CaP risk. The association between calcium supplements and enhanced CaP risk suggests that the calcium component of dairy foods, rather than some other aspect, confers elevated risk. When examining extreme contrasts in

TABLE 8-2. SUMMARY OF COHORT STUDIES OF DIETARY FAT ANIMAL FOODS AND PROSTATE CANCER

				Findings		
Reference	Year	Location(s)	Cases (no.)	Fat intake	Dairy intake	Meat intake
Hirayama et al. (261)	1979	Japan	63 (fatal)	—	—	No association with meat intake
Snowdon et al. (161)	1984	California	99 (fatal)	—	Positive associations with milk (RR, 1.4) and cheese (RR, 1.4) (both NS in multivariate analysis)	Positive association with meat (RR, 1.3; NS in multivariate analysis)
Mills et al. (100)	1989	California	180	—	No association with milk (RR, 0.8)	Positive association with meat, poultry, fish (RR, 1.4; NS)
Severson et al. (173)	1989	Hawaii	174	No association with total fat (RR, 0.9), or saturated fat (RR, 1)	Positive association with butter, margarine, or cheese (RR, 1.5; $p = .05$); no association with milk (RR, 1)	No association with meat (RR, 1)
Hsing et al. (84)	1990	Upper Midwestern and Northeastern United States	149 (fatal)	—	No association with dairy products (RR, 1)	No association with meat (RR, 0.8)
Giovannucci et al. (262)	1993	United States	300 126 advanced	Association with total fat (RR, 1.8; $p = .06$) and animal fat (RR, 1.6; $p = .08$), for advanced cancers only (independent of energy)	—	Association with red meat (RR, 2.6; $p = .02$) for advanced cancers only
Gann et al. (263)	1994	United States	120	—	—	Positive association with red meat (RR, 2.5; $p = .07$)
Le Marchand et al. (104)	1994	Hawaii	198	Positive association with high-fat animal products (RR, 1.6; $p = .05$)	Positive association with milk (RR, 1.4; $p = .05$)	Positive association with beef (RR, 1.6; $p < .05$)
Veierod et al. (163)	1997	Norway	72	No association with total, saturated, or monounsaturated fat	No association with total milk and higher risk with skim relative to whole milk (RR, 2.2; $p < .01$)	Inverse association with meat as a main meal (RR, 0.4; $p = .04$); positive association with main meals with hamburgers, meatballs, and others (RR, 3.1; $p = .02$)
Giovannucci et al. (196)	1998	United States	423 advanced 201 metastatic	—	Positive association with milk Advanced: (RR, 1.6; $p = .002$) Metastatic: (RR, 1.8, $p = .01$)	—

NS, association not statistically significant; RR, relative risk.

risk, achievable because of the high calcium content in supplements, four- to fivefold risk elevations for metastatic CaP were observed between the extreme high (greater than 2,000 mg per day) and low (less than 500 mg per day) intakes of calcium.

Western Dietary Pattern, Hormones, and Prostate Cancer

Evidence suggests that certain endocrinologic patterns are related to risk of CaP, owing to enhanced cell proliferation and angiogenesis and reduced cellular differentiation and apoptosis. Specifically, high levels of T and IGF-1, and low levels of SHBG, IGFBP-3, and 1,25$(OH)_2$D are associated with an increased risk of CaP incidence or progression. Many features of the Western diet and lifestyle appear to yield this "high-risk" hormonal milieu. These relationships, which may affect the progression of CaP at various stages throughout the life cycle, are summarized in Figure 8-2. This dietary pattern consists of high consumption of red meat, dairy products, animal fat, and protein, and is energy dense. Also, diets high in dairy products tend to be high in bioavailable calcium, as calcium from milk is approximately three to four times more bioavailable than is calcium from plant-based foods.

Severe restriction of energy or protein intake lowers IGF-1 levels (198–200). In rodents, IGF-1 appears to mediate some of the anticancer effects of energy restriction (138,201,202). In a cross-sectional study (203), men who consumed less fat had lower plasma T levels. Similar findings were observed in studies in which dietary fat intake was reduced (204,205). However, not all studies have found a relation between fat intake and T levels (89). The intervention studies have not been controlled carefully for total energy intake, however, so it is quite possible that this effect on T levels was primarily related to reduced energy intake.

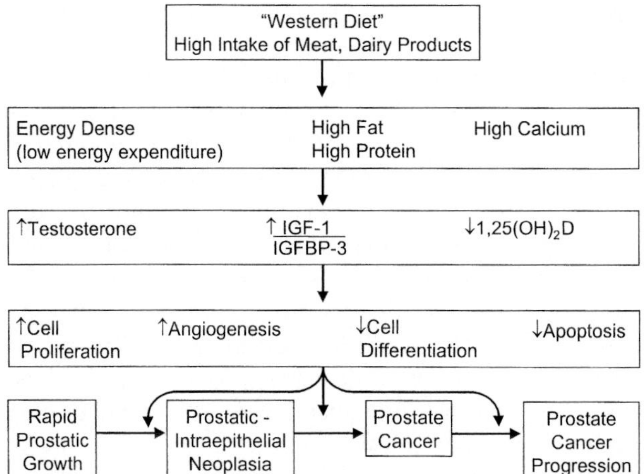

FIGURE 8-2. Summary of the proposed relationships among Western dietary factors, hormonal milieu, cell dynamics, and different stages of prostate carcinogenesis. ↑, increased; ↓, decreased; 1,25$(OH)_2$D, 1,25-dihydroxyvitamin D; IGF-1, insulin-like growth factor 1; IGFBP-3, IGF-binding protein 3.

Important questions about these relationships remain. First, it is unclear whether responses related to relatively short-term adaptations of weeks or months to changes in energy balance, as done in intervention studies, are relevant for nutritional effects for carcinogenesis that can occur over a period of decades. Moreover, the degree of energy restriction required to produce a benefit, as well as the etiologically relevant time period, adolescence or adulthood, or both, is unknown. For example, the endocrinologic effects of energy and protein restriction severe enough to cause growth retardation during adolescence when the prostate gland is growing most rapidly may be sufficient to reduce CaP incidence. However, whether moderate nutritional alterations later in adulthood can impact CaP risk through hormonal mechanisms remains unanswered.

A mechanism underlying the association between milk and calcium intake and CaP is not established, but a plausible mechanism related to vitamin D metabolism has been suggested (196,206). As discussed earlier, 1,25$(OH)_2$D, which is involved in augmenting absorption of calcium, also plays a role in the control of proliferation and differentiation of prostatic epithelial cells. Higher-circulating levels of calcium down-regulate production of 1,25$(OH)_2$D, and, thus, ingestion of higher amounts of calcium suppresses 1,25$(OH)_2$D levels. Milk and dairy products, and calcium supplements are likely to be a dominant factor influencing 1,25$(OH)_2$D levels because of their high concentration of bioavailable calcium. The impact of calcium intake on 1,25$(OH)_2$D levels appears to be substantial enough to influence CaP, although this mechanism remains speculative at this point (196,206).

Unsaturated Fat

An effect of fat may also be related to fatty acid content. Specific fatty acids may induce changes in ligand receptor–binding or modulate receptor activity because of altered cell membrane fatty acid constituents, or may change prostaglandin production (207). Few studies have examined intake of specific fatty acids in relation to CaP. For example, because linoleic acid appears to have a tumor-promoting effect in animal studies, it is important to examine this fatty acid in epidemiologic studies. A recent metaanalysis found that when comparing high to low intake of linoleic acid, the combined RR for CaP was 1.27 [95% confidence interval (CI), 0.97 to 1.66] from case-control studies and 0.83 (95% CI, 0.56 to 1.24) for prospective studies (208). The apparent differences between the animal and human studies may be that a minimum amount of linoleic acid is required to promote tumor growth, but above this threshold, linoleic acid may not be a tumor promoter.

α-Linolenic acid, an omega-3 polyunsaturated fatty acid found in red meat and butter as well as some vegetables, is associated with an increased risk of advanced CaP (191). Prediagnostic blood levels of α-linolenic acid were positively associated with CaP in case-control studies nested within a cohort (207,209). α-Linolenic acid is incorporated into cell membrane phospholipids in which it may influence cell membrane fluidity. Because of its high degree of unsaturation, this fatty acid is quite prone to oxidative attack. Although mechanisms for a role of α-linolenic acid in CaP development remain speculative, the relative consistency of the epidemiologic studies indicates that the impact of this fatty acid on prostate epithelial function should be further studied. Long-chain omega-3 fatty acids, primarily from fish oils, have been hypothesized to lower risk of cancer, including CaP, but human data are quite sparse.

Soy-Based Food Products

One of the major differences between the typical "Asian" and "Western" diets is that soy foods are an important dietary component in many Asian populations but are rarely consumed in the West. Because Asian men tend to be at lower risk for CaP, putative beneficial effects of soy products have been hypothesized. Some *in vitro* work indicates that isoflavones found in high concentrations in soy products, particularly genistein and daidzein, may lower CaP risk. These isoflavones have been shown to inhibit the growth of both androgen-dependent and -independent CaP cell lines. Although the *in vitro* work is promising, data from epidemiologic studies and human intervention trials are very sparse. More research into the role of soy products in human studies is warranted. Even if specific benefits from soy products are not confirmed, increased intake of soy protein as a replacement for meat and dairy sources of protein could still be an important component of a "low-risk" CaP diet, as animal sources of protein have been consistently related to higher risk of CaP.

Retinol and β-Carotene

Several lines of evidence suggest a role for vitamin A or retinol in prostate carcinogenesis. Vitamin A is critical in maintaining normal proliferation and differentiation in many types of cells (210), and retinoids inhibit cancer, including CaP (211), in some animal models (210). However, retinoids have been known to stimulate carcinogenesis in some experimental systems (212,213). Epidemiologic studies have examined intakes and circulating levels for retinol and β-carotene, the major precursor for vitamin A, in relation to risk of CaP. One prospective study showed an inverse association of CaP with retinol intake (101), whereas another prospective study (214) and a case-control study (75) found no consistent association. Circulating retinol levels are tightly regulated and, thus, are not substantially influenced by the normal range of dietary retinol intake. Some epidemiologic studies have found positive associations for retinol intake and CaP risk among older men (158,159,182,214,215). Higher prediagnostic serum vitamin A levels were related to a lower CaP risk in two studies (216,217) but not in others (218,219). In a recent study of U.S. physicians (220), higher prediagnostic retinol levels were related to an elevated risk of CaP, but this finding was limited to nonaggressive CaP.

Two potential anticarcinogenic roles for β-carotene are control of cell growth via conversion into vitamin A and its properties as an antioxidant (221). Some studies show an inverse relationship for intake of β-carotene and CaP (75,183,187,188), although the prospective Health Professionals' Follow-Up Study (214), the Western Electric Study (222), and a randomized intervention trial with a β-carotene arm (223) showed no association. Unlike the Western Electric Study, in which there was a 30-year span between diet assessment and end of follow-up, the null findings in the other two studies, in which the span was less than 10 years, are unlikely to be due to misclassification from changing dietary practices. Serum β-carotene was not associated with CaP in three nested case-control studies (217–219).

Fruits, Vegetables, Tomato Products, and Lycopene

For many cancers, fruits and vegetables appear to confer protection. However, most existing data do not strongly support an important role of fruits and vegetables in reducing CaP risk overall. However, a recent analysis indicated that fructose (fruit sugar), both from fruit directly or as a sweetener, was related to a lower risk of CaP (196). Most other studies have not indicated a benefit of fruits, but these have not examined fructose specifically.

Although overall fruit and vegetable consumption does not appear to be protective, relatively high intakes of one or a few rich sources of specific phytochemicals may have a role. The group of phytochemicals that has received most study is the carotenoids, a group of at least 600 compounds, although only approximately 14 are found in appreciable levels in human tissues. The most common carotenoids in the human diet are β-carotene, α-carotene, lycopene, lutein, and β-cryptoxanthin. In biologic systems, carotenoids react with free radicals and singlet oxygen (224), generated by normal cellular respiration and possibly by exogenous sources, such as cigarette smoking. Antioxidants limit oxidative damage to the cell membrane lipid bilayer and to DNA. Cells have complex, multifaceted systems to limit oxidative damage; it is possible, but not proven, that dietary antioxidants such as carotenoids complement these imperfect systems.

In recent years, focus on lycopene has increased. Lycopene, a carotenoid found primarily in tomatoes, is the most efficient carotenoid in quenching singlet oxygen species (225), and is likely an effective radical scavenger *in vivo* (226). It inhibits proliferation of cancer cells *in vitro* (227),

TABLE 8-3. SUMMARY OF EPIDEMIOLOGIC STUDIES EXAMINING TOMATO INTAKE OR LYCOPENE INTAKE, OR LEVEL AND PROSTATE CANCER RISK

Reference	Year	Location	Years of study	No. of cases	Exposure	Relative risk (RR)[a] (95% CI)
			Diet-based case-control			
Schuman et al. (183)	1982	Minnesota	1976–1979	223	Tomato intake high vs. low	0.70 NS
Le Marchand et al. (234)	1991	Hawaii	1970–1983	452	Lycopene intake quartile 4 vs. 1	0.9 (p = .35, <70 yr) 1.1 (p = .57, ≥70 yr)
Key et al. (235)	1997	United Kingdom	1989–1992	328	Dietary lycopene ≥718 µg vs. <402 µg	0.99 (0.68–1.45) (p = .88)
					Raw tomatoes ≥5/wk vs. ≤3/mo	1.06 (0.55–1.62) (p = .88)
					Cooked tomatoes ≥2/wk vs. <1/mo	0.92 (0.57–1.42) (p = .64)
					Baked beans[b] ≥2/wk vs. <1/mo	0.52 (0.31–0.88) [p(trend) = .075]
Tzonou et al. (236)	1999	Athens, Greece	1994–1997	320	Raw tomatoes 16/mo vs. 8/mo	Inverse [p(trend) = .12[c]]
					Cooked tomatoes 16/mo vs. 8/mo	0.85 (0.75–0.97) [p(trend) = .005]
			Diet-based cohort			
Mills et al. (100)	1989	California Seventh Day Adventists	1974–1982	180	Tomato intake ≥5/wk vs. <1/wk	0.60 (0.37–0.97) (p = .02)
Giovannucci et al. (214)	1995	United States	1986–1992	773	Dietary tomato-based products >10 vs. <1.5 servings/wk	0.65 (0.44–0.95) (p = .01)
					Tomato sauce 2–4 vs. 0 servings/wk	0.66 (0.49–0.90) (p = .001)
Baldwin et al. (abstract) (238)	1996	California	1995	—	Consistent high tomato consumption	0.59 (p = .03)
Cerhan et al. (abstract) (237)	1998	United States	1987–1990	101	Dietary tomatoes quintile 5 vs. 1	0.50 (0.3–0.9) (p = .03)
			Blood-based cohort			
Hsing et al. (217)	1990	Maryland	1974–1985	103	Serum lycopene quartile 4 vs. 1	0.50 (0.20–1.29) (p = .26)
Nomura et al. (239)	1997	Hawaii	1971–1993	142	Serum lycopene quartile 4 vs. 1	1.1 (0.5–2.2) (p = .86)
Gann et al. (220)	1999	United States	1982–1995	581	Plasma lycopene quintile 5 vs. 1	0.56 (0.34–0.91) (p = .05)

[a]Relative risk and 95% confidence interval (CI) or p-value for exposure comparison indicated; in some cases, measures other than the relative risk were given.
[b]Source of highly bioavailable lycopene.
[c]Relative risk not given.

including CaP cell lines induced by stimulation with DHT (228), and *in vivo* (229). In a recent human trial, dietary lycopene provided by tomato juice, spaghetti sauce, and tomato oleoresin resulted in a significant reduction of thiobarbituric acid–reactive substances, which is a measure of lipid oxidation (230). Lycopene is the most abundant carotenoid in plasma (231,232) and in prostate tissue, accounting for 30% of all carotenoids on average (233).

Epidemiologic studies that have evaluated tomato or lycopene intake or level in relation to CaP risk are summarized in Table 8-3. A case-control study conducted in Minnesota (183) found an inverse association between tomato intake and CaP risk, although the study was relatively small and the result was not statistically significant. Another case-control study, conducted in a multiethnic population in Hawaii (234), found no association between consumption of tomatoes and CaP risk. However, the actual intake levels were not reported, and it did not appear that tomato-based products, such as tomato sauce, were specifically considered in this study. A case-control study conducted in the United

Kingdom (235) found no association between raw or cooked tomatoes and risk of CaP. However, the strongest diet-CaP association found was for baked beans (RR, 0.52; 95% CI, 0.31 to 0.88). Tinned baked beans, usually stored in tomato sauce, are a rich source of lycopene. A case-control study conducted in Athens found a slight inverse association between raw tomato consumption and CaP risk (p = .12), and a stronger inverse association with cooked tomatoes (p = .005) (236).

Four prospective dietary studies (100,214,237,238) have reported on the relationship between tomato or lycopene consumption and CaP risk (Table 8-3). In a cohort of 14,000 Seventh-Day Adventist men (100), higher consumption of tomatoes was statistically significantly related to lower risk of CaP. The results remained statistically significant in a multivariate analysis controlling for other food items. The only other food groups related to a lower CaP risk were beans, lentils, and peas. β-Carotene–rich foods were unrelated to risk. In a larger study, the Health Professionals' Follow-Up Study, which had a more comprehensive dietary questionnaire (214), the intake of the carotenoids β-carotene, α-carotene, lutein, and β-cryptoxanthin was not associated with risk of CaP, but high intake of lycopene was related to a statistically significant 21% reduction in risk. Also, high intake of tomatoes and tomato products, which accounted for 82% of lycopene, was associated with a 35% lower risk of CaP and a 53% lower risk of advanced CaP. Tomato sauce had the strongest inverse association with CaP risk [RR, 0.66; 95% CI, 0.49 to 0.90 for two or more servings per week compared to none; p (trend) = .001], and weaker inverse associations were observed with tomatoes and pizza, but not with tomato juice. Of note, the degree of reduction of CaP risk by the tomato-related products (tomato sauce, substantial reduction; tomatoes and pizza, moderate reduction; and tomato juice, no reduction) corresponded with the degree that intake of these items correlated with plasma lycopene levels in a sample of men. Preliminary results from two other cohort studies (237,238) also support an inverse association between tomato or lycopene intake and CaP risk.

Three studies (217,220,239) have reported on the risk between prediagnostic serum carotenoids and risk of CaP. The first report, a study by Hsing et al. (217), was based on serum obtained in 1974 from 25,802 persons in Washington County, Maryland. This study found a 6.2% lower median serum lycopene level in men with CaP diagnosed during a 13-year period compared to age- and race-matched controls. The RR was 0.5 (95% CI, 0.20 to 1.29) between high and low quartiles of lycopene. No other carotenoid was associated with CaP risk in this study. Recent results from the PHS (220) based on 259 cases of aggressive CaP (extraprostatic or Gleason grade greater than or equal to 7 or poorly differentiated) found a statistically significant RR of 0.56 [95% CI, 0.34 to 0.92; p (trend) = .05] when comparing high to low quintiles of plasma lycopene.

A study of prediagnostic levels of serum carotenoids and CaP risk was conducted between 1971 and 1993 in a Japanese-American population in Hawaii (239). No association between serum lycopene levels and risk of CaP was found, but several characteristics of the study may have contributed to the null association. Only 14 cases occurred within the first 5 years of follow-up. In the PHS, which reported a significant inverse association with serum lycopene (220), this finding was strong in the first 7 years but became attenuated over time. Moreover, the Hawaii study included "low virulence" CaP (28% were diagnosed incidentally during surgery for benign prostatic hyperplasia), and both the PHS (plasma-based) and Health Professionals' Follow-Up Study (dietary-based) indicated associations largely limited to "aggressive" CaP. Also, in the Hawaii study, the serum lycopene levels were quite low—that is, the median serum concentration among controls was only 134 ng per mL, compared to 320 ng per mL in the Hsing et al. study (217), 424 ng per mL in the sample of 121 health professionals (214), and 387 ng per mL in the PHS (220). This may indicate either very low intake of lycopene in this population or degradation of lycopene in stored samples. Finally, men of Asian descent appear to have an inherently low susceptibility to CaP (3,5,6,240) and may be the group least likely to benefit from lycopene.

Overall, the epidemiologic data indicate that intake of tomatoes and tomato products may lower risk of CaP, especially aggressive CaP. This benefit may be related to lycopene, but other potential beneficial substances instead of or combined with lycopene cannot be excluded. Although lycopene has the highest concentration of the 14 carotenoids found in human serum, tomato-based products are the major sources of approximately half of them (particularly the more lipophilic carotenoids). Definitive proof may await a randomized trial, but the available data suggest that adequate consumption of tomato and tomato-based products may be prudent. This recommendation is consistent with current guidelines to increase fruit and vegetable consumption to lower risks of cancer and other health-related conditions. The specific use of lycopene-concentrated pills, however, needs to be evaluated in trials before recommendations can be made.

Vitamin E

Vitamin E, or tocopherol, an essential nutrient with antioxidant properties, has been proposed to possess anticancer properties. Some evidence suggests that vitamin E may decrease the growth of CaP cells by inducing apoptosis of cells with damaged DNA (241). Epidemiologic data regarding vitamin E and CaP risk are relatively sparse. In Switzerland, male smokers with low prediagnostic serum levels of vitamin E were at an increased risk of fatal CaP (219). No clear association was seen for serum total, α-, δ-, and γ-tocopherols (the three main tocopherols in the serum), and CaP in nested case-control studies among Japanese-American men (218) and in a U.S. cohort study (217). However, interest in this relationship has reemerged as a result of a randomized trial of β-carotene and vitamin E in the prevention of cancer in Finnish smokers. In that study, a statistically significant 32% reduction in CaP incidence and a 41% reduction in CaP mortality was observed among the men who were randomized to receive vitamin E supplementation compared to those who received a placebo (223). Of note, no association between baseline α-tocopherol levels and CaP risk was noted in this trial (242).

In a recent analysis of 1,896 cases of CaP in the Health Professionals' Follow-Up Study, vitamin E supplementation was not related to a lower risk of CaP (243). This study was very large and had biennially updated measures of vitamin E supplement intake. In a subsample, men reporting vitamin E supplement use had substantially higher levels of plasma tocopherol, validating the self reported exposure. In an analysis of baseline plasma samples in the PHS (220), α-tocopherol was not related to overall risk of CaP, but a slight association was suggested in an analysis limited to 259 aggressive CaP cases [RR, 0.64 for top versus low quintile; *p* (trend) = .11]. This association was slightly stronger for current or ex-smokers (RR, 0.51; 95% CI, 0.26 to 0.98) than for never smokers (RR, 0.84; 95% CI, –0.36 to 1.94).

Although the data regarding vitamin E use and CaP risk are relatively sparse and conflicting, the inverse association observed in a randomized trial is intriguing. Also, studies that have examined smokers have found vitamin E potentially protective in this group. The potential interaction between vitamin E and smoking should be studied, and vitamin E status needs to be taken into account in future studies of smoking and CaP risk.

Selenium

Selenium is essential for the activity of glutathione peroxidase, an important antioxidant enzyme (244). In animal models, selenium, when administered at high levels, reduces carcinogen-induced tumorigenesis (245). In the United States, states having higher soil selenium concentrations have experienced lower incidence and mortality rates from certain malignancies (246). However, studies correlating soil selenium concentration and regional CaP rates within the United States have yielded either weak inverse or null results (246–248). Internationally, a strong inverse association has been observed between CaP mortality and selenium intake ($r = -0.65$, $p = .0001$) and blood selenium levels ($r = -0.72$, $p = .001$).

In epidemiologic studies, selenium intake cannot be easily measured, because the selenium content in foods depends primarily on the concentration of selenium in the soil in which the food plant (or animal feed for meats and dairy products) was cultivated. Data from prospective studies have been relatively sparse for CaP, with less than 100 total cases in the literature having been reported until the past several years. The only relatively large study (n = 51 cases) had been conducted by Knekt et al. (249) in Finland, a region that has a very low soil selenium content. This study found no benefit of selenium on CaP, despite finding strong inverse associations for various other cancers. In a randomized study by Clark et al. (247,250), a striking reduction in CaP risk was observed among men randomized to selenium relative to a placebo (RR, 0.37; $p = .002$). In this study, 13 CaP cases occurred in the selenium-treated group and 35 cases in the placebo group. After restricting the analysis to men with initially normal levels of PSA (less than or equal to 4 ng per mL), only four cases were diagnosed in the selenium-treated group and 16 in the placebo group (RR, 0.26; $p = .009$). Men with PSA values higher than 4 ng per mL also benefited, and the treatment effect of selenium increased as baseline levels of selenium decreased. This study was designed to examine the impact of selenium supplementation on risk of recurrent skin cancer, and CaP was not a primary end point when the study was initiated.

After the report by Clark et al., the relationship between selenium status and CaP risk was examined in a case-control study based on toenail selenium levels nested within a cohort study (251). There were 181 cases of advanced CaP and 181 age-matched control pairs in this subsample of the Health Professionals' Follow-Up Study. Men in the highest quintile of selenium had an RR of 0.35 (0.16 to 0.78) for advanced CaP relative to those in the lowest quintile. To avoid the impact of undiagnosed disease, a 2-year lag was used between the collection of toenail clippings and the start of follow-up.

Other relevant data came from Finland when in 1984 fertilizers were fortified with selenium because of the very low selenium level in the soil. Within a year, selenium levels in representative populations in Finland were noted to rise dramatically by approximately 70% (252). Levels were initially much lower than those in the United States but became comparable to U.S. levels after fortification. Over the next 10 years, CaP incidence rates continued to rise in Finland. This rise could be related to enhanced detection of CaP, but CaP mortality rates have been relatively unchanged, suggesting no impact of selenium. It is unclear why studies in the United States indicate a benefit of selenium (250,251), whereas data from Finland based on the study by Knekt et al. (249) and the experience with supplementation do not support a lowering of CaP risk with higher selenium intake. Although the data from Finland appear to argue against an important role for selenium, resolving the potential impact of selenium as a preventive agent against prostate carcinogenesis should be a top priority, based on the provocative evidence from U.S. studies.

SUMMARY

CaP is a major public health problem in economically developed countries. In the United States, CaP now accounts for 30% of all new cancer diagnoses in men. Even if age-specific incidence rates do not rise, the burden of this cancer is expected to increase as individuals live longer, because rates rise dramatically with age. In addition to being a major cause of mortality, CaP is associated with substantial morbidity and places a huge strain on the health care system.

The causes of CaP are complex, involving interactions among genetic, dietary, hormonal, and lifestyle factors. The definitively established risk factors for CaP, including older age, positive family history, and African-American race or ethnicity, are nonmodifiable. Increasing evidence from diverse sources indicates that normal biologic variations in endocrinologic factors, including the sex steroid, vitamin D, and IGF axes, are major determinants of CaP. The variation in these factors among individuals is in part inherited, but external factors, including nutrition, are likely also to be important. Many of the potential suspected and established risk factors for CaP may act through these endocrinologic axes. Accumulating evidence strongly indicates that, although CaP tends to occur generally very late in the life cycle, a substantial component of the individual risk may be determined by an early age. Thus, it is critical to determine during what stages of prostate carcinogenesis the influence of certain factors is exerted. A better understanding of the interrelationships among hormonal factors and age should be an important focus of future research into CaP etiology.

Although our understanding of potentially modifiable causes of CaP is far from desirable, recent studies suggest potential targets for preventive interventions. Recently identified modifiable factors that eventually may be targets for intervention but require further investigation are the benefits to be derived from higher intake of tomato products or, specifically, the carotenoid lycopene, trace mineral selenium, vitamin E, and other antioxidants. High intake of red meat and dairy products in particular has been consistently related to greater risk of CaP. Although fat or a type of fatty acid may underlie these associations, other components related to this dietary pattern should be evaluated. Calcium from dairy products has been shown to lower $1,25(OH)_2D$ levels that may regulate prostate epithelial cell proliferation and differentiation. Based on these important leads, continued research into the potentially modifiable risk factors for CaP should be a top priority.

REFERENCES

1. Parkin DM, Muir CS, Whelan SL, et al. Cancer incidence in five continents. Lyon: International Agency for Research on Cancer, 1992:45–173.
2. Parker SL, Davis KJ, Wingo PA, et al. Cancer statistics by race and ethnicity. *CA Cancer J Clin* 1998;48:31–48.
3. Haenszel W, Kurihara M. Studies of Japanese migrants. I. Mortality from cancer and other diseases among Japanese in the United States. *J Natl Cancer Inst* 1968;40:43–68.
4. Yu H, Harris RE, Gao YT, et al. Comparative epidemiology of cancers of the colon, rectum, prostate and breast in Shanghai, China versus the United States. *Int J Epidemiol* 1991;20:76–81.
5. Shimizu H, Ross RK, Bernstein L, et al. Cancers of the prostate and breast among Japanese and white immigrants in Los Angeles county. *Br J Cancer* 1991;63:963–966.
6. Shimizu H, Ross RK, Bernstein L. Possible underestimation of the incidence rate of prostate cancer in Japan. *Jpn J Cancer Res* 1991;82:483–485.
7. Armstrong B, Doll R. Environmental factors and cancer incidence and mortality in different countries, with special reference to dietary practices. *Int J Cancer* 1975;15:617–631.
8. Godfrey KM, Barker DJP. Maternal nutrition in relation to fetal and placental growth. *Eur J Obstet Gynecol Reprod Biol* 1995;61:15–22.
9. Tibblin G, Eriksson M, Cnattingius S, et al. High birthweight as a predictor of prostate cancer risk. *Epidemiology* 1995;6:423–424.
10. Ekbom A, Hsieh CC, Lipworth L, et al. Perinatal characteristics in relation to incidence of and mortality from prostate cancer. *BMJ* 1996;313:337–341.
11. Platz EA, Giovannucci E, Rimm EB, et al. Retrospective analysis of birth weight and prostate cancer in the Health Professionals Follow-Up Study. *Am J Epidemiol* 1998;147: 1140–1144.
12. Sakr WA, Haas GP, Cassin BF, et al. The frequency of carcinoma and intraepithelial neoplasia of the prostate in young male patients. *J Urol* 1993;150:379–385.
13. Coffey DS. Physiological control of prostatic growth: an overview. Prostate cancer. UICC Technical Report Series, Geneva: International Union Against Cancer. 1979:4–23.
14. Glantz CM. Cirrhosis and carcinoma of the prostate gland. *J Urol* 1964;91:291–293.
15. Giovannucci E, Rimm EB, Stampfer MJ, et al. Diabetes mellitus and risk of prostate cancer (United States). *Cancer Causes Control* 1998;9:3–9.
16. Geller J, Vazakas G, Fruchtman B, et al. The effect of cyproterone acetate on advanced carcinoma of the prostate. *Surg Gynecol Obstet* 1968;127:748–758.
17. Hovenanian MS, Deming CL. The heterologous growth of cancer of the human prostate. *Surg Gynecol Obstet* 1948; 86:29–35.
18. Noble RL. The development of prostatic adenocarcinoma in Nb rats following prolonged sex hormone administration. *Cancer Res* 1977;37:1929–1933.
19. Pollard M, Luckert PH, Schmidt MA. Induction of prostate adenocarcinomas in Lobund Wistar rats by testosterone. *Prostate* 1982;3:563–568.
20. Hammond GL, Kontturi M, Vihko P, et al. Serum steroids in normal males and patients with prostatic diseases. *Clin Endocrinol* 1978;9:113–121.
21. Ghanadian R, Puah CM, O'Donoghue EPN. Serum testosterone and dihydrotestosterone in carcinoma of the prostate. *Br J Cancer* 1979;39:696–699.
22. Jackson MA, Kovi J, Heshmat MY, et al. Characterization of prostatic carcinoma among blacks: a comparison between a low-incidence area, Ibadan, Nigeria, and a high-incidence area, Washington, DC. *Prostate* 1980;1:185–205.

23. Ahluwalia B, Jackson MA, Jones GW, et al. Blood hormone profiles in prostate cancer patients in high-risk and low-risk populations. *Cancer* 1981;48:2267–2273.
24. Drafta D, Proca E, Zamfir V, et al. Plasma steroids in benign prostatic hypertrophy and carcinoma of the prostate. *J Steroid Biochem* 1982;17:689–693.
25. Meikle AW, Stanish WM. Familial prostatic cancer risk and low testosterone. *J Clin Endocrinol Metab* 1982;54:1104–1108.
26. Zumoff B, Levin J, Strain GW, et al. Abnormal levels of plasma hormones in men with prostate cancer: evidence toward a "two-disease" theory. *Prostate* 1982;3:579–588.
27. Rannikko S, Adlercreutz H. Plasma estradiol, free testosterone, sex hormone binding globulin capacity, and prolactin in benign prostatic hyperplasia and prostatic cancer. *Prostate* 1983;4:223–229.
28. Hulka BS, Hammond JE, DiFerdinando G, et al. Serum hormone levels among patients with prostatic carcinoma or benign prostatic hyperplasia and clinic controls. *Prostate* 1987;11:171–182.
29. Nomura A, Heilbrun LK, Stemmermann GN, et al. Prediagnostic serum hormones and the risk of prostate cancer. *Cancer Res* 1988;48:3515–3517.
30. Barrett-Connor E, Garland C, McPhillips JB, et al. A prospective, population-based study of androstenedione, estrogens, and prostatic cancer. *Cancer Res* 1990;50:169–173.
31. Hsing AW, Comstock GW. Serological precursors of cancer: serum hormones and risk of subsequent prostate cancer. *Cancer Epidemiol Biomarkers Prev* 1993;2:27–32.
32. Carter HB, Pearson JD, Metter EJ, et al. Longitudinal evaluation of serum androgen levels in men with and without prostate cancer. *Prostate* 1995;27:25–31.
33. Gann PH, Hennekens CH, Ma J, et al. Prospective study of sex hormone levels and risk of prostate cancer. *J Natl Cancer Inst* 1996;88:1118–1126.
34. Nomura AMY, Stemmermann GN, Chyou PH, et al. Serum androgens and prostate cancer. *Cancer Epidemiol Biomarkers Prev* 1996;5:621–625.
35. Signorello LB, Tzonou A, Mantzoros CS, et al. Serum steroids in relation to prostate cancer risk in a case-control study (Greece). *Cancer Causes Control* 1997;8:632–636.
36. Vatten LJ, Ursin G, Ross RK, et al. Androgens in serum and the risk of prostate cancer: a nested case-control study from the Janus serum bank in Norway. *Cancer Epidemiol Biomarkers Prev* 1997;6:967–969.
37. Jänne OA, Palvimo JJ, Kallio P, et al. Androgen receptor and mechanisms of androgen action. *Ann Med* 1993;25:83–89.
38. Chamberlain NL, Driver ED, Miesfeld RL. The length and location of CAG trinucleotide repeats in the androgen receptor N-terminal domain affect transactivation function. *Nucleic Acids Res* 1994;22:3181–3186.
39. Edwards A, Hammond HA, Jin L, et al. Genetic variation at five trimeric and tetrameric tandem repeat loci in four human population groups. *Genomics* 1992;12:241–253.
40. Giovannucci E, Stampfer MJ, Krithivas K, et al. The CAG repeat within the androgen receptor gene and its relationship to prostate cancer. *Proc Natl Acad Sci* 1997;94:3320–3323.
41. Kazemi-Esfarjani P, Trifiro MA, Pinsky L. Evidence for a repressive function of the long polyglutamine tract in the human androgen receptor: possible pathogenic relevance for the (CAG)n-expanded neuropathies. *Human Mol Genet* 1995;4:523–527.
42. La Spada AR, Wilson EM, Lubahn DB, et al. Androgen receptor gene mutations in X-linked spinal and bulbar muscular atrophy. *Nature* 1991;352:77–79.
43. Liu CS, Chang YC, Chen DF, et al. Type IV hyperlipoproteinemia and moderate instability of CAG triplet repeat expansion in the androgen-receptor gene. Lipid, sex hormone and molecular study in a Chinese family with Kennedy-Alter-Sung disease. *Acta Neurol Scand* 1995; 92:398–404.
44. Tut TG, Ghadessy FJ, Trifiro MA, et al. Long polyglutamine tracts in the androgen receptor are associated with reduced trans-activation, impaired sperm production, and male infertility. *J Clin Endocrinol Metab* 1997;82: 3777–3782.
45. Irvine RA, Yu MC, Ross RK, et al. The CAG and GGC microsatellites of the androgen receptor gene are in linkage disequilibrium in men with prostate cancer. *Cancer Res* 1995;55:1937–1940.
46. Stanford JL, Just JJ, Gibbs M, et al. Polymorphic repeats in the androgen receptor gene: molecular markers of prostate cancer risk. *Cancer Res* 1997;57:1194–1198.
47. Aaronson S. Growth factors and cancer. *Science* 1991;254: 1146–1153.
48. Rajah R, Valentinis B, Cohen P. Insulin-like growth factor (IGF)-binding protein-3 induces apoptosis and mediates the effects of transforming growth factor-β1 on programmed cell death through a p53 and IGF-independent mechanism. *J Biol Chem* 1997;272:12181–12188.
49. Rechler M. Growth inhibition by insulin-like growth factor (IGF) binding protein-3—what's IGF got to do with it? *Endocrinology* 1997;138:2645–2647.
50. Cohen P, Peehl DM, Rosenfeld RG. The IGF axis in the prostate. *Hormone Metab Res* 1994;26:81–84.
51. Cohen P, Peehl DM, Lamson G, et al. Insulin-like growth factors (IGFs), IGF receptors, and IGF-binding proteins in primary cultures of prostate epithelial cells. *J Clin Endocrinol Metab* 1991;73:401–407.
52. Mantzoros CS, Tzonou A, Signorello LB, et al. Insulin-like growth factor 1 in relation to prostate cancer and benign prostatic hyperplasia. *Br J Cancer* 1997;76:1115–1118.
53. Chan JM, Stampfer MJ, Giovannucci E, et al. Plasma insulin-like growth factor-I and prostate cancer risk: a prospective study. *Science* 1998;279:563–566.
54. Wolk A, Mantzoros CS, Andersson SW, et al. Insulin-like growth factor I and prostate cancer risk: a population-based, case-control study. *J Natl Cancer Inst* 1998;90:911–915.
55. Reichel H, Koeffler HP, Norman AW. The role of the vitamin D endocrine system in health and disease. *N Engl J Med* 1989;320:980–991.
56. Peehl DM, Skowronski RJ, Leung GK, et al. Antiproliferative effects of 1,25-dihydroxyvitamin D_3 on primary cultures of human prostatic cells. *Cancer Res* 1994;54:805–810.
57. Skowronski RJ, Peehl DM, Feldman D. Vitamin D and prostate cancer: 1,25 dihydroxyvitamin D_3 receptors and actions in human prostate cancer cell lines. *Endocrinology* 1993;132:1952–1960.

58. Miller GJ, Stapleton GE, Hedlund TE, et al. Vitamin D receptor expression, 24—hydroxylase activity, and inhibition of growth by 1α,25-dihydroxyvitamin D_3 in seven human prostatic carcinoma cell lines. *Clin Cancer Res* 1995;1:997–1003.
59. Hedlund TE, Moffatt KA, Miller GJ. Stable expression of the nuclear vitamin D receptor in the human prostatic carcinoma cell line JCA-1: evidence that the antiproliferative effects of 1α,25-dihydroxyvitamin D_3 are mediated exclusively through the genomic signaling pathway. *Endocrinology* 1996;137:1554–1561.
60. Bahnson RR, Oeler T, Trump D, et al. Inhibition of human prostatic carcinoma cell lines by 1,25 dihydroxyvitamin D_3 and vitamin D analogs. *J Urol* 1993;149(suppl):471a.
61. Drivdahl RH, Loop SM, Andress DL, et al. IGF-binding proteins in human prostate tumor cells: expression and regulation by 1,25-dihydroxyvitamin D_3. *Prostate* 1995;26:72–79.
62. Esquenet M, Swinnen JV, Heyns W, et al. Control of LNCaP proliferation and differentiation: actions and interactions of androgens, 1α,25-dihydroxycholecalciferol, all-trans retinoic acid, 9-cis retinoic acid, and phenylacetate. *Prostate* 1996;28:182–194.
63. Hsieh T-C, Ng C-Y, Mallouh C, et al. Regulation of growth, PSA/PAP and androgen receptor expression by 1 α,25-dihydroxyvitamin D_3 in the androgen-dependent LNCaP cells. *Biochem Biophys Res Comm* 1996;223:141–146.
64. Schwartz GG, Hill CC, Oeler TA, et al. 1,25-dihydroxy-16-ene-23-yne-vitamin D_3 and prostate cancer cell proliferation in vivo. *Urology* 1995;46:365–369.
65. Lucia MS, Anzano MA, Slayter MV, et al. Chemopreventive activity of tamoxifen, *N*-(4-hydroxyphenyl)retinamide, and the vitamin D analogue Ro24-5531 for androgen-promoted carcinomas of the rat seminal vesicle and prostate. *Cancer Res* 1995;55:5621–5627.
66. Schwartz GG, Hulka BS. Is vitamin D deficiency a risk factor for prostate cancer? (Hypothesis). *Anticancer Res* 1990;10:1307–1311.
67. Corder EH, Guess HA, Hulka BS, et al. Vitamin D and prostate cancer: a prediagnostic study with stored sera. *Cancer Epidemiol Biomarkers Prev* 1993;2:467–472.
68. Gann PH, Ma J, Hennekens CH, et al. Circulating vitamin D metabolites in relation to subsequent development of prostate cancer. *Cancer Epidemiol Biomarkers Prev* 1996;5: 121–126.
69. Morrison NA, Qi JC, Tokita A, et al. Prediction of bone density from vitamin D receptor alleles. *Nature* 1994; 367:284–287.
70. Ingles SA, Ross RK, Yu MC, et al. Association of prostate cancer risk with genetic polymorphisms in vitamin D receptor and androgen receptor. *J Natl Cancer Inst* 1997;89:166–170.
71. Taylor JA, Hirvonen A, Watson M, et al. Association of prostate cancer with vitamin D receptor gene polymorphism. *Cancer Res* 1996;56:4108–4110.
72. Ingles SA, Coetzee GA, Ross RK, et al. Association of prostate cancer with vitamin D receptor haplotypes in African-Americans. *Cancer Res* 1998;58:1620–1623.
73. Ma J, Stampfer MJ, Gann PH, et al. Vitamin D receptor polymorphisms, circulating vitamin D metabolites, and risk of prostate cancer in United States physicians. *Cancer Epidemiol Biomarkers Prev* 1998;7:385–390.
74. Wynder EL, Hebert JR, Kabat GC. Association of dietary fat and lung cancer. *J Natl Cancer Inst* 1987;79:631–637.
75. Ross RK, Shimizu H, Paganini-Hill A, et al. Case-control studies of prostate cancer in blacks and whites in Southern California. *J Natl Cancer Inst* 1987;78:869–874.
76. Fincham SM, Hill GB, Hanson J, et al. Epidemiology of prostatic cancer: a case-control study. *Prostate* 1990;17:189–206.
77. Talamini R, Franceschi S, Barra S, et al. The role of alcohol in oral and pharyngeal cancer in non-smokers, and of tobacco in non-drinkers. *Int J Cancer* 1990;46:391–393.
78. Weir JM, Dunn JE Jr. Smoking and mortality: a prospective study. *Cancer* 1970;25:105–112.
79. Mishina T, Watanabe H, Araki H, et al. Epidemiological study of prostate cancer by matched-pair analysis. *Prostate* 1985;6:423–436.
80. Honda GD, Bernstein L, Ross RK, et al. Vasectomy, cigarette smoking, and age at first sexual intercourse as risk factors for prostate cancer in middle-aged men. *Br J Cancer* 1988;57:326–331.
81. Hiatt RA, Armstrong MA, Klatsky AL, et al. Alcohol consumption, smoking, and other risk factors and prostate cancer in a large health plan cohort in California (United States). *Cancer Causes Control* 1994;5:66–72.
82. Hayes RB, Pottern LM, Swanson GM, et al. Tobacco use and prostate cancer in blacks and whites in the United States. *Cancer Causes Control* 1994;5:221–226.
83. van der Gulden JWJ, Verbeek ALM, Kolk JJ. Smoking and drinking habits in relation to prostate cancer. *Br J Urol* 1994;73:382–389.
84. Hsing AW, McLaughlin JK, Schuman LM, et al. Diet, tobacco use, and fatal prostate cancer: results from the Lutheran Brotherhood Cohort Study. *Cancer Res* 1990; 50:6836–6840.
85. Hsing AW, McLaughlin JK, Olsen JH, et al. Tobacco use and prostate cancer: 26-year follow-up of US veterans. *Am J Epidemiol* 1991;133:437–441.
86. Coughlin SS, Neaton JD, Sengupta A. Cigarette smoking as a predictor of death from prostate cancer in 348,874 men screened for the Multiple Risk Factor Intervention Trial. *Am J Epidemiol* 1996;143:1002–1006.
87. Rodriguez C, Tatham LM, Thun MJ, et al. Smoking and fatal prostate cancer in a large cohort of adult men. *Am J Epidemiol* 1997;145:466–475.
88. Dai WS, Gutai JP, Kuller LH, et al. Cigarette smoking and serum sex hormones in men. *Am J Epidemiol* 1988;128: 796–805.
89. Field AE, Colditz GA, Willett WC, et al. The relation of smoking, age, relative weight, and dietary intake to serum adrenal steroids, sex hormones, and sex hormone-binding globulin in middle-aged men. *J Clin Endocrinol Metab* 1994;79:1310–1316.
90. Daniell HW. A worse prognosis for smokers with prostate cancer. *J Urol* 1995;154:153–157.
91. Hussain F, Aziz H, Macchia R, et al. High grade adenocarcinoma of prostate in smokers of ethnic minority groups and Caribbean island immigrants. *Int J Radiat Oncol Biol Phys* 1992;24:451–461.
92. Giovannucci E, Rimm EB, Ascherio A, et al. Smoking and risk of total and fatal prostate cancer in United States health

professionals. *Cancer Epidemiol Biomarkers Prev* 1999;8: 277–282.

93. Ida Y, Tsujimaru S, Nakamaura K, et al. Effects of acute and repeated alcohol ingestion on hypothalamic-pituitary-gonadal and hypothalamic-pituitary-adrenal functioning in normal males. *Drug Alcohol Depend* 1992;31:57–64.
94. Mendelson JH, Mello NK, Ellingboe J. Effects of acute alcohol intake on pituitary-gonadal hormones in normal human males. *J Pharmacol Exper Therap* 1977;202:676–682.
95. Gordon GG, Altman K, Southren AL, et al. Effect of alcohol (ethanol) administration on sex-hormone metabolism in normal men. *N Engl J Med* 1976;295:793–797.
96. Green JRB. Mechanism of hypogonadism in cirrhotic males. *Gut* 1977;18:843–853.
97. Reichman ME, Judd JT, Longcope C, et al. Effects of alcohol consumption on plasma and urinary hormone concentration in premenopausal women. *J Natl Cancer Inst* 1993; 85:722–727.
98. Ginsburg ES, Mello NK, Mendelson JH, et al. Effects of alcohol ingestion on estrogens in postmenopausal women. *J Am Med Asso* 1996;276:1747–1751.
99. Reference deleted by author.
100. Mills PK, Beeson WL, Phillips RL, et al. Cohort study of diet, lifestyle, and prostate cancer in Adventist men. *Cancer* 1989;64:598–604.
101. Hsing AW, McLaughlin JK, Schuman LM, et al. Diet, tobacco use, and fatal prostate cancer: results from the Lutheran Brotherhood Cohort Study. *Cancer Res* 1990;50: 6836–6840.
102. Hiatt RA, Armstrong MA, Klatsky AL, et al. Alcohol consumption, smoking, and other risk factors and prostate cancer in a large health plan cohort in California (United States). *Cancer Causes Control* 1994;5:66–72.
103. Pollack ES, Nomura AM, Heilbrun LK, et al. Prospective study of alcohol consumption and cancer. *N Engl J Med* 1984;310:617–621.
104. Le Marchand L, Kolonel LN, Wilkens LR, et al. Animal fat consumption and prostate cancer: a prospective study in Hawaii. *Epidemiology* 1994;5:276–282.
105. Cerhan JR, Torner JC, Lynch CF, et al. Association of smoking, body mass, and physical activity with risk of prostate cancer in the Iowa 65+ Rural Health Study (United States). *Cancer Causes Control* 1997;8:229–238.
106. Andersson SO, Baron J, Bergström R, et al. Lifestyle factors and prostate cancer risk: a case-control study in Sweden. *Cancer Epidemiol Biomarkers Prev* 1996;5:509–513.
107. Hayes RB, Brown LM, Schoenberg JB, et al. Alcohol use and prostate cancer risk in US blacks and whites. *Am J Epidemiol* 1996;143:692–697.
108. Whittemore AS, Kolonel LN, Wu AH, et al. Prostate cancer in relation to diet, physical activity, and body size in blacks, whites, and Asians in the United States and Canada. *J Natl Cancer Inst* 1995;87:652–661.
109. Yu H, Harris RE, Wynder EL. Case-control study of prostate cancer and socioeconomic factors. *Prostate* 1988;13: 317–325.
110. Breslow RA ,Weed DL. Review of epidemiologic studies of alcohol and prostate cancer: 1971–1996. *Nutr Cancer* 1998;30:1–13.
111. World Health Organization. Meeting to evaluate research needs and priorities regarding the relationship of vasectomy to cancers of the testis and prostate. Special Programme of Research, Development and Research Training in Human Reproduction. Geneva: World Health Organization, 1991.
112. Giovannucci E, Tosteson TD, Speizer FE, et al. A long-term study of mortality in men who have undergone vasectomy. *N Engl J Med* 1992;326:1392–1398.
113. Massey FJ Jr., Bernstein GS, O'Fallon WM, et al. Vasectomy and health. Results from a large cohort study. *J Am Med Assoc* 1984;252:1023–1029.
114. Hsing AW, Wang RT, Gu FL, et al. Vasectomy and prostate cancer risk in China. *Cancer Epidemiol Biomarkers Prev* 1994;3:285–288.
115. Mettlin C, Natarajan N, Huben R. Vasectomy and prostate cancer risk. *Am J Epidemiol* 1990;132:1056–1061.
116. Hayes RB, Pottern LM, Greenberg R, et al. Vasectomy and prostate cancer in US blacks and whites. *Am J Epidemiol* 1993;137:263–269.
117. Giovannucci E, Tosteson TD, Speizer FE, et al. A retrospective cohort study of vasectomy and prostate cancer in men. *J Am Med Assoc* 1993;269:878–882.
118. Giovannucci E, Ascherio A, Rimm EB, et al. A prospective cohort study of vasectomy and prostate cancer in US men. *J Am Med Assoc* 1993;269:873–877.
119. Rosenberg L, Palmer J, Zauber A, et al. Vasectomy and the risk of prostate cancer. *Am J Epidemiol* 1990;132:1051–1055.
120. Spitz MR, Fueger JJ, Babaian RJ, et al. Vasectomy and the risk of prostate cancer. *Am J Epidemiol* 1991;134:108–109.
121. Platz EA, Yeole BB, Cho E, et al. Vasectomy and prostate cancer: a case-control study in India. *Int J Epidemiol* 1997; 26:933–938.
122. Rosenberg L, Palmer J, Zauber A, et al. The relation of vasectomy to the risk of cancer. *Am J Epidemiol* 1994; 140:431–438.
123. John EM, Whittemore AS, Wu AH, et al. Vasectomy and prostate cancer: results from a multiethnic case-control study. *J Natl Cancer Inst* 1995;87:662–669.
124. Sidney S, Quesenberry CP Jr., Sadler MC, et al. Vasectomy and the risk of prostate cancer in a cohort of multiphasic health-checkup examinees: second report. *Cancer Causes Control* 1991;2:113–116.
125. Nienhuis H, Goldacre M, Seagroatt V, et al. Incidence of disease after vasectomy: a record linkage retrospective cohort study. *BMJ* 1992;304:743–746.
126. Moller H, Knudsen LB, Lynge E. Risk of testicular cancer after vasectomy: cohort study of over 73,000 men. *BMJ* 1994;309:295–299.
127. Zhu K, Stanford JL, Daling JR, et al. Vasectomy and prostate cancer: a case-control study in a health maintenance organization. *Am J Epidemiol* 1996;144:717–722.
128. Skegg D. Vasectomy and prostate cancer: is there a link? *NZ Med J* 1993;106:242–243.
129. Howards SS, Peterson HB. Vasectomy and prostate cancer: Chance, bias, or a causal relationship. *J Am Med Assoc* 1993;269:913–914.
130. Thompson MM, Garland C, Barrett-Connor E, et al. Heart disease risk factors, diabetes, and prostatic cancer in an adult community. *Am J Epidemiol* 1989;129:511–517.

131. Adami HO, McLaughlin J, Ekbom A, et al. Cancer risk in patients with diabetes mellitus. *Cancer Causes Control* 1991;2:307–314.
132. Mishina T, Watanabe H, Araki H, et al. Epidemiological study of prostatic cancer by matched-pair analysis. *Prostate* 1985;6:423–436.
133. La Vecchia C, Negri E, Franceschi S, et al. A case-control study of diabetes mellitus and cancer risk. *Br J Cancer* 1994;70:950–953.
134. Andò S, Rubens R, Rottiers R. Androgen plasma levels in male diabetics. *J Endocrinol Invest* 1984;7:21–24.
135. Nomura AMY, Kolonel LN. Prostate cancer: a current perspective. *Am J Epidemiol* 1991;13:200–227.
136. Giovannucci E. How is individual risk for prostate cancer assessed? *Hematol Oncol Clin North Am* 1996;10:537–548.
137. Norrish AE, Jackson RT, McRae CU. Non-steroidal anti-inflammatory drugs and prostate cancer progression. *Int J Cancer* 1998;77:511–515.
138. Mukherjee P, Sotnikov AV, Mangian HJ, et al. Energy intake and prostate tumor growth, angiogenesis, and vascular endothelial growth factor expression. *J Natl Cancer Inst* 1999;91:512–523.
139. Gann PH, Daviglus ML, Dyer AR, et al. Heart rate and prostate cancer mortality: results of a prospective analysis. *Cancer Epidemiol Biomarkers Prev* 1995;4:611–616.
140. McVary KT, Razzaq A, Lee C, et al. Growth of the rat prostate gland is facilitated by the autonomic nervous system. *Biol Reprod* 1994;51:99–107.
141. Djakiew D. Role of nerve growth factor-like protein in the paracrine regulation of prostate growth. *J Androl* 1992;13: 476–487.
142. Andersson SO, Baron J, Wolk A, et al. Early life risk factors for prostate cancer: a population-based case-control study in Sweden. *Cancer Epidemiol Biomarkers Prev* 1995;4:187–192.
143. Andersson SO, Wolk A, Bergström R, et al. Body size and prostate cancer: a 20-year follow-up study among 135,006 Swedish construction workers. *J Natl Cancer Inst* 1997;89: 385–389.
144. Giovannucci E, Rimm EB, Stampfer MJ, et al. Height, body weight, and risk of prostate cancer. *Cancer Epidemiol Biomarkers Prev* 1997;6:557–563.
145. Herbert PR, Ajani U, Cook N, et al. Adult height and incidence of total malignant neoplasms and prostate cancer: the Physicians' Health Study. *Am J Epidemiol* 1996;143S: 78,309.
146. La Vecchia C, Negri E, Parazzini F, et al. Height and cancer risk in a network of case-control studies from northern Italy. *Int J Cancer* 1990;45:275–279.
147. Wynder EL, Mabuchi K, Whitmore WF. Epidemiology of cancer of the prostate. *Cancer* 1971;28:344–360.
148. Greenwald P, Damon A, Kirmss V, et al. Physical and demographic features of men before developing cancer of the prostate. *J Natl Cancer Inst* 1974;53:341–346.
149. Talamini R, La Vecchia C, Decarli A, et al. Nutrition, social factors and prostatic cancer in a northern Italian population. *Br J Cancer* 1986;53:817–821.
150. Thune I, Lund E. Physical activity and the risk of prostate and testicular cancer: a cohort study of 53,000 Norwegian men. *Cancer Causes Control* 1994;5:549–556.
151. Demark-Wahnefried W, Conaway MR, Robertson CN, et al. Anthropometric risk factors for prostate cancer. *Nutr Cancer* 1997;28:302–307.
152. Pasquali R, Casimirri F, Cantobelli S, et al. Effect of obesity and body fat distribution on sex hormones and insulin in men. *Metabolism* 1991;40:101–104.
153. Amatruda JM, Harman SM, Pourmotabbed G, et al. Depressed plasma testosterone and fractional binding of testosterone in obese males. *J Clin Endocrinol Metab* 1978; 47:268–271.
154. Barrett-Connor E, Khaw KT. Cigarette smoking and increased endogenous estrogen levels in men. *Am J Epidemiol* 1987;126:187–192.
155. Zumoff B. Hormonal abnormalities in obesity. *Acta Med Scand* 1988;723(suppl):153–160.
156. Garn SM, Leonard WR, Hawthorne VM. Three limitations of the body mass index. *Am J Clin Nutr* 1986;44:996–997.
157. Kolonel LN, Yoshizawa CN, Hankin JH. Diet and prostatic cancer: a case-control study in Hawaii. *Am J Epidemiol* 1988;127:999–1012.
158. Graham S, Haughey B, Marshall J, et al. Diet in the epidemiology of carcinoma of the prostate gland. *J Natl Cancer Inst* 1983;70:687–692.
159. West DW, Slattery ML, Robison LM, et al. Adult dietary intake and prostate cancer risk in Utah: a case-control study with special emphasis on aggressive tumors. *Cancer Causes Control* 1991;2:85–94.
160. Lew EA, Garfinkel L. Variations in mortality by weight among 750,000 men and women. *J Chron Dis* 1979;32: 563–576.
161. Snowdon DA, Phillips RL, Choi W. Diet, obesity, and risk of fatal prostate cancer. *Am J Epidemiol* 1984;120:244–250.
162. Chyou PH, Nomura AM, Stemmermann GN. A prospective study of weight, body mass index and other anthropometric measurements in relation to site-specific cancers. *Int J Cancer* 1994;57:313–317.
163. Veierod MB, Laake P, Thelle DS. Dietary fat intake and risk of prostate cancer: a prospective study of 25,708 Norwegian men. *Int J Cancer* 1997;73:634–638.
164. Whittemore AS, Paffenbarger RS Jr., Anderson K, et al. Early precursors of site-specific cancers in college men and women. *J Natl Cancer Inst* 1985;74:43–51.
165. Nomura A, Heilbrun LK, Stemmermann GN. Body mass index as a predictor of cancer in men. *J Natl Cancer Inst* 1985;74:319–323.
166. Severson RK, Grove JS, Nomura AMY, et al. Body mass and prostatic cancer: a prospective study. *BMJ* 1988;297: 713–715.
167. Vena JE, Graham S, Zielezny M, et al. Occupational exercise and risk of cancer. *Am J Clin Nutr* 1987;45:318–327.
168. Albanes D, Blair A, Taylor PR. Physical activity and risk of cancer in the NHANES I population. *Am J Public Health* 1989;79:744–750.
169. Brownson RC, Chang JC, Davis JR, et al. Physical activity on the job and cancer in Missouri. *Am J Public Health* 1991;81:639–642.
170. Hartman TJ, Albanes D, Rautalahti M, et al. Physical activity and prostate cancer in the Alpha-Tocopherol, Beta-Carotene (ATBC) Cancer Prevention Study (Finland). *Cancer Causes Control* 1998;9:11–18.

171. Hsing AW, McLaughlin JK, Zheng W, et al. Occupation, physical activity, and risk of prostate cancers in Shanghai, People's Republic of China. *Cancer Causes Control* 1994; 5:136–140.
172. Oliveria SA, Kohl HW III, Trichopoulos D, et al. The association between cardiorespiratory fitness and prostate cancer. *Med Sci Sports Exerc* 1996;28:97–104.
173. Severson RK, Nomura AMY, Grove JS, et al. A prospective study of demographics, diet, and prostate cancer among men of Japanese ancestry in Hawaii. *Cancer Res* 1989;49: 1857–1860.
174. Polednak AP. College athletics, body size, and cancer mortality. *Cancer* 1976;38:382–387.
175. Paffenbarger RS Jr., Hyde RT, Wing AL. Physical activity and incidence of cancer in diverse populations: a preliminary report. *Am J Clin Nutr* 1987;45(suppl):312–317.
176. Lee IM, Paffenbarger RS Jr., Hsieh CC. Physical activity and risk of prostatic cancer among college alumni. *Am J Epidemiol* 1992;135:169–179.
177. Giovannucci E, Leitzmann M, Spiegelman D, et al. A prospective study of physical activity and prostate cancer in male health professionals. *Cancer Res* 1998;58:5117–5122.
178. Hackney AC. The male reproductive system and endurance exercise. *Med Sci Sports Exerc* 1996;28:180–189.
179. Wheeler GD, Wall SR, Belcastro AN, et al. Reduced serum testosterone and prolactin levels in male distance runners. *J Am Med Assoc* 1984;252:514–516.
180. Kolonel LN, Hankin JH, Lee J, et al. Nutrient intakes in relation to cancer incidence in Hawaii. *Br J Cancer* 1981;44:332–339.
181. Rotkin ID. Studies in the epidemiology of prostatic cancer: expanded sampling. *Cancer Treat Rep* 1977;61:173–180.
182. Talamini R, Franceschi S, La Vecchia C, et al. Diet and prostatic cancer: a case-control study in northern Italy. *Nutr Cancer* 1992;18:277–286.
183. Schuman LM, Mandel JS, Radke A, et al. Some selected features of the epidemiology of prostatic cancer: Minneapolis-St. Paul, Minnesota case-control study, 1976–1979. In: Magnus K, ed. *Trends in cancer incidence: causes and practical implications.* Washington, DC: Hemisphere Publishing Corp, 1982;345–354.
184. Heshmat MY, Kaul L, Kovi J, et al. Nutrition and prostate cancer: a case-control study. *Prostate* 1985;6:7–17.
185. Ewings P, Bowie C. A case-control study of cancer of the prostate in Somerset and East Devon. *Br J Cancer* 1996;74:661–666.
186. Hayes RB, Ziegler RG, Gridley G, et al. Dietary factors and risks for prostate cancer among blacks and whites in the United States. *Cancer Epidemiol Biomarkers Prev* 1999;8:25–34.
187. Ohno Y, Yoshida O, Oishi K, et al. Dietary β-carotene and cancer of the prostate: a case-control study in Kyoto, Japan. *Cancer Res* 1988;48:1331–1336.
188. Mettlin C, Selenskas S, Natarajan NS, et al. Beta-carotene and animal fats and their relationship to prostate cancer risk: a case-control study. *Cancer* 1989;64:605–612.
189. Kaul L, Heshmat MY, Kovi J, et al. The role of diet in prostate cancer. *Nutr Cancer* 1987;9:123–128.
190. Walker ARP, Walker BF, Tsotetsi NG, et al. Case-control study of prostate cancer in black patients in Soweto, South Africa. *Br J Cancer* 1992;65:438–441.
191. Giovannucci E, Rimm EB, Colditz GA, et al. A prospective study of dietary fat and risk of prostate cancer. *J Natl Cancer Inst* 1993;85:1571–1579.
192. Rose D, Boyar A, Wynder E. International comparisons of mortality rates for cancer of the breast, ovary, prostate, and colon, and per capita food consumption. *Cancer* 1986;58: 2363–2371.
193. Decarli A, La Vecchia C. Environmental factors and cancer mortality in Italy: correlational exercise. *Oncology* 1986;43: 116–126.
194. La Vecchia C, Negri E, D'Avanzo B, et al. Dairy products and the risk of prostatic cancer. *Oncology* 1991;48:406–410.
195. Chan JM, Giovannucci E, Andersson SO, et al. Dairy products, calcium, phosphorus, vitamin D, and risk of prostate cancer. *Cancer Causes Control* 1998;9:559–566.
196. Giovannucci E, Rimm EB, Wolk A, et al. Calcium and fructose intake in relation to risk of prostate cancer. *Cancer Res* 1998;58:442–447.
197. Veierod MB, Laake P, Thelle DS. Dietary fat intake and risk of prostate cancer: a prospective study of 25,708 Norwegian men. *Int J Cancer* 1997;73:634–638.
198. Isley WL, Underwood LE, Clemmons DR. Dietary components that regulate serum somatomedin-C concentrations in humans. *J Clin Invest* 1983;71:175–182.
199. Clemmons DR, Underwood LE, Dickerson RN, et al. Use of plasma somatomedin-C/insulin-like growth factor I measurements to monitor the response to nutritional repletion in malnourished patients. *Am J Clin Nutr* 1985;41:191–198.
200. Unterman TG, Vazquez RM, Slas AJ, et al. Nutrition and somatomedin. XIII. Usefulness of somatomedin-C in nutritional assessment. *Am J Med* 1985;78:228–234.
201. Ruggeri BA, Klurfeld DM, Kritchevsky D, et al. Caloric restriction and 7,12-dimethylbenz(a)anthracene-induced mammary tumor growth in rats: alterations in circulating insulin, insulin-like growth factors I and II, and epidermal growth factor. *Cancer Res* 1989;49:4130–4134.
202. Klurfeld DM, Lloyd LM, Welch CB, et al. Reduction of enhanced mammary carcinogenesis in LA/N-cp (corpulent) rats by energy restriction. *Proc Soc Exp Biol Med* 1991;196: 381–384.
203. Howie BJ, Shultz TD. Dietary and hormonal interrelationships among vegetarian Seventh-Day Adventists and non-vegetarian men. *Am J Clin Nutr* 1985;42:127–134.
204. Hill P, Wynder EL, Garbaczewski L, et al. Diet and urinary steroids in black and white North American men and black South African men. *Cancer Res* 1979;39:5101–5105.
205. Hämäläinen E, Adlercreutz H, Puska P, et al. Diet and serum sex hormones in healthy men. *J Steroid Biochem* 1984;20:459–464.
206. Giovannucci E. Dietary influences of 1,25$(OH)_2$ vitamin D in relation to prostate cancer: a hypothesis. *Cancer Causes Control* 1998;9:567–582.
207. Gann PH, Hennekens CH, Sacks FM, et al. Prospective study of plasma fatty acids and risk of prostate cancer. *J Natl Cancer Inst* 1994;86:281–286.
208. Zock PL, Katan MB. Linoleic acid intake and cancer risk: a review and meta-analysis. *Am J Clin Nutr* 1998;68:142–153.

209. Harvei S, Bjerve KS, Tretli S, et al. Prediagnostic level of fatty acids in serum phospholipids: omega-3 and omega-6 fatty acids and the risk of prostate cancer. *Int J Cancer* 1997;71:545–551.
210. Sporn MB, Roberts AB. Role of retinoids in differentiation and carcinogenesis. *J Natl Cancer Inst* 1984;73:1381–1386.
211. Pollard M, Luckert PH. The inhibitory effect of 4-hydroxyphenyl retinamide (4-HPR) on metastasis of prostate adenocarcinoma-III cells in Lobund-Wistar rats. *Cancer Lett* 1991;59:159–163.
212. Schroder EW, Black PH. Retinoids: tumor preventers or tumor enhancers? *J Natl Cancer Inst* 1980;65:671–674.
213. Mayne ST, Graham S, Zheng T. Dietary retinol: prevention or promotion of carcinogenesis in humans? *Cancer Causes Control* 1991;2:443–450.
214. Giovannucci E, Ascherio A, Rimm EB, et al. Intake of carotenoids and retinol in relation to risk of prostate cancer. *J Natl Cancer Inst* 1995;87:1767–1776.
215. Kolonel LN, Hankin JH, Yoshizawa CN. Vitamin A and prostate cancer in elderly men: enhancement of risk. *Cancer Res* 1987;47:2982–2985.
216. Reichman ME, Hayes RB, Ziegler RG, et al. Serum vitamin A and subsequent development of prostate cancer in the first National Health and Nutrition Examination Survey Epidemiologic Follow-up Study. *Cancer Res* 1990;50:2311–2315.
217. Hsing AW, Comstock GW, Abbey H, et al. Serologic precursors of cancer. Retinol, carotenoids, and tocopherol and risk of prostate cancer. *J Natl Cancer Inst* 1990;82:941–946.
218. Nomura AM, Stemmermann GN, Lee J, et al. Serum micronutrients and prostate cancer in Japanese Americans in Hawaii. *Cancer Epidemiol Biomarkers Prev* 1997;6:487–491.
219. Eichholzer M, Stahelin HB, Gey KF, et al. Prediction of male cancer mortality by plasma levels of interacting vitamins: 17-year follow-up of the prospective Basel study. *Int J Cancer* 1996;66:145–150.
220. Gann PH, Ma J, Giovannucci E, et al. Lower prostate cancer risk in men with elevated plasma lycopene levels: results of a prospective analysis. *Cancer Res* 1999;59:1225–1230.
221. Rousseau EJ, Davison AJ, Dunn B. Protection by β-carotene and related compounds against oxygen-mediated cytotoxicity and genotoxicity: implications for carcinogenesis and anticarcinogenesis. *Free Radic Biol Med* 1992;13:407–433.
222. Daviglus ML, Dyer AR, Persky V, et al. Dietary beta-carotene, vitamin C, and risk of prostate cancer: results from the Western Electric Study. *Epidemiology* 1996;7:472–477.
223. Heinonen OP, Albanes D, Virtamo J, et al. Prostate cancer and supplementation with α-tocopherol and β-carotene: incidence and mortality in a controlled trial. *J Natl Cancer Inst* 1998;90:440–446.
224. Sies H, Stahl W. Vitamins E and C, β-carotene, and other carotenoids as antioxidants. *Am J Clin Nutr* 1995;62(suppl): 1315S–1321S.
225. Di Mascio P, Kaiser S, Sies H. Lycopene as the most efficient biological carotenoid singlet oxygen quencher. *Arch Biochem Biophys* 1989;274:532–538.
226. Ribaya-Mercado JD, Garmyn M, Gilchrest BA, et al. Skin lycopene is destroyed preferentially over β-carotene during ultraviolet irradiation in humans. *J Nutr* 1995;125:1854–1859.
227. Levy J, Bosin E, Feldman B, et al. Lycopene is a more potent inhibitor of human cancer cell proliferation than either α-carotene or β-carotene. *Nutr Cancer* 1995;24:257–266.
228. Ripple MO, Henry WF, Rago RP, et al. Prooxidant-antioxidant shift induced by androgen treatment of human prostate carcinoma cells. *J Natl Cancer Inst* 1997;89:40–48.
229. Nagasawa H, Mitamura T, Sakamoto S, et al. Effects of lycopene on spontaneous mammary tumor development in SHN virgin mice. *Anticancer Res* 1995;15:1173–1178.
230. Rao AV, Agarwal S. Bioavailability and in vivo antioxidant properties of lycopene from tomato products and their possible role in the prevention of cancer. *Nutr Cancer* 1998;31:199–203.
231. Ascherio A, Stampfer MJ, Colditz GA, et al. Correlations of vitamin A and E intakes with the plasma concentrations of carotenoids and tocopherols among American men and women. *J Nutr* 1992;122:1792–1801.
232. Kaplan LA, Stein EA, Willett WC, et al. Reference ranges of retinol, tocopherols, lycopene and alpha- and beta-carotene in plasma by simultaneous high-performance liquid chromatographic analysis. *Clin Physiol Biochem* 1987;5:297–304.
233. Clinton SK, Emenhiser C, Schwartz SJ, et al. *cis-trans* lycopene isomers, carotenoids, and retinol in the human prostate. *Cancer Epidemiol Biomarkers Prev* 1996;5:823–833.
234. Le Marchand L, Hankin JH, Kolonel LN, et al. Vegetable and fruit consumption in relation to prostate cancer risk in Hawaii: a reevaluation of the effect of dietary beta-carotene. *Am J Epidemiol* 1991;133:215–219.
235. Key TJA, Silcocks PB, Davey GK, et al. A case-control study of diet and prostate cancer. *Br J Cancer* 1997;76:678–687.
236. Tzonou A, Signorello LB, Lagiou P, et al. Diet and cancer of the prostate: a case-control study in Greece. *Int J Cancer* 1999;80:704–708.
237. Cerhan J, Chiu B, Putnam S, et al. A cohort study of diet and prostate cancer risk. *Cancer Epidemiol Biomarkers Prev* 1998;7:175(abst).
238. Baldwin D, Naco G, Petersen F, et al. The effect of nutritional and clinical factors upon serum prostate specific antigen and prostate cancer in a population of elderly California men [abstract]. Annual meeting of the American Urological Association, New Orleans, Louisiana, 1997.
239. Nomura AMY, Stemmermann GN, Lee J, et al. Serum micronutrients and prostate cancer in Japanese Americans in Hawaii. *Cancer Epidemiol Biomarkers Prev* 1997;6:487–491.
240. Yu H, Harris R, Gao Y, et al. Comparative epidemiology of cancers of the colon, rectum, prostate, and breast in Shanghai, China versus the United States. *Int J Epidemiol* 1991;20:76–81.
241. Sigounas G, Anagnostou A, Steiner M. *dl*-α-tocopherol induces apoptosis in erythroleukemia, prostate, and breast cancer cells. *Nutr Cancer* 1997;28:30–35.
242. Hartman TJ, Albanes D, Pietinen P, et al. The association between baseline vitamin E, selenium, and prostate cancer in the Alpha-Tocopherol, Beta-Carotene Cancer Prevention Study. *Cancer Epidemiol Biomarkers Prev* 1998;7:335–340.
243. Chan JM, Stampfer MJ, Ma J, et al. Supplemental vitamin E intake and prostate cancer risk in a large cohort of men in the United States. *Cancer Epidemiol Biomarkers Prev* 1999; 8:893–899.
244. Combs GF Jr., Combs SB. The nutritional biochemistry of selenium. *Annu Rev Nutr* 1984;4:257–280.

245. Griffin AC. The chemopreventive role of selenium in carcinogenesis. In: Arnott MS, van Eys J, Wang Y-M, eds. *Molecular interrelations of nutrition and cancer.* New York: Raven Press, 1982:401–408.
246. Shamberger RJ, Tytko SA, Willis CE. Antioxidants and Cancer Part VI. Selenium and age-adjusted human cancer mortality. *Arch Environ Health* 1976;31:231–235.
247. Clark LC, Dalkin B, Krongrad A, et al. Decreased incidence of prostate cancer with selenium supplementation: results of a double-blind cancer prevention trial. *Br J Urol* 1998;81:730–734.
248. Schrauzer GN, White DA, Schneider CJ. Cancer mortality correlation studies-III: statistical associations with dietary selenium intakes. *Bioinorg Chem* 1977;7:23–31.
249. Knekt P, Aromaa A, Maatela J, et al. Serum selenium and subsequent risk of cancer among Finnish men and women. *J Natl Cancer Inst* 1990;82:864–868.
250. Clark LC, Combs GF Jr., Turnbull BW, et al. Effects of selenium supplementation for cancer prevention in patients with carcinoma of the skin. A randomized controlled trial. Nutritional Prevention of Cancer Study Group. *JAMA* 1996;276:1957–1963.
251. Yoshizawa K, Willett WC, Morris SJ, et al. Study of prediagnostic selenium level in toenails and the risk of advanced prostate cancer. *J Natl Cancer Inst* 1998;90:1219–1224.
252. Varo P, Alfthan G, Ekholm P, et al. Selenium intake and serum selenium in Finland: effects of soil fertilization with selenium. *Am J Clin Nutr* 1988;48:324–329.
253. Rotkin ID. Studies in the epidemiology of prostatic cancer: expanded sampling. *Cancer Treat Rep* 1977;61:173–180.
254. Graham S. Results of case-control studies of diet and cancer in Buffalo, New York. *Cancer Res* 1983;43(suppl):2409S–2413S.
255. Talamini R, La Vecchia C, Decarli A, et al. Nutrition, social factors, and prostatic cancer in a Northern Italian population. *Br J Cancer* 1986;53:817–821.
256. Ohno Y, Yoshida O, Oishi K, et al. Dietary beta-carotene and cancer of the prostate: a case-control study in Kyoto, Japan. *Cancer Res* 1988;48:1331–1336.
257. Mettlin CJ. Milk drinking, other beverage habits and lung cancer risk. *Int J Cancer* 1989;43:608–612.
258. West DW, Slattery ML, Robison LM, et al. Adult dietary intake and prostate cancer risk in Utah: a case-control study with special emphasis on aggressive tumors. *Cancer Causes Control* 1991;2:85–94.
259. Andersson I, Rossner S. The Gustaf Study: repeated, telephone-administered 24-hour dietary recalls of obese and normal-weight men—energy and macronutrient intake and distribution over the days of the week. *J Am Diet Assoc* 1996;96:686–692.
260. Chan JM, Giovannucci E, Andersson S-O, et al. Dairy products, calcium, phosphorous, vitamin D, and risk of prostate cancer. *Cancer Causes Control* 1998;9:559–566.
261. Hirayama T. Diet and cancer. *Nutr Cancer* 1979;1:67–81.
262. Giovannucci E, Rimm EB, Colditz GA, et al. A prospective study of dietary fat and risk of prostate cancer. *J Natl Cancer Inst* 1993;85:1571–1579.
263. Gann PH, Hennekens CH, Sacks FM, et al. Prospective study of plasma fatty acids and risk of prostate cancer. *J Natl Cancer Inst* 1994;86:281–286.

9

GENETIC EPIDEMIOLOGY OF PROSTATE CANCER

RONALD K. ROSS
GERHARD A. COETZEE

Two great, interrelated mysteries dominate the epidemiology of prostate cancer. The first is that the racial-ethnic and international variation in prostate cancer incidence, with the prostate historically being among the greatest of all cancer sites, is still largely unexplained (1). The second is that this remarkable variation in incidence rates exists despite the fact that occult, subclinical prostate cancer reportedly occurs at very high but relatively comparable rates among those same populations at the extremes and in the middle of the racial-ethnic spectrum in risk of clinical disease (2). Thus, those factors that induce subclinical prostate cancer occur with equal frequency across racial-ethnic groups, whereas those that cause subclinical prostate cancer to progress (or clinical prostate cancer to appear *de novo*) vary greatly across the same groups. Progress has been made in recent years in understanding risk factors, particularly dietary risk factors, for prostate cancer (1), and slower progress is being made in understanding the basis for the strong familial association consistently observed for prostate cancer. However, neither improved understanding of dietary risk factors nor understanding the molecular genetic basis of familial risk has contributed substantively to date in understanding the racial-ethnic comparability of occult disease in the face of huge racial-ethnic variability in clinical disease. Review of progress in these other areas (diet, family history) is made elsewhere in this section. We focus in this chapter on the genetic epidemiology of prostate cancer, emphasizing particularly those aspects with the greatest potential for understanding racial-ethnic variation in incidence and disease progression.

MOLECULAR GENETICS OF PROSTATE CANCER INCIDENCE

The molecular genetics of prostate cancer related to etiology (constitutional or germline genetic risk) have progressed substantially since 1996 primarily through use of the *candidate* gene approach—that is, targeting genes whose functions would predict that they might play an etiologic role. Four areas seem to have been particularly productive to date, and these would appear to offer the greatest opportunities in the near future to improve our understanding of the molecular genetic basis of this disease: (a) androgen metabolic pathways as the major control pathway of cell division in the prostate; (b) vitamin D metabolism pathways as an alternative or complementary control pathway for cell division, as well as a procell differentiation pathway; (c) insulinlike growth factor (IGF) signaling pathways as an alternative or complementary pathway for prostate cell division; and (d) clinical carcinogen metabolic pathways (especially those involving glutathione S-transferases). The latter is probably the least attractive epidemiologically, as nothing in the epidemiology of prostate cancer suggests any strong involvement of chemical carcinogens.

Genes that predispose to cancer are now usually organized into two main categories. The first category includes those single-locus genetic traits that in mutated forms directly cause cancer, typically with a high lifetime penetrance. It is these genes that are responsible for the very strong familial risk patterns seen for some cancers, including cancer of the prostate. The genetic basis for familial prostate cancer is discussed in detail elsewhere in this section and is addressed only minimally here. The other category of genes predisposed to cancer includes those that alter risk by participating in the formation, activation, transport, or metabolism of an endogenous or exogenous carcinogen. These genes have been generally identified by the candidate gene approach—that is, as noted previously, they have been investigated because their function has suggested a possible role in the development of a specific tumor. Mutations or functional polymorphisms in these genes alter risk of cancer indirectly, and typically these altered genes, in contrast to the true hereditary risk genes, carry with them only modest risk alterations. It is these genes that are emphasized below. As the true inherited forms of prostate cancer are rare (estimated to cause at most 9% of all disease), the single inherited susceptibility trait loci, despite the high absolute risk that they carry, account for a relatively small attributable risk. The high-risk alleles of the candidate genes, on the other hand, can be quite common in the population; therefore, despite low absolute risk, they may carry with them a more substantial attributable risk. Moreover, there is a growing consensus that multiple such genes may modify risk in the same etiologic pathway so that in combination these may account for an even larger fraction of all disease.

In seeking candidate genes for prostate cancer, a number of criteria should be applied. Obviously, the candidate gene should be chosen along a plausible biologic pathway. To be evaluated as a potential contributor to prostate cancer risk and to be studied by available epidemiologic means, the gene locus should be polymorphic or have one or more relatively common mutations (or multiple mutations that in combination are reasonably common) in the population. The polymorphisms or mutations, or both, must be shown to be functional—that is, they must change either quantitatively or qualitatively the function of the gene protein product as measured, for example, by *in vitro* transfection-type assays or by assessing biochemical phenotypes *in vivo* (alternatively, nonfunctional polymorphisms have been used epidemiologically with implied linkage to functional differences). Functional significance will reduce the likelihood that an association observed with prostate cancer is simply a chance observation or an artifact of underlying genetic variance between a population of prostate cancer patients and a comparison population that is unrelated to prostate cancer risk *per se*. As racial-ethnic variability is such a powerful feature of prostate cancer epidemiology, variability in the prevalence of the putative high-risk (or low-risk) allele corresponding to the ranking of different racial-ethnic groups in their respective prostate cancer incidence is also desirable. Finally, in studying candidate genes as risk factors for prostate cancer, one must consider the distinct possibility that a particular gene might contain multiple functional allelic loci and that any given individual could have both high and low risk functional loci within the same gene, perhaps resulting in that individual's having an overall risk of prostate cancer associated with that gene that is no different from the population as a whole.

ANDROGEN METABOLISM PATHWAYS

As there is substantial indirect evidence for a role of androgens in prostate cancer etiology, there is also strong rationale to investigate genetic control of androgen metabolism in relationship to prostate cancer risk (3). The primary role of androgens in regulating cell division in the prostate is undisputed and, in and of itself, makes a compelling argument for investigation of a role of androgen metabolic pathways in prostate cancer etiology (4). However, other evidence speaks to a likely role for androgens as well. Although it has historically been difficult to produce experimental models of prostate cancer with histologic or morphologic features that closely mimic the human disease and there still exist relatively few such models, those models that do exist uniformly require androgens for tumor induction or tumor progression, or both (5,6). Although proponents for an androgen role in prostate cancer development point to the fact that men with conditions of substantial androgen deficiency, such as eunuchs or men with constitutional 5α-reductase deficiency (the enzyme required for metabolic activation of testosterone in the prostate), not only have underdeveloped prostates but also have never been reported to develop prostate cancer, there has never in actuality been a systematic epidemiologic study of this question.

The difficulties in proving that high endogenous hormone levels (e.g., in blood or urine), such as androgens, cause a particular disease or that low levels protect against it have been the topic of previous detailed reviews (7). The most important of these include sporadic and episodic variations in the hormones under study, the imprecision of the laboratory assays to measure these hormones, and the usually unknown relationship between blood and urine levels (i.e., accessible biologic "compartments" for human studies) and target tissue levels, which are usually inaccessible on an individual basis and always inaccessible in large-scale population-based epidemiologic studies. Nonetheless, the best-designed prospective study on this issue (i.e., a study designed in such a way that baseline blood or urine samples are available on a large cohort of healthy men who are then followed for prostate cancer development) found that men in the highest quartile of circulating testosterone levels had a 2.4-fold increased risk of prostate cancer compared to men in the lowest quartile after allowing for levels of sex hormone–binding globulin, which is a protein that binds testosterone and makes it unavailable to target tissues (8).

There is evidence that androgens may explain a significant part of the racial-ethnic variation in prostate cancer incidence and mortality. African-American men have higher exposure to testosterone than their white and Asian counterparts (9,10). This exposure difference appears to start in the *in utero* period, because African-American women at any given point in early pregnancy have testosterone levels that exceed those of white women by 50% or more (11). This observation led Henderson and colleagues to speculate that these high testosterone exposures *in utero* might contribute to high prostate cancer rates later in life by permanently altering the *gonadostat*—that is, the hypothalamic-pituitary-testicular axis in African-Americans relative to whites—or by permanently altering the sensitivity of androgen target tissues in African-Americans relative to whites (12). Whatever the contribution of this *in utero* testosterone exposure, high testosterone levels in African-American men compared to whites also occur in young adulthood (9) but gradually decline through midlife (10). For men in their early 20s, this difference may be as large as 15% or more, but for men in their early 40s, circulating testosterone levels in African-American men average only roughly 3% higher than in whites (10). Nonetheless, differences of these magnitudes are sufficient to explain much of the excess risk of prostate cancer in African-Americans (9). An extension of this thinking would hypothesize higher testosterone levels in Asian populations, such as China or Japan. There is no evidence to support this notion. However, it is now well established that such Asian men have substantially reduced circulating levels of androstanediol glucuronide, a biochemical correlate of 5α-reductase activity (13,14). In fact, this observation provided a substantial part of the rationale for the ongoing national chemoprevention trial for prostate cancer using the 5α-reductase inhibitor finasteride (13).

The relationship between genetic control of androgen metabolic pathways and prostate cancer risk is just beginning to be understood. As there are literally hundreds of genes directly or indirectly involved in this pathway, a totally complete and detailed understanding of this relationship likely will not be forthcoming in the foreseeable future. Genes of particular interest currently include

1. Those involved in androgen biosynthesis. Among endogenous human androgens, testosterone and dihydrotestosterone are the most potent biologically, and of these two, testosterone produced primarily in the testes throughout life is by far the more abundant. Other androgens, such as dihydroepiandrosterone and its sulfate conjugate produced primarily in the adrenals, have some bioactivity in prostate cells, but they are qualitatively and, for the prostate at least, quantitatively unimportant. Among the genes involved in androgen biosynthesis in the prostate, only two have undergone preliminary evaluation directly or indirectly in relationship to prostate cancer. The CYP17 gene encodes a cytochrome p450 isozyme involved in key points in testosterone biosynthesis in the testes. The 3β-hydroxysteroid dehydrogenase type II gene encoding type II 3β-hydroxysteroid dehydrogenase catalyzes the conversion of androstenedione to testosterone in the testes and also (perhaps as a different isozyme) is one of the two enzymes involved in the inactivation of the highly bioactive androgen dihydrotestosterone in the prostate (it is discussed below in the context of this latter function).
2. Those involved in androgen transport and signal transduction. These genes encode products that transport androgens in blood (sex hormone–binding globulin) and in the prostate [the androgen receptor (AR)] and affect expression of target genes. The latter has been reasonably well-studied epidemiologically in relationship to prostate cancer.
3. Those involved in androgen metabolic activation [steroid 5α-reductase type II gene (SRD5A2)], and inactivation (e.g., 3α-hydroxysteroid dehydrogenase, type II 3β-hydroxysteroid dehydrogenase, and CYP3A4 genes). The former gene has been explored somewhat in relationship to prostate cancer risk, whereas the latter three are in the very initial stages of exploration.
4. Those downstream genes that are transactivated by the AR, such as the prostate-specific antigen gene. There have not yet been any reports related to this category of genes, many of which remain to be identified.

An overview of genetic control of androgen stimulation of the prostate is provided in Figure 9-1.

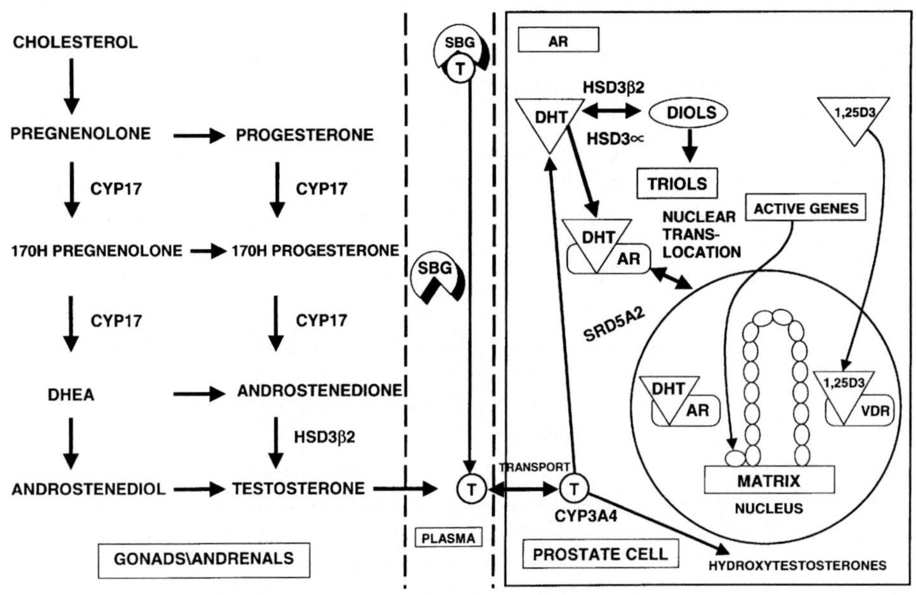

FIGURE 9-1. A diagram demonstrating the sites of activity of the gene products of certain candidate genes in the androgen metabolism and Vitamin D signaling pathways. AR, androgen receptor; DHT, dihydrotestosterone; HSD3α, 3α-hydroxysteroid dehydrogenase; HSD3β2, 3β-hydroxysteroid dehydrogenase type 2; SBG, sex hormone binding globulin; SRD5A2, steroid 5α-reductase type II; T, testosterone; $1{,}25D_3$, 1,25 dihydroxy vitamin D_3. (Adapted from Ross RK, Pike MC, Coetzee GA, et al. Androgen metabolism and prostate cancer: establishing a model of genetic susceptibility. *Cancer Res* 1998;58:4497–4504.)

Androgen Biosynthesis

The CYP17 gene encodes one of the p450 isozymes (cytochrome p450c17) that catalyzes key steps in testosterone biosynthesis in the testes and the adrenals (15). The gene, located on chromosome 10, contains a single base pair polymorphism near the promoter region that creates a recognition site for the restriction enzyme MspA1. This polymorphism results in two alleles, designated as A1 and A2, and is hypothesized to alter rate of transcription. This notion is supported by the observation that young women homozygous for the A2 allele have higher circulating estradiol levels (the enzyme also catalyzes steps in the biosynthesis of estrogens) than women homozygous for the A1 allele (16,17). Moreover, at least one study has shown this polymorphism to be related to risk of both male pattern baldness in men and polycystic ovarian disease in women, which are disorders strongly correlated with abnormal patterns of androgen biosynthesis and metabolism (15). No studies have yet been published on the relationship of this polymorphism to prostate cancer risk within or between racial-ethnic groups, but this would appear to be a strong candidate gene for further evaluation.

Androgen Transport

The AR gene, located on the long arm of the X chromosome, encodes a transcription factor, the AR, that serves multiple functions in prostatic epithelium, including binding of androgens (dihydrotestosterone and, with lesser affinity, testosterone), translocation of androgens to the nucleus for DNA binding, and transactivation of genes with androgen response elements in their promoter regions (18). Coetzee and Ross first proposed a specific role for the AR gene in prostate cancer risk mediated by a trinucleotide $(CAG)_n$ repeat polymorphism in exon 1 (19). They hypothesized that the length of this repeat might be inversely related to prostate cancer risk. The hypothesis was based primarily on observations related to Kennedy's disease (spinal and bulbar muscular atrophy), an adult-onset motor neuron disease. Kennedy's disease is an X-linked genetic disorder, and the single genetic defect causing this disorder is an expansion of the same CAG microsatellite (20). Men with Kennedy's disease have, on average, a doubling of the CAG repeat stretch that in men without the disorder has a range of 8 to approximately 36. Coetzee and Ross noted that men with this disorder, in addition to the neuromuscular problem characteristic of the disease, also showed evidence of suboptimal androgenization with testicular atrophy accompanied by reduced sperm production and reduced fertility and low virilization (21,22). They hypothesized that, because a doubling of this repeat length appeared to cause reduced androgen activity, differences in androgen activity might also occur within the normal size range of repeats—that is, low repeat length being associated with lower prostate androgen activity mediated through the AR than high repeat length. The hypothesis received indirect support from the correlation observed between CAG repeat length distribution and prostate cancer incidence rates among healthy men representing different racial-ethnic groups (19,23). Thus, African-American men with very high prostate cancer incidence have a relatively low average number of repeats, whereas Asian men (Chinese or Japanese) with low prostate cancer incidence have a relatively high number, and white men at intermediate risk have an intermediate range of repeats.

Subsequently, the hypothesis received further support from both clinical observations and *in vitro* experimental results. Clinically, men with impaired sperm production and associated infertility are more likely than otherwise healthy men to have CAG repeat lengths in the long end of the normal range (24). Moreover, not only do AR genes with the expanded CAG repeat lengths cloned from patients with Kennedy's disease have reduced androgen transactivation activity in transfection assays (despite normal binding of androgens to the receptor), but there is also a negative correlation between CAG repeat length and transactivation with AR genes cloned from healthy men (25). In fact, total elimination of the CAG repeat causes a marked elevation in transactivation *in vitro* (26). Ingles et al. eventually tested this hypothesis directly and demonstrated in a population-based case-control study among white residents of Los Angeles County that a low number of CAG repeat sequences are associated with a high risk of prostate cancer and that this association was particularly noteworthy for men who presented with advanced disease (27). This observation has been independently confirmed through two other studies (28,29). The results of these three studies are summarized in Table 9-1.

Details of the familial risk patterns observed with prostate cancer are discussed elsewhere in Chapter 10. Most studies have found a *skip pattern* of familial prostate cancer risk across generations—that is, that men with prostate cancer–affected brothers have approximately twice the risk of men with prostate cancer–affected fathers (whose risk is nonetheless still higher than the general population) (30,31). Although the AR gene is on the X chromosome, and this inheritance pattern suggests a possible X-linked disorder, there is no direct evidence of AR gene linkage in multiplex prostate cancer families (32). Nonetheless, a second polymorphic marker in the AR gene, a *Stu*I restriction fragment–length polymorphism, which, like the $(CAG)_n$ microsatellite, is located in exon 1 and has been reported preliminarily to be associated with familial prostate cancer. An excess proportion of the S1 allele (cut by the restriction enzyme) was found by Crocitto et al. among prostate cancer patients with an affected brother (12 of 14; 86%) compared to men without such a family history (118 of 204; 58%) (33).

Androgen Metabolism and Inactivation

Metabolic activation of testosterone to dihydrotestosterone in the prostate is regulated by a single enzyme, steroid 5α-

TABLE 9-1. SUMMARY OF STUDIES OF THE $(CAG)_N$ REPEAT OF THE ANDROGEN RECEPTOR GENE AND PROSTATE CANCER RISK

Reference	CAG comparison	Subgroup	Relative risk	95% CI
Stanford et al. (27)	≥22	Reference		
	<22	Family Hx positive	1.6	0.6, 4.1
	<22	Short GGN (≤16)	2.1	1.1, 3.8
	<22	<60 yr	1.5	0.96, 2.3
Ingles et al. (28)	≥20	Reference		
	<20	"Advanced"	2.4	1.02, 5.49
Giovannucci et al. (29)	≥26	Reference		
	≤18	"High grade or stage"	2.14	1.14, 4.01

CI, confidence interval; Hx, history.

reductase type II (34). This enzyme is encoded by the SRD5A2 gene on chromosome 2p. Germline mutations of SRD5A2 are rare, but in inbred kindreds, in which homozygous mutations occur, lead to substantially altered phenotype. Boys with the mutated gene are phenotypically female at birth. With increased testosterone production at puberty, these boys have development of secondary sex characteristics but sustain no substantial prostate development (35).

Several polymorphic markers of SRD5A2 have been preliminarily evaluated in relationship to prostate cancer risk and also in terms of prevalence of variant alleles across racial-ethnic groups. These studies have been conducted primarily in the laboratory of Reichardt and colleagues (36–39). The initial work by this laboratory was to evaluate the importance of SRD5A2 to prostate cancer risk focused on a $(TA)_n$ dinucleotide repeat in the 3' untranslated region (UTR) of the gene (37). Interest in this marker was stimulated primarily by the observation that there were unique alleles in Asians and African-Americans (especially a series of expanded repeat alleles unique to African-Americans) that in preliminary analyses appeared to convey increased prostate cancer risk (37). However, an expanded data set evaluated by Reichardt's group and an independent data set evaluated by others (40) were unable to find any consistent relationship between this marker and prostate cancer risk.

Reichardt's laboratory has also identified a series of seven missense mutations in SRD5A2 (resulting in an altered amino acid), several of which seem promising in terms of predicting prostate cancer risk (36). In particular, a valine-to-leucine substitution mutation at codon 89 (V89L) correlates with circulating levels of androstanediol glucuronide, the biochemical index of whole-body 5α-reductase activity, with valine homozygotes having levels approximately 40% higher than leucine homozygotes, with valine-leucine heterozygotes having intermediate levels (38). Consistent with these biochemical results, Japanese and Chinese men have a much lower prevalence of valine homozygotes (29%) than African-Americans (59%) or whites (57%) but a much higher prevalence of leucine homozygotes (22%) than these other two groups (3% and 4%, respectively) (38).

A second missense mutation has already been preliminarily evaluated in relationship to prostate cancer risk, with complex results. This mutation, an alanine-to-threonine substitution at codon 49, is substantially less common than the V89L mutation. However, Reichardt and colleagues have shown that African-American and Latino men who carry a T allele are at very high risk of advanced prostate cancer (relative risks of 10.6 and 4.5, respectively), with associated *p* values of .001 and .040, compared to alanine homozygotes (39). Risk levels are also modestly elevated for localized disease for these two groups. Preliminary data for Japanese and white men, however, do not support a comparable elevated risk associated with presence of a T allele in these racial groups. Reichardt's laboratory has provided *in vitro* support for functional changes in 5α-reductase activity induced by these mutations (39). Using a site-directed mutagenesis approach, they have demonstrated, for example, that the alanine-to-threonine substitution at codon 49 enzyme has a fivefold higher V_{max} for testosterone conversion than the wild type, whereas the V89L mutation shows a roughly 33% reduction in activity.

The 3β-hydroxysteroid dehydrogenase type II (HSD3B2) gene encodes type II 3β-hydroxysteroid dehydrogenase that, together with 3α-hydroxysteroid dehydrogenase, is one of the principal enzymes initiating inactivation of dihydrotestosterone in the prostate (40). This enzyme (most likely a different isoform) also catalyzes the final step in the biosynthetic pathway for testosterone in the testes. The HSD3B2 gene is located on the short arm of chromosome 1, and a complex, highly polymorphic dinucleotide repeat $[(TG)_n (TA)_n (CA)_n]$ has been identified in intron 3 (41). Twenty-five distinct alleles of this polymorphism have been identified in a screen of 312 healthy individuals with substantial heterogeneity across racial-ethnic groups at the extremes of prostate cancer risk (42). No functional relevance has been attached to this marker, however, in terms of differential rates of dihydrotestosterone degradation or testosterone biosynthesis. It is probable that full-scale sequencing of the gene in individuals of different racial-ethnic groups, especially those with variant biochemical phenotypes (e.g., high or low circulating testosterone or high or low circulating androstanediol glucuronide), will establish additional missense mutations or polymorphisms, which can then undergo more rigorous epidemiologic investigations.

Another candidate gene in the androgen-deactivation component of the androgen metabolism pathway is CYP3A4, whose product is involved in oxidation of testosterone to a series of biologically inactive metabolites in the prostate, including 2β-, 6β-, and 15β-hydroxytestosterone (43). Rebbeck and colleagues have conducted the only study of this gene to date related to human prostate cancer (44). They compared genotype frequency in a series of high-grade or advanced-stage prostate cancer, or both, to a series of low-grade or early-stage tumors, or both, using an A to G mutation in a regulatory element in the 5' region of the CYP3A4 gene (44). This mutation has been hypothesized to explain some of the substantial individual variations observed in oxidative testosterone metabolism (45). In this study, men carrying the variant allele (CYP3A4-V) were substantially more likely to have advanced stage tumors than men with wild-type genotype, especially men who were relatively old (older than 63 years of age) and without a family history of prostate cancer (44). Forty-six percent of men with advanced tumors in this group carried a variant allele, compared to just 5% of men in the group with early-stage disease (odds ratio, 9.5; $p < .001$) (44).

VITAMIN D METABOLISM PATHWAYS

The hypothesis that vitamin D activity might modify prostate cancer risk is built around a series of epidemiologic observations and experimental results. The epidemiologic evidence alone is not compelling, based initially on the ecologic observation that prostate cancer mortality rates are correlated with latitude of residence on a geographic basis that, in turn, is inversely correlated with exposure to ultraviolet radiation, the major inducer of endogenously synthesized vitamin D (45,46). In one prospective study conducted in Northern California, men who developed prostate cancer had significantly lower levels of 1,25-dihydroxyvitamin D, the active form of vitamin D, than men who did not regardless of the level of 25-hydroxyvitamin D, the vitamin D parent compound (47). However, other prospective studies, including the Physicians' Health Study, found no such overall relationship (48). A case-control study in North Carolina also found no relationship between 1,25-dihydroxyvitamin D levels and prostate cancer risk but did find that high levels of vitamin D–binding protein were associated with increased risk (45). As only unbound vitamin D is bioavailable, this finding may be compatible with a protective influence of vitamin D.

Although cutaneous production of vitamin D induced by sunlight exposure is the principal source of circulating vitamin D, vitamin D–fortified foods represent an additional important source. Most epidemiologic studies have found no clear relationship between dietary sources of vitamin D and prostate cancer risk when dietary fat (a strong dietary correlate of vitamin D and probable prostate cancer risk factor) is taken into account (49). In the prospective Physicians' Health Study, a positive association was observed between estimated dietary intake of calcium and prostate cancer risk that the authors speculated might be due to a suppressive effect of calcium on conversion of 25-hydroxyvitamin D to 1,25-dihydroxyvitamin D (50). More details on the relationship between dietary sources of vitamin D and prostate cancer risk can be found in Chapter 8.

Experimental data provide more substantial support for a protective influence of vitamin D on prostate cancer risk. 1,25-Dihydroxyvitamin D is a potent inhibitor of prostatic cell proliferation *in vitro* (51) and also promotes differentiation of prostate epithelial cells, thereby making them less susceptible to malignant transformation (51,52). As prostate cells themselves produce substantial amounts of 1,25-hydroxyvitamin D, cell proliferation modulation by vitamin D can be regulated in an autocrine or paracrine manner (53). Vitamin D experimentally also contributes to prostate cancer progression, reducing metastatic potential and prostate cancer volume in rat models (54,55). Vitamin D decreases metalloproteinases that degrade cell matrix, allowing prostate cancer invasion (56).

Vitamin D activity is mediated through the vitamin D receptor (VDR) (Fig. 9-1). The VDR gene is located on chromosome 12 and contains eight exons (57). A number of polymorphisms have been identified in the VDR gene. Several restriction fragment–length polymorphisms exist in and around the 3' UTR of the VDR gene. One of these, a *Bsm*I restriction enzyme polymorphism in intron 8 that has been associated with indices of bone mineral density (58), and a polymorphic polyA microsatellite in the 3' UTR has been studied preliminarily in relation to prostate cancer risk (27,59). The polyA microsatellite is bimodal, so that alleles can be classified as long or short polyA stretches. In a small population-based case-control study of prostate cancer in non-Latino whites in Los Angeles County involving 57 men younger than age 65 with prostate cancer and 169 population controls of similar age, Ingles et al. reported that men with at least one long A allele had a 4.6-fold increase in risk [95% confidence interval (CI), 1.3, 15.8] of prostate cancer compared to men homozygous for short A alleles (27). This effect was more pronounced for advanced disease (of the 26 patients tested with advanced disease, all had at least one long A allele vs. 36 of 169 controls). The comparable odds ratio for localized disease (prostate cancer that had not invaded the prostate cancer capsule) was 2.3 (95% CI, 0.7, 9.9) (27). Ingles et al. have shown that in whites (but not African-Americans), the *Bsm*I restriction site is in tight linkage disequilibrium with the polyA locus, so that prostate cancer risk levels associated with *Bsm*I alleles are comparable to those observed for the polyA locus (long A linked with the *Bsm*I b allele) (58). Another restriction fragment–length polymorphism in the 3' UTR, a *Taq*I that recognizes a silent single nucleotide substitution, is also in linkage disequilibrium with both the *Bsm*I and polyA loci (60). Taylor et al., in a case-control study of whites, showed that individuals with a *Taq*I T allele have a threefold increase in prostate cancer risk compared to individuals who are tt homozygotes (59).

Only one study has been conducted of the VDR gene and prostate cancer risk in African-Americans, and no studies have been reported to date in Asians. Ingles et al. examined VDR genotypes in 151 African-American prostate cancer patients (49 advanced, 102 localized) and 174 African-American controls (61). As noted earlier, this group of investigators had demonstrated that, in African-Americans, there is at best only weak linkage disequilibrium in the 3' UTR region of the gene. To study the polymorphic markers of interest in African-Americans, they devised a direct *Bsm*I/polyA haplotyping assay. African-American individuals with one or more *Bsm*IB/long polyA (L) haplotypes had a twofold or more increase in risk of advanced prostate cancer compared to individuals with no BL haplotypes (61).

One other study evaluated a VDR gene polymorphism in conjunction with circulating vitamin D levels and prostate cancer risk (62). The *Bsm*I genotype was associated with a substantial increase in prostate cancer risk, but only in men with low circulating levels of 25-hydroxyvitamin D.

INSULINLIKE GROWTH FACTOR SIGNALING PATHWAYS

IGF signaling pathways have received much attention recently, not only with regard to prostate cancer risk, but also as a common major etiologic pathway for multiple cancer sites (63). IGF-1 stimulates cell proliferation and reduces apoptosis (programmed cell death) *in vitro* in both normal and malignant prostate epithelium (64,65). The first indication that IGF-1 might be associated with prostate cancer was from a small case-control study demonstrating that IGF-1 levels were substantially higher in the prostate cancer patients than controls (66). However, a case-control study design is not ideal to test this hypothesis, because the presence of the cancer may alter IGF-1 levels. By far, the best study of this relationship to date was conducted in the context of the Physicians' Health Study, a prospective study in which nearly 15,000 men who provided blood samples at baseline have been systematically followed for prostate cancer and other chronic disease occurrence (67). After approximately 7 years of follow-up, 152 prostate cancer patients and 152 age- and smoking-matched controls were analyzed. In multivariate analysis controlling for levels of IGF-binding protein (IGFBP) 3 (the major IGFBP in the circulation), men in the second, third, and fourth quartiles of IGF-1 had 1.9, 2.8, and 4.3 times the risk of prostate cancer compared to men in the lowest quartile [p (trend) = .001]. The molecular genetics of IGF-biosynthesis and -binding as they relate to prostate cancer risk are unstudied but of obvious interest to further understand this relationship. A $(CA)_n$ dinucleotide repeat has been described in the promoter region of the IGF-1 gene, and allelic variation is correlated with circulating IGF-1 levels (68). Several polymorphisms of unknown functional relevance have also been described in the IGFBP 3 gene (69).

CHEMICAL CARCINOGEN METABOLIC PATHWAYS

Many human chemical carcinogens require metabolic activation *in vivo* to reach their full carcinogenic potential. This metabolic activation is regulated by a large series of enzymes, including many of the large family of cytochrome p450 isozymes, which collectively have been designated *phase I enzymes*. On the other hand, another series of enzymes designated *phase II* are largely responsible for deactivating chemical carcinogens *in vivo* and facilitating excretion. Many of the genes that encode these enzymes are polymorphic, with established functional differences among genotypes defined by these polymorphic markers. The role of these enzymes in modifying cancer risk after an environmental exposure is the subject of much current scientific interest. Nonetheless, this area of research has received little attention related to prostate cancer risk, as no specific environmental chemical exposure has ever been linked convincingly to prostate cancer, and the epidemiology of the disease does not support a strong environmental risk component. For example, there is no strong link to urbanization, no consistent relationship with socioeconomic status, and no accepted association with broad or specific categories of occupation or industry (1).

One of the phase II enzymes, glutathione S-transferase P1 (GSTP1), has been preliminarily investigated in relationship to prostate cancer in a tissue-based study. Lee and colleagues found that only 3 of 91 prostate cancers analyzed expressed GSTP1, suggesting that reduced activity of this phase II detoxifying enzyme might be involved in prostate carcinogenesis (71). Moreover, this group of investigators found that reduced expression was uniformly associated with hypermethylation of regulatory sequences of GSTP1 [*hypermethylation* is an alternative epigenetic mechanism to mutation or loss of heterozygosity (LOH) in "silencing" genes] (71). The significance of these findings in prostate cancer development remains unclear but is clearly worthy of further exploration.

MOLECULAR GENETICS OF PROGRESSION OF PROSTATE CANCER

It is widely believed that cancer progression involves sequential *genetic* steps, each having the pivotal features of somatic (as opposed to germline) genetic change that provides the cells with a selective growth advantage over their neighboring cells. In some cancers, these steps likely occur in a series, as proposed for colorectal cancer (72), or in others progression proceeds down alternative parallel paths with different potential for invasion and aggressiveness, as proposed for bladder cancer (73). However, the molecular genetics of progression are not well understood for prostate cancer, and no clear single pathway of required genetic changes has yet emerged. This lack of knowledge is particularly troublesome for prostate cancer because, as noted earlier, rates of occult, subclinical prostate cancer are very high, yet only a small proportion of these lesions progress to meaningful, clinically relevant disease with the potential to invade, metastasize, and kill. It is very likely that progression has a strong genetic component, and, hence, the identification of genetic markers for the transition to advanced disease carries tremendous public health implications.

A somatic change at a candidate genetic locus for tumor progression is often indicated by a LOH, in which a large part of or a whole chromosome is lost from the cell. Such events normally point to the possible location of a tumor suppressor gene (i.e., a gene that functions normally in maintaining normal cell growth; LOH results in loss of a wild-type allele, after which the remaining allele must be inactivated at random; by mutation; or by an epigenetic event, such as methylation). After each event (LOH and mutation), cell clones with a growth advantage are selected. Growth advantage is bestowed because the one allele only or the mutant, or both, are unable to suppress cell growth. In prostate cancer, chromosomes 8p, 10q, and 16q show LOH in a high percentage of tumors, indicating the likely presence of prostate tumor suppressor genes in these regions (74,75). Losses in 18q (76) and 17q (77) are less commonly found.

Another indication of loci of tumor suppression is revealed by the technique of *in vitro* chromosome transfer. This technique has shown that some regions in chromosomes 8 and 11 suppress prostate cell metastases (78,79), whereas chromosome region 12pter-12q13 suppresses prostate tumorigenicity (80).

Somatic alterations in chromosomes related to prostate cancer have also been studied more recently by comparative genomic hybridization analyses [summarized in (81)]; genetic losses and gains are eloquently revealed by this technique. Chromosome arms that are lost more often in hormone-resistant (typically more advanced in the end-fatal prostate cancer) than in primary prostate tumors are 1p, 10q, 19p, 19q, 20p, and 20q, whereas gains are recorded in 8q, 18q, and Xq. The gain in Xq is most likely due to amplification in the AR gene located on Xq12 (see below).

As in cancer etiology, candidate genes based on gene function have been investigated in prostate cancer progression primarily by hunting for the presence of somatic mutations. In prostate cancer, candidate gene mutations have been detected in *Mxi*-1 (82), *KAI*1 (83), *TP53* (84), *RB* (85), and in the DNA polymerase β gene (86). Evidence that these genes might be "progression" genes is based on the observation that the mutations are considerably more common in metastatic lesions than in localized primary tumors.

To fully understand prostate cancer progression requires the development of a disease progression model showing how multiple genes can be altered in combination to allow a cell to change from a normal one to one with metastatic potential. None of the previously mentioned somatic changes has yet been put into such a disease progression pathway owing to, in part, their unknown functions or relatively low frequencies of occurrence.

Prostate tumors, for the most part, depend on androgen stimulation for growth, and even resistance to androgen ablation seems to be a consequence of deregulated androgen signaling rather than total loss of androgen sensitivity (see below). Thus, genetic changes in genes involved in androgen metabolic pathways, such as the AR locus, potentially provide a unifying mechanism to explain how prostate cancer progresses to advanced disease (87). Importantly, the AR gene is X-linked, and, therefore, only a single copy is present in male cells. LOH is therefore irrelevant in the case of the AR gene in men.

In recent years, it has become increasingly apparent that abnormal AR gain of function genetic alterations contribute to at least a subset of advanced prostate cancer. The expression of the AR is also maintained in all advanced prostate cancer (88–91), and AR-negative prostate tumors may not exist, indicating that the AR maintains a role during prostate cancer progression. Somatic mutations that increase AR activity or broaden AR ligand specificity have been identified in prostate tumors and prostate cancer–derived cell lines [references in (92)]. Even androgen antagonists (e.g., hydroxyflutamide) are able to activate certain mutant ARs (92–95). In addition, amplification of the AR gene has been identified in up to 30% of locally recurrent prostate tumors [see below and (96)].

Somatic mutations in the AR occur in a subset of advanced prostate tumors, but the exact frequency has not been determined accurately (97). Furthermore, the relationships of these mutations to androgen ablation therapies remain vague. Initial studies indicated that AR gene mutations in clinical prostate cancer might be an uncommon occurrence. However, earlier investigations assessed only exons 2 through 8 of the gene. As exon 1 comprises 58% of the AR coding sequence and is difficult to polymerase chain reaction amplify, owing to GC-rich stretches, the low frequencies of AR mutations reported in these studies might be due to this incomplete screening (97). Recent advances, such as the discovery and development of polymerases with higher efficiencies and greater temperature stabilities than the traditional Taq polymerase, or the use of additives (TritonX100 or dimethyl sulfoxide, or both), have allowed for the efficient amplification of all areas of the AR. In one study in which the entire AR coding sequence was investigated, Tilley et al. found mutations in 11 of 25 (44%) primary tumors (87). They were either missense or nonsense mutations, and 50% occurred in exon 1. Several additional somatic mutations have since been found in exon 1 (W. D. Tilley et al., *personal communication*). These results indicate that a relatively large proportion of prostate tumors, at least in advanced stage, may contain AR mutations. More work is needed to determine accurately the frequency of AR mutations in prostate cancer especially across different stages of disease.

The role(s) of the altered AR becomes critical in maximizing the efficacy of treatment of the disease. The most effective primary treatment for advanced prostate cancer is the so-called hormone deprivation therapy, which results in a reduction in testosterone levels or an inhibition of the effects of the hormone on prostate cells, or both. However, this treatment is not a cure, and men die of prostate cancer as a result of the inevitable failure of hormone deprivation treatments (98).

Hormone manipulation as primary prostate cancer therapy can be divided into two main strategies—namely, partial and complete androgen blockades. Partial androgen blockade is achieved by the suppression of testicular androgens either by castration or by high-dose treatment with either estrogen or luteinizing hormone releasing hormone analogs. Although this strategy does not reduce serum testosterone levels completely, nor does it suppress adrenal androgens, it nonetheless results in tumor regression in 80% to 85% of men with metastatic prostate cancer. Complete androgen blockade is normally achieved through the additional use of competitive AR inhibitors. This strategy inhibits androgen action at the level of the receptor and, as a result, is indiscriminate of the androgen source. Although some evidence supports the use of competitive AR inhibitors, such as hydroxyflutamide, to produce complete androgen blockade as an effective form of hormone treatment for prostate cancer, the high cost of the drugs and the poor tolerance by some men have discouraged their universal use in the treatment of advanced prostate cancer. A treatment modality in which gonadal androgen blockade is followed some time later by flutamide treatment (*deferred flutamide treatment*) has been proposed (99). Such a strategy provides enhanced disease control in patients with localized prostate cancer due to the greater density of androgen-dependent tumor cells after gonadal androgen ablation. Thus, standard treatment for localized or advanced prostate cancer often involves some type of hormonal manipulation with partial or complete androgen blockade (simultaneously or deferred). As the target for each of these treatments is the AR, these regimens themselves may impose selective pressure for genetic alterations at the AR locus.

In the case of partial androgen blockade, evidence indicates that cells with AR gene amplifications selected for by low androgen levels might cause hormone-refractory disease. Koivisto et al. (96) identified significant amplification of the AR gene in 30% of recurrent prostate tumors. Amplification was found only in patients in whom recurrence was diagnosed after an average of 30 months of partial blockade with estrogen therapy or orchiectomy. These results suggest that AR amplification emerged during androgen-deprivation therapy by facilitating tumor cell growth in low androgen concentrations. AR gene amplification was associated with substantially increased messenger RNA levels, as determined by *in situ* hybridization. AR amplification also occurred more often in tumors that initially responded to endocrine treatment and whose response lasted for at least one year. Clearly, cell clones with AR amplifications seem to be selected for as a consequence of partial androgen blockade.

In the case of complete androgen blockade, evidence indicates that refractory tumors arise through a related mechanism as a consequence of gain of function mutations in the AR gene. One of the first clues that AR point mutations might be selected for in hormone-refractory disease came from the recognition of the clinical phenomenon known as *flutamide withdrawal syndrome*. After an initial period of response to complete androgen blockade, tumors eventually become refractory, but approximately 10% to 75% of these prostate cancer patients experience a significant tumor response or stabilization brought about by the discontinuation of antiandrogens, such as flutamide (100–102). Although the precise mechanism for this paradoxic response in hormone-refractory prostate cancer to flutamide withdrawal is not entirely clear, evidence suggests that it might be due to specific mutations in the AR. Such mutations must result in a gain of function to allow for flutamide-dependent growth selection, as the alternative (i.e., loss of function mutations) is highly unlikely to result in the emergence of androgen-independent growth (because there would be no selective growth advantage for cells harboring an inactive AR during androgen-dependent phases of tumor growth).

Thus, it is possible to view the AR gene as a protooncogene that, when functioning normally, orchestrates both the development and differentiation of the prostate under normal endocrine control. However, during tumorigenesis, the AR gene acquires gain of function mutations or undergoes gene amplification, or both, providing cancer cells with a selective growth advantage under conditions that previously precluded normal prostate epithelial proliferation.

Even in cases in which no AR involvement is suspected (e.g., advanced hormone-independent prostate cancers) and no AR amplification events or mutations have been detected, the AR could still be involved in an androgen-independent manner. For example, peptide growth factors, such as IGF, keratinocyte growth factor, and epidermal growth factor, are all able to activate AR-mediated signaling (103,104). In addition, activators of protein kinase A (forskolin, which acts by increasing cyclic adenosine monophosphate) also activate the AR in the absence of androgens (105), and even widely used luteinizing hormone releasing hormone analogs (used in prostate cancer hormone therapies) weakly activate the AR in the absence of androgens and strongly in their presence (106). Recently, it was found that androgen-independent induction of the AR-responsive gene, prostate-specific antigen, occurs via cross-talk between the AR and protein kinase A signal transduction pathways (107). Alternate mechanisms for hormone-independent prostate cancer are proposed to involve AR signaling via Her2/neu (108,109) or mitogen-activated protein kinase 1–activated phosphorylation steps (110). These studies indicate that androgen-independent cancer does not, *ipso facto*, mean AR independence.

The mechanistic reasons as to why prostate epithelial cells may remain AR dependent even in advanced disease is not clear; however, it could be due, in part, to the type and level of "downstream" gene activation mediated by the AR. A number of androgen-regulated genes have been identified and include PSA (111), prostate-specific membrane antigen (112), epidermal growth factor receptor (113), fibroblast growth factor 2 (114), calreticulin (115), IGFBP 3 (116) and 5 (117), the homeobox gene Nkx3.1 (118,119), apolipoprotein D (120), the AR coactivator ARA70 (119), the AR itself (121,122), and kallikreinlike genes (123). Exactly how these different genes with vastly different functions fit into a proliferation or apoptosis model, or both, however, is not clear. Also, possible differences in the expression profile of these genes in hormone-responsive versus -independent tumors are currently not known, nor are the implications of altered AR transactivation selected for during different hormone treatment strategies. A recent study showed that the AR transduces the androgen signal by influencing the expression of genes involved in the G1 to S transition of the cell cycle (124), including cdk1 and cdk2 (119).

The exact mechanism(s) behind the inevitable failure of androgen ablation therapies in most patients remains largely unknown, however, and hormone-independent prostate cancer has a dismal prognosis. As a result, oncologists faced with making difficult decisions as to how best to treat metastatic hormone–independent prostate cancer are left with few effective options. If it is true that in most cases of hormone-refractory disease, tumor growth remains AR dependent, a treatment strategy that targets specifically the AR might have utility. The aim would be to ablate the AR signaling axis, enabling inhibition of both ligand-dependent and -independent AR signaling. Examples of such approaches are the use of AR antisense or AR-dominant negative constructs in gene therapy protocols. Development of such novel therapies may help in effectively treating this devastating disease.

REFERENCES

1. Ross RK, Schottenfeld D. Prostate cancer. In: Schottenfeld D, Fraumeni JF, eds. *Cancer epidemiology and prevention,* 2nd ed. New York: Oxford University Press, 1996.
2. Yatani R, Chigusa I, Akazaki K, et al. Geographic pathology of latent prostatic carcinoma. *Int J Cancer* 1982;29:611–616.
3. Ross RK, Pike MC, Coetzee GA, et al. Androgen metabolism and prostate cancer: establishing a model of genetic susceptibility. *Cancer Res* 1998;58:4497–4504.
4. Coffey DS. Physiological control of prostatic growth: an overview. In: *Prostate cancer*. 1979.
5. Noble RL. The development of prostatic adenocarcinoma in Nb rats following prolonged sex hormone administration. *Cancer Res* 1977;37:1929–1933.
6. Gingrich JR, Barrios RJ, Morton RA, et al. Metastatic prostate cancer in a transgenic mouse. *Cancer Res* 1996;56: 4096–4102.
7. Bernstein L, Ross RK. Endogenous hormones and breast cancer risk. *Epidemiol Rev* 1993;15:48–65.
8. Gann PH, Hennekens CH, Ma J, et al. Prospective study of sex hormone levels and risk of prostate cancer. *J Natl Cancer Inst* 1996;88:1118–1126.
9. Ross RK, Bernstein L, Judd H, et al. Serum testosterone levels in healthy young black and white men. *J Natl Cancer Inst* 1986;76:45–48.
10. Ellis L, Nyburg H. Racial/ethnic variation in male testosterone levels: a probable contributor to group differences in health. *Steroids* 1992;57:72–75.
11. Henderson BE, Bernstein L, Ross RK, et al. The early *in utero* estrogen and testosterone environment of blacks and whites: potential effects on male offspring. *Br J Cancer* 1988;57:216–218.
12. Ross RK, Henderson BE. Do diet and androgens alter prostate cancer risk via a common etiologic pathway? *J Natl Cancer Inst* 1994;86:252–254.
13. Ross RK, Bernstein L, Lobo RA, et al. 5-Alpha reductase activity and risk of prostate cancer among Japanese and US white and black males. *Lancet* 1992;339:887–889.
14. Lookingbill DP, Demers LM, Wang C, et al. Clinical and biochemical parameters of androgen action in normal healthy Caucasian versus Chinese subjects. *J Clin Endocrinol Metab* 1991;72:1242–1248.
15. Carey AH, Waterworth D, Patel K, et al. Polycystic ovaries and premature male pattern baldness are associated with one allele of the steroid metabolism gene CYP17. *Hum Mol Genet* 1994;3:1873–1876.
16. Feigelson HS, Coetzee GA, Kolonel LN, et al. A polymorphism in the CYP17 gene increases the risk of breast cancer. *Cancer Res* 1997;57:1063–1065.

17. Haiman CA, Hankinson SE, Spiegelman D, et al. The relationship between a polymorphism in CYP17 with plasma hormone levels and breast cancer. *Cancer Res* 1999;59:1015–1020.
18. Clark JH, Schräder WT, O'Malley B. Mechanisms of action of steroid hormones. In: Wilson JD, Foster DW, eds. *Williams textbook of endocrinology*. Philadelphia: WB Saunders, 1992.
19. Coetzee GA, Ross RK. Prostate cancer and the androgen receptor. *J Natl Cancer Inst* 1994;86:872–873.
20. La Spada AR, Wilson EM, Lubahn DB, et al. Androgen receptor gene mutations in X-linked spinal and bulbar muscular atrophy. *Nature* 1991;352:77–79.
21. Arbizu T, Santamaria J, Gomex JM, et al. A family with adult spinal and bulbar muscular atrophy X-linked inheritance and associated with testicular failure. *J Neurol Sci* 1983;59:371–382.
22. Nagashima T, Seko K, Hirose K, et al. Familial bulbo-spinal muscular atrophy associated with testicular atrophy and sensory neuropathy (Kennedy-Alter-Sung syndrome). Autopsy case report of two brothers. *J Neurol Sci* 1988;87:141–152.
23. Edwards A, Hammond HA, Jin L, et al. Genetic variation at five trimeric and tetrameric tandem repeat loci in four human population groups. *Genomics* 1992;12:241–253.
24. Tut T, Ghadessy FJ, Trifiro MA, et al. Long polyglutamine tracts in the androgen receptor are associated with reduced trans-activation, impaired sperm production, and male infertility. *J Clin Endocrinol Metab* 1997;82:3777–3782.
25. Chamberlain NL, Driver ED, Miesfeld RL. The length and location of CAG trinucleotide repeats in the androgen receptor N-terminal domain affect transactivation function. *Nucleic Acids Res* 1994;22:3181–3186.
26. Chamberlain NL, Whitacre DC, Miesfeld RL. Delineation of two distinct type 1 activation functions in the androgen receptor amino-terminal domain. *J Biol Chem* 1996;271: 26772–26778.
27. Ingles SA, Ross RK, Yu MC, et al. Association of prostate cancer risk with genetic polymorphisms in vitamin D receptor and androgen receptor. *J Natl Cancer Inst* 1997;89:166–170.
28. Stanford JL, Just JJ, Gibbs M, et al. Polymorphic repeats in the androgen receptor gene: molecular markers of prostate cancer risk. *Cancer Res* 1997;57:1194–1198.
29. Giovannucci E, Stampfer MJ, Krithivas K, et al. The CAG repeat within the androgen receptor gene and its relationship to prostate cancer. *Proc Natl Acad Sci U S A* 1997;94:3320–3323.
30. Monroe KR, Yu MC, Kolonel LN, et al. Evidence of an X-linked genetic component to prostate cancer risk. *Nat Med* 1995;1:827–829.
31. Narod SA, Dupont A, Cusan L, et al. The impact of family history on early detection of prostate cancer. *Nat Med* 1995;1:99–101.
32. Sun S, Narod SA, Aprikian A, et al. Androgen receptor and familial prostate cancer. *Nat Med* 1995;1:848–849.
33. Crocitto LE, Irvine RA, Ross RK, et al. Association of allelic variation at the androgen receptor locus with prostate cancer risk in African-American high-risk families (submitted).
34. Wilson JD, Griffin JE, Russell DW. Steroid 5 α-reductase 2 deficiency. *Br J Cancer* 1993;14:577–593.
35. Thigpen AE, Davis DL, Gautier T, et al. The molecular basis of steroid 5-alpha-reductase deficiency in a large Dominican kindren. *N Engl J Med* 1992;327:1216–1219.
36. Reichardt JKV, Makridakis N, Henderson BE, et al. Genetic variability of the human SRD5A2 gene: implications for prostate cancer risk. *Cancer Res* 1995;55:3973–3975.
37. Ross RK, Coetzee GA, Reichardt J, et al. Does the racial-ethnic variation in prostate cancer risk have a hormonal basis? *Cancer* 1995;75:1778–1782.
38. Makridakis N, Ross RK, Pike MC, et al. A prevalent missense substitution that modulates activity of prostatic steroid 5α-reductase. *Cancer Res* 1997;57:1020–1022.
39. Reichardt JKV, Makridakis NM, Ross RK, et al. A missense mutation in the SRD5A2 gene with a significant population-attributable risk for clinically apparent prostate-cancer through increased dihydrotestosterone biosynthesis (in press).
40. Geissler WM, Davis DL, Wu L, et al. Male pseudohermaphroditism caused by mutations of testicular 17β-hydroxysteroid dehydrogenase 3. *Nat Genet* 1994;7:34–39.
41. Verreault H, Dufort I, Simard J, et al. Dinucleotide repeat polymorphisms in the HSD3B2 gene. *Hum Mol Genet* 1994;3:384.
42. Devgan SA, Henderson BE, Yu MC, et al. Genetic variation of 3β-hydroxysteroid dehydrogenase type II in three racial/ethnic groups: implications for prostate cancer risk. *Prostate* 1997;33:9–12.
43. Waxman DJ, Attisano C, Guengerich FP, et al. Human liver microsomal steroid metabolism: identification of the major microsomal steroid hormone 6β-hydroxylase cytochrome P-450 enzyme. *Arch Biochem Biophys* 1988;263:424–436.
44. Rebbeck TR, Jaffe JM, Walker AH, et al. Modification of clinical presentation of prostate tumors by a novel genetic variant in CYP3A4. *J Natl Cancer Inst* 1998;90:1225–1229.
45. Schwartz GG. Multiple sclerosis and prostate cancer: What do their similar geographies suggest? *Neuroepidemiology* 1992;11:244–254.
46. Hanchette CL, Schwartz GG. Geographic patterns of prostate cancer mortality. Evidence for a protective effect of ultraviolet radiation. *Cancer* 1992;70:2861–2869.
47. Corder EH, Friedman GD, Vogelman JH, et al. Seasonal variation in vitamin D, vitamin D-binding protein, and dehydroepiandrosterone: risk of prostate cancer in black and white men. *Cancer Epidemiol Biomarkers Prev* 1995; 4:655–659.
48. Gann PH, Ma J, Hennekens CH, et al. Circulating vitamin D metabolites in relation to subsequent development of prostate cancer. *Cancer Epidemiol Biomarkers Prev* 1996;5:121–126.
49. Giovannucci E. Dietary influences of 1,25$(OH)_2$ vitamin D in relation to prostate cancer: a hypothesis. *Cancer Causes Control* 1998;9:567–582.
50. Giovannucci E, Rimm EB, Wolk A, et al. Calcium and fructose intake in relation to risk of prostate cancer. *Cancer Res* 1998;58:442–447.
51. Peehl DM, Skowronski RJ, Leung GK, et al. Antiproliferative effects of 1,25-dihydroxyvitamin D_3 on primary cultures of human prostatic cells. *Cancer Res* 1994;54:805–810.
52. Schwartz GG, Hill CC, Oeler TA, et al. 1,25-Dihydroxy-16-ene-23-yne-vitamin D_3 and prostate cancer cell proliferation *in vivo*. *Urology* 1995;46:365–369.

53. Schwartz GG, Whitlatch LW, Chen TC, et al. Human prostate cells synthesize 1,25-dihydroxyvitamin D_3 from 25-hydroxyvitamin D_3. *Cancer Epidemiol Biomarkers Prev* 1998; 7:391–396.
54. Lokeshwar BL, Schwartz GG, Selzer MG, et al. Inhibition of prostate cancer metastasis in vivo: a comparison of 1,26-dihydroxyvitamin D (calcitriol) and EB1089. *Cancer Epidemiol Biomarkers Prev* 1999;8:241–248.
55. Johnson CS, McElwain MC, Light BW, et al. Anti-proliferative effects of vitamin D and its analogs in rodent tumor models. In: Norman AW, Bouillon R, Thomasset M, eds. *Vitamin D: chemistry, biology and clinical applications of the steroid hormone*. 1997:451–458.
56. Schwartz GG, Wang MH, Zhang M, et al. 1α,25-dihydroxyvitamin D (calcitriol) inhibits the invasiveness of human prostate cancer cells. *Cancer Epidemiol Biomarkers Prev* 1997;6:727–732.
57. Saijo T, Ito M, Takeda E, et al. A unique mutation in the vitamin D receptor gene in three Japanese patients with vitamin D-dependent rickets type II: utility of single-strand confirmation polymorphism analysis for heterozygous carrier detection. *Am J Human Genet* 1991;49:668–673.
58. Morrison NA, Yeoman R, Kelly PJ, et al. Contribution of trans-acting factor alleles to normal physiological variability: vitamin D receptor gene polymorphism and circulating osteocalcin. *Proc Natl Acad Sci U S A* 1992;89:6665–6669.
59. Taylor JA, Hirvonen A, Watson M, et al. Association of prostate cancer with vitamin D receptor gene polymorphism. *Cancer Res* 1996;56:4108–4110.
60. Ingles SA, Haile RW, Henderson BE, et al. Strength of linkage disequilibrium between two vitamin D receptor markers in five ethnic groups: implications for association studies. *Cancer Epidemiol Biomarkers Prev* 1997;6:93–98.
61. Ingles SA, Coetzee GA, Ross RK, et al. Association of prostate cancer with vitamin D receptor haplotypes in African-Americans. *Cancer Res* 1998;58:1620–1623.
62. Ma J, Stampfer MJ, Gann PH, et al. Vitamin D receptor polymorphisms, circulating vitamin D metabolites, and risk of prostate cancer in United States physicians. *Cancer Epidemiol Biomarkers Prev* 1998;7:385–390.
63. Burroughs KD, Dunn SE, Barrett JC, et al. Insulin-like growth factor-I: a key regulator of human cancer risk. *J Natl Cancer Inst* 1999;91:579–581.
64. Cohen P, Peehl DM, Rosenfeld RG. The IGF axis in the prostate. *Hormone Metab Res* 1994;26:81–84.
65. Cohen P, Peehl DM, Lamson G, Rosenfeld RG. Insulin-like growth factors (IGFs), IGF receptors, and IGF-binding proteins in primary cultures of prostate epithelial cells. *J Clin Endocrinol Metab* 1991;73:401–407.
66. Mantzoros CS, Tzonou A, Signorello LB, et al. Insulin-like growth factor 1 in relation to prostate cancer and benign prostatic hyperplasia. *Br J Cancer* 1997;76:1115–1118.
67. Chan JM, Stampfer MJ, Giovannucci E, et al. Plasma insulin-like growth factor-I and prostate cancer risk: a prospective study. *Science* 1998;279:563–566.
68. Rosen CJ, Kurland ES, Vereault D, et al. Association between serum insulin growth factor-I (IGF-I) and a simple sequence repeat in IGF-I gene: implications for genetic studies of bone mineral density. *J Clin Endocrinal Metab* 1998;83:2286–2290.
69. Sun G, Chagnon M, Bouchard C. A common polymorphism in the human insulin-like growth factor binding protein 3 gene. *Mol Cell Probes* 2000;14:55–56.
70. Zou T, Fleisher AS, Kong D, et al. Sequence alterations of insulin-like growth factor binding protein 3 in neoplastic and normal gastrointestinal tissues. *Cancer Res* 1998;58: 4802–4804.
71. Lee WH, Morton RA, Epstein JI, et al. Cytidine methylation of regulatory sequences near the pi-class glutathione S-transferase gene accompanies human prostatic carcinogenesis. *Proc Natl Acad Sci U S A* 1994;91:11733–11737.
72. Vogelstein B, Kinzler KW. The multistep nature of cancer. *Trends Genet* 1993;9:138–141.
73. Spruck CH III, Ohneseit PF, Gonzalez-Zulueta M, et al. Two molecular pathways to transitional cell carcinoma of the bladder. *Cancer Res* 1994;54:784–788.
74. Carter BS, Ewing CM, Ward WS, et al. Allelic loss of chromosomes 16q and 10q in human prostate cancer. *Proc Natl Acad Sci U S A* 1990;87:8751–8755.
75. Bova GS, Carter BS, Bussemakers MJ, et al. Homozygous deletion and frequent allelic loss of chromosome 8p22 loci in human prostate cancer. *Cancer Res* 1993;53:3869–3873.
76. Latil A, Baron JC, Cussenot O, et al. Genetic alterations in localized prostate cancer: identification of a common region of deletion on chromosome arm 18q. *Genes Chromosomes Cancer* 1994;11:119–125.
77. Gao X, Zacharek A, Salkowski A, et al. Loss of heterozygosity of the BRCA1 and other loci on chromosome 17q in human prostate cancer. *Cancer Res* 1995;55:1002–1005.
78. Ichikawa T, Ichikawa Y, Dong J, et al. Localization of metastasis suppressor gene(s) for prostatic cancer to the short arm of human chromosome 11. *Cancer Res* 1992;52: 3486–3490.
79. Ichikawa T, Nihei N, Suzuki H, et al. Suppression of metastasis of rat prostatic cancer by introducing human chromosome 8. *Cancer Res* 1994;54:2299–2302.
80. Berube NG, Speevak MD, Chevrette M. Suppression of tumorigenicity of human prostate cancer cells by introduction of human chromosome del(12)(q13). *Cancer Res* 1994;54:3077–3081.
81. Nupponen N, Visacorpi T. Molecular biology of progression of prostate cancer. *Eur Urol* 1999;35:351–354.
82. Eagle LR, Yin X, Brothman AR, Williams BJ, et al. Mutation of the MXI1 gene in prostate cancer. *Nat Genet* 1995;9:249–255.
83. Dong JT, Lamb PW, Rinker-Schaeffer CW, et al. KAI1, a metastasis suppressor gene for prostate cancer on human chromosome 11p11.2. *Science* 1995;268:884–886.
84. Navone NM, Troncoso P, Pisters LL, et al. p53 protein accumulation and gene mutation in the progression of human prostate carcinoma. *J Natl Cancer Inst* 1993;85: 1657–1669.
85. Bookstein R, Rio P, Madreperla SA, et al. Promoter deletion and loss of retinoblastoma gene expression in human prostate carcinoma. *Proc Natl Acad Sci U S A* 1990;87:7762–7766.
86. Dobashi Y, Shuin T, Tsuruga H, et al. DNA polymerase beta gene mutation in human prostate cancer. *Cancer Res* 1994;54:2827–2829.
87. Tilley WD, Buchanan G, Hickey TE, et al. Mutations in the androgen receptor gene are associated with progression

of human prostate cancer to androgen independence. *Clin Cancer Res* 1996;2:277–285.
88. Van der Kwast TH, Schalken J, De Winter JA, et al. Androgen receptors in endocrine-resistant human prostate cancer. *Int J Cancer* 1991;48:189–193.
89. Hobisch A, Culig Z, Radmayr C, et al. Distant metastases from prostatic carcinoma express androgen receptor protein. *Cancer Res* 1995;55:3068–3072.
90. Tilley WD, Lim-Tio SS, Horsfall DJ, et al. Detection of discrete androgen receptor epitopes in prostate cancer by immunostaining: measurement by color video image analysis. *Cancer Res* 1994;54:4096–4102.
91. Sadi MV, Barrack ER. Image analysis of androgen receptor immunostaining in metastatic prostate cancer. Heterogeneity as a predictor of response to hormonal therapy. *Cancer* 1993;71:2574–2580.
92. Veldscholte J, Ris-Stalpers C, Kuiper GG, et al. A mutation in the ligand binding domain of the androgen receptor of human LNCaP cells affects steroid binding characteristics and response to anti-androgens. *Biochem Biophys Res Commun* 1990;173:534–540.
93. Tan J, Sharief Y, Hamil KG, et al. Dehydroepiandrosterone activates mutant androgen receptors expressed in the androgen-dependent human prostate cancer xenograft CWR22 and LNCaP cells. *Mol Endocrinol* 1997;11:450–459.
94. Taplin ME, Budley GJ, Shuster TD, et al. Mutation of the androgen-receptor gene in metastatic androgen-independent prostate cancer. *N Engl J Med* 1995;332:1393–1398.
95. Fenton MA, Shuster TD, Fertig AM, et al. Functional characterization of mutant androgen receptors from androgen-independent prostate cancer. *Clin Cancer Res* 1997;3:1383–1388.
96. Koivisto P, Kononen J, Palmberg C, et al. Androgen receptor gene amplification: a possible molecular mechanism for androgen deprivation therapy failure in prostate cancer. *Cancer Res* 1997;57:314–319.
97. Bentel JM, Tilley WD. Androgen receptors in prostate cancer. *J Endocrinol* 1996;151:1–11.
98. Wilson JD. The promiscuous receptor: prostate cancer comes of age. *N Engl J Med* 1995;332:1440–1441.
99. Fowler JE, Pandey P, Seaver LE, et al. Prostate specific antigen after gonadal androgen withdrawal and deferred flutamide treatment. *J Urol* 1995;154:448–453.
100. Dupont A, Gomez JL, Cusan L, et al. Response to flutamide withdrawal in advanced prostate cancer in progression under combination therapy. *J Urol* 1993;150:908–913.
101. Scher HI, Kelly WK. Flutamide withdrawal syndrome: its impact on clinical trials in hormone-refractory prostate cancer. *J Clin Cancer* 1993;11:1566–1572.
102. Sartor O, Cooper M, Weinberger M, et al. Surprising activity of flutamide withdrawal, when combined with aminoglutethimide, in treatment of "hormone-refractory" prostate cancer. *J Natl Cancer Inst* 1994;86:222–227.
103. Culig Z, Hobisch A, Cronauer MV, et al. Activation of the androgen receptor by polypeptide growth factors and cellular regulators. *World J Urol* 1995;13:285–289.
104. Culig Z, Hobisch A, Hittmair A, et al. Expression, structure, and function of androgen receptor in advanced prostatic carcinoma. *Prostate* 1998;35:63–70.
105. Nazareth LV, Weigel NL. Activation of the human androgen receptor through a protein kinase A signaling pathway. *J Biol Chem* 1996;27:19900–19907.
106. Culig Z, Hobisch A, Hittmair A, et al. Synergistic activation of androgen receptor by androgen and luteinizing hormone-releasing hormone in prostatic carcinoma cells. *Prostate* 1997;32:106–114.
107. Sadar MD. Androgen-independent induction of prostate-specific antigen gene expression via cross-talk between the androgen receptor and protein kinase A signal transduction pathways. *J Biol Chem* 1999;274:7777–7783.
108. Craft N, Shostak Y, Carey M, et al. A mechanism for hormone-independent prostate cancer through modulation of androgen receptor signaling by the HER-2/neu tyrosine kinase. *Nat Med* 1999;5:280–285.
109. Yeh S, Lin HK, Kang HY, et al. From HER2/Neu signal cascade to androgen receptor and its coactivators: a novel pathway by induction of androgen target genes through MAP kinase in prostate cancer cells. *Proc Natl Acad Sci U S A* 1999;96:5458–5463.
110. Abreu-Martin MT, Chari A, Palladino AA, et al. Mitogen-activated protein kinase kinase kinase 1 activates androgen receptor-dependent transcription and apoptosis in prostate cancer. *Mol Cell Biol* 1999;19:5143–5154.
111. Cleutjens CB, Steketee K, van Eekelen CC, et al. Both androgen receptor and glucocorticoid receptor are able to induce prostate-specific antigen expression, but differ in their growth-stimulating properties of LNCaP cells. *Endocrinology* 1997;138:5293–5300.
112. Wright GLJ, Grob BM, Haley C, et al. Upregulation of prostate-specific membrane antigen after androgen-deprivation therapy. *Urology* 1996;48:326–334.
113. Brass AL, Barnard J, Patai BL, et al. Androgen up-regulates epidermal growth factor receptor expression and binding affinity in PC3 cell lines expressing the human androgen receptor. *Cancer Res* 1995;55:3197–3203.
114. Saric T, Shain SA. Androgen regulation of prostate cancer cell FGF-1, FGF-2, and FGF-8: preferential down-regulation of FGF-2 transcripts. *Growth Factors* 1998;16:69–87.
115. Zhu N, Pewitt EB, Cai X, et al. Calreticulin: an intracellular Ca++-binding protein abundantly expressed and regulated by androgen in prostatic epithelial cells. *Endocrinology* 1998;139:4337–4344.
116. Marcelli M, Haidacher SJ, Plymate SR, et al. Altered growth and insulin-like growth factor-binding protein-3 production in PC3 prostate carcinoma cells stably transfected with a constitutively active androgen receptor complementary deoxyribonucleic acid. *Endocrinology* 1995;136:1040–1048.
117. Gregory CW, Kim D, Ye P, et al. Androgen receptor up-regulates insulin-like growth factor binding protein-5 (IGFBP-5) expression in a human prostate cancer xenograft. *Endocrinology* 1999;140:2372–2381.
118. Prescott JL, Blok L, Tindall DJ. Isolation and androgen regulation of the human homeobox cDNA, NKX3.1. *Prostate* 1998;35:71–80.
119. Gregory CW, Hamil KG, Kim D, et al. Androgen receptor expression in androgen-independent prostate cancer is associated with increased expression of androgen-regulated genes. *Cancer Res* 1998;58:5718–5724.

120. Hall RE, Aspinall JO, Horsfall DJ, et al. Expression of the androgen receptor and an androgen-responsive protein, apolipoprotein D, in human breast cancer. *Br J Cancer* 1996;74:1175–1180.
121. Lindzey J, Grossmann M, Kumar MV, et al. Regulation of the 5'-flanking region of the mouse androgen receptor gene by cAMP and androgen. *Mol Endocrinol* 1993;7:1530–1540.
122. Wolf DA, Herzinger T, Hermeking H, et al. Transcriptional and posttranscriptional regulation of human androgen receptor expression by androgen. *Mol Endocrinol* 1993;7:924–936.
123. Wolf DA, Schultz P, Fittler F. Transcriptional regulation of prostate kallikrein-like genes by androgen. *Mol Endocrinol* 1992;6:753–762.
124. Knudsen KE, Arden KC, Cavenee WK. Multiple G1 regulatory elements control the androgen-dependent proliferation of prostatic carcinoma cells. *J Biol Chem* 1998;273:20213–20222.

10

FAMILIAL PROSTATE CANCER

WILLIAM B. ISAACS
JIANFENG XU

Over the past decade, conceptual and technologic advancements in molecular genetics have led to the elucidation of the molecular mechanisms responsible for inherited predisposition for a number of common human cancers. Genes such BRCA1 and -2, VHL, APC, and hMSH2, in which changes as small as single-nucleotide substitutions result in greatly increased organ-specific cancer risk, have been identified through studies of familial breast, renal, and colorectal cancers, respectively. Likewise, major efforts are under way worldwide to identify and characterize hereditary prostate cancer (HPC) genes through the study of prostate cancer families. Multiple loci suspected to harbor such genes have been identified to date, and efforts to clone the specific genes are in progress. A primary goal of these efforts is the development of genetic tests to determine which individuals carry high-risk prostate cancer alleles.

Although the specific genes responsible for HPC are largely unknown, it is clear that a positive family history of prostate cancer is one of the strongest risk factors yet identified for this disease. Indeed, the usefulness of family history to identify men at elevated risk for prostate cancer has been repeatedly demonstrated with the magnitude of this increase in risk depending on variables such as age of diagnosis and number of affected relatives. Once HPC genes are identified and characterized, the ability to determine HPC gene carrier status by genetic testing will enable a more quantitative and reliable assessment of risk associated with family history. This chapter reviews the evidence for an inherited form of prostate cancer and summarizes the progress to date in the search for prostate cancer susceptibility genes.

COMMON VERSUS RARE PROSTATE CANCER SUSCEPTIBILITY GENES

Disease susceptibility genes can be defined as any gene that possesses allelic variants that are associated with increased (or decreased) disease risk in carriers compared to noncarriers of such variants. Studies of genetic susceptibility for common cancers have indicated that at least two major classes of cancer susceptibility genes exist that vary substantially in character, including the magnitude of their effect and their frequency in the population. One class of such genes has relatively common risk-modifying alleles, although the increases in risk conferred by these genes tend to be moderate and may be strongly influenced by environmental factors. Polymorphic variants of genes such as the glutathione S-transferases, N-acetyl transferases, and members of the cytochrome P450 family, often identified through case-control studies, are examples of this important class of cancer risk–modifying genes. Examples of the second class of genes include BRCA1, VHL, and APC, which are genes with disease-causing alleles that are rare (e.g., 0.0001 to 0.0010) yet confer greatly increased risk for carriers (e.g., 40% to 90% lifetime risk for carriers). These rare, highly penetrant genes have typically been discovered through studies of families with distinctive phenotypes, usually characterized by frequent occurrences of early-onset organ-specific carcinogenesis. In some cases (e.g., for colorectal and kidney cancer), the identification of these types of genes has provided critical insight into the molecular pathways underlying not only inherited cancers, but also sporadic cancers, as the same gene may be mutated somatically in these latter cancers and in the germ line in the inherited disease (1,2). Although it is likely that for prostate cancer, and for common cancers in general, the former class of genes may be more important in terms of overall contribution to inherited risk on a population basis (due to the higher frequency of risk-modifying alleles), on an individual and mechanistic basis, the rare, highly penetrant BRCA1-like genes may play a particularly prominent role.

GENETIC EPIDEMIOLOGY

Family Studies

Familial clustering of disease is a useful but not conclusive indicator of an underlying genetic etiology. Morganti and colleagues (3) were perhaps the first to document, more than 40 years ago, the tendency of prostate cancer to cluster in families. Importantly, in 1960, a study in the Utah Mormon population by Woolf (4) suggested that the likelihood of dying from prostate cancer was increased for men with affected first-degree relatives. Two large studies are of particular interest in addressing the issue of familial clustering of prostate cancer. Cannon-Albright et al. (5) published a genetic epidemiologic study on prostate cancer also in the Utah Mormon population. Notably, prostate cancer showed the fourth strongest degree of familial clustering after lip, skin melanoma, and ovarian cancer. Prostate cancer had a higher familiarity than colon and breast carcinoma, two solid tumors that are well recognized as having a genetic or familial component.

A case-control study of patients treated for prostate cancer at Johns Hopkins was carried out by Steinberg et al. (6) to assess the extent of familial aggregation in prostate cancer. Cancer pedigrees were obtained on 691 men with prostate cancer and 640 spouse controls. The only consistent risk factor for prostate cancer found in this study was a positive family history. Men with a father or brother affected were twice as likely to develop prostate cancer as men with no relatives affected. In addition, there was a trend of increasing risk with increasing number of affected family members such that men with two or three first-degree relatives affected had a five- and 11-fold increased risk of developing prostate cancer. Cox proportional hazards analysis in the case relatives revealed that risk was particularly increased to relatives of younger probands (less than 55 years). Evidence for aggregation of prostate cancer in families has been provided by many additional studies using either retrospective or cohort study designs (7–20). Five major findings emerged from these studies:

1. There is an increased risk for developing prostate cancer among the first- and second-degree relatives of prostate cancer patients.
2. The risk for developing prostate cancer among the first- and second-degree relatives increases with an increase in the number of affected individuals in the families.
3. The risk for developing prostate cancer among the first- and second-degree relatives increases with a decrease in the age at diagnosis of index prostate cancer cases.
4. Family history as an important risk factor for prostate cancer appears to be independent of ethnicity or race.
5. Having an affected brother tends to increase risk to a greater extent than does having a father with prostate cancer.

This latter tendency—that is, the increased risk associated with having an affected brother as compared to an affected father—prompted several authors to suggest a recessive or X-linked mode of inheritance for prostate cancer (see below).

Segregation Analyses

Whereas these studies consistently indicate a significant role for familial clustering as a risk factor for prostate cancer, both genetic components and common environmental risk factors shared within a family can lead to a significant finding in family studies. An estimation of contributions made by genetics as compared to environmental contributions can be determined through twin studies (see below) and complex segregation analyses. By testing the fit of several explicit models of inheritance (e.g., a major Mendelian gene model, an environmental model, or polygene model, or all) to the distribution of a disease in families, complex segregation analysis can identify the specific model that best describes the transmission of the disease in families. Three complex segregation analyses of prostate cancer have been reported, and each is consistent with the hypothesis that there is an autosomal dominant susceptibility gene (21–23). However, gene frequencies estimated by these studies vary appreciably (from 0.003 to 0.010), as do estimated gene penetrances (63% to 89% lifetime risk), presumably reflecting the different populations studied [families of radical prostatectomy patients in the Carter (21) and Schaid (23) studies vs. a population-based study by Gronberg (22)].

Twin Studies

The goal of twin studies is to compare the similarities (concordance rate) of a trait or disease in monozygotic and dizygotic twins as a means to dissect the genetic and environmental components of a familial aggregation. Twin studies by Gronberg et al. (24) and Page et al. (25) have observed higher concordance rates of prostate cancer in monozygotic twins compared to those of dizygotic twins, implicating a genetic contribution for familial aggregation of prostate cancer. More recently, in a large study of more than 44,000 Scandinavian twin pairs, Lichtenstein et al. (26) reported a statistically significant effect of heritable factors for prostate cancer. Somewhat surprisingly, these authors suggested that heritable factors accounted for a larger proportion of prostate cancer (42%) than either breast or colorectal cancer.

Familial versus Hereditary Prostate Cancer

Based on their results of case-control and segregation analyses, Carter et al. (27) proposed an operational definition of HPC that emphasized the factors of age of onset of disease and the number of affected family members as critical defining characteristics of a hereditary form of the disease. This group proposed the following definition of HPC: three or more affected individuals within one nuclear family, affected individuals in three successive generations on either the proband's paternal or maternal lineages, or clustering of two or more individuals affected less than 55 years. Does this exclude families with only two members, affected at an older age, from the possibility of having a genetic form of the disease? The answer is definitely not, as there can certainly be families segregating high penetrance susceptibility alleles that are limited in numbers of affected individuals simply by having a small family size and a small number of male members. In addition, weaker genetic effects (e.g., those attributed to more common, low penetrance genes) may be very important in such smaller clusters and, in fact, may be more readily detected in studies of a large number of smaller prostate cancer families (e.g., affected sibling pairs). However, an important point for consideration, in terms of susceptibility gene mapping, is that a substantial proportion of families with only two first-degree relatives affected are quite likely to occur by chance, owing to the very high disease prevalence of prostate cancer. Obviously, the likelihood of chance clustering decreases as the number of affected men in a nuclear family increases, and it is not surprising that most of the rare high-penetrance cancer susceptibility genes that have been identified to date through linkage studies have been identified in large extended pedigrees with many affected members.

Clinical and Pathologic Characterization of Hereditary Prostate Cancer

To determine whether any differences might distinguish HPC from its sporadic counterpart, a number of clinical features of prostate cancer were examined by Carter et al. in patients with or without a family history of prostate cancer (28). Clinical stage at presentation, preoperative prostate-specific antigen level, final pathologic stage, and prostate weight were examined in a series of approximately 650 patients divided among three categories: those having HPC (as defined earlier), those with no other family members affected (i.e., sporadic), or those in whom there were other family members affected but not to the extent found in families classified as hereditary. No unique clinical or pathologic characteristic distinguished HPC in this group of patients in this study.

This lack of difference between hereditary and sporadic prostate cancer extends to the incidence of multifocality found for each of these categories. Based on studies of individuals harboring other cancer susceptibility alleles, in which multiple cancer foci are often observed in target organs, one might predict that prostate cancer would tend to be more multifocal in patients with a hereditary form of the disease. In a study by Bastacky et al. (29), this was not found to be the case, however. As has been previously observed, prostate cancer in general is multifocal, and no difference was observed between sporadic and hereditary cases in this respect. Keetch et al. (9) examined the pathologic characteristics of prostate cancers from men undergoing radical prostatectomy for treatment of clinically localized disease as a function of family history. The only difference observed was that familial cancers tended to have a slightly lower Gleason score (6.6 vs. 7.6).

Several studies have examined the effect of family history on outcome of prostate cancer after treatment. Bova et al. (30) found no differences in progression rates as measured by prostate-specific antigen elevation in a cohort of men classified as having HPC compared to men with sporadic disease. Similarly, in a Swedish population study, Gronberg et al. (31) found no significant differences in either overall or prostate cancer–specific survival between familial and sporadic prostate cancer cases. The spectrum of tumor grades at diagnosis in familial cases did not differ from that in a population with prostate cancer unselected for family history. These results led the authors to conclude that no differences in treatment between men with or without a positive family history of prostate cancer are justified at this time. In contrast, Kupelian et al. (32,33) did observe a significant tendency for men with a positive family history to progress more rapidly after either surgical or radiation treatment for clinically localized disease. Additionally, Rodriguez et al. (34) made the observation that men with a family history of prostate cancer are more likely to die from their disease [rate ratio (RR), 1.60; 95% confidence interval, 1.31 to 1.97]. Obviously, additional studies are needed to address this important question, particularly as our ability to define the phenotype of HPC becomes more refined.

GENE IDENTIFICATION STUDIES

Linkage Studies as an Approach to Identify Prostate Cancer Susceptibility Alleles

With strong evidence for a genetic component in the etiology of prostate cancer and evidence for a major susceptibility gene, mapping the gene(s) using linkage approaches is a natural next step. This approach provided the mapping data that led to the identification of multiple cancer susceptibility genes, including BRCA1 and -2 in breast cancer, VHL in renal cell carcinoma, and APC and the DNA mismatch repair genes in colorectal cancer (2). However, linkage analysis of prostate cancer has proved to be a difficult undertaking for the following reasons. First, as prostate cancer is diagnosed late in life, even in the case of onset disease, individuals in the parental generation of the probands are usually deceased, and individuals in the offspring generations are usually too young to manifest the phenotype, thus making many pedigrees only marginally informative for linkage analysis. Second, segregation analyses notwithstanding, there are likely multiple modes of inheritance (dominant, recessive, and X-linked) and multiple genes (i.e., genetic and allelic heterogeneity) involved in prostate cancer susceptibility, largely decreasing the power of individual studies to detect the effect of any single major gene. Third, with such a high prevalence of disease and such a strong environmental component, phenocopies (nongene carriers with disease) are likely to be common. Fourth, incomplete and age-dependent penetrance of prostate cancer genes may decrease the power to detect linkage. In spite of these difficulties, tremendous effort has been extended in this area, and at least six different loci have been implicated by linkage studies in the past several years.

A Genome-Wide Screen Resulted in the Identification of HPC1 at *1q24-25*

The first genome-wide screen for prostate cancer susceptibility genes was performed on 66 prostate cancer families ascertained at The Johns Hopkins Hospital (35). Each of these families met an operational definition of HPC—that is, having at least three cases of prostate cancer in the first-degree relatives (see earlier). The average age at diagnosis in these families was 65, which is more than 5 years less than the average age of diagnosis in the United States. A total of 341 dinucleotide repeat markers covering the genome with approximately 10-cM resolution (on the average, 1 cM in genetic distance is equivalent to approximately one million base pairs in physical distance) were genotyped and analyzed in these families. Two-point parametric linkage analysis identified seven regions with lod score greater than 1, in which *lod* is defined as the logarithm of odds ratio in favor of linkage versus no linkage. The highest lod score observed was 2.75 at marker D1S218, which maps to the long arm of chromosome 1 (*1q24-25*). The other regions implicated were 1q33-42, 4q26-27, 5p12-13, 7p21, 13q31-33, and Xq27-28.

The region of highest lod score was further studied in 25 additional HPC families, 13 collected at Johns Hopkins and the remaining 12 families from Sweden. The overall two-point lod score in the total 91 families was 3.65 at the recombination fraction (θ) of 0.18 with marker D1S2883 at *1q24-25*. Significant evidence for locus heterogeneity was obtained by an admixture test with an estimate of 34% of families linked to the region. In other words, only approximately one-third of the families in this study could be explained by HPC1; the remaining two-thirds are presumably due to the action of different genes. Under the assumption of heterogeneity (i.e., that only a subset of families are linked to HPC1, and that other genes account for the remaining families), the maximum multipoint lod score was 5.43. The nonparametric (i.e., model-free) analysis provided consistent results, with a peak multipoint NPL score of 4.71 (p = 1E − 5). This locus was termed *HPC1* (35).

In an attempt to understand the clinical characteristics of prostate cancer potentially linked to HPC1 locus, Gronberg et al. (36) studied a subset of 74 HPC families ascertained at Johns Hopkins. The 74 families were divided into two groups, either potentially linked (33 families) or unlinked (44 families), on the basis of haplotype analysis in the region of HPC1. The mean age at diagnosis of prostate cancer for men in potentially linked families was significantly lower than for men in potentially unlinked families (63.7 vs. 65.9 years, p = .01). Higher-grade cancers (grade 3) were more common in potentially linked families, and advanced-stage diseases were found in 41% of the case patients in potentially linked families, compared with 31% in potentially unlinked families.

Stratification analyses were performed in an attempt to characterize HPC families that are most likely to be linked to HPC1 (37). Results from these stratified analyses showed several interesting findings: (a) Evidence for linkage to HPC1 was mainly from families with mean age at diagnosis less than 65. (b) Evidence for linkage at HPC1 is stronger in families with at least five affected family members than that of families with three and four affected family members. (c) Stronger evidence for linkage at HPC1 was observed in the families with male to male disease transmission.

Replication Studies of Hereditary Prostate Cancer 1

The results of the replication of the *1q24-25* linkage by other research groups have been inconsistent. Three independent studies corroborated linkage to HPC1. Cooney et al. (38) reported a linkage study of *1q24-25* in 59 prostate cancer families, each with two or more affected individuals. The peak NPL score was 1.58 at D1S466 (p = .057) in the total 59 families but was 1.72 (p = .045) in the subset of 20 families that met the criteria for HPC families. Hsieh et al. (39) reported further evidence to support HPC1. In 92 unrelated families having three or more affected individuals, the NPL score was 1.71 (p = .046). The evidence for linkage was stronger in the 46 families with mean age at diagnosis younger than 67. The NPL score was 2.04 (p = .023). The strongest replication study of HPC1 to date was reported by Neuhausen et al. (40). These authors presented positive evidence for linkage in 41 large HPC families ascertained in Utah. The peak two-point lod was 1.73 (p = .005) in the total families and a two-point lod of 2.82 (p = .0003) in early age of onset of families. Finally, in a study of 144 HPC families collected at Mayo Clinic, Berry et al. (41) did not find evidence for linkage at HPC1 region in the total sample but found evidence for HPC1 linkage in a subset of 102 families with male to male disease transmission. The peak NPL score was 1.99 (p = .03) at D1S212.

Three other groups, however, reported no clear evidence for linkage of HPC1 in their study populations. Goode et al. (42) reported no evidence for linkage in this region in 150 high-risk prostate cancer families, using either a parametric lod score approach assuming homogeneity or nonparametric analysis. Even for the 21 white families in this study population with five or more affected family members and mean age at diagnosis 65 years or younger, the lod scores at $\theta = 0$ remained less than –4. Berthon et al. (43) reported results of a genome-wide screen and results from the *1q24-25* region in 47 French and German families. For the three markers in the 1q region, they found negative two-point lod scores assuming a dominant model. No results were reported for the families with early age of diagnosis or a large number of affected individuals. Eeles et al. (44) reported a linkage study of *1q24-25* in 136 prostate cancer families ascertained in the United Kingdom, Quebec, and Texas, 76 of which have three or more affected individuals. They found negative NPL scores in this region in the total sample but positive NPL scores in a subset of 35 families with four or more affected members.

Multiple factors, such as genetic locus heterogeneity, proportion of families with an early mean age at diagnosis, with a large number of affected family members, and with male to male disease transmission, may explain the difference among the different linkage studies. In light of the previously mentioned difficulties of prostate cancer linkage analysis, the number of families from any single study population may provide only limited power to detect any linkage. To increase the power to detect linkage, a collaborative effort was made to examine the HPC1 locus in a worldwide study. This was accomplished by a combined analysis for six markers in the *1q24-25* regions in 772 HPC families ascertained by members of the International Consortium for Prostate Cancer Genetics from North America, Australia, Finland, Norway, Sweden, and the United Kingdom (45). Overall, there was some evidence for linkage with a peak parametric multipoint lod score assuming heterogeneity (hlod) of 1.40 ($p = .01$) at *D1S212*. This evidence was also observed using a nonparametric approach. However, the estimated proportion of families linked to the locus (α) was only 0.06 (1-lod support interval from 0.01 to 0.12). Further parametric analyses revealed a significant effect of the presence of male to male disease transmission within the families. In the subset of 491 such families, the peak hlod was 2.56 ($p = .0006$) and α was 0.11 (1-lod support interval from 0.04 to 0.19), compared to hlods of 0 in the remaining 281 families. Within the male to male disease transmission families, the α increased with early mean age of diagnosis (younger than 65 years, $\alpha = 0.19$, with 1-lod support interval from 0.06 to 0.34) and number of affected family members (greater than or equal to 5, $\alpha = 0.15$, with 1-lod support interval from 0.04 to 0.28). The highest α was observed for the 48 families that met all three criteria (peak hlod = 2.25, $p = .001$, and $\alpha = 0.29$, with 1-lod support interval from 0.08 to 0.53). These results support the finding of a prostate cancer susceptibility gene linked to *1q24-25*, albeit in a defined subset of prostate cancer families. Whereas *HPC1* accounts for only a small proportion of all HPC families, it appears to play a more prominent role in the subset of families with multiple members affected at an early age and with male to male disease transmission. As with any HPC gene, determination of the true impact of HPC1 on familial prostate cancer will not be possible until the gene is cloned and mutations characterized (e.g., frequency and penetrance).

Evidence for a Prostate Cancer Susceptibility Gene on the X Chromosome

In a combined study population of 360 prostate cancer families collected at four different sites in North America, Finland, and Sweden, a linkage to Xq27-28 was observed, which was termed HPCX (46). This region had been previously implicated in the genome-wide scan by Smith et al (35). The peak two-point lod score was 4.6 at *DXS1113*, and the peak multipoint lod score was 3.85 between *DXS1120* and *DXS297*. Significant evidence for locus heterogeneity was observed. The proportion of families linked to *HPCX* was estimated to be 16% in the combined study population and was similar in each separate family collection. The linkage of a prostate cancer gene to the X chromosome is consistent with the results of several population-based studies, suggesting an X-linked mode of inheritance of prostate cancer (4,10–12,19,20). The most obvious implication of this finding is that in some prostate cancer families men can inherit this gene only from their mother, and men can transmit the gene only to their daughters. This finding, along with the indication of autosomal disease transmission in other prostate cancer families, emphasizes the need to include queries of prostate cancer in the maternal side of the family when ascertaining family history of this disease.

PCaP—Another Susceptibility Locus on Chromosome 1

By the combination of genome-wide screening and fine mapping on a selection of 47 French and German families, Berthon et al (43) reported prostate cancer susceptibility locus at 1q42-43 (*PCaP*). The maximum two-point lod score was 2.7 with marker D1S2785. Multipoint parametric analysis yielded an hlod of 2.2, and nonparametric analysis yielded an NPL score of 3.1. They estimated that 50% of the 47 families were linked to the locus.

CaPB—A Locus That May Predispose to Both Prostate and Brain Cancer

Based on initial results of a genome-wide screen in 70 prostate cancer families and candidate-region mapping in 71 additional families, Gibbs et al. (47) reported linkage to 1p36. Further evaluation of this data set revealed the exciting observation of an association between 1p36 linkage and the presence of brain cancer in a subset of the linked prostate cancer families. The overall two-point lod score was 3.22 at D1S507 for 12 families with a history of prostate cancer and a blood relative with primary brain cancer. In the younger age group (mean age at diagnosis, less than 66 years), a maximum two-point lod of 3.65 at D1S407 was observed. This linkage was rejected in both early- and late-age-onset families without a history of brain cancer. Interestingly, tumors of the central nervous system were the only cancers found to be in excess in a study of other cancers in multiplex prostate cancer families reported by Isaacs et al (48).

Hereditary Prostate Cancer 20: Linkage in a Novel Subset of Prostate Cancer Families

Berry et al. (49) found evidence for linkage to chromosome 20q13 while conducting a genome-wide search on 162 North American families with three or more members affected with prostate cancer. Two-point parametric lod scores greater than 1 were observed at multiple sites with the highest two-point lod score of 2.69 for marker D20S196. The maximum multipoint NPL score for the entire data set was 3.02 (p = .002) at D20S887. The strongest evidence of linkage was evident with the pedigrees having fewer than five family members affected with prostate cancer, a later average age of diagnosis, and no male to male transmission. The group of patients having all three of these characteristics (n = 19) had a multipoint NPL score of 3.69 (p = .0001). These results would suggest that HPC20 may account for a subset of families that are distinct from the groups more likely to be linked to previously identified loci.

BRCA1 and *-2* and Risk of Prostate Cancer

As a result of various epidemiologic studies over the past four decades, a link between prostate and breast cancer etiology has been suspected for many years (50–52). Anderson and Badzioch (53) observed an increase in breast cancer risk as a function of family history of prostate cancer in families ascertained through male or female probands having breast cancer. However, an examination of a large number of prostate cancer families for other cancers by Isaacs et al. (48) found only tumors of the central nervous system to be in significant excess; the number of breast cancer cases was not significantly elevated in this study. More recent studies have demonstrated an association between *BRCA1* and *-2* mutations and increased risk of prostate cancer in carriers (54–57). The most direct evidence for a role of these genes in prostate cancer susceptibility comes from an observation of Ashkenazi men known to harbor *BRCA1* or *-2* gene mutations (57). In this cohort, the rate of prostate cancer diagnosis by age 70 was 16%, compared to 3.8% for nonmutation carriers. Furthermore, in an extensive study of other cancers in BRCA2 carriers from the Breast Cancer Linkage Consortium (58), a strong association with prostate cancer was seen (estimated RR, 4.65; 95% confidence interval, 3.48 to 6.22) for mutation carriers, particularly for men younger than 65 years (RR, 7.33). Other studies examining a role for these genes in prostate cancer have been less supportive of a prominent effect, although these studies have been mainly restricted to the Ashkenazi-Jewish population. Lehrer et al. (59) reported an absence of *BRCA1* and *-2* founder mutations in Ashkenazi prostate cancer cases, although only a limited number of these men reported a positive family history of the disease. Langston et al. (60) found a *BRCA1* 185delAG mutation in an affected member of a Jewish prostate cancer family, although no other family members were tested. A study of multiplex Ashkenazi-Jewish prostate cancer families did not find elevated rates of common mutations in *BRCA1* or *-2* (61). A similar finding was reported by Nastiuk et al. (62), who determined the rate of founder BRCA1 and -2 mutations in early-onset prostate cancer to be the same as the general Ashkenazi population. Finally, a comprehensive search for mutations in prostate cancer families that had at least two breast or ovarian cancer, or both, cases revealed no inactivating mutations in either BRCA1 or -2 (63). Overall, whereas there is compelling evidence that mutations in BRCA1 and BRCA2 increase risk for prostate cancer, the contribution of these genes to familial clustering of prostate cancer in general appears too small.

SUMMARY AND FUTURE DIRECTIONS

Although many questions remained unanswered, the extensive effort that has been put forth in recent years has provided a critical foundation for the eventual understanding of hereditary factors and prostate cancer risk. A summary of established concepts includes the following:

1. A positive family history of prostate cancer is an important risk factor for the disease; this risk appears to be stronger in men with multiple first-degree relatives affected at an early age.
2. No single gene explains the majority of familial clustering of prostate cancer. To date, linkage studies in a large number of prostate cancer families have implicated at least five different loci, and more will undoubtedly be identified.
3. The etiology of familial clustering of prostate cancer is most likely highly complex, with different factors being relatively more important in different families. These factors include (a) a strong genetic influence, owing to the effect of a BRCA1-like gene in some families; (b) a weaker genetic influence in other families, perhaps in the context of shared environmental factors; and (c) owing to high disease prevalence, many small clusters have a high likelihood of being due to chance. This etiologic heterogeneity greatly complicates the analysis of the respective contributions of each of these factors to familial prostate cancer.

4. To address these difficulties, efforts should be made to stratify prostate cancer families by clinical and epidemiologic variables and, in doing so, hopefully reduce the etiologic heterogeneity to more manageable levels. This means the establishment of extensive family databases incorporating not only genotypic data but clinical and epidemiologic variables as well.
5. Finally, the emerging ability to carry out systematic, high density genome-wide single nucleotide polymorphism scans to evaluate haplotype sharing among affected individuals, and the association of various gene polymorphisms with prostate cancer risk, should provide unique insight into the mechanisms of susceptibility for this disease.

REFERENCES

1. Knudsen AG. All in the (cancer) family. *Nature Genetic* 1993;5:103–104.
2. Fearon ER. Human cancer syndromes: clues to the origin and nature of cancer. *Science* 1997;278:1043–1050.
3. Morganti G, Cianferrari L, Cresseri A, et al. Recherches clinico-statistiques et genetiques sur les neoplasies de la prostate. *Acat Genet Statis* 1956;6:304–305.
4. Woolf CM. An investigation of familial aspects of carcinoma of the prostate. *Cancer* 1960;13:739–744.
5. Cannon L, Bishop DT, Skolnick M, et al. Genetic epidemiology of prostate cancer in the Utah Mormon genealogy. *Cancer Surveys* 1982;1:47–69.
6. Steinberg GD, Carter BS, Beaty TH, et al. Family history and the risk of prostate cancer. *Prostate* 1990;17:337–347.
7. Meikle AW, Stanish WM. Familial prostatic cancer risk and low testosterone. *J Clin Endocrinol Metab* 1982;54:1104–1108.
8. Spitz MR, Currier RD, Fueger JJ, et al. Familial patterns of prostate cancer: a case-control analysis. *J Urol* 1991;146: 1305–1307.
9. Keetch DW, Humphrey PA, Smith DS, et al. Clinical and pathological features of hereditary prostate cancer. *J Urol* 1996;155:1841–1843.
10. Narod SA, Dupont A, Cusan L, et al. The impact of family history on early detection of prostate cancer [letter]. *Nat Med* 1995;1:99–101.
11. Monroe KR, Yu MC, Kolonel LN, et al. Evidence of an X-linked or recessive genetic component to prostate cancer risk [see comments]. *Nat Med* 1995;1:827–829.
12. Hayes RB, Liff JM, Pottern LM, et al. Prostate cancer risk in U.S. blacks and whites with a family history of cancer. *Int J Cancer* 1995;60:361–364.
13. Whittemore AS, Wu AH, Kolonel LN, et al. Family history and prostate cancer risk in black, white, and Asian men in the United States and Canada. *Am J Epidemiol* 1995;141: 732–740.
14. Lesko SM, Rosenberg L, Shapiro S. Family history and prostate cancer risk. *Am J Epidemiol* 1996;144:1041–1047.
15. Ghadirian P, Howe GR, Hislop TG, et al. Family history of prostate cancer: a multi-center case-control study in Canada. *Int J Cancer* 1997;70:679–681.
16. Aprikian AG, Bazinet M, Plante M, et al. Family history and the risk of prostatic carcinoma in a high risk group of urological patients. *J Urol* 1995;154:404–406.
17. Goldgar DE, Easton DF, Cannon-Albright LA, et al. Systematic population-based assessment of cancer risk in first-degree relatives of cancer probands. *J Natl Cancer Inst* 1994;86:1600–1608.
18. Gronberg H, Damber L, Damber JE. Familial prostate cancer in Sweden. A nationwide register cohort study. *Cancer* 1996;77:138–143.
19. Schuurman AG, Zeegers MP, Goldbohm RA, et al. A case-cohort study on prostate cancer risk in relation to family history of prostate cancer. *Epidemiology* 1999;10:192–195.
20. Cerhan JR, Parker AS, Putnam SD, et al. Family history and prostate cancer risk in a population-based cohort of Iowa men. *Cancer Epidemiol Biomarkers Prev* 1999;8:53–60.
21. Carter BS, Beaty TH, Steinberg GD, et al. Mendelian inheritance of familial prostate cancer. *Proc Natl Acad Sci U S A* 1992;89:3367–3371.
22. Gronberg H, Damber L, Damber JE, et al. Segregation analysis of prostate cancer in Sweden: support for dominant inheritance. *Am J Epidemiol* 1997;146:552–557.
23. Schaid DJ, McDonnell SK, Blute ML, et al. Evidence for autosomal dominant inheritance of prostate cancer. *Am J Hum Genet* 1998;62:1425–1438.
24. Gronberg H, Damber L, Damber JE. Studies of genetic factors in prostate cancer in a twin population. *J Urol* 1994; 152:1484–1487.
25. Page WF, Braun MM, Partin AW, et al. Heredity and prostate cancer: a study of World War II veteran twins. *Prostate* 1997;33:240–245.
26. Lichtenstein P, Holm NV, Verkasalo PK, et al. Environmental and heritable factors in the causation of cancer—analyses of cohorts of twins from Sweden, Denmark, and Finland [see comments]. *N Engl J Med* 2000;343:78–85.
27. Carter BS, Bova GS, Beaty TH, et al. Hereditary prostate cancer: epidemiologic and clinical features [review]. *J Urol* 1993;150:797–802.
28. Carter BS, Bova GS, Beaty TH, et al. Hereditary prostate cancer: epidemiologic and clinical features. *J Urol* 1993; 150:797–802.
29. Bastacky SI, Wojno KJ, Walsh PC, et al. Pathological features of hereditary prostate cancer. *J Urol* 1995;153:987–992.
30. Bova GS, Partin AW, Isaacs SD, et al. Biological aggressiveness of hereditary prostate cancer: long-term evaluation following radical prostatectomy. *J Urol* 1998;160:660–663.
31. Gronberg H, Damber L, Tavelin B, et al. No difference in survival between sporadic, familial and hereditary prostate cancer. *Br J Urol* 1998;82:564–567.
32. Kupelian PA, Klein EA, Witte JS. Re: Biological aggressiveness of hereditary prostate cancer: long-term evaluation following radical prostatectomy [letter]. *J Urol* 1999;161: 1585–1586.
33. Kupelian PA, Klein EA, Witte JS, et al. Familial prostate cancer: A different disease? *J Urol* 1997;158:2197–2201.
34. Rodriguez C, Calle EE, Miracle-McMahill HL, et al. Family history and risk of fatal prostate cancer. *Epidemiology* 1997;8:653–657.
35. Smith JR, Freije D, Carpten JD, et al. Major susceptibility locus for prostate cancer on chromosome 1 suggested by a

genome-wide search [see comments]. *Science* 1996;274: 1371–1374.

36. Gronberg H, Isaacs SD, Smith JR, et al. Characteristics of prostate cancer in families potentially linked to the hereditary prostate cancer 1 (HPC1) locus [see comments]. *JAMA* 1997;278:1251–1255.
37. Gronberg H, Xu J, Smith JR, et al. Early age at diagnosis in families providing evidence of linkage to the hereditary prostate cancer locus (HPC1) on chromosome 1 [published erratum appears in *Cancer Res* 1998;58:3191]. *Cancer Res* 1997;57:4707–4709.
38. Cooney KA, McCarthy JD, Lange E, et al. Prostate cancer susceptibility locus on chromosome 1q: a confirmatory study [see comments]. *J Natl Cancer Inst* 1997;89:955–959.
39. Hsieh CL, Oakley-Girvan I, Gallagher RP, et al. Re: Prostate cancer susceptibility locus on chromosome 1q: a confirmatory study [letter; comment]. *J Natl Cancer Inst* 1997; 89:1893–1894.
40. Neuhausen SL, Farnham JM, Kort E, et al. Prostate cancer susceptibility locus HPC1 in Utah high-risk pedigrees. *Hum Mol Genet* 1999;8:2437–2442.
41. Berry R, Schaid DJ, Smith JR, et al. Linkage analyses at the chromosome 1 loci 1q24-25 (HPC1), 1q42.2-43 (PCAP), and 1p36 (CAPB) in families with hereditary prostate cancer. *Am J Hum Genet* 2000;66:539–546.
42. Goode EL, Stanford JL, Chakrabarti L, et al. Linkage analysis of 150 high-risk prostate cancer families at 1q24-25. *Genet Epidemiol* 2000;18:251–275.
43. Berthon P, Valeri A, Cohen-Akenine A, et al. Predisposing gene for early-onset prostate cancer, localized on chromosome 1q42.2-43. *Am J Hum Genet* 1998;62:1416–1424.
44. Eeles RA, Durocher F, Edwards S, et al. Linkage analysis of chromosome 1q markers in 136 prostate cancer families. The Cancer Research Campaign/British Prostate Group U.K. Familial Prostate Cancer Study Collaborators. *Am J Hum Genet* 1998;62:653–658.
45. Xu J. Combined analysis of hereditary prostate cancer linkage to 1q24-25: results from 772 hereditary prostate cancer families from the International Consortium for Prostate Cancer Genetics. *Am J Hum Genet* 2000;66:945–957.
46. Xu J, Meyers D, Freije D, et al. Evidence for a prostate cancer susceptibility locus on the X chromosome. *Nat Genet* 1998;20:175–179.
47. Gibbs M, Stanford JL, McIndoe RA, et al. Evidence for a rare prostate cancer-susceptibility locus at chromosome 1p36. *Am J Hum Genet* 1999;64:776–787.
48. Isaacs SD, Kiemeney LA, Baffoe-Bonnie A, et al. Risk of cancer in relatives of prostate cancer probands. *J Natl Cancer Inst* 1995; 87:991–996.
49. Berry R, Schroeder JJ, French AJ, et al. Evidence for a prostate cancer-susceptibility locus on chromosome 20. *Am J Hum Genet* 2000;67:82–91.
50. Ekman P, Pan Y, Li C, et al. Environmental and genetic factors: a possible link with prostate cancer. *Br J Urol* 1997;79[Suppl 2]:35–41.
51. McCahy PJ, Harris CA, Neal DE. Breast and prostate cancer in the relatives of men with prostate cancer. *Br J Urol* 1996;78:552–556.
52. Thiessen EU. Concerning a familial association between breast cancer and both prostatic and uterine malignancies. *Cancer* 1974;34:1102–1107.
53. Anderson DE, Badzioch MD. Familial breast cancer risks. Effects of prostate and other cancers. *Cancer* 1993;72:114–119.
54. Easton DF, Steele L, Fields P, et al. Cancer risks in two large breast cancer families linked to BRCA2 on chromosome 13q12-13. *Am J Hum Genet* 1997;61:120–128.
55. Ford D, Easton DF, Bishop DT, et al. Risks of cancer in BRCA1-mutation carriers. Breast Cancer Linkage Consortium. *Lancet* 1994;343:692–695.
56. Sigurdsson S, Thorlacius S, Tomasson J, et al. BRCA2 mutation in Icelandic prostate cancer patients. *J Mol Med* 1997;75:758–761.
57. Struewing JP, Hartge P, Wacholder S, et al. The risk of cancer associated with specific mutations of BRCA1 and BRCA2 among Ashkenazi Jews [see comments]. *N Engl J Med* 1997;336:1401–1408.
58. The Breast Cancer Linkage Consortium. Cancer risks in BRCA2 mutation carriers. *J Natl Cancer Inst* 1999;91: 1310–1316.
59. Lehrer S, Fodor F, Stock RG, et al. Absence of 185delAG mutation of the BRCA1 gene and 6174delT mutation of the BRCA2 gene in Ashkenazi Jewish men with prostate cancer. *Br J Cancer* 1998;78:771–773.
60. Langston AA, Stanford JL, Wicklund KG, et al. Germ-line BRCA1 mutations in selected men with prostate cancer [letter]. *Am J Hum Genet* 1996;58:881–884.
61. Wilkens EP, Freije D, Xu J, et al. No evidence for a role of BRCA1 or BRCA2 mutations in Ashkenazi Jewish families with hereditary prostate cancer. *Prostate* 1999;39:280–284.
62. Nastiuk KL, Mansukhani M, Terry MB, et al. Common mutations in BRCA1 and BRCA2 do not contribute to early prostate cancer in Jewish men. *Prostate* 1999;40:172–177.
63. Sinclair CS, Berry R, Schaid D, et al. BRCA1 and BRCA2 have a limited role in familial prostate cancer. *Cancer Res* 2000;60:1371–1375.

11

RACE AND RISK

OLIVER SARTOR
ISAAC J. POWELL

The definition of *race* is unclear and controversial. The definition of race varies as a function of time and geography, a fact fully appreciated when reviewing governmental actions over the past century. There is no genetic or biologic definition of race that is at this time broadly accepted in the scientific literature. Heterogeneity is particularly characteristic of populations in the United States. "Caucasians" are derived from a multitude of regions (e.g., Sweden and Italy) that may or may not share a common genetic and cultural heritage. "African-American" populations are descended from diverse indigenous populations that inhabit a large and culturally distinct continent. In many statistical analyses, "African-Americans" and "Caucasians" are frequently classified as categoric variables, a fact that does not adequately reflect the genetic, phenotypic, and cultural heterogeneity known to all researchers in the field. No single solution completely obviates these problems.

Despite difficulties in the definition and well-described variations in populations, certain variables may be more prevalent among one "racial" group as opposed to another. Genetically, this has been documented by variations in the frequency of certain alleles or polymorphisms. In addition to genetic elements, there are a number of epigenetic and nongenetic factors that potentially distinguish one racial group from another. These factors include diet, hormonal status, life expectancy, socioeconomic status (SES), literacy, health-seeking behavior, fear of cancer, and nihilistic views of cancer treatment. Each of these issues can potentially affect prostate cancer outcomes. The importance of these factors in race-related prostate cancer risk is often difficult to dissect. All researchers in the field acknowledge that certain factors may alter prostate cancer risk and cancer-specific mortality. Cause and effect relationships are much more difficult to ascertain.

An important issue in any study of race and prostate cancer is to acknowledge that the patient and tumor represent two independent but interrelated variables. In particular, when examining data on the stage at presentation, it is often impossible to distinguish whether the tumor was more extensive because of more aggressive growth or because the diagnosis was made at a different time in the natural history of the disease. This conundrum cannot be readily answered without examining growth rates of tumors in individual patients over time.

EPIDEMIOLOGY OF RACIAL VARIATIONS: PROBLEMS AND PITFALLS

When assessing the incidence and prevalence of prostate cancer, several unique features related to the disease must be taken into account. Prostate cancer is a frequent finding when prostate glands are carefully examined at autopsy. Estimates indicate that as many as 57% of men older than the age of 80 will have prostate cancer if the gland is step sectioned and examined microscopically (1). Only a fraction of these men are diagnosed with prostate cancer in their lifetime. Consequently, the vast majority of men with microscopic organ-confined prostate cancer has latent or clinically irrelevant disease. In a study published at the very beginning of the prostate-specific antigen (PSA) era, the lifetime risk of microscopic prostate cancer for a 50-year-old man was estimated at 42%. Fewer than 10% of these men, however, were estimated to have a clinical diagnosis of prostate cancer in their lifetime, and fewer than 3% of men were estimated to die from this disease (2). These percentages and their ratios are critical to keep in mind when assessing studies of prostate cancer. In particular, because the definition of *clinically* detected cancer is simply that a living patient is diagnosed with prostate cancer, "incidence" studies of prostate cancer are subject to significant variations not encountered in studies of other human malignancies.

The number of men clinically diagnosed with prostate cancer is highly dependent on the intensity of the diagnostic search as well as the number of specialists qualified to diagnose and treat the disease. The intensity of the diagnostic search for prostate cancer has changed dramatically in recent years with the introduction of PSA as a screening tool for the early diagnosis of cancer (3).

Although controversial in terms of long-term benefits, unequivocal data indicate that PSA-driven biopsies can detect cancer at a nonpalpable and asymptomatic stage. Dramatic differences in the incidence of prostate cancer are documented in the post-PSA era as compared to the pre-PSA era in regions where this test has been used as a screening tool. The incidence of prostate cancer is increased in men undergoing a transurethral resection of the prostate. Men having a transurethral resection of the prostate are much more likely to be diagnosed with prostate cancers than are men not undergoing this procedure (4,5). Men undergoing multiple biopsies are much more likely to be diagnosed with prostate cancer than are men undergoing a single biopsy. Standard practice today dictates multiple biopsies, whereas in the past only single biopsies were typically performed. Taken together, the number of men diagnosed with prostate cancer varies with the intensity of the diagnostic search. These facts underscore the importance of comparing prostate cancer incidence in studies using similar indications for biopsy and methodologies of detection whenever possible. International studies rarely meet these criteria (6). To make this point clearly, we note that epidemiologic studies conducted in the United States during the mid-1990s cannot be readily compared to countries not using PSA-based prostate cancer screening. More commonly, subtle distinctions between manuscripts exist. Populations at risk and methodologies for detection must often be compared on a study-by-study basis.

RACE AND INCIDENCE OF PROSTATE CANCER

The risk of clinically diagnosed prostate cancer varies dramatically from country to country (7,8). In fact, the variations in international incidence for prostate cancer are one of the highest of any human cancer. Proper interpretation of variations in risk is dependent on the variables and caveats noted earlier. Direct comparisons are often difficult (or impossible), given marked differences in the intensities of diagnostic procedures and the availability of urology specialists. Regardless of the methodologies involved, however, it would appear that northern Europeans and white residents of the United States have a considerably increased risk of prostate cancer in comparison to Asians or Asian-Americans (Fig. 11-1). The reasons for these international differences are undoubtedly multifactorial. Access to medical care and variations in diagnostic abilities make interpretation of racial and ethnic incidence calculations problematic in the context of international data.

Analyzing studies from a single country over time provides a more readily analyzable data set when evaluating racial factors and their contribution to alterations in prostate cancer risk. To assess risk of prostate cancer among different populations in the United States, it is optimal to use population-based data derived from both the pre- and post-PSA eras. In the United States, this data is available from the SEER program (Surveillance, Epidemiology, and End Results Program of the National Cancer Institute). Using SEER data (Fig. 11-2), African-Americans have a higher risk of invasive prostate cancer as compared to other ethnic groups in the United States (9,10). Among African-American men, the overall age-adjusted incidence increased from 106.3 per 100,000 in 1973, to 134.68 per 100,000 in 1983, to 271.6 per 100,000 in 1993. Among white individuals in the United States, the age-adjusted rate of prostate cancer increased from 62.6 per 100,000 in 1973, to 83.9 per 100,000 in 1983, to 163.9 per 100,000 in 1993. The peak incidence of prostate cancer in the United States occurred in 1993 for African-Americans and in 1992 for white individuals. Since that time, the incidence has been declining for both groups of men.

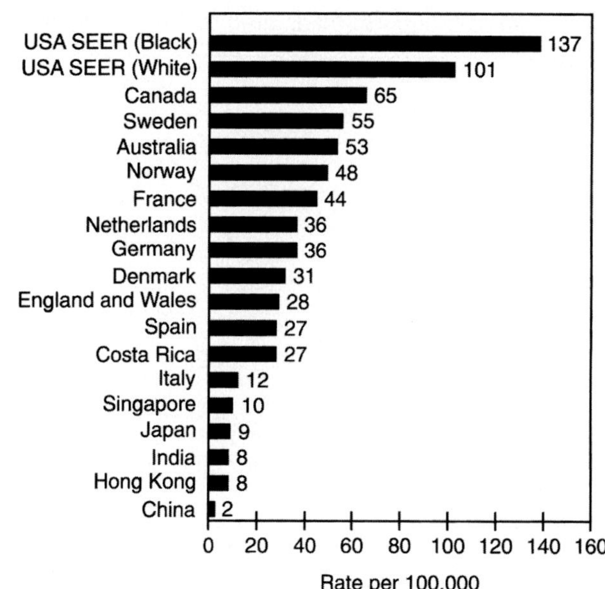

FIGURE 11-1. Incidence of prostate cancer in selected countries per age-adjusted 100,000 population of men in 1988 to 1992. SEER, Surveillance, Epidemiology, and End Results Program. (Adapted from Stanford JL, Stephenson RA, Coyle LM, et al., eds. *Prostate cancer trends 1973–1995, SEER Program*. Bethesda, MD: National Cancer Institute, 1999:NIH Pub. No. 99-4543.)

In the SEER assessment of racial or ethnic patterns of cancer (10) in the United States from 1988 to 1992, the incidence of prostate cancer in African-Americans was 180.6 per 100,000 (Table 11-1). This contrasts to Japanese-Americans having an incidence of 88 and white men having an incidence of 134.7. Although data are more limited, Chinese men had rates of 46 (8). These data clearly indicate on an age-adjusted basis that the incidence of prostate cancer in the United States is more than twice as high in African-American populations as compared to populations of Asian-Americans.

Using a series of assumptions that take into account life expectancy and competing risk factors for death, African-American men are calculated to have a 1.12-fold higher risk

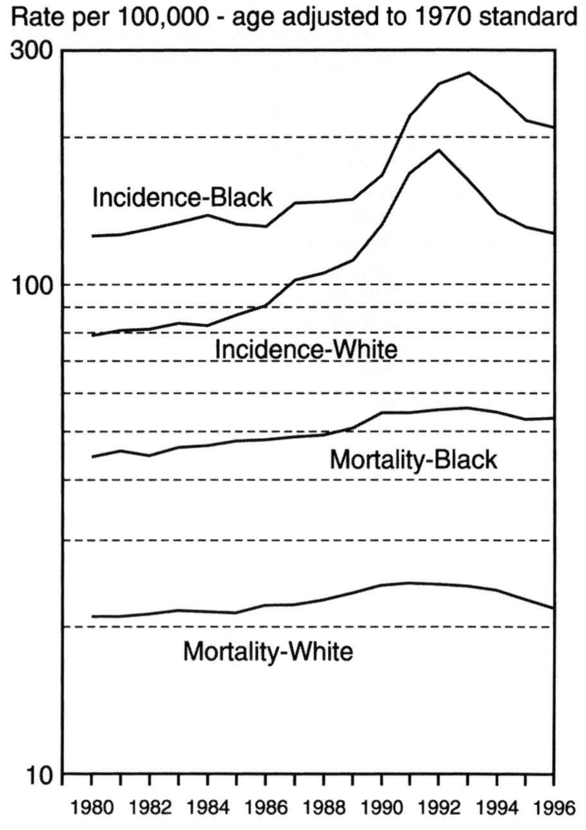

FIGURE 11-2. Incidence and mortality rates for prostate cancer in the United States as a function of race (1980 to 1996). (Adapted from Ries LAG, Kosary CL, Hankey BF, et al., eds. *SEER cancer statistics review, 1973–1996*. Bethesda, MD: National Cancer Institute, 1999.)

for prostate cancer in their lifetimes as compared to white individuals (11). Using a different set of assumptions (in the pre-PSA era), African-Americans are calculated to have a 1.8-fold increased risk as compared to white Americans (12). Regardless of the methodology of the calculations, African-Americans are at increased risk for prostate cancer as compared to the average citizen of the United States.

TABLE 11-1. INCIDENCE AND MORTALITY RATES FOR PROSTATE CANCER BY ETHNIC GROUP IN THE UNITED STATES FROM 1988–1992 (PER AGE-ADJUSTED 100,000 MALE POPULATION)

	Whites	African-Americans	Japanese	Chinese
Incidence	134.7	180.6	88.0	46.0
Mortality	24.1	53.7	11.7	6.6
Mortality/incidence ratio	0.18	0.30	0.13	0.14

Adapted from Ries LAG, Kosary CL, Hankey BF, et al., eds. *SEER cancer statistics review, 1973–1996*. Bethesda, MD: National Cancer Institute, 1999.

International data also suggest a high incidence of prostate cancer among men of sub-Saharan African descent. This increased incidence is unlikely to be accounted for by variations in diagnostic intensity. For instance, a study of prostate cancer in Jamaica (13) indicates that Jamaican men have an even higher prostate cancer incidence than African-Americans. The average age-adjusted incidence of prostate cancer in Kingston, Jamaica has been calculated at 304 per 100,000 men in a study conducted during 1989 to 1994. A recent report of prostate cancer incidence in Nigeria suggested that the magnitude of risk in that population has been grossly underestimated in the past. Osegbe (14) prospectively studied Nigerian men aged 45 years and older with prostate symptoms and suggested that the incidence of prostate cancer in Nigerians may very well approximate that found in the United States, a rate that is 13-fold greater than previously reported in this population. Taken together, these data suggest that men of sub-Saharan African descent are at a high risk of being diagnosed with prostate cancer in their lifetime.

RACE AND RISK OF PROSTATE CANCER DEATH

Understanding the death rates from prostate cancer is more complex than for most other tumors. Patients are older when diagnosed, and many patients have long periods between diagnosis and death; the possibility that deaths in prostate cancer patients may be incorrectly attributed to prostate cancer is substantial (15,16). Data from a large health maintenance organization indicate that approximately 54% of men diagnosed with prostate cancer in the pre-PSA era will die from their disease (16). A recent study analyzing data from men diagnosed with organ-confined prostate cancer indicates that 21.5% of men between age 65 and 74 will die from prostate cancer when treated expectantly and followed for 10 or more years (17). Studies such as this clearly demonstrate the substantial potential for misclassifying deaths in men diagnosed with prostate cancer, a factor still not fully resolved in the vast majority of epidemiologic studies. Death certificates are notoriously inaccurate. Patients dying as a consequence of prostate cancer and its complications are often not fully distinguished from patients diagnosed with prostate cancer but dying from other causes.

Significant country to country variability is reported for prostate cancer mortality rates (Table 11-2). In general, men of northern Europe have a higher incidence and mortality rate of prostate cancer as compared to men in southern Europe (7). Asians and men from the Middle East have a relatively low death rate from prostate cancer as compared to northern Europeans and white individuals living in the United States. African-Americans are noted to have one of the highest rates in the world of deaths attributed to cancer of the prostate (7).

In the United States, there is considerable variability of mortality rates based on racial or ethnic heritage with a hierar-

TABLE 11-2. INTERNATIONAL MORTALITY RATES FOR PROSTATE CANCER 1986–1988 (PER AGE-ADJUSTED 100,000 MALE POPULATION)

Country	Mortality rate	Mortality/U.S. ratio
Norway	21.2	1.35
Denmark	17.7	1.13
Germany	16.7	1.06
Canada	16.7	1.06
Australia	16.6	1.06
United States	15.7	1.00
Portugal	12.8	0.82
Italy	11.8	0.75
Singapore[a]	4.8	0.31
Japan	3.5	0.22
Korea[a]	0.5	0.003
Thailand[a]	0.2	0.001

[a]1986–1987 only.
Adapted from Harras A, Edwards BK, Blot WJ, et al., eds. *Cancer rates and risks*. Bethesda, MD: National Cancer Institute, 1996:NCI Pub. No. 96-691.

chy that resembles the incidence of prostate cancer. African-American men have a clearly higher risk of prostate cancer death (approximately twofold) as compared to white individuals (Fig. 11-2). In 1973, 1983, and 1993, the age-adjusted mortality rates from prostate cancer were 39.5, 46.6, and 56.2 (respectively) per 100,000 African-Americans. For white individuals, mortality rates in 1973, 1983, and 1993 were 20.3, 21.6, and 24.3 (respectively). The peak death rate among white individuals was calculated at 24.7 per 100,000 in 1993. By 1996, the death rate had declined to 22 per 100,000. Among African-American men, the peak mortality rate was 56.2 per 100,000 in 1993. By 1996, this had decreased to 53.7 per 100,000. The decrease in mortality rates since the peak was greater among white individuals (11.1%) than among African-Americans (4.5%) (9). The cause for this decrease in mortality is unclear and thought to be multifactorial. Early detection and more aggressive treatments of early disease better treatment are often invoked as explanations for this decrease in mortality.

Although calculations vary considerably with underlying assumptions and the timing of study, recent SEER data suggest that the lifetime risk of a white individual's dying from prostate cancer in the United States is approximately 3.5%; for African-Americans, the estimate is 4.3% (9). This represents a 1.23-fold increased risk of dying for African-American men. Taken together, African-American men have both a higher risk of diagnosis and dying from prostate cancer as compared to white Americans.

SEER data collected from the United States from 1988 to 1992 (see Table 11-1) indicate that the age-adjusted African-American mortality rate from prostate cancer was 53.7 per 100,000. This contrasts to a rate of 24.1 in whites and 11.7 in Japanese-Americans (9). Chinese-Americans have 6.6 deaths per 100,000. These data again indicate that Asian-Americans have a lower rate of prostate cancer death in comparison to other major ethnic groups in the United States.

Findings from Autopsy Series

Despite wide variations in the clinical incidence of prostate cancer in various international studies, much smaller racial variations in age-adjusted prevalence rates of prostate cancer are documented in autopsy series. Several studies have analyzed microscopic prostate cancer in biracial populations in the United States. In a comprehensive study of 500 men in New Orleans, the prevalence of latent prostate cancer was found to be essentially the same in both African-American and white populations (18). In a more recent study from the Detroit area focusing only on men under the age of 50, similar findings were reported (19). Interestingly, the prevalence of high-grade prostatic intraepithelial neoplasia (PIN) was noted to be much more prevalent in African-American men. It was further noted that high-grade PIN was closely associated with the presence of aggressive prostate cancer (19). Thus, high-grade PIN may be linked to the higher incidence of clinically significant prostate cancer among African-American men.

Appropriately controlled international studies of prostate cancer in autopsy series are relatively rare. In a well-conducted study using serially step-sectioned prostates and microscopic examination (20), age-adjusted prevalence of prostate cancer was noted to be similar in African-Americans (36.9%) as compared to whites in the United States (34.6%). These rates were somewhat higher than Japanese in Japan (20.5%) and Japanese migrants in Hawaii (25.6%). In a separate series using "blinded" observers and standardized methods (21), men from Hong Kong and Singapore were noted to have a lower incidence of latent cancers as compared to Western Europeans and blacks from Jamaica. These variations, however, were considerably smaller than the documented variations in the "clinical" incidence of prostate cancer.

Taken together, autopsy studies of prostate cancer, which carefully examine for evidence of prevalent disease, are much less striking in variation as compared to studies of both clinical incidence and death. These data indicate that although the initiating factors for pathologic prostate cancer are relatively constant in various racial and ethnic populations, additional factors determining clinical prostate cancer rates are much more variable. Various studies of migrating ethnic groups have implicated environmental factors. Most of these studies have been conducted in migrating Asian populations. When Japanese men migrate from Japan to the United States (22,23) or to Brazil (24), the incidence of prostate cancer more closely resembles that of the population in which they settle as compared to their native land. Some studies indicate that age of immigration is irrelevant to subsequent risk of prostate cancer (22). Other studies indicate that Japanese men born in the United States are at higher risk as compared

TABLE 11-3. INCIDENCE AND MORTALITY RATES FOR PROSTATE CANCER IN THE UNITED STATES AS A FUNCTION OF AGE AND RACE (PER 100,000 MEN FOR THE YEARS 1992–1996)

	Incidence		Mortality	
Age (yr)	Whites	African-Americans	Whites	African-Americans
35–39	0.3	0.3	0.0	0.1
40–44	3.3	7.9	0.2	0.6
45–49	21.0	49.1	0.8	3.0
50–54	96.6	197.6	3.5	10.6
55–59	260.8	507.6	11.0	34.0
60–64	548.9	969.8	30.4	91.8
65–69	920.9	1397.8	69.4	188.2
70–74	1212.1	1878.6	139.5	379.2
75–79	1211.5	1804.2	249.2	576.3
80–84	1123.1	1551.2	431.9	967.4

Adapted from Ries LAG, Kosary CL, Hankey BF, et al., eds. *SEER cancer statistics review, 1973–1996.* Bethesda, MD: National Cancer Institute, 1999.

to immigrants (23). Factors influencing the incidence of prostate cancer in immigrants are very poorly understood at this time. Investigators have speculatively implicated many factors, such as diet; however, appropriate controls for diagnostic intensity and availability of urologic specialists have not been adequately examined in these studies.

Interactions between Age and Race

Age-adjusted prostate cancer incidence and mortality rates are informative but tell only a portion of the overall story. Prostate cancer risk rises rapidly with age. In fact, increases in incidence and death as a function of age are more striking for prostate cancer than any other major adult malignancy in the United States (7,9). Deaths from prostate cancer are rare under the age of 50 and markedly increase in each decade thereafter (Table 11-3). The risk of death has increased almost 1,000-fold for patients older than age 85 as compared to those younger than age 50. As noted previously, African-American men have higher incidence and mortality rates from prostate cancer. In addition, prostate cancer and prostate cancer–related deaths occur at substantially younger ages in African-Americans as compared to white individuals (9). Median age at diagnosis and death for men diagnosed with prostate cancer are younger for African-American as compared to white populations in the United States. Reliable population-based data from Asian men residing in the United States are more difficult to accurately ascertain.

PROSTATE-SPECIFIC ANTIGEN AND RACE IN MEN WITHOUT PROSTATE CANCER

PSA is a serine protease synthesized in both benign and malignant prostate tissue. In addition to being a tumor marker, serum PSA levels are powerful predictors of future prostate cancer risk in studies performed in a predominantly white population (25). Interestingly, a variety of studies indicate that African-American men without prostate cancer have an increased serum PSA relative to white populations in the United States. In a series of almost 500 men with a prostate biopsy that was negative for malignancy, multivariate regression analyses indicated that African-American men had both higher PSAs and a higher PSA density (serum PSA per cc prostate gland) in comparison to white men (26). These studies have subsequently been independently confirmed (27). The finding that PSA density is elevated in African-American men suggests either higher rates of PSA synthesis, lower rates of PSA clearance from the circulation, or higher rates of leakage from the prostate gland to the blood stream. Little data are available to address these separate hypotheses.

In large prostate cancer screening studies, in which the vast majority of men did not have a prostate biopsy, African-Americans were noted to have higher PSA values as compared to white individuals (28,29). Community-based studies suggest that age-related PSA levels for Japanese-Americans are lower as compared to white individuals residing in the continental United States (30).

A comparison of reports suggests that PSA may have a greater predictive value for detection of prostate cancer among African-American men as compared to American white men [see (31,32)]. Other studies, however, indicate that race is not an independent predictor of a positive prostate biopsy (33) in men with an abnormal digital rectal exam and a PSA in the normal range.

ETIOLOGY OF RACIAL DIFFERENCES IN PROSTATE CANCER RISK

To determine the relationship between race and prostate cancer risk, one must examine issues that relate to the etiology and pathogenesis of prostate cancer. These factors are relatively poorly understood. Age and family history are well-described risk factors, but the relationship between these clinical variables and prostate cancer risk is poorly understood. Epidemiologic studies have linked prostate cancer risk to genetic polymorphisms, diet, and hormonal status. Each of these putative risk factors is discussed in the context of race in the sections below (Table 11-4).

Genetics, Race, and Incidence of Prostate Cancer

Genetics and prostate cancer risk have been an area of intense investigation over the past several years, using a variety of techniques. Surprisingly few observations have

TABLE 11-4. POTENTIAL FACTORS INCREASING PROSTATE CANCER RISK IN AFRICAN-AMERICAN MEN

Genetic polymorphisms: androgen receptor exon one CAG repeats
Diet: high-fat diet
Hormones:
  Increased androgens *in utero*
  Increased androgens in young adults

come from these studies that might shed light on the relationship between prostate cancer and increased racial risk.

Comparative genomic hybridization is a molecular cytogenetic method that assays tumor tissue for somatic chromosomal gains and deletion. An advantage of this technique for a comparative ethnic study is that the entire genome can be examined for chromosomal aberrations. Recent studies have been conducted in prostate cancer using comparable pathologic stage groupings in African-American men and white men. It was concluded that no significant racial differences could be detected by comparative genomic hybridization (34). This study supports the concept that any genetic differences in prostate cancer between the races must be explained by subtle genomic changes, not alterations at the chromosomal level.

Investigators have studied hereditary prostate cancer (HPC) in high-risk prostate cancer families from North America and Sweden; two of these families were African-American. Of the 91 families studied, approximately one-third showed linkage to a putative HPC gene (HPC1) located in chromosomal region 1q24-25, including both African-American families (35). Whether African-Americans have a higher risk of carrying the putative HPC1 gene is speculative at this time. A larger study is under way to recruit African-American families to further substantiate the relationship between this chromosomal region and HPC in African-American men. Investigations by Cooney et al. (36) confirm that chromosome 1q24-25 is likely to contain a prostate cancer susceptibility gene. Six African-American families are reported in their study; these families contributed disproportionally to the linkage observation studies.

A variety of chromosomal regions have been examined in relationship to prostate cancer. Multiple chromosomes have been implicated in studies of microdissected prostate cancer. Alteration of the 8p terminal region has been identified as a region of interest by a number of investigators. Macoska et al. (37) examined correlation of chromosome 8p changes in 135 patients of various ethnic origins. Tumors from radical prostatectomy specimens were examined after matching for stage and grade. These alterations were associated with both more advanced cancer and higher recurrence of disease. Preliminary studies suggest the possibility that 8p terminal loss may be more prevalent among African-American men than white men.

The androgen receptor is an X-linked steroid receptor superfamily member that mediates signal transduction for all androgenic hormones in man (testosterone, dihydrotestosterone, androstenedione, and others). Like all steroid receptor family members, three functional domains have been defined: a ligand-binding region, a DNA-binding region, and a transactivation domain. The androgen receptor gene has a highly polymorphic microsatellite in the first exon; a CAG repeat normally varies from 9 to 31 in length (38). This CAG repeat region encodes for a variable number of glutamines in the receptor's transactivation domain. Because the androgen receptor gene is X-linked, the androgen receptor gene product is derived from only one allele in each male cell. Studies using transfected androgen receptors with varying lengths of first exon CAG repeats indicate that increased repeat length is associated with less efficient ligand-triggered signal transduction (39). In Kennedy's syndrome, an X-linked neurodegenerative disorder, the androgen receptor has a marked increase in CAG repeat length. Patients with this syndrome have a decreased pituitary responsiveness to androgen administration (40), a finding compatible with decreased androgen receptor function.

Increased prostate cancer risk is associated with decreased androgen receptor CAG repeat length in some, but not all, studies. In the first reported study using a non-Hispanic white population, an approximate twofold increased risk was associated with CAG repeat lengths of less than 20 as compared to greater than or equal to 20 (41). Furthermore, men having less than 20 CAG repeats presented with more advanced disease. In a second study incorporating 587 patients and 588 controls, Giovannucci and colleagues (42) reported an approximately 1.5-fold increased risk for men with less than 19 CAG repeats and compared to men with a CAG repeat length of greater than 25. Furthermore, in this study, men with shorter CAG repeats were more likely to be diagnosed with cancer that had spread beyond the prostate and poorly differentiated tumors. Shorter CAG repeats were at particularly high risk for fatal prostate cancer. Thus, in a large and well-controlled study, decreased CAG repeats were associated with more advanced and more aggressive cancers. In a third study (43) of white men, shorter CAG repeat length was not statistically associated with increased prostate cancer risk unless linked with a shortened GGN repeat (less than or equal to 16). The GGN repeat represents a second polymorphism in the androgen receptor. Another study noted that men with a shorter CAG repeat length had an earlier onset of the disease (44).

The androgen receptor exon one CAG repeat length varies in a racially defined manner. African-American men have a shorter CAG repeat length than do white men (38,45). In particular, African-American populations have a much higher proportion of men with a CAG repeat length of less than 20. In men without an elevation in PSA and without abnormalities on prostate exam, 58% of the African-

American population had less than 20 CAG repeats as compared to 26% in a white population (46). These data strongly indicate that CAG repeat length is a potentially causative factor in the increased risk of prostate cancer in the African-American population. Interestingly, men in the Asian population have a higher average number of CAG repeats than do white men (45). Taken together, the average number of CAG repeats in three major racial populations varies in a manner that is proportional to that population's incidence of prostate cancer. Although additional studies are needed, this genetic polymorphism may substantially contribute to the racial variations in prostate cancer risk.

A recent study of the type II 5α-reductase gene in African-American and white men suggests that an alanine-to-threonine substitution at codon 49 significantly increases clinically significant prostate cancer risk in African-American and Hispanic populations. This alanine-to-threonine substitution at codon 49 enzyme variant is associated with a higher *in vitro* V_{max} for the conversion of testosterone to dihydrotestosterone (47). These potentially important data need confirmation in additional studies.

Diet, Race, and Prostate Cancer Risk

Environmental factors, such as diet, may play a significant role in explaining the racial or ethnic differences of prostate cancer incidence. A number of dietary factors, especially fat, lycopene, and soy products, have been implicated in alterations of prostate cancer risk.

Accumulating evidence from a number of studies over the past several decades indicates that a diet high in fat content is associated with prostate cancer risk. The relationship between fat consumption and prostate cancer is complex, and all studies are not necessarily consistent with one another. Furthermore, the putative mechanisms whereby fat influences prostate cancer are subject to considerable controversy. Initial studies were derived from international populations (48,49). More recently, there has been increasing appreciation that studying cancer risk and diet in the international setting is seriously confounded by many other variables, including, but not limited to, genetics and access to specialty medical care (50).

A number of large and careful prospective studies performed in single- (51) and multi-ethnic (52) cohorts indicate that the increased fat consumption is associated with increased prostate cancer risk. These studies also indicate that the increased risk related to fat consumption was related primarily to animal fat intake. Other carefully controlled studies indicate that increased risk of prostate cancer is primarily related to energy intake rather than fat consumption, *per se* (53–55). Some (56), but not all (57), studies indicate that fat consumption is higher in African-Americans than in other ethnic groups in the United States. Dietary factors and prostate cancer risk have been specifically studied in both African-American and white populations by Hayes and colleagues (58). In these studies, using a case-control design in three geographic regions of the United States, diets high in animal fat were associated with a statistically significant increased risk of prostate cancer in African-Americans but not in white individuals. Additional analysis, however, revealed that high animal fat intake was associated with initial diagnosis of advanced prostate cancer in both races (58). These data suggest that dietary increases in animal fats could potentially contribute to the increased incidence and mortality of prostate cancer in African-American men.

Whittemore et al. (59) have studied prostate cancer in relation to diet among African-American, white, and Asian individuals in the United States and Canada for the years 1987 through 1991. These studies indicated a positive statistically significant association of prostate cancer risk and total fat intake among all ethnic groups combined. In particular, this association was attributable to energy from saturated fats; after adjusting for saturated fat, risk was associated only weakly with monounsaturated fat and was unrelated to protein, carbohydrates, polyunsaturated fat, and total food energy consumption. Fat intake and the percentage of energy from fat differed appreciably among different ethnicity; African-Americans were higher than that of white individuals who, in turn, were followed by the Japanese- and Chinese-Americans. Crude estimates suggest that the differences in saturated fat intake account for approximately 10% of African-American to white differences and 10% to 15% of white to Asian-American differences in prostate cancer incidence (59). Similar conclusions were drawn after analyses of studies conducted in Hawaii (60). Thus, although high-fat diets may be a contributory factor to increased prostate cancer risk, it is clear that other factors also contribute to the differences observed in population-based studies.

Giovannucci et al. (61) recently reported on a prospective study of 47,894 initially cancer-free health professionals regarding dietary intake and prostate cancer risk. A semiquantitative food frequency questionnaire, assessing dietary intake, was used to assess specific food and nutrient intake. A total of 812 new cases of prostate cancer were documented over a 6-year period. In this cohort study, intake of lycopene was associated with a reduced prostate cancer risk. Four foods accounted for 82% of lycopene intake in these studies. These included tomatoes, tomato sauces, tomato juices, and pizza. When analyzing combined intake of these foods, prostate cancer risk was reduced by 35% for those with the highest rates of consumption. When solely analyzing cases of advanced prostate cancer (nonorgan confined), risk was reduced by more than 50%. Further data supporting the concept that reduced lycopenes may be associated with elevated prostate cancer risk are derived from plasma studies of carotenoids (62). Low plasma lycopenes were strongly related to subsequent prostate cancer risk. Men living in southern Europe, particularly in the countries bordering the Mediterranean, are reported to have a relatively low incidence of clinical prostate cancer (7) and a higher intake of tomato products (63). The relationship between lycopene intake and ethnic variation in prostate cancer risk is provocative and needs confirmation in additional studies.

Increased soy intake has been associated with decreased risk of prostate cancer (64,65). A series of isoflavones (i.e., genistein, daidzein, and their metabolites) have potential anticancer activity in model systems. Japanese diets are high in soy products, such as tofu and natto. A number of investigators have speculated that high-soy intake contributes to the relatively low incidence of prostate cancer in Japanese men. Controlled studies are needed in this area.

Hormones, Race, and Prostate Cancer

The hormonal dependency of prostate growth and development is well established. Multiple animal models indicate that prostate cancer growth can be increased by androgens and decreased by antiandrogens. The effects of hormonal manipulations on human prostate cancer growth were initially demonstrated by Huggins and colleagues in the 1940s (66). Today, hormonal deprivation is well established as an effective modality in the treatment of prostate cancer. In contrast to the well-accepted role of androgen blockade in the treatment of prostate cancer, the role of androgens in the development of human prostate cancer is poorly defined. It is stated at times that eunuchs do not develop prostate cancer; however, no meaningful studies of this population have been published. Multiple prospective epidemiologic studies have evaluated serum concentrations of various sex hormones in adult men to evaluate the attractive hypothesis that higher serum androgen levels are associated with increased risk of prostate cancer. Although a review of these studies is beyond the scope of this chapter, suffice it to say that a recent review concluded that, with the possible exception of androstanediol-glucuronide, no significant differences are found in circulating sex-steroid levels between men who subsequently developed prostate cancer and men who remained free of this disease (67).

Studies of hormone levels in adults may or may not be relevant to prostate cancer risk. Studies in another hormonally dependent neoplasm (breast cancer) indicate that cancer risk may be influenced by factors at one age but not at another. Childbirth before age 30 reduces breast cancer risk; childbirth after age 30 has little protective effect. Taken together, factors influencing cancer development may be age specific in their effects.

Studies of prostate cancer risk and hormonal levels have primarily been conducted in adult subjects. The relationship between hormonal levels at younger ages (fetal, childhood, adolescent) and prostate cancer risk has not been carefully studied. Although racial differences in androgens are not clearly present in mature adult men, African-Americans have higher circulating testosterone levels than white individuals *in utero* (68) and in young adulthood (69). The relationships between these age-specific differences in testosterone and prostate cancer risk have yet to be fully explored in appropriately designed studies.

RACE AND PROSTATE CANCER MORTALITY

To determine the relationship between prostate cancer, race, and mortality, one must first consider the relationship between variables known to alter the risk of death from prostate cancer. These variables include factors related to both the cancer and the patient. Stage at presentation, PSA, Gleason's score, treatment, and co-morbidities are all variables implicated in deaths of patients with prostate cancer. Some of these factors have been implicated in the increased rate of deaths from this disease in African-Americans (Table 11-5).

Several sources of bias are notable in this literature. Research reports often contain data derived from specialty practices as compared to populations. Patients selected for radiation therapy or radical prostatectomy are inherently a subset of the overall population. We also note that factors that relate to the patient (as compared to the cancer) are often underestimated and frequently underreported in many research reports. The significance of a prostate cancer cannot be determined by a study of the cancer alone. In particular, co-morbidities are rarely discussed in the urologic literature. To make this point clearly, we note that a low-grade, organ-confined prostate cancer poses a significant health risk for a healthy 50-year-old but little risk for an 80-year-old with congestive heart failure. Discussions of race and risk of prostate cancer death need to include factors that relate to both the tumor and patient. These factors are discussed in the following sections.

Stage and Race

Clinical stage is simply a measure of the extent of tumor spread at the time of diagnosis. Poor prognosis strongly correlates with advanced stage at presentation. Typically, stage is determined by a combination of imaging techniques and physical examinations with or without biopsies. Multiple comparative studies of clinical stages at presentation clearly indicate that African-Americans with prostate cancer are diagnosed with more advanced disease as compared to other ethnic groups in the United States (70,71). This is true for studies published

TABLE 11-5. POTENTIAL FACTORS CONTRIBUTING TO INCREASED MORTALITY RELATED TO PROSTATE CANCER IN AFRICAN-AMERICAN MEN

Incidence: increased incidence in African-Americans
Tumor stage: higher stage at diagnosis in African-Americans
Tumor differentiation: higher Gleason sum at diagnosis in African-Americans
Therapy: African-Americans less likely to receive curative therapies

before and after the introduction of PSA as a screening test. More African-Americans have frank metastatic disease at the time of presentation, and less African-Americans have organ-confined disease (70,71). Because the prognosis of cancer patients is closely linked to the extent of cancer spread at diagnoses, these data clearly demonstrate that higher prostate cancer death rates in African-Americans may be attributable to a higher proportion of patients with advanced disease at the time of the initial diagnosis. Whether this is due to a delay in diagnosis or to more aggressive spread of cancers cannot be determined with certainty from the available data.

Tumor Grade and Race

Gleason score is a semiquantitative description of tumor cell morphology closely linked to prognoses. Studies comparing cancerous tissue derived from African-American tissue as compared to white individuals indicate that African-Americans are more likely to be diagnosed with more aggressive histologic variants of prostate cancer. The reasons for these findings are obscure but have clear prognostic importance.

Data from a Veterans Administration study looking at prostate biopsies from 796 consecutive men showed that African-Americans with local prostate were 1.66-fold more likely to have high-grade (Gleason 8 to 10) tumors than were white individuals (72). Additional studies have confirmed these findings in specialty practices. Thus, we find that the populations known to have a higher death rate from prostate cancer also have more aggressive phenotypes as assessed by histologic findings.

In a comprehensive study evaluating prostate cancer Gleason score and outcome, the percentage of tumors having Gleason score 4 and higher conferred important prognostic information (73). When investigators have examined the components of Gleason sum 7 in radical prostatectomy specimens stratified by race, African-American men had a greater percentage of 4 plus 3 components in radical prostatectomy specimens than did white men. These differences are particularly evident for patients 55 years of age and younger (74).

Whether the increased Gleason score in African-American men is due to increased histologic aggressiveness at the beginning of the tumor growth or because tumors are diagnosed later cannot be determined with certainty. Some data (72) suggest that on a stage-matched basis, African-Americans have a greater percentage of high-grade tumors, implying that tumors are inherently more aggressive in the African-American population than in white individuals living in the United States.

PROSTATE-SPECIFIC ANTIGEN AND RACE IN MEN WITH PROSTATE CANCER

PSA is an independent risk factor in the prognosis of patients treated for prostate cancer. Multiple studies demonstrate that patients with higher PSA values have higher rates of relapse after a variety of local therapies. Higher PSA values are typically noted in African-Americans as compared to white individuals at the time of prostate cancer diagnosis. In a Veterans Administration hospital study evaluating patients with local, regional, and metastatic disease (irrespective of treatment administered), African-Americans with both local and regional diseases were noted to have higher PSA values at diagnosis than were white men (72).

In a large study of 2,219 patients receiving either radiotherapy or radical prostatectomy at the Cleveland Clinic, African-Americans had a statistically significant higher PSA at the time of diagnosis as compared to white men (75). In a large multicenter study of 709 patients with no evidence of metastatic disease enrolled into Radiation Therapy Oncology Group trials, Vijayakumar et al. (76) reported that African-Americans have higher PSAs at diagnosis than do white individuals. Other studies in smaller radiation oncology settings have supported these findings (77) but suggest that these findings are restricted to African-Americans with no private insurance coverage. These authors concluded that differences in PSA values may be related to differences in SES and that African-Americans, uninsured through the majority of their lives, sought care at a later stage of disease.

In studies of patients undergoing radical prostatectomy, Moul et al. (78) studied data on 541 men (408 white individuals and 131 African-Americans) and reported that the preoperative PSA concentration was significantly higher in African-American men as compared to white individuals for all stage, grade, and age categories. On careful analysis, higher tumor volume within each tumor stage was noted among African-American men, indicating that stage for stage, these men were diagnosed with higher tumor volumes than were white individuals. Interestingly, follow-up studies by the same group indicate that racial differences in PSA persisted despite rigorous adjustment for both tumor volume and gland size. This finding is consistent with African-Americans' having a higher PSA density derived from either benign (*vide supra*) or malignant tissue.

Powell et al. (79) examined radical prostatectomy specimens of clinically localized prostate cancer from 759 patients (333 African-Americans and 426 white individuals). For the age group 50 to 59 years, African-American men had significantly higher mean and median PSA values, higher Gleason scores, and more advanced disease than did white individuals. For the age group 60 to 69 years, the median PSA level among African-American men was significantly greater than among white individuals (however, the mean was not different). For ages greater than 70 years, African-American men and white individuals demonstrated similar mean and median PSA values (79).

In summary, a series of studies indicates that PSA values are higher in African-American than white individuals at the time that prostate cancer is diagnosed. Even when controlling for stage at presentation, racial differences persist.

Whether this is secondary to factors relating to volume of disease or increased PSA secretion from benign or malignant, or both, prostatic epithelium cannot be ascertained from these studies. Some data support each of these hypotheses. Comparative data from Asian populations are lacking at this time.

TREATMENT AND RACE

African-Americans are less likely to receive radical prostatectomy or radiation therapy for localized prostate cancer as compared to white individuals in the United States (80). These data, derived from SEER databases over an extended period of time, indicate that even when African-American men are diagnosed with potentially curable cancers, potentially curative therapy is delivered less often to this population. The reasons for these findings are unclear; access to urologists, differences in insurance, co-morbidities, and patient choice are all invoked as potential explanations. These data clearly indicate that undertreatment of potentially curable disease may contribute to the excess prostate cancer–specific mortality observed in African-American populations.

FACTORS POTENTIALLY CONTRIBUTING TO ADVANCED STAGE AT DIAGNOSIS IN AFRICAN-AMERICANS

Data reviewed earlier indicate that the increased mortality rate of prostate cancer in African-Americans may very well be secondary to increased incidence as well as more advanced cancer at the time of the initial diagnosis. Factors contributing to these findings are undoubtedly multifactorial and include issues such as SES, literacy, screening behavior, tumor aggressiveness, and angiogenesis (Table 11-6).

SES has been implicated in the mortality rates of numerous diseases, including cancer. These findings have been verified in studies performed throughout the world (81), including in countries thought to have more equitable access to care than in the United States (82,83). SES interacts with human disease through multiple mechanisms. Low SES is known to restrict access to various medical specialists and treatments; however, this explains only a part of the relationship between SES and mortality (84). Furthermore, SES influences factors such as health insurance coverage, which, in turn, influence stage of cancer at diagnosis (85). Many of the relationships between prostate cancer, race, and SES have been poorly studied to date (86). Although the number of studies in this area is relatively small, some authors have hypothesized that racial differences in survival among men in the United States can be largely explained by differences in the distribution of factors that relate to SES (87).

TABLE 11-6. POTENTIAL FACTORS CONTRIBUTING TO INCREASED STAGE AT DIAGNOSIS IN AFRICAN-AMERICAN MEN

Lower socioeconomic status
Lower literacy
Less access to cancer screening
More aggressive tumors

Whether PSA-based screening for prostate cancer enhances overall survival is controversial; however, data suggest that PSA testing can detect cancer at a stage when the patient is asymptomatic and the physical exam unremarkable. Furthermore, the possibility of being offered curative therapy is markedly increased by PSA-based screening programs. Although population-based statistics are difficult to assemble, the available data suggest that African-American men are less often represented in large prostate cancer screening programs as compared to men in other ethnic groups in the United States (88). Less screening activity in the African-American population may significantly contribute to advanced stage at diagnosis during the PSA era.

Literacy is often an unrecognized factor in issues that relate to health care. Literacy assessments in patients with prostate cancer indicate that low literacy correlates with advanced stages at diagnosis (89). Additional data indicate that African-Americans were more likely to fall in a low literacy category than were white individuals. Interestingly, in this study, literacy level was more important than race in predicting stage at presentation. Low literacy educational tools have been successfully used to enhance preventive medical (vaccine) interventions in low-literate populations (90). Similar approaches may be successful in prostate cancer early detection as well.

FACTORS AFFECTING CANCER GROWTH RATES

Although risk of prostate cancer and fat consumption has been studied intensively over the past several decades, surprisingly little data are available regarding dietary fat and prostate cancer progression rates. Recent studies from Quebec indicate that saturated fat intake is associated with shortened disease-specific survival (91). In these studies (controlling for age, stage, and grade of cancers), high saturated fat consumption increased the risk of prostate cancer death more than threefold (91), suggesting that high-fat diets may promote prostate cancer growth rates. Thus, it is conceivable that high-fat diets may contribute to both the increased incidence (as discussed earlier) and death rates observed in African-American populations.

A variety of studies have correlated angiogenesis and tumor growth rates. Studies have shown that overexpression of the eIF4E gene up-regulates angiogenic growth factors, such as the vascular-endothelial growth factor and fibroblast growth factor 2. Williams et al. (92) examined race-specific relationships between the translation initiation factor eIF4E and angiogenesis in prostate tumors from white and African-American men matched for age, eIF4E expression, tumor stage, and tumor grade. Their findings suggested that microvessel density was higher in prostate tumors from African-American men than in tumors from white men. These findings suggest that angiogenesis may be differentially regulated in African-Americans with prostate cancer, a finding of potential importance in understanding prostate cancer growth rates.

SUMMARY

The relationship between prostate cancer and race is complex and multifaceted. Incidence and death rates vary in a race-related manner. Although international variation in clinical incidence rates is effected by dramatic differences in health-care systems, it is also clear that prostate cancer rates are higher in men derived from sub-Saharan ancestry and is relatively low in men derived from Asian populations. White individuals typically occupy an intermediate position between these two extremes. Incidence variations may be explained by a combination of genetic, hormonal, and dietary factors. Mortality variations are even more complex and involve interactions between the incidence rate, stage at diagnosis, and treatment.

REFERENCES

1. Scott R, Mutchnik D, Laskowski T, et al. Carcinoma of the prostate in elderly men: incidence, growth characteristics, and clinical significance. *J Urol* 1969;101:602–607.
2. Scardino PT. Early detection of prostate cancer. *Urol Clinc North Am* 1989;16:635–655.
3. Hankey BF, Feuer EJ, Clegg LX, et al. Cancer surveillance series: interpreting trends in prostate cancer—part I: evidence of the effects of screening in recent prostate cancer incidence, mortality, and survival rates. *J Natl Cancer Inst* 1999;91:1017–1024.
4. Potosky AL, Kessler L, Gridley G, et al. Rise in prostatic cancer incidence associated with increased use of transurethral resection. *J Natl Cancer Inst* 1990;82:1624–1628.
5. Merrill RM, Feuer EJ, Warren JL, et al. Role of transurethral resection of the prostate in population-based prostate cancer incidence rates. *Am J Epidemiol* 1999;150:848–860.
6. Angwafo FF. Migration and prostate cancer: an international perspective. *J Natl Med Assoc* 1998;11[Suppl]:S720–S723.
7. Landis SH, Murray T, Bolden S, et al. Cancer statistics 1998. *CA Cancer J Clin* 1998;48:6–29.
8. Hsing AW, Tsao L, Devesa SS. International trends and patterns of prostate cancer incidence and mortality. *Int J Cancer* 2000;85:60–67.
9. Ries LAG, Kosary CL, Hankey BF, et al., eds. *SEER cancer statistics review, 1973–1996.* Bethesda, MD: National Cancer Institute, 1999.
10. Miller BA, Kolonel LN, Berstein L, et al., eds. *Racial/ethnic patterns of cancer in the United States 1988–1992.* Bethesda, MD: National Cancer Institute, 1996:NIH Pub. No. 96-4101.
11. Merrill RM, Weed DL, Feuer EJ. The lifetime risk of developing prostate cancer in white and black men. *Cancer Epidemiol Biomarkers Prev* 1997;6:763–768.
12. Seidman H, Mushinski MH, Gelb SK, et al. Probabilities of eventually developing or dying of cancer in the United States. *CA Cancer J Clin* 1985;35:36–56.
13. Glover FE Jr., Coffey DS, Douglas LL, et al. The epidemiology of prostate cancer in Jamaica. *J Urol* 1998;159:1984–1986.
14. Osegbe DN. Prostate cancer in Nigerians: facts and nonfacts. *J Urol* 1997;157:1340–1343.
15. Feuer EJ, Merrill RM, Hankey BF. Cancer surveillance series: interpreting trends in prostate cancer—part II: cause of death misclassification and the recent rise and fall in prostate cancer mortality. *J Natl Cancer Inst* 1999;91:1025–1032.
16. Satariano WA, Ragland KE, Van Den Eeden SK. Cause of death in men diagnosed with prostate carcinoma. *Cancer* 1998;83:1180–1188.
17. Brasso K, Friis S, Juel K, et al. Mortality of patients with clinically localized prostate cancer treated with observation for 10 years or longer: a population based registry study. *J Urol* 1999;161:524–528.
18. Guileyardo JM, Johnson WD, Welsh RA, et al. Prevalence of latent prostate carcinoma in two U.S. populations. *J Natl Cancer Inst* 1980;65:311–316.
19. Sakr WA, Haas GP, Cassin BF, et al. The frequency of carcinoma and intraepithelial neoplasia of the prostate in young male patients. *J Urol* 1993;150:379–385.
20. Yatani R, Chigusa I, Akazaki K, et al. Geographic pathology of latent prostatic carcinoma. *Int J Cancer* 1982;29:611–616.
21. Breslow N, Chan CW, Dhom G, et al. Latent carcinoma of prostate of autopsy in seven areas. *Int J Cancer* 1977;20:680–688.
22. Shimizu H, Ross RK, Bernstein L, et al. Cancers of the prostate and breast among Japanese and white immigrant in Los Angeles county. *Br J Cancer* 1991;63:963–966.
23. Cook LS, Goldoft M, Schwartz SM, et al. Incidence of adenocarcinoma of the prostate in Asian immigrants to the United States and their descendants. *J Urol* 1999;161:152–155.
24. Tsugane S, deSouza JM, Costa ML Jr., et al. Cancer incidence rates among Japanese immigrants in the city of Sao Paulo, Brazil, 1969–78. *Cancer Causes Control* 1990;1:189–193.
25. Gann PH, Hennekens CH, Stampfer MJ. A prospective evaluation of plasma prostate-specific antigen for detection of prostatic cancer. *JAMA* 1995;4:289–294.
26. Henderson RJ, Eastham JA, Culkin DJ, et al. Prostate-specific antigen (PSA) and PSA density: racial differences in men without prostate cancer. *J Natl Cancer Inst* 1997;89:134–138.
27. Abdalla I, Ray P, Ray V, et al. Comparison of serum prostate-specific antigen levels and PSA density in African-American, white, and Hispanic men without prostate cancer. *Urology* 1998;51:300–305.
28. Smith DS, Bullock AD, Catalona WJ, et al. Racial differences in a prostate cancer screening study. *J Urol* 1996;4:1366–1369.

29. Weinrich MC, Jacobsen SJ, Weinrich SP, et al. Reference ranges for serum prostate-specific antigen in black and white men without cancer. *Urology* 1998;52:967–973.
30. Oesterling JE, Kumamoto Y, Tsukamoto T, et al. Serum prostate-specific antigen in a community-based population of healthy Japanese men: lower values than for similarly aged white men. *Br J Urol* 1995;75:347–353.
31. Powell J, Heibrun L, Littrup P, et al. Outcome of African American men screened for prostate cancer, the DEED (Detroit Education and Early Detection) study. *J Urol* 1997;158:146–149.
32. Brawer MK, Chetner MP, Beatie J, et al. Screening for prostate carcinoma with prostate specific antigen. *J Urol* 1992; 147:841–845.
33. Kubricht WS, Kattan MW, Sartor O, et al. Race is not independently associated with a positive prostate biopsy in men suspected of having prostate cancer. *Urology* 1999;53:553–556.
34. Cher M, Lewis PE, Banerjee M, et al. A similar pattern of chromosome attractions in prostate cancers from African Americans and Caucasian Americans. *Clin Cancer Res* 1998; 4:1273–1278.
35. Smith JR, Freije D, Carpten JD. Major susceptibility locus for prostate cancer on chromosome 1 suggested by a genome-wide search. *Science* 1996;2743:1371–1374.
36. Cooney KA, McCarthy JD, Lange E, et al. Prostate cancer susceptibility locus on chromosome 1q: confirmation study. *J Natl Cancer Inst* 1997;89:955–959.
37. Macoska JA, Trybus TM, Benson PD, et al. Evidence for three tumor suppressor gene loci on chromosome 8p in human prostate cancer. *Cancer Res* 1995;55:5390–5395.
38. Edwards A, Hammond HA, Jin L, et al. Genetic variation at five trimetric and tetrameric tandem repeat loci in four human populations. *Genomics* 1992;12:241–253.
39. Chamberlain NL, Driver ED, Miesfeld RL. The length and location of CAG trinucleotide repeats in the androgen receptor N-terminal domain affect transactivation function. *Nuclear Acids Res* 1994;22:3181–3186.
40. Sobue G, Doyu M, Morishimi T, et al. Aberrant androgen action and increased size of the tandem CAG repeat in androgen receptor gene in X-linked recessive bulbospinal neuronopathy. *J Neurol Sci* 1994;121:167–171.
41. Ingles SA, Ross RK, Yu MC, et al. Association of prostate cancer risk with genetic polymorphisms in vitamin D receptor and androgen receptor. *J Natl Cancer Inst* 1997;89:166–170.
42. Giovannucci E, Stampfer MJ, Krithivas K, et al. The CAG repeat within the androgen receptor gene and its relationship to prostate cancer. *Proc Natl Acad Sci* 1997;94:3320–3323.
43. Stanford JL, Just JJ, Gibbs M, et al. Polymorphic repeats in the androgen receptor gene: molecular markers of prostate cancer risk. *Cancer Res* 1997;57:1194–1198.
44. Hardy DO, Scher HI, Bogenreider T, et al. Androgen receptor CAG repeat lengths in prostate cancer: correlation with age of onset. *J Clin Endocrinol Metab* 1996;12:4400–4405.
45. Irvine RA, Yu MC, Ross RK, et al. The CAG and GGC microsatellites of the androgen receptor gene are in linkage disequilibrium in men with prostate cancer. *Cancer Res* 1995;9:1937–1940.
46. Sartor O, Zheng Q, Eastham J. Androgen receptor gene CAG repeat length varies in a race-specific fashion in men without prostate cancer. *Urology* 1999;53:378–380.
47. Makridakis NM, Ross RK, Pike MC, et al. Association of mis-sense substitution in SRD5A2 gene with prostate cancer in African-American and Hispanic men in Los Angeles, USA. *Lancet* 1999;354:975–978.
48. Correa P. Epidemiological correlations between diet and cancer frequency. *Cancer Res* 1981;41:3685–3690.
49. Rose DP, Boyar AP, Wynder EL. International comparisons of mortality rates for cancer of the breast, ovary, prostate, and colon, and per capita food consumption. *Cancer* 1986;11:2363–2371.
50. Willett WC. Dietary fat intake and cancer risk: a controversial and instructive story. *Semin Cancer Biol* 1998;4:245–253.
51. Giovannucci E, Rimm EB, Colditz GA, et al. A prospective study of dietary fat and risk of prostate cancer. *J Natl Cancer Inst* 1993;19:1571–1579.
52. Le Marchand L, Kolonel LN, Wilkens LR, et al. Animal fat consumption and prostate cancer: a prospective study in Hawaii. *Epidemiology* 1994;3:276–282.
53. Anderssen SO, Wolk A, Bergstrom R, et al. Energy, nutrient intake and prostate cancer risk: a population based case-control study in Sweden. *Int J Cancer* 1996;6:716–722.
54. Rohan TE, Howe GR, Burch JD, et al. Dietary factors and risk of prostate cancer: a case-control study in Ontario, Canada. *Cancer Causes Control* 1995;2:145–154.
55. Meyer F, Bairati I, Fradet Y, et al. Dietary energy and nutrients in relation to preclinical prostate cancer. *Nutr Cancer* 1997;2:120–126.
56. Patterson BH, Harlan LC, Block G, et al. Food choices of whites, blacks, and Hispanics: data from the 1987 National Health Interview Survey. *Nutr Cancer* 1995;23:105–119.
57. Swanson CA, Gridley G, Greenberg RS, et al. A comparison of diets of blacks and whites in three area of the United States. *Nutr Cancer* 1993;2:153–165.
58. Hayes RB, Ziegler RG, Gridley G, et al. Dietary factors and risks for prostate cancer among blacks and white in the United States. *Cancer Epidemiol Biomarkers Prev* 1999;1:25–34.
59. Whittemore AS, Kolonel LN, Wu AH, et al. Prostate cancer in relation to diet, physical activity, and body size in blacks, whites, and Asians in the United States and Canada. *J Natl Cancer Inst* 1995;9:652–661.
60. Hankin JH, Zhoa LP, Kolonel LN. Attributable risk of breast, prostate, and lung cancer in Hawaii due to saturated fat. *Cancer Causes Control* 1992;1:17–23.
61. Giovannucci E, Ascherio A, Rimm EB, et al. Intake of carotenoids and retinol in relation to risk of prostate cancer. *J Natl Cancer Inst* 1995;23:1767–1776.
62. Gann PH, Ma J, Giovannucci E, et al. Lower prostate cancer risk in men with elevated plasma lycopene levels: results of a prospective analysis. *Cancer Res* 1999;6:1225–1230.
63. Mancini M, Parfitt VJ, Rubba P. Antioxidants in the Mediterranean diet. *Can J Cardiol* 1995;11[Suppl G]:105G–109G.
64. Jacobsen BK, Knutsen SF, Fraser GE. Does high soy milk intake reduce prostate cancer incidence? The Adventist Health Study. *Cancer Causes Control* 1998;6:553–557.
65. Serverson RK, Nomura AM, Grove JS, et al. A prospective study of demographics, diet, and prostate cancer among men of Japanese ancestry in Hawaii. *Cancer Res* 1989; 7:1857–1860.
66. Huggins C, Hodges CV. Studies on prostatic cancer. I. The effects of castration, of estrogen, and of androgen injection

on serum phosphatases in metastatic carcinoma of the prostate. *Cancer Res* 1941;1:293–297.

67. Eaton NE, Reeves GK, Appleby RN, et al. Endogenous sex hormones and prostate cancer: a quantitative review of prospective studies. *Br J Cancer* 1999;80:930–934.
68. Henderson BE, Bernstein L, Ross RK, et al. The early in utero estrogen and testosterone environment of blacks and white: potential effects on male offspring. *Br J Cancer* 1988;57:216–218.
69. Ross R, Bernstein L, Judd H, et al. Serum testosterone levels in healthy young black and white men. *J Natl Cancer Inst* 1986;76:45–48.
70. Stanford JL, Stephenson RA, Coyle LM, et al. *Prostate cancer trends 1973–1995, SEER Program.* Bethesda, MD: National Cancer Institute, 1999.
71. Polednak AP. Stage at diagnosis of prostate cancer in Connecticut by poverty and race. *Ethn Dis* 1997;7:215–220.
72. Fowler JE Jr., Bigler SA. A prospective study of the serum prostate specific antigen concentrations and Gleason histologic scores of black and white men with prostate carcinoma. *Cancer* 1999;86:836–841.
73. Stamey TA, McNeal JE, Yemoto CM, et al. Biological determinants of cancer progression in men with prostate cancer. *JAMA* 1999;281:1395–1400.
74. Sakr WA, Tefilli MV, Grignon DJ, et al. Gleason score 7 prostate cancer: a heterogeneous entity? Correlation with pathologic parameters and disease-free survival. *Urology* 2000;56:730–734.
75. Sohayda CJ, Kupelian PA, Altsman KA, et al. Race as an independent predictor of outcome after treatment for localized prostate cancer. *J Urol* 1999;162:1331–1336.
76. Vijayakumar S, Winter K, Sause W, et al. Prostate-specific antigen levels are higher in African-American than in white patients in a multicenter registration study: results of RTOG 94-12. *Int J Radiat Oncol Biol Phys* 1998;40:17–25.
77. Vijayakumar S, Weichselbaum R, Vaida F, et al. Prostate-specific antigen levels in African-Americans correlate with insurance status as an indicator of socioeconomic status. *Cancer J Sci Am* 1996;4:225.
78. Moul JW, Sesterhenn IA, Connelly RR, et al. Prostate-specific antigen values at the time of prostate cancer diagnosis in African-American men. *JAMA* 1995;274:1277–1281.
79. Powell IJ, Banarjee M, Sakr W, et al. Should African-American men be tested for prostate carcinoma at an earlier stage than white men? *Cancer* 1999;85;472–477.
80. Harlan L, Brawley O, Pommerenke F, et al. Geographic, age, and racial variation in the treatment of local/regional carcinoma of the prostate. *J Clin Oncol* 1995;13:93–100.
81. Fein O. The influence of social class of health status: American and British research on health inequalities. *J Gen Intern Med* 1995;10:577–586.
82. Mackillop WJ, Zhang-Salomons J, Groome PA, et al. Socioeconomic status and cancer survival in Ontario. *J Clin Oncol* 1997;4:1680–1690.
83. Schrijvers CT, Coebergh JW, van der Heijden LH, et al. Socioeconomic variation in cancer survival in the Southeastern Netherlands, 1980–1989. *Cancer* 1995;75:2946–2953.
84. Adler NE, Boyce WT, Chesney MA, et al. Socioeconomic inequalities in health. No easy solution. *JAMA* 1993;24: 3140–3145.
85. Roetzheim RG, Pal N, Tennant C, et al. Effects of health insurance and race on early detection of cancer. *J Natl Cancer Inst* 1999;16:1409–1415.
86. Dale W, Vijayakumar S, Lawlor EF, et al. Prostate cancer, race, and socioeconomic status: inadequate adjustment for social factors in assessing racial differences. *Prostate* 1996; 5:271–281.
87. Dayal HH, Polissar L, Dahlberg S. Race, socioeconomic status, and other prognostic factors for survival from prostate cancer. *J Natl Cancer Inst* 1985;5:1001–1006.
88. DeAntoni EP, Crawford ED, Oesterling JE, et al. Age- and race-specific references ranges for prostate-specific antigen from a large community-based study. *Urology* 1996;48;234–239.
89. Bennett CL, Ferreira MR, Davis TC, et al. Relation between literacy, race, and stage of presentation among low-income patients with prostate cancer. *J Clin Oncol* 1998;9:3101–3104.
90. Jacobson TA, Thomas DM, Morton FJ, et al. Use of a low-literacy patient education tool to enhance pneumococcal vaccination rates. A randomized controlled trial. *JAMA* 1999;282:646–650.
91. Fradet Y, Meyer F, Bairati I, et al. Dietary fat and prostate cancer progression and survival. *Eur Urol* 1999;35:388–391.
92. Williams BJ, Tyler K, Stage C, et al. The influence of elF4E on angiogenesis in prostate tumors from African American men. *J Urol* 1999;161:3505(abst).

12

CONSERVATIVE MANAGEMENT OF LOCALIZED PROSTATE CANCER

GERALD W. CHODAK

Counseling patients with localized prostate cancer has become an increasingly difficult challenge because of the growing number of treatment options and the absence of randomized studies. Ultimately, the choice for an individual becomes a trade-off between the risks and benefits. Unlike almost all solid tumors, prostate cancer often grows slowly, enabling the patient to die of other causes without suffering from their disease. Thus, in some cases, the relative benefits of localized treatment, such as radical prostatectomy, radiation therapy, brachytherapy, and cryosurgery, may be small or possibly nonexistent. Therefore, all patients need information about the natural history of their disease when no local therapy is administered. This approach has been assigned such terms as *watchful waiting* or *conservative therapy*. Of the two, the latter is far more appropriate and potentially easier to consider, given the public's fear of cancer. Over the past several years, improved information has become available about the long-term outcomes from this approach. Nevertheless, there are also shortcomings, creating a need for caution when presenting the data to patients. A critical review seems both timely and necessary.

The traditional approach to discussing outcomes from different treatments divides patients into three groups based on Gleason score. This score still represents the best predictor of long-term survival. Until recently, outcomes were thought to be similar for tumors with Gleason scores of 2, 3 and 4; 5, 6, and 7; and 8, 9, and 10. As a result, most outcome studies divided patients into these three groups. However, an important study by Albertson and coworkers (1) showed that the long-term survival for men with Gleason 6 was significantly worse than it was for Gleason 5 and better than for Gleason 7. As a result, comparing studies of different treatments, in which the Gleason 5 to 7 tumors are reported together, has the possibility of introducing so much bias that the comparisons are not really valid. Stated differently, such an analysis has so much uncertainty that firm conclusions really cannot be made.

This problem is illustrated in two large studies, one involving men managed conservatively and another involving men treated by radical prostatectomy. Both studies used the technique of a pooled analysis (2,3). This involves obtaining the original case data from published studies, combining patients with similar outcomes to minimize confidence intervals, and then preparing new Kaplan-Meier survival curves. Of the possible techniques available for comparing different treatments, a randomized prospective study will yield the most reliable estimate of difference in outcomes. Next comes a pooled analysis, followed by a metaanalysis of published data, case-controlled studies, and, finally, an individual cohort series.

The first pooled analysis study included 828 patients from six nonrandomized reports of men diagnosed with localized prostate cancer between 1985 and 1992 who were treated conservatively (2). These data were assessed for potential biases, such as the impact of delayed local therapy, in a small subset, the inclusion of men with Tol (A1) cancers, the old age of the cohort, and the use of patients from four countries, and none appeared to bias the results. Patients were divided into three groups, Gleason 2 to 4, 5 to 7, and 8 to 10, according to the existing convention at that time. The 10-year cancer-specific survival was 87% (81% to 91%, confidence interval) for men with Gleason 2 to 4 cancers, 87% (80% to 92%) for men with Gleason 5 to 7 cancers, and only 34% (19% to 50%) for men with Gleason 8 to 10 cancers. There were two major conclusions from his study. First, at 10 years, the vast majority of men with Gleason 2 to 4 tumors did not die of their disease. This means that those men with a life expectancy of 10 years or less and a Gleason 2 to 4 cancer may gain very little from aggressive therapy, because the disease is not very life threatening. Approximately 15% to 20% of cancers may fall into this group. Equally important, the data demonstrate that poorly differentiated cancer is extremely life threatening, with two-thirds dying of their disease in 10 years and perhaps half of the survivors having metastatic disease over that interval. Although the risk of dying for men with intermediate-grade cancers appears quite moderate, the lack of information about the distribution of Gleason 5, 6, or 7 cancer makes the results for this group uncertain in light of the subsequent report by Albertsen that was described earlier (1).

A follow-up study using the same technique of pooled analysis was reported by Gerber and associates on a cohort of 2,758 men with localized cancer from eight centers located in three countries (3). Although the follow-up was shorter, this study still permits some useful comparisons with the conservative therapy study. The 10-year cancer-specific survival was 87% to 98% for Gleason 2 to 4 cancers, 74% to 85% for Gleason 5 to 7 cancers, and 65% to 86% for Gleason 8 to 10 cancers. One implication from these two reports is that approximately 13 men with Gleason 2 to 4 cancers must be treated surgically to prevent one cancer death. These two studies also provide important insight into the potential impact of radical prostatectomy in men with poorly differentiated prostate cancer. They suggest that the difference in survival could be approximately 30% in 10 years, an observation that clearly needs to be confirmed in a randomized study. They also show that the minimal impact of treating well-differentiated prostate cancer is at least at 10 years.

Unfortunately, deficiencies in these two studies limit the ability to make very firm conclusions. The limitations include possible patient selection biases, differences in follow-up, and the absence of both a central pathology review and uniform review of the cause of death. Nevertheless, in the absence of a randomized study, these reports provide some insight into the range of outcomes that might be expected with these two treatments. Another large study that looked at the impact of conservative therapy included data on more than 59,000 men with prostate cancer who were obtained from the Surveillance, Epidemiology, and End Results Program (4). These patients, aged 50 to 79 years, were diagnosed and treated by conservative therapy, radical prostatectomy, or external beam radiation therapy between 1983 and 1992. The end points included overall survival and prostate cancer–specific survival. The results were analyzed using the Kaplan-Meier method. The large sample size in each group resulted in very narrow confidence intervals. At 10 years, the cancer-specific survival after conservative therapy was 94% (91% to 95%) for men with Gleason 2 to 4 cancers but only 45% (40% to 51%) for men with Gleason 8 to 10 tumors. The Gleason 2 to 4 tumors treated conservatively had essentially the same results as the men treated by radiation therapy. This reconfirms the findings from the pooled analysis studies that the impact of local therapy is probably quite small after 10 years of follow-up. Although surgery resulted in a slightly higher survival than the other two treatments, the groups are not really comparable, because the Gleason score for the conservative and radiation groups was obtained from the prostate biopsy, whereas the Gleason score for the surgery group was obtained from the radical prostatectomy specimen. Upgrading is known to occur in approximately 30% of the surgery specimens. Therefore, any comparison of surgery to other therapies has a significant probability of bias in favor of the surgery group.

Based on the comparison of radiation and conservative therapy for men with high Gleason scores in this study, with an estimated 8% higher survival with radiation at 10 years, approximately 12 men have to be treated with radiation to prevent one cancer death.

In the men with Gleason 5 to 7 tumors, conservative therapy actually was slightly better than radiation therapy. However, as explained previously, such a comparison is invalid, because the distribution of Gleason 5, 6, or 7 cancers within each group is not described. Because the outcomes for these three grades differ, no valid conclusions are possible for the moderately differentiated group.

Despite the large cohort of patients, the level of confidence associated with these results is uncertain. Potential problems include nonuniform review of the biopsies, variable follow-up, uncertainty over the reliability of the cause of death, potential variations in the radiation therapy dose and technique, and the timing and use of hormone therapy in the men treated with radiation therapy. Perhaps the only valid conclusion from this study is that, if there is any benefit from radiation therapy using the techniques available during that time period in men with Gleason 2 to 4 cancers, then that benefit is likely to be extremely small, at least at 10 years after diagnosis. Perhaps longer follow-up will show greater differences. Although there was no detectable difference between radiation and conservative therapy for the men with Gleason 5, 6, or 7 cancer, again no conclusion is justified, because these tumors were not evaluated separately.

In addition to providing important information about the difference in outcomes for Gleason 5, 6, and 7 cancers, Albertsen and his associates are credited with providing the 15-year outcomes for men with localized prostate cancer who were treated conservatively (1). They developed a competing risk analysis for men between the ages of 55 and 74 years, estimating the probability of dying from prostate cancer or other causes, or being alive, stratified by Gleason score. This work is particularly important, because it is the only report on conservative management to show the outcomes separately for Gleason 5, 6, and 7 cancers.

The study was performed by searching the Connecticut Tumor Registry for men aged 55 to 74 years who were diagnosed with localized prostate cancer between 1971 and 1984 and either did not receive local treatment, such as radiation, surgery, or brachytherapy, or received immediate or delayed hormone therapy. The most important aspect of this study is that all of the biopsy specimens were re-reviewed by one pathologist. The authors found that at 15 years the chances of dying from prostate cancer were 4% to 7% for men with Gleason 2 to 4 cancer, 6% to 11% for men with Gleason 5 cancer, 18% to 30% for men with Gleason 6 cancer, 42% to 70% for men with Gleason 7 cancer, and 60% to 87% for men with Gleason 8 to 10 cancer. These data further demonstrate the low probability of suffering from prostate cancer over a 15-year period for Gleason 2 to 5 cancer. Even for Gleason 6 cancers, the risk is not very high, especially in men aged older than 70 years, because they have a much higher risk of dying from other causes. These data also clearly demonstrate the high risk posed by this disease in men whose tumor has a high Gleason score (7 to 10). Even at 5 years, men with high-grade prostate cancer have a significant risk of dying from their disease, regardless of whether they are 55 or 74 years of age.

Despite the methods used to minimize bias, the study is still a retrospective review and, therefore, subject to the same selection biases of other nonrandom studies. Nevertheless, the results are remarkably consistent for the well and poorly differentiated cancers compared to the other studies cited.

One additional large, single-institution cohort study reported 15-year survival results for men with To to T2 prostate cancer (5). The patients were diagnosed in Sweden between 1977 and 1984 either by fine-needle aspiration or by examining surgical specimens obtained from men undergoing surgery for benign prostatic hypertrophy. The mean age at diagnosis was 72 years. Although the study was retrospective, all the cases were re-reviewed for this report. Some men with high-grade cancers were excluded and received local therapy. All patients were followed until death. The average follow-up was 168 months, and it included a bone scan every 6 to 12 months. All death certificates were also reviewed. The results showed that only 12% developed metastases, and 11% died of prostate cancer. The 15-year cancer-specific survival for the entire group was 72% to 89%. Death from prostate cancer occurred in 6%, 17%, and 56% of men with well, moderate, and poorly differentiated cancers; however, survival curves were not provided. As a result, this study does not permit easy comparisons with other reports.

Although this report has received considerable attention, it too suffers from several valid criticisms. These include the use of cytology rather than histology to make the diagnosis, the small number of poorly differentiated cancers, and the inclusion of 72 of 300 patients with Tol cancers (similar to the old A1 cancers that carry very small risk).

SUMMARY

Until randomized studies are completed, patients will have to rely on data from uncontrolled reports, such as those described previously. Although caution is needed, there is a recurring pattern of behavior of well-differentiated localized tumors treated conservatively with a very small percentage dying from their disease even by 10 to 15 years after diagnosis. At the same time, the mortality is quite high for the poorly differentiated cancers. Perhaps the greatest problem in using these data to counsel patients diagnosed in the year 2001 is that none of the studies includes men diagnosed by PSA, which represents the most common means of diagnosis at the present time. Because the estimated lead time bias of PSA-detected cancers is approximately 3 years, the natural history of newly diagnosed prostate cancers is likely to be even longer than those included in the studies cited. Nevertheless, the counseling problem is not alleviated, because the average age at diagnosis is declining, and many men have a life expectancy much greater than the 15 years for which data currently exists. Longer follow-up will be needed for the well and moderately differentiated cancers before these results are available. Regardless of these outcomes, however, conservative management is a reasonable treatment option for men with localized prostate cancer and Gleason scores of 2 to 6.

REFERENCES

1. Albertsen PC, Hanley JA, Gleason DF, et al. Competing risk analysis of men aged 55–74 years at diagnosis managed conservatively for clinically localized prostate cancer. *JAMA* 1998;280:975–980.
2. Chodak GW, Thisted RA, Gerber GS, et al. Results of conservative management of clinically localized prostate cancer. *N Engl J Med* 1994;330:242–248.
3. Gerber GS, Thisted RA, Scardino PT, et al. Results of radical prostatectomy in men with clinically localized prostate cancer. *JAMA* 1996;276:615–619.
4. Lu-Yao GL, Yao SL. Population-based study of long-term survival in patients with clinically localized prostate cancer. *Lancet* 1997;349:906–910.
5. Johansson JE, Holmberg L, Johansson S, et al. Fifteen-year survival in prostate cancer. *JAMA* 1997;277:467–471.

13

CLINICAL EPIDEMIOLOGY: INCIDENCE RATES, DATABASES, AGE, AND CO-MORBIDITY

PETER C. ALBERTSEN

Prostate cancer is the most common non–skin cancer among American men and is the second leading cause of cancer death after lung cancer in men in the United States. The American Cancer Society (ACS) estimates that 198,100 men will be diagnosed with prostate cancer in the United States in 2001, and 31,500 men will die from this disease (1). Worldwide, prostate cancer is the sixth most common cancer in terms of incidence and the fourth most common cancer among men. The lifetime incidence of prostate cancer in developed countries is approximately 14.3%, compared to only 4.3% in third-world nations (1). An older population and more aggressive screening most likely explain these differences. Although the incidence of prostate cancer is relatively high, prostate cancer represents only 5.6% of all cancer deaths among men. These statistics reflect the relatively good prognosis of many men diagnosed with this disease.

From a public health perspective, prostate cancer represents a significant disease burden. Approximately 19% of men diagnosed with prostate cancer will die from their disease. As the life expectancy for a 65-year-old man continues to increase, the burden posed by prostate cancer will also increase. The aging of the post–World War II generation will cause the absolute number of prostate cancer cases to increase dramatically in the next few decades. This absolute increase in incidence and mortality is obscured in age-adjusted incidence and mortality rates reported by several large cancer agencies. It is therefore important to understand how cancer statistics are generated and reported.

HOW ARE CANCER DATABASES CREATED?

In the United States, a major source of information concerning newly diagnosed cancer cases is from data generated by the National Cancer Institute's Surveillance, Epidemiology, and End Results (SEER) program (2). This program was created in 1971 as part of the National Cancer Act and is charged to collect, analyze, and disseminate information that is useful in preventing, diagnosing, and treating cancer. The SEER program is comprised of 11 large tumor registries that together conduct surveillance of approximately 14% of the U.S. population. The tumor registries of five states, Connecticut, Hawaii, Iowa, New Mexico, and Utah, and five standard metropolitan regions, Atlanta, Detroit, San Francisco–Oakland, Seattle–Puget Sound, and Los Angeles County, plus four counties in the San Jose–Monterey region south of San Francisco, comprise the SEER program. Each of these registries is responsible for obtaining detailed information concerning every patient diagnosed with cancer who resides in these defined geographic regions. Legislative statutes mandate the reporting of newly diagnosed cancer in every SEER region.

Information regarding cancer deaths is derived from a different source. The National Center for Health Statistics compiles detailed information concerning all deaths that occur within the United States. Most state health departments and vital statistics offices use the standard death certificate format recommended by the World Health Assembly. The death certificate consists of two parts. Part I contains three lines for physicians to record the train of medical events leading directly to the patient's death. Part II contains one line for physicians to record any "other significant conditions." Specifically, physicians are asked to record "conditions contributing to death but not related to cause." The National Center for Health Statistics codes information available on death certificates using a standard coding algorithm that is part of the *International Classification of Diseases 9* system. The general principle of the coding algorithm states that when more than one condition is entered on the certificate, the condition entered alone on the lowest used line of part I should be selected only if it could give rise to all of the conditions entered above it. Whether information on part I of the certificate appears incomplete or is unlikely to be the definitive cause of death, information on part II may be used. This most often occurs for poorly defined conditions, such as senility, various trivial conditions, surgical procedures, and multiple malignancies. Details of the coding rules can be found in Chapter 4 of the *International Classification of Diseases and Related Health Problems* (3).

To better understand the relationship between prostate cancer incidence and mortality, it is useful to determine the agreement between the underlying cause of death from death certificates among men diagnosed with prostate cancer before and after the introduction of testing for prostate-specific antigen (PSA) (4). The *International Classification of Diseases 9* coding rules concerning the underlying cause of death favor over- rather than underreporting prostate cancer deaths when compared with hospital medical record review. This occurs most frequently when other cancers were present or when a patient died after surgery to treat prostate cancer. However, a high level of agreement exists between the underlying cause of death from information available in hospital medical records and on death certificates for men with prostate cancer. Moreover, cause of death determination does not appear to have changed after the introduction of testing for PSA.

HOW ARE CANCER INCIDENCE AND MORTALITY RATES REPORTED?

More than any other cancer, prostate cancer is a disease of the elderly. In developed countries, 82% of cases occur in men older than 65 years. Therefore, the absolute number of new cases depends on the absolute number of older men alive in the population being studied. Western countries generally have a proportionately greater number of elderly people compared with developing nations. As more men live longer lives, the number of men at risk for developing prostate cancer increases. This will be especially true during the next several decades when the post–World War II generation ages.

Cancer statistics can be reported using several different methods. One method is simply to tally the number of new cancer cases and cancer deaths that occur during a specific time period, such as 1 year. Although this technique provides some information concerning the magnitude of prostate cancer within a population, it does not account for the number of patients at risk for developing this disease. Because of this problem, and differences in the age structure between populations, cancer researchers frequently express cancer statistics as an *age-adjusted rate*. By adjusting the incidence rates by the number and age structure of the population at risk, epidemiologists can determine whether the incidence of prostate cancer (expressed per unit of population) is increasing, decreasing, or remaining constant. Furthermore, this method allows epidemiologists to make meaningful comparisons between different populations of men separated by either time or geography. Normally, the Bureau of Vital Statistics adjusts the incidence rates to fit the U.S. population age distribution present during a census year. The standard used by the SEER program is the age distribution recorded in the 1970 census of the United States. Incidence rates and mortality rates are normally expressed as an age-adjusted rate per 100,000 men.

HOW ARE CANCER INCIDENCE AND MORTALITY RATE PROJECTIONS CALCULATED?

The ACS prepares estimates of incidence and mortality rates annually for all major cancers (1). These rates are published each January and provide detailed information on the projected number of new cancer cases and cancer deaths occurring in the United States. The information is derived from data collected by the U.S. Census Bureau and the National Cancer Institute's SEER program. Estimates of new cancer cases are calculated using a three-step procedure. First, the annual age-specific cancer incidence rates for a 15-year period are multiplied by the age-appropriate U.S. Census Bureau population projections for the same years to estimate the number of cases diagnosed annually for a 15-year period. These annual cancer case estimates are then fitted to an autoregressive quadratic model. This model is used to predict the following year's rate.

Because of the unavoidable delay in assembling cancer incidence data from tumor registries that participate in the SEER system, accurate cancer incidence rates are only available for time periods that precede the current year by approximately 3 years. Therefore, the estimates provided by the ACS are actually statistical projections 3 years into the future. For example, ACS estimates of new prostate cancer cases published in 2001 were based on SEER public use data available only through 1997. Because of the rapid rise in the number of new cases reported during the early 1990's, the ACS projections initially underestimated and then overestimated the true incidence derived from SEER data. Because of these dramatic changes in the projected rates, the ACS published an adjustment to the 1997 estimates in the July/August issue of *CA: A Cancer Journal for Clinicians* that reduced the projected number of new cases for 1997 from 334,500 to 209,900 (5). These new estimates were based on an assumption that incidence rates would continue to decline during the next few years. For 2001, the ACS projects that 198,100 men will be diagnosed with prostate cancer and 31,500 men will die from their disease, but because of the huge fluctuations in incident prostate cancers in recent years, these figures should be interpreted cautiously.

The rapid rise in the ACS projections concerning the incidence of prostate cancer that occurred after the introduction of testing for PSA led many clinicians to speak of a prostate cancer epidemic. In hindsight, the recent changes in prostate cancer incidence rates reflect a *cull* phenomenon that can occur after the introduction of a new, more sensitive screening tool. PSA testing has led to the discovery of a large number of previously unsuspected cases, especially among men in their seventh decade. This cull effect is confirmed by the observation that incidence rates have fallen most dramatically among older men who have undergone repeated testing for PSA. Stephenson has reported that PSA testing appears to be related to age and that since 1992 the incidence rates for older men have fallen more rapidly than for younger men. The fraction of men undergoing PSA testing increases as a function of their age, from 17% of men in their fifth decade to 75% of men in their ninth decade (6).

HOW DOES PROSTATE CANCER COMPARE WITH OTHER COMMON CANCERS?

Prostate cancer is only one of several cancers that afflict older Americans. Estimates for 2001 suggest that 31% of cancers diagnosed in men will be prostate, 14% will be lung and bronchus, and 10% will be colon and rectal cancer (Fig. 13-1) (1). Deaths from prostate cancer, however, occur less frequently than from other common cancers. Estimates for 2001 suggest that 31% of cancer deaths in men will be from lung cancer, 11% from prostate cancer, and 10% from colon and rectal cancer (Fig. 13-2).

Common cancers present at different ages. Between 1990 and 1994, the median age at diagnosis for prostate cancer was 71 years; for colon and rectal cancer, the median age at diagnosis was 72 years, but for female breast cancer, by comparison, it was 64 years. The median age at death during this same period was 78 years for prostate cancer, 74 years for colon and rectal cancers, and 68 years for female breast cancer. Therefore, the median time from diagnosis to disease-specific death was 7 years for prostate cancer, 2 years for colon and rectal cancer, and 4 years for female breast cancer. The number of life years lost for these dis-

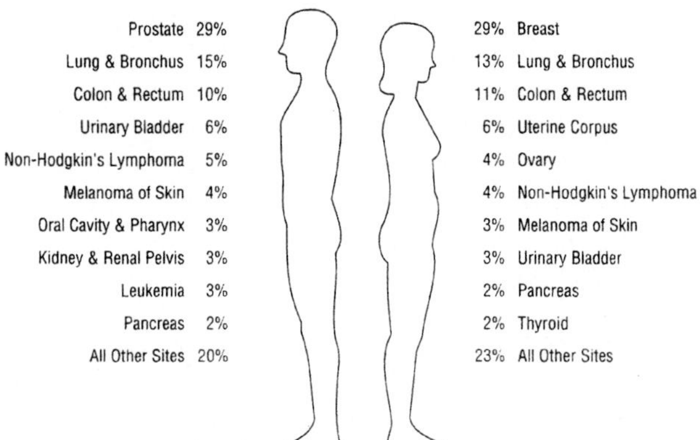

FIGURE 13-1. Estimated new cancer cases, ten leading sites by gender, United States, 1999. Excludes basal and squamous cell skin cancers and *in situ* carcinomas except urinary bladder. (From Landis SH, Murray T, Boled S, et al. Cancer statistics, 1999. *CA Cancer J Clin* 1999;49:16, with permission.)

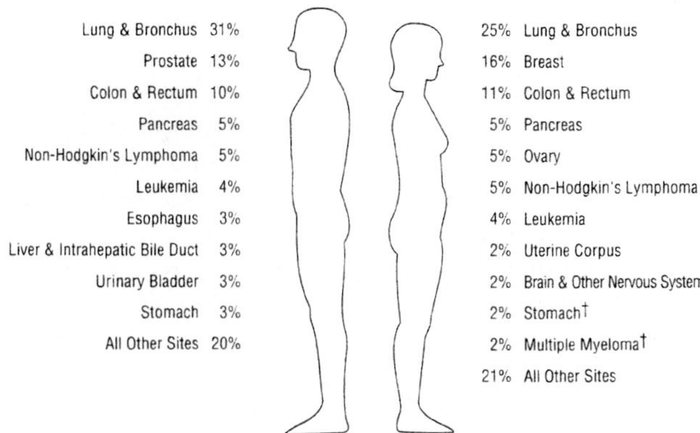

FIGURE 13-2. Estimated cancer deaths, ten leading sites by gender, United States, 1999. Excludes basal and squamous cell skin cancers and *in situ* carcinomas except urinary bladder. †These two cancers received a ranking of 10; they have the same number of deaths and contribute the same percentage. (From Landis SH, Murray T, Boled S, et al. Cancer statistics, 1999. *CA Cancer J Clin* 1999;49:16, with permission.)

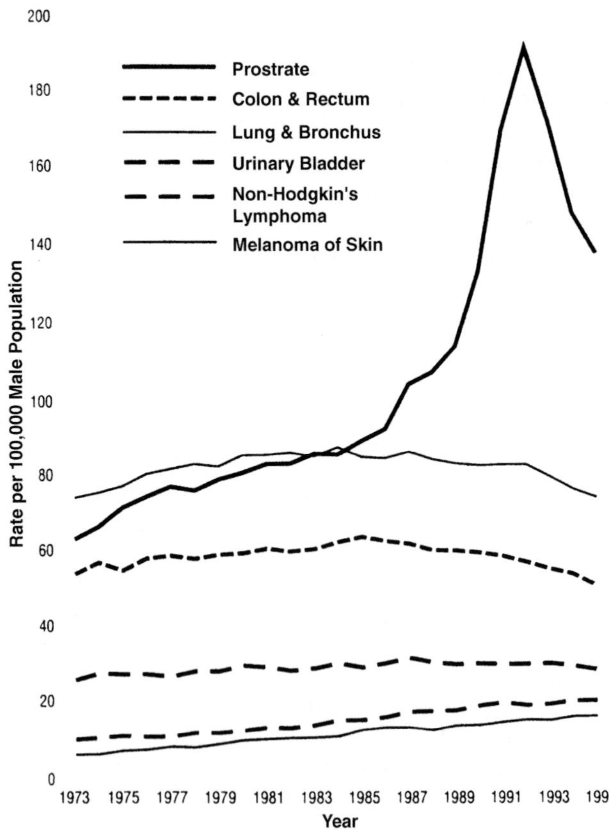

FIGURE 13-3. Age-adjusted cancer incidence rates for men by site, United States, 1973 to 1995. Rates are per 100,000 population and are age-adjusted to the 1970 U.S. standard population. (From Landis SH, Murray T, Boled S, et al. Cancer statistics, 1999. *CA Cancer J Clin* 1999;49:19, with permission.)

eases is 8 years for prostate cancer, 10 years for colon and rectal cancers, and 17 years for breast cancer. By comparison, the average number of life years lost to cardiovascular disease is 12 years.

HOW HAVE PROSTATE CANCER INCIDENCE RATES CHANGED?

Over the past three decades, incidence rates for prostate cancer have changed dramatically. During the period 1973 to 1986, they rose linearly, but they increased much more rapidly from 1987 to 1992. Since then, the rates have been falling and are now approaching values originally seen during the earlier portion of the 1990s (Fig. 13-3). During the 5 years preceding 1992, the age-adjusted incidence rate of prostate cancer increased 84% from 102.9 cases per 100,000 men in 1987 to 189.4 per 100,000 men in 1992. The two largest increases were observed in 1990 and 1991. Since 1992, there has been a precipitous drop in the number of new cases, such that by 1995, the most current year for which accurate numbers are available, the incidence rates were 168.7 per 100,000, a value just slightly above that recorded for 1990 (Fig. 13-4). The incidence rate curves over time for African-American and white individuals have a similar shape, except that the peak incidence rate for African-Americans occurred 1 year later than the peak for white individuals (Fig. 13-5). The incidence of prostate cancer in African-Americans is almost double that seen among white individuals.

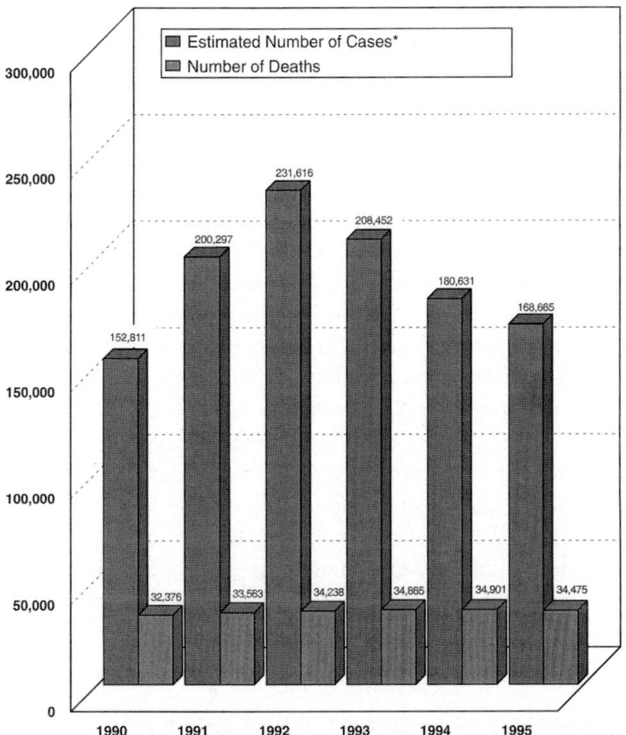

FIGURE 13-4. Prostate cancer incidence and mortality in the United States, 1990 to 1995. SEER, Surveillance, Epidemiology, and End Results. (From Stanford JL, Stephenson RA, Coyle LM, et al. *Prostate cancer trends 1973–1995, SEER program*. Bethesda, MD: National Cancer Institute, 1998:NIH Pub. No. 99-4543, with permission.)

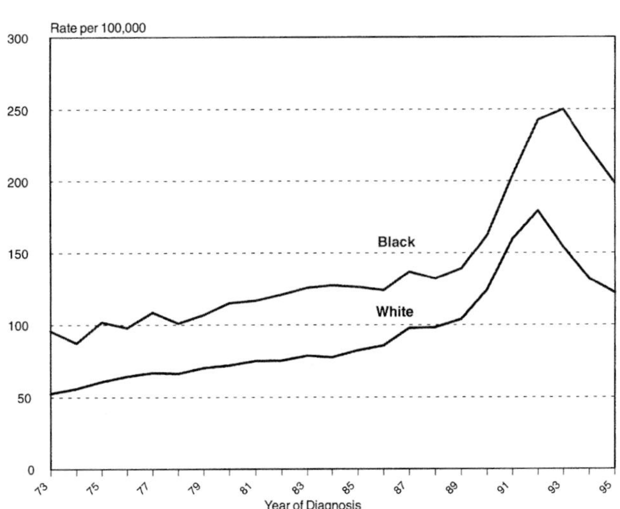

FIGURE 13-5. Prostate cancer Surveillance, Epidemiology, and End Results (SEER) program incidence rates, 1973 to 1995. Rates are age adjusted to the 1970 U.S. standard. Rates from 1973 to 1987 are based on data from the nine standard SEER registries. Data from San Jose and Los Angeles are included in the rate calculations for 1988 to 1995. (From Stanford JL, Stephenson RA, Coyle LM, et al. *Prostate cancer trends 1973–1995, SEER program*. Bethesda, MD: National Cancer Institute, 1998:NIH Pub. No. 99-4543, with permission.)

HOW DO PROSTATE CANCER INCIDENCE RATES VARY BY AGE AT DIAGNOSIS?

Despite widespread screening efforts targeted at men aged 50 to 65 years, age-specific incidence rates still suggest that prostate cancer is a disease of older men. For the two decades leading up to 1993, the age-specific incidence rates were highest for men aged 75 years and older, followed by that for men aged 65 to 74 years (7). Since 1993, the rate has decreased sharply among men aged 75 years and older, so that the highest rate of prostate cancer now occurs among men aged 65 to 74 years. Prostate cancer is still relatively uncommon among men under the age of 65, but the annual rate among this group more than tripled between 1989 and 1992. The rate has decreased slightly since 1992 (Fig. 13-6).

Before the introduction of testing for PSA, the mean age at diagnosis for men with prostate cancer was 72 years for white individuals and 70 years for African-Americans. Since then, the mean age has been falling. As of 1994, the mean age at diagnosis among white individuals was 69 years and 67 years among African-Americans. Thus, as a result of testing for PSA, prostate cancer is being diagnosed approximately 2.5 years earlier than it was a decade ago. As a consequence, all

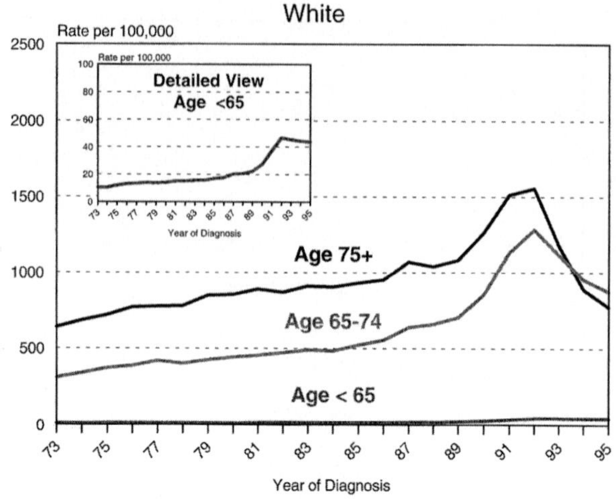

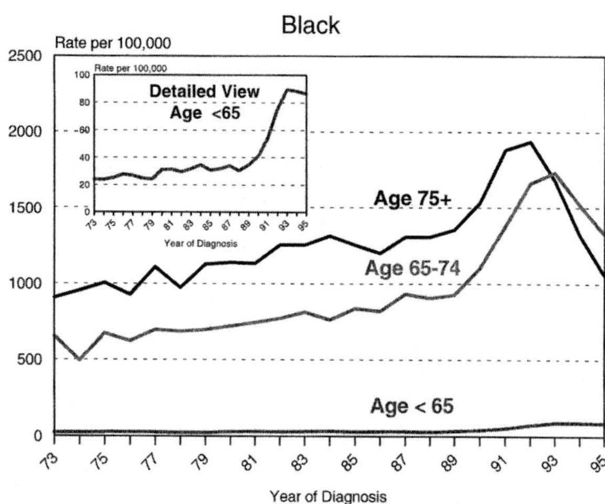

FIGURE 13-6. Prostate cancer Surveillance, Epidemiology, and End Results (SEER) program incidence rates by age at diagnosis, 1973 to 1995. Rates are age adjusted to the 1970 U.S. standard. Rates from 1973 to 1987 are based on data from the nine standard SEER registries. Data from San Jose and Los Angeles are included in the rate calculations for 1988 to 1995. (From Stanford JL, Stephenson RA, Coyle LM, et al. *Prostate cancer trends 1973–1995, SEER program*. Bethesda, MD: National Cancer Institute, 1998:NIH Pub. No. 99-4543, with permission.)

comparisons with historical case series concerning longevity postcancer diagnosis must account for a 2.5-year lead time. To attribute increased longevity to earlier diagnosis and treatment, researchers must see a survival improvement of at least this amount after radical surgery or radiation.

HOW HAS THE STAGE OF INCIDENCE CASES OF PROSTATE CANCER CHANGED SINCE 1990?

The SEER program reports a summary cancer stage for all patients with newly diagnosed disease. For prostate cancer, four categories are used: localized, regional, distant, and unknown. Before the introduction of PSA testing, patients with localized cancer accounted for the major proportion of incident cases. Relatively modest increases were recorded for regional and distant-stage disease. After 1986, the stage-specific incidence rates began to increase rapidly for all stages except for distant-stage disease. From 1986 to 1991, the incidence of localized disease increased 75%, whereas incidences of regional and unstaged disease rose 144% and 161%, respectively. The incidence of distant-stage disease remained essentially unchanged.

The introduction of testing for PSA has had a profound effect on the incidence of distant-stage disease. Since 1991, the age-adjusted incidence rate for distant disease has fallen dramatically and is now approximately half of what it was at the beginning of the 1990s. Although a decreasing rate of distant disease is an indicator that early detection may subsequently lead to decreased mortality, this fact alone is not sufficient to demonstrate the efficacy of prostate cancer screening and treatment. The efficacy of early detection and treatment requires a significant decline in mortality rates. Although prostate cancer mortality rates have shown a modest decline during the last few years, the drop has not been of a sufficient magnitude to confirm the value of early detection and treatment. Given the long natural history of prostate cancer, if PSA screening is effective, the associated earlier detection of prostate cancer combined with curative treatment of localized disease will not yield large population-based improvements in mortality until the mid 2000s.

Screening for cancer can produce significant stage shifts and still not result in significant reductions in mortality rates. In the 1960s, for example, a number of organizations within the United States advocated lung cancer screening by chest x-ray, because data from several large case series suggested a shift in stage and an increase in patient survival (8). Controversy surrounding screening ended only after clinical trials demonstrated that routine chest x-rays did not result in a decline in mortality from lung cancer. The recent Japanese and Canadian experiences with neuroblastoma screening are other examples of cancer screening programs that yielded a favorable stage shift and an apparent increased survival without evidence of decreased mortality (9,10). Further evaluation of screening tests for catecholamine metabolites has demonstrated that there are two kinds of neuroblastoma, a benign form that will never progress, and an aggressive, usually fatal form that is unlikely to be found at a curable stage even with screening. Neuroblastoma screening has caused a significant number of children to undergo unnecessary treatment. It is plausible that a similar phenomenon for older adult men is occurring due to PSA screening for prostate cancer.

HOW HAS THE GRADE OF PROSTATE CANCER CHANGED SINCE 1990?

The past two decades have witnessed a change in the distribution of cancer grade among men with newly diagnosed prostate cancer. The SEER program classifies prostate cancer into four differentiation grade categories: well, moderate, poor, and undetermined. Well differentiated includes tumors with Gleason scores 2 to 4 and moderately differentiated includes tumors with Gleason scores 5 to 6, whereas poorly differentiated includes tumors with Gleason scores 7 to 10. Between 1974 and 1984, the rate of well- and poorly differentiated tumors increased slowly, whereas the age-adjusted incidence of moderately differentiated tumors grew more rapidly. After 1989, with the introduction of widespread testing for PSA, there was a dramatic increase in the number of moderately differentiated tumors, such that the number of new cases in this grade category was two to three times higher than the number of well- and poorly differentiated tumors. Since 1991, moderately differentiated tumors have represented half of all newly diagnosed cases, whereas well- and poorly differentiated tumors have each accounted for approximately 20% of new cases.

Coding rules used by the SEER program may explain some of these changes. According to SEER conventions, the most accurate pathology grade is used when recording the grade of newly diagnosed cancers. For patients undergoing radiation therapy or conservative management, the grade of tumor is based on needle biopsy or the transurethral resection specimen that resulted in diagnosis. For patients undergoing radical prostatectomy, the results of the surgical pathology report replace the results obtained on biopsy. As a result, some of the tumors that are well differentiated initially may be upgraded to moderately differentiated tumors so that trends in tumor stage and grade must take into account trends in prostate cancer treatment. It is unclear whether these changes account for the majority of the changes observed for moderately differentiated disease.

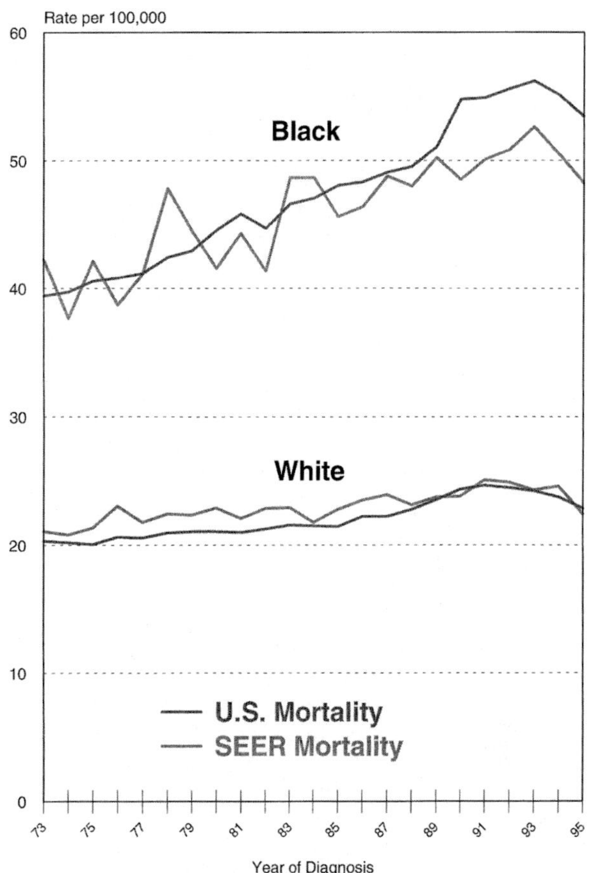

FIGURE 13-7. Prostate cancer mortality rates, 1973 to 1995. Rates are age adjusted to the 1970 U.S. standard. Rates from 1973 to 1987 are based on data from the nine standard prostate cancer Surveillance, Epidemiology, and End Results (SEER) program registries. Data from San Jose and Los Angeles are included in the rate calculations for 1988 to 1995. (From Stanford JL, Stephenson RA, Coyle LM, et al. *Prostate cancer trends 1973–1995, SEER program*. Bethesda, MD: National Cancer Institute, 1998:NIH Pub. No. 99-4543, with permission.)

HOW HAVE PROSTATE CANCER MORTALITY RATES CHANGED SINCE 1990?

During the past two decades, the mortality rate from prostate cancer has gradually increased for both white individuals and African-Americans. Since then, the number of deaths has been stable. In absolute terms, 33,565 men died from prostate cancer in 1991 compared with a projection of 31,500 deaths in 2001 (Fig. 13-4). When viewed in relative terms, however, the data suggest a different trend. Among white men, the age-adjusted mortality rate rose from 20.3 deaths per 100,000 men in 1973 to 24.7 deaths per 100,000 men in 1991. Rates for African-American men were more than twice as high. Since then, however, rates have declined in both populations (Fig. 13-7). The National Cancer Institute recently reported data showing that the prostate cancer death rate in the United States fell between 1991 and 1995 from a crude rate of 26.5 to 17.3 deaths per 100,000 men in the overall population (11). The percentage decline was the greatest for young, white men and smallest for older men and African-Americans.

The differences between absolute and relative age-adjusted rates are explained, in part, by the increasing number of men dying from prostate cancer but also by the even greater increase in the number of older men still alive in the U.S. population. The increase in the size of the population at risk (the denominator) has been proportionally more rapid than the increase in the number of men dying from prostate cancer (the numerator).

There has been a small decline in the age-adjusted mortality rate during the past few years. After increasing steadily from 1973 to 1990, the mortality rate from prostate cancer fell by 6.3% from 1991 to 1995 (2). The age-specific fall was the greatest for men younger than age 75 years (7.4%) and lowest for men older than 75 years (3.8%). Men older than age 75 years account for two-thirds of all prostate cancer deaths (Fig. 13-8). This is the first recorded fall in the mortality rate from prostate cancer since the 1930s, when cancer statistics were first collected. Many urologists attribute this decline in prostate cancer

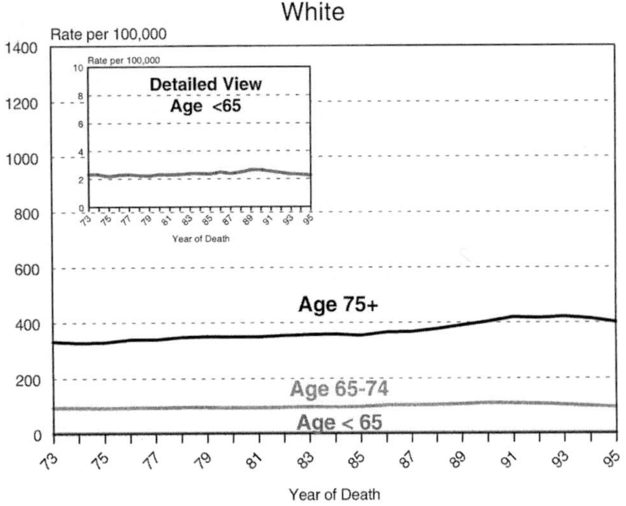

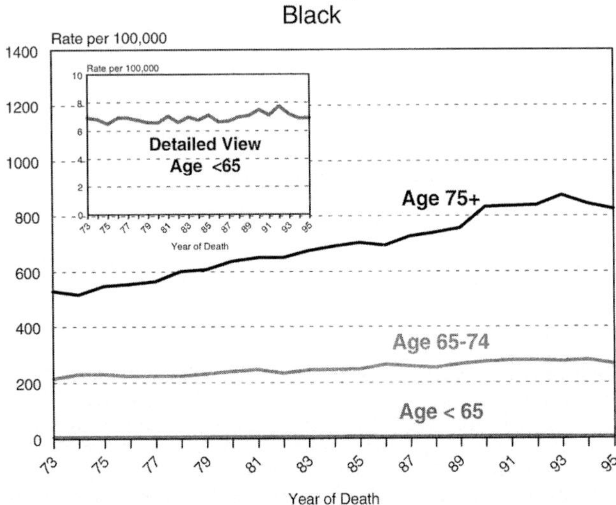

FIGURE 13-8. Prostate cancer U.S. mortality rates by age at death, 1973 to 1995. Rates are age adjusted to the 1970 U.S. standard. (From Stanford JL, Stephenson RA, Coyle LM, et al. *Prostate cancer trends 1973–1995, SEER program*. Bethesda, MD: National Cancer Institute, 1998:NIH Pub. No. 99-4543, with permission.)

mortality to early diagnosis through PSA screening. There are several equally plausible explanations that can account for a decline of this magnitude.

The discrepancy between a 19% lifetime incidence of prostate cancer and a 3.6% lifetime mortality from prostate cancer indicates that the majority of prostate cancers do not result in death. Most prostate cancers occur in older men, and, because the progression rate is often slow, most men with prostate cancer die of other causes before their prostate cancer causes death. Autopsy series have revealed that approximately one-third of men older than age 50 years have asymptomatic prostate cancer (12). By age 80 years, approximately 60% to 70% of men will have microscopic evidence of disease. Why most of these cancers do not become clinically significant remains unknown.

CAN THE RECENT DECLINE IN PROSTATE CANCER MORTALITY RATES BE ATTRIBUTED TO SCREENING AND TREATMENT?

Virtually all physicians and public health experts agree that prostate cancer is a significant health problem, and, therefore, efforts to prevent and control this disease should be part of the American public health agenda. To promote testing for PSA as a method of screening for prostate cancer, public health officials seek to determine whether PSA testing satisfies several important criteria. These include the following four criteria:

1. Is testing for PSA an accurate and relatively inexpensive method of identifying prostate cancer?
2. Does early detection of prostate cancer improve clinical outcome?
3. Are there potentially harmful consequences associated with the diagnosis and treatment of prostate cancer?
4. From a public health perspective, does screening for prostate cancer do more good than harm?

Many researchers have evaluated the performance of PSA testing when used as a tool to screen for prostate cancer. Unfortunately, because most men with normal PSA results do not undergo prostate biopsy, the true sensitivity and specificity of screening for prostate cancer using PSA remains uncertain. Catalona and colleagues reported a sensitivity of 80% when PSA is used to screen healthy men for prostate cancer (13). The specificity, however, is not nearly so high. Men with benign prostate hypertrophy and prostatitis frequently have false-positive results. PSA values are elevated in 25% to 46% of men with benign prostate hypertrophy, and only 28% to 35% of men testing positive for PSA will be found to have prostate cancer on biopsy (14,15). Recently, researchers have explored whether measurements of the ratio of free to complexed PSA can improve the specificity of testing for PSA. This approach has yielded modest improvements in specificity in the range of results between 4 and 10 ng per mL (16).

Attempts to determine the impact of screening large segments of the population are confounded by another significant problem. Because prostate cancer is a relatively slow-growing malignancy that frequently strikes older men, many men can be diagnosed with prostate cancer but never succumb to this disease. Screening large numbers of healthy patients risks identifying a large number of latent cancers that are not destined to progress to death during the patient's lifetime but may result in treatment with associated morbidity and mortality. Dugan and colleagues estimate that, based on prostate cancer volume-doubling times, 0.3% to 14.5% of cancers identified by testing for PSA are clinically insignificant (17), but others would argue this figure to be substantially higher.

The value of screening for prostate cancer using PSA testing ultimately rests on the clinical outcomes of those men who underwent testing. Numerous publications have focused on the relative merits of various strategies, such as PSA density, PSA velocity, and tumor ploidy, to identify men with clinically significant prostate cancer. These articles hold little value if screening does not significantly improve either longevity or quality of life. Some clinicians justify screening for PSA solely on the basis that the test can detect organ-confined disease. This finding alone is not sufficient to justify a screening program. Men undergoing screening must have outcomes that are superior to those men who are not screened. Clinical trials support the efficacy of breast, cervical, and colorectal cancer screening (18). Similar evidence is still lacking for prostate cancer, although a large national trial is ongoing. Observational studies of screening by alternative strategies, such as digital rectal examination alone, report no benefit (19,20).

IF TESTING FOR PROSTATE-SPECIFIC ANTIGEN IS EFFECTIVE, WHEN SHOULD A DECLINE IN PROSTATE CANCER MORTALITY BECOME EVIDENT?

Although it is tempting to attribute the recent modest decline in the age-adjusted prostate cancer mortality rate to the aggressive detection and treatment programs initiated throughout the country during the past decade, epidemiologists remind us that age-adjusted rates are falling for other common cancers affecting American men. In 2001, 52% of male cancer deaths will be from cancers of the lung, prostate, colon, and rectum. Between 1991 and 1995, mortality rates for American men decreased 6.7% for lung cancer, 6.3% for prostate cancer, and 7% for colorectal cancer (21). The drop in the number of deaths from lung cancer accounts for more than half of the overall drop in cancer mortality among men during this period. This fall can most likely be attributed to a decline in smoking, rather than early detection and treatment. Although the fall in colorectal cancers may be attributed to screening and treatment, an equally plausible possibility is that the decline is owing to primary prevention strategies, such as a decrease in the fat content of the average diet.

An explanation for the fall in prostate cancer rates remains elusive. Some experts claim that the fall is a consequence of screening and treatment (11,22). The SEER registries, however, document that the largest declines in prostate cancer mortality in the United States have occurred in regions of the country in which aggressive screening and treatment have been promoted least (21). In Connecticut, for example, where prostate cancer testing for PSA was not widely adopted until the early 1990s, the age-adjusted mortality rate was 23.5 per 100,000 men during the period 1991 to 1995. In Seattle, where prostate cancer was aggressively promoted during the late 1980s and was followed by a significantly higher rate of radical prostatectomy, prostate cancer mortality rates were 25.1 per 100,000 men during the same period (21,23). Given the long natural history of prostate cancer, aggressive screening and treatment programs cannot possibly yield large population-based improvements in mortality rates until the mid 2000s.

HOW DOES PATIENT AGE IMPACT THE DIAGNOSIS AND TREATMENT OF PROSTATE CANCER?

Incidence and prevalence data highlight the strong correlation between age and mortality from prostate cancer. Although older men have a relatively high incidence of prostate cancer, death from this disease occurs less frequently when compared with other competing hazards, such as heart disease and other cancers (Table 13-1). Because of the relatively low chance of dying from prostate cancer, especially when diagnosed at a very early stage, some physicians have argued against diagnosing and treating men who have a life expectancy of less than 10 years (24,25). Based on 1991 life expectancy tables, this occurs at approximately age 73 years for men in average health (Table 13-2). Men diagnosed with localized prostate cancer in their mid-seventies face a low probability of dying from their disease as compared to other causes.

HOW ARE OUTCOMES ASSESSED AFTER TREATMENTS FOR PROSTATE CANCER?

Researchers and clinicians can use several different experimental approaches to assess the impact of treating prostate cancer. Prostate cancer therapies are usually designed to achieve two goals, an increase in longevity while maintaining quality of life. Although randomized, experimental pro-

TABLE 13-1. LEADING CAUSES OF DEATH FOR U.S. MEN IN 1991

	Age 55 to 74 yr (%)	Age 75+ yr (%)
All causes	100	100
Heart disease	35	38
Cancer other than prostate	30	17
Lung disease	5	6
Cerebrovascular disease	4	7
Prostate cancer	3	4
Diabetes	2	2
Accidents	2	2
Pneumonia	2	5
Liver cirrhosis	2	—
Arterial disease	2	2
Suicide	1	—
Nephritis	—	1
Atherosclerosis	—	1

TABLE 13-2. LIFE EXPECTANCY AT SINGLE YEARS OF AGE FOR MEN OF ALL RACES

Age (yr)	Life expectancy (yr)
65	14.6
66	13.9
67	13.3
68	12.7
69	12.1
70	11.6
71	11.0
72	10.5
73	10.0
74	9.5
75	9.0
76	8.6
77	8.1
78	7.7
79	7.3
80	6.9
81	6.5
82	6.1

tocols are the ideal way to evaluate new and existing diagnostic tests and procedures, this intervention approach is not always practical, especially for chronic diseases, such as prostate cancer, that require many years of follow-up. The choice of study design depends on the question that is being addressed and usually entails a selection between an experimental design, in which patients are assigned to a treatment, or a nonexperimental design, in which data are assembled after patients select their own treatment.

Many physicians use case-series reports to document clinical outcomes after a specific medical intervention. Although these reports provide some insight concerning treatment efficacy, data from case series frequently suffer from numerous confounding factors and biases that limit their usefulness when generalizing results to the population of patients seen in community practice. Because data from case series lack a comparison group, patients and clinicians are often unable to differentiate between the impact of treatment and the natural progression of the disease or the impact of competing medical problems. It is often assumed that the majority of patients receiving treatment were destined to die from their disease in the absence of treatment. Researchers reporting case series usually do not provide information concerning the likely outcome if the patients had not received therapy. Without this comparison information, however, it is impossible to assess the relative increase in longevity or improvement in quality of life offered by the treatment being evaluated.

In 1996, for example, Gerber et al. published a multiinstitutional pooled analysis of men with clinically localized disease treated by radical prostatectomy between 1970 and 1993 (26). They reported excellent 10-year disease-specific survival estimates of 94%, 80%, and 77% for men with well- (Gleason score 2 to 4), moderately (Gleason score 5 to 7), and poorly (Gleason score 8 to 10) differentiated disease. Initial review of these data suggests that radical prostatectomy is most efficacious among men with well-differentiated disease and least efficacious among men with poorly differentiated disease. Unfortunately, no comparison population is available to determine the relative increased survival achieved by the patients undergoing treatment compared to those patients receiving no treatment.

More recently, Shipley et al. published a multiinstitutional pooled analysis of men with clinically localized prostate cancer treated with radiation therapy between 1988 and 1995 (27). They reported excellent 5-year disease-specific survival estimates of 95.1% for all men treated with radiation. Those patients with Gleason score 2 to 4 tumors and a PSA level less than 10 ng per mL at diagnosis had an 81% 5-year probability of being disease free. Men with Gleason score 5 to 6 tumors had an 86% 5-year probability of being disease free, whereas men with Gleason score 7 to 10 tumors had a 79% 5-year disease-free survival.

Although not an ideal comparison population, we analyzed the long-term outcome of 767 men followed conservatively for newly diagnosed localized prostate cancer (28). The 10-year disease-specific survival for this group of patients was 94%, 71%, and 30%, respectively, for men with well-, moderately, and poorly differentiated disease. These results are identical to those reported by Gerber et al. and better than those reported by Shipley et al. for men with Gleason score 2 to 4 tumors, suggesting that radical prostatectomy or radiation therapy may not provide a significant survival advantage among these patients. Conversely, results among patients treated conservatively were much worse for men with poorly differentiated disease, suggesting the possibility that radical prostatectomy or radiation therapy may offer a significant survival advantage among this group of patients. For men with Gleason score 5 to 7 tumors, a group of men frequently targeted for aggressive intervention, disease-specific survival outcomes appear to be relatively similar. Gerber reported a 10-year disease-specific survival of 80% (95% confidence interval, 74% to 85%). Shipley et al. reported a 5-year, no evidence of disease outcome of 86% (95% confidence interval, 78% to 95%) for men with Gleason 5 to 6 tumors. Data from our study suggest a 10-year disease-specific survival of 72% (95% confidence interval, 67% to 76%) for men with Gleason 5 to 7 tumors. Because all three series of cases are subject to significant selection biases, and many of the Connecticut patients were inadequately staged, it is impossible to determine whether radical prostatectomy or radiation therapy offers a significant survival advantage among this group of patients.

HOW ARE COMPARISON POPULATIONS SELECTED FOR CASE-SERIES ANALYSES?

When making comparisons between the relative efficacy of different treatment strategies, researchers frequently compare the outcomes of patients treated in the contemporary era with historical controls. Unfortunately, patients diagnosed with cancers in one era are rarely comparable to those in another. Helgesen, for example, recently reported the outcomes associated with the treatment of 80,901 men diagnosed with prostate cancer in Sweden during the period 1960 through 1988 (29). They demonstrated a significant survival improvement during this period despite the absence of any effective therapeutic interventions. These findings are most likely consistent with an increase in the detection of nonlethal tumors coupled with the significant effect of lead-time bias associated with tumor identification after transurethral resection of the prostate. As noted earlier, a similar effect has been noted after the introduction of widespread PSA testing in the United States. By advancing the date of diagnosis, clinicians guarantee a survival advantage to contemporary patients that is independent of treatment when compared to historical controls from the pre-PSA era.

Comparison populations selected from contemporary patients also exhibit significant selection biases. Men who choose surgery, for example, are frequently healthier than those patients who select alternative strategies. Barry et al. showed that the men undergoing radical prostatectomy at the Mayo Clinic or at the University of Utah had a survival that was superior to an age-matched series of contemporary patients who had not been diagnosed with prostate cancer (30). It is unlikely that surgery improved these patients' longevity such that they would have a survival advantage over patients not diagnosed with prostate cancer.

HOW DOES CLASSIFICATION BIAS IMPACT PROSTATE CANCER OUTCOMES?

As noted earlier, the National Cancer Institute's SEER program uses the best information available when recording tumor stage and grade. For men undergoing radical prostatectomy, staging information often includes an assessment of pelvic lymph nodes. Tumor grade and stage are often coded upward after a review of the higher-volume surgical pathology, available through prostatectomy, and a histologic review of pelvic nodes. These differences in the methods of assessing tumor stage and grade introduce a classification bias that is often referred to as the *Will Rogers* phenomenon. Feinstein et al. originally described this phenomenon in an article concerning survival of lung cancer patients (31). By reclassifying some patients into higher categories, the average survival of all categories of patients will appear to improve, even though none of the individual patient's survivals has improved. A similar phenomenon occurs when prostate cancer patients are restaged from local disease to regional or distant disease after surgical exploration. Surgical patients will appear to have an improved survival compared to similar patients receiving external beam radiation therapy or brachytherapy, or are simply managed conservatively. The descriptive title of this effect is based on a famous joke by Will Rogers, who commented when all the "Oklahomans" moved to California during the Great Depression of the 1930s, the average intelligence quotient of both states went up!

Classification biases can also result, depending on how researchers assemble patient cohorts for study. Traditional population-based studies usually analyze patient outcomes related to date of diagnosis. Aus et al. proposed an alternative approach. They assembled a cohort of 301 Swedish patients identified by the Swedish Cancer Registry as those having localized disease at the time of diagnosis who died in Goteborg during the period 1988 to 1990 (32). As a consequence of selecting patients according to their date of death, Aus et al. selected patients with different characteristics over different time periods. Men with aggressive tumors were diagnosed relatively recently, whereas men with more indolent tumors were diagnosed from an earlier era. Because the population at risk changed in size and in age distribution, and the incidence of disease increased during the accrual period, the results were biased in favor of selecting men with more aggressive disease (33). As a consequence, their estimates of the 15-year survival outcomes from prostate cancer are much higher than those reported by others, including Johansson et al., Chodak et al., and Albertsen et al. (34–36).

HOW DO CO-MORBIDITIES IMPACT OUTCOMES OF PATIENTS WITH PROSTATE CANCER?

Because prostate cancer is frequently a slowly progressive disease, competing medical hazards play a significant role in determining long-term clinical outcomes. The presence of co-morbid conditions confounds comparisons of case-series reports of different treatment alternatives, in part because they contribute to differing survival outcomes, but also because they result in selection biases. Healthier patients tend to choose more aggressive treatment strategies than patients who have significant heart disease, pulmonary problems, or other coexisting serious health problems.

Several instruments have been developed to assist physicians in classifying the extent of co-morbid disease. None was specifically designed for use in prostate cancer patients. The index of coexistent disease developed by Greenfield et al. was designed to predict the functional status of patients after hospitalization and includes measures of the activities of daily living (37). It has been tested on patients with breast cancer and hip fractures. Charlson et al. developed a co-morbidity scoring system for use in patients entering clinical trials (38). The index developed by Kaplan and Feinstein was designed to classify initial co-morbidity among patients with diabetes mellitus who participated in a long-term outcome analysis (39).

When deciding between different treatment recommendations, physicians currently estimate patient potential life expectancy by incorporating information based on patient age, modified by a subjective estimate of the impact of co-morbidity. By using formal instruments, researchers and clinicians can potentially control for co-morbidity when evaluating survival data from large series. Such instruments were recently tested among men with newly diagnosed, clinically localized prostate cancer to determine whether these three systems could be used to stratify men into groups with distinctly different prognoses, according to the presence or absence of competing medical hazards (40). Results showed that Gleason score and a co-morbidity index were the two most powerful predictors of long-term survival. Figure 13-9 demonstrates the cumulative mortality for all causes of death for 411 men who died during a 15-year follow-up period in this study. Men with no co-morbidities at diagnosis demonstrated an apparent survival advantage over those with minimal, moderate, and severe co-morbidities. Only 62% to 68% of men with no co-morbidities at diagnosis died within 10 years of diagnosis, depending on which instrument was used. Men with minimal or moderate co-morbid conditions had a 70% to 80% death rate 10 years after diagnosis. Men with severe co-morbidities, on the other hand, had a cumulative mortality exceeding 90% within 10 years of diagnosis.

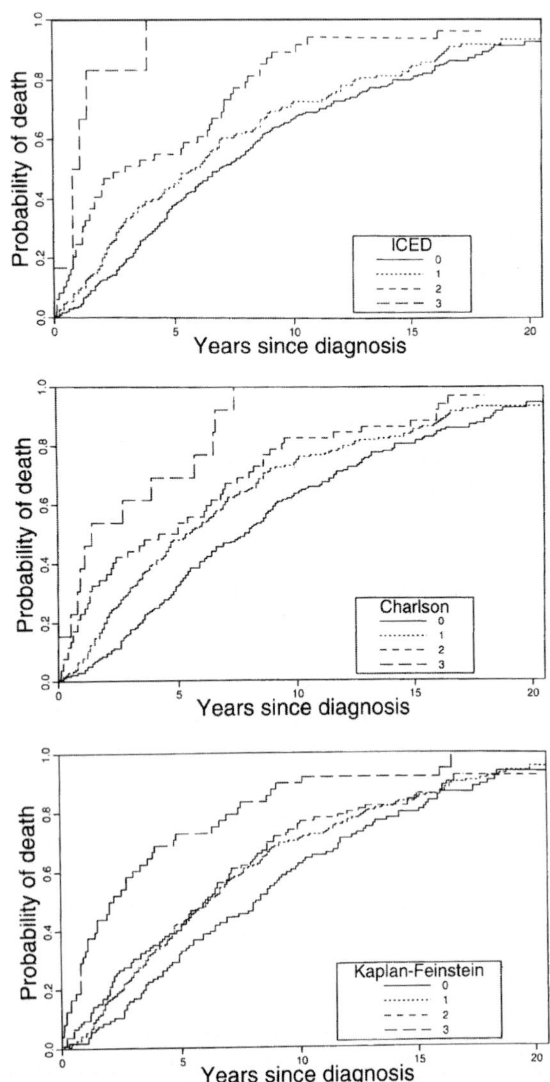

FIGURE 13-9. Cumulative mortality from all causes of death stratified by severity of co-morbidities at diagnosis, as measured by each of the three instruments tested. Data are not adjusted for patient age or Gleason sum. ICED, index of coexistent disease. (From Albertsen PC, Fryback DG, Storer BE, et al. The impact of co-morbidity on life expectancy among men with localized prostate cancer. *J Urol* 1996;156:127–132, with permission.)

In addition to showing an increased probability of dying from competing medical hazards, these results demonstrated that the presence of co-morbid disease has an impact on prostate cancer–specific mortality. After adjusting for age and Gleason score, patients with higher co-morbidity scores had a higher cumulative mortality over a 10-year follow-up period. These findings suggest that cause-specific survival analyses may not adequately control for the impact of competing medical hazards.

HOW CAN RESEARCHERS ACCOUNT FOR THE IMPACT OF COMPETING MEDICAL HAZARDS?

Physicians reporting results from research studies, such as randomized trials, population-based analyses, and case series, can select from several potential outcomes. Historically, overall survival has been the primary outcome used to evaluate treatment efficacy in oncology. This metric has the distinct advantage of being very precise and is advantageous to patients by allowing them to estimate their average probability of surviving using different treatment alternatives.

However, there are three major disadvantages to using overall survival as an outcome metric. First, long-term survival does not separate the impact of prostate cancer from that of competing medical problems. As a result, patients and clinicians have difficulty separating the impact of treatment from the impact of co-morbidities. Second, because prostate cancer is a chronic disease extending over many years, death is a relatively rare event, especially when follow-up is less than 5 to 10 years. Because modern screening efforts identify patients very early in the course of their disease, survival is not a particularly useful measure over a short amount of time. Finally, overall survival is a relatively crude measure and does not incorporate quality of life. As a consequence, researchers frequently turn to alternative outcome measures.

Cause-specific survival analysis is an analytic methodology, designed to minimize the impact of competing medical hazards and, instead, focus specifically on the impact of treatment on prostate cancer mortality. This technique provides researchers with better estimates of treatment efficacy

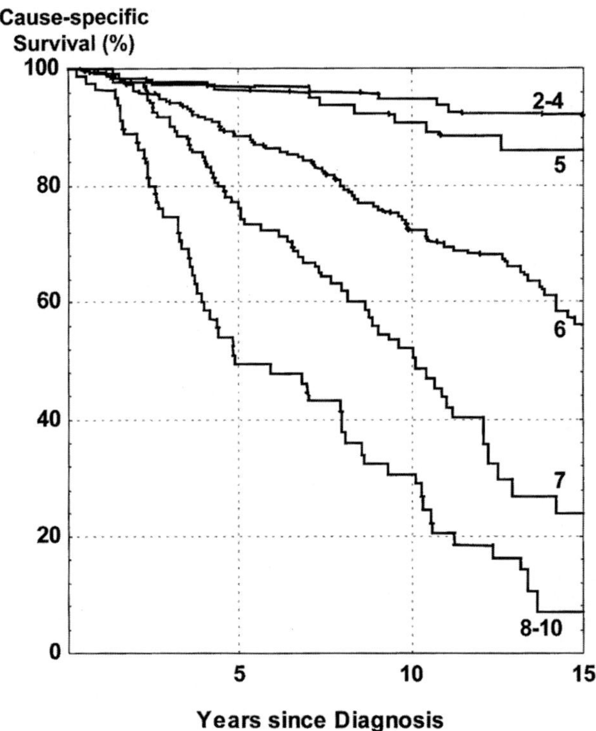

FIGURE 13-10. Cause-specific survival of 767 men diagnosed with localized prostate cancer and managed conservatively, stratified by Gleason score. (From Albertsen PC, Hanley JA, Murphy-Setzko M. Statistical considerations when assessing outcomes after treatment for prostate cancer. *J Urol* 1999;162:439–444, with permission.)

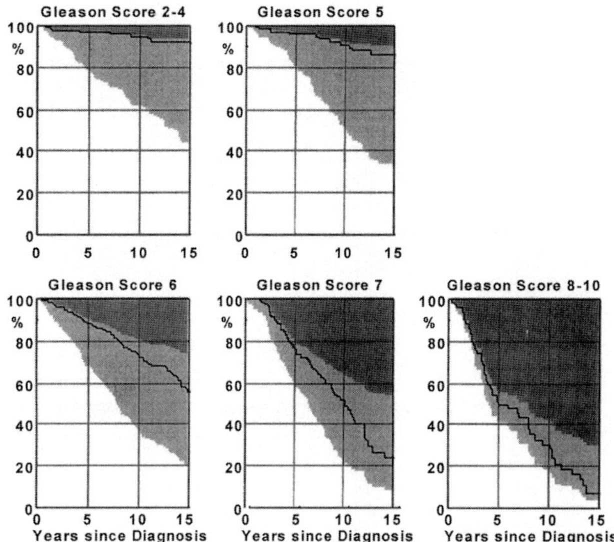

FIGURE 13-11. Competing risk survival compared with cause-specific survival for 767 men diagnosed with localized prostate cancer and managed conservatively stratified by Gleason score. Cumulative mortality from prostate cancer is shown by the dark upper band; cumulative mortality from other causes is shown by the lighter middle band. The percentage of men surviving is shown by the lowest white band. Cause-specific survival is shown by the staircase solid line. Note that, because competing mortality is substantial, the complement of cause-specific survival (i.e., the portion above the solid line) overestimates the percentage of men who actually die of their prostate cancer. (From Albertsen PC, Hanley JA, Murphy-Setzko M. Statistical considerations when assessing outcomes after treatment for prostate cancer. *J Urol* 1999;162:439–444, with permission.)

and is frequently used when a comparison population is absent. By eliminating deaths from competing medical hazards, researchers may provide overly optimistic estimates of treatment efficacy, especially among older patients.

For example, a cause-specific survival analysis was recently conducted on a sample of 767 men diagnosed with prostate cancer in Connecticut during the period 1971 to 1984 and was managed conservatively for their localized disease (41). Figure 13-10 shows these data stratified by Gleason score. The results suggest relatively good outcomes for men with Gleason 2 to 5 disease and poorer outcomes for men with Gleason scores 6 to 10 disease. Patients viewing these data might assume that their 15-year survival with low-grade prostate cancer is more than 80%. Figure 13-11 shows the same data displayed using a competing-risk analysis. In this figure, the cumulative mortality from prostate cancer for the entire cohort is presented as a dark band, whereas the cumulative mortality from competing disease hazards is presented as a lighter band. The percentage of men alive is shown in the white band. The corresponding cause-specific survival curve is superimposed for comparison. For men with relatively lethal tumors (Gleason scores 7 to 10), the results of a cause-specific analysis and a competing-risk analysis are comparable, especially during the first 5 years after diagnosis. For men with lower-grade disease, however, competing medical hazards pose a significantly greater threat than prostate cancer. Cause-specific survival analysis overstates the percentage of patients who actually die from their disease, a concept known as the *case fatality rate*. Figure 13-11 demonstrates this effect. The single black line, documenting the cause-specific survival analysis, falls significantly below the break between the dark and lighter bands, which documents the actual percentage of men who died from prostate cancer. This distortion increases with each year of follow-up and is more pronounced in older men.

HOW CAN PATIENTS BEST INTERPRET OUTCOMES ASSOCIATED WITH THE TREATMENT OF PROSTATE CANCER?

Many patients select their initial treatment for prostate cancer after a discussion with their physicians. Information concerning the impact of competing medical hazards is rarely provided. Figure 13-12 provides results from the retrospective analysis of 767 prostate cancer patients described earlier (42). The figure demonstrates that few men with Gleason scores 2 to 4 tumors, identified by prostate biopsy, had progression leading to death from prostate cancer

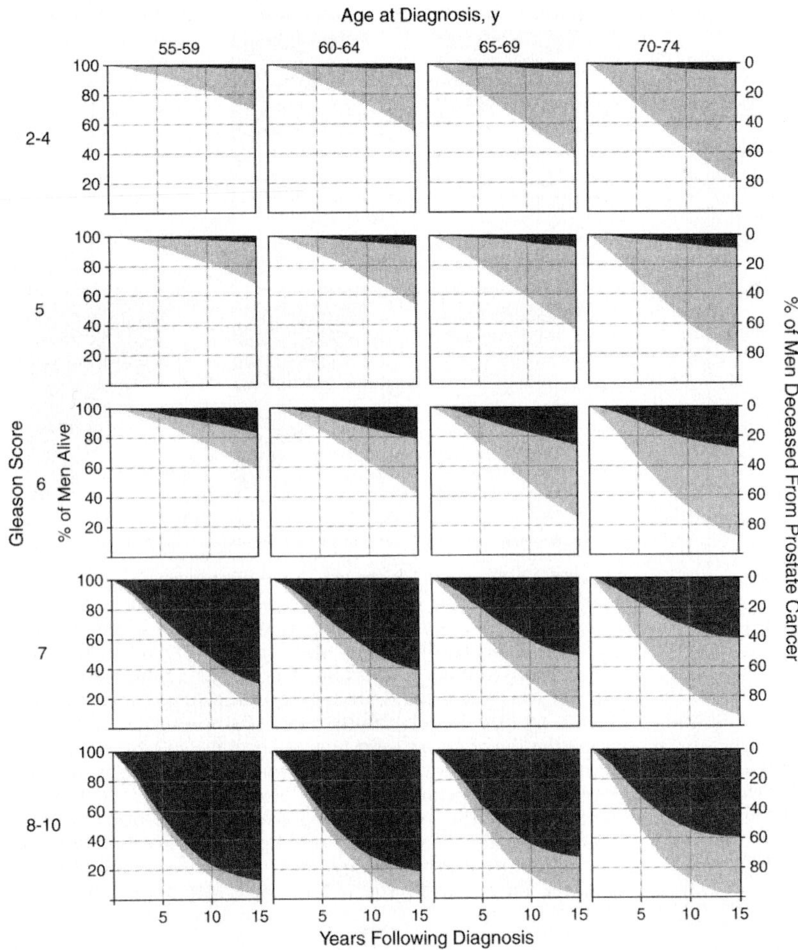

FIGURE 13-12. Survival (*white lower band*) and cumulative mortality from prostate cancer (*dark gray upper band*) and other causes (*light gray middle band*) up to 15 years after diagnosis, stratified by age at diagnosis and Gleason score. Percentage of men alive can be read from the left-hand scale, and percentage of men who have died from prostate cancer or from other causes during this interval can be read from the right-hand scale. (From Albertsen PC, Hanley JA, Gleason DF, et al. Competing risk analysis of men aged 55 to 74 years at diagnosis managed conservatively for clinically localized prostate cancer. *JAMA* 1998;280:975–980, with permission.)

within 15 years. A majority of the younger men are still alive and face a small possibility of death from prostate cancer in the future. In contrast, most older men with Gleason scores 2 to 4 tumors identified on biopsy have died of competing medical hazards rather than prostate cancer.

Compared to men with well-differentiated tumors, men with Gleason score 5 and 6 tumors experienced a higher risk of death from prostate cancer when managed conservatively. However, more than half of the younger men who had Gleason 5 and 6 tumors are still alive after 15 years, whereas a majority of the older men have died from competing medical hazards.

Men with Gleason score 7, and especially those men with Gleason scores 8 to 10 tumors, experienced a very high rate of death from prostate cancer, regardless of their age at diagnosis. Very few of these men are still alive. Most have died from prostate cancer, except for approximately one-third of the oldest men, who died from competing medical hazards. By presenting the data to highlight the probability of dying from prostate cancer versus dying from other competing medical hazards, patients and clinicians can decide whether prostate cancer poses a significant threat to survival, and these data should help in selecting among treatment options.

SUMMARY

The diagnosis and treatment of prostate cancer poses difficult management questions. Some clinicians recommend aggressive treatment strategies, whereas others suggest a more conservative approach. The controversy stems in part from the absence of data from randomized clinical trials that document a net benefit of one treatment modality over another. From a clinician's perspective, the safest approach is to recommend an aggressive treatment, such as surgery or radiation therapy. If it succeeds, the clinician claims a cure; if it fails, he or she has done everything possible. For patients, however, the choice of therapy should depend on their assessment of the risks of disease progression versus the potential efficacy and risks associated with aggressive treatment options.

Data gathered concerning the incidence of prostate cancer and the mortality associated with this disease should provide clinicians with a better understanding of the burden posed by this disease from a public health perspective. Data gathered concerning the clinical outcomes associated with different treatment strategies should help patients select among competing treatment strategies. Only by better understanding the strengths and weaknesses of different study designs and the potential confounding caused by patient co-morbidities and tumor stage and grade can patients and clinicians recognize which treatments will truly provide an increase in longevity and quality of life.

REFERENCES

1. Greenlee RT, Hill-Harmon MB, Murray T, et al. Cancer statistics, 2001. *CA Cancer J Clin* 2001;51:15–36.
2. Ries LAG, Kosary CL, Hankey BF, et al., eds. *SEER cancer statistics review, 1973–1995.* Bethesda, MD: National Cancer Institute, 1998:NIH Publication 98-2789.
3. World Health Organization. International statistical classification of diseases and health related problems (10th revision). Geneva: World Health Organization 1993;2:30.
4. Albertsen PC, Walters S, Hanley JA. A comparison of cause of death determination among men previously diagnosed with prostate cancer and dying in either 1985 or 1995. *J Natl Cancer Inst* 2000;163(2):519–523.
5. Wingo PA, Landis S, Ries LAG. An adjustment to the 1997 estimate for new prostate cancer cases. *CA Cancer J Clin* 1997;47:239–242.
6. Stephenson RA. Population-based prostate cancer trends in the PSA era: data from the Surveillance, Epidemiology and End Results (SEER) program. In: *1998 Monographs in Urology.* Montverde, FL: Medical Directions Publishing Company, 1998.
7. Potosky AL, Miller BA, Albertsen PC, et al. The role of increasing detection in the rising incidence of prostate cancer. *JAMA* 1995;273:548–552.
8. Collins MM, Barry MJ. Controversies in prostate cancer screening: analogies to the early lung cancer screening debate. *JAMA* 1996;276:1976–1979.
9. Woods WG, Tuchman M, Robison LL, et. al. The utility of screening for neuroblastoma; a population-based study. *Lancet* 1996;348:1682–1687.
10. Nishi M, Miyake H, Takeda T, et al. Mass screening for neuroblastoma targeting children age 14 months in Sapporo city: a preliminary report. *Cancer* 1998;82:1973–1977.
11. Mettlin CJ, Murphy GP. Why is the prostate cancer death rate declining in the United States? *Cancer* 1998;82:249–251.
12. Franks LM. Latency and progression in tumors: the natural history of prostatic cancer. *Lancet* 1956;2:1037–1039.
13. Catalona WJ, Richie JP, Ahmann FR, et al. Comparison of digital rectal examination and serum prostate specific antigen in the early detection of prostate cancer: results of multicenter clinical trial of 6,630 men. *J Urol* 1994;151:1283–1290.
14. Sershon PD, Barry MJ, Oesterling JE. Serum prostate-specific antigen discriminates weakly between men with benign prostatic hyperplasia and patients with organ-confined prostate cancer. *Eur Urol* 1994;25:281–287.
15. Catalona WJ, Smith DS, Ratliff TL, et al. Detection of organ-confined prostate cancer is increased through prostate-specific antigen-based screening. *JAMA* 1993;270:948–954.
16. Catalona WJ, Partin AW, Slawin KM, et al. Use of percentage of prostate-specific antigen to enhance the differentiation of prostate cancer from benign disease. *JAMA* 1998;279:1542–1547.
17. Dugan JA, Bostwick DG, Myers RP, et al. The definition and preoperative prediction of clinically insignificant prostate cancer. *JAMA* 1996;275:288–294.
18. Preventive Services Task Force. *Guide to clinical preventive services,* 2nd ed. Baltimore: Williams & Wilkins, 1995.
19. Friedman GD, Hiatt RA, Queensberry CP Jr., et al. Case-controlled study of screening for prostatic cancer by digital rectal examinations. *Lancet* 1991;337:1526–1529.
20. Gerber GS, Thompson IM, Thisted R, et al. Disease-specific survival following routine prostate cancer screening by digital rectal examination. *JAMA* 1993;269:61–64.
21. Stanford JL, Stephenson RA, Coyle LM, et al. *Prostate cancer trends 1973–1995, SEER program.* Bethesda, MD: National Cancer Institute, 1999:NIH Pub. No. 99-4543.
22. Walsh PC, Brooks JD. The Swedish prostate cancer paradox. *JAMA* 1997;277:497–498.
23. Lu-Yao GL, McLerran D, Wasson J, et al. An assessment of radical prostatectomy. Time trends, geographic variation, and outcomes. *JAMA* 1993;269:2633–2636.
24. Brendler CB, Walsh PC. The role of radical prostatectomy in the treatment of prostate cancer. *CA Cancer J Clin* 1992;42:212–222.
25. Lange PH. The next era for prostate cancer: controlled clinical trials. *JAMA* 1993;269:95–96.
26. Gerber GS, Thisted RA, Scardino PT, et al. Results of radical prostatectomy in men with clinically localized prostate cancer. *JAMA* 1996;276:615–619.
27. Shipley WU, Thames HD, Sandler HM, et al. Radiation therapy for clinically localized prostate cancer. *JAMA* 1999;281:1598–1604.
28. Albertsen PC, Hanley JM, Gleason DF, et al. A competing risk analysis of men aged 55 to 74 years at diagnosis managed conservatively for clinically localized prostate cancer. *JAMA* 1998;280:975–980.
29. Helgesen F, Holmberg L, Johansson JE, et al. Trends in prostate cancer survival in Sweden, 1960 through 1988: evidence of increasing diagnosis of nonlethal tumors. *J Natl Cancer Inst* 1996;88:1216–1221.
30. Barry MJ, Albertsen PC, Bagshaw MA, et al. Outcomes for men with clinically nonmetastatic prostate cancer managed with radical prostatectomy, external beam radiotherapy, or expectant management: a retrospective analysis with standardized assessments of stage, grade and comorbidity. *Cancer* 2001 (*in press*).
31. Feinstein AR, Sosin DM, Wells CK. The Will Rogers phenomenon. Stage migration and new diagnostic techniques as a source of misleading statistics for survival in cancer. *N Engl J Med* 1985;312:1604–1608.
32. Aus G, Hugosson J, Norlen L. Long-term survival and mortality in prostate cancer treated with noncurative intent. *J Urol* 1995;154:460–465.
33. Abrahamsson PA, Adami HO, Taube A, et al. Letter to the editor. *J Urol* 1996;155:296–297.
34. Johansson JE, Holmberg L, Johansson S, et al. Fifteen-year survival in prostate cancer. A prospective, population-based study in Sweden. *JAMA* 1977;277:467–471.
35. Chodak GW, Thisted RA, Gerber GS, et al. Results of conservative management of clinically localized prostate cancer. *N Engl J Med* 1994;330:242–248.

36. Albertsen PC, Fryback DG, Storer BE, et al. Long-term survival among men with conservatively treated localized prostate cancer. *JAMA* 1995;274:626–631.
37. Greenfield S, Apolone G, McNeil BJ, et al. The importance of co-existent disease in the occurrence of postoperative complications and one-year recovery in patients undergoing total hip replacement. Comorbidity outcomes after hip replacement. *Med Care* 1993;31:141–154.
38. Charlson ME, Pompie P, Ales KL, et al. A new method of classifying prognostic comorbidity in longitudinal studies: development and validation. *J Chron Dis* 1987;40:373–383.
39. Kaplan MH, Feinstein AR. The importance of classifying initial co-morbidity in evaluating the outcomes of diabetes mellitus. *J Chron Dis* 1974;27:387–404.
40. Albertsen PC, Fryback DG, Storer BE, et al. The impact of co-morbidity on life expectancy among men with localized prostate cancer. *J Urol* 1996;156:127–132.
41. Albertsen PC, Hanley JA, Murphy-Setzko M. Statistical considerations when assessing outcomes following treatment for prostate cancer. *J Urol* 1999;162:439–444.
42. Albertsen PC, Hanley JA, Gleason DF, et al. Competing risk analysis of men aged 55 to 74 years at diagnosis managed conservatively for clinically localized prostate cancer. *JAMA* 1998;280:975–980.

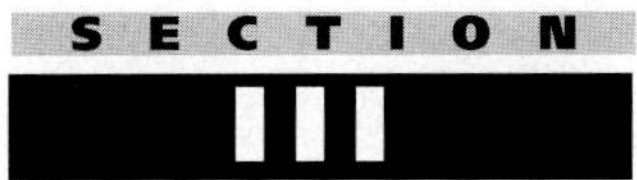

DIAGNOSIS AND STAGING

14

SCREENING FOR PROSTATE CANCER: PROSTATE-SPECIFIC ANTIGEN, DIGITAL RECTAL EXAMINATION, AND FREE, DENSITY, AND AGE-SPECIFIC DERIVATIVES

ARNOLD D. BULLOCK
GERALD L. ANDRIOLE

SCREENING FOR PROSTATE CANCER

Prostate cancer control has become a major health concern, and this issue will maintain its prominence with the overall aging of the population. Prostate cancer is the most commonly diagnosed cancer in men; it represents 41% of all malignant male cancers diagnosed (1). Prostate cancer is the second-leading cancer killer of American men (1). African-American men are disproportionately affected with prostate cancer, with incidence rates nearly twice that of white Americans and a mortality rate that is 120% higher than white Americans (Fig. 14-1) (2,3). The American man has roughly a one in nine chance of developing clinically detectable prostate cancer.

The increased public awareness and interest in prostate cancer, in conjunction with the widespread use of screening tests, has "pushed" prostate cancer prevalence to staggering levels. The increased awareness has resulted from information in the lay press, recognition of prominent public figures who are living with or have died from prostate cancer, and an increasingly informed American public (4). Between 1985 and 1995, there was a threefold rise in the incidence of prostate cancer, with 85,000 men and 244,000 men, respectively, diagnosed in the United States (5). Although heralded as a major breakthrough in cancer management by many, the relatively new detection modalities, leading to our increased ability to detect prostate cancer, have been a source of controversy. There are varied groups in the scientific and lay community who are strongly opposed to random, mass prostate cancer screening. The two issues surrounding this controversy regard the appropriateness of detecting asymptomatic prostate cancer and the economic cost of this technology when applied to the general public (6,7).

Compared to mammogram-based breast cancer screening, prostate-specific antigen (PSA)–based prostate cancer screening has a higher positive predictive value (PPV) and a lower direct cost. There is little dispute that screening is effective at detecting a higher percentage of earlier stage disease, but is it reasonable? The basis of this question is twofold. First, prostate cancer has a broad spectrum of biologic potentials, and most prostate cancers do not lead to serious morbidity or death. Second, there are no randomized, controlled studies demonstrating disease-specific mortality reduction from any test or procedure.

Unlike the natural history of most other cancers, which are normally more rapidly and uniformly fatal if left untreated, the natural history of prostate cancer covers a wide spectrum of potential biologic activity. This variance of aggressiveness has led to common descriptions of "latent" and "clinical" prostate cancers. *Latent* cancer is clinically silent, unlikely to result in any morbidity, and most commonly seen in autopsy series (8). *Clinical* cancer may progress to symptoms, morbidity, and death if not adequately managed in its early stage (9). The natural history of prostate cancer is poorly understood, for the prevalence of histologic (latent) disease far exceeds the prevalence of clinically detectable disease. Autopsy studies in men age 50 years and older, without a clinical history of prostate cancer, demonstrate a 30% incidence of occult disease on serial-step sections of the gland. In men aged 80 years, this prevalence rate increases to 70% (10). Similar findings are found in cystoprostatectomy specimens, removed in the management of transitional cell carcinoma of the bladder (11). Approximately 20% to 25% of these cancers are estimated to be clinically significant (12). Slightly fewer than 3% of men will actually die from prostate cancer. Although

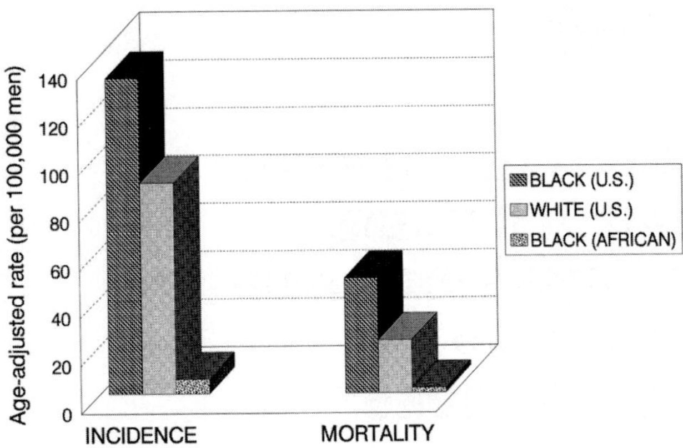

FIGURE 14-1. Prostate cancer: age-adjusted incidence and mortality.

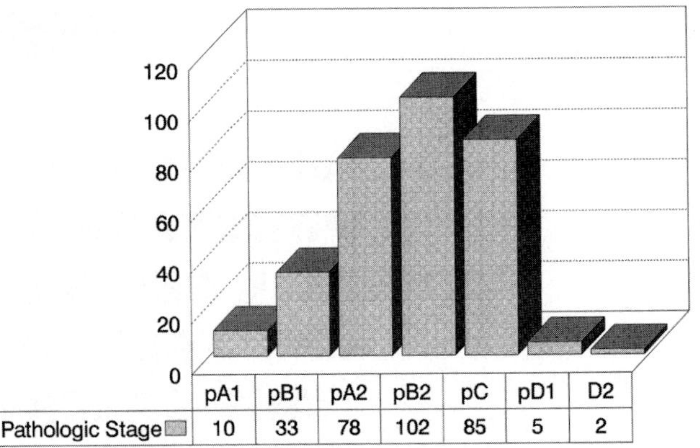

	pA1	pB1	pA2	pB2	pC	pD1	D2
Pathologic Stage	10	33	78	102	85	5	2

FIGURE 14-2. Pathologic staging of cancers detected by screening. (From Catalona WJ, Smith DJ, Ratliff TL, et al. Detection of organ-confined prostate cancer is increased through prostate-specific antigen–based screening. *JAMA* 1993;270:948–954.)

a number of pathologic parameters (grade, stage, and volume) can predict the behavior of cancers in general, most clinically detected prostate cancers are of moderate grade, and there are no accurate available means to predict the aggressiveness in an individual with certainty (13,14).

One of the arguments against screening asymptomatic men is that the advanced testing detects large numbers of men with latent, clinically indolent disease. The diagnosis and treatment of these men with disease, destined to remain clinically silent, would result in unnecessary high costs and physical and psychological morbidity (15). This concern has been supported by a few studies reporting low rates of prostate cancer–specific mortality in men diagnosed with localized prostate cancer treated with a *watchful waiting* strategy (16,17). Significant flaws were found in the studies showing low prostate cancer–specific mortality rates with an observation protocol. Dr. Walsh was the first to outline these flaws in the decision analysis of the benefits of treating prostate cancer (18). He repeated the analysis using data from several series of conservatively managed prostate cancer patients (17) and from a series of patients with clinically localized prostate cancer treated with brachytherapy in the same model. These decision analyses showed a marked benefit of therapy over watchful waiting (19,20). Other studies from Sweden have demonstrated a high mortality rate from clinically localized prostate cancer managed conservatively in a population-based study examining all deaths within a geographically defined area (21).

Contrary to the speculation that screening would detect large numbers of men with clinically indolent disease, large prostate cancer screening studies have shown a small percentage of the cancers detected to be low-stage and low-grade. In the Washington University PSA study of more than 20,000 volunteers, only 3.2% of the cancers detected were stage A1, and 10.5% of the cancers were stage B1 (Fig. 14-2) (22). Among men selected for radical prostatectomy, nonpalpable tumors detected with PSA were more predictable for advanced pathologic extent than incidental cancer after transurethral resection of the prostate (TURP). Their particular pathologic characteristics suggest that they include clinically significant tumors that would progress, if untreated, to palpable and, eventually, metastatic disease (23). PSA progression in men with incidental cancer has been previously demonstrated to be predicted more reliably by residual cancer on needle biopsy after TURP than by pathologic appearance of the tumor in the resected specimen (23). In view of this progressive behavior, cancer detected by PSA should be considered clinically significant, particularly in men with a life expectancy of at least 10 years.

Resolution of the prostate cancer screening controversy is pending the conclusion of several ongoing, randomized, controlled trials comparing various diagnostic and treatment strategies for prostate cancer (24,25). There exist suggestive data from cancer surveillance series of the National Cancer Data Base (26) and the National Cancer Institute (27), demonstrating an improved prognosis and lower mortality with screen-detected cases. Clinical highlights from the 1999 National Clinical Data Base report an average 1% per year decline in the annual prostate cancer death rate in the United States since 1990. The percentage of patients diagnosed with stage IV disease decreased from 25.3% to 21.2% over the period 1984 to 1990 (26). According to Feuer et al. of the National Cancer Institute (27), "The following findings are consistent with a screening effect: (a) the recent decrease since 1991 in the incidence of distant stage disease, after not having been perturbed by screening; (b) the decline in the incidence of earlier stage disease beginning the following year (1992); (c) the recent increases and decreases in prostate cancer incidence and mortality by age that appear to indicate a calendar period effect; and (d) trends in the incidence of distant stage disease by tumor grade and trends in the survival of patients with distant stage disease by calendar year that provide suggestive evidence of the tendency of screening to detect slower growing tumors." Hence, the decline in the incidence of distant-stage disease holds the promise that testing for PSA may lead to a sustained decline in prostate cancer mortality.

Merrill and Stephenson (28) also reported on a downward trend in mortality in patients with prostate cancer detected during the PSA-screening era. In their assessment of the influence of PSA on mortality rates, they used the data from the Surveillance, Epidemiology, and End Results (SEER) program and found that cancer mortality due to prostate cancer decreased from 37% in 1988 to 30% in 1995, largely as a result of a sharp increase in non–prostate cancer mortality rates. The overall trend in prostate cancer mortality rates increased from 1988 to 1992 and then decreased. The increase and decrease in rates occurred across categories of age, race, grade, and number of cancer primaries. They concluded that PSA screening influenced the increase and decrease in prostate cancer. However, population data are complex, and it is difficult to confidently attribute relatively small changes in mortality to any one cause (29).

Historically, the clinical diagnosis of prostate cancer has been insensitive for detecting organ-confined disease. The diagnosis was usually made when a person presented to a urologist with voiding symptoms or an unrelated urologic problem. When diagnosed typically by digital rectal examination (DRE) findings, approximately 30% of patients had disseminated disease. The median duration of survival of men with this stage of disease is less than 3 years (30). An additional 30% of such patients had pathologic evidence of tumor extension beyond the confines of the prostate at the time of presentation, and evidence of disease progression generally occurs within 10 years, irrespective of therapy (31,32). Therefore, only 40% of the patients will present with localized disease when the diagnosis is made based on "case finding" in the evaluation of symptoms. Of these, 10% have minimal cancer that is found on simple prostatectomy, and most clinicians believe that it does not require aggressive management (30). Therefore, without screening, fewer than one-third of all men presenting with carcinoma are suitable candidates for curative therapy.

It is, therefore, clear that routine clinical approaches to the identification of men with prostate cancer are woefully inadequate. Most patients present with locally advanced or metastatic disease, and even among those with favorable clinical parameters, cancer progression, with its long, drawn-out morbidity and negative effects on the quality of life, occurs all too often.

In general, the morbidity of cancer can potentially be reduced by three means: (a) reduce the risk of the disease, (b) improve the curative therapy, and (c) improve the early detection of significant, curable disease. Although it is speculated that diet and environmental toxins may predispose one to the disease, there are no definitive means to reduce the risk of developing prostate cancer. The Prostate Cancer Prevention Trial is a large, prospective 7-year study to determine whether the use of finasteride will lower the risk of prostate cancer. It will take several more years for this study to provide final results. The Southwest Oncology Group initiated a multicenter Selenium and Vitamin E Cancer Prevention Trial study that is a 12-year project to define the potential benefit of selenium and vitamin E in the reduction in prostate cancer incidence and aggressiveness. The second option in the battle to reduce prostate cancer–related mortality is to improve the efficacy of therapy. There are many options in the clinical armamentarium for managing prostate cancer in all stages. For those with localized disease, the modifications in radical prostatectomy and radiation therapy have lowered morbidity rates. However, there remains a controversy as to these approaches' actual rates of decreasing cancer mortality. Once metastasis has occurred, there are no available therapies that will provide true cure, and palliation with hormonal ablation therapy is the standard of care. If the disease cannot be prevented or cured in its advanced stage, then the remaining alternative is to detect it at an earlier, more curable stage. Screening is performed in the belief that detection of a disease in its early stages, when cure is possible, will lead to treatment that will result in less morbidity or mortality than had the disease gone undetected. Although there is recent heightened public awareness of prostate cancer and screening, the rationale for screening was presented by Hugh Hampton Young in the 1930s (33):

> If patients could be examined early and if doctors would be suspicious of even small areas or nodules that are hard, many cases of cancer of the prostate would be brought to radical operation and cured. It behooves all elderly males to undergo occasional examination in which the prostate is carefully palpated.

Several medical organizations, including the American Cancer Society and the American Urologic Society, have recommended screening for prostate cancer for large numbers of men presenting with incurable, advanced-stage disease. The diagnosis of early-stage, organ-confined prostate cancer necessitates an examination of a large number of the "at-risk" population while they are asymptomatic. *Screening* is the "application of the testing and examination process to an entire population" of "apparently well" people.

Early detection is similar to screening, because its goal is also to detect and treat prostate cancer in time to reduce mortality from the disease. The difference between screening and early detection is that early detection targets a population considered at risk because of signs, symptoms, environmental exposure, genetic background, or other established risk factors. With early detection, individual patients seek out prostate programs; with screening, health initiatives are developed to seek out appropriate patients to be screened. The problem with prostate cancer is that the environmental and genetic risk factors are not fully defined, and there are no specific symptoms in early-stage disease. Both terms are used interchangeably in the literature, but their distinction from a health policy perspective is important economically.

The cost of screening entire populations is overwhelming. The cost of screening in the United States is projected to be $5 billion per year (34), and the first-year costs of treatment and treatment-related complications in a widespread screening program are predicted to range from $5.2 billion to $14.1 billion (35). In Sweden, an analysis suggested that the 2-year financial impact of complete (direct, indirect, and intangible costs) screening would be $131 to $174 million, a staggering amount for a country with only 2 million men older than the age of 40 (36). The psychological costs to society should be considered, both for false-positive and false-negative tests. The number of lives and life years saved and a measure of quality of life must mitigate the economic cost.

Because tumors are diagnosed before symptoms develop, the length of survival may seem increased due to lead-time bias (37). If the patient eventually dies of the disease without any prolongation of life, then screening provides no benefit. Similarly, length-time bias can appear to show that screening is beneficial, because it detects slower-growing, less aggressive tumors; the more aggressive tumors are not diagnosed through screening, for the symptoms lead patients to seek medical attention. The best method of evaluating the impact of a screening program is the randomized, controlled study. The best end point is cancer-specific mortality, which avoids both lead-time bias and length-time bias inherent in other outcome variables.

For screening to be considered useful, the disease under study must meet certain conditions:

1. The disease must be a serious health problem.
2. There should be effective treatment of the low-stage disease being studied that reduces morbidity and mortality.
3. The screening tests should be simple, quick, reproducible, inexpensive, and safe, and they should have high sensitivity and specificity.

Prostate cancer fulfills some of the conditions required of a disease that might be managed by population screening. Although prostate cancer does not meet all of these criteria, prostate cancer screening is an option presently available to possibly reduce the number of life years lost. There are approximately 40,000 men in the United States who die per year from this disease. For the properly informed patient with at least a 10-year life expectancy, it would seem that early detection efforts, using DRE and serum PSA determination, are beneficial. Considerable controversy abounds about early detection and screening and will continue until definitive proof of decreased prostate cancer mortality, as a result of effective early detection and treatment regimens, is demonstrated. Until then, all men with at least a 10-year life expectancy should be counseled as to the potential benefits and risks.

WHO SHOULD BE SCREENED?

There are certainly some groups of men at higher risk of developing prostate cancer, and these men should be informed of their increased risk and encouraged to be screened for the disease. The two groups considered at high risk include African-American men and men with a family history of the disease. Prostate cancer in African-Americans has to be considered in the context of the broader problem of cancer, in general, in African-Americans. African-Americans are disproportionately affected by cancer of all kinds in terms of incidence and mortality rates (3). African-American men have cancer and mortality rates well above those of white men, whereas African-American women have incidence rates marginally below and mortality rates above those of white women. The prostate cancer incidence in African-Americans is twofold greater than in white Americans, and the prostate cancer mortality rate is 120% greater. One reason for the lower survival rates is a tendency for African-Americans to have cancer diagnosed at a more advanced stage (38–40). In a study of 861 consecutive cases of prostate cancer diagnosed at one Veterans Administration hospital in the pre–PSA-screening era, Brawn et al. (41) found that 52% of African-Americans and 26% of whites had stage D disease, and the higher rate of advanced disease in African-Americans was seen throughout a 22-year observation period. A proportional hazards (Cox) model showed an overall poorer survival in African-Americans as a result of staging differences (41). Similarly, Aziz et al. (39) showed that 55% of African-Americans versus 23% of whites ($p < .001$) were first seen with stage D disease, and this resulted in a difference in median survival of 3.2 years versus 4.8 years ($p = .007$), respectively. Similar advanced-stage results were obtained by others (43,44). In a retrospective review of three Radiation Therapy Oncology Group trials, Roach et al. (45) demonstrated that a significantly higher percentage of African-Americans had elevated serum acid phosphatase levels at diagnosis as compared to whites, 42% and 21%, respectively, and this is consistent with a higher rate of advanced disease in African-Americans. The African-American–white difference in the proportion of metastatic cancers in other large series was 35.4% versus 22.1% from the Connecticut Tumor Registry data (46), 28% versus 19% from the 1974 to 1986 SEER program data (43), and 37.1% versus 23.0% in the American College of Surgeons' surgery of cases diagnosed in 1983 (44). Given these results, one can conclude that the stage at diagnosis is partially responsible for the disparity in survival between the two groups (Fig. 14-3).

Despite the greater morbidity experienced by African-Americans with prostate cancer, they have a lower rate of participation in cancer screening efforts. The reasons for the lower participation include a lower knowledge base regarding cancer detection and treatments, fear of the medical "research" institution, and a generally greater optimistic view of the risk of developing cancer and a pessimistic outlook on cancer cure. With a widespread belief among African-Americans that cancer would present with symptoms, urinary symptoms are a predictor for participation in prostate cancer screening among African-American men (47). More

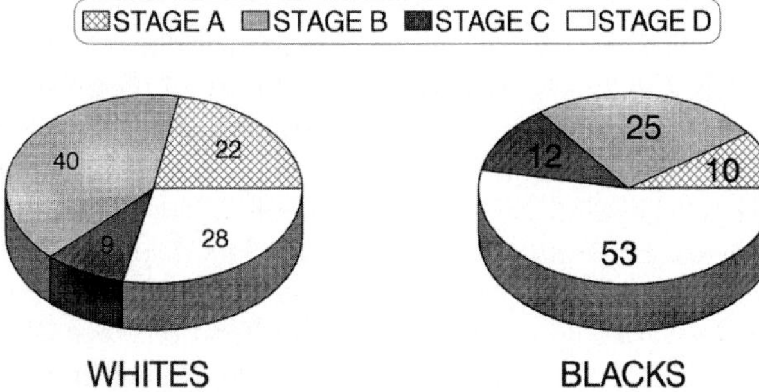

FIGURE 14-3. Clinical stage at initial diagnosis of prostate cancer—pre–prostate-specific antigen screening era. (Adapted from reference 41.)

African-American men will participate in prostate cancer screening after educational seminars about the disease (3,48,49). Targeted efforts in public education and screening may be useful in promoting early detection of prostate cancer in African-American men.

The disproportion in staging may be even more pronounced when stratified by the age at diagnosis, in addition to race. Targonski et al. (50) showed that the percentage of localized disease in whites remains fairly stable, despite age at diagnosis, but African-Americans younger than age 65 have a lower rate of localized disease (45%) as compared to African-Americans older than the age of 75 (54%). Data from the SEER program for the period 1981 to 1985 in four areas are used to show a higher ratio of advanced to localized disease at various ages in African-Americans and whites (38). It has been suggested that African-Americans and others at high risk for prostate cancer be screened at the age of 40 years. The SEER prostate cancer incidence data from 1981 to 1985 revealed a cancer incidence of 16.6 per 100,000 for African-Americans between the ages of 40 and 49; in whites in this age group, the incidence was 3.7 per 100,000 (38). From these data, 6,250 African-American men of this age would need to be screened to detect one case of prostate cancer. If African-American men between the ages of 40 and 44 years were screened, there would be one case in 37,037 men screened. Similarly, studies at Howard University Medical Center demonstrated that only 1.2% of their patients were younger than 50 years (51). At Washington University, a study on the benefits of screening high-risk younger men is in progress. With nearly 1,000 men aged 40 to 49 years screened, the positive screen rate (suspicious DRE or PSA greater than 4 ng per mL, or both) in an African-American is 2.64% and 2.09% in a younger white individual. Family history in our small sample group appears to be insignificant in the younger whites, but a positive family history in a younger African-American increases the positive screen rate to 6.12%. This remains only half the screen rate in men older than 50 years.

A positive family history is one of the strongest known risk factors for prostate carcinoma, in addition to age and race. Gronberg et al. (52) showed that both patient age at the time of prostate carcinoma diagnosis and the number of men affected in the families influenced the risk of developing prostate carcinoma significantly. Using data from a population-based cohort study, including 5,706 sons of Swedish men who had been diagnosed with prostate carcinoma, they found that unaffected men in families with two or more cases of prostate carcinoma have a very high risk of developing prostate carcinoma at a young age. The cumulative risks in these families are 5%, 15%, and 30% by ages 60, 70, and 80 years, respectively, compared with only 0.45%, 3%, and 10%, respectively, at the same ages in the general population (52). These same two family-based factors were found in a similar study by Matikainen et al. (53) Men from prostate cancer families with an average age of onset of under 60 years had a significantly higher frequency of PSA positivity (28.6%, p = .01), as well as cancers (14.3%, p = .02), than those with a later age of onset (53).

SCREENING TESTS

Digital Rectal Examination

The DRE remains a cornerstone in the diagnosis of prostate cancer, owing to its ease, lack of cost, low risk, and contribution to detection of cancer in men with normal PSA levels. With its low position in the pelvis, below the bladder neck, the anatomic position of the prostate allows palpation of the posterior wall by the finger placed per rectum. The DRE is used to diagnose benign prostatic hyperplasia (BPH) and macroscopic prostate cancer and to evaluate its extent. However, DRE is only moderately sensitive in diagnosing small, early-stage prostate cancer, and it is not sensitive in detecting disease minimally extended beyond the capsule. The DRE is useful toward prostate cancer detection, because most cancers arise in the peripheral zone of the prostate. The test is obviously limited in that some tumors are microscopic, and others arise in the transitional zone within the inner aspects of the prostate and are less amenable to digital detection.

The DRE has been used for centuries and has the Latin term *palpatio per anum*. The use of the DRE in the diagnosis and staging of prostate cancer was accurately described by Marion in 1921 (54):

> Prostate cancer is generally easy to differentiate from BPH. The consistency of the prostatic mass is distinctive and, rather than elastic, hard and almost always irregular. The form instead of being regular rounded is frequently uneven. Finally, instead of feeling a distinctive border, one feels a continuation with the surrounding tissue, many times on the superior and external borders. Sometimes the mass is regular and limited but hard as wood. This is cancer. Sometimes one feels no mass but a simple hard nodule without precise delineation in the tissue.
>
> The diagnosis becomes delicate when one deals with an early cancer and is only characteristic by the feeling of a few

hard nodules in a mass that has all the specifications of BPH. They may be BPH but are very suspicious, especially if they do not disappear by rectal massage. The diagnosis in the early stage of the disease is very delicate and even experienced urologists are sometimes obliged to reserve their diagnosis for a certain time.

Although nodularity is obviously a significant finding on DRE, the classic study by Jewett (55) showed that only 50% of the lesions palpated by this clinical expert and considered suspicious were actually cancer on biopsy. In more recent studies, only 26% to 34% of men with suspicious findings on DRE have positive biopsies for cancer (56–58). The most widely used test for the detection of prostate cancer is also the most subjective. Differing skills among examiners, varied indication for the examination, selection of patients based on symptoms and age, and an increasing suspicion of subtle abnormalities have resulted in wide variability in the sensitivity and specificity of the DRE in cancer detection in men. Detection rates of 0.8% to 25.0% have been reported, along with PPVs of 6.3% to 50.0% (58–66).

In a multicenter prostate cancer screening study of 6,630 men aged 50 years or older, 15% had an abnormal DRE, and one-fifth had cancer diagnosed on sextant biopsy. In this study by Catalona et al. (67), the cancer detection rate was 3.2%, and the PPV of the DRE was 21%. This compares with other studies showing a PPV ranging from 22% to 39% and a detection rate for prostate cancer by DRE ranging from 0.13% to 3.20% (68). In a series at the University of Washington, carcinoma has been detected in 24 of 185 men (13%) with asymmetry as their only abnormality and 112 of 456 (24.6%) with prostatic induration. In contrast, 79 of 150 (52.7%) with clearly palpable nodules or areas of marked induration strongly suggestive of carcinoma actually demonstrated malignancy (69).

The sensitivity of the DRE in the detection of prostate cancer is low, and the results of this subjective test vary widely with the indication for the examination, selection of patients based on symptoms and age, and clinical experience of the examiner. Despite the shortcomings of the DRE, in terms of low sensitivity and specificity, up to 25% of prostate cancers are still detected by DRE in men with normal PSA levels. Therefore, a suspicious DRE should be followed by a prostate ultrasound and biopsy, unless it is clinically inappropriate, owing to overall poor patient health (70). A routine annual DRE is recommended by the American Cancer Society, American Urological Association, and American Medical Association. In a survey conducted in the United States by the American Cancer Society, this practice was found to be followed by 97% of family practitioners and internists (71).

Prostate-Specific Antigen Testing

PSA is an organ-specific, kallikreinlike, serine protease produced by the columnar epithelial cells that line ducts of the prostate gland and periurethral glands (72,73). PSA is metabolized by the liver and has a serum half-life of approximately 2 to 3 days. Secreted into the lumen of the prostatic ducts, it is in high concentration in seminal fluid, in which it is involved in liquefaction of the seminal coagulum (74). PSA is believed to leak from the prostatic-ductal system into the prostatic stroma and then into the blood stream. Prostate cancer cells actually produce less PSA and PSA messenger RNA than do normal prostate epithelial cells and BPH (72,75,76). It remains unclear why there are higher PSA-serum concentrations in the setting of prostate cancer.

The combination of DRE and serum PSA has been shown to be effective for detecting early prostate cancer in various outpatient settings. PSA testing provides the means to detect cancer in men with normal DRE that may otherwise present as so-called incidental cancer at TURP for apparently benign disease or later in the course of its natural history as locally advanced or metastatic disease (23). Numerous studies have demonstrated PSA screening as the best single modality for the detection of early-stage prostate cancer.

Originally designed as a demonstration project, the American Cancer Society National Prostate Cancer Detection Project (ACS-NPCDP) was established in 1987 to demonstrate the feasibility of early detection of prostate cancer as a cancer-control strategy. The project was aimed at testing the efficacy variables, such as sensitivity, specificity, and predictive value, of several detection tools, including the unproven PSA and transrectal ultrasound (TRUS). To test the range of application of these emerging technologies, the project involved a multidisciplinary group of investigators from private medical practices, community hospitals, university hospitals, and cancer centers (77). The cancer detection rates across five annual examinations averaged 2%, with a high of 2.7% with the first examination. More than 70% of the tumors were sensitive to detection by PSA at every annual examination. Most sensitive in the first year, by the fifth year of serial study, the DRE was sensitive to only 25% of the cancers detectable by other means. The results of this early detection study were compared with the outcome patterns of prostate cancers diagnosed via contemporary means and documented in the National Cancer Database. In this comparative review of 204 completely staged cancers of the ACS-NPCDP, only 8.3% of ACS-NPCDP cancers were clinically advanced (American Joint Committee on Cancer stage III or IV) at the time of diagnosis, in contrast to 34% of comparable National Cancer Database cases (78). This project was one of the first to demonstrate the potential benefit of PSA testing for early detection of prostate cancer. However, because one-third of the men diagnosed with cancers had a PSA level less than 4 ng per mL, it also revealed one of the flaws with PSA screening.

At Washington University, Dr. Catalona has directed one of the largest single-institution studies with approximately 30,000 community volunteers enrolled in one of three screening projects. Based on the initial screen, approximately 10% of the men had a PSA greater than 4 ng per mL, and 8% to 10% had suspicious DREs. The PPV for detecting carcinoma ranged from 25% to 33% across the studies. More than 90% of the tumors detected showed clinicopathologic features of significant cancer (79).

In an evaluation of the use of the PSA, Candas et al. (80) also reviewed screening records of 11,817 first-screen visits and 46,751 annual follow-up visits performed since 1988. PSA was above 3 ng per mL in 16.6% and 15.6% of men at first and follow-up visits, respectively. Prostate cancer was found in 2.9% of men invited for screening at first visit and in only 0.4% of men at follow-up visits, for a 7.1-fold decrease at follow-up visits done up to 11 years. PSA alone was the basis for the diagnosis of 90.5% and 90.0% of the cancers detected at the first and follow-up visits, respectively; this compares to 41.1% and 25.0% of cancers detected by DRE alone. In their study, PSA used as a prescreening tool (followed by DRE and TRUS, when elevated) was effective in detecting 99% of cancers at a localized stage.

There have been numerous other studies supporting the ability to detect prostate cancer in earlier stages with PSA screening. In summary, studies show that 8% to 15% of screened men aged 50 years and older will have a PSA level greater than 4 ng per mL and the PPV of an elevated PSA with the initial biopsy ranges from 30% to 37% (22,59,67,80–82). These PPVs are higher than the mammography PPVs of approximately 20% (83). In a referral population, the PPV of an elevated PSA level for an ultrasound-guided biopsy of the prostate is in an even higher range of 35% to 54% (59,84,85). The probability of detecting prostate cancer at various stages is dependent on the serum PSA concentration and DRE findings (Table 14-1).

The racial differences in prostate cancer incidence persist in screened populations of men. In an evaluation of 18,527 white and 949 African-American men 50 years of age or older screened by DRE and PSA, African-American men had a higher prevalence of elevated PSA (13.1% vs. 8.9%) and cancer (5.1% vs. 3.2%) than white men (86). A PSA greater than 4 ng per mL detected more cancers than the DRE. The PPV for prostate cancer of PSA and DRE was greater in African-American men than in white men (48% vs. 34%, and 38% vs. 22%, respectively) (82). In our screened population, the African-American men had a higher prevalence of clinically localized disease, but there was not a significant difference in pathologically advanced cancer among the men in both racial groups who underwent a radical prostatectomy (86). This dramatic improvement over the racial disparity seen in clinical cancer registry studies provides support for an optimistic outlook on a future resolution of the racial mortality differential.

TABLE 14-1. PATHOLOGIC STAGING: CANCER DISTRIBUTION BY PROSTATE-SPECIFIC ANTIGEN (PSA) AND DIGITAL RECTAL EXAMINATION (DRE)

Detection modality	Staged No.	Stage A, B No.	% Stage A, B
PSA <4.1 ng/mL			
DRE suspicious	79	68	86.1
PSA 4.1–10.0 ng/mL			
DRE benign	94	74	78.7
DRE suspicious	70	46	65.7
PSA >10 ng/mL			
DRE benign	31	18	58.1
DRE suspicious	42	17	40.5

From Washington University PSA screening study, with permission.

Serial screening for prostate cancer can significantly reduce the risk of developing advanced disease. Using a cohort of data from the 77,700 volunteers in the Prostate Cancer Awareness Week longitudinal study, Crawford et al. (87) showed a dramatically lower rate of metastatic disease in men who had at least two negative screenings. From 1992 to 1996 in this study, more than 60% of the cancers were detected within the first year of screening, and most of the remaining cancers were diagnosed with the second screening. Although rare, some men were diagnosed with advanced-stage disease in years 3 and 4, presumably due to failure to evaluate prior abnormal tests or interim development of rapidly growing tumors between screenings. In contrast to the high rate of clinically advanced prostate cancer at the time of diagnosis in the pre-PSA era, in serial screening studies at Washington University, 98% of the screen-detected cancers are clinically localized (Fig. 14-4).

PSA has been found to be the single best test for detecting prostate cancer, but it is nonspecific—that is, up to three-fourths of men with an abnormal PSA may not have prostate cancer. Numerous factors can alter the serum PSA level and interfere with its reliability as a test for cancer. Increases in serum PSA levels are caused by disruption of the prostatic epithelium by any disease processes. In addition to malignancy, BPH, urinary tract infections, prostatitis, prostatic stones, and instrumentation of the lower

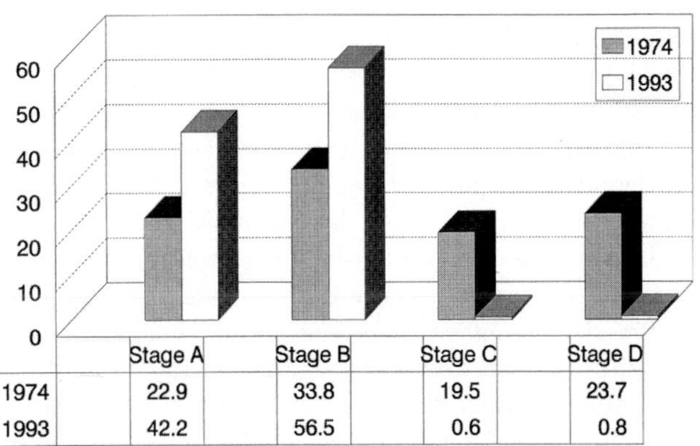

FIGURE 14-4. Clinical stage of clinically diagnosed versus screen-detected prostate cancers. (From Brawn PN, Johnson EH, Kuhl DL, et al. Stage at presentation and survival of white and black patients with prostate carcinoma. *Cancer* 1993;71:2569–2573; and Washington University PSA Screening Study, with permission.)

urinary tract can cause increases in PSA. Manipulation of the prostate by DRE and ejaculation may lead to transient increases in the PSA (88). Transrectal needle biopsy can significantly increase the PSA for up to 1 month postbiopsy. These effects are usually transient and not clinically significant, unless the PSA is on the border of a cutoff point.

Serum PSA concentrations may also be decreased by hormonal therapies, including finasteride (a 5α-reductase inhibitor). Finasteride prevents the conversion of testosterone to dihydrotestosterone, and in the prostate, the dihydrotestosterone level decreases by 90%. Although the individual variation in serum-PSA reduction ranges from 21% to 81%, the average PSA reduction is 50%. The serum-PSA decrease occurs within 6 months of therapy with little decrease thereafter. Despite the reduction in the total PSA (tPSA), finasteride does not effect the total to free PSA (fPSA) ratio (89). Using the data from the placebo arm of the Proscar Long-Term Efficacy and Safety Study, it has been shown that the average PSA increases by 10% over a 4-year period in an untreated group of men with lower urinary tract symptoms (90). There was no evidence that treatment with finasteride hindered the diagnosis of prostate cancer, for there was no difference in the diagnosis of cancer between the placebo group and the treatment group, when simple prostatectomy (TURP) diagnosed cancers were excluded. Because there was a higher rate of BPH-related surgery in the placebo arm, there was a slightly higher rate of prostate cancer detected in the placebo arm if prostatectomy specimens were included. In the placebo arm, the men with prostate cancer had a greater rise in their PSA over a 4-year period compared to those without cancer with an average PSA increase of 16% and 10%, respectively. In comparison, the men in the finasteride-treated arm had the expected average PSA reduction of 50%. In the treated arm, those with prostate cancer had less of a PSA reduction compared to those without evidence of prostate cancer with PSA changes of 41% and 57%, respectively. Based on this data from the Proscar Long-Term Efficacy and Safety Study, Andriole et al. (91) suggested that differential PSA response to treatment with finasteride might be used as an adjunct in differentiating BPH from prostate cancer in men with an elevated PSA.

Although PSA screening carries indisputable potential for the earlier diagnosis of prostate cancer, it also carries the drawback of a high rate of false-positive results. Because TRUS imaging does not reliably identify every small focus of cancer, effectively, every individual testing positive (PSA greater than 4 ng per mL) will require a TRUS-guided biopsy to rule out cancer. Approximately 15% of screened populations of men older than 50 years test PSA positive, but only 2% to 5% prove positive, in fact, on biopsy. Thus, between two-thirds and four-fifths of men will be worried that they may have cancer until the biopsy result is known. The psychological effects and sequelae of this period of anxiety are unknown, but approximately 3% of those testing false-positive and undergoing biopsy will experience significant morbidity from the procedure (e.g., sepsis or bleeding). Several methods called *PSA derivatives* have been proposed to enhance the clinical efficacy of PSA in the identification of patients with prostate cancer. The following are practical considerations for using PSA derivatives.

Prostate-Specific Antigen Velocity

PSA velocity (PSAV) (or *slope*) is defined as the change in PSA value over a period of time. It is hypothesized that PSA will rise more rapidly in men with significant cancers than in men with benign prostates. PSAV can be used as an absolute rate of change or as a percentage rate of change. The acceptable rate of change has not been determined, but Carter et al. (92–94) have suggested a value of 0.75 ng per mL per year as indicative of prostate cancer. Based on the observations by Schmid et al. (95) on the PSA doubling time in untreated prostate cancer, Brawer et al. (96,97) selected an annual percent change of 20% over the baseline as suspicious for cancer.

During a 13-year observation period of 9,671 patients, Ito et al. (98) found that 62% of patients demonstrated a PSA abnormality for more than 1 year (average, 2.8) before prostate cancer diagnosis. Prostate cancer that was diagnosed within 1 year after a PSA value became abnormal was not associated with bone metastasis. Concerning the relationship between PSAV and clinical stage, the proportion of stage B cancer was 86% in the subjects whose PSAV level before diagnosis was 0.18 ng per mL per year or less, and it was only 29% in those with PSAV levels of 4.5 ng per mL per year or more.

Carter et al. (93,94) performed PSA testing on sera collected as part of the Baltimore Longitudinal Aging Study and reported that an annual PSA-level increase of 0.75 ng per mL indicated men who would develop prostate cancer. This optimal annual rate of change of 0.75 ng per mL yielded a sensitivity of nearly 80% and a specificity of 66% for men with PSA values less than 4 ng per mL. The serum saved in the Baltimore Longitudinal Aging Study was collected over many years, and the assumptions made by Carter were based on PSA changes annualized over a minimum of 7 years. Pearson and Carter (92) demonstrated that, in men with prostatic carcinoma, there was a transition from a linear to an exponential phase of PSAV beginning 7.3 years before the diagnosis in men with localized disease and 9.2 years before the diagnosis in men with advanced-stage disease. Use of PSAV may save 10% to 30% of biopsies among men with elevated serum PSA and prior negative biopsy but may miss 5% to 20% of cancers (92).

Porter et al. (99) reported on a series with 1- and 2-year intervals between PSA measurements. With 1-year intervals, men with prostate carcinoma could not be differentiated with any PSAV parameter, including 0.75 ng per mL per year change, 20% increase, median PSAV, or median percent PSA increase per year. With the 2-year interval PSA measurements, there remained no use of PSAV manipulation in the diagnosis of men with prostate cancer. Littrup et al. (100) analyzed the results of the ACS-NPCDP, and they found that with greater intervals between PSA determinations, PSAV could be used to separate men with and without prostate cancer. They determined that a PSAV of greater than 1 ng per mL per year predicted cancer, and percent change in PSA did not enhance cancer detection.

In his ongoing study of PSA screening, Brawer (96) reported a diagnosis of prostate cancer in 17% of those men whose PSA increased by more than 20% over 1 year. Komatsu et al. (101) showed that when specimens were drawn 15 to 183 days (mean 80 days) apart, a greater than 20% increase was seen in 36.5% of men, and more than a 0.75 ng per mL increase in PSA was seen in 10% of patients. In the short term, the degree of biologic variation in serum PSA levels is significant with and without prostate disease. The use of percent change in PSA appears to be ineffective in predicting prostate cancer. An absolute PSA change of 0.75 ng per mL to 1.00 ng per mL per year can be predictive of prostate cancer, but, owing to the variability of PSA among men with benign prostates, at least three measurements separated by at least 18 months are needed to reliably calculate PSAV. In view of this requirement, PSAV is not a very useful tool for the early detection of prostate cancer or the elimination of a large percentage of unnecessary biopsies.

Prostate-Specific Antigen Density

PSA density (PSAD) (also referred to as *PSA index*) is calculated by dividing the serum PSA (ng per mL) by the prostate volume. It is conjectured that PSAD adjusts for increases in serum PSA that occur owing to benign prostatic enlargement. Stamey et al. (102) first reported that prostate cancer contributes ten times more to the serum PSA than BPH, volume for volume. Because prostatic enlargement occurs in the transition zone and most serum PSA leak occurs from the transition zone, calculating a PSAD using the transition zone volume [PSA transition zone density (PSATZD)] may be more predictive of prostate cancer than using the total prostate volume.

There have been several reports on improved stratification between patients with BPH and prostatic carcinoma using PSAD (103,104). In a study of 41 men with prostate cancer and 20 men with BPH, Benson and colleagues (105) found the mean PSAD in those with cancer to be significantly greater than in BPH. In a larger study of 595 patients referred for PSA values between 4.1 and 10.0 ng per mL, Benson et al. (106) were unable to differentiate the patients with and without cancer by PSA value in this intermediate range, but there was a strongly significant difference ($p < .0001$) in PSAD between those with positive and negative biopsies in this same group of men. The PSAD in men with, versus without, prostatic carcinoma was 0.297 and 0.208, respectively. In a similar study by Brawer et al. (97), PSAD was significantly different between those with and without cancer, but only in the men biopsied for PSA values between 4.1 and 10.0 ng per mL. In those with PSA values less than 4 ng per mL and greater than 10 ng per mL, PSAD was not a useful tool in differentiating benign disease from carcinoma.

In a comparative study of the various PSA derivatives, Kikuchi et al. (107) performed sextant biopsies on 147 men with PSA levels between 4.1 and 10.0 ng per mL. According to ROC curve analysis, PSATZD had the most useful validity in the differentiation between prostate carcinoma and benign prostatic enlargement. At the sensitivity of 90%, PSATZD would have prevented unnecessary biopsies in 68 of 117 patients who were without prostate carcinoma, whereas PSA, fPSA to tPSA ratio, and PSA complexed with alpha-1 antichymotrypsin (PSA-ACT) would have prevented unnecessary biopsies in 25, 28, and 25 patients, respectively. In an evaluation of the benefits of PSATZD and fPSA to tPSA ratio value, Horniger et al. (108) used an ROC curve analysis to show that by using a PSATZD of more than 0.22 ng per mL per cc as a biopsy criterion, 24.4% of negative biopsies could be avoided. In comparison, ROC curve analyses for fPSA showed that by using percent fPSA (%fPSA) less than 20% as a biopsy criterion, 45.5% of negative biopsies could be eliminated. When combining these two diagnostic tests, 54.2% of negative biopsies could be avoided.

A PSAD value of 0.15 retains the sensitivity of the test but reduces the number of biopsies by 24% to 42%. In men with a tPSA of 4 to 10 ng per mL and a prior negative biopsy, the performance characteristics may be even better. Thirty-one percent of rebiopsies may be prevented, while missing 10% of prostate cancers (109).

A cutoff of 0.3 ng per mL for PSATZD in men with normal DRE reduced the number of biopsies by 51%, while detecting one out of eight cancers. Sensitivity and specificity were 88% and 57%, respectively. These studies were of referral populations, and studies of screening populations have not shown a significant benefit of PSATZD in the detection of prostate cancer.

Total PSAD and PSATZD are not ideal primary screening modalities, owing to the fact that they require a TRUS of the prostate (an invasive and costly procedure) for a more objective measurement of volume. Additionally, TRUS-calculated volumes are not precise, and this may limit the accuracy of the calculated PSA densities. The PSATZD is better for prostate glands with a volume of 30 cc or more. PSAD seems to be most useful in patients with an elevated PSA who have had a previous negative biopsy.

Age-Specific Prostate-Specific Antigen Range

Age-specific PSA reference ranges (ASRR) were established based on the rationale that, as the prostate enlarges with age, PSA levels will also increase with age, whether or not cancer is present. Although the incidence of prostate cancer rises markedly in men older than the age of 60 years, the assumption is that using a higher tPSA cut point for older men is unlikely to result in higher morbidity or mortality from the disease. The use of age-specific PSA levels also presumes that it is more important to diagnose prostate cancer in younger men, because a longer life expectancy places them at greater risk of disease progression, metastases, and death due to more "at risk" years. By raising the upper limits of normal for older men, it was hypothesized that the number of biopsies in this population would be reduced, while not compromising prostate cancer detection among younger men.

The original upper limit of normal, 4 ng per mL, was determined by the Hybritech Company based on analyses of levels in 860 men and women without prostate cancer (110). The age-specific cut points advocated were established based on the ninety-fifth percentile for PSA levels among age-stratified cohorts of men without prostate cancer.

In the initial studies by Oesterling (111), adjusting the PSA cutoff from 4.0 to 4.5 ng per mL for men in the 60- to 69-year age group would eliminate 15% of biopsies, while missing 3% of cancers. Of the cancers missed, 95% were considered of "little clinical significance." Among men ages 70 to 79 years, 44% percent of biopsies could be prevented, but at the expense of missing 47% of cancers. In a larger review of 4,597 men with clinically localized prostate cancer, Partin and Oesterling et al. (112) used age-specific PSA cut points of 2.5, 3.5, 4.5, and 6.5 ng per mL for the age groups of 40 to 49, 50 to 59, 60 to 69, and 70 to 79 years, respectively. With these age-specific cut points, an additional 18% (74 men) of younger men (under the age of 60 years) could have been diagnosed by PSA screening. Among these 74 additional younger men, 19% had "unfavorable pathology." Using these reference ranges, 22% (191 of 252) of the cancers in older men would have been missed. Of these missed cancers, fewer than 3% were T1c, and 95% of these undetected T1c cancers were of "favorable pathologic status." ASRR were recommended over the standard 4 ng per mL cut point by this group at The Johns Hopkins University, based on their finding of an increased detection of more potentially curable cancer in the young and decreased detection of more favorable tumors in older men.

However, several other investigators (113–116) found that disturbing numbers of clinically serious cancers and cancers of advanced stage are missed in older men, using similar age-specific reference ranges. The percentage of avoided biopsies was also not as significant in follow-up studies. Using ASRR in men aged 60 to 79 years with negative DRE, Borer et al. (113) found that 73 of 1,280 (5.7%) biopsies would have been avoided, but 15 of the 73 (20.5%) men who avoided biopsy had cancer. In contrast to the studies by Oesterling et al., 60% (9 of 15) of the missed cancers had unfavorable histology. In similar studies of men aged 60 years and older, the avoided biopsy rate ranged from 6% to 15%, but 12% to 30% of histologically significant cancers were missed (117–120). In these other studies by Dalkin (117), Crawford (118), Anderson (119), and Oesterling (120), between 60% and 71% of the cancers that went undetected using ASRR were considered to be of unfavorable histology.

This concept that the elderly are more likely to have clinically insignificant tumors has not been borne out; studies have shown that in the PSA range of 4 to 10 ng per mL, older men are more likely to have detectable prostate cancer, and the grade of the cancers might worsen with age. Sung et al. (121) reviewed the findings of 210 men aged 70 years and older referred for prostate ultrasound and biopsy, and the men aged 80 years and older had higher cancer incidence, grade, and stage. The overall cancer detection rate was 56.8%, but the cancer rate in men aged 80 and older was 81%. These elderly men had twice the rate of poorly differentiated cancer than the men aged 70 to 79 years (64.7% versus 33.0%), and they also had a larger proportion of high-stage cancer. However, although the patients aged 80 years and older were less likely to respond well to treatment, none of the patients aged 80 years and older died of prostate cancer. Owing to these findings, age-adjusted PSA reference ranges seem to have limited clinical use.

In considering the use of ASRR, the racial differences in prostate cancer detection at various ages is also considered. In the study by Borer et al. (113), a statistically significantly higher cancer detection rate was found in African-Americans as compared to whites in all age groups studied. For African-American men aged 60 to 69 years, the use of ASRR would have excluded only 1 of 309 biopsies performed over the 4.7-year study period.

Because serum PSA levels show a tendency to rise with age, a given individual screened by PSA testing will be more likely to test positive simply by virtue of being older. Although the incidence of prostate cancer also rises steeply with age, it is probably more important to diagnose the disease in younger men, because their greater life expectancy gives them more years "at risk" of developing disease progression and metastases. Although both of the above statements may be true, they do not justify an intent to avoid detection of potentially aggressive prostate cancer in older men. They have led to further studies regarding the potential benefits of using lower PSA cut points in younger men for the early detection of potentially curable and significant cancer in men under the age of 60 years.

Using a Lower Prostate-Specific Antigen Cutoff

The ideal cutoff point to define a serum PSA level as "normal" has not been determined. Currently, a PSA value of greater than 4 ng per mL is the most widely held standard considered normal, but recent studies have shown that up to 25% of men with prostate cancer have a PSA value of less than 4 ng per mL. Cooner and associates (59) reported that 52 of 263 (20%) men with prostate cancer had a normal PSA (under 4 ng per mL), and 32% of the men with cancer in a study by Brawer (96) had normal PSA levels. In most PSA screenings, studies that have evaluated men with serum PSA concentrations between 0 and 4 ng per mL, the cancer detection rate ranges from 4% to 9% with a negative DRE and 10% to 17% with a positive DRE. At Washington University, Colberg et al. (122) found a cancer detection rate of 7% among 111 men with normal DRE and serum PSA levels between 2.8 and 4.0 ng per mL. In a more recent study at Washington University, Smith et al. (123), on the use of a lower PSA cutoff (PSA between 2.6 and 4.0 ng per mL) in men age 50 years and older with benign DRE, showed that African-American men were younger (60 vs. 63 years old, $p = .005$) and presented with slightly higher PSA levels (3.3 vs. 3.1 ng per mL, $p = .03$) than white men. Consistent with most other screening studies with various PSA cutoffs, African-Americans had a twofold higher detection rate (13 of 29; 45%) than did white (93 of 362; 26%) men ($p = .03$), and the overall cancer detection rate was 27%. In controlling for age, tPSA, PSAD, %fPSA, and number of prior screening visits, race remained a significant predictor of cancer (adjusted odds ratio, 3.4). Based on the widely differing results of these two studies at the same institution, the use of a lower PSA cutoff remains controversial.

Free Prostate-Specific Antigen

PSA exists in several different molecular forms in the serum and in seminal fluid. tPSA consists of all immunodetectable PSA in the serum and is comprised of primarily fPSA and PSA-ACT. PSA also exists complexed to alpha-2 macroglobulin (PSA-MG), to protein C inhibitor, to alpha-1 antichymotrypsin, and to interalpha-trypsin. Only the free form and the ACT-complexed form are measurable by currently available immunoassays (124). PSA-ACT is the predominant form (60% to 95%) of PSA in the serum, whereas 5% to 30% of the immunodetectable PSA is the free, noncomplexed form. ACT is known to react with PSA in a 1 to 1 molar ratio, and the serum concentrations of ACT and MG (the main protease inhibitors that bind with PSA) are 10^5 to 10^6 times greater than the serum concentration of PSA (125). Why all the serum PSA is not complexed to ACT or MG remains unknown. fPSA levels are measured using monoclonal antibodies to epitope E (one of five major epitope sites on the PSA molecule), which remains fully exposed on the fPSA molecule but is blocked when complexed. There are also monoclonal antibodies that can be independently used to measure PSA-ACT and tPSA.

Stenman and associates (126) were the first to demonstrate that men with prostate cancer tend to have higher ratios of PSA-ACT to tPSA than men without prostate cancer. In a study of men with prostate cancer (n = 67), BPH (n = 30), and controls (n = 10), they found that the proportion of PSA-ACT to the tPSA increased with increasing PSA, and this same ratio was seen in the men with prostate carcinoma. In a follow-up study, Christensson et al. (127) confirmed the significantly higher PSA-ACT to tPSA ratio in prostate cancer as compared to BPH, and they also demonstrated that there is a significantly lower fPSA to tPSA ratio in cancer patients as compared to those with BPH (0.18 vs. 0.28, respectively; $p < .0001$). With this new modality, the specificity increased from 55%, using a tPSA cutoff of greater than 4 ng per mL, to 73% using an fPSA to tPSA ratio cutoff of 0.18 ng per mL. The potential benefit of the fPSA was further confirmed by Luderer and colleagues (128), who found that 73% of the men with cancer, as compared to 29% of the men with BPH, had fPSA to tPSA ratios of less than 15% ($p < .0001$). They suggested that a cutoff ratio of 20% would increase specificity from 37% to 52%, but the sensitivity would decrease from 93% to 87%.

Catalona et al. (129) were the first to demonstrate that the fPSA level was dependent on cancer status and prostate size. In a study of 113 men aged 50 years and older with tPSA concentrations between 4 and 10 ng per mL, 63 men had BPH, 20 men had prostate cancer with normal-sized prostates, and 30 men had prostate cancer with enlarged glands. The median %fPSA in men with BPH was 19%, with cancer in the normal-sized glands being 9% and cancer in the enlarged gland being 16%. In this initial study by Catalona et al., they suggested a cutoff of 23.4%, and this would result in a 31% increase in specificity without any compromise to sensitivity (greater than 90%). In men with normal-sized prostates, the cutoff could potentially be much lower.

More recent studies have evaluated larger numbers of men in the sample population. In a multicenter trial conducted at seven university medical centers (130), 773 men aged 50 to 75 years with benign DRE and serum PSA levels between 4 and 10 ng per mL were evaluated in a prospective blinded study of the optimal fPSA cutoff. There was no difference in tPSA concentrations between the men with benign versus malignant prostates (tPSA 5.6 vs. 5.9, respectively). The %fPSA was able to differentiate the group of men with benign disease (mean fPSA of 18%) from those with cancer (12% mean fPSA). A fPSA to tPSA cutoff of 25% detected 95% of cancers while avoiding 20% of unnecessary biopsies. The few cancers associated with an fPSA greater than 25% were more often in older patients and of lower grade and volume. Use of a cutoff of 22% would have avoided 29% of the biopsies, but 10% of the cancer would have been missed. The lower the fPSA, the higher the risk of detectable carcinoma. %fPSA has an inverse correlation with tumor aggressiveness—that is, a lower %fPSA is suggestive of a more aggressive form of prostate cancer.

The optimal cut point for fPSA has not been determined, for this cut point is a balance between optimal sensitivity relative to specificity. This should be based on prostate size, DRE findings, tPSA concentration, and biopsy history. To achieve the goal of minimizing the number of benign biopsies in older men without compromising cancer detection in younger men, several different cut points have been suggested. A %fPSA cut point of 25% among men with tPSA values between 4 and 10 ng per mL eliminates 34% of unnecessary biopsies in men aged 70 to 75 years, 19% in men aged 60 to 69 years, and 11% in men aged 50 to 59 years. This occurs at the cost of missing 2%, 6%, and 9%, respectively, in these various age groups. The 25% cutoff maintains a 95% sensitivity in African-Americans and whites (131). Another system recommends using a higher cut point for %fPSA in men with a tPSA of 2.5 to 4.0 ng per mL. For these men, a %fPSA cutoff of 27% led to the avoidance of 18% of biopsies while missing 10% of cancers.

Human Glandular Kallikrein 2

Human glandular kallikrein 2 (hK2) is related to PSA as a serine protease, and it shares approximately 80% of sequence homology. Similar to PSA, it is produced by the prostate columnar epithelium under the regulation of androgens. It forms complexes with alpha-l antichymotrypsin and alpha-2 macroglobulin. Preliminary studies suggest that the ratio of total hK2 to fPSA provides improved specificity over percentage of fPSA (132). In men with tPSA in the range of 2.5 to 10.0 ng per mL, hK2 concentrations were not different between groups of men with prostate cancer and BPH. However, hK2 to fPSA ratio was a stronger predictor of prostate cancer than the fPSA to tPSA ratio. At 95% specificity in men with tPSA between 2.5 and 10.0 ng per mL, the hK2 to fPSA ratio identified 30% of patients who had cancer. In another study, Becker et al. (133,134) found that the total hK2 serum concentrations were significantly different between groups of men with BPH, localized prostate cancer, and advanced prostate cancer. hK2 concentrations were less than 0.05 ng per mL in all 50 healthy volunteers, and hK2 was greater than 0.05 in 28 of 54 men (52%) with BPH (p <.001). One hundred of 136 (74%) men with localized prostate cancer had hK2 levels greater than 0.05 ng per mL, as compared to 55 of 57 (96%) men with advanced malignancy (p <.0001). Becker et al. also confirmed the ability of the hK2 to fPSA ratio to differentiate the benign groups from those with cancer. The potential benefits of hK2 in a clinical practice are yet unproven, and further studies with larger patient populations are in progress.

SUMMARY

Prostate cancers are known to be present in approximately 30% to 40% of men older than age 60 years, but only a small proportion of cancers known to be present become clinically evident, and more men die with prostate cancer than of it. The risk of a 50-year-old man with a 25-year life expectancy having microscopic cancer is 42%, having clinically evident cancer is 9.5%, and dying of prostate cancer 2.9% (135). In 50- to 60-year-old men, carrying out a rectal examination and PSA test will detect clinically suspicious areas within the prostate in approximately 5%, and approximately 10% will have an elevated PSA. Eventually, after such screening, around 4% of men with an otherwise normal prostate will be found to have prostate cancers. A high false-negative rate of screening with the standard DRE and PSA regimen, leading to large numbers of unnecessary prostate biopsies, has remained a major problem with prostate cancer screening. Differing screening protocols and testing intervals were recommended to improve cost efficiency while maintaining detection rate. Various methods have been proposed to increase the specificity of PSA, including ASRR, PSAD, PSAV, and %fPSA. The use of rectal examination may increase the number of tumors found, but compliance is reduced when a DRE is a required part of the protocol. The use of the various PSA derivatives will reduce the number of unnecessary biopsies, but at the expense of missing some tumors.

Ross and Carter et al. (136) compared seven different PSA-screening strategies using outcome measures of numbers of prevented prostate cancer deaths, PSA tests, and prostate biopsies per 1,000 men aged 40 through 80 years. Compared with annual PSA testing beginning at age 50 years, the strategy of PSA testing at ages 40 and 45 years, followed by biannual testing beginning at age 50 years, was estimated to simultaneously reduce prostate cancer mortality and number of PSA tests and biopsies performed per 1,000 men. Specifically, compared with no screening, the standard strategy prevents 3.2 deaths, with an additional 10,500 PSA tests and 600 prostatic biopsies, whereas the earlier but less frequent strategy prevents 3.3 deaths, with an additional 7,500 PSA tests and 450 prostate biopsies. Strategies using lowered PSA thresholds and age-specific PSA were not more efficient than using a PSA greater than 4 ng per mL. Their conclusion was that the standard strategy of annual PSA screening beginning at age 50 years appears to be less effective and more resource intensive compared with a strategy that begins earlier but screens biennially instead of annually. In a similar study of screening strategies using a computer model, Etzioni et al. (137) also concluded that biennial PSA screening is a cost-effective alternative to annual screening for prostate cancer. They found that biennial screening with PSA greater than 4 ng per mL was projected to reduce the number of screens and false-positive tests by almost 50%, relative to annual screening, while retaining 93% of years of life saved.

In a multicenter study, Catalona et al. (138) compared several PSA derivatives for their use in cancer detection and their ability to predict pathologic stage after radical prostatectomy in patients with clinically localized, stage T1c cancer. This blinded, prospective study showed that %fPSA and age-specific PSA cutoffs enhanced PSA specificity for cancer detection, but %fPSA maintained significantly higher sensitivities. Age-specific PSA cutoffs missed 20% to 60% of cancers in men older than 60 years. %fPSA and PSAD performed equally well for detection (95% sensitivity), if cutoffs of 25% fPSA or 0.078 PSAD were used, respectively. The commonly used PSAD cutoff of 0.15 detected only 59% of cancers. %fPSA and PSAD also produced similar results for prediction of the postradical prostatectomy pathologic stage. Patients with cancer with higher %fPSA values (greater than 15%) or lower PSAD values (0.15 or less) tended to have less aggressive disease. Because %fPSA and PSAD provided comparable results, their conclusion was that %fPSA may be used in place of PSAD for biopsy decisions and in algorithms for prediction of less aggressive tumors, because the determination of %fPSA does not require ultrasound. Finne et al. (139) have suggested that the specificity of PSA screening might be improved using an artificial neural network (multilayer perceptron) and logistic regression models based on tPSA, the proportion of fPSA, DRE, and prostate volume in men with tPSA levels in the range 4 to 10 ng per mL.

Of more concern, we remain uncertain as to how effective aggressive local treatment is in altering the natural history of the disease. The effectiveness of these treatment modalities will continue to be confounded by inappropriate "attribution" of cause of death, the detection of men with better prognosis, distant-metastatic disease responsive to hormonal ablation, and changes in social factors, such as diet. Screening will identify some men with cancer who will not benefit from treatment. Although it is yet unproven whether screening would be followed by a reduction in morbidity and mortality, recent data suggest a screening effect has been observed in the United States with an increase in incidence, a decrease in men with distant metastases, and a small decrease in prostate cancer mortality. Future changes may incorporate molecular markers that might aid identification of men best treated aggressively, because of a risk of progression. Tests to identify genetic predisposition may also allow targeted screening. New treatments and early chemoprevention or dietary strategies will again shift the ground on which these arguments are being disputed.

REFERENCES

1. Boring CC, Squires TS, Tong T. Cancer statistics, 1993. *CA Cancer J Clin* 1993;43:7–26.
2. Mettlin C, Jones GW, Murphy GP. Prostate cancer in blacks: an update form the American College of Surgeons patterns of care studies. *J Surg Oncol* 1989;40:232–236.
3. Bullock AD, Morton RA. Prostate cancer in African-Americans. In: Lytton B, Catalona WJ, Lipshultz LI, Bloom D, eds. *Advances in Urology*, vol. 8. New York: Mosby–Year Book, 1995:131–156.
4. Mokulis J, Thompson I. Screening for prostate cancer: pros, cons, and reality. *Cancer Control* 1995;2:15–21.
5. Boring CC, Squires TS, Tong T. Cancer statistics, 1996. *CA Cancer J Clin* 1996;46:5–27.
6. Chodak GW. Screening for prostate cancer in 1993: Is it appropriate, or not? *Semin Urol* 1993;11:47–49.
7. Littrup PJ, Goodman AC, Mettlin CJ. The benefit and cost of prostate cancer early detection. *CA Cancer J Clin* 1993; 43:134–149.
8. Franks LM. Latency and progression in tumors: the natural history of prostatic cancer. *Lancet* 1956;1:60–63.
9. Dhom G. Epidemiologic aspects of latent and clinically manifest carcinoma of the prostate. *J Cancer Res Clin Oncol* 1983;106:210–218.
10. Holund B. Latent prostate cancer in consecutive autopsy series. *Scand J Urol Nephrol* 1980;14:29–35.
11. Kabalin JN, McNeal JE, Price HM, et al. Unsuspected adenocarcinoma of the prostate in patients undergoing cystoprostatectomy for other causes: incidence, histology and morphometric observations. *J Urol* 1989;141:1091–1094.
12. Scardino PT, Weaver R, Hudson MA. Early detection of prostate cancer. *Hum Pathol* 1992;23:211–222.
13. Stamey TA, Freiha FS, McNeal JE, et al. Localized prostate cancer: relationship of tumor volume to clinical significance for treatment of prostate cancer. *Cancer* 1993;71(Suppl 3):933–938.
14. Aihara M, Wheeler TM, Ohori M, et al. Heterogeneity of prostate cancer in radical prostatectomy specimens. *Urology* 1994;43:60–66.
15. Optenberg SA, Thompson IM. Economics of screening for carcinoma of the prostate. *Urol Clin North Amer* 1990;17: 719–737.
16. Johansson JE, Adami HO, Anderson SO, et al. High 10-year survival rate in patients with early untreated prostate cancer. *JAMA* 1992;267:2191–2196.
17. Chodak GW, Thisted RA, Gerber GS, et al. Results of conservative management of clinically localized prostate cancer. *Cancer* 1993;72:310–322.
18. Walsh PC. A decision analysis of alternative treatment strategies for clinically localized prostate cancer. *J Urol* 1993;150:1330–1332.
19. Scardino PT, Beck JR, Miles BJ. Conservative management of prostate cancer. *N Engl J Med* 1994;330:1831.
20. Beck JR, Kattan MY, Miles BJ. A critique of the decision analysis for clinically localized prostate cancer. *J Urol* 1994;152:1894–1899.
21. Aus G. Prostate cancer: mortality and morbidity after non-curative treatment with aspects on diagnosis and treatment. *Scand J Urol Nephrol* 1994;167(Suppl):9–41.
22. Catalona WJ, Smith DJ, Ratliff TL, et al. Detection of organ-confined prostate cancer is increased through prostate-specific antigen-based screening. *JAMA* 1993;270:948–954.
23. Feneley MR. Does screening for prostate cancer identify clinically important disease? *Ann R Coll Surg Engl* 1999; 81:207–214.
24. Gohagan JK, Prorok PC, Kramer BS, et al. Prostate cancer screening in the prostate, lung, colorectal and ovarian cancer screening trial of the National Cancer Institute. *J Urol* 1994;152:1905–1909.

25. Wilt TJ, Brawer MK. The Prostate Cancer Intervention Versus Observation Trial: a randomized trial comparing radical prostatectomy versus expectant management for the treatment of clinically localized prostate cancer. *J Urol* 1994;152:1910–1914.
26. Fremgen AM, Bland KI, McGinnis LS, et al. Clinical highlights from the National Cancer Data Base, 1999. *CA Cancer J Clin* 1999;49:145–158.
27. Feuer EJ, Merrill RM, Hankey BF. Cancer surveillance series: interpreting trends in prostate cancer II: cause of death misclassification and the recent rise and fall in prostate cancer mortality. *J Natl Cancer Inst* 1999;91:1025–1032.
28. Merrill RM, Stephenson RA. Trends in mortality rates in patients with prostate cancer during the era of prostate specific antigen screening. *J Urol* 2000;163:503–510.
29. Hankey BF, Feuer EJ, Clegg LX, et al. Cancer surveillance series: interpreting trends in prostate cancer—part I: evidence of the effects of screening in recent prostate cancer incidence, mortality, and survival rates. *J Natl Cancer Inst* 1999;91:1017–1024.
30. Crawford ED. A controlled trial of leuprolide with and without flutamide in prostate carcinoma. *N Engl J Med* 1989;321:419–424.
31. Smith J, Haynes T, Middleton R. Impact of external irradiation on local symptoms and survival free of disease in patients with pelvic lymph node metastasis from adenocarcinoma of the prostate. *J Urol* 1984;131:705–707.
32. Menck HR, Garfinkel L, Dodd GD. Preliminary report of the National Cancer Data Base. *Cancer* 1991;41:7–18.
33. Young HH. *A surgeon's autobiography*. New York: Harcourt Brace, 1940:131.
34. Goluboff ET, Olsson CA. Urologists on a tight-rope: coping with a changing economy. *J Urol* 1994;151:1–4.
35. Kramer BS, Brown ML, Prorok PC, et al. Prostate cancer screening: what we know and what we need to know. *Ann Intern Med* 1993;119:914–923.
36. Carlsson P, Pedersen KV, Varenhorst E. Costs and benefits of early detection of prostatic cancer. *Health Policy* 1990;16: 241–253.
37. Love RR, Camilli AE. The value of screening. *Cancer* 1998;48(Suppl 2):489–494.
38. Mebane C, Tyson G, Horm J. Current status of prostate cancer in North American black males. *J Natl Med Assoc* 1980;82:782–788.
39. Aziz H, Rotman M, Thelmo W, et al. Radiation-treated carcinoma of the prostate. *Am J Clin Oncol* 1988;11:166–171.
40. Myers NM, Hankey BF. *Cancer patient survival experience*. Bethesda, MD: National Institutes of Health, 1980: Pub. No. 80-2184.
41. Brawn PN, Johnson EH, Kuhl DL, et al. Stage at presentation and survival of white and black patients with prostate carcinoma. *Cancer* 1993;71:2569–2573.
42. Levine RL, Wilchinsky M. Adenocarcinoma of the prostate: a comparison of the disease in blacks versus whites. *J Urol* 1979;121:761–762.
43. Natarajan N, Murphy GP, Mettlin C. Prostate cancer in blacks: an update from the American College of Surgeons' patterns of care studies. *J Surg Oncol* 1989;40:232–236.
44. *The 1987 annual cancer statistics review including cancer trends, 1950–1985*. Bethesda, MD: National Cancer Institute, 1987: Pub. No. 88-2789.
45. Roach M, Krall J, Keller JW, et al. The prognostic significance of race and survival from prostate cancer based on patients irradiated on Radiation Therapy Oncology Group protocols (1976–1985). *Int J Radiat Oncol Biol Phys* 1992;24:441–449.
46. Polednak AP, Flannery JT. Black versus white racial differences in clinical stage at diagnosis and treatment of prostate cancer in Connecticut. *Cancer* 1992;70:2152–2158.
47. Weinrich SP, Weinrich M, Mettlin C, et al. Urinary symptoms as a predictor for participation in prostate cancer screening among African-American men. *Prostate* 1998;37: 215–222.
48. Weinrich SP, Boyd MD, Weinrich M, et al. Increasing prostate cancer screening in African-American men with peer-educator and client-navigator interventions. *J Cancer Educ* 1998;13:213–219.
49. Barber KR, Shaw R, Folts M, et al. Differences between African-American and Caucasian men participating in a community-based prostate cancer screening program. *J Community Health* 1998;23:441–451.
50. Targonski PV, Guinan P, Phillips CW. Prostate cancer: the stage disadvantage in the black male. *J Natl Med Assoc* 1991;83:1094–1096.
51. Heshmat MY, Kovi J, Rao MS, et al. Review of prostatic surgical procedures at a predominately black hospital: a 22-year study. *J Natl Med Assoc* 1992;84:677–680.
52. Gronberg H, Wiklund F, Damber JE. Age specific risks of familial prostate carcinoma: a basis for screening recommendations in high risk populations. *Cancer* 1999;86:477–483.
53. Matikainen MP, Schleutker J, Morsky P, et al. Detection of subclinical cancers by prostate-specific antigen screening in asymptomatic men from high-risk prostate cancer families. *Clin Cancer Res* 1999;5:1275–1279.
54. Marion G, ed. *Traite d' urologie II*. Paris: Masson, 1921:1050.
55. Jewett JJ. Significance of the palpable prostatic nodule. *JAMA* 1956;160:838–839.
56. Thompson IM, Ernst JJ, Gangai MP, et al. Adenocarcinoma of the prostate: results of routine urological screening. *J Urol* 1984;132:690–692.
57. Chodak GW, Keller P, Schoenberg H. Routine screening for prostate cancer using the digital rectal examination. *Prog Clin Biol Res* 1988;269:87–98.
58. Lee F, Littrup PJ, Torp-Pedersen ST, et al. Prostate cancer: comparison of transrectal US and digital rectal examination for screening. *Radiology* 1988;168:389–394.
59. Cooner W, Mosley R, Rutherford CJ, et al. Prostate cancer detection in a clinical urologic practice by ultrasonography, digital rectal examination and prostate specific antigen. *J Urol* 1990;143:1146–1152.
60. Chodak GW, Schoenberg HW. Progress and problems in screening for carcinoma of the prostate. *World J Surg* 1989;13:60–64.
61. Faul P. [Preventive testing and rational diagnosis of prostatic neoplasms]. *Med Welt* 1978;29:1191–1193.
62. Gilbertsen VA. Cancer of the prostate gland: results of early diagnosis and therapy undertaken for cure of the disease. *JAMA* 1976;215:81–84.
63. Jenson CB, Shahon DB, Wangensteen OH. Evaluation of annual examinations in the detection of cancer: special refer-

ence to cancer of the gastrointestinal tract, prostate, breast and female reproduction tract. *JAMA* 1960;174:1783–1788.
64. Reference deleted by author.
65. Mueller EJ, Crain TW, Thompson IM, et al. An evaluation of serial digital rectal examinations in screening for prostate cancer. *J Urol* 1988;140:1445.
66. Thompson IM, Rounder JB, Teaque JL, et al. Impact of routine screening for adenocarcinoma of the prostate on stage distribution. *J Urol* 1987;137:424.
67. Catalona WJ, Richie JP, Ahmann FR, et al. Comparison of digital rectal examination and serum prostate specific antigen in the early detection of prostate cancer: results of a multicenter clinical trial of 6630 men. *J Urol* 1994;151: 1283–1290.
68. Bentvelsen FM, Schroder FH. Modalities available for screening for prostate cancer. *Eur J Cancer* 1993;29a:804–811.
69. Kirby RS, Christmas TJ, Brawer M. Screening for prostate cancer. In: Kirby RS, Brawer MK, Christmas TJ, eds. *Prostate cancer*. New York: Mosby–Year Book, 1996.
70. Basler JW, Thompson IM. Lest we abandon digital rectal examination as a screening test for prostate cancer [editorial; comment]. *J Natl Cancer Inst* 1998;90:1761–1763.
71. American Cancer Society. 1989 Survey of physicians' attitudes and practices in early cancer detection. *CA Cancer J Clin* 1990;40:77–80.
72. Wang M, Valenzuela L, Murphy G, et al. Purification of a human prostate specific antigen. *Invest Urol* 1979;17:159–163.
73. Lilja H. A kallikrein-like serine protease in prostatic fluid cleaves the predominant seminal vesicle protein. *J Clin Invest* 1985;76:1899–1903.
74. Schelhammer P, Wright G. Biomolecular and clinical characteristics of PSA and other candidate prostate tumor markers. *Urol Clin North Am* 1993;20:597–606.
75. Papsidero LD, Kuriyama M, Wang MC, et al. Prostate antigen: a marker for human prostate epithelial cells. *J Natl Cancer Inst* 1981;66:37–42.
76. Qiu SD, Young CY, Bilhartz DL, et al. In situ hybridization of prostate-specific antigen mRNA in human prostate. *J Urol* 1990;144:1550–1556.
77. Mettlin C, Lee F, Drago J, et al. The American Cancer Society National Prostate Cancer Detection Project: findings on the detection of early prostate cancer in 2,425 men. *Cancer* 1991;67:2949–2958.
78. Mettlin C, Murphy GP, Babaian RJ, et al. The results of a five-year early prostate cancer detection intervention. Investigators of the American Cancer Society National Prostate Cancer Detection Project. *Cancer* 1996;77:150–159.
79. Smith DS, Humphrey PA, Catalona WJ. The early detection of prostate carcinoma with prostate specific antigen: the Washington University experience. *Cancer* 1997;80: 1852–1856.
80. Candas B, Cusan L, Gomez JL, et al. Evaluation of prostatic specific antigen and digital rectal examination as screening tests for prostate cancer. *Prostate* 2000;45:19–35.
81. Brawer MK, Chetner MP, Beatie J, et al. Screening for prostatic carcinoma with prostate specific antigen. *J Urol* 1992;147:841–845.
82. Smith DS, Bullock AD, Catalona WJ. Racial differences in operating characteristics of prostate cancer screening tests. *J Urol* 1997;158:1861–1865.
83. Moskowitz M. Cost-benefit determinations in screening mammography. *Cancer* 1987;60:1680–1683.
84. Rommel FM, Augusta VE, Breslin JA, et al. The use of prostate specific antigen and prostate specific antigen density in the diagnosis of prostate cancer in a community based urology practice. *J Urol* 1994;151:88–93.
85. Brawer MK, Lange PH. PSA in the screening, staging and follow-up of early-stage prostate cancer: a review of recent developments. *World J Urol* 1989;7:7–11.
86. Smith DS, Bullock AD, Catalona WJ, et al. Racial differences in a prostate cancer screening study. *J Urol* 1996; 156:1366–1369.
87. Crawford ED. Prostate cancer awareness week: September 22 to 28, 1997. *CA Cancer J Clin* 1997;47:288–296.
88. Yuan JJ, Coplen DE, Petros JA, et al. Effects of rectal examination, prostatic massage, ultrasonography and needle biopsy on serum prostate specific antigen levels. *J Urol* 1992;147:810–814.
89. Keetch DW, Andriole GL, Ratliff TL, et al. Comparison of percent free prostate specific antigen levels in men with benign prostatic hyperplasia treated with finasteride, terazosin or watchful waiting. *Urology* 1997;50:901–905.
90. McConnell JD, Bruskewitz R, Walsh P, et al. The effects of finasteride on the risk of acute urinary retention and the need for surgical treatment among men with benign prostatic hyperplasia. *N Engl Med* 1998;338:557–563.
91. Andriole GL, Guess HA, Epstein JI, et al. Treatment with finasteride preserves usefulness of prostate-specific antigen in the detection of prostate cancer: results of a randomized, double-blind, placebo-controlled clinical trial. PLESS Study Group. Proscar Long-term Efficacy and Safety Study. *Urology* 1998;52:195–201.
92. Pearson JD, Carter HB. Natural history of changes in prostate specific antigen in early stage prostate cancer. *J Urol* 1994;152:1743–1748.
93. Carter HB, Morrell CH, Pearson JD, et al. Estimation of prostatic growth using serial prostate-specific antigen measurements in men with and without prostate disease. *Cancer Res* 1992;52:3323–3328.
94. Carter HB, Pearson JD, Metter EJ, et al. Longitudinal evaluation of prostate-specific antigen levels in men with and without prostate disease. *JAMA* 1992;267:2215–2220.
95. Schmid HP, McNeal JE, Stamey TA. Observations on the doubling time of prostate cancer: The use of serial prostate-specific antigen in patients with untreated disease as a measure of increasing cancer volume. *Cancer* 1993;71: 2031–2040.
96. Brawer MK, Beatie J, Wener MH, et al. Screening for prostatic carcinoma with prostate specific antigen: results of the second year. *J Urol* 1993;150:106–109.
97. Brawer MK. How to use prostate-specific antigen in the early detection or screening for prostatic carcinoma. *CA Cancer J Clin* 1995;45:148–164.
98. Ito K, Kubota Y, Suzuki K, et al. Correlation of prostate-specific antigen before prostate cancer detection and clinicopathologic features: evaluation of mass screening populations. *Urology* 2000;55:705–709.
99. Porter JR, Hayward R, Brawer MK. The significance of short-term PSA change in men undergoing ultrasound-guided prostate biopsy. *J Urol* 1994;151(Suppl):293A.

100. Littrup PJ, Kane RA, Mettlin CJ, et al. Cost-effective prostate cancer detection. *Cancer* 1994;74:3146–3158.
101. Komatsu K, Wehner N, Prestigiacomo AF, et al. Variation of serum prostate specific antigen in 814 men from a screening population: Intra-individual assay variation is greater than the repeat assay variation. *J Urol* 1994;151(Suppl):401A.
102. Stamey T, Yang N, Hay AR, et al. Prostate-specific antigen as a serum marker for adenocarcinoma of the prostate. *N Engl J Med* 1987;317:909–916.
103. Habib GK, Bissas A, Neil WA, et al. Flow cytometric analysis of cellular DNA in human prostate cancer: Relationship to 5-alpha reductase activity of the tissue. *Urol Res* 1989; 17:239.
104. Gormley GI, Stoner E, Bruskewitz RC, et al. The effects of finasteride in men with benign prostatic hyperplasia. *N Engl J Med* 1992;327:1185.
105. Benson M, Whang I, Pantuck A, et al. Prostate specific antigen density: a means of distinguishing benign prostatic hypertrophy and prostate cancer. *J Urol* 1992;147:815–816.
106. Benson M, Whang I, Olsson C, et al. The use of prostate-specific antigen density to enhance the predictive value of intermediate levels of serum prostate-specific antigen. *J Urol* 1992;147:817–821.
107. Kikuchi E, Nakashima J, Ishibashi M, et al. Prostate specific antigen adjusted for transition zone volume: the most powerful method for detecting prostate carcinoma. *Cancer* 2000;89:842–849.
108. Horninger W, Reissigl A, Klocker H, et al. Improvement of specificity in PSA-based screening by using PSA-transition zone density and percent free PSA in addition to total PSA levels. *Prostate* 1998;37:133–137.
109. McMurtry J, Keetch DW, Smith DS, et al. PSA density versus PSA slope as predictors of prostate cancer in patients with initially negative prostatic biopsies. *J Urol* 1994;151: 401A.
110. Myrtle JF, Klimley PG, Ivor LP, et al. Clinical utility of prostate-specific antigen (PSA) in the management of prostate cancer. In: *Advances in Cancer Diagnostics.* San Diego: Hybritech, 1986.
111. Oesterling JE, Jacobson SJ, Chute CG, et al. The establishment of age-specific reference ranges for prostate-specific antigen. *J Urol* 1993;149:510A.
112. Partin AW, Criley SR, Subong EN, et al. Standard versus age-specific prostate specific antigen reference ranges among men with clinically localized prostate cancer: a pathological analysis. *J Urol* 1996;155:1336–1339.
113. Borer JG, Sherman J, Solomon MC, et al. Age specific prostate specific antigen reference ranges: population specific. *J Urol* 1998;159:444–448.
114. Catalona WJ, Hudson MA, Scardino PT, et al. Selection of optimal prostate specific antigen cutoffs for early detection of prostate cancer: receiver operating characteristics curves. *J Urol* 1994;152:2037.
115. Reissigl A, Pointer J, Horninger W, et al. Comparison of different prostate-specific antigen cutpoints for early detection of prostate cancer: results of a large screening study. *Urology* 1995;46:662–665.
116. Pettaway J, Brawer MK. Age specific versus 4.0 ng/mL as a PSA cutoff in the screening population: impact on cancer detection. *J Urol* 1995;153:465A.
117. Dalkin BL, Ahmann FR, Kopp JB. Prostate specific antigen levels in men older than 50 years without clinical evidence of prostatic carcinoma. *J Urol* 1993;150:1837–1839.
118. Crawford ED, DeAntoni EP, Stone NN, et al. Prostate cancer awareness week demonstrates continued value to early detection strategies. *J Urol* 1995;153:312A.
119. Anderson JR, Strickland D, Corbin D, et al. Age specific reference ranges for serum prostate-specific antigen. *Urol* 1995;46:54–57.
120. Oesterling JE, Jacobsen SJ, Chute CG, et al. Serum prostate-specific antigen in a community-based population of healthy men: establishment of age-specific reference ranges. *JAMA* 1993;270:860–864.
121. Sung JC, Kabalin JN, Terris MK. Prostate cancer detection, characterization, and clinical outcomes in men aged 70 years and older referred for transrectal ultrasound and prostate biopsies. *Urology* 2000;56:295–301.
122. Colberg JW, Smith DS, Catalona WJ. Prevalence and pathologic extent of prostate cancer in men with prostate specific antigen levels of 2.9–4.0 ng/mL. *J Urol* 1993;149: 507.
123. Smith DS, Carvalhal GF, Mager DE, et al. Use of lower prostate specific antigen cutoffs for prostate cancer screening in black and white men. *J Urol* 1998;160:1734–1738.
124. McCormack RT, Rittenhouse HG, Finlay JA, et al. Molecular forms of prostate-specific antigen and the human kallikrein gene family. *Urology* 1995;45:729–744.
125. Christensson A, Laurell CB, Lilja H. Enzmatic activity of the prostate-specific antigen and its reactions with extracellular serine proteinase inhibitors. *Eur J Biochem* 1990;194: 755–763.
126. Stenman UH, Leinonen J, Alfthan H, et al. A complex between prostate-specific antigen and alpha-1 antichymotrypsin is the major form of prostate-specific antigen in serum of patients with prostatic cancer: Assay of the complex improves clinical sensitivity for cancer. *Cancer Res* 1991;51:222–226.
127. Christensson A, Bjork T, Bilsson O, et al. Serum prostate specific antigen complexed to alpha-1 antichymotrypsin as an indication of prostate cancer. *J Urol* 1993;150:100–105.
128. Luderer AA, Chen YT, Soriano TF, et al. Measurement of the proportion of free to total prostate specific antigen in the diagnostic gray zone of total prostate-specific antigen. *Urology* 1995;46:187–194.
129. Catalona WJ, Smith DS, Wolfert RL, et al. Evaluation of percentage of free serum prostate specific antigen to improve specificity of prostate cancer screening. *JAMA* 1995;274:1214–1220.
130. Catalona WJ, Partin AW, Slawin KM, et al. Use of percentage of free prostate-specific antigen to enhance differentiation of prostate cancer from benign prostatic disease: a prospective multicenter clinical trial. *JAMA* 1998;279: 1542–1547.
131. Catalona WJ, Partin AW, Slawin KM, et al. Percentage of free PSA in black versus white men for detection and staging of prostate cancer: a prospective multicenter clinical trial. *Urology* 2000;55:372–376.
132. Partin AW, Catalona WJ, Finlay JA, et al. Use of human glandular kallikrein 2 for the detection of prostate cancer: preliminary analysis. *Urology* 1999;54:839–845.

133. Becker C, Piironen T, Pettersson K, et al. Clinical value of human glandular kallikrein 2 and free and total prostate specific antigen in serum from a population of men with prostate specific antigen levels 3.0 ng/ml or greater. *Urology* 2000;55:694–699.
134. Becker C, Piironen T, Kiviniemi J, et al. Sensitivity and specific immunodetection of human glandular kallikrein 2 in serum. *Clin Chem* 2000;46:198–206.
135. Neal DE, Leung HY, Powell PH, et al. Unanswered questions in screening for prostate cancer. *Eur J Cancer* 2000;36:1316–1321.
136. Ross KS, Carter HB, Pearson JD, et al. Comparative efficiency of prostate-specific antigen screening strategies for prostate cancer detection. *JAMA* 2000;284:1399–1405.
137. Etzioni R, Cha R, Cowen ME. Serial prostate specific antigen screening for prostate cancer: a computer model evaluates competing strategies. *J Urol* 1999;162:741–748.
138. Catalona WJ, Southwick PC, Slawin KM, et al. Comparison of percent free PSA, PSA density, and age-specific PSA cutoffs for prostate cancer detection and staging. *Urology* 2000;56:255–260.
139. Finne P, Finne R, Auvinen A, et al. Predicting the outcome of prostate biopsy in screen-positive men by a multilayer perceptron network. *Urology* 2000;56:418–422.

15

SERUM TUMOR MARKERS IN PROSTATE CANCER

DANIEL W. LIN
ROBERT L. VESSELLA
PAUL H. LANGE

Serum tumor markers have a critical role in the evaluation and management of prostate cancer (CaP). One of the earliest tumor markers in oncology was acid phosphatase, described by Gutman and Gutman in 1938 (1). Subsequent development of methods for measuring unique acid phosphatase isoenzymes, such as prostatic acid phosphatase, increased the clinical use of this marker. However, for many reasons, there were too many false-positive and false-negative results, and the use of this marker became limited. Acid phosphatase has been all but replaced by another enzyme nearly exclusively produced by the prostate, namely *prostate-specific antigen* (PSA), which was first identified by Hara et al. (2) in 1971 in human seminal plasma and later described in prostate tissue in 1979 by Wang et al. (3). During the past 15 years, PSA has become indispensable in the management of CaP, and it is probably the best tumor marker in all of human oncology. Other tumor markers have recently shown promise in CaP and include prostate-specific membrane antigen, human glandular kallikrein 2 (hK2), and other more recently discovered novel proteins or proteases.

This chapter briefly describes (a) the principles and nomenclature of tumor markers; (b) the biology and clinical application of PSA, prostate-specific membrane antigen, hK2, and other markers; and (c) the future of tumor markers in CaP.

PRINCIPLES OF TUMOR MARKERS

The performance of tumor markers, in large part, is measured by the sensitivity, specificity, positive-predictive value, and negative-predictive value. *Sensitivity* is the percentage of the patients in the population being screened with the disease for whom the test is positive, whereas the *specificity* of a test is the percentage of patients in the population being screened without the disease for whom the test is negative. Ideally, the sensitivity and specificity would be very high; however, perhaps the most meaningful parameter in large-scale CaP tumor marker studies is the *positive-predictive value*—that is, the probability that the patient actually has the disease if the test is positive (4). The equations for these terms are given in Table 15-1.

CaP represents a particularly challenging case in tumor marker detection because of the high prevalence of the disease (and, thus, the denominator in calculations of sensitivity and specificity). It has been shown in postmortem studies that the prevalence of CaP increases with age, from approximately 25% in the third decade to 65% in the seventh decade of life (5). Nevertheless, most of these lesions are innocuous or so-called "autopsy cancer" and should not or cannot be detected clinically because they are so small. Moreover, if a tumor marker identified all CaP as soon as it developed, an undesirable situation would arise, as clearly not all these cancers need to be treated. Operationally, almost all studies in CaP tumor markers define patients with CaP as those who have a positive biopsy result and patients without the disease as those who have a negative biopsy result or who do not appear to have the disease on digital rectal examination (DRE) or serum PSA determination.

Although the ideal tumor marker would be produced exclusively by a specific malignancy 100% sensitive in its detection and 100% specific for that disease, other characteristics realistically are desirable. These other marker attributes would include fast, inexpensive, and reproducible results. Additionally, the marker's measurable extent or intensity would be detectable at early stages of disease and would increase linearly with tumor volume, thereby allowing for direct correlation with the disease course and offering prognostic information, as well as vital surveillance data. Finally, the ideal tumor marker would have a relatively short half-life, so that therapeutic intervention could be assessed accurately and quickly (6). Obviously, the ideal tumor marker is not yet available in CaP, but PSA and the

TABLE 15-1. EQUATIONS FOR SENSITIVITY, SPECIFICITY, POSITIVE AND NEGATIVE PREDICTIVE VALUES, AND OVERALL ACCURACY

Test outcome	Disease-present	Disease-absent
Positive	a	b
Negative	c	d
Total	(a + c)	(b + d)

Sensitivity $= \frac{a}{a + c}$

Specificity $= \frac{d}{b + d}$

Positive-predictive value $= \frac{a}{a + b}$

Negative-predictive value $= \frac{d}{d + c}$

Overall accuracy $= \frac{a + d}{a + b + c + d}$

other exciting markers are pushing the envelope toward that ideal.

PROSTATE-SPECIFIC ANTIGEN

Since its discovery, a great deal of information has been accumulated about the biology and biochemistry of PSA. It is known to be a 6-kilobase gene product of chromosome 19 with an overall molecular weight of 34,000 (3,7). The PSA gene and protein structure are similar to those of other kallikriens, most notably an 82% amino acid homology with hK2, which is a substance also preferentially located in prostate tissue (8). However, unlike the glandular kallikreins, which are trypsinlike proteases, the enzymatic activity of PSA is chymotrypsinlike, such that it slowly hydrolyzes peptide bonds behind certain tyrosines and leucine residues. Also, like most enzymes, it is known that PSA has a precursor form (or zymogen) whose exact identity is still unknown; hK2 has been shown *in vitro* to be critical in the process of activating proPSA to active PSA (9) (see Human Glandular Kallikrein 2).

Extensive knowledge of both the synthesis and physiologic properties of PSA has been gathered in the last decade. The PSA gene is an androgen-regulated gene, as evidenced by the androgen-responsive element in the promoter region (10). Synthesized in the epithelial cells, PSA is secreted into the lumen of prostate ducts and is present in high concentrations in the seminal plasma. PSA may reach the serum by diffusion from luminal cells through the epithelial basement membrane and prostatic stroma, in which it can pass through the capillary basement membrane or "leak" into the lymphatics or bloodstream. PSA enzymatically cleaves the major sperm-trapping gel proteins, semenogelin I and II and fibronectin, thereby liquifying the seminal coagulum and releasing the spermatozoa (11).

Histologically, early work assumed that PSA was produced exclusively by prostate tissue; however, it is now known that PSA, although predominantly in prostatic tissue, is also produced, albeit in small amounts, by a variety of other tissues. Immunohistochemical studies have shown that PSA is present in normal and hyperplastic benign prostate tissue and in primary and metastatic CaP. It appears that the concentration of PSA within the cells is greatest in the normal prostate, less in benign prostatic hyperplasia (BPH), and significantly reduced in CaP; also, it is apparently inversely proportional to histologic grade (12). PSA has also been shown to be produced by periurethral glands and probably other glands of cloacal origin, including residual glands in women. Additionally, PSA seems to be produced in certain conditions by other tissues in very small amounts, most notably in breast cancers and, recently, in breast milk (13). PSA in nonprostatic tissues may reflect end-organ responses to circulating steroids, based on the discovery of androgen-responsive elements in the PSA gene promoter regions and glandular tissues, in which PSA has been found (14,15). To date, production of PSA by nonprostatic sources has not been reported to interfere with its value as a serum tumor marker; thus, for clinical and practical purposes, PSA can be considered to be histologically exclusive to the prostate.

Like other serine proteases, serum PSA exists mostly in the complexed and inactive form; however, a smaller fraction remains in a "free" but inactivated form. The two major complexing proteins are alpha-2 macroglobulin and alpha-1 antichymotrypsin. Alpha-2 macroglobulin engulfs epitopes on the PSA molecule and has not been considered in total PSA measurements, although an assay has recently been developed to measure PSA alpha-2 macroglobulin complex (16). It has been speculated that approximately 40% of PSA is bound to alpha-2 macroglobulin. The remaining PSA is either bound to alpha-1 antichymotrypsin or exists in a free form. Given the higher serum concentrations of alpha-2 macroglobulin and alpha-1 antichymotrypsin (greater than 1,000 times in excess compared with PSA in serum) and the presence of a free or unbound PSA, it has been postulated that this free or unbound PSA may represent the zymogen or "nicked" form, or a combination of forms yet unidentified (17,18). Because the complex with alpha-1 antichymotrypsin still allows PSA to expose a limited number of antigenic sites, both the complexed and free form are measurable in commercial assays (see Prostate-Specific Antigen Immunoassays).

The clinical characteristics of PSA have also been subject of exhaustive research. The half-life of PSA in serum has been reported to be between 2.2 and 3.2 days (19,20), with clearance after first-order kinetics; thus, the serum concentrations of total PSA may take several weeks to return to baseline levels after certain procedures, such as radical prostatectomy. The definition of the normal reference range (0.1 to 4.0 ng per mL) for PSA is somewhat arbitrary, given that all healthy men have some detectable level of PSA in their serum. Furthermore, BPH exists to a varying degree in all aging men, and CaP is found in up to 40% of older men, although often unrecognized. Subsequent studies have shown that PSA may be minimally elevated (4 to 10 ng per mL) in up to 20% of patients with BPH. Additionally, elevated PSA levels are seen in patients with other nonmalignant pertubations of the prostate, including prostatitis, and, temporarily, in patients undergoing cystoscopy or needle biopsies of the prostate. It has been reported that PSA changes with ambulatory status (20) and also that it may temporarily change after ejaculation (21). Although studies have found no diurnal variation (22–24), there is some physiologic variation, as reported by Prestigiacomo and Stamey, that requires further study but is probably not more than 20% to 30% (25).

Prostate-Specific Antigen Immunoassays

In 1986, the U.S. Food and Drug Administration approved the first commercial immunoassay (Hybritech) for PSA as an aid in the clinical management of patients with CaP. Since then, dozens of other commercial and research immunoassays have been developed—initially, to total PSA, and more recently, to the free PSA component. The number of assays for the quantitation of PSA serum levels is by order of magnitude, greater than for any other cancer marker. The types of assays now available range from very highly sophisticated assay designs that are run on automated random access immunoassay systems to very simplistic assays suitable for the small "on-site" medical practice office.

An aspect of PSA immunoassay design that has received considerable attention in the past several years is one of standardization. Stamey and colleagues were the first to advocate the standardization of PSA immunoassays and, subsequently, convened scientific forums to discuss approaches and solutions (26–28). PSA immunoassay standardization was considered critical, because differences in assay design and reagents had shown that not all of the commercial immunoassays were reporting similar PSA values in comparison studies of patient serum. This finding was attributed, in part, to the fact that some assays were not equimolar with regard to quantitating accurate levels of total PSA when there existed significant variability of the free PSA component (29). One solution was to design future immunoassays using monoclonal antibody reagents, with those designs tested for equimolarity and for current immunoassays to adapt a reference standard consisting of 90% PSA complexed with alpha-1 antichymotrypsin, 10% free PSA, which is often referred to as the *Stamey 90:10* standard (27). To the credit of all participants in these forums, great strides have been made by most of the manufacturers in the last 2 to 3 years in taking steps toward PSA assay standardization.

Another issue of interest has been the discussion on the use of ultrasensitive PSA assays—that is, those having the ability to accurately report total PSA levels below 0.1 ng per mL. The first of the commercial assays with this level of performance was the Abbott IMx PSA assay (30), but many others have followed in recent years. It would not be difficult to find commercial immunoassays with significant accuracy at or approaching the 0.01 ng per mL level and research assays up to an order of magnitude below that level. The use of such low levels of detection is limited to the posttreatment monitoring of patients for biochemical recurrence. Data from a few laboratories, including our own, have repeatedly demonstrated that one can obtain 1 to 3 years of lead time in predicting a clinical recurrence by monitoring PSA levels with ultrasensitive assays, with detection limits below 0.01 ng per mL (17). However, the debate remains as to how to use this information in the management of the patient.

A final comment is warranted on the potential artifact of high PSA levels attributed to what is referred to as the *human antimouse antibody* (HAMA) effect. It is well recognized that in patient sera, the presence of heterophile and multispecificity antibodies has the potential to interfere with immunoassays in general (31,32). Over the past several years, we have been presented with a small number of patients who have elevated PSA levels on either diagnostic workup or during monitoring posttherapy of an undefined nature. In a high proportion of these undefined PSA elevations, an analysis of the patient's serum revealed a detectable level of host antibodies that would bind to mouse antibodies (i.e., the HAMA effect). Because many of the commercial immunoassays use a pair of mouse monoclonal antibodies for the detection of the antigen (e.g., PSA) in a sandwichlike design, host antibodies that are reactive to these mouse antibodies form a cross-linked "sandwich," even in the absence of the antigen for which the assay is designed. Accordingly, the assay reports an elevation that is false. One manner in which this can be partly ascertained is to ask the reference laboratory performing the PSA test to run another marker test (e.g., carcinoembryonic antigen), using an identical assay design from that manufacturer. If this irrelevant marker is also elevated, the possibility of a HAMA effect should be considered, and the assay manufacturer's tech support unit contacted for advice. In recognition of this potential problem, some manufacturers are taking steps to block HAMA reactivity in their assays, but this practice is not universal. The reasons why some individuals have HAMA are often difficult to define, but we have seen this associated with farmers, pet mouse owners, and patients who have been involved in research clinical trials that used mouse monoclonal antibodies *in vivo*. However, we should emphasize that this phenomenon is rare; most "unexplained" PSA elevations are from "natural" causes (e.g., BPH or CaP).

Prostate-Specific Antigen in Diagnosis and Screening

Undoubtedly, PSA has made the most impact in its ability to diagnose CaP and in its use as a screening tool (33). As previously stated, false-positive tests are common in a screened population, because approximately 20% of patients with clinically localized CaP have PSA levels below 4 ng per mL within what is now considered the normal PSA range (34). Despite the fact that PSA is not cancer specific, the positive-predictive value for CaP in otherwise asymptomatic men is approximately 30%. Results have been promising using PSA alone, as well as in using PSA combined with DRE for diagnosis in screened and unscreened populations. More important, it would appear that more organ-confined, and presumably curable, cancers are diagnosed with either PSA alone or PSA and DRE than if DRE were used alone. Catalona and associates (35) found in their screening trials that if cancer was detected on initial screening, then the tumor was pathologically organ confined in approximately 65% of patients, and if it was detected on serial evaluation, then the organ-confined rates increased to 75%, which is significantly better than the approximately 50% or less that are organ confined when screening is performed with DRE alone. Also, most of the 25% that were not organ confined had only capsular penetration, and evidence would suggest that many of these are cured by surgery alone. Furthermore, evidence is mounting that cancers detected by these modern diagnostic techniques (i.e., PSA with or without DRE initially, and transrectal ultrasound with biopsy, if abnormal) are what would be defined as *significant* cancers, or greater than 0.5 cc, as defined by Epstein (36) and Stamey (37). Using this definition, reportedly 75% to 85% of tumors found in large screening studies are significant (38,39).

Because of the significant number of false-positives resulting from the overlap in concentration of serum PSA between men with BPH and men with CaP, especially in the low abnormal range of 4 to 10 ng per mL, multiple modifications have been made to enhance the specificity of PSA testing. These modifications include age-specific PSA (40), race-specific PSA, PSA density (41), PSA velocity (42), transition-zone PSA density (43), and PSA isoforms (44,45). Although there have been multiple reports challenging the use of these modifications in their ability to perform better than PSA alone, PSA isoforms seem to have withstood many challenges and have particular usefulness in management of biopsy-negative patients with elevated PSA, especially in the range of 4 to 10 ng per mL. A complete discussion of PSA in screening and diagnosis is explored in detail in Chapter 14.

Prostate-Specific Antigen in Staging

Before the PSA era, numerous studies evaluated the efficacy of staging CaP patients for extraprostatic spread and pelvic lymph node involvement by using pedal lymphangiography, computed tomographic scanning, and magnetic resonance imaging. In general, these staging studies have failed to differentiate local from extraprostatic disease and do not detect approximately 50% of pelvic lymph node metastases (46) with both high false-negative and false-positive results. For this reason, most investigators do not recommend these studies as part of routine staging evaluations in newly diagnosed CaP.

With the advent of PSA, an additional preoperative parameter is available for staging in CaP. In CaP series, serum PSA levels have been shown to correlate well with increasing clinical stage, tumor volume, DNA ploidy, and pathologic stage (20,47–50). Significantly increased PSA concentrations are seen with advancing stage of the disease; however, there is tremendous overlap in PSA levels between stages of disease that precludes the use of PSA alone for preoperative staging. Several series have shown that 70% to 80% of men with serum PSA concentrations lower than 4 ng per mL have organ-confined disease, 50% of those with levels higher than 10 ng per mL have extracapsular extension, and most men with levels higher than 50 ng per mL have positive lymph nodes at surgery (51).

The reasons for the inaccuracy of PSA alone to predict stage of disease are severalfold. PSA is produced by prostate epithelial cells, as previously stated, but the ratio of stromal to epithelial PSA in BPH can vary by as much as threefold, thereby leading to false-positive elevations in PSA. Furthermore, the perturbations of the basement membrane (and, therefore, presumably of the propensity to "leak" PSA) can occur with inflammation and possibly with prostatic intraepithelial neoplasia. Last, in CaP, the decreasing concentration of cellular PSA with increasing grade combines with the increasing volume (and presumably increasing "leak") to influence serum PSA levels in unpredictable ways (47).

Recent reports have combined PSA with other preoperative variables, such as tumor grade and clinical stage, considerably enhancing its ability to predict the probability of metastatic or locally advanced disease (49,52–54). Despite the usefulness of this combination of preoperative variables, multivariate analysis has shown that PSA is the strongest predictor. Probability tables and nomograms based on the parameters of preoperative clinical stage, serum PSA level, and Gleason grade have been generated from data on large numbers of men who have undergone radical prostatectomy. One such nomogram is illustrated in Figure 15-1. In this nomogram, with a preoperative serum PSA level of 4 ng per mL, there is a 73% predicted probability that the tumor will be organ confined if the clinical stage is T1, T2a, or T2b and the grade is low, but only a 23% probability if the grade is high or the clinical stage is T3. Similar nomograms and tables have been constructed to predict the probability of lymph nodal metastasis, information often used to decide whether it is worthwhile to perform a pelvic lymphadenectomy (55,56).

Combinations of PSA and other preoperative parameters are being used, perhaps more frequently, to provide probabilities that can be used to advise patients to pursue definitive treatment for their CaP (surgery vs. radiotherapy) or to pursue a "watch and wait" strategy. For example, Epstein and colleagues (36) defined *insignificant disease* as

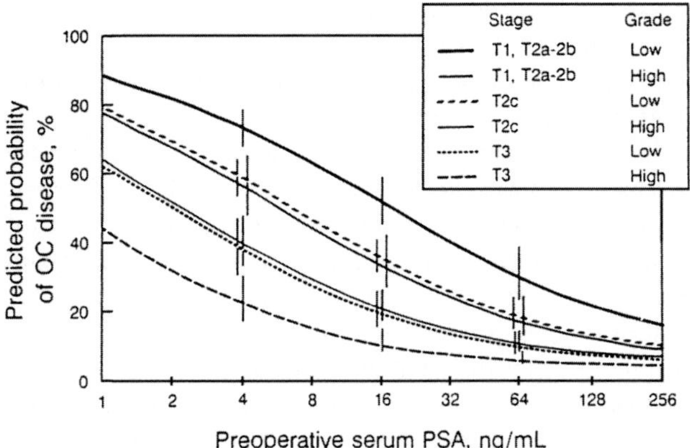

FIGURE 15-1. Predicted probability of organ-confined (OC) disease as a function of preoperative prostate-specific antigen (PSA) (ng per mL), clinical stage, and clinical grade. Ninety-five percent confidence intervals are included for PSA values of 4, 16, and 64 ng per mL. Low grade includes clinical grades 1 and 2. High grade includes clinical grades 3 and 4. (From Kleer E, Larson-Keller JJ, Zincke H, et al. Ability of preoperative serum prostate-specific antigen value to predict pathological stage and DNA ploidy: influence of clinical stage and tumor grade. *Urology* 1993;41:207–216, with permission.)

the presence of less than 0.5 cc of organ-confined cancer in a radical prostatectomy specimen and determined those preoperative parameters that best predicted this cancer. They found that the best combination of preoperative variables for predicting insignificant cancer was as follows: a PSAD lower than 0.1, biopsies with fewer than three cores involved with cancer and no more than 50% of any one core involved, and no cores with Gleason grade greater than 4 or 5. In the retrospective experience of these authors, men who fulfill these preoperative criteria have a 65% chance of having insignificant cancer in the radical prostatectomy specimen, and those who do not meet these criteria have a 92% chance that the cancer is significant.

Prostate-Specific Antigen after Radical Prostatectomy

Theoretically, serum PSA should be undetectable after radical prostatectomy, because the curative intent of such surgery is to remove all the prostatic tissue (including normal, BPH, and adenocarcinoma). Therefore, men with recurrent disease, either local or systemic, will have a detectable serum PSA level. There are rare reports of local recurrences after radical prostatectomy with undetectable serum PSA (57,58), but these are so uncommon that this phenomenon is of little consequence.

Determination of the lower detection limit of serum PSA is still an evolving field surrounded by much controversy and complexity, as mentioned in this chapter and elsewhere (17). Here, it is sufficient to state that the clinical cancer detection limit for the most popular PSA assays (Hybritech Tandem-R or Abbott IMx PSA assay) is between 0.1 and 0.2 ng per mL. Using these detection limits, many studies have shown that a persistently elevated or rising PSA level is a reliable and almost invariable sign of persistent or recurrent disease after radical prostatectomy. Importantly, this sign usually occurs months to years before clinical signs of recurrence (59).

Clearly, the probability tables and nomograms for staging using preoperative PSA and other parameters are clinically useful, but the need for improvement is evident. In the diagnostic "gray" zone of 4 to 10 ng per mL, the confidence intervals are still quite wide. Additional data need to be accumulated incorporating other parameters, including those parameters that are already well known, such as DNA ploidy and biopsy volume of cancer. Perhaps more promising is the wealth of parameters newly discovered from the basic science laboratory, such as prostase (60), p21 (61), and angiogenesis (62). The complexity in using all of these parameters certainly is daunting; however, efforts are already under way on several fronts to conquer the challenges of staging CaP through artificial neural networking (63–65).

Most large radical prostatectomy series are now using postradical prostatectomy PSA levels as a surrogate end point for clinical outcome. In general, approximately 25% to 40% of men will have PSA elevations after surgery (66–68). Partin and associates (69) reported a 13% and 23% progression-free likelihood at 5 and 10 years postradical prostatectomy, respectively, when defining progression as an elevated serum PSA only. Stein and colleagues reported that the overall freedom from PSA relapse at 5 and 10 years was 71% and 61%, respectively (70). The Johns Hopkins data were updated, reporting on 1,997 men with a median follow-up of 5.3 years, reporting a 15% biochemical recurrence (59). Moreover, approximately 30% to 50% of men with elevated PSA after radical prostatectomy have cancer in biopsies of the prostatic fossa, even though the DRE results are normal (71). This finding has led many to recommend PSA alone in follow-up after radical prostatectomy instead of PSA plus DRE (72,73).

The pattern of PSA elevation after radical prostatectomy, together with other pathologic parameters, has significance with regard to the site of recurrence and the rate of progression. Several studies have investigated the significance of a detectable serum PSA level within one year of radical prostatectomy, reporting 60% to 100% progression rates in this population regardless of nadir PSA levels (48,69,70). Usually, if the PSA level does not return to an undetectable level after surgery, then systemic recurrence (with or without local recurrence) is likely. Among those patients whose PSA falls to undetectable levels after surgery, the rate of rise (PSA velocity) or the PSA doubling time (PSADT) has clinical significance. Pound and colleagues (59) most recently reported on 315 men with biochemical recurrence after radical prostatectomy and followed them for clinical evidence of progression. They found that time to biochemical failure (fewer than 2 years vs. more than 2 years) after radical prostatectomy and PSADT (fewer than

10 months vs. more than 10 months) were independent parameters affecting metastasis-free survival. Men with rapid PSA elevations (fewer than 2 years), a Gleason score of 5 to 7, and a PSADT higher than 10 months demonstrated a 76% probability of remaining free of metastatic disease for 5 years after initial PSA elevation, compared to men with a shorter PSADT (fewer than 10 months) who had only a 35% chance of remaining free of metastatic disease for 5 years after biochemical failure. This confirms earlier work by Patel and associates (74), who suggested that PSADT is a useful predictor of the type of eventual recurrence after radical prostatectomy, reporting that shorter PSADTs (fewer than 6 months) were more indicative of distant disease when compared with local recurrence.

The value of adjuvant radiation therapy either immediately after radical prostatectomy or at the time of PSA recurrence cannot be definitively proven until randomized studies are complete; however, multiple studies have yielded preliminary data (75–78). In general, most men with elevated PSA after radical prostatectomy experience a decrease in their PSA levels with adjuvant radiotherapy and, in approximately 50%, the PSA levels may become undetectable. However, the durability of such response is usually very low and is related to the pattern of PSA relapse and site of recurrence. Men whose PSA values never reach undetectable levels postradical prostatectomy, or whose PSADT is very high, rarely have durable suppression and probably should not receive adjuvant radiation, whereas patients with slow PSADT may benefit from adjuvant radiotherapy. For example, in the Johns Hopkins series, there was a 10% response to radiation therapy (undetectable serum PSA for more than 2 years) for men with isolated elevations of PSA and a 29% response for those with documented local recurrence (and presumably slow PSADT) (69).

The significance of PSA levels after radical prostatectomy has prompted the development of more sensitive PSA assays. These assays will not only detect recurrence earlier, but also shorten the time to cure—that is, the time after which, if PSA remains normal, the patient can be reassured that he is cured. Indeed, several investigators have already shown that these more sensitive PSA assays can reveal clinically useful information (79,80). Of course, with increasing sensitivity often comes decreased specificity and the concern that elevated PSA levels could result from factors other than persistent disease, such as cross-reacting substances, very small normal prostate remnants, or periurethral glands that make PSA and secrete it into the urethral lumen (81). These issues are addressed in this chapter.

Prostate-Specific Antigen after Primary Radiotherapy

The changes in serum PSA levels during and after radiotherapy have been the subject of increasing scrutiny. During radiotherapy, PSA levels often rise, presumably as a result of cellular damage, inflammation, and disruption of the basement membrane with resultant release of PSA into the circulation (82). Zagars and associates (83) reported a mean increase above the baseline of 2.2 ng per mL in 82% of men during radiation therapy; however, they stated that this modest increase in PSA should not be misinterpreted for disease progression. Most radiotherapists do not routinely obtain PSA determinations during the course of radiation treatments.

Several studies have investigated the rate of decline in serum PSA after radiation treatments (84–87). Although the serum half-life of PSA after radical prostatectomy has been calculated to be approximately 2 to 3 days (20,88), it has been reported to be between 1.9 and 4.2 months by multiple groups (85–87,89). Currently, the best estimate for mean PSA half-life after radiation treatments is 2 months (85). The factors that influence this rate of decline include pretherapy serum PSA value, tumor volume, volume of normal prostate, degree of differentiation, dose and delivery of therapy, and the effect of radiation dose on the testes and androgen production (51,85). The time to PSA nadir has been variably reported in the literature. Few studies demonstrate continued decreases in postradiation PSA beyond 12 months (90). The M. D. Anderson group suggested that approximately 95% of men have a significant decline in serum PSA, and, in approximately 80%, the PSA levels fall to normal range by 6 months (85). Stamey and colleagues (91) reported that only 8% of men continued to show decline in serum PSA after one year. The data from these investigations predict that serum PSA values will be undetectable in 10% to 30% of men, and they will stabilize at levels below normal in 40% to 70% at 3 years postradiation (51).

The PSA level necessary to prove disease-free states and the definition of PSA failure after radiation therapy have been controversial subjects. A consensus meeting sponsored by the American Society of Therapeutic Radiation Oncology recommended that, pending further research on PSA, recurrence after radiation therapy be defined as three consecutive rises above the nadir level with follow-up every 6 months (92). An absolute nadir PSA level, although recognized as a prognostic factor, was not defined. PSA nadirs have been reported between 0.5 ng per mL (93,94) and not more than 4.0 ng per mL. One report from Massachusetts General Hospital reported that after a median of 4-year follow-up, a nadir of less than or equal to 0.5 ng per mL was associated with a 93% freedom of PSA failure, a nadir of 0.6 to 1.0 ng per mL with 41%, and a nadir of greater than 1 ng per mL with 37% (94). Another recent report revealed similar results with respect to PSA nadir (95).

Given these data on PSA nadir and biochemical failure, the pretreatment PSA level becomes an important issue. Shipley and colleagues (95) recently reported on 1,765 men with stage T1b, T1c, and T2 tumors in a multiinstitutional pooled analysis of biochemical failure after external beam radiation therapy alone. Estimated rates of freedom from PSA failure, using the current American Society of Therapeutic Radiation Oncology definition, were 81% for patients with pretreatment PSA of less than 10 ng per mL, 68% for 10 to 20 ng per mL, 51% for 20 to 30 ng per mL, and 31% for those greater than 30 ng per mL. The mean follow-up on these patients was only 5 years; extended follow-up is needed to evaluate the durability of the results. Additionally, only 44% of the men in this study reached a nadir PSA of less than 0.5 ng per mL, 26% reached 0.5 to 0.9 ng per mL, 17% at 1.0 to 1.9 ng per mL, and 13% greater than 2 ng per mL. Given the relative minority of patients who are in the pretreatment (PSA level) and posttreatment (PSA nadir) subset to derive lasting benefit from radiation monotherapy, as measured by PSA nadirs, other strategies are being investigated using combination and conformal therapy (90).

The question remains What is the source or sources of detectable PSA after radiation treatment? Presumably, sources would include radio-resistant CaPs, *de novo* growth of new tumors, BPH or normal prostates, or metastatic diseases at the time of radiation treatment. Grob et al. (96) performed *in situ* immunohistochemistry for PSA on biopsy specimens 12 months after radiation treatment and found that benign glands did not stain for PSA, and only glands histologically consistent with CaP displayed PSA staining. This finding is tempered by the rarely reported positive prostate biopsy after radiation treatment in the setting of an undetectable PSA (97). Regardless of the source of detectable PSA after radiotherapy, a rising level portends poor prognosis, as evidenced by several studies (98). The ultimate percentage of durable undetectable levels of PSA after radiotherapy is reported to be between 20% and 60%, with one study reporting, at best, 10% undetectable levels at the 10-year follow-up (99).

Prostate-Specific Antigen after Androgen Ablation

Because the production and secretion of PSA are androgen-dependent, serum PSA levels have been used as surrogate markers for the efficacy of androgen-ablation therapy. Contrary to radiotherapy, which primarily affects only the dividing cell population (i.e., the CaP cells), androgen-ablation therapy is proposed to affect all the prostatic epithelial cells and, thus, all the PSA-producing cells. However, CaP is a heterogeneous population of androgen-dependent, as well as androgen-independent, cells. Consequently, a low or even undetectable PSA level does not necessarily indicate cure or significant destruction of cells (100).

Most studies have observed a rapid decline of serum PSA after androgen-deprivation therapy, sometimes to undetectable levels within the first 6 months of therapy (101,102). One study demonstrated a decrease in serum PSA levels greater than 80% within the first month after initiation of androgen ablation (103). In one large series, 55%, 32%, and 13% of patients reached their PSA nadir within 3 and 6 months and after 6 months, respectively (104). However, ongoing studies address how the degree of PSA response, absolute PSA nadir, and durability of response affect outcome.

There have been several studies investigating the prognostic value in both the slope of PSA response and nadir value in serum PSA after androgen-ablation therapy. Stamey and associates (101) reported that, despite the dramatic initial decrease in PSA after androgen deprivation among virtually all patients, after 2 years, only 9% of patients still had undetectable serum PSA levels, and 22% were within normal limits, but 72% (many of whom had excellent PSA responses during the first 6 months) had rising PSA levels within the second 6 months of therapy. Others have shown that a PSA decline greater than 50% during the first month of therapy and maintenance of a normal level of PSA at 6 months or a decline to below normal levels within the first 6 months of therapy predicted a favorable response or stable disease versus progression among men with stage D2 CaP (101,102). Another study by Miller and colleagues (105) reported longer survival (mean, 42 months) if the nadir PSA was lower than 4 ng per mL than if the nadir did not reach 4 ng per mL (mean, 10 months). Presumably, these rises in PSA are reflective of androgen-insensitive CaP.

Similarly, PSA levels are now being used as response criteria for many experimental trials in hormone-refractory cancer (106), although the relationship between PSA levels and symptoms is not always linear (100). Myers and colleagues (107) at the National Cancer Institute reported that after suramin treatment, a 75% decrease from baseline PSA was indicative of a significantly better survival than for patients who did not have a similar decrease. Hudes and colleagues (108) also reported that declines of greater than 50% of baseline had increased survival when patients were treated with a combination of estramustine and vinblastine sulfate. More recently, Pienta and associates (109) analyzed the PSA response in 42 patients with hormone-refractory CaP undergoing chemotherapy with etoposide and estramustine. Seventy-five percent of patients who showed a greater than 50% decline in baseline PSA had soft tissue disease response or improved bone scans. A study from Memorial Sloan Kettering Cancer Center also used multivariate analysis, showing that a greater than 50% decline in PSA and the natural log of lactate dehydrogenase were the most significant variables that predicted survival in a data set from 110 patients enrolled in seven different treatment programs with various cytotoxic agents used alone or in combination (110) (Fig. 15-2). Although there have been other studies that do not show significant similar prognostic information with regards to PSA response (111), PSA is still the most clinically available tool for predicting response in patients receiving chemotherapy. Trials are under way to prove definitively the value of PSA as a surrogate end point for survival.

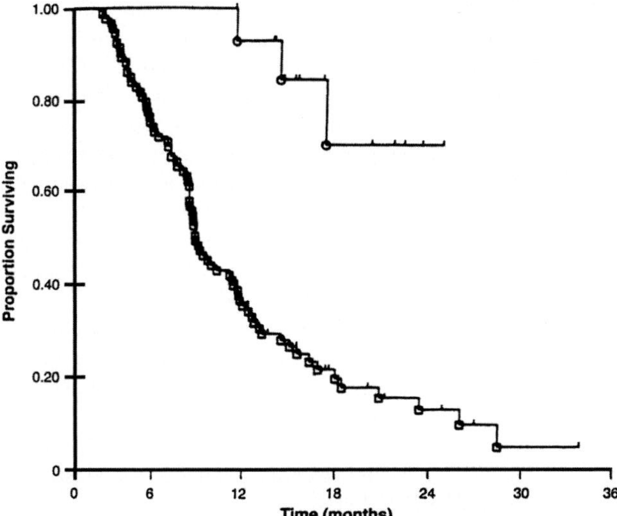

FIGURE 15-2. Overall survival for patients with greater than 50% decline in prostate-specific antigen (PSA) (*open circles*) versus less than 50% decline in PSA from baseline. (From Kelly WK, Scher HI, Mazumdar M, et al. Prostate-specific antigen as a measure of disease outcome in metastatic hormone-refractory prostate cancer. *J Clin Oncol* 1993;11:607–615, with permission.)

HUMAN GLANDULAR KALLIKREIN 2

hK2 is a member of the human tissue kallikrien gene family, which also includes pancreatic or renal kallikrein and PSA (hK3). hK2 and PSA possess approximately 80% homology (112) and can be found in high concentrations and almost exclusively in prostatic tissue (113). However, whereas PSA is generally expressed less in poorly differentiated prostate tumors than in well-differentiated tumors or benign tissue, hK2 appears to be expressed the highest in poorly differentiated CaP cells, suggesting that hK2 may be more tumor associated than PSA (113). Furthermore, both PSA and hK2 exist in different molecular forms ("pro," "free," and "complexed" forms) and contain androgen-responsive elements in their gene promoter regions (114).

Despite their structural similarity, PSA and hK2 differ in their proposed enzymatic function and physiologic roles. PSA has chymotrypsinlike activity, whereas hK2 has trypsinlike specificity. It has been found that hK2 can autoactivate by cleaving pro-hK2 to hK2 (115). More important, several investigators have found that hK2 activates pro-PSA to active PSA *in vitro* (9,116,117). This active PSA can then be complexed to alpha-1 antichymotrypsin, alpha-2 macroglobulin, and other protease inhibitors. Last, hK2 has been shown to activate the zymogen form of urokinase-type plasminogen activator *in vitro* (9,118). Urokinase-type plasminogen activator has been associated with cancer aggressiveness specifically in CaP, suggesting another role of hK2 in CaP biology (119,120).

Several recent studies have evaluated the use of hK2 as a tumor marker for CaP separately or in combination with various forms of PSA (free vs. total). Higher hK2 to free PSA ratios and hK2 to total PSA ratios have also been shown in higher-grade disease (121,122). In one published study, hK2 was detectable in 90 patients with PSA levels between 4 and 10 ng per mL. The hK2 to free PSA ratio had a better specificity without loss of sensitivity for CaP than total PSA or the free PSA to total PSA ratio within the range of PSA 4 to 10 ng per mL, suggesting that hK2 in combination with free PSA may offer a new diagnostic means for CaP detection (121). Further studies are now under way to investigate the use of reverse transcriptase-polymerase chain reactions for hK2 in staging and prognosis (123,124). As new assays for this interesting protein become available, more large-scale clinical trials will certainly shed light on the use of hK2, the molecular forms of hK2, and various combinations of hK2 and PSA in early detection, staging, and monitoring of patients with CaP.

PROSTATE-SPECIFIC MEMBRANE ANTIGEN

An antibody, designated 7E11-C5.3, to the then-unknown PSMA protein was derived by Horoszewicz et al. (125,126) from the immunization of mice with a membrane preparation of the CaP cell line LNCaP. Subsequently, investigation at the messenger RNA (mRNA) level revealed that PSMA mRNA undergoes alternative splicing, resulting in a 266 base pair deletion near the 5' end of the molecule (127). This truncated form was referred to as PSMA'. Then, 9 years after generation of the 7E11-C5.3 antibody, Carter et al. (128) identified the PSMA protein as an N-acetylated alpha-linked acidic dipeptidase. By a variety of analytic methods, there have been preliminary data suggesting that the PSMA protein is often associated with more aggressive disease, but clearly more studies are necessary. Several studies have demonstrated that the detection of PSMA mRNA by reverse transcriptase-polymerase chain reactions in the blood and lymph nodes correlates with the presence of putative CaP cells that have escaped the confines of the prostate (129–131). Unfortunately, detection of the PSMA protein in the blood as a marker for CaP has been a difficult task that remains under intense investigation.

FUTURE TUMOR MARKERS

Much of the recent progress in CaP research involves the identification of novel genes and their cognate proteins. One promising technology involves the use of complementary DNA microarrays to measure relative expression of thousands of different genes in tissue samples. These microarrays have already been widely used to measure gene expression in other systems (132,133). One novel serine protease, prostase, has been recently discovered after constructing prostate complementary DNA libraries and analysis by expressed sequence tags (60). Further analysis has shown that prostase is prostate specific and androgen regulated. Additionally, prostase shares 35% amino acid homology with PSA and 78% homology with porcine enamel matrix serine proteinase 1, an enzyme involved in the disruption of intracellular junctions and degradation of enamel matrix proteins. The homology between prostase and enamel matrix serine proteinase 1 is intriguing in view of the high propensity of prostate carcinoma to metastasize to bone (60).

As the molecular revolution continues to blossom, we can only expect to discover many more prostate-specific or "preferential" genes and proteins. It is likely that some of these will be clinically important serum markers for CaP (134).

REFERENCES

1. Gutman AB, Gutman EB. "Acid" phosphatase occurring in serum of patients with metastasizing carcinoma of prostate gland. *J Clin Invest* 1938;17:473.
2. Hara M, Koyanagi Y, Inoue Y, et al. Some physico-chemical characteristics of gamma-seminoprotein, an antigenic component specific for human seminal plasma: forensic immunological study of body fluids and secretion, VII [in Japanese]. *Nipon Hoigaku Zasshi* 1971;25:322.
3. Wang M, Valenzuela L, Murphy G, et al. Purification of human prostate specific antigen. *Invest Urol* 1979;17:159.
4. Cooner WH. Definition of the ideal tumor marker. *Urol Clin North Am* 1993;20:575.
5. Sakr WA, Haas GP, Cassin BJ, et al. The frequency of carcinoma and intraepithelial neoplasia of the prostate in young males. *J Urol* 1993;150:379.
6. Montie JE, Meyers SE. Defining the ideal tumor marker for prostate cancer. *Urol Clin North Amer* 1997;24:247.
7. Lundwall A, Lilja H. Molecular cloning of human prostate-specific antigen cDNA. *FEBS Lett* 1987;214:317.
8. Schedlich LJ, Bennets BH, Morris BJ. Primary structure of a human glandular kallikrein gene. *DNA* 1987;6:429.
9. Takayama TK, Fujikawa K, Davie EW. Characterization of the precursor of prostate-specific antigen. Activation by trypsin and by human glandular kallikrein. *J Biol Chem* 1997;272:21582.
10. Reigman PH, Vlietstra RJ, Van der Korput JA, et al. The promoter of the prostate-specific antigen gene contains a functional androgen responsive element. *Mol Endocrin* 1991;5:1921.
11. Lilja H. A kallikrein-like serine protease in prostatic fluid cleaves the predominant seminal vesicle protein. *J Clin Invest* 1985;76:1899.
12. Epstein JI. PSA and PAP as immunohistochemical markers in prostate cancer. *Urol Clin NA* 1993;20:757.
13. Yu H, Diamandis EP, Sutherland DJ. Immunoreactive prostate-specific antigen levels in female and male breast tumors and its association with steroid hormone receptors and patient age. *Clin Biochem* 1994;27:75.
14. Graves HC. Nonprostatic sources of prostate-specific antigen: a steroid hormone-dependent phenomenon. *Clin Chem* 1995;41:7.
15. Yu H, Diamandis EP, Zarghami N, et al. Induction of prostate specific antigen production by steroids and tamoxifen in breast cancer cell lines. *Breast Cancer Res Treat* 1994;32:291.
16. Espana F, Sanchez-Cuenca J, Estelles A, et al. Quantitative immunoassay for complexes of prostate-specific antigen with alpha-2-macroglobulin. *Clin Chem* 1996;42:545.
17. Vessella RL, Lange PH. Issues in the assessment of PSA immunoassay. *Urol Clin North Am* 1993;20:607.
18. Noldus J, Chen Z, Stamey TA. Isolation and characterization of free form prostate specific antigen (f-PSA) in sera of men with prostate cancer. *J Urol* 1997;158:1606.
19. Oesterling JE, Chan DW, Epstein JI, et al. Prostate specific antigen in the preoperative and postoperative evaluation of localized prostatic cancer treated with radical prostatectomy. *J Urol* 1988;139:766.
20. Stamey TA, Yang N, Hay AR, et al. Prostate-specific antigen as a serum marker for adenocarcinoma of the prostate. *N Engl J Med* 1987;317:909.
21. Simak R, Madersbacher S, Zhang Z, et al. The impact of ejaculation on serum prostate specific antigen. *J Urol* 1993;150:895.
22. El-Shirbiny AM, Nilson T, Pawar HN. Serum PSA hourly change/24 hours compared with prostatic acid phosphatase. *Urology* 1990;35:88.
23. Dejter SW Jr., Martin JS, McPherson RA, et al. Daily variability in human serum PSA and prostatic acid phosphatase: a comparative evaluation. *Urology* 1988;32:288.
24. Mermall H, Sothern RB, Kanabrocki EL, et al. Temporal (circadian) and functional relationship between prostate-specific antigen and testosterone in healthy men. *Urology* 1995;46:45.
25. Prestigiacomo AF, Stamey TA. Clinical usefulness of free and complexed PSA. *Scand J Clin Lab Invest* 1995; 55[Suppl 221]:32.
26. Graves HCB, Wehner K, Stamey TA. Comparison of a polyclonal and monoclonal immunoassay for PSA: need for an international antigen standard. *J Urol* 1990;144:1516.
27. Stamey TA. Second Stanford conference on international standardization of PSA immunoassays. September 1 and 2, 1994. *Urology* 1995;45:173.
28. Stamey TA, Chen Z, Prestigiacomo AF. Standardization of immunoassays for prostate-specific antigen: a different view based on experimental observations. *Cancer* 1995;74:1662.
29. Vessella RL, Lange PH. Issues in the assessment of prostate-specific antigen immunoassays. *Urol Clin North Am* 1997; 24:261.
30. Vessella RL, Noteboom J, Lange PH. Evaluation of the Abbott IMx automated immunoassay of PSA. *Clin Chem* 1992;38:2044.
31. Schroff RW, Foon KA, Beatty SM, et al. Human antimurine immunoglobulin responses in patients receiving monoclonal antibody therapy. *Cancer Res* 1985;45:879.
32. Boscato LM, Stuart MC. Heterophilic antibodies: a problem for all immunoassays. *Clin Chem* 1988;34:27.
33. Oesterling JE. Prostate specific antigen: a critical assessment of the most useful tumor marker for adenocarcinoma of the prostate. *J Urol* 1991;145:907.
34. Pound CR, Partin AW, Epstein JI, et al. PSA following anatomical radical retropubic prostatectomy: patterns of recurrence and cancer control. *Urol Clin North Am* 1997;24:395.

35. Catalona WJ, Smith DS, Ratliff TL, et al. Detection of organ-confined prostate cancer is increased through PSA-based screening. *JAMA* 1993;270:948.
36. Epstein JI, Walsh PC, Carmichael M, et al. Pathologic and clinical findings to predict tumor extent of nonpalpable (Stage T1c) prostate cancer. *JAMA* 1994;271:368.
37. Stamey TA, Freiha FS, McNeal JE, et al. Localized prostate cancer: relationship of tumor volume to clinical significance for the treatment of prostate cancer. *Cancer* 1993;71:993.
38. Smith DS, Catalona WJ. The nature of prostate cancer detected through PSA based screening. *J Urol* 1994;152: 1732.
39. Ohori M, Wheeler TM, Dunn JK, et al. The pathological features and prognosis of prostate cancer detectable with current diagnostic tests. *J Urol* 1994;152:1714.
40. Oesterling JE, Cooner WH, Jacobsen SJ, et al. Influence of patient age on the serum PSA concentration: an important clinical observation. *Urol Clin North Am* 1993;20:671.
41. Seaman E, Whang M, Olsson CA, et al. PSA density (PSAD): role in patient evaluation and management. *Urol Clin North Am* 1993;20:653.
42. Carter HB, Pearson JD. PSA velocity: a new concept for the diagnosis of early prostate cancer. *Urol Clin North Am* 1993;20:665.
43. Zlotta AR, Djavan B, Margerger M, et al. Prostate specific antigen density of the transition zone: a new effective parameter for prostate cancer prediction. *J Urol* 1997;157: 1315.
44. Lilja H. Significance of different molecular forms of serum PSA. The free, noncomplexed form of PSA versus that complexed to alpha-1-antichymotrypsin. *Urol Clin North Am* 1993;20:681.
45. Catalona WJ, Smith DS, Wolfert RL, et al. Evaluation of percentage of free serum PSA to improve specificity of prostate cancer screening. *JAMA* 1995;274:1214.
46. Rees MA, Resnick MI, Oesterling JE. Use of prostate-specific antigen, Gleason score, and digital rectal examination in staging patients with newly diagnosed prostate cancer. *Urol Clin North Am* 1997;24:379.
47. Partin AW, Carter HB, Chan DW, et al. Prostate specific antigen in the staging of localized prostate cancer: influence of tumor differentiation, tumor volume and benign hyperplasia. *J Urol* 1990;143:747.
48. Lange PH, Ercole CJ, Lightner DJ, et al. The value of serum prostate specific antigen determinations before and after radical prostatectomy. *J Urol* 1989;141:873.
49. Kleer E, Larson-Keller JJ, Zincke H, et al. Ability of preoperative serum PSA value to predict pathologic state and DNA ploidy. *Urology* 1993;41:207.
50. Haapianen RK, Permi EJ, Rannikko SA, et al. Prostate tumor markers as an aid in staging of prostate cancer. *Br J Urol* 1990;65:264.
51. Partin AW, Oesterling JE. The clinical usefulness of prostate specific antigen: update 1994. *J Urol* 1994;152:1358.
52. Bluestein DL, Bostwick DG, Bergstralh EJ, et al. Eliminating the need for bilateral pelvic lymphadenectomy in select patients with prostate cancer. *J Urol* 1994;151:1315.
53. Partin AW, Yoo J, Carter HB, et al. The use of PSA, clinical stage and Gleason score to predict pathologic stage in men with localized prostate cancer. *J Urol* 1993;150:110.
54. Sands ME, Zagars GK, Pollack A, et al. Serum prostate-specific antigen, clinical stage, pathologic grade, and the incidence of nodal metastasis in prostate cancer. *Urology* 1994;44:215.
55. Partin AW, Walsh PC. The use of prostate specific antigen, clinical stage and Gleason score to predict pathological stage in men with localized prostate cancer [Letter]. *J Urol* 1994;152:172.
56. Narayan P, Gajendran V, Taylor SP, et al. The role of transrectal ultrasound-guided biopsy-based staging, preoperative serum prostate-specific antigen, and biopsy Gleason score in prediction of final pathologic diagnosis in prostate cancer. *Urology* 1995;46:205.
57. Takayama T, Krieger JN, True LD, et al. Recurrent prostate cancer despite undetectable prostate-specific antigen. *J Urol* 1992;148:1541.
58. Goldrath DE, Messing EM. Prostate specific antigen: not detectable despite tumor progression after radical prostatectomy. *J Urol* 1989;142:1082.
59. Pound CR, Partin AW, Eisenberger MA, et al. Natural history of progression after PSA elevation following radical prostatectomy. *JAMA* 1999;281:1591.
60. Nelson PS, Gan L, Ferguson C, et al. Molecular cloning and characterization of prostase, an androgen-regulated serine protease with prostate-restricted expression. *Proc Natl Acad Sci* 1999;96:3114.
61. Osman I, Drobnjak M, Fazzari M, et al. Inactivation of the p53 pathway in prostate cancer impact on tumor progression. *Clin Cancer Res* 1999;5:2082.
62. Brawer MK, Jonsson E, Gibbons RP, et al. Extent of prostate neovascularity predicts progression in patients with pathologic stage C adenocarcinoma treated with radical prostatectomy. *J Urol* 1994:289A.
63. Narayan P, Tewari A. Systematic biopsy-based staging of prostate cancer: scientific background, individual variables, combination of parameters, and current integrative models. *Semin Urol Oncol* 1998;16:172.
64. Tewari A, Narayan P. Novel staging tool for localized prostate cancer: a pilot study using genetic adaptive neural networks. *J Urol* 1998;160:430.
65. Wei JT, Zhang Z, Barnhill SD, et al. Understanding artificial neural networks and exploring their potential applications for the practicing urologist. *Urology* 1998;52:161.
66. Catalona WJ, Smith DS. 5-year tumor recurrence rates after anatomical radical retropubic prostatectomy for prostate cancer. *J Urol* 1994;152:1837.
67. Zincke H, Oesterling JE, Blute ML, et al. Long-term (15 years) results after radical prostatectomy for clinically localized (stage T2c or lower) prostate cancer. *J Urol* 1994;152:1850.
68. Trapasso JG, deKernion JB, Smith RB, et al. The incidence and significance of detectable levels of serum PSA after radical prostatectomy. *J Urol* 1994;152:1821.
69. Partin AW, Pound CR, Clemens JQ, et al. Serum PSA after anatomic radical prostatectomy: the Johns Hopkins experience after 10 years. *Urol Clin North Am* 1993;20:713.
70. Stein A, deKernion JB, Dorey F. Prostate-specific antigen related to clinical status 1 to 14 years after radical retropubic prostatectomy. *Br J Urol* 1991;67:626.
71. Takayama TK, Lange PH. Radiation therapy for local recurrence of prostate cancer after radical prostatectomy. *Urol Clin North Am* 1994;21:687.

72. Holzbeierlein JM, Smith JA. Value of digital rectal exam after radical prostatectomy in detecting recurrence. *J Urol* 1999;161:923A.
73. Obek C, Neulander E, Sadek S, et al. Is there a role for digital rectal examination in the followup of patients after radical prostatectomy? *J Urol* 1999;162:762.
74. Patel A, Dorey F, Franklin J, et al. Recurrence patterns after radical retropubic prostatectomy: clinical usefulness of prostate specific antigen doubling times and log slope prostate specific antigen. *J Urol* 1997;158:1441.
75. Lange PH, Lightner DJ, Medini E, et al. The effects of radiation therapy after radical prostatectomy in patients with elevated PSA levels. *J Urol* 1990;144:927.
76. Schild SE, Buskirk SJ, Robinow JS, et al. The results of radiotherapy for isolated elevation of serum PSA levels following radical prostatectomy. *Int J Radiat Oncol Biol Phys* 1992;23:141.
77. Link P, Freiha FS, Stamey TA. Adjuvant radiation therapy in patients with detectable prostate specific antigen following radical prostatectomy. *J Urol* 1991;145:532.
78. Hudson MA, Catalona WJ. Effect of adjuvant radiation therapy on PSA following radical prostatectomy. *J Urol* 1990;143:1174.
79. Ellis WJ, Vessella RL, Noteboom JL, et al. Early detection of recurrent prostate cancer with an ultrasensitive chemiluminescent prostate-specific antigen assay. *Urology* 1997; 50:573.
80. Vessella RL. Trends in immunoassay of PSA: serum complexes and ultrasensitivity. *Clin Chem* 1993;39:2035.
81. Takayama TK, Vessella RL, Brawer MK, et al. Urinary PSA levels after radical prostatectomy. *J Urol* 1994;151:82.
82. Vijayakumar S, Quadri SF, Sen S, et al. Measurement of weekly prostate specific antigen levels in patients receiving pelvic radiotherapy for nonprostatic malignancies. *Int J Radiat Oncol Biol Phys* 1995;32:189.
83. Zagars GK, Sherman NE, Babaian RJ. Prostate-specific antigen and external beam radiation therapy in prostate cancer. *Cancer* 1991;67:412.
84. Zagars GK. Serum PSA as a tumor marker for patients undergoing definitive radiation therapy. *Urol Clin North Am* 1993;20:737.
85. Zagars GK, Pollack A. The fall and rise of prostate-specific antigen: kinetics of serum prostate-specific antigen levels after radiation therapy for prostate cancer. *Cancer* 1993; 72:832.
86. Kaplan LD, Cox RS, Bagshaw MA. A model of prostatic carcinoma tumor kinetics based on prostate specific antigen levels after radiation therapy. *Cancer* 1991;66:400.
87. Ritter MA, Messing EM, Shanahan TG, et al. Prostate-specific antigen as a predictor of radiotherapy response and patterns of failure in localized prostate cancer. *J Clin Oncol* 1992;10: 1208.
88. Oesterling JE, Chan DW, Epstein JL, et al. Prostate-specific antigen in the pre-operative and postoperative evaluation of localized prostatic cancer treated with radical prostatectomy. *J Urol* 1988;139:766.
89. Meek AG, Park TL, Oberman E, et al. A prospective study of PSA levels in patients receiving radiotherapy for localized carcinoma of the prostate. *Int J Radiat Oncol Biol Phys* 1990;19:733.
90. Schellhammer PF, El-Mahdi AM, Kuban DA, et al. Prostate-specific antigen after radiation therapy. *Urol Clin North Am* 1997;24:407.
91. Stamey TA, Kabalin JN, Ferrari M. Prostate specific antigen in the diagnosis and treatment of adenocarcinoma of the prostate. III. Radiation treated patients. *J Urol* 1989;141:1084.
92. American Society for Therapeutic Radiology and Oncology Consensus Panel. Consensus statement: guidelines for PSA following radiation therapy. *Int J Radiat Oncol Biol Phys* 1997;37:1035.
93. Critz FA, Levinson AK, Williams WH, et al. Prostate specific antigen nadir achieved by men apparently cured of prostate cancer by radiotherapy. *J Urol* 1999;161:1199.
94. Tibbs MK, Zeitman AL, Dallwo KC, et al. Biochemical outcome following external beam radiation therapy for T1-2 prostate carcinoma: the importance of achieving an undetectable nadir PSA. *Int J Radiat Oncol Biol Phys* 1995; 32[Suppl 1]:230.
95. Shipley WU, Thames HD, Sandler HM, et al. Radiation therapy for clinically localized prostate cancer. *JAMA* 1999;281:1598.
96. Grob BM, Schellhammer PF, Brassil DN, et al. Changes in immunohistochemical staining of PSA, PAP, and TURP-27 following irradiation therapy for clinically localized prostate cancer. *Urology* 1994;44:525.
97. Kabalin JN, Hodge KH, McNeal JE, et al. Identification of residual cancer in the prostate following radiation therapy: role of transrectal ultrasound guided biopsy and prostate specific antigen. *J Urol* 1989;142:326.
98. Kaplan ID, Cox RS, Bagshaw MA. Prostate-specific antigen after external beam radiotherapy for prostatic cancer: followup. *J Urol* 1993;149:519.
99. Schellhammer PE, El-Mahdi AM, Wright GL, et al. Prostate-specific antigen to determine progression-free survival after radiation therapy for localized carcinoma of prostate. *Urology* 1993;42:13.
100. Leo ME, Bilhartz DL, Bergstrahl EJ, et al. Prostate specific antigen in hormonally treated stage D2 prostate cancer: Is it always an accurate indicator of disease status? *J Urol* 1991;145:802.
101. Stamey TA, Kabalin JN, Ferrari M, et al. Prostate specific antigen in the diagnosis and treatment of adenocarcinoma of the prostate: IV. Anti-androgen treated patients. *J Urol* 1989;141:1088.
102. Zanetti G, Trinchieri A, Del Nero A, et al. Prognostic significance of prostate-specific antigen in endocrine treatment for prostatic carcinoma. *Eur Urol* 1992;21:96.
103. Arai Y, Yoshiki T, Yoshida O. Prognostic significance of specific antigen in endocrine treatment for prostatic cancer. *J Urol* 1990;144:1415.
104. Matzkin H, Eber P, Todd B, et al. Prognostic significance of changes in prostate-specific markers after endocrine treatment of stage D2 prostate cancer. *Cancer* 1992;70:2302.
105. Miller JI, Ahman FR, Drach GW, et al. The clinical usefulness of serum PSA after hormonal therapy of metastatic prostate cancer. *J Urol* 1992;147:956.
106. Smith DC, Pienta KJ. The use of prostate-specific antigen as a surrogate end point in the treatment of patients with hormone refractory prostate cancer. *Urol Clin North Am* 1997;24:433.

107. Myers C, Cooper M, Stein C, et al. Suramin: a novel growth factor antagonist with activity in hormone-refractory metastatic prostate cancer. *J Clin Oncol* 1992;10:881.
108. Hudes GR, Greenberg R, Kreigel RL, et al. Phase II study of estramustine and vinblastine, two microtubule inhibitors, in hormone refractory prostate cancer. *J Clin Oncol* 1992; 10:1754.
109. Pienta KJ, Redman B, Hussain M. Phase II evaluation of oral estramustine and oral etoposide in hormone refractory adenocarcinoma of the prostate. *J Clin Oncol* 1994;12: 2005.
110. Kelly WK, Scher HI, Mazumdar M, et al. Prostate-specific antigen as a measure of disease outcome in metastatic hormone-refractory prostate cancer. *J Clin Oncol* 1993;11:607.
111. Sridhara R, Eisenberber MA, Sinibaldi VJ, et al. Evaluation of prostate-specific antigen as a surrogate marker for response of hormonerefractory prostate cancer to suramin therapy. *J Clin Oncol* 1995;13:2944.
112. Young CY, Andrews PE, Montgomery BT, et al. Tissue-specific and hormonal regulation of human prostate-specific glandular kallikrein. *Biochemistry* 1992;31:818.
113. Darson MF, Pacelli A, Roche P, et al. Human glandular kallikrein 2 expression in prostatic intraepithelial neoplasia and adenocarcinoma: a novel prostate cancer marker. *Urology* 1997;49:857.
114. Reigman PH, Vlietstra RJ, Van der Korput HA, et al. Identification and androgen-regulated expression of two major human glandular kallikrein-1 (hGK-1) mRNA species. *Mol Cell Endocrinol* 1991;76:181.
115. Mikolajczyk SD, Millar LS, Marker KM, et al. Ala217 is important for the catalytic function and autoactivation of prostate-specific human kallikrein 2. *Eur J Biochem* 1997; 246:440.
116. Kumar A, Mikolajczyk SD, Goel AS, et al. Expression of pro form of prostate-specific antigen by mammalian cells and its conversion to mature, active form by human kallikrein 2. *Cancer Res* 1997;57:3111.
117. Lovgren J, Rajakoski K, Karp M, et al. Activation of the zymogen form of prostate-specific antigen by human glandular kallikrein 2. *Biochem Biophys Res Commun* 1997;238: 549.
118. Frenette G, Tremblay RR, Lazure C, et al. Prostatic kallikrein hK2, but not prostate-specific antigen activates single-chain urokinase-type plasminogen activator. *Int J Cancer* 1997;71:897.
119. Achbarou A, Kaiser S, Tremblay G, et al. Urokinase overproduction results in increased skeletal metastasis by prostate cancer cells in vivo. *Cancer Res* 1994;54:2372.
120. Lyon PB, See WA, Xu Y, et al. Diversity and modulation of plasminogen activator activity in human prostate carcinoma cell lines. *Prostate* 1995;27:179.
121. Kwiatkowski MK, Recker F, Piironen T, et al. In prostatism patients the ratio of human glandular kallikrein to free PSA improves the discrimination between prostate cancer and benign hyperplasia within the diagnostic "gray zone" of total PSA 4 to 10 ng/ml. *Urology* 1998;52:360.
122. Becker C, Lilja H, Piironen T, et al. hK2 measurements in a randomly selected, population based screening for prostate cancer. *J Urol* 1999;161:1233A.
123. Erdamar S, Nguyen C, Shariat S, et al. pT30N0 prostate cancer patients with RT-PCR-hK2-L-positive lymph nodes are at higher risk for recurrence. *J Urol* 1999;161:912A.
124. Van Nguyen C, Dickason R, Song W. RT-PCR for hK2 mRNA: a new assay for detecting circulating prostate cells. *J Urol* 1997;157:112.
125. Horoszewicz JS, Leong SS, Kawinski E, et al. LNCaP model of human prostatic carcinoma. *Cancer Res* 1983;43:1809.
126. Horoszewicz JS, Kawinski E, Murphy GP. Monoclonal antibodies to new antigenic marker in epithelial prostatic cells and serum of prostatic cancer patients. *Anticancer Res* 1987;7:927.
127. Su SL, Huang IP, Fair WR, et al. Alternatively spliced variants of prostate-specific membrane antigen RNA: ratio of expression as a potential measurement of progression. *Cancer Res* 1995;55:1441.
128. Carter RE, Feldman AR, Coyle JT. Prostate-specific membrane antigen is a hydrolase with substrate and pharmacologic characteristics of a neuropeptidase. *Proc Natl Acad Sci U S A* 1996;93:749.
129. Cama C, Olsson CA, Raffo AJ, et al. Molecular staging of prostate cancer. A comparison of the application of an enhanced reverse transcriptase polymerase chain reaction assay for prostate specific antigen versus prostate specific membrane antigen. *J Urol* 1995;153:1373.
130. Israeli RS, Miller WH, Su SL, et al. Sensitive detection of prostatic hematogenous tumor cell dissemination using prostate specific antigen and prostate specific membrane-derived primers in the polymerase chain reaction. *J Urol* 1995;153:573.
131. Fair WR, Israeli RS, Wang Y, et al. Neoadjuvant androgen-deprivation therapy (ADT) before radical prostatectomy results in a significantly decreased incidence of residual micrometastatic disease as detected by nested RT-PCR with PSM primers. *J Urol* 1995;153:391A.
132. Shalon D, Smith SJ, Brown PO. A DNA microarray system for analyzing complex DNA samples using two-color fluorescent probe hybridization. *Genome Res* 1996;6:639.
133. Schena M, Shalon D, Heller R, et al. Parallel human genome analysis: microarray-based expression monitoring of 1000 genes. *Proc Natl Acad Sci U S A* 1996;93:10614.
134. Gundy AP. Rapid research response emphasized in unique prostate cancer program. *JAMA* 1997;277:945.

16

SYSTEMATIC BIOPSY OF THE PROSTATE: APPLICATIONS FOR DETECTION, STAGING, AND RISK ASSESSMENT

JOSEPH C. PRESTI, JR.

The systematic sextant biopsy of the prostate under transrectal ultrasound (TRUS) guidance was introduced just over 10 years ago and has revolutionized our ability to detect prostate cancer (CaP) (1). Before transrectal systematic sampling, prostate biopsies were usually performed with a transperineal approach, using a manually fired 14-gauge needle under digital guidance, and were directed at palpable nodules. Transrectal biopsy approaches were later introduced, and although having a higher complication rate from infection than transperineal approaches, the improved accuracy in needle placement outweighed the slightly increased complication rate. The introduction of prostate-specific antigen (PSA) into clinical practice in the 1980s greatly enhanced our ability to detect CaP, and it quickly became evident that many patients with CaP only had elevations in serum PSA levels without any lesions appreciated on digital rectal examination (DRE). Many investigators then reported on the application of TRUS-guided biopsies in these patients (elevated PSA level and normal DRE). Many of these patients had hypoechoic lesions visualized by TRUS, and biopsy of these lesions demonstrated cancer in approximately one-third of the patients. The development of a spring-loaded biopsy gun, using 18-gauge needles in conjunction with the refinement of TRUS imaging, enabled the safe performance of transrectal systematic sampling. The superiority of this biopsy scheme over conventional lesion-directed biopsies is well established (2). In addition to cancer detection, systematic biopsy of the prostate also provides information pertaining to tumor grade, volume assessment, local staging of the disease, and risk of relapse after therapy. Each of these applications is reviewed.

CANCER DETECTION

As described earlier, the introduction of systematic prostate biopsy has facilitated our ability to detect CaP. Today, six biopsies are usually performed in the parasagittal line halfway between the lateral border and midline of the prostate on both right and left sides from the base, midgland, and apex (Fig. 16-1). Recently, several investigators have questioned whether additional biopsies are warranted. It seems naïve to assume that six biopsies of the prostate are appropriate for all prostate sizes and configurations. Although this may be adequate sampling in some prostates, it may be inadequate in larger prostates. Several investigators have demonstrated that CaP detection rates are inversely proportional to prostate size. In a referral population undergoing systematic sextant biopsies, one study demonstrated a 23% cancer detection rate in men with prostates greater than or equal to 50 cc in size, compared to 38% in men with prostates smaller than 50 cc (3). In a large prospective study of 1,974 men with a normal DRE and TRUS and an elevated PSA who underwent systematic sextant biopsy, cancer detection rates incrementally decreased with incremental increases in prostate size (4).

The majority of CaPs originates in the peripheral zone (PZ) of the prostate, and most biopsy schemes focus on sampling this area (5). Recently, interest has grown in exploring schemas using additional biopsy approaches. In general, studies on new biopsy schemes have used one of two approaches: (a) prospective evaluations of different biopsy schemes on referral-based populations and (b) computer modeling of biopsy schemes. Each of these approaches is now reviewed.

Prospectively Evaluated Schemes

Since 1997, several investigators have prospectively evaluated new systematic biopsy regimens in referral-based populations. One group studied a five-region technique of systematic biopsy in a series of 119 patients (6). The five regions included the standard sextant biopsy regimen

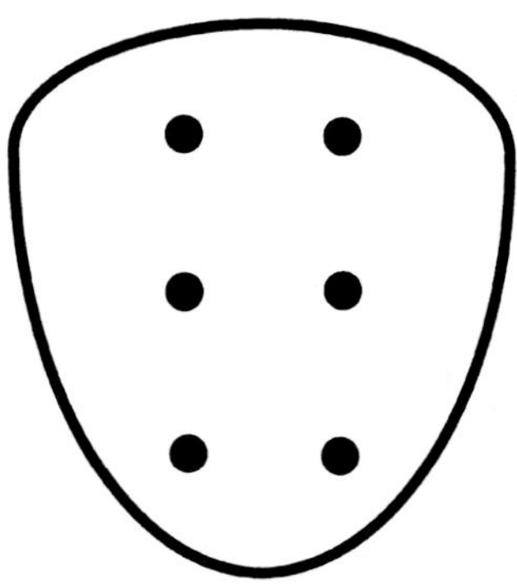

FIGURE 16-1. Standard sextant biopsy scheme of the peripheral zone of the prostate in the coronal plane on right and left sides at the base (*top*), midgland, and apex (*bottom*).

obtained halfway between the lateral border and midline of the prostate on both right and left sides (regions 2 and 4) but, in addition, obtained two biopsies from each lateral aspect of the prostate (regions 1 and 5) and three biopsies from the midline at the apex, midgland, and base (region 3). Of the 119 patients, 48 (40%) had cancer on the biopsy, of which 17 (35% of cancers detected) were only detected in regions 1, 3, and 5. Of note, only two cancers were detected by the three centrally placed biopsies of region 3. With respect to complications, these investigators reported an 80% incidence of gross hematuria, which they attributed to the region 3 biopsies that probably penetrated the urethra (Table 16-1).

Another group prospectively evaluated an eight- or ten-biopsy regimen, depending on gland size, in 512 patients (7). In this protocol, all patients underwent eight biopsies of the PZ, four from each lobe at the apex, midgland, base, and lateral midgland. When prostate length exceeded 4 cm, two additional biopsies were obtained from the transition zone (TZ). When comparing the standard sextant biopsy regimen with the extended biopsy regimen, overall cancer detection rates increased from 85% to 97%. If lesion-directed biopsies had been added to the standard sextant biopsy regimen, then cancer detection rates would have increased to 93% (Table 16-1).

TABLE 16-1. DETECTION RATES IN SEVERAL BIOPSY SERIES

Series	Number of biopsies	% of cancers detected
Prospectively evaluated schemes		
Eskew et al. (6) (n = 48)	6	65
	13	100
Norberg et al. (7) (n = 276)	6	85
	8	96
Chang et al. (10) (n = 121)	6	82
	10	96
Computer modeling schemes		
Bauer et al. (21) (n = 201)	6	73
	6 (lateral)	95
	10	99
	14	99
	16	100
Chen et al. (22) (n = 180)	4	59
	6	63
	8	65
	13	74
	18	77

Note: *n* denotes number of cancers in each series.

Another approach taken by one group has been to investigate the use of performing two consecutive sets of sextant biopsies of the prostate in a single office visit in 137 consecutive patients in a referral-based population (8). A total of 43 cancers were detected in the entire study population (31% cancer detection rate). Using the first sextant biopsy set as the reference set, 30 cancers were detected (70% of all cancers), so the second biopsy set increased the detection rate by 30%. However, if the second biopsy set had been used as the reference, then 40 cancers were detected (93% of all cancers), whereas the first biopsy set would have only increased the detection rate by 7%. The benefit of this type of approach needs further study, with a larger patient cohort, as sextant sampling, presumably from similar locations, resulted in wide variation in detection rates (70% vs. 93%).

Because the majority of carcinomas arises in the PZ, it seemed logical to us that systematic biopsies should focus on better sampling this zone. Stamey had suggested moving the standard sextant biopsies more laterally to better sample the anterior extension of the PZ (Fig. 16-2) (9). The work of Eskew et al. (6) and Norberg et al. (7), as well as the report by Dr. Stamey, prompted us to prospectively evaluate the use of adding four lateral biopsies of the PZ to the routine sextant biopsy regimen (Fig. 16-3). Two hundred and seventy-three consecutive patients referred for an abnormal DRE or with PSA greater than or equal to 4 ng per mL, or both, underwent TRUS and systematic biopsies along with lesion-directed biopsies (10). Sextant biopsies were obtained in the midlobar parasagittal plane, halfway between the lateral edge and midline of the prostate gland, at the base, midgland, and apex. The lateral PZ biopsies

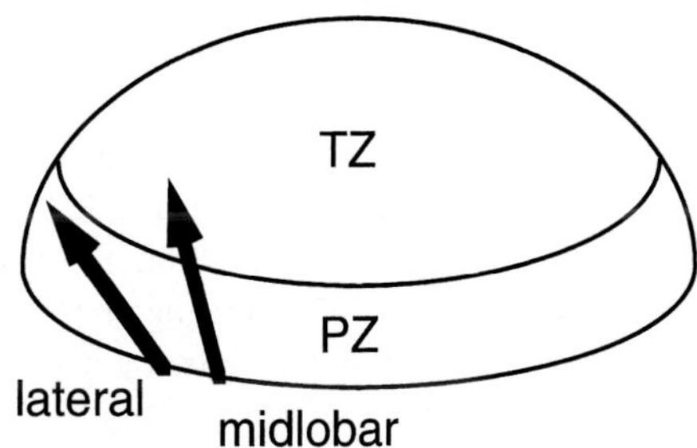

FIGURE 16-2. Transverse diagram of the prostate demonstrating the needle trajectory in the standard midlobar plane and in the laterally directed plane. Notice that the laterally directed biopsy actually samples more peripheral zone (PZ) than the midlobar biopsy, which also samples some transition zone (TZ).

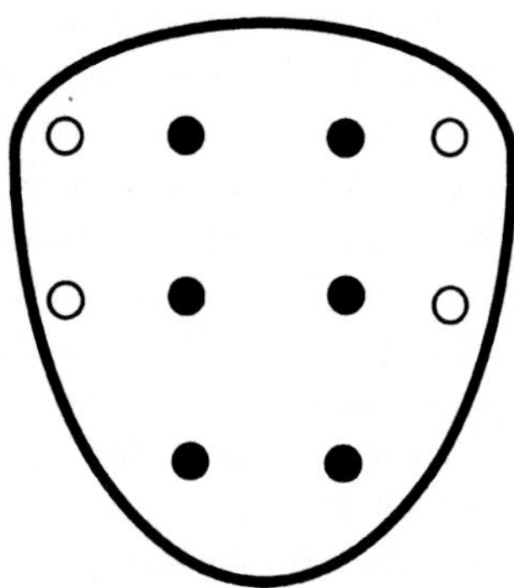

FIGURE 16-3. Ten-biopsy scheme of the peripheral zone of the prostate in the coronal plane using the standard sextant scheme (*closed circles*) and additional biopsies obtained from the lateral aspect of the peripheral zone at the base and midgland (*open circles*).

were performed by positioning the probe just medial to the lateral edge of the prostate. The lateral PZ biopsies were obtained at the midgland and base only as apical biopsies are, in fact, lateral as the prostate narrows in this area. Forty-four percent (121 of 273) of the patients had cancer on biopsy. Although the routine sextant biopsies detected 82% of the cancers, 77% (17 of 22) of the missed cancers were detected by the lateral PZ biopsies. Lateral PZ biopsies increased cancer detection rates by 14% (Table 16-1). In the subset of the 147 patients with lesions on TRUS imaging, cancer was found in 50% (74 of 147); routine sextant biopsies detected 76% (56 of 74) of the cancers, whereas the lateral PZ biopsies detected 80% (59 of 74). This finding is striking when considering that this comparison is between a four-biopsy regimen (lateral biopsy) and a six-biopsy regimen (sextant biopsy). Fifteen of these 74 patients (20%) had positive lateral PZ biopsies with negative sextant biopsies. Lesion-directed biopsies uniquely identified only one cancer. Our conclusions from this study were that the performance of ten biopsies of the PZ increased cancer detection rates by 14% and nearly eliminated the need for lesion-directed biopsies, thus minimizing the operator dependence of the TRUS examination.

Recently, we have begun investigating the use of each of the specific biopsy sites in our ten-biopsy scheme of the PZ (11). Preliminary analysis of 483 patients from our referral-based population revealed cancer in 42%. Traditional sextant biopsies missed 20% of the cancers. In evaluating our ten-biopsy scheme of the PZ, the least efficient location for the systematic biopsies was the midlobar base biopsy. Eliminating these midlobar base biopsies from the systematic ten-biopsy regimen and, thus, converting it to an eight-biopsy regimen would have only minimally decreased the detection rate of this regimen (96% to 95%). This eight-biopsy scheme maintained a detection rate of 95% when stratified for DRE result (abnormal vs. normal) and PSA level (less than or equal to 10 ng per mL vs. greater than 10 ng per mL). The two most efficient six-biopsy regimens were the apex, midlobar midgland, and lateral base regimen, and the apex, lateral midgland, and lateral base regimen. Both resulted in an 88% detection rate. When controlling for prostate size, these detection rates were lower for prostates larger than 50 cc in size (76% and 80%, respectively). We also observed that the detection rate of the laterally directed sextant regimen (apex, lateral midgland, and lateral base) was superior to the detection rate of the standard midlobar sextant regimen [89% vs. 80%, $p = .027$ (McNemar's test)]. Explanations for the increased yield from laterally directed PZ biopsies might include (a) laterally directed biopsies might more extensively sample the PZ (Fig. 16-2), or (b) CaP may more commonly reside in the lateral aspect of the PZ. Our conclusions from this study were that six systematic biopsies of the PZ were inadequate. A minimum of eight systematic biopsies of the PZ including the apex, midlobar midgland, lateral midgland, and lateral base should be performed routinely.

Approximately 25% to 30% of CaPs originate in the TZ of the prostate (12). Appropriate indications for TZ biopsies remain an area of debate. One retrospective series demonstrated a low unique cancer detection rate in TZ biopsies when performed in all patients (TZ biopsy only site of positive biopsy in 2% of patients with cancer) (13). A prospective evaluation of the performance of two TZ biopsies in all patients was performed by one group and demonstrated a low unique cancer detection rate for the TZ biopsies. For all patients, TZ biopsies were the only positive site in 2.9% (8 of 279) of cancers, and, if considering only patients with a normal DRE, then TZ biopsies were the unique site of cancer in 4.1% (6 of 145) of cancers (14). As the prostate enlarges, preferential zonal growth tends to occur in the TZ. We thus believed it important to control for prostate size in determining the need for TZ biopsies. Recently, we prospectively evaluated 213 consecutive patients from a referral-based population who had calculated prostate sizes larger than 50 cc (15). All patients underwent the conventional sextant biopsies of the PZ and, in addition, underwent additional sextant biopsies of the TZ for a total of 12 biopsies. The PZ biopsy specimens were obtained in the parasagittal plane midway between the lateral border and the midline of the gland. Three specimens were obtained from each lobe at the apex, midportion, and base of the gland. The TZ biopsies were obtained just lateral to midline, and the needles were advanced into the gland to approximately 1.5 cm from the anterior capsule before firing the gun to minimize sampling of the PZ. Three cores were obtained from each side at the apex, midportion, and base of the prostate. Fifty-five cases of carcinoma were found for a 26% detection rate. The TZ biopsies detected cancer in 30 of the 55 patients (55%), compared to the 47 patients detected by the PZ biopsies (85%). Only seven cancers (13% of cancers) were detected by the additional TZ biopsies. Subsequently, an additional prospective evaluation of TZ biopsies has been reported (16). This study obtained two biopsies of the TZ and did not control for prostate size. Seven of 151 (5%) of the cancers were only detected by the TZ biopsies. Results were stratified for race; however, no racial differences were observed in the yield of TZ biopsies.

Most investigators agree that TZ biopsies are indicated in patients with a high suspicion of CaP who have had negative prior systematic biopsies. One retrospective series demonstrated that in this scenario, 19% (9 of 47) of patients with cancer demonstrated cancer only in the TZ biopsies (17). Other investigators have retrospectively demonstrated similar detection rates in this population, specifically 14% (8 of 58) of patients with cancer in one series and 10% (2 of 19) of patients with cancer in another series (18,19).

Computer Modeling Schemes

Several investigators have used computer simulations and modeling to better refine systematic biopsy schemes of the prostate. One approach uses step-sectioned radical prostatectomy specimens. Data are obtained from well-mapped specimens, including total prostate volume measurements, as well as total tumor volume measurements. Computer-generated prostate models with varying tumor sizes are then created, and systematic sampling is then simulated. Different biopsy schemes can be tested to determine their efficiency for cancer detection. One study demonstrated that systematic sextant biopsies could miss cancers as large as 6 cc (20). Limitations of simulated models, as described here, include the fact that tumors must typically be simulated as spheres within the prostate, and the differential zonal incidence of carcinoma is often neglected. Additionally, as most data for these models are derived from radical prostatectomy specimens, the means of cancer detection that resulted in a patient's undergoing surgery must be acknowledged. In the study mentioned previously, cancers were detected by a lesion-directed approach alone. Such models may not be useful in refining cancer detection schemes for T1c lesions. If sextant sampling was used to detect the cancers in a given radical prostatectomy series used to construct a computer model, then the applicability of these models in studying novel biopsy regimens using sites outside the traditional sextant regions is unknown. Despite this possible limitation, a recent computer model has demonstrated the use of altering the standard systematic sextant biopsy by directing the biopsy needles into the more lateral aspect of the PZ (21). Cancer detection rates increased by 23% with this simple manipulation. Additional biopsies resulted in only a modest increase in cancer detection rates (Table 16-1). Another computer model has also demonstrated increasing cancer detection rates by increasing the number of systematic biopsies; however, reported detection rates demonstrate significant variations between series (Table 16-1) (22).

Another computer-assisted approach involved the retrospective review of 156 consecutive patients diagnosed with T1c CaP (23). In this model, a computer randomly deleted one of the biopsies from the right and left lobes and then evaluated the number of cancers that would have been missed if only four biopsies had been obtained. This model demonstrated that between 4% and 19% of the cancers would have been missed if only four, rather than six, biopsies were performed. One confounding issue, which the authors point out, is that if a four-biopsy regimen were used, then the four sites would most likely not correspond to four of the six sites from the sextant regimen. However, this model also seems to support the concept that the clinically positive biopsy rate may depend, in part, on the extent of gland sampling.

Recently, one group attempted to define the number of biopsies required for a given prostate size and patient age to detect a clinically significant cancer (24). This complex computer model gives consideration to tumor and host factors, including an estimate of tumor doubling time of 4 years, and assumes that a tumor volume of 20 cc results in the death of the host. Other assumptions of this model include a spherical tumor size and a random distribution of the tumor throughout the entire volume of the prostate. This model demonstrated that, for a given age of patient, the number of biopsies required increases with increasing prostate size. A 55-year-old man with a 20-, 30-, or 40-cc prostate was recommended to undergo 10, 15, and 20 biopsies, respectively. A 60-year-old man with comparable prostate sizes was recommended to undergo 7, 10, and 13 biopsies, respectively. As described previously, this model makes several assumptions; however, the introduction of host factors (age related to life expectancy) is novel.

Further work is needed to define the optimal systematic biopsy strategy. Six biopsies are probably not adequate for most prostates. The number and position of systematic biopsies would most likely vary with prostate size, configuration, and PSA levels. Sampling error would be greatest in large prostates or in the presence of small tumors. If only a limited number of biopsies were obtained in these two scenarios, then false-negative results might be obtained. Other variables that might need to be considered include race and family history. It is possible that cancers in patients with a genetic predisposition may have different biopsy needs (perhaps from a higher rate of multifocality) than those without significant risk factors.

TUMOR GRADE ESTIMATES

Accurate determination of tumor grade significantly contributes to the management of CaP patients. As noted earlier for cancer detection, needle biopsy of the prostate represents a sampling of the gland, and accurate prediction of tumor grade within the prostate may be hindered by sampling error. In general, in several series correlating tumor grade on the biopsy with the grade of tumor in the radical prostatectomy specimen, needle biopsies exactly correlate with the prostatectomy in 31% to 59% of cases (25–28). The magnitude of this grading error is greater than or equal to 2 points in the Gleason sum in 26% to 38% of cases, with the needle biopsy more likely underestimating the tumor grade in comparison to the radical prostatectomy specimen.

Two approaches toward better estimating the tumor grade have been used. One group investigated the use of the number of core biopsies obtained in predicting tumor grade on the prostatectomy specimen. A community-based retrospective analysis of 124 prostatectomy specimens demonstrated that four to six biopsy cores accurately predicted the final pathologic grade within one Gleason grade in 75% of cases (29). Further increase in the number of cores obtained failed to improve the results. This study was, however, limited because of the lack of a referee pathologist reading the specimens and the lack of a standardized systematic biopsy scheme.

An approach taken by another group of investigators has been to explore the use of repeat biopsy on patients before radical prostatectomy (30). A group of 51 patients who had been diagnosed with CaP at an outside facility underwent repeat sextant biopsy of the PZ before radical prostatectomy. Error rates between the highest grade in the needle biopsy and that of the prostatectomy specimen were compared to another group of 226 patients who only had one set of biopsies performed. In the single biopsy group, 38% were upgraded to a Gleason score of greater than or equal to 7 when comparing the needle biopsy grade to the prostatectomy grade, whereas in the two-biopsy group, 19% were upgraded. This study was strengthened by the use of a referee pathologist who reviewed all biopsy and prostatectomy histology; however, systematic sextant PZ biopsies were routinely used only in the rebiopsy group at the second setting. Similar studies are warranted in patients who undergo extended biopsy schemes, as outlined previously in the section Cancer Detection.

TUMOR VOLUME ESTIMATES

The progression of most, if not all, cancers is linked to cell division and tumor growth (31). This observation has led to the hypothesis that the biologic behavior of a given CaP is directly related to the tumor volume. Careful step-sectioned histopathologic analyses of radical prostatectomy specimens have demonstrated a direct correlation between measured tumor volume and probability of extracapsular extension (ECE), seminal vesicle invasion, and lymph node metastases (32,33). ECE is rare in tumors smaller than 4 cc in size and is almost uniformly present in tumors larger than 12 cc. Risk of seminal vesicle invasion and lymph node metastases, although also related to tumor volume, are difficult to ascertain as a result of verification bias (patients with these features identified preoperatively are not taken to surgery). The importance of preoperative identification of tumor volume is clear from the previous discussion; however, estimates of tumor volume must be based on clinically available information.

Some investigators have demonstrated the use of measuring the length of the core needle biopsy involved with cancer as contributing to the prediction of tumor volume. This correlation appears to be highest for large cancers. A large degree of involvement of the core biopsies with cancer is strongly suggestive of high-stage disease (34,35). A threshold of 3 mm of core length involvement on one core biopsy reliably predicts cancer volumes of 0.5 cc or larger (36). However, the converse is not always true; focal cancer on the needle biopsy is not always associated with an insignificant cancer volume at radical prostatectomy. In a series of 33 consecutive radical prostatectomy patients who were identified as having focal CaP on needle biopsy (single focus smaller than 3 mm in length on only one biopsy without any Gleason pattern 4 or 5), only two patients had a measured tumor volume of less than 0.5 mL in the radical prostatectomy specimen (37). Such attempts at quantifying length of needle core involvement are labor intensive and subject to interpretative variability. One study demonstrated no advantage in quantifying the total length of cancer involvement on all needle biopsies over the percentage of core biopsies involved (correlation coefficients of 0.47 and 0.49, respectively) (38). Another study demonstrated that PSA density, in conjunction with the maximum length of cancer involvement in any one core, was the most valuable means of predicting insignificant cancer at radical prostatectomy (39).

A recent study has suggested that the performance of additional systematic biopsies may more accurately assess tumor volume. A scheme using ten biopsies (conventional sextant biopsies in the PZ bilaterally from the apex, mid, and base of the gland and adding bilateral biopsies of the TZ and laterally directed biopsies of the PZ in the midgland) more accurately predicted tumor volume than sextant biopsies alone (correlation coefficients of 0.56 and 0.39, respectively) (40).

LOCAL STAGING ASSESSMENT AND RISK OF RELAPSE AFTER RADICAL PROSTATECTOMY

Analysis of the number of positive biopsies has been suggested, by several investigators, to contribute to the prediction of ECE at radical prostatectomy. This type of information might, in fact, differ from the quantitation of core length involvement, as it represents a "mapping" of the prostate. This regional sampling of the prostate may be a surrogate to tumor volume and, thus, may contribute to the prediction of ECE or risk of treatment failure, or both.

In one series, 100 radical prostatectomy patients were analyzed and several preoperative clinical parameters were studied in their ability to predict ECE and recurrence (41).

Several parameters correlated with ECE, including a palpable nodule larger than one-half of one lobe, a PSA greater than 25 ng per mL, a PSA density greater than or equal to 0.6, perineural invasion on the needle core, and the involvement of greater than or equal to 67% of the core biopsies obtained. The same parameters correlated with serologic recurrence, but, in addition, the presence of bilaterally positive biopsies and the presence of Gleason scores greater than or equal to 7 on the biopsy also contributed to predicting recurrence.

Another series analyzed 102 radical prostatectomy specimens and evaluated the role of systematic sextant biopsies in predicting ECE (42). Patients with three or fewer positive biopsies had a lower risk of ECE than did those with four or more positive biopsies (20% vs. 76%). Patients with four or more positive sextant biopsies and a Gleason score greater than or equal to 7 had a much higher risk of ECE than those with fewer positive biopsies and lower-grade tumors (greater than 80% vs. less than 40%, respectively).

One series reported on 257 consecutive radical prostatectomy patients and demonstrated that the number of positive sextant biopsies, preoperative PSAs, and Gleason scores correlated with ECE (p <.0001, p = .0135, and p = .0004, respectively) (43). In addition, the number of positive sextant biopsies, preoperative PSAs, and Gleason scores correlated with positive surgical margins (p <.0001, p = .0120, and p = .0008, respectively). With respect to serologic recurrence, patients with fewer than three positive biopsies and a Gleason score less than 7 were at a low risk to recur irrespective of preoperative PSA levels (14% risk with a mean follow-up of 2 years). In a multivariate analysis, the number of positive sextant biopsies was the most powerful predictor of serologic recurrence, followed by Gleason score and preoperative PSA (p = .0052, p = .0306, and p = .1472, respectively)

Another series of 480 patients demonstrated that the probability of having organ-confined CaP at radical prostatectomy decreased with the increasing percentage of positive sextant biopsies (44). Patients with fewer than 33%, between 33% and 50%, and greater than or equal to 50% of positive biopsies had an 84%, 62%, and 38% probability of being organ confined, respectively. Patients with fewer than 50% of systematic biopsies positive demonstrated a disease-free survival of more than 80% at 2 years.

We previously reported on 104 patients who had undergone systematic sextant biopsy before radical prostatectomy (45). In our study, we performed a side-for-side analysis and demonstrated that the risk of ECE was 8% and 14% on sides containing no or one of three positive biopsies, whereas it was 37% and 43% in sides containing two or three positive biopsies, respectively. For a given side of the prostate, if two of three systematic biopsies demonstrated cancer, then the positive-predictive value in predicting ECE was approximately 40%, whereas, if less than two systematic biopsies was positive, the negative-predictive value was approximately 90%. Thus, in planning nerve sparing at the time of radical prostatectomy, patients with less than two positive biopsies on a given side are optimal candidates for ipsilateral nerve preservation.

We reported on a different patient population consisting of 109 patients who had undergone systematic sextant biopsy before radical prostatectomy (46). No patients in this series received neoadjuvant or adjuvant therapy. This study correlated preoperative clinical parameters, including the number of positive systematic biopsies, preoperative PSA levels, and Gleason scores with a risk of serologic recurrence. We demonstrated that patients who had four or more positive sextant biopsies were at a significantly higher risk of failure after radical prostatectomy than patients with three or fewer positive biopsies [relative risk (RR), 2.3; p = .02]. In a multivariate Cox regression model, systematic biopsy results and tumor grades were the most powerful predictors of serologic relapse (RR, 2.3; p = .026 and RR, 1.9; p = .046, respectively). Additional work is needed in this population to determine the site of serologic failure. It will be critical to distinguish between those patients who are failing locally from those who are failing distantly.

More recently, we wished to determine whether the number of positive sextant biopsies contributed to the prediction of positive surgical margins at radical prostatectomy (47). Consecutive patients (n = 108) who had a radical retropubic prostatectomy and systematic sextant biopsies were retrospectively evaluated. Twenty-two of 108 patients (20.4%) had a positive surgical margin because of extension of the tumor through the capsule. Patients with three or more positive biopsies were at higher risk of having a positive surgical margin (p = .009). Patients with bilaterally positive biopsies at either the base or midprostate were more likely to have a positive surgical margin. The risk of a positive surgical margin was not significantly determined by the primary Gleason grade, Gleason score, or preoperative PSA. Multivariable logistic-regression models were created that consistently demonstrated that the number of positive biopsies was the best predictor of margin status.

Future studies in this area should explore the use of the extended biopsy schemes (eight to ten PZ biopsies) in predicting ECE, margin status, and risk of relapse. Such schemes may be more powerful in their prediction of such end points if systematic biopsy does indeed act as a surrogate for tumor volume.

CONCLUSION

Systematic biopsy of the prostate has greatly enhanced our ability to detect CaP. Defining the optimal systematic biopsy regimen for cancer detection in a given prostate size and shape is currently being refined. Sextant biopsies are probably inadequate in most cases, and more extended PZ biopsy schemes definitely increase cancer detection rates. More recently, greater attention has focused on the ability of systematic biopsy to provide additional information with respect to tumor volume, grade, stage, and risk assessment. Future work will investigate the use of extended systematic biopsy schemes in the prediction of these clinical parameters in conjunction with tumor grade, PSA levels, DRE, and imaging.

REFERENCES

1. Hodge KK, McNeal JE, Stamey TA. Ultrasound guided transrectal core biopsies of the palpably abnormal prostate. *J Urol* 1989;142:66–70.
2. Hodge KK, McNeal JE, Terris MK, et al. Random systematic versus directed ultrasound guided transrectal core biopsies of the prostate. *J Urol* 1989;142:71–75.
3. Uzzo RG, Wei JT, Waldbaum RS, et al. The influence of prostate size on cancer detection. *Urology* 1995;46:831–836.
4. Karakiewicz PI, Bazinet M, Aprikian AG, et al. Outcome of sextant biopsy according to gland volume. *Urology* 1997;49:55–59.
5. McNeal JE, Redwine EA, Freiha FS, et al. Zonal distribution of prostatic adenocarcinoma: correlation with histologic pattern and direction of spread. *Am J Surg Pathol* 1988;12:897–906.
6. Eskew LA, Bare RL, McCullough DL. Systematic 5 region prostate biopsy is superior to sextant method for diagnosing carcinoma of the prostate. *J Urol* 1997;157:199–203.
7. Norberg M, Egevad L, Holmberg L, et al. The sextant protocol for ultrasound-guided core biopsies of the prostate underestimates the presence of cancer. *Urology* 1997;50:562–566.
8. Levine MA, Ittman M, Melamed J, et al. Two consecutive sets of transrectal ultrasound guided sextant biopsies of the prostate for the detection of prostate cancer. *J Urol* 1998; 159:471–476.
9. Stamey TA. Making the most out of six systematic sextant biopsies. *Urology* 1995;45:2–12.
10. Chang JJ, Shinohara K, Bhargava V, et al. Prospective evaluation of lateral biopsies of the peripheral zone for prostate cancer detection. *J Urol* 1998;160:2111–2114.
11. Presti JC Jr., Chang JJ, Bhargava V, et al. The optimal systematic prostate biopsy scheme should include eight rather than six biopsies: results of a prospective clinical trial. *J Urol* 2000;163:163–166.
12. McNeal JE, Villers AA, Redwine EA, et al. Capsular penetration in prostate cancer: significance for natural history and treatment. *Am J Surg Pathol* 1990;14:240–247.
13. Terris MK, Pham TQ, Issa MM, et al. Routine transition zone and seminal vesicle biopsies in all patients undergoing transrectal ultrasound guided prostate biopsies are not indicated. *J Urol* 1997;157:204–206.
14. Bazinet M, Karakiewicz PI, Aprikian AG, et al. Value of systematic transition zone biopsies in the early detection of prostate cancer. *J Urol* 1996;155:605–606.
15. Chang JJ, Shinohara K, Hovey RM, et al. Prospective evaluation of systematic sextant transition zone biopsies in large prostates for cancer detection. *Urology* 1998;52:89–93.
16. Fowler JE Jr., Bigler SA, Kilambi NK, et al. Results of transition zone biopsy in black and white men with suspected prostate cancer. *Urology* 1999;53:346–350.
17. Lui PD, Terris MK, McNeal JE, et al. Indications for ultrasound guided transition zone biopsies in the detection of prostate cancer. *J Urol* 1995;153:1000–1003.
18. Keetch DW, Catalona WJ. Prostatic transition zone biopsies in men with previous negative biopsies and persistently elevated serum prostate specific antigen values. *J Urol* 1995; 154:1795–1797.
19. Fleshner NE, Fair WR. Indications for transition zone biopsy in the detection of prostatic carcinoma. *J Urol* 1997; 157:556–558.
20. Daneshgari F, Taylor GD, Miller GJ, et al. Computer simulation of the probability of detecting low volume carcinoma of the prostate with six random systematic core biopsies. *Urology* 1995;45:604–609.
21. Bauer JJ, Zeng J, Weir J, et al. Three-dimensional computer-simulated prostate models: lateral prostate biopsies increase the detection rate of prostate cancer. *Urology* 1999;53:961–967.
22. Chen ME, Troncoso P, Tang K, et al. Comparison of prostate biopsy schemes by computer simulation. *Urology* 1999; 53:951–960.
23. Karakiewicz PI, Aprikian AG, Meshref AW, et al. Computer-assisted comparative analysis of four-sector and six-sector biopsies of the prostate. *Urology* 1996;48:747–750.
24. Vashi AR, Wojno KJ, Gillespie B, et al. A model for the number of cores per prostate biopsy based on patient age and prostate gland volume. *J Urol* 1998;159:920–924.
25. Catalona WJ, Stein AJ, Fair WR. Grading errors in prostatic needle biopsies: relation to the accuracy of tumor grade in predicting pelvic lymph node metastases. *J Urol* 1982;127: 919–922.
26. Babaian RJ, Grunow WA. Reliability of Gleason grading system in comparing prostate biopsies with total prostatectomy specimens. *Urology* 1985;25:564–567.
27. Bostwick DG. Gleason grading of prostatic needle biopsies. Correlation with grade in 316 matched prostatectomies. *J Surg Pathol* 1994;18:796–803.
28. Cookson MS, Fleshner NE, Soloway SM, et al. Correlation between Gleason score of needle biopsy and radical prostatectomy specimen: accuracy and clinical implications. *J Urol* 1997;157:559–562.
29. Thickman D, Speers WC, Philpott PJ, et al. Effect of number of core biopsies of the prostate on predicting Gleason score of prostate cancer. *J Urol* 1996;156:110–113.
30. Fleshner NE, Cookson MS, Soloway SM, et al. Repeat transrectal ultrasound-guided prostate biopsy: a strategy to improve reliability of needle biopsy grading in patients with well differentiated prostate cancer. *Urology* 1998;52:659–662.
31. Cohen SM, Ellwein LB. Cell proliferation in carcinogenesis. *Science* 1990;249:1007–1111.
32. McNeal JE, Villers AA, Redwine EA, et al. Histologic differentiation, cancer volume and pelvic lymph node metastasis in adenocarcinoma of the prostate. *Cancer* 1990;66:1225–1233.
33. McNeal JE. Cancer volume and site of origin of adenocarcinoma in the prostate: relationship to local and distant spread. *Hum Pathol* 1992;23:258–266.
34. Terris MK, McNeal JE, Stamey TA. Detection of clinically significant prostate cancer by transrectal ultrasound-guided systematic biopsies. *J Urol* 1992;148:829–832.

35. Hammerer P, Huland H, Sparenberg A. Digital rectal examination, imaging, and systematic sextant biopsy in identifying operable lymph node-negative prostatic carcinoma. *Eur Urol* 1992;22:281–287.
36. Dietrick DD, McNeal JE, Stamey TA. Core cancer length in ultrasound-guided systematic sextant biopsies: a preoperative evaluation of prostate cancer volume. *Urology* 1995;45:987–992.
37. Weldon VE, Tavel FR, Neuwirth H, et al. Failure of focal prostate cancer on biopsy to predict focal prostate cancer: the importance of prevalence. *J Urol* 1995;154:1074–1077.
38. Cupp MR, Bostwick DG, Myers RP, et al. The volume of prostate cancer in the biopsy specimen cannot reliably predict the quantity of cancer in the radical prostatectomy specimen on an individual basis. *J Urol* 1995;153:1543–1548.
39. Goto Y, Ohori M, Arakawa A, et al. Distinguishing clinically important from unimportant prostate cancers before treatment: value of systematic biopsies. *J Urol* 1996;156:1059–1063.
40. Egevad L, Norberg M, Mattson S, et al. Estimation of prostate cancer volume by multiple core biopsies before radical prostatectomy. *Urology* 1998;52:653–658.
41. Ravery V, Boccon-Gibod LA, Dauge-Geffroy MC, et al. Systematic biopsies accurately predict extracapsular extension of prostate cancer and persistent/recurrent detectable PSA after radical prostatectomy. *Urology* 1994;44:371–376.
42. Peller PA, Young DC, Marmaduke DP, et al. Sextant prostate biopsies. A histopathologic correlation with radical prostatectomy specimens. *Cancer* 1995;75:530–538.
43. Huland H, Hammerer P, Henke RP, et al. Preoperative prediction of tumor heterogeneity and recurrence after radical prostatectomy for localized prostatic carcinoma with digital rectal examination, prostate specific antigen and the results of 6 systematic biopsies. *J Urol* 1996;155:1344–1347.
44. D'Amico AV, Whittington R, Malkowicz SB, et al. Combined modality staging of prostate carcinoma and its utility in predicting pathologic stage and postoperative prostate specific antigen failure. *Urology* 1997;49:23–30.
45. Borirakchanyavat S, Bhargava V, Shinohara K, et al. Systematic sextant biopsies in the prediction of extracapsular extension at radical prostatectomy. *Urology* 1997;50:373–378.
46. Presti JC Jr., Shinohara K, Bacchetti P, et al. The positive fraction of systematic biopsies predicts risk of relapse after radical prostatectomy. *Urology* 1998;52:1079–1084.
47. Tigrani V, Bhargava V, Shinohara K, et al. Number of positive systematic sextant biopsies predicts surgical margin status at radical prostatectomy. *Urology* 1999;54:689–693.

17

PATHOLOGY

JONATHAN I. EPSTEIN

PROSTATIC INTRAEPITHELIAL NEOPLASIA

Definition and Terminology

In 1986, McNeal published an article on a premalignant lesion of the prostate that he termed *intraductal dysplasia* (1). This lesion consists of architecturally benign prostatic acini or ducts lined by cytologically atypical cells (Fig. 17-1). Although prostatic intraepithelial neoplasia (PIN) is characterized by nuclear atypia, there are often accompanying architectural abnormalities, including flat, tufting, papillary, and cribriform patterns (2). Intraductal dysplasia was initially subcategorized into three grades. Grade 1 intraductal dysplasia (mild dysplasia) was characterized by increased nuclear size with increased variability of nuclear size, along with irregular focal crowding and multilayering. In grade 2 intraductal dysplasia (moderate dysplasia), there were similar features to grade 1 dysplasia, with the additional finding of hyperchromatism and occasional small prominent nucleoli. The hallmark of grade 3 intraductal dysplasia (severe dysplasia) was the finding of numerous large prominent nucleoli. Over the ensuing years, the diagnostic criteria proposed by McNeal have generally been adopted as the accepted method of grading cytologically atypical lesions within the prostate. However, various criticisms of the term *intraductal dysplasia* were raised, and other nomenclatures were championed. The opposition for the term *dysplasia* is that it is often used to describe abnormalities in embryogenesis such as *dysplastic kidney*. Others note that the atypical lesions within the prostate often do not occur within large ducts but within acini. The most widely used synonym for intraductal dysplasia is PIN. This term has some advantages, given that it is relatively recent and has not been used by different authors to denote different lesions. Using the PIN terminology, PIN1 equals mild dysplasia, PIN2 equals moderate dysplasia, and PIN3 equals severe dysplasia. Most authorities, including this author, use the terms high-grade PIN to encompass both PIN2 and PIN3 and low-grade PIN for PIN1.

Incidence of Prostatic Intraepithelial Neoplasia in Prostates with and without Infiltrating Cancer

Much of the indirect evidence that associates PIN with carcinoma of the prostate has come from studies examining differences between prostate glands with carcinoma and prostate glands without carcinoma (3). Studies addressing these differences antedated the use of the terminology low-grade PIN and high-grade PIN, and rather used PIN1, PIN2, and PIN3.

Prostatic Intraepithelial Neoplasia 1

The exact incidence of PIN1 in glands with and without carcinoma is difficult to determine from the literature. Studies by McNeal and Bostwick (1) and Troncoso (4) report only the dominant grade of PIN or the worst grade of PIN, such that the number of cases with PIN1 were often obscured by cases with higher-grade PIN. Another explanation of why these studies underrepresented the incidence of PIN1 in benign glands is that most of these studies used autopsy specimens, in which subtle and focal degrees of PIN1 would not be identifiable.

Histologic identification of the mildest forms of atypia in almost any organ system is extremely subjective and carries with it the least clinical significance. In a subsequent work by McNeal, the following quotation summarizes his consideration of PIN1: "There is not a sharp line of demarcation between grade 1 dysplasia and mild degrees of deviation from normal histology" (5). We have demonstrated that, even among genitourinary pathologists, there is a lack of consensus as to the distinction between PIN1 and variations of normal histology (6). For this reason and the lack of its clinical significance, to be described later, we do not comment on low-grade PIN in diagnostic reports.

Prostatic Intraepithelial Neoplasia 2

As with PIN1, it is difficult to determine the incidence of PIN2 in glands with and without carcinoma, because several of the larger studies have only reported the worst grade of PIN in a gland. Consequently, glands with PIN3 and PIN2 would not be recorded as showing PIN2. The frequency of PIN2 in benign prostates ranges from 11% to 68%. The figure that I believe is most credible is that 68% of benign glands without infiltrating cancer contain PIN2 (7). This figure was derived from well-fixed cystoprostatectomy specimens, in contrast to prostates studied at autopsy. There are no data reporting the incidence of PIN2 in prostates with cancer that are not confounded by the incidence of PIN3, which is often the worst PIN seen in these glands.

Prostatic Intraepithelial Neoplasia 3

It appears that between 15% and 18% of glands without carcinoma may have foci of PIN3. The incidences of PIN3 in prostates with carcinoma differ to a greater extent, ranging from approximately 33% in autopsy studies, to 72% in surgical specimens performed for transitional cell carcinoma, to 100% in radical prostatectomy specimens performed for carcinoma of the prostate.

Relationship of Prostatic Intraepithelial Neoplasia to Carcinoma of the Prostate

Histologic and Morphometric Evidence

In addition to an increased incidence of higher-grade PIN, it has also been noted that the size of PIN foci and the number of PIN foci are increased in prostate glands with carcinoma as compared to glands without carcinoma (3). Also, with increasing amounts of PIN there is a greater number of multifocal carcinomas. This observation follows whether PIN is a precursor to some carcinomas, because with more precursor lesions one would expect that there would be more early carcinomas. The finding of zones of high-grade PIN, from which there appears to be budding off glands of carcinoma, is further histologic evidence that PIN is a precursor to some prostate carcinomas. McNeal has designated these foci as *transitive glands*, although most other investigators prefer the term *PIN with microinvasive carcinoma* (7). Several studies have also noted an increase of PIN in the peripheral zone of the prostate corresponding to the site of origin for most adenocarcinomas of the prostate (3). All these findings would be expected if PIN were a precursor lesion to carcinoma of the prostate.

Montironi has studied the histologic features of PIN more rigorously with computer-assisted morphometric measurements (8). The following features were intermediate in PIN as compared to epithelial cells in benign prostate glands and cancer: nuclear size, nuclear size variability, nucleolar size, nucleolar number, and nucleolar eccentricity. Other parameters investigated included nuclear stratification and nuclear crowding.

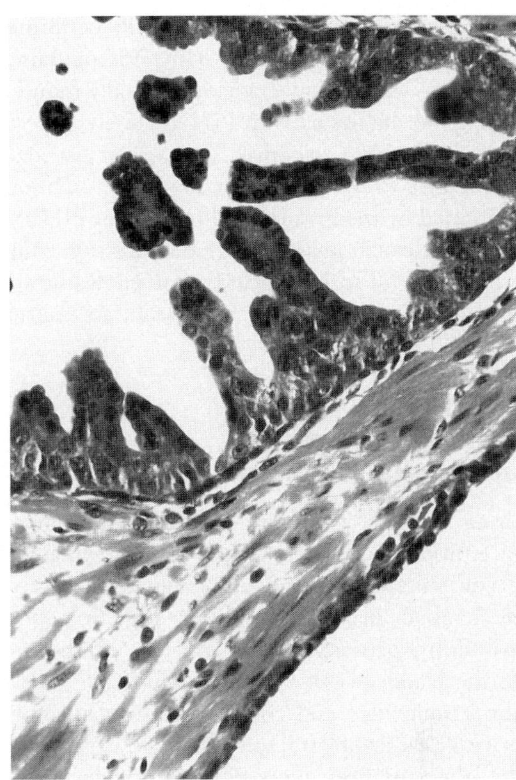

FIGURE 17-1. High-grade prostatic intraepithelial neoplasia (PIN). Note the cytologically atypical cells with prominent nucleoli in the architecturally benign gland. Contrast cytology in PIN to benign glands in upper right and left corners.

Histochemical, Immunohistochemical, and Genetic Evidence

There is a growing body of data demonstrating that the expression of various biomarkers is either (a) the same in PIN and carcinoma, as opposed to benign prostate glands, or (b) intermediate between benign glands and carcinoma (3,9,10).

In many cases, ploidy results in high-grade PIN, also parallel those seen in carcinomas. Studies that have used image analysis techniques rather than flow cytometry have, in general, demonstrated ploidy patterns in PIN that are intermediate between benign glands and cancer (3). In general, diploid high-grade PIN may be associated with adjacent tumors that are either diploid or aneuploid. In contrast, carcinomas adjacent to aneuploid foci of high-grade PIN are almost invariably aneuploid as well.

Relationship of Prostatic Intraepithelial Neoplasia to Cancer: Influence of Location and Tumor Grade

Intermediate-grade multifocal carcinomas, as well as peripherally located low- or intermediate-grade carcinomas, are associated with adjacent PIN to a much higher extent than are low-grade transition zone adenocarcinomas (11–13). These low-grade, centrally located adenocarcinomas tend to be the tumors that are incidentally found in transurethral resections of the prostate (TURP) performed for presumed prostatic hyperplasia. This finding raises the question as to whether low-grade, incidentally found carcinomas may not be linked with PIN as closely as peripherally located palpable carcinomas. This weaker association of high-grade PIN to transition zone low-grade carcinomas is also supported by the histologic differences of PIN as compared to these carcinomas. Low-grade transition zone adenocarcinomas tend to have bland cytologic features, often lacking nuclear enlargement or nucleoli, in contrast to high-grade PIN.

Mimickers of Prostatic Intraepithelial Neoplasia

PIN must, on one hand, be distinguished from several benign entities, and, on the other, be differentiated from variants of infiltrating carcinoma. Benign mimickers of PIN include a variant of normal histology with Roman bridge and cribriform patterns seen at the base of the prostate toward the bladder (14). Clear-cell cribriform hyperplasia can also mimic PIN and consists of crowded cribriform glands with clear cytoplasm, sometimes growing as a nodule and, in other instances, more diffusely, usually within the transition zone (15). It has been recognized that otherwise typical basal cell hyperplasia may show prominent nucleoli, along with mitotic activity (16). Because of the prominent nucleoli, these lesions may be mistaken for PIN.

In some cases, it is impossible to distinguish a focus of cribriform PIN from cribriform Gleason pattern 3 adenocarcinoma (14). Although the distinction between cribriform Gleason pattern 3 and cribriform PIN may be difficult, from a diagnostic standpoint, this is usually not critical. Almost always, when there is cribriform Gleason pattern 3, the cribriform glands are accompanied by small, infiltrating glands of cancer, in which the diagnosis of infiltrating tumor can be made. Only when cribriform glands are so large or back to back, or both, that they are inconsistent with cribriform PIN should infiltrating cribriform carcinoma be diagnosed on hematoxylin and eosin–stained sections in the absence of small infiltrating glands. Immunohistochemistry with antibodies to high-molecular-weight keratin can be used in difficult cases to differentiate these two entities. In the setting of numerous cribriform glands, in which the differential diagnosis is cribriform PIN versus cribriform carcinoma, a negative reaction in all of the glands is diagnostic of carcinoma; positive staining, even if patchy, verifies the lesion as cribriform PIN.

A more difficult distinction is between cribriform PIN and the rarer ductal (endometrioid) adenocarcinoma of the prostate (17–19). Ductal adenocarcinomas are aggressive tumors often of advanced pathologic stage and associated with a poor prognosis. Consequently, their distinction from cribriform PIN is critical.

Significance of Prostatic Intraepithelial Neoplasia on Biopsy Material

As discussed earlier, the finding of low-grade PIN (PIN1) is common in entirely benign prostates and subjective and difficult to distinguish from normal or slightly reactive epithelium (6). Consequently, we do not comment on low-grade PIN on biopsy material. Furthermore, when low-grade PIN is diagnosed on needle biopsy, studies have shown that the likelihood of cancer's being detected on repeat biopsy is no higher than in men whose initial biopsies reveal benign prostate tissue (20,21).

The incidence of high-grade PIN on needle biopsy in the absence of carcinoma is controversial, varying from 1.5% to 16.5% (22–27). In our material, the incidence is 5.5% (26). Although variable patient populations might account for some of these differences, the most likely etiology is different thresholds for diagnosing high-grade PIN. In men with high-grade PIN on biopsy, the reported likelihood of cancer's being detected on subsequent biopsy is between 33% and 50% (21,28–32). There are conflicting data as to whether an abnormal rectal examination, abnormal ultrasound, or elevated serum prostate-specific antigen (PSA) level identifies patients who are more likely to have carcinoma on follow-up biopsies. It does not appear that high-grade PIN by itself gives rise to elevated serum PSA values (33). One rationale for combining PIN2 and PIN3 into "high-grade PIN" is that even genitourinary pathologists cannot reproducibly distinguish between PIN2 and PIN3 (6). It is not surprising that ultrasound does not discriminate between cases with only PIN from those with PIN and carcinoma, because it has been demonstrated that high-grade PIN may appear indistinguishable from cancer as a hypoechoic lesion (34). It has been demonstrated that when cancer is found on repeat biopsy, it may be anywhere in the gland, not only at the initial site in which the high-grade PIN was found (35). Consequently, repeat sextant biopsies should be performed when high-grade PIN is found on needle biopsy. When high-grade PIN is found on a biopsy that also contains cancer, the PIN is of no clinical significance.

There is relatively scant information as to the significance of finding high-grade PIN on transurethral resection (TUR) (36–38). The current management of a patient with high-grade PIN on TUR, is in large part determined by the patient's age. In an elderly patient with high-grade PIN on TUR after ruling out a clinically significant tumor on rectal examination, probably no further management would be instigated. The finding of high-grade PIN on TUR in a younger individual would trigger a more aggressive workup to rule out a clinically significant tumor. This might include, in addition to rectal examination, the performance of transrectal ultrasound and sextant biopsies.

Treatment of Prostatic Intraepithelial Neoplasia

Several studies have demonstrated that the extent and prevalence of high-grade PIN are substantially decreased in prostates that have been treated with androgen deprivation for 3 months before radical prostatectomy (39,40). These findings indicate that the dysplastic cells of high-grade PIN are hormone dependent, as are normal secretory cells. As high-grade PIN appears to be a precursor to many prostate cancers, hormone deprivation may become a means of preventing or decreasing the risk of malignant transformation. Whether less potent methods of hormone therapy, such as 5α–reductase inhibitors, also inhibit high-grade PIN is unknown. Another possibility that must also be considered is that the apparent decrease in PIN lacks biologic significance; despite the lack of morphologic PIN, the cells could still harbor a genetic predisposition to progress into carcinoma.

Prostatic Intraepithelial Neoplasia versus Carcinoma *In Situ*

Based on much of the data presented herein, high-grade PIN appears to be a precursor to some forms of carcinoma of the prostate. For these reasons, some individuals believe that high-grade PIN should be termed *carcinoma* in situ (CIS). However, the one piece of evidence that we do have for premalignant lesions in other organs that is lacking in the prostate is the natural history of high-grade PIN. With the prostate, there is currently no capability of monitoring a PIN focus to determine whether (a) there is not already infiltrating carcinoma at that site or (b) when infiltrating carcinoma evolves, has it done so in the immediate vicinity of the PIN focus? There are a few reports of prostatic lesions seen on ultrasound in which PIN was found on biopsy, and then the patient was followed for relatively short periods of time, subsequently to be shown to have infiltrating carcinoma (41). High-grade PIN has also been reported on fine-needle aspiration biopsy, in which the patient was followed and later demonstrated to have infiltrating carcinoma (42). Although these cases were interpreted as showing evolution from PIN to carcinoma, more likely, the infiltrating component was already present at the time of the initial biopsy or aspiration and was not sampled. Because we do not know, when high-grade PIN is found on biopsy material what percentage of patients develop infiltrating carcinoma over a given follow-up interval, most authorities do not use the term *CIS of the prostate.* The term has implications that these lesions will develop into infiltrating carcinoma at a sufficiently high frequency that may lead some aggressive clinicians to treat these lesions in a radical fashion. Given that there is still controversy as to whether even infiltrating adenocarcinoma of the prostate should always be treated aggressively, it is doubtful that these potential precursor lesions should be treated by aggressive therapy until their natural history is better understood. These same arguments against the use of CIS reflect the one negative aspect of the term PIN, because its relationship to carcinoma will generally be assumed to parallel that seen within cervical intraepithelial neoplasia of the cervix by virtue of their similar terminology. However, our understanding of the natural history of cytologically atypical lesions within the prostate is not nearly as well defined as in the cervix.

Given the information presented previously, one might assume that PIN is a universal precursor lesion to prostatic adenocarcinomas. However, there are some data that raise questions regarding the relationship of PIN to carcinomas. In a recent study by Sakr et al. from Wayne State University, the onset of high-grade PIN was noted to have occurred later than the onset of carcinoma (43). This is at odds to what one would expect if PIN were a precursor lesion to all prostate cancers. Furthermore, 70% of the prostates with early carcinomas lacked any high-grade PIN within the entirely embedded prostate gland. In addition, even in those prostate glands, in which there existed early cancer and high-grade PIN, only in one-third of the cases was the PIN adjacent to cancer. Other evidence against PIN's being a universal precursor to prostatic carcinomas is that transition zone cancers uncommonly show adjacent PIN.

ADENOCARCINOMA

Location

Almost all stage T2 and T3 (palpable) tumors and 85% of stage T1c tumors are primarily peripherally up against the edge of the prostate (44–46). Tumors diagnosed on TUR (stage T1a and T1b) and 15% of stage T1c cases are predominantly located in the transition zone (i.e., periurethrally or anteriorly). Tumors that appear to be unilateral on rectal examination are bilateral in approximately 70% of cases when examined pathologically. Adenocarcinoma of the prostate is multifocal in more than 85% of cases (45). In many of these cases of bilateral or multifocal, or both, tumors, the other tumors are small, low grade, and clinically insignificant.

Spread of Tumor

The prostate lacks a discrete histologic capsule, such that the term *capsular invasion*, describing tumors extending into the "capsule," has no validity (47). Although we and others used to diagnose tumors out of the prostate as showing *capsular penetration*, we currently refer to tumors out of the prostate as exhibiting *extraprostatic extension.* Cases without extraprostatic extension are considered *organ confined.* Peripherally located adenocarcinomas of the prostate tend to extend out of the prostate via perineural space invasion (48). Perineural invasion in a radical prostatectomy specimen by itself does not worsen the prognosis, because perineural invasion merely represents extension of a tumor along a plane of decreased resistance and not invasion into lymphatics (49). Extraprostatic extension preferentially occurs posteriorly and posterolaterally, paralleling the location of most adenocarcinomas.

Further local spread of tumors may lead to seminal vesicle invasion, which is diagnosed when a tumor extends into the muscular wall of the seminal vesicle. The most common route of seminal vesicle invasion is by the extension of a tumor out of the prostate at the base of the gland (50). The tumor then extends into the periseminal vesicle soft tissue and eventually into the seminal vesicles. Less commonly, there may be direct extension through the ejaculatory ducts into the seminal vesicles or direct extension from the base of the prostate into the wall of the seminal vesicles. Least commonly, there may be discrete metastases to the seminal vesicle, which one study found to have a better prognosis (51).

Tumor Volume

In general, prostate cancer tumor volume correlates with tumor aggressiveness (52). Extraprostatic extension is uncommon in tumors smaller than 0.5 cc. Tumors that are smaller than 4 cc uncommonly reveal lymph node metastases or seminal vesicle invasion. Tumor volume is also proportional to the grade. The location and grade of the tumor also modulate the effect of tumor volume (52,53). For example, periurethrally located (i.e., transition zone) tumors, as a result of their lower grade and greater distance from the edge of the gland, tend to achieve larger volumes than peripheral zone tumors before they exhibit extraprostatic extension.

Grade

The most widely used grading system for prostate cancer is the Gleason system (54,55). There are several unique aspects of the Gleason grading system. First, the Gleason grading system is solely based on the architectural pattern (Fig. 17-2). Cytologic features are not factored in. The second unique feature of the Gleason grading system is that the overall grade is not based on the highest grade within the tumor. Gleason and the Veterans' Administration Cooperative Study found that the prognosis of prostate cancer was intermediate between that of the most predominant pattern of cancer and the second most predominant pattern. Consequently, the Gleason grading system factors in the most prevalent pattern (Gleason pattern 1) and the second most prevalent pattern (Gleason pattern 2). These two patterns are added together to arrive at a *Gleason score.* Synonyms for Gleason score include *Gleason sum* and *combined Gleason grade.*

Gleason patterns 1 and 2 tumors are composed of relatively circumscribed nodules of uniform, single, separate, closely packed medium sized glands (Figs. 17-3 and 17-4).

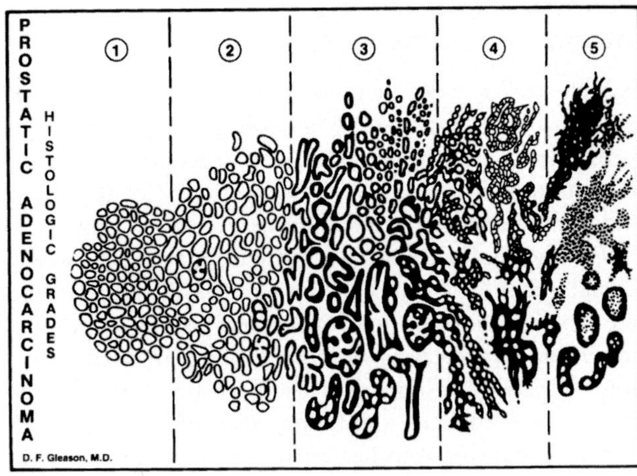

FIGURE 17-2. Schematic diagram of Gleason grading system.

Gleason pattern 3 tumor infiltrates in and among the nonneoplastic prostate, and the glands have marked variation in size and shape, with smaller glands than seen in Gleason patterns 1 or 2 (Fig. 17-5). Gleason pattern 4 glands are no longer single and separate as seen in patterns 1 to 3. In Gleason pattern 4, one may also see large irregular cribriform glands as opposed to the smoothly circumscribed smaller nodules of cribriform Gleason pattern 3 (Fig. 17-6). Gleason pattern 5 tumor shows no glandular differentiation, composed of solid sheets, cords, single cells, or solid nests of

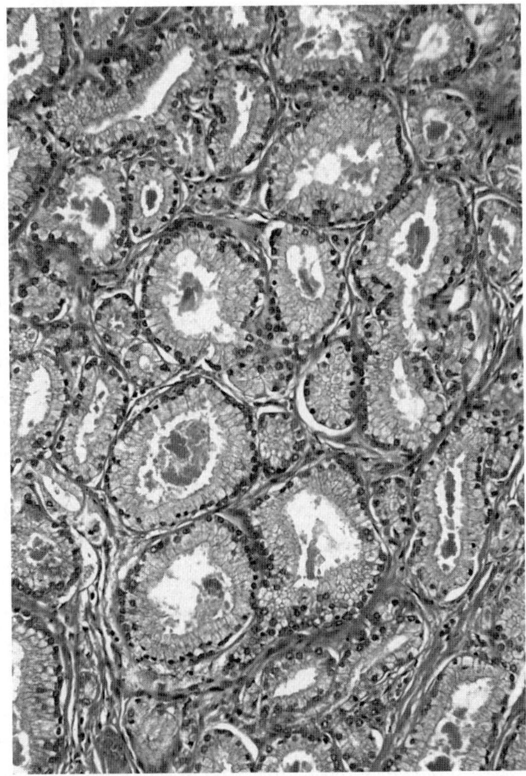

FIGURE 17-3. Gleason pattern 1 tumor consists of closely packed uniform large glands.

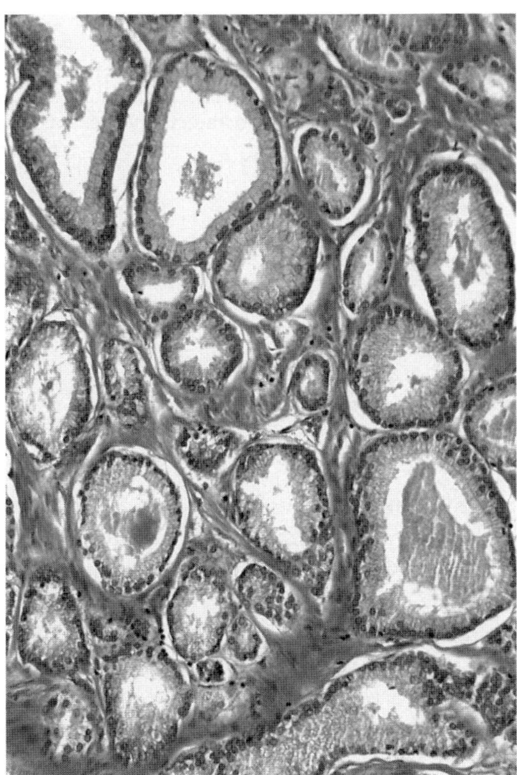

FIGURE 17-4. Gleason pattern 2 tumor has similar large, fairly uniform, pale-staining glands with greater separation and minimal variation of gland size and shape between glands as compared to Gleason pattern 1. (From Epstein JI. *Interpretation of prostate biopsies*, 2nd ed. New York: Raven Press, 1995, with permission.)

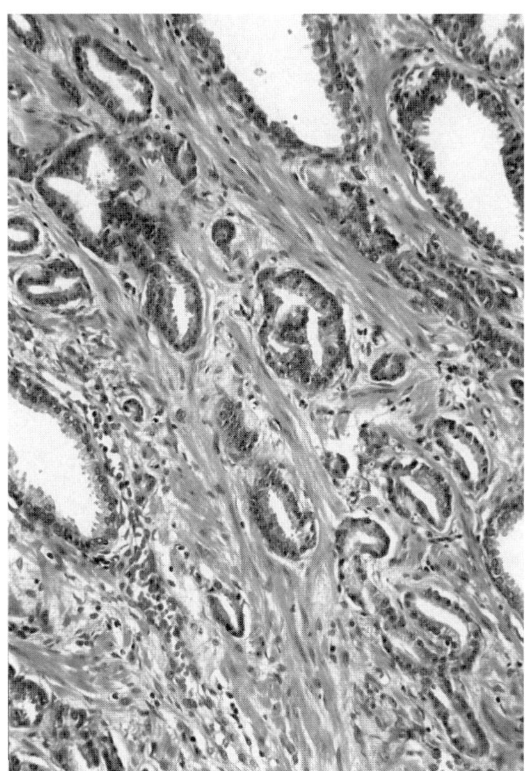

FIGURE 17-5. Gleason pattern 3 with a greater variability in gland size as compared to a lower-grade tumor. At least some of the glands are smaller than seen in Gleason patterns 1 and 2. The glands infiltrate in between larger benign glands (*upper right*).

tumor with central comedonecrosis (Fig. 17-7). The following combination of Gleason scores results in groups of similar prognosis: Gleason score 2 to 4 (well differentiated), Gleason score 5 to 6 (moderately differentiated), Gleason score 7 (moderately poorly differentiated), and Gleason 8 to 10 (poorly differentiated) (56).

A point to note in the Gleason schematic diagram is that there are no sharp demarcations between the various Gleason patterns. Rather, there is a gradual transition from one pattern into the other. One could, therefore, see how a tumor that straddles between a Gleason pattern 3 and Gleason pattern 4 could, by one pathologist, be read out as a Gleason pattern 3 (on the poorly differentiated side), whereas another pathologist would read it out as a Gleason pattern 4 (on the better-differentiated side). Furthermore, different pathologists may have different thresholds as to, for example, how many poorly formed glands are needed to diagnose Gleason pattern 4.

Distribution of Gleason Patterns

The distribution of the various Gleason patterns may be skewed depending on the type of surgical specimen. In radical prostatectomy specimens seen at The Johns Hopkins Hospital, only 6% of cases are assigned a Gleason score of 2 to 4 and 9.7% a Gleason score of 8 to 9 (57). The majority of cases is Gleason scores 5 to 6 (53.8%) or Gleason score 7 (30.5%). In contrast, Gleason scores 2 to 4 tumors are more frequently seen on TUR (53). This discrepancy reflects the prevalence of Gleason scores 2 to 4 tumors in the transition zone (i.e., periurethral region), in which the tumors tend to be fairly small and of low stage. In signing out a radical prostatectomy specimen, one usually assigns the grade to the dominant tumor (i.e., index tumor). Smaller, multifocal low-grade cancers are not incorporated within the grade of index tumor. Low-grade carcinomas are also infrequently seen on needle biopsy (1%), as it is uncommon for the needle biopsy to sample these anteriorly located small tumors (58). At the other end of the spectrum, high-grade tumors uncommonly come to radical prostatectomy, as many of these tumors are advanced and not amenable to surgery.

Prognosis

Gleason's data with 2,911 patients and subsequent studies with long-term follow-up have demonstrated a good correlation between Gleason score and prognosis (55,59). When stage of disease is factored in with the grade, prognostication is enhanced (55). Gleason score correlates

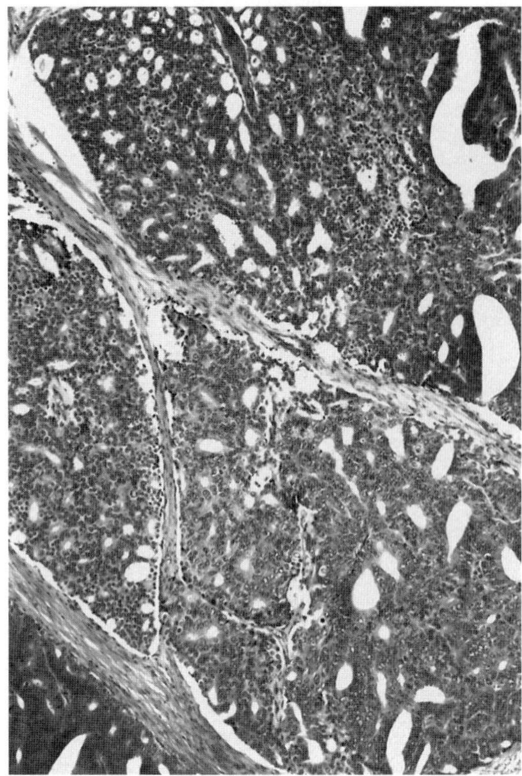

FIGURE 17-6. Gleason pattern 4 consisting of large irregular cribriform glands.

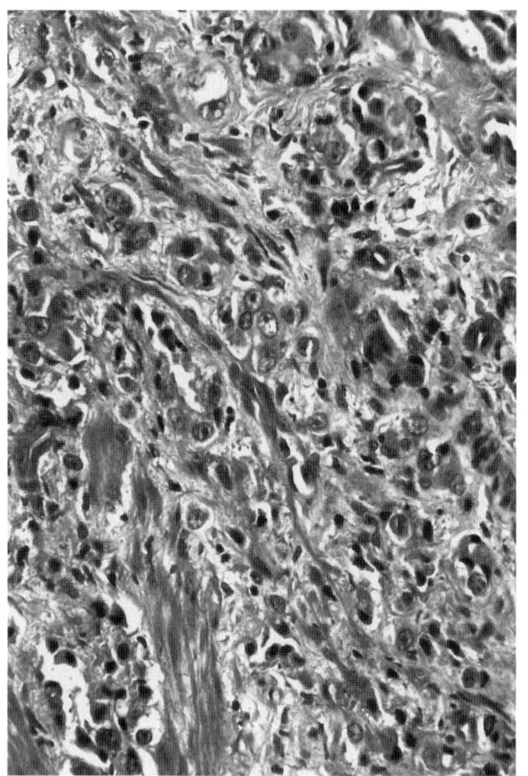

FIGURE 17-7. Gleason pattern 5 composed of solid nests of cells without gland formation.

TABLE 17-1. CORRELATION OF RADICAL PROSTATECTOMY GLEASON GRADE WITH P STAGE AND MARGINS IN 988 MEN (1994–1998)

	Radical prostatectomy Gleason score			
Stage	5–6 (%)	7 (%)	8–10 (%)	Total (%)
Organ-confined	78	43	13	66
Focal EPE	11	17	4	13
Established EPE	9	25	33	15
SV invasion	1	7	17	3
Node metastases	1	8	33	3
Positive margins	5	10	20	7

EPE, extraprostatic extension; SV, seminal vesicles.

with all prognostic variables seen at radical prostatectomy and with prognosis after radical prostatectomy (Table 17-1). Gleason score 7 tumors behave significantly worse than Gleason scores 5 to 6 tumors and should not be combined as "intermediate-grade carcinoma" (56,57,60). Gleason score 7 tumors do, however, fare better than Gleason scores 8 to 9 tumors. Biopsy Gleason scores can also be combined with serum PSA values and clinical stage to predict organ-confined versus non–organ-confined disease and risk of progression after radical prostatectomy (61,62).

Correlation between Biopsy and Radical Prostatectomy Specimen

There have been several studies correlating core biopsy and radical prostatectomy grade (58,63,64). In a recent study, needle biopsies were graded at various institutions throughout the country and then regraded by various staff pathologists at The Johns Hopkins Hospital before patients underwent radical prostatectomy (58). Whereas 87 of 390 (23%) of needle biopsies were assigned a Gleason score of 2 to 4 on the outside, only four (1%) of these needle biopsies were graded as Gleason scores 2 to 4 at Hopkins. Of the 87 cases graded as Gleason scores 2 to 4 at outside institutions, 18 had focal extraprostatic extension, 26 had more extensive extraprostatic disease, and four had either seminal vesicle invasion or lymph node metastases. Although the few cases on biopsy graded by Hopkins pathologists as Gleason scores 2 to 4 were organ confined at the time of radical prostatectomy, the prostatectomy grade in all of these cases was Gleason scores 5 to 6.

This widespread undergrading of needle biopsies has potentially serious implications. Some clinicians, when they receive a needle biopsy report of adenocarcinoma of the prostate with a Gleason score of 2 to 4, will assume that these are low-grade indolent tumors and potentially follow these patients conservatively. However, 55% of the tumors that were assigned a Gleason score of 2 to 4 on needle biopsy by outside institutions were not organ confined at

TABLE 17-2. CORRELATION OF GLEASON SCORE BETWEEN BIOPSY AND RADICAL PROSTATECTOMY (BOTH GRADED AT THE JOHNS HOPKINS HOSPITAL)

	Radical prostatectomy score				
Biopsy score	2–4	5–6	7	8–9	Total
2–4	—	5	1	—	6
5–6	2	225	126	4	357
7	—	16	91	13	120
8–9	—	—	3	13	16
Total	2	246	221	30	499

Note: Dark shade corresponds to an exact match. Light shade reflects discordance by one category.

the time of radical prostatectomy. This misconception that low-grade cancer on needle biopsy correlates with indolent behavior in part relates to several publications that have demonstrated that low-grade carcinomas on TURPs behave fairly indolently if present in limited quantity (65). Low-grade cancer on TURP often represents sampling of low-grade transition zone cancers that, if limited in extent, have, in general, an indolent course (66). However, the finding of low-grade cancer on needle biopsy almost always reflects undergrading of the needle biopsy or sampling error, in which a higher-grade tumor was not biopsied (58,67). Whether the Gleason score is 2 to 4 or 5 to 6 on needle biopsy should not alter therapeutic decisions.

In a large study performed at The Johns Hopkins Hospital, a Gleason score of 5 to 6 on biopsy corresponded to the same grade in the radical prostatectomy in 64% of the cases (58) (Table 17-2). When the Gleason score was 7 or higher on biopsy, the radical prostatectomy grade was the same in 87.5% of the cases. In general, adverse findings on needle biopsy accurately predict adverse findings in the radical prostatectomy specimen, whereas favorable findings on the needle biopsy do not necessarily predict favorable findings in the radical prostatectomy specimens, in large part owing to sampling error.

Some pathologists do not assign a grade to small foci of prostate cancer on needle biopsy. We found that the grade assigned to very small cancers on biopsy (less than 1 mm) was just as accurate as compared to cases with more extensive cancer on biopsy (58). We therefore assign both a primary and secondary Gleason pattern to even tiny foci of cancer on needle biopsy. The sampling error between cases with a limited amount of cancer on needle biopsy compared to those with a greater amount of cancer on needle biopsy is not as great, as in cases with greater amounts of cancer on needle biopsy samples, compared to the entire tumor in the radical prostatectomy specimen. One core of prostatic tissue is approximately 1 of 10,000 of the prostate gland. Even cases with fairly extensive cancer on needle biopsy are sampling only a small fraction of the tumor. There is also a practical reason to assigning a primary and secondary pattern to limited cancer on needle biopsy. We have seen some cases signed out as "Gleason grade 4," when the pathologist meant to convey that the tumor was high-grade (i.e., Gleason pattern 4). However, the urologist interpreted it to mean a Gleason score of 4 (i.e., Gleason grade 2 + 2 = 4). By assigning both a primary and secondary pattern, even in cases with a limited amount of cancer, the urologist is clear as to the grade of the tumor.

Sources of Discrepancies between Radical Prostatectomy and Biopsy Grade

In the Hopkins study, we identified four sources of discrepancy between biopsy and radical prostatectomy grade (58). Pathology error was most frequently seen when pathologists assigned a Gleason score of 4 or less on a needle biopsy that, in fact, was a Gleason score of 5 to 6. The other source of discrepancy between biopsy and radical prostatectomy grade was borderline cases. As mentioned earlier, in the description of the Gleason grading system, there are some cases that are right at the interface between two different patterns, in which there will be interobserver variability and possibly even intraobserver variability.

The other common source of discrepancy is sampling error. The more common type of sampling error is when there is a higher-grade component present within the radical prostatectomy specimen that is not sampled on needle biopsy. This typically occurs when a needle biopsy tumor is graded as a Gleason grade 3 + 3 = 6. In the radical prostatectomy, there exists Gleason pattern 4, which was not sampled on the biopsy, resulting in a prostatectomy grade of Gleason grade 3 + 4 = 7. Reverse sampling is less common. In this situation, there is a minute amount of a pattern that is not incorporated in the radical prostatectomy grade, yet it happened to have been sampled on needle biopsy. An example of this would be a tumor that on biopsy is accurately graded as a Gleason grade 3 + 4 = 7. The radical prostatectomy tumor is 99% Gleason pattern 3, with just a minute amount of Gleason pattern 4. The grade assigned to the radical prostatectomy tumor is Gleason grade 3 + 3 = 6.

Interobserver Reproducibility

In a recent study, 46 needle biopsies with adenocarcinoma of the prostate of varying grades were sent to ten different urologic pathologists (68). Gleason scores were grouped according to the following: 2 to 4, 5 to 6, 7, and 8 to 10. In 82.6% of the cases, at least seven of the ten pathologists agreed on the group. Thirty-eight needle biopsies, in which there was greater than or equal to 70% consensus among urologic pathologists, were then sent to 41 different community-based pathologists. Of the cases in which there was a consensus score by the urologic pathologists of 5 to 6, only approximately one-half of the time was the score of 5 to 6 by the general pathologists. In the remaining half of the cases, the tumors were undergraded as Gleason scores 2 to 4. Of the nine cases with a consensus score of Gleason score 7, only approximately half of the cases were correctly assigned a Gleason score of 7 by the general pathologists. Again, there was undergrading, with 43% of the cases being called a Gleason score of 5 to 6 and 5% of the cases being called a Gleason score of 2 to 4. Even with the 16 cases having a consensus Gleason score 8 to 10, there was undergrading, with 17% called a Gleason score of 7 and 6% called a Gleason score of 5 to 6.

We have demonstrated that education programs for pathologists can result in more accurate Gleason grading. Using a web-based tutorial and test, in which we now have more than 1,000 completions on the site, we demonstrated that pathologists were able to significantly improve grading of needle biopsies (69) (http://www.pathology.jhu.edu/prostate).

Evolution in Grade over Time

Some men with low-grade cancers will, after several years, develop high-grade tumors (70). It is unclear whether the residual low-grade cancer progressed or whether there was subsequent development of a multifocal, more aggressive tumor. Although in general, larger tumors are high grade and small tumors low grade, exceptions occur (71). There is a tendency to hypothesize that tumors begin as low-grade tumors and, on reaching a certain size, dedifferentiate into higher-grade lesions, accounting for the relationship between size and grade. Alternatively, high-grade tumors may be high grade at their inception, yet, because of their rapid growth, are detected at an advanced size. Similarly, low-grade tumors may evolve so slowly that they tend to be detected at lower volumes.

Assessment of Needle Biopsies

The diagnosis of adenocarcinoma of the prostate on biopsy is based on a constellation of architectural, cytologic, and ancillary findings that differ from the surrounding benign glands (Fig. 17-8) (72). The underdiagnosis of limited adenocarcinoma of the prostate on needle biopsy is one of the most frequent problems in prostate pathology. It is not uncommon to have several needle biopsy cores of prostatic tissue in which there are only a few malignant glands, which may be difficult to diagnose. There are also numerous benign mimickers of adenocarcinoma of the prostate (14). The most common benign lesions seen on needle biopsy that are mistaken for carcinoma include atrophy, adenosis, and nonspecific granulomatous prostatitis. In some of these cases, the use of antibodies to high-molecular-weight cytokeratin may resolve the diagnosis (73). Benign glands contain basal cells and are labeled with these antibodies, whereas prostate cancer shows no staining. In approximately 5% of needle biopsies, there will be findings suspicious, but not diagnostic of, carcinoma (22–26,74,75). Pathologists should sign out atypical cases descriptively as a "focus of atypical glands" rather than use ambiguous terminology, such as "atypical hyperplasia." A comment should be added in the report describing why the focus is suspicious for cancer yet not diagnostic, with a recommendation for repeat biopsy. In this way, there is no confusion in the urologist's mind that he or she is dealing with a lesion that is likely to be infiltrating cancer, yet the pathologist is not comfortable establishing the diagnosis. Repeat biopsy will reveal prostate cancer in approximately 50% of cases (24,76–78). The risk of finding cancer on repeat biopsy is independent of serum PSA levels and findings on digital rectal examination. If repeat biopsy is negative, then this does not exclude the presence of carcinoma, because prostatic needle biopsies are associated with fairly high false-negative rates (79). We have seen numerous cases in which the first biopsy was called atypical and a repeat biopsy was entirely benign, whereupon review of the initial biopsy, it was diagnostic of cancer. It is incumbent on the pathologist in these cases to have the initial biopsy sent off for consultation or try to resolve the initial biopsy with ancillary techniques, such as immunoperoxidase with antibodies to high-molecular-weight keratin. We have shown that in subsequent biopsies after an atypical biopsy, the chance of detecting cancer is highest in the region of the atypical site (80). We recommend that the repeat biopsy sample three cores from this site. The next most frequent site of finding cancer at repeat biopsy, after an atypical biopsy, is

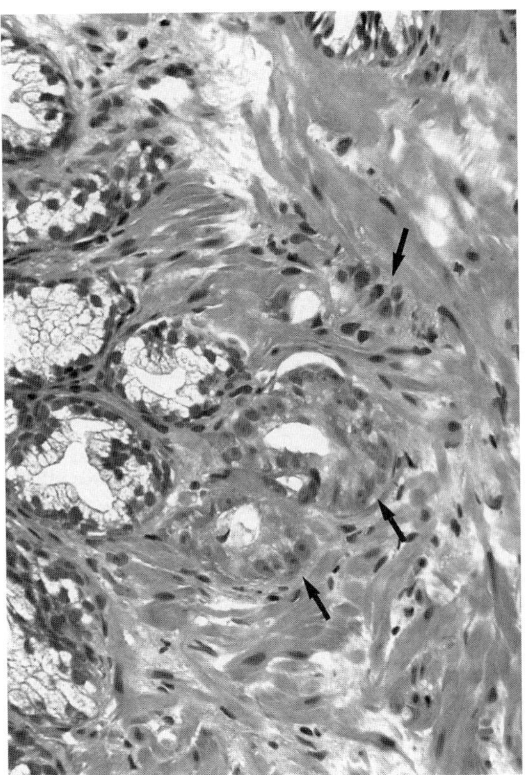

FIGURE 17-8. Minimal cancer on needle biopsy consisting of small, crowded glands infiltrating among larger, benign glands. Note the enlarged nuclei with prominent nucleoli in cancer (*arrows*) as compared to the benign glands (*left*).

TABLE 17-3. CORRELATION BETWEEN NUMBER OF POSITIVE BIOPSY CORES AND PATHOLOGIC STAGE

Number of positive cores	Percent of cases with extraprostatic extension (each number represents a different study)
1	10, 38, 40
2	33, 38, 47
3	38, 54, 60
<4	44
4	69, 77
≥4	70, 75
5	63, 100
5–6	83
6	83, 100

the adjacent contralateral and adjacent ipsilateral areas; we advise that two cores be sampled from each of these sites. One core should be sampled from each remaining sextant, because cancer may also be found away from the initial atypical site. We advocate that biopsies taken from different areas of the prostate should be submitted to the pathologist in separate containers so that rebiopsy of atypical cases can be directed in this more concentrated fashion into and around the region of the initial atypical biopsy.

There are multiple ways in which pathologists may record the extent of cancer on needle biopsy. These include the number of positive cores, the total millimeters of cancer, the total percent of cancer, and the maximal percent of cancer per core. All these measurements have been correlated with measurements of tumor aggressiveness, such as tumor volume, stage, progression, and margins of resection. An equal number of studies claim the superiority of one technique over the other. We recommend that pathologists record the number of cores containing cancer, as the presence of multiple positive cores correlates with adverse findings at radical prostatectomy (26,81–84) (Table 17-3). Pathologists should also record the millimeters of cancer or percent of cancer on biopsy, as these carry prognostic significance. It is important to recognize that limited adenocarcinoma of the prostate on needle biopsy does not necessarily reflect limited cancer within the prostate due to sampling error.

When perineural invasion is seen on needle biopsy, the likelihood of finding extraprostatic extension in the prostatectomy specimen has been reported to range from 32% to 93% (average, 59%) (83,85–90). The absence of perineural invasion on biopsy does not indicate organ-confined disease, with extraprostatic extension reported in 26% to 49% of cases. There are conflicting studies as to whether perineural invasion on needle biopsy provides independent prediction of extraprostatic extension beyond that provided by biopsy Gleason grade and preoperative serum PSA levels. Perineural invasion by prostate cancer on needle biopsy has been shown to predict lymph node metastases and seminal vesicle invasion (86,91). If the urologist, at the time of radical prostatectomy, excises the neurovascular bundle on the same side from which the biopsy demonstrates cancer with perineural invasion came, the incidence of positive margins will decrease from 51.3% to 33.8% (88). Because the finding of perineural invasion on needle biopsy provides prognostic information and is readily performed by the pathologist, it should be recorded on the pathology report.

Assessment of Transurethral Resection Specimens

The staging system that is recommended for tumors that are incidentally found on TURPs done for presumed benign prostatic hypertrophy (BPH) is based on the percentage of the specimen involved by tumor, with 5% being the cutoff between stage T1a and T1b (92). All stage T1b tumors will be detected by processing between six and eight cassettes of a TUR specimen. By processing eight to ten cassettes, more than 90% of stage T1a lesions will be identified (93–96). Depending on the institution, all TUR tissues may be examined in relatively young men (65 years or younger), in whom aggressive therapy for stage T1a disease might be pursued (66). High-grade tumor, which we define as Gleason score of 7 or higher, of any quantity is classified as stage T1b disease.

Radical Prostatectomy Specimens

There are several ways in which radical prostatectomy specimens may be submitted, in part depending on whether tissue is being harvested for research purposes (97–102). Most prostate cancers are peripherally located (i.e., posterior and posterolateral). By examining differences between the left and right halves of the gland, one can usually visualize prostate cancer as a more solid, homogeneous, yellowish-white tissue. In contrast, the normal peripheral zone has a spongier, microcystic appearance. One can submit only those sections containing gross tumor, along with routine margin sections, the apex, and base of the seminal vesicles (100). We recommend submitting the whole prostate if the prostate is small. In cases with no grossly evident tumor, either the entire prostate is submitted or, if it is large, the posterior halves are submitted. By submitting the posterior halves, sampling of the transition zone will also be accomplished. We do not believe it is necessary to perform whole-mount sections. Whole-mount sections add nothing to that of processing specimens in a routine fashion. The handling of radical prostatectomies using whole-mount sections is much more cumbersome, requiring specialized processing techniques, storage facilities, materials, and dedicated technicians. Furthermore, using whole-mount techniques requires a greater fixation period, resulting in a further delay in the diagnosis.

Only 25% of men with seminal vesicle invasion and none with lymph node metastases are progression-free at 10

TABLE 17-4. KAPLAN-MEIER ESTIMATES OF RISK OF PROGRESSION WITH NEGATIVE SEMINAL VESICLES AND NEGATIVE LYMPH NODES

Prostatectomy pathology	5-yr postprostatectomy (%)	10-yr postprostatectomy (%)
Gleason sum 2–4	0	4
Gleason sum 5–6	3	19
Gleason sum 7	25	50
Gleason sum 8–10	43	66
Organ-confined	0	17
Focal penetration	10	33
Established penetration	24	43
Margins negative	6	22
Margins positive	27	46
Gleason sum 5–6 (OC and MAR–)[a]	1	8
Gleason sum 5–6 (FCP and MAR±) or (ECP and MAR–)[a]	2	23
Gleason sum 5–6 (ECP and MAR+)[a]	15	28
Gleason sum 7 (OC and MAR–)	3	32
Gleason sum 7 (FCP and MAR±) or (ECP and MAR–)	17	52
Gleason sum 7 (ECP and MAR+)	50	58

ECP, established capsular penetration; FCP, focal capsular penetration; MAR+, margins positive; MAR–, margins negative; MAR±, margins positive or negative; OC, organ-confined.
[a]Excluding tumors with Gleason pattern 4.

years after radical prostatectomy (56). The presence of extraprostatic extension and its extent also influence progression (Table 17-4). Pathologists frequently underdiagnose extraprostatic extension. When a tumor penetrates the prostatic gland, it induces a dense desmoplastic response in the periprostatic adipose tissue, in which it can be difficult to judge whether the tumor has extended out of the gland or is within the fibrous tissue of the prostate. Positive margins are another important parameter and disproportionally occur toward the apex (56,103,104). Only approximately 50% of men with positive margins progress after radical prostatectomy (Table 17-4) (56). A major source of this discrepancy is that even in cases in which margins histologically appear to be positive, additional tissue removed from the site does not always show tumor (105). Artifactually positive margins relate to the scant tissue surrounding the prostate, which may easily be disrupted during surgery or the pathologic evaluation of the gland. Margins designated as "close" but negative are not associated with an increased risk of postoperative progression (106).

Gleason grade, extraprostatic extension, and margins of resection are all strong, independent predictors of progression (elevated postoperative serum PSA level). A more refined prognostication is not needed for men with Gleason scores 2 to 4, because these men are almost all invariably cured by surgery (Table 17-4). Men with Gleason scores 8 to 10 have a poor prognosis after prostatectomy (Table 17-4), with nodal metastases as the major prognostic determinant. Of cases with negative seminal vesicles and lymph nodes, Gleason scores 5 to 7 account for 88% of tumors removed by radical prostatectomy and can be stratified into prognostic groups depending on the status of extraprostatic extension and margins (Table 17-4). Tumor volume correlates well with pathologic stage, Gleason grade, and progression after radical prostatectomy (60). However, it has been demonstrated that tumor volume does not independently predict postradical prostatectomy progression once grade and pathologic stage are accounted for (107,108). Consequently, it is not essential that tumor volume be calculated for clinical purposes in radical prostatectomy specimens. Rather, there should be some overall subjective indication of tumor volume to identify those cases with a minute amount of tumor with an excellent prognosis and those with an extensive tumor and a worse prognosis.

Subtypes of Prostatic Adenocarcinoma

Subtypes of prostate cancer, which have a more aggressive course than ordinary prostate cancer, include prostatic ductal adenocarcinoma, mucinous adenocarcinoma of the prostate, and small cell carcinoma.

Although most adenocarcinomas of the prostate are of acinar origin, between 0.4% and 0.8% of prostatic adenocarcinomas arise within prostatic ducts (17–19). These tumors are characterized by tall, pseudostratified columnar cells, in contrast to the single layer of cuboidal cells seen in ordinary (acinar) prostate adenocarcinoma (Fig. 17-9). Ductal adenocarcinomas may be papillary, cribriform, or solid, or composed of individual glands. Prostatic duct adenocarcinomas may be the sole component yet more frequently are admixed with tumors showing acinar differentiation, seen in approximately 5% of prostatic adenocarcinomas. Prostatic duct adenocarcinomas arise in large primary periurethral prostatic ducts, in which they may grow as exophytic lesions

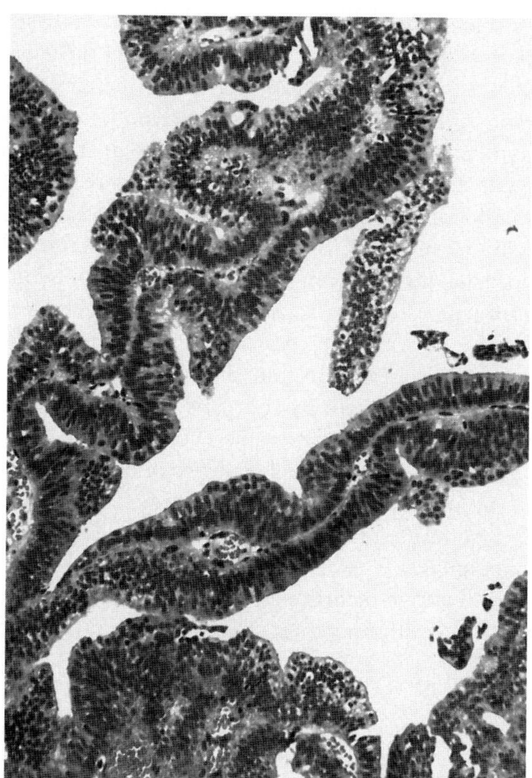

FIGURE 17-9. Ductal adenocarcinoma of the prostate with papillary fronds lined by tall, pseudostratified columnar cells. (From Epstein JI. *Interpretation of prostate biopsies*, 2nd ed. New York: Raven Press, 1995, with permission.)

into the urethra, most commonly in and around the verumontanum. At cystoscopy, these lesions closely resemble papillary transitional cell carcinomas. Often in these cases, the digital rectal examination is normal, and patients present with either obstructive symptoms or gross or microscopic hematuria. Tumors arising in the more peripheral prostatic ducts may or may not have a urethral component and may be palpable on rectal examination.

Because of the histologic resemblance to endometrial carcinoma, as well as the tendency to arise around the verumontanum (a Müllerian remnant), prostatic duct adenocarcinomas were initially considered to be of endometrial origin and were designated as endometrioid carcinomas of the prostate. Subsequent studies have refuted the existence of an endometrial carcinoma of the prostate, showing them to be reactive with prostate-specific acid phosphatase (PSAP) and PSA. Further evidence that these are not endometrial adenocarcinomas is that some of the tumors will respond to hormone therapy and the intimate mingling of ductal and acinar components seen in some tumors. Previous studies have suggested a poor prognosis with conservative management of prostatic duct adenocarcinoma, with an average survival of 36 months (18). Even if treated by radical prostatectomy, the prognosis is poor (19). Compared to acinar carcinomas of similar clinical stage, ductal cancers are larger and occupy a larger proportion of the gland. They show advanced final pathologic stage with 93% having extraprostatic extension, 43% positive margins, 43% seminal vesicle invasion, and 29% positive lymph nodes. They also have a higher short-term risk of progression after radical prostatectomy. When diagnosed on needle biopsy, they are associated with more advanced pathologic stage and increased risk of postradical prostatectomy progression than acinar carcinomas (109).

Mucinous adenocarcinoma of the prostate gland is one of the least common morphologic variants of prostatic carcinoma (110,111). A lack of precision in the definition of these mucinous neoplasms has resulted in reports that have overstated the incidence of this lesion. Using criteria developed for mucinous carcinomas of other organs, the diagnosis of mucinous adenocarcinoma of the prostate gland should be made when at least 25% of the tumor resected contains lakes of extracellular mucin. Histologically, mucinous adenocarcinomas of the prostate are predominantly intermediate-grade tumors, in which a cribriform pattern tends to predominate in the mucinous areas (Fig. 17-10). In contrast to bladder adenocarcinomas, mucinous adenocarcinoma of the prostate rarely contains signet cells. Some carcinomas of the prostate will have a signet ring cell appearance, yet the vacuoles do not contain intracytoplasmic mucin (112). Only a few cases of prostate cancer have been reported with mucin-positive signet cells (113,114).

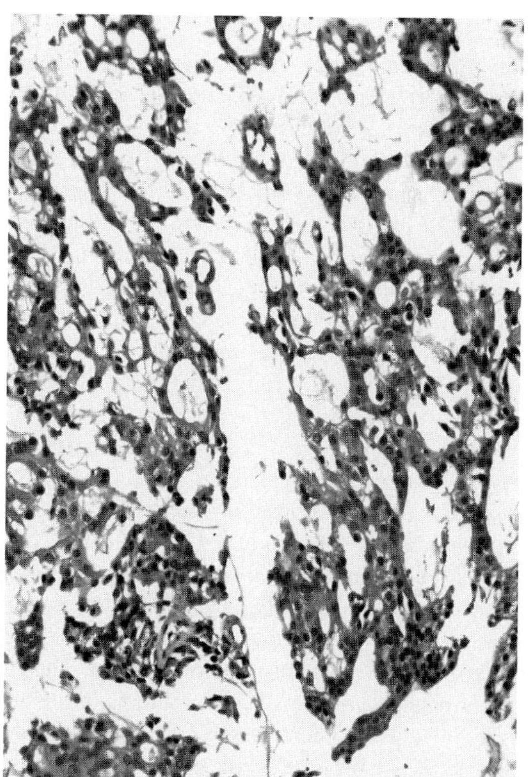

FIGURE 17-10. Mucinous adenocarcinoma of the prostate with cribriform glands floating within mucinous lakes. (From Epstein JI. *Interpretation of prostate biopsies*, 2nd ed. New York: Raven Press, 1995, with permission.)

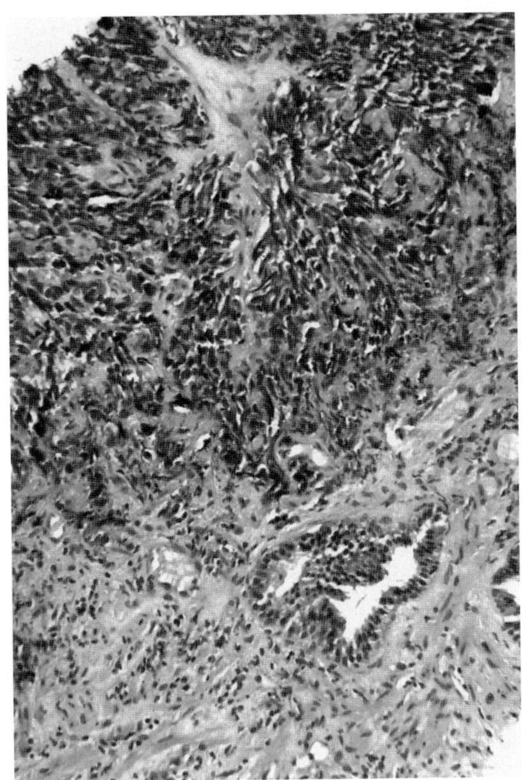

FIGURE 17-11. Mixed small cell (top) and adenocarcinoma of the prostate (bottom). (From Epstein JI. *Interpretation of prostate biopsies*, 2nd ed. New York: Raven Press, 1995, with permission.)

Bladder adenocarcinomas, either when the sole component or admixed with transitional cell elements, may, in a minority of cases, show cross-reactive staining with antisera to PSAP (115). Prostate adenocarcinomas, which are mucinous, behave aggressively (110,111). In the largest reported series, 7 of 12 patients died of the tumor (mean, 5 years), and five were alive with the disease (mean, 3 years). Although these tumors are not as hormonally responsive as their nonmucinous counterparts, some respond to androgen withdrawal. They have a propensity to develop bone metastases and increased serum acid phosphatase and PSA levels with advanced disease.

The most virulent variant of prostate cancer is small cell carcinoma of the prostate (116). In approximately 50% of the cases, the tumors are mixed small cell carcinoma and adenocarcinoma of the prostate (Fig. 17-11). Although most small cell carcinomas of the prostate lack clinically evident hormone production, they account for the majority of prostatic tumors with clinically evident adrenocorticotropic hormone or antidiuretic hormone production. The average survival of patients with small cell carcinoma of the prostate is less than a year. There is no difference in prognosis between patients with pure small cell carcinomas and those with mixed glandular and small cell carcinomas. The appearance of a small cell component within the course of adenocarcinoma of the prostate usually indicates an aggressive terminal phase of the disease, with the manifestations and patterns of tumor spread still resembling those of typical adenocarcinoma of the prostate. The heterogeneity of prostatic small cell tumors suggests that they arise from multipotential prostatic-epithelial cells that may express divergent differentiation. It is important to recognize that neuroendocrine differentiation in the prostate is not restricted to small cell carcinoma. Neuroendocrine cells in the normal prostate contain serotonin and, less frequently, calcitonin, somatostatin, or human chorionic gonadotropin (hCG). In histologically typical adenocarcinomas of the prostate, it is common to find similar cells that label with antibodies to serotonin, adrenocorticotropic hormone, calcitonin, hCG, or neuron-specific enolase (117,118). Most of these cases have no clinical evidence of ectopic hormonal secretion, and there are conflicting studies as to the prognostic significance of neuroendocrine expression in ordinary prostate cancer.

Individual case reports exist on variants of prostatic adenocarcinoma with oncocytic changes and lymphoepithelial features (119,120).

OTHER CARCINOMAS INVOLVING THE PROSTATE

Transitional Cell Carcinoma

Primary transitional cell carcinoma of the prostate without bladder involvement accounts for 1% to 4% of all prostate carcinomas (121). In cases of primary transitional cell carcinoma of the prostate, stromal invasion is almost always identified (122). In a minority of primary transitional cell carcinomas of the prostate, an adenocarcinoma component may also be identified. Primary transitional cell carcinomas of the prostate show a propensity to infiltrate the bladder neck and surrounding soft tissue, such that more than 50% of the patients present with stage T3 or T4 tumors. Twenty percent of the patients present with distant metastases, with bone, lung, and liver being the most common sites. In contrast to adenocarcinoma of the prostate, bone metastases tend to be osteolytic. Treatment of stage T3 disease with radiation results in a 5-year survival rate of approximately 34%. In the minority of cases with tumors localized to the prostate (T2), radical surgery has resulted in long-term disease-free survival in several patients.

More commonly, transitional cell carcinoma involves prostatic ducts and acini in patients with a history of flat CIS of the bladder who have been treated over a period of months to years with intravesical topical chemotherapy (123–126). Between 35% and 45% of cystoprostatectomies performed for transitional cell carcinoma contain prostatic involvement. However, this number is dependent on the amount of histologic sampling of the prostate tissue and may be much higher in completely mapped specimens

(127). Although the intravesical therapy may effectively rid the bladder of tumor, the chemotherapy may not treat effectively the prostatic urethra and does not reach the underlying prostatic ducts and acini. To rule out extension of tumor into the prostate, patients who are treated conservatively for CIS of the bladder undergo periodic deep transurethral biopsies of the prostatic urethra and underlying prostate. The finding of intraductal transitional cell carcinoma usually leads to radical cystoprostatectomy. If cystoprostatectomy is performed and only intraductal transitional cell carcinoma is present, the prostatic involvement does not worsen the prognosis, which is determined by the stage of the bladder tumor (128). Intraductal transitional cell carcinoma of the prostate appears to involve the prostate via direct extension from the overlying urethra that is usually involved by CIS. Intraductal and infiltrating transitional cell carcinoma involving the prostate tends to be seen in higher-stage bladder tumors, in which the patients have a poor prognosis attributable to either the advanced bladder or prostatic disease. A minority of these cases will have a low-stage bladder tumor and a poor prognosis, demonstrating the adverse effect of prostatic stromal infiltration (128). It is therefore prognostically important to identify prostatic stromal invasion in cases with intraductal transitional cell carcinoma, especially in patients with a low-stage bladder tumor.

Finally, one may find direct invasion from a bladder transitional cell carcinoma into the stroma of the prostate, in which there is no *in situ* component within the prostatic ducts. This situation is associated with a dramatic decrease in the prognosis of transitional cell carcinoma of the bladder and is equivalent in survival to cases with local metastases. In some of these cases, it is difficult to differentiate between a poorly differentiated transitional cell carcinoma of the bladder and a Gleason pattern 5 prostatic adenocarcinoma. Because in some cases antisera to PSA are more sensitive in identifying prostatic tumors, and PSAP gives superior results in other cases, both antisera should be used in establishing whether the tumor is of prostatic origin. Even when PSA and PSAP are used, the lack of immunoreactivity in a poorly differentiated tumor within the prostate, especially if present in limited amount, does not exclude the diagnosis of a poorly differentiated prostatic adenocarcinoma. In addition, immunohistochemical stains can be done for high-molecular-weight cytokeratin, cytokeratin 7, and cytokeratin 20, which preferentially label urothelial carcinoma and are uncommonly expressed in adenocarcinoma of the prostate (129,130). With only a few exceptions, immunoperoxidase staining for PSA and PSAP is very specific for prostatic tissue (131).

Squamous Cell Carcinoma

Pure primary squamous carcinoma of the prostate is rare (0.5% of prostate tumors) and is associated with a poor survival (132). These tumors develop osteolytic metastases, do not respond to hormone therapy, and do not develop elevated serum PSA with metastatic disease. More commonly, squamous differentiation occurs in the primary and metastatic deposits of adenocarcinomas that have been treated with hormone or radiation therapy (133–135). After therapy, the prostate may develop squamous metaplasia only in benign glands or, in some cases, in some of the neoplastic glands as well, resulting in an adenosquamous carcinoma. The metastases may be adenosquamous carcinoma or pure squamous carcinoma; in some cases, the squamous component may be PSA or PSAP positive (136). There have also been rare reports of adenosquamous carcinoma of the prostate in which there was no previous therapy.

MESENCHYMAL TUMORS

Benign Mesenchymal Tumors and Tumorlike Lesions

Benign soft tissue tumors of the prostate are rare, the most common being leiomyoma. The difficulty in diagnosing a leiomyoma of the prostate is that one often may find small stromal nodules with the histologic appearance of a leiomyoma in prostates with nodular hyperplasia (137). These stromal nodules, although they contain abundant smooth muscle, lack the well-organized fascicles of a leiomyoma and do not have the other degenerative features commonly seen in leiomyomas, such as hyalinization, necrosis, and calcification. Large, single, symptomatic leiomyomas of the prostate are rare, most presenting with lower urinary obstructive symptoms (138). Hemangiomas involving the prostate have also been described (139).

There are two spindle cell lesions occurring in the genitourinary tract that are benign, yet resemble sarcomas. Postoperative spindle cell nodules in men have been found in the prostate, bladder, and prostatic urethra. Cystoscopically, they manifest as an ulcer, ill-defined tumor, or nodule. As the name implies, they follow a prior surgical procedure. On average, the TUR precedes the spindle cell nodule by 3 months, with a range of 2 to 15 months. There is a wide age range of 29 to 79 years (median, 60 years). Often, these nodules are incidentally found, yet may result in hematuria or obstructive symptoms. These lesions are usually small (5 to 9 mm). These lesions may be infiltrative and destroy surrounding smooth muscle. Another spindle cell tumor occurring in this region arises without a prior history of surgery. These lesions have been reported under a multitude of names, most commonly *nodular fasciitis of bladder*, *pseudosarcomatous myofibroblastic proliferation*, *inflammatory pseudotumor*, or *pseudosarcomatous fibromyxoid tumor*. These lesions occur within even a wider range, from 2 to 73 years, with a median age of 28 years. Most cases have been described within the bladder, with an occasional case found within the prostate. These lesions range from 1.5 to 9.0 cm. These lesions may, as with postoperative spindle cell nodules, invade into the bladder wall. Postoperative spindle cell nodules and pseudosarcomatous fibromyxoid tumors are benign, with only a rare recurrence after incomplete excision (140–142).

Sarcomas

Sarcomas (excluding those of specialized prostatic stroma) of the prostate account for 0.1% to 0.2% of all malignant prostatic tumors. Rhabdomyosarcoma is the most frequent mesenchymal tumor within the prostate and is seen almost exclusively in childhood. Rhabdomyosarcomas of the prostate occur from infancy to early adulthood, with an average age at diagnosis of 5 years (143). Most patients present with stage 3 disease, in which there is gross residual disease after incomplete resection or biopsy only. A smaller but significant proportion of patients presents with distant metastases. A localized tumor that may be completely resected is only rarely present. Histologically, most prostate rhabdomyosarcomas are of the embryonal subtype. Because of their large size at the time of diagnosis, the distinction between rhabdomyosarcoma originating in the bladder and that arising in the prostate is often impossible. After the development of effective chemotherapy for rhabdomyosarcomas, those few patients with localized disease (stage 1) or microscopic residual regional disease (stage 2) stand an excellent chance of being cured. Although the majority of patients with gross residual disease (stage 3) remains without evidence of disease for a long period of time, approximately 15% to 20% die of their tumor. The prognosis for patients with metastatic tumor (stage 4) is more dismal, with most patients dying of the tumor.

Leiomyosarcomas are the most common sarcomas involving the prostate in men (144). The majority of patients is between 40 and 70 years of age, although in some series, up to 20% of leiomyosarcomas have occurred in young adults or children. Leiomyosarcomas have ranged in size from 2 to 24 cm, with a mean size of 9 cm. After local excision or resection of prostatic leiomyosarcomas, the clinical course tends to be characterized by multiple recurrences. Metastases, when present, are usually found in the lung and liver. The average survival with leiomyosarcoma of the prostate is between 3 and 4 years.

Other rare mesenchymal tumors of the prostate that are malignant or have the potential for malignancy are malignant peripheral nerve sheath tumors, angiosarcomas, hemangiopericytomas, malignant fibrous histiocytomas, specialized stromal tumors of the prostate, and pheochromocytomas (145–149).

MISCELLANEOUS BENIGN TUMORS OR TUMORLIKE CONDITIONS

Other benign lesions reported in the prostate include ganglioneuromas, carcinoid tumors, mucinous metaplasia, xanthomas, and Paneth's cell metaplasia (150–154). *Prostatic cystadenomas* are large, tumorlike lesions with the appearance of BPH (155). They have been reported to arise in the retrovesical space, either attached to the prostate by a pedicle or apparently separate from the prostate. Occasionally, these lesions are intraprostatic and are differentiated from nodular hyperplasia only when they are composed of a well-circumscribed nodule occupying one side of an otherwise nonhyperplastic gland. A variant of adenosis that may be confused with intermediate high-grade adenocarcinoma of the prostate is sclerosing adenosis of the prostate (156).

MISCELLANEOUS MALIGNANT TUMORS OR TUMORLIKE CONDITIONS

The following malignant tumors have been rarely described in the prostate: Wilms' tumor, rhabdoid tumor, and basaloid carcinomas (adenoid cystic carcinoma) (157–159). Other malignant tumors of the prostate include cases of malignant mixed tumors resembling those of the salivary gland and endodermal sinus tumor (160,161).

Carcinosarcomas, which are typically composed of adenocarcinoma of the prostate admixed with a sarcomatous component, have also been reported within the prostate and have a dismal prognosis (162).

Primary prostatic lymphoma without lymph node involvement appears to be much less common than secondary infiltration of the prostate (163). Most reported lymphomas have been of the large cell and small cleaved-cell types with a diffuse pattern. Lymphomas with a nodular pattern involving the prostate are seen infrequently. The entire spectrum of malignant lymphomas seen at other sites may become manifest in the prostate, including undifferentiated lymphomas, angiotropic lymphomas, Hodgkin's lymphoma, myelomas, and T-cell lymphomas, as well as a case of pseudolymphoma (164–166). Malignant lymphoma involving the prostate appears to carry a poor prognosis regardless of patient age, stage at presentation, histologic classification (with the exception of small lymphocytic lymphoma), or treatment regimen. The poor prognosis of prostatic lymphoma is related to the generalized disease that eventually results rather than to prostatic involvement.

The most common form of leukemic involvement of the prostate is that of chronic lymphocytic leukemia (small lymphocytic lymphoma), although monocytic, granulocytic, and lymphoblastic leukemias have also been described in the prostate (167). Most patients are known leukemics or have the diagnosis established at the time of assessment for urinary symptoms. It is often unclear whether the prostatic leukemic infiltrate in chronic lymphocytic leukemia is an incidental finding in patients with BPH or the cause of their obstructive symptoms. Men with chronic lymphocytic leukemia involving the pelvic lymph nodes or the prostate may have an indolent course and still benefit from radical prostatectomy (168).

Excluding hematopoietic neoplasms, the prostate even at autopsy is rarely involved by metastatic tumor. Metastases from malignant melanoma and carcinoma of the lung predominate (169).

TREATMENT CHANGES IN THE PROSTATE

Radiation

Radiation changes in the prostate are usually seen in patients who have been irradiated for adenocarcinoma of the prostate (170). The prostate may also be affected when radiotherapy is administered to the bladder for transitional cell carcinoma.

Radiation atypia alters the cytology of prostatic epithelium with relative sparing of the overall glandular architecture. Radiated adenocarcinoma of the prostate may show a decrease in the number of neoplastic glands or no recognizable difference from nonradiated cancer. Radiation atypia in benign glands can be distinguished from carcinoma in difficult cases with the help of basal cell specific antibodies, such as high-molecular-weight cytokeratin. These antibodies can demonstrate the presence of a basal cell layer in benign glands with radiation effect (171). Carcinoma, when present in a biopsy performed 12 to 18 months after radiotherapy, is a powerful predictor of local or distant postradiation failure (172). Some studies have demonstrated that the morphologic appearance of the cancer after radiotherapy correlates with prognosis (173).

Hormonal Therapy

Within the last few years, some urologists have treated men with combination endocrine therapy consisting of a luteinizing hormone releasing hormone agonist and flutamide before radical prostatectomy (174–179). The histology of the normal and neoplastic tissue may be significantly altered with this therapy, making the assessment of these specimens difficult. The major effects of combination endocrine therapy on benign prostate tissue are the presence of atrophic changes with immature squamous and transitional cell metaplasia and basal cell hyperplasia (180–185). Histologically, the changes seen in adenocarcinoma are more problematic, in which the altered cancer glands can resemble benign atrophy, histiocytes, or inflammation (180–185). These altered epithelial cells retain their keratin immunoreactivity. In a few cases, we have not been able to identify residual carcinoma after combined endocrine therapy. When signing out these cases, we state that although no residual carcinoma is seen, the identification of carcinoma after combined endocrine therapy may be extremely difficult, and we cannot entirely exclude the possibility of a residual tumor. One of the problems with evaluating carcinomas that have been treated with hormone therapy is that the grade often appears artifactually higher. Evidence to support that the apparently higher grade is artifactual comes from evaluation of the prehormone therapy needle biopsies, which often appear lower grade. Furthermore, the treated cancers are predominantly diploid and have low proliferation rates. There is controversy as to whether pathologists can accurately grade treated cancers taking into account the hormone effect. The majority of investigators believes that treated carcinomas cannot be assigned an accurate Gleason grade. However, if there are other areas of the tumor that do not show a pronounced hormone effect, then these areas can be Gleason graded.

PREDICTIVE FACTORS

Pathologists are currently called on to address two markers for clinical patient management (186). These are DNA ploidy and microvessel density as a measure of neoangiogenesis. Although most studies have shown that ploidy correlates with pathologic stage and tumor behavior, there are conflicting studies as to whether ploidy offers independent prognostic information beyond that of routinely measured parameters. Consequently, ploidy is not currently recommended for routine clinical use (187,188). One situation in which there is evidence that ploidy may be of prognostic importance, is in patients undergoing radical prostatectomy who have nodal metastases. Some studies have demonstrated that patients who have undergone radical prostatectomy with positive nodes, who have diploid tumors, do significantly better than patients with nondiploid tumors (189). There have been two studies from the group at Albany showing that ploidy results on the needle biopsy independently predict tumor upgrading in the corresponding radical prostatectomy specimen and postradical prostatectomy recurrence (190,191). However, in a more recent joint study with the same group of investigators at Albany, we found that, in the setting of accurate Gleason grading of the needle biopsies, ploidy does not provide additional staging or grading prognostic information in the radical prostatectomy specimen (192). Consequently, the role of ploidy on needle biopsy may be to provide prognostic information in situations in which an individual questions accuracy of the grade assigned to the cancer on needle biopsy.

Many, although not all, studies have demonstrated that quantitation of the microvascular density within prostate cancer is prognostic (186,193). There are conflicting studies as to whether microvessel density characterized on needle biopsy is predictive of pathologic stage (194,195).

There has been a tremendous proliferation of other putative prostate cancer biomarkers in recent years (186). The vast majority of these markers is experimental, with relatively few studies on a limited number of patients. Even the better prognostic attributes are limited by technical difficulty, lack of standardization, poor reproducibility, and little overall added performance to that of standard available parameters, such as grade, serum PSA levels, clinical stage, pathologic stage, and margin status. Nonetheless, the future holds many possibilities, with physicians having the responsibility for the rational use of new technology in a cost-effective manner.

REFERENCES

1. McNeal JE, Bostwick DG. Intraductal dysplasia: a premalignant lesion of the prostate. *Hum Pathol* 1986;17:64–71.
2. Bostwick DG, Amin MB, Dundore P, et al. Architectural patterns of high-grade prostatic intraepithelial neoplasia. *Hum Pathol* 1993;24:298–310.
3. Häggman MJ, Macoska JA, Wojno KJ, et al. The relationship between prostatic intraepithelial neoplasia and prostate cancer: critical issues. *J Urol* 1997:158:12–22.
4. Troncoso P, Babaian RJ, Ro JY, et al. Prostatic intra-epithelial neoplasia and invasive prostatic adenocarcinoma in cystoprostatectomy specimens. *Urology* 1989;34[Suppl]:52–56.
5. McNeal JE. Significance of duct-acinar dysplasia in prostatic carcinogenesis. *Urology* 1989;34[Suppl]:9–15.
6. Epstein JI, Grignon DJ, Humphrey PA, et al. Interobserver reproducibility in the diagnosis of prostatic intraepithelial neoplasia. *Am J Surg Pathol* 1995;19:873–886.
7. McNeal JE, Villers A, Redwine EA, et al. Microcarcinoma in the prostate: its association with duct-acinar dysplasia. *Hum Pathol* 1991;22:644–652.
8. Montironi R, Scarpelli M, Magi Galluzzi C, et al. Aneuploidy and nuclear features of prostatic intraepithelial neoplasia (PIN). *J Cell Biochem* 1992;50[Suppl]:47–53.
9. Bostwick DG, Pacelli A, Lopez-Beltran A. Molecular biology of prostatic intraepithelial neoplasia. *Prostate* 1996;29:117–134.
10. Busch PC, Egevad L, Haggman M. Precancer of the prostate. *Cancer Surveys* 1998;32:149–179.
11. Greene DR, Wheeler TM, Egawa S, et al. A comparison of the morphological features of cancer arising in the transition zone and in the peripheral zone of the prostate. *J Urol* 1991;146:1069–1076.
12. NcNeal JE, Price HN, Redwine EA, et al. Stage A versus stage B adenocarcinoma of the prostate: morphological comparison and biological significance. *J Urol* 1988;139:61–65.
13. Quinn BD, Cho KR, Epstein JI. Relationship of severe dysplasia to stage B adenocarcinoma of the prostate. *Cancer* 1990;65:2328–2337.
14. Epstein JI. *Interpretation of prostate biopsies*, 2nd ed. New York: Raven Press, 1995.
15. Ayala AG, Srigley JR, Ro JY, et al. Clear cell cribriform hyperplasia of prostate. Report of 10 cases. *Am J Surg Pathol* 1986;10:665–671.
16. Epstein JI, Armas OA. Atypical basal cell hyperplasia of the prostate. *Am J Surg Pathol* 1992;16:1205–1214.
17. Bostwick DG, Kindrachuk RW, Rouse RV. Prostatic adenocarcinoma with endometrioid features. Clinical, pathologic, and ultrastructural findings. *Am J Surg Pathol* 1985;9:595–609.
18. Epstein JI, Woodruff J. Prostatic carcinomas with endometrioid features: a light microscopic and immunohistochemical study of ten cases. *Cancer* 1986;57:111–119.
19. Christensen W, Walsh PC, Epstein JI. Prostatic duct adenocarcinoma: findings at radical prostatectomy. *Cancer* 1991;67:2118–2124.
20. Brawer MK, Bigler SA, Sohlberg OE, et al. Significance of prostatic intraepithelial neoplasia on prostate needle biopsy. *Urology* 1991;38:103–107.
21. Keetch DW, Humphrey PA, Stahl D, et al. Morphometric analysis and clinical follow-up of isolated prostatic intraepithelial neoplasia in needle biopsy of the prostate. *J Urol* 1995;154:347–351.
22. Bostwick DG, Qian J, Frankel K. The incidence of high grade PIN in needle biopsies. *J Urol* 1995;154:1791–1794.
23. Cheville JC, Reznicek MJ, Bostwick DG. The focus of "atypical glands, suspicious for malignancy" in prostatic needle biopsy specimens. Incidence, histologic features, and clinical follow-up of cases diagnosed in a community practice. *Am J Clin Pathol* 1997;108:633–640.
24. Renshaw AA, Santis WF, Richie JP. Clinicopathological characteristics of prostatic adenocarcinoma in men with atypical prostate needle biopsies. *J Urol* 1998;159:2018–2022.
25. Orozco R, O'Dowd G, Kunnel B, et al. Observations on pathology trends in 62,537 prostate biopsies obtained from urology private practices in the United States. *Urology* 1998;51:186–195.
26. Wills ML, Hamper UM, Partin AW, et al. Incidence of high-grade prostatic intraepithelial neoplasia in sextant needle biopsy specimens. *Urology* 1997;49:367–373.
27. Hu JC, Palapattu GS, Kattan MW, et al. The association of selected pathological features with prostate cancer in a single-needle biopsy accession. *Hum Pathol* 1998;29:1536–1538.
28. Davidson D, Bostwick D, Qian J, et al. Prostatic intraepithelial neoplasia is a risk factor for adenocarcinoma: predictive accuracy in needle biopsies. *J Urol* 1995;154:1295–1299.
29. Weinstein MH, Epstein JI. Significance of high grade prostatic intraepithelial neoplasia (PIN) on needle biopsy. *Hum Pathol* 1993;24:624–629.
30. Raviv G, Janssen T, Zlotta AR, et al. Prostatic intraepithelial neoplasia: influence of clinical and pathological data on the detection of prostate cancer. *J Urol* 1996;156:1050–1055.
31. Langer JE, Rovner ES, Coleman BG, et al. Strategy for repeat biopsy of patients with prostatic intraepithelial neoplasia detected by prostate needle biopsy. *J Urol* 1996;155:228–231.
32. Aboseif S, Shinohara K, Weidner N, et al. The significance of prostatic intraepithelial neoplasia. *Br J Urol* 1995;76:355–359.
33. Ronnette BM, Carmichael MJ, Carter HB, et al. Does prostatic intraepithelial neoplasia result in elevated serum prostate specific antigen levels? *J Urol* 1993;150:386–389.
34. Hamper UM, Sheth S, Walsh PC, et al. Stage B adenocarcinoma of the prostate: transrectal US and pathologic correlation of non-malignant hypoechoic peripheral zone lesions. *Radiology* 1991;180:101–104.

35. Shepherd D, Keetch DW, Humphrey PA, et al. Repeat biopsy strategy in men with isolated prostatic intraepithelial neoplasia on prostate needle biopsy. *J Urol* 1996;156:460–463.
36. Gaudin PB, Sesterhenn IA, Wojno KJ, et al. Incidence and clinical significance of high-grade prostatic intraepithelial neoplasia in TURP specimens. *Urology* 1997;49:558–563.
37. Harvei S, Skjorten FJ, Robsahm TE, et al. Is prostatic intraepithelial neoplasia in the transition/central zone a true precursor of cancer? A long-term retrospective study in Norway. *Br J Cancer* 1998;78:46–49.
38. Pacelli A, Bostwick DG. Clinical significance of high-grade prostatic intraepithelial neoplasia in transurethral resection specimens. *Urology* 1997;50:355–359.
39. Ferguson J, Zincke H, Ellison E, et al. Decrease of prostatic intraepithelial neoplasia following androgen deprivation therapy in patients with stage T3 carcinoma treated by radical prostatectomy. *Urology* 1994;44:91–95.
40. Vaillancourt L, Têtu B, Fradet Y, et al. Effect of neoadjuvant endocrine therapy (combined androgen blockade) on normal prostate and prostatic carcinoma. A randomized study. *Am J Surg Pathol* 1996;20:86–93.
41. Lee F, Torp-Pedersen ST, Carroll JT, et al. Use of transrectal ultrasound and prostate-specific antigen in diagnosis of prostatic intra-epithelial neoplasia. *Urology* 1989;34[Suppl]: 4–8.
42. Markham CW. Prostatic intra-epithelial neoplasia: detection and correlation with invasive cancer and fine-needle biopsy. *Urology* 1989;34[Suppl]:57–61.
43. Sakr WA, Haas GP, Cassin BF, et al. The frequency of carcinoma and intraepithelial neoplasia of the prostate in young male patients. *J Urol* 1993;150:379–385.
44. Epstein JI, Walsh PC, Carmichael M, et al. Pathological and clinical findings to predict tumor extent of non-palpable (stage T1c) prostate cancer. *JAMA* 1994;271:368–374.
45. Byar DP, Mostofi FK, and the Veterans Administrative Cooperative Urologic Research Groups. Carcinoma of the prostate: prognostic evaluation of certain pathologic features in 208 radical prostatectomies. *Cancer* 1972;30:5–13.
46. McNeal JE. Origin and development of carcinoma in the prostate. *Cancer* 1969;23:24–34.
47. Ayala AG, Ro JY, Babaian R, et al. The prostatic capsule: Does it exist? Its importance in the staging and treatment of prostatic carcinoma. *Am J Surg Pathol* 1989;13:21–27.
48. Villers AA, McNeal JE, Redwine EA, et al. The role of perineural space invasion in the local spread of prostatic adenocarcinoma. *J Urol* 1989;142:763–768.
49. Hassan MO, Maksem J. The prostatic perineural space and its relation to tumor spread. *Am J Surg Pathol* 1980;4:143–148.
50. Epstein JI, Carmichael M, Walsh PC. Adenocarcinoma of the prostate invading the seminal vesicle: definition and relation of tumor volume, grade, and margins of resection to prognosis. *J Urol* 1993;149:1040–1045.
51. Ohori M, Scardino PT, Lapin SL, et al. The mechanisms and prognostic significance of seminal vesicle involvement by prostate cancer. *Am J Surg Pathol* 1993;17:1252–1261.
52. McNeal JE. Cancer volume and site of origin of adenocarcinoma of the prostate: relationship to local and distant spread. *Hum Pathol* 1992;23:258–266.
53. Christensen WN, Partin AW, Walsh PC, et al. Pathologic findings in stage A2 prostate cancer: relation of tumor volume, grade and location to pathologic stage. *Cancer* 1990;65:1021–1027.
54. Gleason DF, Mellinger GT, the Veterans Administration Cooperative Urological Research Group. Prediction of prognosis for prostatic adenocarcinoma by combined histologic grading and clinical staging. *J Urol* 1974;111:58–64.
55. Gleason DF, the Veterans Administration Cooperative Urological Research Group. Histologic grading and clinical staging of prostatic carcinoma. In: Tannenbaum M, ed. *Urologic pathology: the prostate*. Philadelphia: Lea & Febiger, 1977:171–197.
56. Epstein JI, Pizov G, Walsh PC. Correlation of pathologic findings progression following radical retropubic prostatectomy. *Cancer* 1993;71:3582–3593.
57. Epstein JI, Partin AW, Sauvageot J, et al. Prediction of progression following radical prostatectomy: a multivariate analysis of 721 men with long-term follow-up. *Am J Surg Pathol* 1996;20:286–292.
58. Steinberg DM, Sauvageot J, Piantadosi S, et al. Correlation of prostate needle biopsy and radical prostatectomy Gleason grade in academic and community settings. *Am J Surg Pathol* 1997;21:566–576.
59. Sogani PC, Israel A, Lieberman PH, et al. Gleason grading of prostate cancer: a predictor of survival. *Urology* 1985; 25:223–227.
60. McNeal JE, Villers AA, Redwine EA, et al. Histologic differentiation, cancer volume, and pelvic lymph node metastasis in adenocarcinoma of the prostate. *Cancer* 1990;66:1225–1233.
61. Partin AW, Kattan MW, Subong EN, et al. Combination of prostate-specific antigen, clinical stage, and Gleason score to predict pathological stage of localized prostate cancer. A multi-institutional update. *JAMA* 1997;277:1445–1451.
62. Kattan MW, Eastham JA, Stapleton AMF, et al. A preoperative nomogram for disease recurrence following radical prostatectomy for prostate cancer. *J Nat Cancer Inst* 1998;90: 766–771.
63. Spires SE, Cibull ML, Wood DP Jr., et al. Gleason histologic grading in prostatic carcinoma. Correlation of 18-gauge core biopsy with prostatectomy. *Arch Pathol Lab Med* 1994;118:705–708.
64. Bostwick DG. Gleason grading of prostatic needle biopsies. Correlation with grade in 316 matched prostatectomies. *Am J Surg Pathol* 1994;18:796–803.
65. Albertsen PC, Fryback DG, Storer BE, et al. Long-term survival among men with conservatively treated localized prostate cancer. *JAMA* 1995;274:626–631.
66. Matzkin H, Patel JP, Aaltwein JE, et al. Stage T_{1A} carcinoma of prostate. *Urology* 1994;43:11–21.
67. Epstein JI, Steinberg GD. The significance of low grade prostate cancer on needle biopsy: a radical prostatectomy study of tumor grade, volume, and stage of the biopsied and multifocal tumor. *Cancer* 1990;66:1927–1932.
68. Allsbrook W, Lane R, Lance C, et al. Interobserver reproducibility of Gleason's grading system. Urologic pathologists. *Hum Pathol* 2001;32:74–80.
69. Kronz JD, Silberman MA, Allsbrook W Jr., et al. Use of a web-based tutorial improves practicing pathologists' Glea-

son grading of prostate cancer on needle biopsies. *Cancer* 2001;89:1818–1823.
70. Brawn PN. The dedifferentiation of prostate carcinoma. *Cancer* 1983;52:246–251.
71. Epstein JI, Carmichael MJ, Partin AW. Small high grade adenocarcinomas of the prostate in radical prostatectomy specimens performed for non-palpable disease: pathogenic and clinical implications. *J Urol* 1994;151:1587–1592.
72. Epstein JI. Diagnostic criteria of limited adenocarcinoma of the prostate on needle biopsy. *Hum Pathol* 1995;26:223–229.
73. Wojno KJ, Epstein JI. The utility of basal cell specific anti-cytokeratin antibody (34 beta E12) in the diagnosis of prostate cancer: a review of 228 cases. *Am J Surg Pathol* 1995;19:251–260.
74. Kahane H, Sharp JW, Shuman GB, et al. Utilization of high molecular weight cytokeratin on prostate biopsies in an independent laboratory. *Urology* 1995;45:981–986.
75. Weinstein MH, Greenspan DL, Bhagavan B, et al. Diagnoses rendered on prostate needle biopsies in community hospitals. *Prostate* 1998;35:50–55.
76. Iczkowski KA, MacLennan GT, Bostwick DG. Atypical small acinar proliferation suspicious for malignancy in prostate needle biopsies. Clinical significance in 33 cases. *Am J Surg Pathol* 1997;21:1489–1495.
77. Roehrborn CG, Pickens GJ, Sanders JS. Diagnostic yield of repeated transrectal ultrasound-guided biopsies stratified by specific histopathologic diagnoses and prostate-specific antigen levels. *Urology* 1996;47:347–352.
78. Chan TY, Epstein JI. Follow-up of atypical prostate needle biopsies. *Urology* 1999;53:351–355.
79. Keetch DW, Catalona WJ, Smith DS. Serial prostatic biopsies in men with persistently elevated serum prostate specific antigen values. *J Urol* 1994;151:1571–1574.
80. Allen EA, Kahane H, Epstein JI. Repeat biopsy strategies for men with atypical diagnoses on initial prostate needle biopsy. *Urology* 1998;52:803–807.
81. Peller PA, Young DC, Marmaduke DP, et al. Sextant prostate biopsies: a histopathologic correlation with radical prostatectomy specimens. *Cancer* 1995;75:530–538.
82. Huland H, Hammerer P, Henke RP, et al. Preoperative prediction of tumor heterogeneity and recurrence after radical prostatectomy for localized prostatic carcinoma with digital rectal examination, prostate specific antigen and the results of 6 systematic biopsies. *J Urol* 1996;155:1344–1347.
83. Ravery V, Boccon-Gibod LA, Dauge-Geffroy MC, et al. Systemic biopsies accurately predict extracapsular extension of prostate cancer and persistent/recurrent detectable PSA after radical prostatectomy. *Urology* 1994;44:371–376.
84. Badalament RA, Miller MC, Peller PA, et al. An algorithm for predicting nonorgan confined prostate cancer using the results obtained from sextant core biopsies with prostate specific antigen level. *J Urol* 1996;156:1375–1380.
85. Vargas SO, Jiroutek MJ, Welch WR, et al. Perineural invasion in prostate needle biopsy specimens: Correlation with extraprostatic extension at resection. *Am J Clin Pathol* 1999;111:223–228.
86. Egan AJ, Bostwick DG. Prediction of extraprostatic extension of prostate cancer based on needle biopsy findings: Perineural invasion lacks significance on multivariate analysis. *Am J Surg Pathol* 1997;21:1496–1500.
87. Rubin MA, Strawderman M, Bassily N, et al. Prostate cancer staging: evaluation of nomogram predicting unfavorable pathology. *J Urol* 1999;161[Suppl]:242.
88. Holmes GF, Walsh PC, Pound CR, et al. Excision of the neurovascular bundle at radical prostatectomy in cases with perineural invasion on needle biopsy. *Urology* 1999;53:752–756.
89. Bastacky SI, Walsh PC, Epstein JI. Relationship between perineural tumor invasion in needle biopsy and radical prostatectomy capsular penetration in clinical stage B adenocarcinoma of the prostate. *Am J Surg Pathol* 1993;17:336–341.
90. de la Taille A, Katz A, Bagiella E, et al. Perineural invasion on prostate needle biopsy: an independent predictor of final pathologic stage. *Urology* 1999;54:1039–1043.
91. Stone NN, Stock RG, Parikh D, et al. Perineural invasion and seminal vesicle involvement predict lymph node metastasis in men with localized carcinoma of the prostate. *J Urol* 1998;160:1722–1726.
92. Cantrell BB, DeKlerk DP, Eggleston JC, et al. Pathological factors that influence prognosis in stage A prostatic cancer. The influence of extent versus grade. *J Urol* 1981;125:516–520.
93. Murphy WM, Dean PJ, Brasfield JA, et al. Incidental carcinoma of the prostate. How much sampling is adequate? *Am J Surg Pathol* 1986;10:170–174.
94. Newman AJ, Graham MA, Carlton CE, et al. Incidental carcinoma of the prostate at the time of transurethral resection: importance of evaluating every chip. *J Urol* 1982;128: 948–950.
95. Rohr LR. Incidental adenocarcinoma in transurethral resections of the prostate: partial versus complete microscopic examination. *Am J Surg Pathol* 1987;11:53–58.
96. Vollmer RT. Prostate cancer and chip specimens: complete versus partial sampling. *Hum Pathol* 1986;17:285–290.
97. Furman J, Murphy WM, Rice L, et al. Prostatectomy tissue for research. *Am J Clin Pathol* 1998;110:4–9.
98. Egevad L, Engström K, Busch C. A new method for handling radical prostatectomies enabling fresh tissue harvesting, whole mount sections, and landmarks for alignment of sections. *J Urol Pathol* 1998;9:17–28.
99. Hoedemaeker RF, Ruijter ETG, Winter R, et al. Processing radical prostatectomy specimens. a comprehensive and standardized protocol. *J Urol Pathol* 1998;9:211–222.
100. Hall GS, Kramer CE, Walsh PC, et al. Evaluation of radical prostatectomy specimens: a comparative analysis of various sampling methods. *Am J Surg Pathol* 1992;16:315–324.
101. Bova GS, Fox W, Epstein JI. Methods of radical prostatectomy specimen processing: A novel technique for harvesting fresh prostate cancer tissue and review of processing techniques. *Mod Pathol* 1993;6:201–207.
102. Renshaw AA, Chang H, D'Amico AV. An abbreviated protocol for processing radical prostatectomy specimens. *J Urol Pathol* 1996;5:183–192.
103. Stamey TA, Villers AA, McNeal JE, et al. Positive surgical margins at radical prostatectomy: importance of the apical dissection. *J Urol* 1990;143:1166–1173.
104. Wieder JA, Soloway MS. Incidence, etiology, location, prevention and treatment of positive surgical margins after radical prostatectomy for prostate cancer. *J Urol* 1998;160: 299–315.

105. Epstein JI. Evaluation of radical prostatectomy capsular margins of resection: the significance of margins designated as negative, closely approaching, and positive. *Am J Surg Pathol* 1990;14:626–632.
106. Epstein JI, Sauvageot J. Do close but negative margins in radical prostatectomy specimens increase the risk of postoperative progression? *J Urol* 1997;157:241–243.
107. Epstein JI, Carmichael M, Partin AW, et al. Is tumor volume an independent predictor of progression following radical prostatectomy? A multivariate analysis of 185 clinical stage B adenocarcinomas of the prostate with five years follow-up. *J Urol* 1993;149:1478–1481.
108. Wheeler TM, Dillioglugil Ö, Kattan MW, et al. Clinical and pathological significance of the level and extent of capsular invasion in clinical stage T1-2 prostate cancer. *Hum Pathol* 1998;29:856–862.
109. Brinker DA, Potter SE, Epstein JI. Ductal adenocarcinoma of the prostate diagnosed on needle biopsy: correlation with clinical and radical prostatectomy findings and progression. *Am J Surg Pathol* 1999;23:1471–1479.
110. Epstein JI, Lieberman PH. Mucinous adenocarcinoma of the prostate. Mucinous adenocarcinomas of the prostate gland. *Am J Surg Pathol* 1985;9:299–307.
111. Ro JY, Grignon J, Ayala AG, et al. Mucinous adenocarcinoma of the prostate: histochemical and immunohistochemical studies. *Hum Pathol* 1990;21:593–600.
112. Ro JY, Naggar A, Ayala AG, et al. Signet-ring cell carcinoma of prostate. *Am J Surg Pathol* 1988;12:453–460.
113. Hejka AG, England DM. Signet ring cell carcinoma of prostate. Immunohistochemical and ultrastructural study of a case. *Urology* 1989;34:155–158.
114. Uchijima Y, Ito H, Takahashi M, et al. Prostate mucinous adenocarcinoma with signet ring cell. *Urology* 1991;36: 267–268.
115. Epstein JI, Kuhajda FP, Lieberman PH. Prostate specific acid phosphatase immunoreactivity in adenocarcinomas of the urinary bladder. *Hum Pathol* 1986;17:939–942.
116. Tetu B, Ro JY, Ayala AG, et al. Small cell carcinoma of prostate. Part 1: a clinicopathologic study of 20 cases. *Cancer* 1987;59:1803–1809.
117. Fetissof F, Bertrand G, Guilloteay D, et al. Calcitonin immunoreactive cells in prostate gland and cloacal derived tissues. *Virchows Arch* 1986;409:523–533.
118. Purnell DM, Heatfield BM, Trump BF. Immunocytochemical evaluation of human prostatic carcinomas for carcinoembryonic antigen, nonspecific cross-reacting antigen, B-chorionic gonadotrophin, and prostate-specific antigen. *Cancer Res* 1984;44:285–292.
119. Pinto JA, Gonzalez JE, Granadillo MA. Primary carcinoma of the prostate with diffuse oncocytic changes. *Histopathology* 1994;25:286–288.
120. Bostwick DG, Adlakha K. Lymphoepithelioma-like carcinoma of the prostate. *J Urol Pathol* 1994;2:319–325.
121. Sawczuk I, Tannenbaum M, Olsson CA, et al. Primary transitional cell carcinoma of prostatic periurethral ducts. *Urology* 1985;25:339–343.
122. Greene LF, O'Dea MJ, Dockerty MB. Primary transitional cell carcinoma of the prostate. *J Urol* 1976;116:761–763.
123. Schellhammer PF, Bean MA, Whitmore WF Jr. Prostatic involvement by transitional cell carcinoma: pathogenesis, patterns, and prognosis. *J Urol* 1977;118:399–403.
124. Mahadevia PS, Koss LG, Tar IJ. Prostatic involvement in bladder cancer: prostate mapping in 20 cystoprostatectomy specimens. *Cancer* 1986;58:2096–2102.
125. Matzkin H, Soloway MS, Hardeman S. Transitional cell carcinoma of the prostate. *J Urol* 1991;146:1207–1212.
126. Wood DP, Montie JE, Pontes JE, et al. Transitional cell carcinoma of the prostate in cystoprostatectomy specimens removed for bladder cancer. *J Urol* 1989;141:346–349.
127. Sakamoto N, Tsuneyoshi M, Naito S, et al. An adequate sampling of the prostate to identify prostatic involvement by urothelial carcinoma in bladder cancer patients. *J Urol* 1993;149:318–321.
128. Esrig D, Freeman JA, Elmajian DA, et al. Transitional cell carcinoma involving the prostate with a proposed staging classification for stromal invasion. *J Urol* 1996;156:1071–1076.
129. Vallorosi CJ, Bassily NH, Montie JE, et al. Coordinate expression of cytokeratins 7 and 20 in distinguishing bladder transitional cell carcinoma from prostate adenocarcinoma. *J Urol* 1999;161[Suppl]:53.
130. Genega EM, Hutchison B, Reuter VE, et al. Immunophenotype of intermediate and high grade prostatic and urothelial carcinoma. *Mod Pathol* 1999;12:98A.
131. Epstein JI. PSAP and PSA as immunohistochemical markers. *Urol Clin North Am* 1993;20:757–770.
132. Little NA, Wiener JS, Walther PJ, et al. Squamous cell carcinoma of the prostate: 2 cases of a rare malignancy and review of the literature. *J Urol* 1993;149:137–139.
133. Devaney DM, Dorman A, Leader M. Adenosquamous carcinoma of the prostate: a case report. *Hum Pathol* 1991;22: 1046–1050.
134. Miller VA, Reuter V, Scher HI. Primary squamous cell carcinoma of the prostate after radiation seed implantation for adenocarcinoma. *Urology* 1995;46:111–113.
135. Braslis KG, Davi RC, Nelson E, et al. Squamous cell carcinoma of the prostate: a transformation from adenocarcinoma after the use of a luteinizing hormone-releasing hormone agonist and flutamide. *Urology* 1995;45:329–331.
136. Acetta PA, Gardner WA. Squamous metastases from prostatic adenocarcinoma. *Prostate* 1982;3:515–521.
137. Moore RA. Benign hypertrophy of the prostate: a morphologic study. *J Urol* 1943;50:680–710.
138. Michaels MM, Brown HE, Favino CJ. Leiomyoma of prostate. *Urology* 1974;3:617–620.
139. Sudarasivarao D, Banerjea S, Nagewswararao A, et al. Hemangioma of the prostate: a case report. *J Urol* 1973; 110:708–709.
140. Ro JY, El-Naggar AK, Amin MB, et al. Pseudosarcomatous fibromyxoid tumor of the urinary bladder and prostate: immunohistochemical, ultrastructural, and DNA flow cytometric analyses of nine cases. *Hum Pathol* 1993;24:1203–1210.
141. Huang WL, Grignon DJ, Swanson D, et al. Postoperative spindle cell nodule of the prostate and bladder. *J Urol* 1990;143:824–826.
142. Proppe KH, Scully RE, Rosai J. Postoperative spindle cell nodules of genitourinary tract resembling sarcomas. A report of eight cases. *Am J Surg Pathol* 1984;8:101–108.
143. Hays DM, Raney RB, Lawrence W, et al. Bladder and prostatic tumors in the intergroup rhabdomyosarcoma study (IRSI): results of therapy. *Cancer* 1982;50:1472–1482.

144. Cheville JC, Dundore PA, Nascimento AG, et al. Leiomyosarcoma of the prostate. Report of 23 cases. *Cancer* 1995;76:1422–1427.
145. Chin W, Fay R, Ortega P. Malignant fibrous histiocytoma of prostate. *Urology* 1986;27:363–365.
146. Reyes JW, Shinozuka H, Garry P, et al. A light and electron microscopy study of a hemangiopericytoma of the prostate with local extension. *Cancer* 1977;40:1122–1126.
147. Schuppler J. Malignant neurolemmoma of prostate gland. *J Urol* 1971;106:903–905.
148. Smith DM, Manivel C, Kappa D, et al. Angiosarcoma of the prostate: report of 2 cases and review of the literature. *J Urol* 1986;135:382–384.
149. Gaudin PB, Rosai J, Epstein JI. Sarcomas and related proliferative lesions of specialized prostatic stroma. *Am J Surg Pathol* 1998;22:148–162.
150. Nassiri M, Ghazi C, Stivers JR, et al. Ganglioneuroma of the prostate. A novel finding in neurofibromatosis. *Arch Pathol Lab Med* 1994;118:938–939.
151. Sebo TJ, Bostwick DG, Farrow GM, et al. Prostatic xanthoma: a mimic of prostatic adenocarcinoma. *Hum Pathol* 1994;25:386–389.
152. Grignon DJ, O'Malley FP. Mucinous metaplasia in the prostate gland. *Am J Surg Pathol* 1993;17:287–290.
153. Egan MAJ, Youngkin TP, Bostwick DG. Mixed carcinoid-adenocarcinoma of the prostate with spindle cell carcinoid: the spectrum of neuroendocrine differentiation in prostatic neoplasia. *Pathology Case Reviews* 1996;1:65–69.
154. Weaver MG, Abdul-Karim FW, Srigley J. Paneth cell-like change of the prostate gland. A histological, immunohistochemical, and electron microscopic study. *Am J Surg Pathol* 1992;16:62–68.
155. Lim DJ, Hayden RT, Murad T, et al. Multilocular prostatic cystadenoma presenting as a large complex pelvic cystic mass. *J Urol* 1993;149:856–859.
156. Sakamoto N, Tsuneyoshi M, Enjoji M. Sclerosing adenosis of the prostate. Histopathologic and immunohistochemical analysis. *Am J Surg Pathol* 1991;15:660–667.
157. Ekfors TO, Aho HJ, Kekomaki M. Malignant rhabdoid tumor of the prostate region: immunohistological and ultrastructural evidence for epithelial origin. *Virchows Arch* 1985;406:381–388.
158. Casiraghi O, Martinez-Madrigal F, Mostofi FK, et al. Primary prostatic Wilms' tumor. *Am J Surg Pathol* 1991;15: 885–890.
159. Yang XJ, McEntee M, Epstein JI. Distinction of basaloid carcinoma of the prostate from benign basal cell lesions by using immunohistochemistry for BCL-2 and KI-67. *Hum Pathol* 1998;28:1447–1450.
160. Manrique JJ, Albores-Saavedra J, Orantes A, et al. Malignant mixed tumor of the salivary gland type, primary in the prostate. *Am J Clin Pathol* 1978;70:932–937.
161. Tay HP, Bidair M, Shabaik A, et al. Primary yolk sac tumor of the prostate in a patient with Klinefelter's syndrome. *J Urol* 1995;153:1066–1069.
162. Lauwers GY, Schevchuk M, Armenakas N, et al. Carcinosarcoma of the prostate. *Am J Surg Pathol* 1993;17:342–349.
163. Bostwick DG, Mann RB. Malignant lymphoma involving the prostate. A study of 13 cases. *Cancer* 1985;56:2932–2938.
164. Hollenberg GM. Extraosseous multiple myeloma simulating primary prostatic neoplasm. *J Urol* 1978;119:292–294.
165. Peison B, Benisch B, Nicora B, et al. Acute urinary obstruction secondary to pseudolymphoma of prostate. *Urology* 1977;10:478–479.
166. Ben-Ezra J, Sheibani K, Kendrick FE, et al. Angiotropic large cell lymphoma of the prostate gland: an immunohistochemical study. *Hum Pathol* 1986;17:964–967.
167. Dajai YF, Burke M. Leukemic infiltration of the prostate: a case study and clinicopathologic review. *Cancer* 1976;38: 2442–2446.
168. Eisenberger CF, Walsh PC, Eisenberger MA, et al. Incidental non-Hodgkin's lymphoma in patients with localized prostate cancer. *Urology* 1999;53:175–179.
169. Zein TA, Huben R, Lane W, et al. Secondary tumors of the prostate. *J Urol* 1985;133:615–616.
170. Bostwick DG, Egbert BM, Fajardo LF. Radiation injury of the normal and neoplastic prostate. *Am J Surg Pathol* 1982;6:501–551.
171. Brawer MK, Nagle RB, Pitts W, et al. Keratin immunoreactivity as an aid to the diagnosis of persistent adenocarcinoma following prostatic irradiation. *Cancer* 1989;63:454–460.
172. Scardino PT, Frankel JM, Wheeler TM, et al. The prognostic significance of post-irradiation biopsy results in patient with prostatic cancer. *J Urol* 1986;135:510–516.
173. Crook JM, Bahadur YA, Robertson SJ, et al. Evaluation of radiation effect, tumor differentiation, and prostate specific antigen staining in sequential prostate biopsies after external beam radiotherapy for patients with prostate carcinoma. *Cancer* 1997;79:79–81.
174. Labrie F, Cusan L, Gomez J-L, et al. Down-staging of early prostate cancer before radical prostatectomy: the first randomized trial of neoadjuvant therapy with flutamide and LHRH agonist. *Urology Symposium* 1994;44:29–37.
175. Macfarlane MT, Abi-Aad A, Stein A, et al. Neoadjuvant hormonal deprivation in patients with locally advanced prostate cancer. *J Urol* 1993;150:132–134.
176. Oesterling JE, Andrews PE, Suman VJ, et al. Preoperative androgen deprivation therapy: artificial lowering of serum prostate specific antigen without downstaging the tumor. *J Urol* 1993;149:779–782.
177. Pummer K, Crawford ED, Daneshgari F, et al. Hormonal pretreatment does not affect the final pathologic stage in locally advanced prostate cancer. *Urology Symposium* 1994;44:38–42.
178. Soloway MS, Sharifi R, Wajsman Z, et al. Randomized prospective study comparing radical prostatectomy alone versus radical prostatectomy preceded by androgen blockade in clinical stage B2 (T2bNxMO) prostate cancer. *J Urol* 1995;154:424–428.
179. Van Poppel H, De Ridder D, Elgamal AA, et al. Neoadjuvant hormonal therapy before radical prostatectomy decreased the number of positive surgical margins in stage T2 prostate cancer: interim results of a prospective randomized trial. *J Urol* 1995;154:429–434.
180. Armas OA, Aprikian AG, Melamed J, et al. Clinical and pathobiological effects of neoadjuvant total androgen ablation therapy on clinically localized prostatic adenocarcinoma. *Am J Surg Pathol* 1994;18:979–991.
181. Murphy WM, Soloway MS, Barrows GH. Pathologic changes associated with androgen deprivation therapy for prostate cancer. *Cancer* 1991;68:821–828.

182. Smith DM, Murphy WM. Histologic changes in prostate carcinomas treated with leuprolide (LHRH effect). *Cancer* 1994;73:1472–1477.
183. Smith DM, Murphy WM. Histologic changes in prostate carcinomas treated with leuprolide (luteinizing hormone-releasing hormone effect). Distinction from poor tumor differentiation. *Cancer* 1994;73:1472–1477.
184. Têtu B, Srigley JR, Boivin JC, et al. Effect of combination endocrine therapy (LHRH Agonist and Flutamide) on normal prostate and prostatic adenocarcinoma. A histopathologic and immunohistochemical study. *Am J Surg Pathol* 1991;15:111–120.
185. Vaillancourt L, Têtu B, Fradet Y, et al. Effect of neoadjuvant endocrine therapy (combined androgen blockade) on normal prostate and prostatic carcinoma. A randomized study. *Am J Surg Pathol* 1996;20:86–93.
186. Bostwick DG. Practical clinical application of predictive factors in prostate cancer. A review with an emphasis on quantitative methods in tissue specimens. *Analyt Quant Cytol Histol* 1998;20:323–342.
187. Adolfsson J. Prognostic value of deoxyribonucleic acid content in prostate cancer: a review of current results. *Int J Cancer* 1994;58:211–216.
188. Shankey TV, Kallioniemi OP, Koslowski JM, et al. Consensus review of the clinical utility of DNA content cytometry in prostate cancer. *Cytometry* 1993;14:497–500.
189. Seay TM, Blute ML, Zincke H. Long-term outcome in patients with pTxN+ adenocarcinoma of prostate treated with radical prostatectomy and early androgen ablation. *J Urol* 1998;159:356–364.
190. Ross JS, Figge H, Bui HX, et al. Prediction of pathologic stage and postprostatectomy disease recurrence by DNA ploidy analysis of initial needle biopsy specimens of prostate cancer. *Cancer* 1994;74:2811–2818.
191. Ross JS, Sheehan CE, Ambros RA, et al. Needle biopsy DNA ploidy status predicts grade shifting in prostate cancer. *Am J Surg Pathol* 1999;23:296–301.
192. Brinker DA, Ross JS, Tran TA, et al. Can ploidy of prostate carcinoma diagnosed on needle biopsy predict radical prostatectomy stage and grade? *J Urol* 1999;162:2036–2039.
193. Rubin MA, Buyyounouski M, Bagiella E, et al. Microvessel density in prostate cancer: lack of correlation with tumor grade, pathologic stage, and clinical outcome. *Urology* 1999;53:542–547.
194. Brinker DA, Partin AW, Epstein JI, et al. Does angiogenesis (microvessel density) of prostate carcinoma diagnosed on needle biopsy correlate with radical prostatectomy stage. *J Urol* 1999;161[Suppl]:238.
195. Bostwick DG, Wheeler TM, Blute M. Optimized microvessel density analysis improves prediction of cancer stage from prostate needle biopsies. *Urology* 1996;48:47–57.

18

COMBINED-MODALITY STAGING IN PREDICTING PROSTATE-SPECIFIC ANTIGEN OUTCOME AFTER DEFINITIVE LOCAL THERAPY FOR MEN WITH CLINICALLY LOCALIZED PROSTATE CANCER

ANTHONY V. D'AMICO

During the past 10 years, it has become increasingly apparent that by combining the pretreatment serum prostate-specific antigen (PSA), biopsy Gleason score, and the American Joint Commission on Cancer Staging (AJCC) T stage, a reliable prediction of pathologic stage can be made preoperatively (1). Although patients with pathologically organ-confined prostate cancer at the time of radical prostatectomy (RP) are the most likely to achieve long-term disease-specific survival, patients with microscopic extracapsular extension (ECE), established ECE, and seminal vesicle involvement are less likely to remain disease free. Patients in the worse prognostic category are those with positive pelvic lymph nodes (2). Yet within each prognostic group, there are those patients who are long-term survivors and those who die of prostate cancer. The ideal outcome predictor of the pretreatment clinical predictors would be cause-specific survival (CSS), but follow-up times of databases in this era of PSA diagnosis are too short to critically evaluate this important end point. Therefore, as an intermediate end point, PSA failure-free survival is evaluated.

The method used to define PSA failure-free survival is the methodology of *combined-modality staging*. This methodology has been previously defined (3) as a technique for identifying "the least common denominator" of clinical factors needed to optimize the prediction of posttherapy outcome. The methodology uses a multivariable analysis whose strength is to eliminate clinical predictors that reproduce information about posttherapy outcome already provided by the established clinical indicators (i.e., PSA, biopsy Gleason score, and the AJCC clinical T stage). Using this methodology, when a new test becomes available, the predictive value of the test can be evaluated in conjunction with the currently established prognostic factors to see whether new information about posttherapy outcome is provided by the test.

PROSTATE-SPECIFIC ANTIGEN, BIOPSY GLEASON SCORE, AND 1992 AMERICAN JOINT COMMISSION ON CANCER STAGING CLINICAL STAGE FOR PREDICTING PROSTATE-SPECIFIC ANTIGEN OUTCOME

Using a combined-modality staging approach, three risk groups for postoperative or postradiation PSA failure can be established from a review of the literature (4–17) in patients with clinically localized disease and are based on the known prognostic factors: PSA, biopsy Gleason score, and 1992 AJCC T stage.

Low risk: higher than 85% 5-year PSA failure-free survival

1992 AJCC clinical stage T1c,2a, PSA of 10 ng per mL or less, and biopsy Gleason score of 6 or less

Intermediate risk: approximately 50% 5-year PSA failure-free survival

1992 AJCC clinical stage T2b, or PSA higher than 10 but no more than 20 ng per mL, or biopsy Gleason score 7

High risk: approximately 33% 5-year PSA failure-free survival

1992 AJCC stage T2c disease, or PSA higher than 20 ng per mL, or biopsy Gleason score of 8 or higher

Patients presenting with bladder outlet obstructive symptoms and being diagnosed on the basis of a transurethral resec-

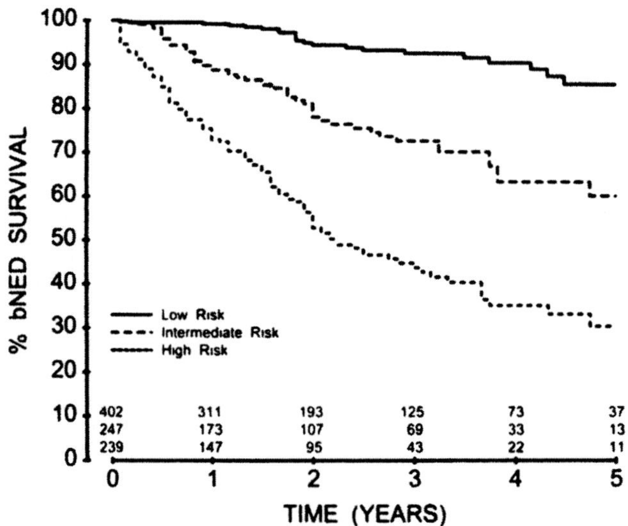

FIGURE 18-1. Biochemical no evidence of disease (bNED) as a function of a risk group for 888 surgically managed patients at the Hospital of the University of Pennsylvania.

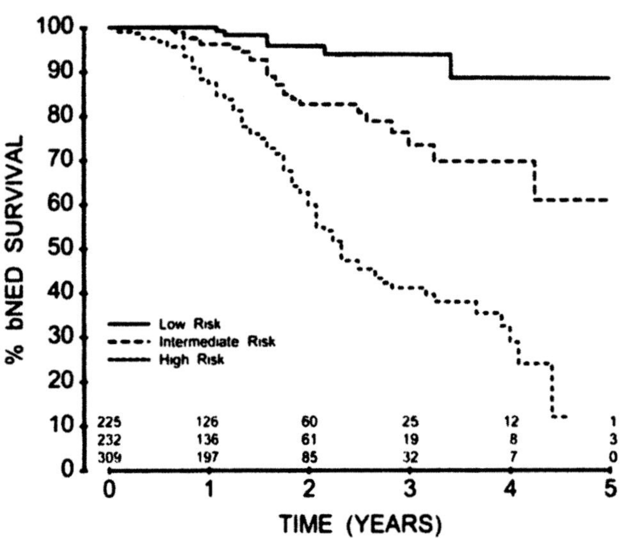

FIGURE 18-2. Biochemical no evidence of disease (bNED) as a function of a risk group for 766 radiation-managed patients at the Joint Center for Radiation Therapy.

tion of the prostate are becoming less common but would be grouped as low risk if T1a and intermediate risk if T1b.

Figures 18-1 and 18-2 display the estimates of PSA failure-free survival for 888 patients managed with a radical retropubic prostatectomy at the Hospital of the University of Pennsylvania (HUP) and 766 patients managed using conformal external beam radiation therapy (RT) at the Joint Center for Radiation Therapy (JCRT) at Harvard Medical School, using the risk stratification scheme defined earlier. The median follow-up for the surgically and radiation-managed patients was 38 (range, 8 to 100) months and 38 (range, 8 to 75) months, respectively.

Recently, a multiinstitutional pooled analysis of 1,607 men with clinical stage T1b,2NXM0 prostate cancer was performed by Shipley and colleagues (18), providing further validation of the ability of the pretreatment PSA level to predict PSA outcome after radical external beam RT, as shown in Figure 18-3. Specifically, 81%, 68%, 51%, and 31% of patients with a pretreatment PSA level less than 10 ng per mL, greater than or equal to 10 to 20 ng per mL, greater than or equal to 20 to 30 ng per mL, and greater than or equal to 30 ng per mL were estimated using a Kaplan-Meier analysis to be PSA failure free at 5 years, using the American Society for Therapeutic Radiol-

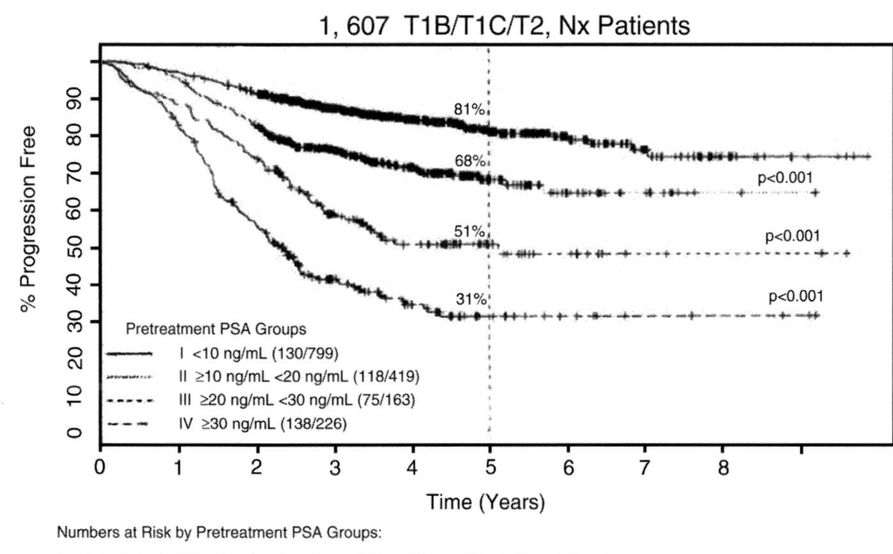

FIGURE 18-3. Multiinstitutional pooled analysis of the estimated prostate-specific antigen (PSA) failure-free survival (% progression free) after radical external beam radiation therapy stratified by the pretreatment PSA level. Nx, clinical node negative.

ogy and Oncology consensus definition for PSA failure after RT.

It is clear from these figures that the majority of low-risk patients is doing well at 5 years after RP or external beam RT. Conversely, most patients with high-risk but clinically localized disease are estimated to have failed biochemically by 5 years. Therefore, just on the basis of PSA, biopsy Gleason score, and AJCC clinical T stage, it is fair to say that most low-risk patients are unlikely to require more than local therapy for potential cure, whereas high-risk patients are unlikely to remain disease free after only local therapy. A more difficult group about which to make definitive statements regarding potential cure after local therapy is in the intermediate-risk population, in that a little more than half of these patients remain PSA failure free by 5 years. In this risk group, the ability of several clinical parameters has been evaluated to assess whether a clinically significant stratification of PSA failure-free survival can be obtained. The first parameter that is explored is the percent of positive prostate biopsies.

INTERMEDIATE RISK GROUP: THE ROLE OF PERCENT-POSITIVE BIOPSIES IN PREDICTING PROSTATE-SPECIFIC ANTIGEN OUTCOME

The fraction of prostate biopsies found to contain prostate cancer is information that is readily available for all patients with PSA-detected or clinically palpable prostate cancer. Studies investigating the ability of the fraction of positive prostate biopsies ×100 (percent-positive biopsies) to predict pathologic end points after RP suggest a role for this clinical factor in predicting tumor volume (19), ECE (20,21), seminal vesicle invasion (SVI) (22), lymph node involvement (23), and the percent Gleason grades 4 and 5 disease in the RP specimen (24). Whether the percent of positive prostate biopsies provides information in addition to that already embodied in the known prognostic factors in predicting PSA control after RP has been recently elucidated.

Several investigators have attempted to establish whether the number of biopsies containing adenocarcinoma provides further information about PSA outcome after RP. In particular, Presti and colleagues (25) performed a Cox regression multivariable analysis evaluating the clinical use of the fraction of systematic biopsies (1 to 3 vs. 4 to 6), pretreatment PSA level (less than or equal to 20 ng per mL vs. greater than 20 ng per mL), and biopsy Gleason score (2 to 6 vs. 7 to 10) to predict time to postoperative PSA failure. They had 109 patients in their analysis and used two consecutive rises in PSA greater than 0.1 ng per mL as the definition of PSA failure. They found that both the biopsy Gleason score and fraction of systematic biopsies were predictive of PSA outcome after RP. In addition, Huland and colleagues (26) recently reported on 318 consecutive patients treated using RP for localized prostate cancer. In their multivariable analysis, performed after a median follow-up of 42 months, they found the number of biopsies with predominant grade 4 or 5 disease, followed by the number of positive biopsies and the pretreatment PSA level, were the significant independent predictors of time to postoperative PSA failure.

To provide clinical use, D'Amico and colleagues evaluated the percent-positive biopsies within the previously established risk group categorization based on the pretreatment PSA, biopsy Gleason score, and 1992 AJCC clinical T-stage. They also defined a specific categorization of the percent-positive biopsy data for evaluation before their analysis to provide ease in clinical application. The categorization selected corresponded to 1 to 2 (less than 34%), 3 (34% to 50%), or 4 to 6 (greater than 50%) positive biopsies in the case of a standard sextant sampling. When analyzed in this manner, the percent-positive biopsy data were found to be an independent predictor of time to PSA failure after RP, after controlling for the previously defined risk stratification schema based on the known prognostic factors (27). The stratification of PSA outcome after RP provided by the percent-positive biopsies was also clinically significant in that, for the study and the validation cohorts, the vast majority (78% to 80%) of the intermediate-risk patients could be categorized into a high- or low-risk category for PSA outcome after RP. That result translated into a marked improvement in the physician's ability to counsel patients in the intermediate-risk category regarding outcome after RP. Specifically, Figures 18-4 and 18-5 show the clinically relevant stratification obtained using the percent-positive biopsy parameter in the intermediate-risk patients for the study and validation cohorts.

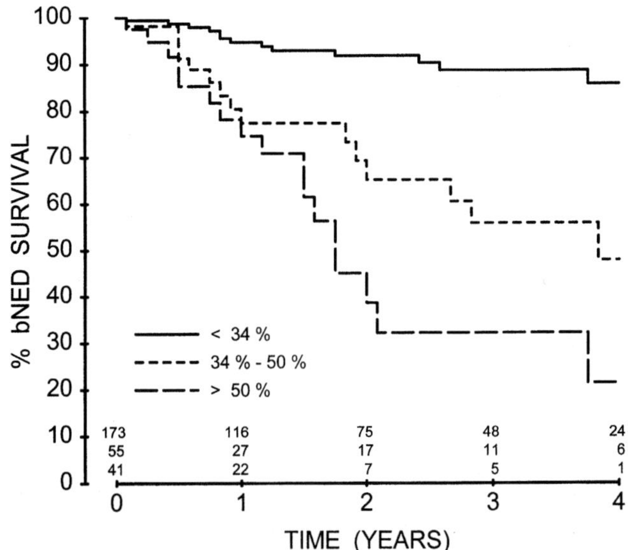

FIGURE 18-4. Estimated biochemical no evidence of disease (bNED) for intermediate-risk patients managed using radical prostatectomy at the Hospital of the University of Pennsylvania stratified by the percent-positive biopsies.

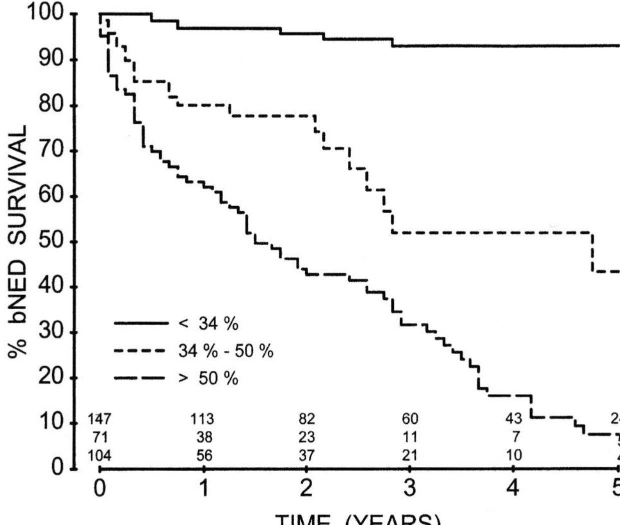

FIGURE 18-5. Biochemical no evidence of disease (bNED) for intermediate-risk patients managed using radical prostatectomy at the Brigham and Women's Hospital stratified by the percent-positive biopsies.

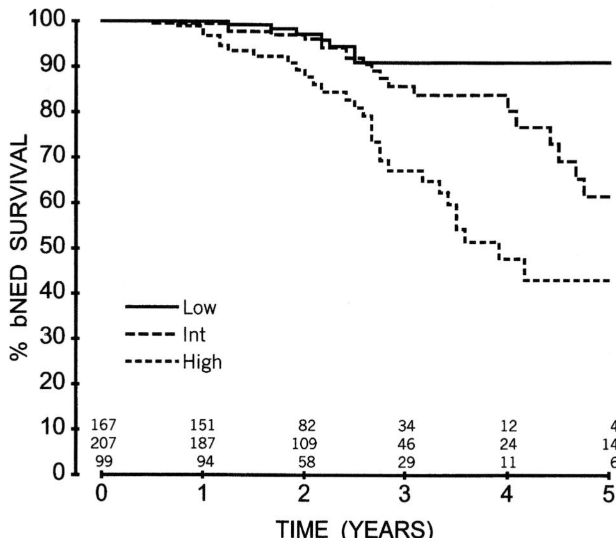

FIGURE 18-6. Biochemical no evidence of disease (bNED) for intermediate-risk patients managed using external beam radiation therapy at the Joint Center for Radiation Therapy stratified by the percent-positive biopsies. Int, intermediate.

Recently, the percent of positive prostate biopsies has also been shown to provide information in addition to that already embodied in the known prognostic factors in predicting PSA control after external beam RT (28). Specifically, 473 men treated using three-dimensional conformal external beam RT at the JCRT between 1989 and 1998 who had PSA-detected or clinically palpable prostate cancer comprised the study population. Random sextant biopsies were obtained in 301 (64%) of the study patients. The remaining 36% of patients had less than six (18%) or more than six (18%) biopsies. Specifically, 60 (12%), 28 (6%), 33 (7%), 27 (6%), 10 (2%), and 14 (3%) patients had four, five, seven, eight, nine, and ten or more biopsies obtained, respectively. Figure 18-6 illustrates the ability of the previously described risk group system 4 that was based on the pretreatment PSA level, biopsy Gleason score, and 1992 AJCC clinical T stage to stratify patients according to PSA outcome. Specifically, 5 years after RT, 91%, 62%, and 43% of low-, intermediate-, and high-risk patients, respectively, had not experienced PSA failure as defined by the American Society for Therapeutic Radiology and Oncology consensus panel. All pairwise comparisons were significant, with a p value less than or equal to .001.

Figure 18-7 illustrates the clinically relevant stratification provided by the percent-positive biopsies information in the previously defined intermediate-risk group based on the pretreatment PSA level, biopsy Gleason score, and the 1992 AJCC clinical T stage. Specifically, patients in the intermediate-risk subgroups that also had less than 34% of the biopsies positive improved their risk stratification for PSA outcome by one category to low risk. Conversely, patients with greater than 50% positive biopsies performed less well than expected and comparable to the high-risk patients.

Of particular importance, however, is that the majority of patients (158 of 207, 76%) in the intermediate-risk group could be classified into a 30% or 85% 5-year PSA control high- or low-risk cohort, respectively, using the preoperative prostate biopsy data. Therefore, of the 473 study patients, all but 49 (10%) were classified into high- or low-risk groups regarding PSA outcome after RT, using the percent-positive prostate biopsies, PSA level, biopsy Gleason score, and the 1992 AJCC clinical T stage.

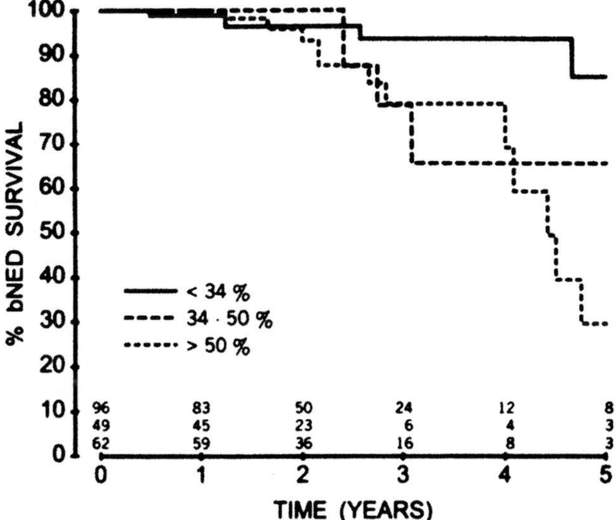

FIGURE 18-7. Prostate-specific antigen (PSA) outcome after external beam radiation therapy stratified using the risk group system that was based on the pretreatment PSA level, biopsy Gleason score, and 1992 American Joint Commission on Cancer Staging clinical T stage. bNED, biochemical no evidence of disease.

Therefore, the percent of positive prostate biopsies is information that is routinely available on newly diagnosed prostate cancer patients. This information has been previously shown in RP-managed patients (27) and has also recently been shown in RT-managed patients to provide a clinically significant improvement in predicting PSA outcome in intermediate-risk patients, in whom improved outcome prediction is most needed. Therefore, the percent-positive prostate biopsies should be considered in conjunction with the PSA level, biopsy Gleason score, and 1992 AJCC clinical T stage when counseling patients with newly diagnosed and clinically localized prostate cancer about PSA outcome after RP or RT.

ROLE OF ENDORECTAL COIL MAGNETIC RESONANCE IMAGING IN PREDICTING PROSTATE-SPECIFIC ANTIGEN OUTCOME

The reliability of the endorectal coil magnetic resonance imaging (erMRI) to predict pathologic stage has been shown to be related to the technique and experience level of the individual MR radiologist (29). In experienced hands and select patients, the erMRI scan has been shown to have an accuracy of approximately 80% (30,31) in predicting pathologic stage. A detailed examination of the clinical use of erMRI in predicting time to PSA failure after RP in 1,025 consecutive men with clinically localized or PSA-detected prostate cancer was performed by D'Amico and colleagues (32) after controlling for the PSA level, biopsy Gleason score, 1992 AJCC clinical T stage, and percent-positive biopsies. A prospective evaluation using a Cox regression time to PSA failure analysis was performed to evaluate the role of erMRI in predicting PSA outcome after RP at an academic institution, in which an expert prostate MR radiologist is located. The main outcome measure was actuarial biochemical no evidence of disease (bNED). The erMRI did not add clinically meaningful information for the vast majority of the patients (834 of 1,025; 81%) after accounting for the prognostic value of the PSA level, biopsy Gleason score, clinical T stage, and the percent-positive biopsies. In the remaining 191 patients, who were in the intermediate-risk group based on the established prognostic factors (PSA, biopsy Gleason score, AJCC clinical T stage, and percent-positive biopsies), the erMRI provided a clinically and statistically relevant stratification of 5-year PSA outcome. Specifically, the relative risk of PSA failure was 3.6 (95% confidence interval, 2.0 to 6.3) in patients whose erMRI was read as having extracapsular, as opposed to organ-confined, disease, and the 5-year bNED rate was 33% versus 72% (p <.0001), respectively, as shown in Figure 18-8. Despite expert MR radiologic interpretation, the erMRI was found to be of potential clinical value in fewer than 20% of the cases in this study after accounting for the established prognostic factors. Although further study on

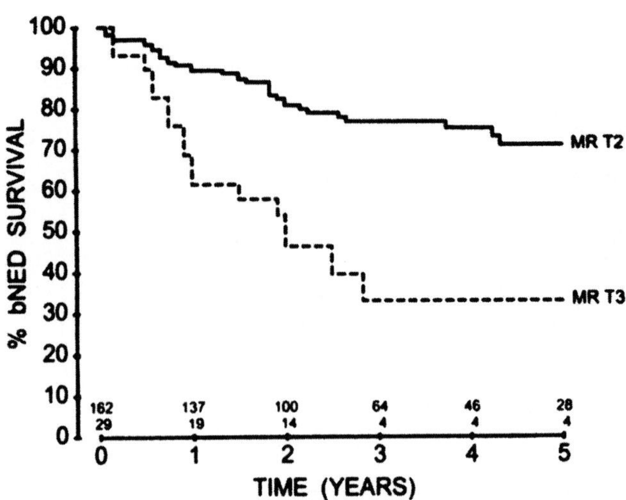

FIGURE 18-8. Biochemical no evidence of disease (bNED) for intermediate-risk patients stratified by the endorectal coil magnetic resonance (MR) imaging stage.

the value of erMRI in predicting clinical outcome after RP should be performed in this select cohort, the routine use of erMRI cannot be justified on the basis of these data.

NOMOGRAMS FOR PROSTATE-SPECIFIC ANTIGEN FAILURE-FREE SURVIVAL BASED ON PRETREATMENT CLINICAL FACTORS

Using the pretreatment PSA level, biopsy Gleason score, and 1992 AJCC clinical T stage, Partin and colleagues (1) have compiled tables predicting the probability of organ-confined, focal and established ECE, SVI, and lymph node disease using a 4,133-pooled patient database acquired between April 1982 and June 1996. Although useful, it has become increasingly apparent that not all patients with pathologic organ-confined disease remain without PSA failure, particularly if their preoperative PSA was greater than 10 ng per mL or biopsy Gleason score was at least 7 (13). Moreover, not all patients with established ECE or SVI fail biochemically within 5 years postoperatively (3,12). Therefore, in an attempt to more closely approximate the clinically relevant end point of survival, the reporting of PSA failure-free survival has been used. Specifically, Kattan and colleagues (33) have established a tool based on the pretreatment PSA, biopsy Gleason score, and 1992 AJCC clinical stage to predict PSA failure-free survival at 5 years postoperatively, as shown in Figure 18-9.

In addition, nomograms have been derived (34) expressing 2-year PSA failure rates with 95% confidence intervals as a function of the pretreatment PSA, biopsy Gleason score, and 1992 AJCC clinical stage for patients undergoing RP or RT. The time point of 2 years was chosen in an attempt to identify patients with early PSA failure. Patients with early PSA failure have been previously shown to present with dis-

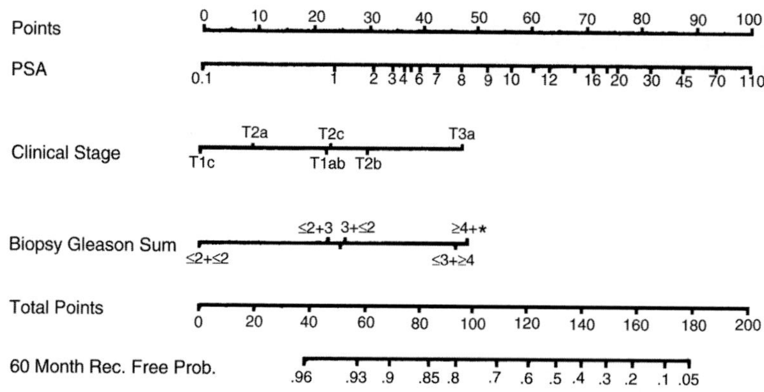

Instructions for physician: Locate the patient's PSA on the PSA axis. Draw a line straight upwards to the points axis to determine how many points towards recurrence the patient receives for his PSA. Repeat this process for the clinical stage and biopsy Gleason sum axes, each time drawing straight upward to the points axis. Sum the points achieved for each predictor and locate this sum on the total points axis. Draw a line straight down to find the patient's probability of remaining recurrence free for 60 months assuming he does not die of another cause first.

Note: *this nomogram is not applicable to a man who is not otherwise a candidate for radical prostatectomy. You can use this only on a man who has already selected radical prostatectomy as treatment for his prostate cancer.*

Instruction to patient: "Mr. X, if we had 100 men exactly like you we would expect between <predicted percentage from nomogram – 10%> and <predicted percentage + 10%> to remain free of their disease at 5 years after radical prostatectomy, and recurrence after 5 years is very rare."

FIGURE 18-9. Preoperative nomogram for estimating 5-year prostate-specific antigen (PSA) failure-free survival after radical prostatectomy.

tant failure as their most common site of first failure (3,10) and, therefore, are more likely to harbor occult micrometastatic disease at the time of local therapy. Realizing that metastatic prostate cancer is currently not a curable disease, the finding of early PSA failure, given time, is likely to translate into a decrement in cause-specific and overall survival. The tables for 2-year PSA failure-free survival are shown in Tables 18-1 and 18-2 for a group of 892 men managed with RP at the HUP and 762 men managed using three-dimensional conformal external beam RT at the JCRT, respectively. In addition, Table 18-3 provides the probability of PSA failure at 2 years and 95% confidence intervals stratified by the known prognostic factors and the percent-positive biopsy groups. Using these four clinical pretreatment parameters, more than 90% of all patients with clinically localized prostate cancer can be definitively stratified into high or low risk of PSA failure within 5 years of RP.

Only recently has data from both the surgically (35) and radiation-managed (36) patients provided a connection between PSA failure after RP or RT and time to distant failure. Specifically, Pound and colleagues (35) from The Johns Hopkins Hospital showed that the predictors of time to distant failure after RP include time to PSA failure after RP, the PSA doubling time, and the prostatectomy Gleason score, in which less than 2 years, less than 10 months, and greater than or equal to 8, respectively, were more strongly associated with distant failure. Similarly, Smith and colleagues (36) from the M. D. Anderson Cancer Center have shown similar results for patients managed with RT, in which the time to PSA failure was less than 1 year, the PSA doubling time was less than 1 year, or the biopsy Gleason score was greater than 7.

SUMMARY

1. The ideal end point for deciding on management for a patient with clinically localized adenocarcinoma of the prostate is CSS.
2. Follow-up of mature databases in the PSA era is too short to report CSS, but accurate 5-year estimates of PSA failure-free survival after RP or RT and stratified by the PSA level, biopsy Gleason score, and 1992 AJCC clinical T stage are now available.
3. The combination of the pretreatment PSA, biopsy Gleason score, and 1992 AJCC T stage can select patients with clinically localized disease very likely* (greater than 85%) and very unlikely† (less than 33%) to be without PSA failure at 5 years after local therapy. An intermediate group‡ remains for which more information is needed.
4. Intermediate-risk patients with one or two cores positive of six have 5-year PSA failure-free rates equivalent to the low-risk patients. Those patients with four or more positive biopsies of six have an estimated 5-year PSA failure-free survival similar to the high-risk patients.

---

*AJCC clinical stage T1c,2a, PSA less than or equal to 10 ng per mL, and biopsy Gleason score less than or equal to 6.

†AJCC clinical stage T2c, or PSA greater than 20 ng per mL, or biopsy Gleason score greater than or equal to 8.

‡AJCC clinical stage T2b, or PSA greater than 10 but not more than 20 ng per mL, or biopsy Gleason score 7.

TABLE 18-1. PERCENT PROSTATE-SPECIFIC ANTIGEN (PSA) FAILURE AT 2 YEARS AND THE 95% CONFIDENCE INTERVALS STRATIFIED BY THE PRETREATMENT PSA, 1992 AMERICAN JOINT COMMISSION ON CANCER STAGING CLINICAL STAGE, AND THE BIOPSY GLEASON SCORE FOR THE 892 SURGICALLY MANAGED PATIENTS AT THE HOSPITAL OF THE UNIVERSITY OF PENNSYLVANIA

Biopsy Gleason score	T1c (%)	T2a (%)	T2b (%)	T2c (%)
		PSA 0.0–4.0 ng/mL		
2–4	4 (2–7)	5 (3–7)	8 (4–13)	10 (6–17)
5	8 (5–11)	9 (6–11)	15 (8–21)	18 (12–25)
6	10 (6–15)	11 (8–14)	19 (11–27)	24 (17–31)
7	14 (8–20)	15 (11–19)	25 (15–35)	31 (22–40)
8–10	24 (13–37)	26 (16–36)	42 (24–59)	50 (34–65)
		PSA 4.1–10.0 ng/mL		
2–4	5 (3–8)	6 (4–9)	10 (5–16)	13 (8–20)
5	10 (6–14)	11 (8–13)	18 (11–25)	22 (16–30)
6	13 (8–18)	14 (11–17)	24 (15–32)	29 (22–37)
7	17 (11–24)	19 (14–23)	31 (20–42)	37 (28–46)
8–10	29 (17–44)	32 (20–44)	50 (31–67)	58 (43–72)
		PSA 10.1–20.0 ng/mL		
2–4	7 (4–12)	8 (5–13)	15 (8–23)	18 (11–29)
5	14 (9–20)	15 (11–19)	25 (17–34)	31 (23–40)
6	18 (11–26)	20 (15–25)	33 (22–43)	39 (31–48)
7	24 (15–34)	26 (20–33)	42 (29–54)	49 (40–59)
8–10	39 (24–58)	43 (29–58)	63 (44–80)	72 (56–84)
		PSA 20.1–50.0 ng/mL		
2–4	18 (10–34)	20 (12–36)	33 (19–54)	40 (25–64)
5	31 (18–52)	34 (23–53)	52 (36–73)	61 (46–81)
6	40 (24–63)	43 (30–63)	63 (47–83)	72 (60–88)
7	50 (32–74)	53 (39–75)	75 (58–91)	82 (71–95)
8–10	72 (48–94)	76 (57–94)	92 (77–99)	96 (88–100)

ASSESSMENT OF OUTCOME PREDICTION MODELS FOR PATIENTS WITH LOCALIZED PROSTATE CANCER MANAGED WITH RADICAL PROSTATECTOMY OR EXTERNAL BEAM RADIATION THERAPY

The 1992 AJCC clinical and pathologic staging systems for prostate cancer (37) remain the gold standards. To date, no preoperative clinical staging system has been able to provide reliable and reproducible information on which clinical decisions can be based before treatment, regarding the likelihood of cure after RP or external beam RT. Recently, several pretreatment clinical staging systems (1,38–40) have been proposed that combine the pretreatment PSA, biopsy Gleason score, and 1992 AJCC clinical stage in various ways in an attempt to optimize the prediction of time to PSA failure after external beam RT. A single study by Movsas and colleagues (41) at Fox Chase Cancer Center evaluated the predictive value of these various staging systems using a cohort of 421 prostate cancer patients managed with external beam RT. They concluded that all models were statistically significant predictors of postradiation PSA failure.

In a subsequent study by D'Amico and colleagues (42), the PSA outcome of 1,441 prostate cancer patients (976 treated with RP, 465 treated with external beam RT) was used to compare the predictive value of the proposed clinical staging systems. The requirement in that analysis was that a single model provided a statistically and clinically relevant stratification of PSA failure-free survival after RP or RT. The staging systems evaluated are shown below.

I. Standard paradigm:	PSA (continuous) Biopsy Gleason score (2 to 6 vs. 7 to 10) Clinical stage (T1 vs. T2)
II. Risk score (continuous) for patients with either T1 or T2 disease:	1.2 $\log_e$ (PSA) + 1.21 (Gleason risk) Gleason risk = 0 for biopsy Gleason 2 to 6 Gleason risk = 1 for biopsy Gleason 7 to 10
III. Volume of cancer (V_{Ca}) and PSA:	V_{Ca} <0.5 cm^3 V_{Ca} ≥0.5 and ≤4.0 cm^3 and PSA <10 ng per mL V_{Ca} ≥0.5 and ≤4.0 cm^3 and PSA ≥10 ng per mL V_{Ca} >4.0 cm^3
IV. PSA and Gleason 1:	PSA ≤20 ng per mL and biopsy Gleason 2 to 6

	PSA ≤20 ng per mL and biopsy Gleason 7 to 10
	or
	PSA >20 ng per mL and biopsy Gleason 2 to 6
	PSA >20 ng per mL and biopsy Gleason 7 to 10
V. PSA and Gleason 2:	PSA ≤4 ng per mL
	PSA >4 and ≤20 ng per mL and biopsy Gleason 2 to 6
	PSA >4 and ≤20 ng per mL and biopsy Gleason 7 to 10
	PSA >20 ng per mL

Cox regression multivariable analysis (43) was used to evaluate the ability of each staging system to predict time to posttreatment PSA failure. In surgically managed patients, PSA failure was defined as two consecutive detectable PSA values after a nondetectable value with the *time of failure* defined as the time of the first detectable value. A similar definition was used in radiation-managed patients with two rising PSA values after PSA nadir or a PSA nadir greater than 1 ng per mL. To increase the likelihood that the best staging system would be chosen, two different comparative measures were used to assess the ability of each staging system to predict time to posttherapy PSA failure. In particular, Akaike's Information Criterion (AIC) (44) and the Schwartz Bayesian Criterion (SBC) (45) estimates and their standard deviations were calculated for each clinical staging system using each data set. A smaller numeric value of the AIC or SBC estimates suggested an improved ability of the staging system to predict time to posttherapy PSA failure. The numeric difference between the AIC and SBC estimates for two most-predictive staging systems was then further tested to ascertain whether the numeric difference was large enough to be statistically significantly different. This analysis involved pairwise comparisons of the AIC and SBC estimates for the two staging systems, using a formal bootstrap technique (46) with 2,000 replications that were used to evaluate the relative ability of the two clinical staging systems to predict time to posttherapy PSA failure.

The results of this analysis concluded that both the staging system, based on the risk score, and calculated volume of prostate cancer (cV_{Ca}) optimized the prediction of time to posttherapy PSA failure after RP or RT. The cV_{Ca} system, however, provided a more clinically useful stratifica-

TABLE 18-2. PERCENT PROSTATE-SPECIFIC ANTIGEN (PSA) FAILURE AT 2 YEARS AND THE 95% CONFIDENCE INTERVALS STRATIFIED BY THE PRETREATMENT PSA, 1992 AMERICAN JOINT COMMISSION ON CANCER STAGING CLINICAL STAGE, AND THE BIOPSY GLEASON SCORE FOR THE 762 RADIATION-MANAGED PATIENTS AT THE JOINT CENTER FOR RADIATION THERAPY

Biopsy Gleason score	T1c (%)	T2a (%)	T2b (%)	T2c (%)
		PSA 0–4 ng/mL		
2–4	3 (1–5)	4 (2–7)	5 (3–9)	6 (3–9)
5	7 (4–10)	8 (5–12)	11 (7–16)	12 (7–17)
6	10 (6–14)	12 (8–17)	16 (10–23)	17 (11–24)
7	14 (9–20)	18 (11–25)	23 (15–34)	25 (17–35)
8–10	29 (17–46)	36 (21–55)	45 (27–68)	48 (29–69)
		PSA 4.1–10.0 ng/mL		
2–4	4 (2–6)	5 (2–8)	6 (3–10)	7 (3–11)
5	8 (5–11)	10 (6–14)	13 (8–18)	14 (9–20)
6	11 (7–15)	14 (9–19)	18 (12–26)	20 (13–27)
7	16 (11–23)	20 (13–28)	26 (17–37)	28 (19–39)
8–10	33 (20–50)	40 (24–59)	50 (31–72)	52 (33–74)
		PSA 10.1–20.0 ng/mL		
2–4	4 (2–8)	5 (3–10)	7 (4–13)	8 (4–14)
5	9 (6–14)	12 (7–17)	16 (10–22)	17 (11–24)
6	14 (9–19)	17 (11–24)	22 (15–31)	24 (17–33)
7	20 (13–27)	25 (16–34)	32 (22–44)	34 (24–46)
8–10	39 (25–57)	47 (30–67)	58 (38–79)	61 (40–81)
		PSA 20.1–50.0 ng/mL		
2–4	7 (3–14)	9 (4–18)	12 (6–23)	13 (7–24)
5	16 (10–24)	20 (13–30)	26 (16–37)	27 (17–39)
6	23 (15–32)	28 (20–39)	36 (25–49)	38 (27–51)
7	32 (23–42)	39 (28–51)	49 (36–64)	51 (38–66)
8–10	58 (41–76)	67 (49–85)	78 (58–93)	80 (62–94)

TABLE 18-3. TWO-YEAR PROSTATE-SPECIFIC ANTIGEN (PSA) FAILURE PROBABILITIES (95% CONFIDENCE INTERVALS) STRATIFIED BY THE PRETREATMENT PSA LEVEL, 1992 AMERICAN JOINT COMMISSION ON CANCER STAGING CLINICAL T STAGE, BIOPSY GLEASON SCORE, AND THE PERCENT-POSITIVE BIOPSIES

Gleason score	%+ bxs	T1c	T2a	T2b	T2c
		PSA 0–4 ng/mL			
2–4	<34	2 (1, 3)	2 (1, 3)	2 (1, 4)	2 (1, 5)
	34–50	4 (2, 9)	6 (4, 12)	5 (3, 11)	6 (3, 12)
	>50	6 (3, 12)	8 (5, 15)	7 (3, 14)	8 (4, 16)
5	<34	2 (1, 4)	2 (1, 4)	3 (1, 5)	3 (2, 6)
	34–50	6 (3, 11)	6 (4, 12)	8 (4, 13)	8 (5, 15)
	>50	8 (4, 15)	8 (5, 15)	10 (5, 18)	11 (6, 19)
6	<34	2 (1, 5)	2 (1, 5)	3 (1, 6)	3 (2, 7)
	34–50	7 (4, 13)	7 (5, 13)	9 (5, 15)	9 (6, 17)
	>50	9 (5, 18)	10 (7, 18)	12 (6, 20)	13 (8, 22)
7	<34	2 (1, 6)	3 (2, 6)	4 (2, 7)	4 (2, 8)
	34–50	8 (5, 15)	9 (6, 16)	11 (6, 18)	11 (7, 20)
	>50	11 (6, 21)	12 (8, 21)	14 (7, 23)	15 (9, 25)
8–10	<34	4 (2, 8)	4 (2, 8)	5 (2, 9)	5 (3, 10)
	34–50	12 (6, 23)	12 (7, 24)	15 (7, 27)	16 (8, 29)
	>50	15 (8, 31)	16 (10, 31)	20 (10, 34)	21 (12, 37)
		PSA 4.1–10.0 ng/mL			
2–4	<34	4 (2, 7)	4 (3, 7)	6 (3, 9)	7 (3, 10)
	34–50	13 (7, 22)	13 (8, 23)	16 (8, 26)	17 (9, 29)
	>50	17 (9, 29)	18 (10, 30)	21 (11, 33)	22 (12, 36)
5	<34	6 (3, 10)	7 (4, 10)	9 (4, 12)	9 (5, 13)
	34–50	17 (10, 27)	18 (13, 28)	22 (12, 31)	23 (15, 33)
	>50	23 (14, 35)	24 (17, 35)	29 (16, 38)	30 (20, 42)
6	<34	7 (4, 12)	8 (4, 12)	10 (4, 13)	11 (6, 16)
	34–50	20 (12, 31)	21 (15, 31)	26 (15, 35)	27 (18, 37)
	>50	27 (16, 40)	28 (20, 39)	33 (20, 43)	35 (24, 45)
7	<34	9 (4, 14)	10 (5, 14)	11 (5, 16)	12 (7, 18)
	34–50	24 (14, 36)	25 (18, 26)	30 (17, 40)	31 (20, 42)
	>50	31 (18, 45)	33 (23, 45)	38 (23, 49)	40 (28, 51)
8–10	<34	13 (5, 22)	13 (7, 23)	16 (7, 25)	18 (9, 27)
	34–50	32 (17, 51)	34 (21, 52)	40 (21, 55)	41 (25, 58)
	>50	41 (24, 62)	43 (28, 62)	50 (28, 66)	51 (34, 68)
		PSA 10.1–20.0 ng/mL			
2–4	<34	10 (4, 15)	11 (5, 16)	13 (5, 18)	14 (6, 20)
	34–50	26 (13, 42)	27 (16, 42)	32 (16, 46)	34 (18, 51)
	>50	33 (18, 51)	35 (21, 52)	41 (21, 56)	43 (25, 60)
5	<34	14 (7, 19)	17 (8, 22)	18 (8, 22)	18 (10, 24)
	34–50	35 (20, 50)	37 (25, 49)	43 (25, 53)	44 (29, 57)
	>50	69 (43, 87)	46 (32, 59)	53 (33, 62)	53 (33, 62)
6	<34	17 (8, 23)	17 (10, 24)	21 (9, 25)	22 (12, 28)
	34–50	40 (23, 56)	42 (30, 55)	49 (29, 59)	50 (34, 62)
	>50	50 (31, 65)	52 (38, 64)	60 (38, 67)	61 (46, 70)
7	<34	19 (9, 27)	21 (11, 27)	24 (11, 30)	25 (13, 33)
	34–50	46 (26, 62)	48 (34, 61)	55 (33, 65)	57 (39, 68)
	>50	56 (36, 72)	59 (44, 71)	66 (43, 74)	68 (52, 76)
8–10	<34	26 (11, 40)	26 (14, 40)	33 (14, 44)	34 (17, 47)
	34–50	58 (33, 79)	60 (40, 79)	68 (40, 81)	70 (47, 84)
	>50	69 (43, 87)	72 (51, 86)	79 (52, 88)	80 (60, 89)
		PSA 20.1–50.0 ng/mL			
2–4	<34	24 (10, 30)	24 (11, 35)	31 (12, 39)	31 (13, 43)
	34–50	54 (27, 75)	56 (32, 76)	64 (33, 79)	65 (37, 83)
	>50	65 (36, 84)	67 (42, 85)	75 (42, 86)	76 (49, 89)
5	<34	32 (15, 44)	33 (17, 44)	39 (18, 47)	41 (20, 50)

(*continued*)

TABLE 18-3. *continued*

Gleason score	%+ bxs	T1c	T2a	T2b	T2c
		PSA 20.1–50.0 ng/mL			
	34–50	67 (39, 84)	69 (47, 84)	76 (48, 85)	78 (53, 88)
	>50	78 (50, 90)	80 (58, 90)	86 (60, 91)	87 (68, 93)
6	<34	37 (17, 49)	38 (21, 50)	45 (21, 53)	46 (25, 56)
	34–50	73 (45, 88)	75 (54, 88)	82 (55, 89)	84 (61, 92)
	>50	83 (57, 93)	85 (67, 93)	90 (68, 94)	91 (76, 95)
7	<34	42 (19, 55)	44 (24, 57)	51 (24, 59)	54 (28, 62)
	34–50	79 (50, 92)	81 (60, 92)	87 (60, 93)	88 (67, 94)
	>50	88 (63, 96)	90 (73, 96)	94 (74, 96)	95 (82, 97)
8–10	<34	55 (24, 73)	57 (29, 74)	64 (29, 75)	65 (35, 78)
	34–50	89 (59, 98)	91 (68, 98)	87 (60, 93)	88 (67, 94)
	>50	95 (73, 99)	96 (81, 99)	98 (83, 99)	99 (89, 100)

Note: Numbers in parentheses represent 95% confidence intervals.
%+ bxs, percent-positive biopsies.

tion of PSA outcome, in that a distinct group of men estimated to be at a very low (less than 15%) or very high risk (greater than 67%) of post-RP or post-RT PSA failure by 4 years could be defined.

The cV_{Ca} clinical staging system was also compared to the 1992 AJCC pathologic stage for surgically managed patients by the same investigators using a surgical database (Brigham and Women's Hospital) that was independent of the surgical database (HUP) used to establish the cV_{Ca} staging system. The results of that study found that the 1992 AJCC pathologic stage and the cV_{Ca}-PSA clinical stage were significant predictors of time to postoperative PSA failure (p = .0001) using a Cox regression analysis. Further analyses using the AIC and SBC comparative measures of the 1992 AJCC pathologic stage and cV_{Ca}-PSA clinical stage ability to predict postoperative PSA failure found the cV_{Ca}-PSA staging system to provide a more clinically useful prediction of time to postoperative PSA failure. Specifically, the cV_{Ca}-PSA staging system was able to identify surgically managed patients with pathologic AJCC stage T2 disease who did poorly (3-year freedom from PSA failure = 22%).

In summary, the clinical staging system based on the cV_{Ca} provided a clinically and statistically useful stratification of PSA outcome after RP or external beam RT. Lankford and colleagues at M. D. Anderson Cancer Center have documented the ability of the cV_{Ca} to stratify PSA outcome in radiation-managed patients with a pretreatment PSA between 4 and 20 ng per mL in a statistically superior fashion to the PSA level, PSA density, biopsy Gleason score, and prostatic acid phosphatase (47). Validation studies by other investigators are under way.

PROSTATE-SPECIFIC ANTIGEN OUTCOME AFTER RADICAL PROSTATECTOMY, EXTERNAL BEAM RADIATION THERAPY, OR INTERSTITIAL RADIATION THERAPY FOR CLINICALLY LOCALIZED PROSTATE CANCER USING COMBINED-MODALITY STAGING

Recommendations for treatment of clinically localized adenocarcinoma of the prostate should be made using the results of evidence-based medicine. To date, there are no completed

TABLE 18-4. *P* VALUES FROM THE COX REGRESSION ANALYSES EVALUATING THE ABILITY OF A TREATMENT MODALITY TO PREDICT THE TIME TO POSTTHERAPY PROSTATE-SPECIFIC ANTIGEN FAILURE, STRATIFIED BY RISK GROUP

Treatment	Low risk	Intermediate risk	High risk
RP at HUP	—	—	—
RT at JCRT	.98	.13	.27
	RR = 1.1 (0.5–2.7)	RR = 0.8 (0.5–1.2)	RR = 0.9 (0.7–1.1)
Implant	.28	.001	.001
	RR = 1.8 (0.6–5.2)	RR = 3.9 (1.9–7.7)	RR = 2.7 (1.6–4.4)
Implant + hormones	.60	.22	.006
	RR = 0.8 (0.2–2.5)	RR = 1.6 (0.7–3.6)	RR = 2.6 (1.3–5.2)

HUP, Hospital of the University of Pennsylvania (baseline group); JCRT, Joint Center for Radiation Therapy; RT, radiation therapy.
Note: The relative risk (RR) is defined as the proportional increase in prostate-specific antigen failure expected with a given treatment modality when compared to radical prostatectomy (RP). This value is shown with a 95% confidence interval.

prospective randomized trials comparing definitive local treatment options for this disease. Retrospective comparisons (48,49) stratified by the known prognostic factors and using actuarial analyses have been published comparing RP to external beam RT. However, a direct comparison of the results of ultrasound-guided interstitial prostate RT with or without neoadjuvant androgen-deprivation therapy to RP or RT stratified by the pretreatment prognostic factors using the combined modality staging approach outlined here has not been previously reported.

Table 18-4 lists the *p* values from the Cox regression multivariable analyses evaluating the effect of the treatment type on time to posttherapy PSA failure stratified by risk group. The relative risks of PSA failure with a 95% confidence interval are also listed. No significant difference ($p \geq .25$) in outcome was noted in low-risk patients (T1c,2a and PSA less than or equal to 10 and Gleason less than or equal to 6) across all treatment modalities. The 95% confidence intervals for the relative risk of PSA failure for those patients managed with RT or implant with or without neoadjuvant androgen-deprivation therapy, compared to RP, included a relative risk of 1.0. High-risk patients (T2c, PSA greater than 20, or Gleason greater than or equal to 8), however, treated using RP or RT, did significantly better ($p \leq .012$) than those managed with implant with or without neoadjuvant androgen deprivation. Specifically, high-risk patients managed with implant therapy had at least a 2.2-fold increased risk of PSA failure compared to those treated with RP, even if neoadjuvant androgen-deprivation therapy was used. Intermediate-risk patients (T2b, Gleason 7, or PSA greater than 10 and less than or equal to 20) did significantly worse ($p \leq .003$) if managed by implant alone but fared equivalently ($p = .18$) to those patients managed with RP if a median of 3 months of androgen deprivation was also administered. Intermediate-risk patients, managed with implant therapy alone, had a 3.1-fold increased risk of PSA failure compared to those patients managed with RP.

For the purpose of illustration, estimates of bNED outcome with pairwise *p* values evaluating the comparisons between treatment types were calculated using the actuarial method of Kaplan and Meier (50) and are graphically displayed by risk group in Figures 18-10, 18-11, and 18-12. The use of the combined-modality staging methodology can be appreciated here, where randomized data on outcome after various treatments are lacking. Yet, when controlling for the known prognostic factors (PSA, biopsy Gleason score, and AJCC T stage), implant therapy alone appears to be inferior to RP or RT in patients with PSA greater than 10 ng per mL, biopsy Gleason score greater than or equal to 7, or 1992 AJCC clinical stage greater than or equal to T2b.

SUMMARY

1. Low-risk patients had equivalent estimates of 5 years' bNED outcome after treatment with RP, RT, or implant with or without neoadjuvant androgen deprivation.
2. Intermediate- and high-risk patients treated with RP or RT did statistically better than those treated by implant.
3. Whether the use of 3 months of neoadjuvant androgen-suppression therapy before implant therapy in intermediate-risk patients produces equivalent clinical control rates to RP or RT requires longer follow-up to ascertain.

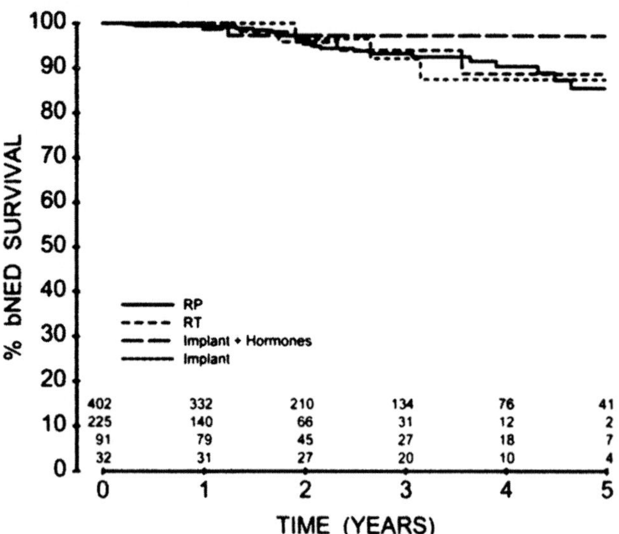

FIGURE 18-10. Biochemical no evidence of disease (bNED) outcome for low-risk patients stratified by treatment modality. All pairwise *p* values are >.25. RP, radical prostatectomy; RT, radiation therapy.

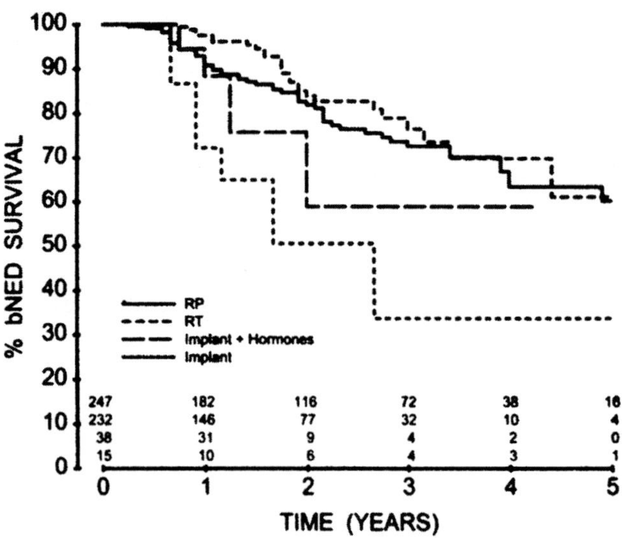

FIGURE 18-11. Biochemical no evidence of disease (bNED) outcome for intermediate-risk patients. Pairwise *p* values: radical prostatectomy (RP) vs. radiation therapy (RT), .26; RP vs. implant + androgen ablation, .18; RP vs. implant, .003; RT vs. implant + androgen ablation, .009; RT vs. implant, .0002; and implant + androgen ablation vs. implant, .14.

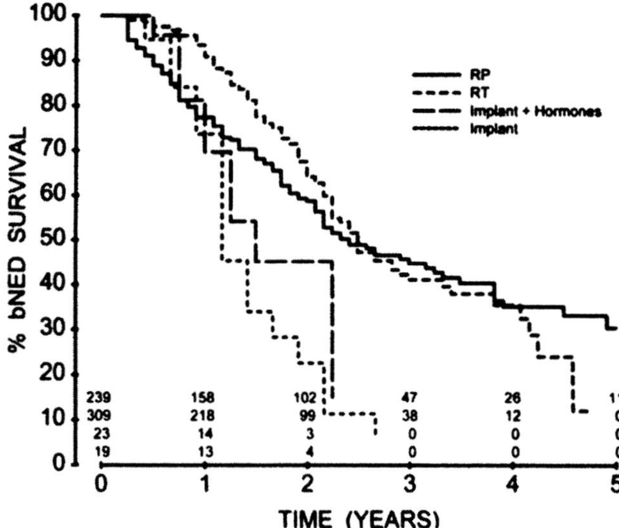

FIGURE 18-12. Biochemical no evidence of disease (bNED) outcome for high-risk patients. Pair-wise *p* values: radical prostatectomy (RP) vs. radiation therapy (RT), .25; RP vs. implant + androgen ablation, .012; RP vs. implant, .0005; RT vs. implant + androgen ablation, .0007; RT vs. implant, <.0001; and implant + androgen ablation vs. implant, .41.

4. Prospective randomized trials are needed to verify these findings.

COMBINED-MODALITY STAGING USING THE PREOPERATIVE PROSTATE-SPECIFIC ANTIGEN LEVEL AND POSTOPERATIVE PATHOLOGIC FINDINGS TO PREDICT PROSTATE-SPECIFIC ANTIGEN OUTCOME IN MEN WITH CLINICALLY LOCALIZED PROSTATE CANCER

Time to Prostate-Specific Antigen Failure Analyses

Using the methodology of combined-modality staging, a Cox regression analysis was performed on 862 surgically managed patients at HUP evaluating the ability of the preoperative PSA, pathologic Gleason score, pathologic stage, and pathologic margin status to predict time to postoperative PSA failure (51). Results from the Cox regression multivariable analysis confirmed the independent prognostic significance of the preoperative PSA (p = .0001), pathologic stage ($p \leq .002$), prostatectomy Gleason score (p = .034), and margin status (p = .0001) in predicting time to postoperative PSA failure.

Postoperative Prostate-Specific Antigen Failure Stratified by Prostate-Specific Antigen and Pathologic Data

Table 18-5 is a compilation of the 2-year PSA failure rates and the respective 95% confidence intervals stratified by preoperative PSA group (less than or equal to 4, greater than or equal to 4 to 10, greater than or equal to 10 to 20, greater than 20 ng per mL), prostatectomy Gleason score (2 to 4, 5 to 6, 7, and 8 to 10), and pathologic stage (organ confined and margin negative, organ confined and margin positive, focal ECE and margin negative, focal ECE and margin positive, established ECE and margin negative, established ECE and margin positive, SVI and margin negative, and SVI and margin positive). Two-year PSA failure rates ranged from 4% to 25% in men with pathologic organ-confined disease. Conversely, 59% to 99% of men with SVI and positive surgical margins sustained PSA failure by 2 years postoperatively.

In a previous study by Partin and colleagues (10), it was suggested that early postoperative PSA failure translated into distant failure as a site of first failure in the majority of patients. This finding was further supported by Cadeddu and colleagues (52), who showed that the ability of post-prostatectomy external beam RT to cause a rising postoperative PSA to become undetectable decreased dramatically as the interval to postoperative PSA failure shortened. In particular, only 6% of patients responded if PSA failure occurred within the first postoperative year, supporting the existence of micrometastatic disease outside the surgical bed. Therefore, the 2-year PSA failure probabilities presented in Table 18-5 could be used to select patients at high risk for harboring occult micrometastatic disease. In an attempt to improve cure rates in these select men, entry into postoperative adjuvant therapy trials would be an option.

Kattan and colleagues (53) have also performed a similar analysis on 996 patients with clinical stage T1a to T3c prostate cancer managed using an RP at the Baylor College of Medicine between 1983 and 1997. In their patient cohort with a median follow-up of 37 (1 to 168) months, a *nomogram* was defined, as shown on Figure 18-13, to predict the 7-year recurrence-free probability as a function of the preoperative PSA, prostatectomy Gleason score, pathologic T and N stage, extent of capsular invasion, and margin status. What remains to be done is the execution and analysis of adjuvant therapy clinical trials using the results provided by such nomograms to identify the patients in need of systemic therapy to improve their chance of long-term disease-free survival.

COMBINED-MODALITY STAGING USING POSTOPERATIVE PROSTATE-SPECIFIC ANTIGEN KINETICS AND THE PROSTATECTOMY GLEASON SCORE TO PREDICT PROSTATE-SPECIFIC ANTIGEN OUTCOME IN MEN WITH CLINICALLY LOCALIZED PROSTATE CANCER

An analysis of 1,997 patients with clinical stage T1 and -2 prostate cancer, managed with an RP by Dr. Patrick Walsh at The Johns Hopkins University, was performed to aid in

TABLE 18-5. PERCENT PROSTATE-SPECIFIC ANTIGEN (PSA) FAILURE AT 2 YEARS AND THE 95% CONFIDENCE INTERVALS STRATIFIED BY THE PREOPERATIVE PSA, PATHOLOGIC STAGE, PROSTATECTOMY GLEASON SCORE, AND MARGIN STATUS

P (pathologic) Gleason score	POC margin −	POC margin +	$PECE_{foc}$ margin −	$PECE_{foc}$ margin +	$PECE_{est}$ margin −	$PECE_{est}$ margin +	PSVI margin −	PSVI margin +
PSA 0–4 ng/mL								
2–4	4 (2–7)	8 (3–15)	8 (3–14)	14 (5–26)	18 (6–34)	32 (12–55)	36 (14–64)	59 (26–86)
5–6	6 (4–8)	12 (7–19)	12 (6–18)	22 (14–30)	26 (16–39)	46 (34–60)	51 (32–71)	76 (58–91)
7	7 (4–10)	13 (6–24)	13 (7–19)	24 (15–34)	29 (19–42)	50 (36–66)	55 (37–75)	79 (61–94)
8–10	9 (5–17)	17 (8–36)	17 (8–32)	31 (18–51)	38 (21–61)	61 (41–84)	66 (42–90)	89 (70–99)
PSA 4.1–10.0 ng/mL								
2–4	5 (2–8)	9 (3–17)	9 (3–17)	17 (6–29)	21 (7–39)	37 (14–61)	41 (16–70)	65 (30–90)
5–6	7 (5–9)	13 (8–22)	13 (7–21)	25 (16–34)	30 (19–44)	52 (40–65)	56 (37–77)	81 (65–94)
7	8 (5–12)	15 (8–27)	15 (9–22)	28 (18–38)	33 (22–47)	56 (42–71)	61 (43–80)	85 (70–96)
8–10	11 (6–19)	20 (10–40)	20 (10–36)	36 (21–56)	43 (25–67)	67 (47–87)	72 (49–93)	92 (77–99)
PSA 10.1–20.0 ng/mL								
2–4	6 (2–10)	11 (4–21)	11 (4–22)	21 (8–37)	26 (9–49)	45 (18–70)	50 (20–78)	75 (38–95)
5–6	9 (6–12)	17 (10–34)	17 (9–27)	31 (21–42)	38 (24–53)	61 (49–73)	66 (46–85)	89 (77–97)
7	10 (6–15)	19 (10–34)	19 (11–28)	34 (24–46)	41 (28–56)	66 (52–79)	70 (53–87)	91 (81–98)
8–10	14 (7–24)	25 (13–48)	25 (13–44)	44 (26–66)	52 (32–76)	77 (58–93)	81 (60–97)	96 (87–99)
PSA 20.1–50.0 ng/mL								
2–4	11 (4–21)	21 (7–40)	21 (7–42)	37 (14–62)	44 (17–76)	69 (33–92)	74 (34–95)	93 (60–99)
5–6	17 (11–26)	31 (18–49)	31 (16–51)	52 (34–71)	60 (41–82)	84 (71–95)	88 (69–98)	99 (94–100)
7	19 (11–29)	34 (19–57)	34 (20–53)	56 (39–74)	64 (47–83)	87 (75–96)	91 (77–98)	99 (96–100)
8–10	25 (13–45)	43 (23–73)	43 (23–72)	67 (44–90)	76 (54–96)	94 (82–99)	96 (84–99)	99 (98–100)

$PECE_{est}$, pathologic extracapsular extension, established; $PECE_{foc}$, pathologic extracapsular extension, focal; POC, pathologic organ-confined; PSVI, pathologic seminal vesical invasion.

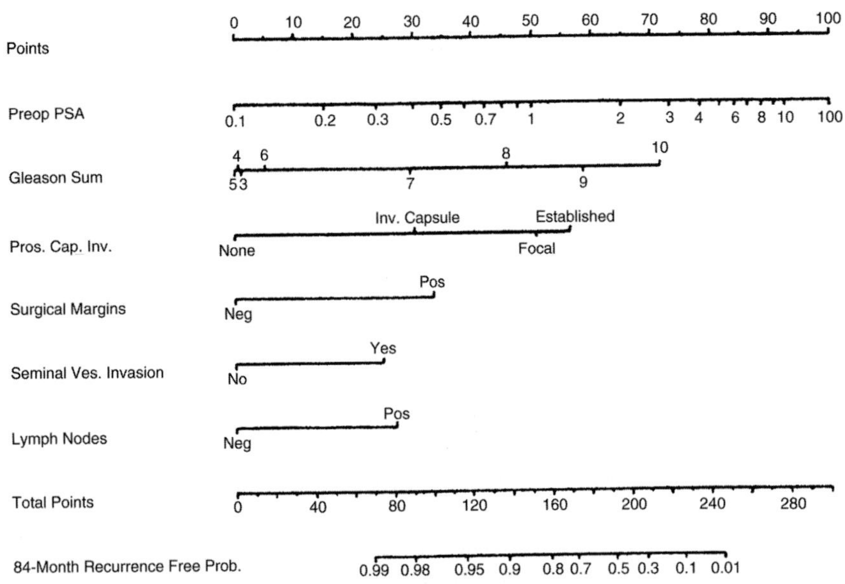

Instructions for physician: Locate the patient's PSA on the PSA axis. Draw a line straight upwards to the points axis to determine how many points towards recurrence the patient receives for his PSA. Repeat this process for the other axes, each time drawing straight upward to the points axis. Sum the points achieved for each predictor and locate this sum on the total points axis. Draw a line straight down to find the patient's probability of remaining recurrence free for 84 months assuming he does not die of another cause first.

Instruction to patient: "Mr. X, if we had 100 men exactly like you we would expect between <predicted percentage from nomogram – 10%> and <predicted percentage + 10%> to remain free of their disease at 7 years after radical prostatectomy, and recurrence after 7 years is very rare."

FIGURE 18-13. Postoperative nomogram for estimating the 7-year freedom from prostate-specific antigen (PSA) failure after radical prostatectomy. Cap, capsule; Inv, invasion; Prob, probability; Ves, vesicle.

counseling patients after RP as to the likelihood of remaining without evidence of metastatic disease after RP (34). They performed a multivariable analysis and found that the prostatectomy Gleason score (less than or equal to 7 vs. greater than or equal to 8), PSA doubling time (less than or equal to 10 months vs. greater than or equal to 10 months), and the time to postoperative PSA failure (less than or equal to 2 years vs. greater than 2 years) were predictive of distant failure. Specifically, for men with all three of these factors, 82% remained without evidence of metastatic disease at 7 years after PSA failure. Time to distant failure was the only predictor of CSS. Specifically, the median survival for men who developed distant disease within 3 years, 4 to 7 years, or greater than 7 years postoperatively was 4, 5, and greater than 5 years (not reached at median follow-up of 5.3 years) after the documentation of distant disease, respectively.

SUMMARY

1. Using combined-modality staging, patients at high risk for early (less than 2 years) postoperative PSA failure can be identified and offered adjuvant systemic therapy (e.g., hormonal or chemohormonal therapy) in the setting of a clinical trial.
2. Patients with at least a 50% chance of PSA failure within 2 years postoperatively were generally those with
   a. SVI independent of the margin status
   b. Established ECE with a positive margin
   c. Established ECE with a negative margin and a preoperative PSA greater than 20 ng per mL
   d. Established ECE with a negative margin and a PSA greater than 10 ng per mL but not more than 20 ng per mL and a prostatectomy Gleason score greater than or equal to 8
   e. Focal ECE and a positive margin and a preoperative PSA greater than 20 ng per mL
3. A prostatectomy Gleason score greater than or equal 8, time to PSA failure less than or equal to 2 years after RP, and a PSA doubling time less than or equal to 10 months are predictive of the probability and the time to distant failure, whereas the time to distant failure is a predictor of time to death from prostate cancer.

REFERENCES

1. Partin AW, Kattan MW, Subong ENP, et al. Combination of prostate specific antigen, clinical stage, and Gleason score to predict pathologic stage of localized prostate cancer: a multi-institutional update. *JAMA* 1997;277:1445–1451.
2. Walsh PC, Partin AW, Epstein JI. Cancer control and quality of life following anatomical radical retropubic prostatectomy: results at 10 years. *J Urol* 1994;152:1831–1836.
3. D'Amico AV, Whittington R, Malkowicz SB, et al. A multivariate analysis of clinical and pathological factors which predict for prostate-specific antigen failure after radical prostatectomy after prostate cancer. *J Urol* 1995;154:131–138.
4. Zagars GK, Pollack A, Kavadi VS, et al. Prostate specific antigen and radiation therapy for clinically localized prostate cancer. *Int J Radiat Oncol Biol Phys* 1995;32:293–306.
5. Pisansky TM, Kahn MJ, Rasp GM, et al. A multiple prognostic index predictive of disease outcome after irradiation for clinically localized prostate cancer. *Cancer* 1997;79:337–344.
6. Lee WR, Hanks GE, Schultheiss TE, et al. Localized prostate cancer treated by external-beam radiotherapy alone: serum prostate-specific antigen–driven outcome analysis. *J Clin Oncol* 1995;13:464–469.
7. Pisansky TM, Cha SS, Earle JD, et al. Prostate specific antigen as a pretherapy prognostic factor in patients treated with radiation therapy for clinically localized prostate cancer. *J Clin Oncol* 1993;11:2158–2166.
8. Zietman AL, Coen JJ, Shipley WU, et al. Radical radiation therapy in the management of prostatic adenocarcinoma: the initial prostate specific antigen value as a predictor of treatment outcome. *J Urol* 1994;151:640–645.
9. Hanks GE, Lee WR, Schultheiss TE. Clinical and biochemical evidence of control of prostate cancer at 5 years after external beam radiation. *J Urol* 1995;154:456–459.
10. Partin AW, Piantadosi S, Sanda MG, et al. Selection of men at high risk for disease recurrence for experimental adjuvant therapy following radical prostatectomy. *Urology* 1995;45:831–838.
11. Lerner SE, Blute ML, Bergstralh EJ, et al. Analysis of risk factors for progression in patients with pathologically organ confined prostate cancers after radical retropubic prostatectomy. *J Urol* 1996;156:137–143.
12. Zietman AL, Edelstein RA, Coen JJ, et al. Radical prostatectomy for adenocarcinoma of the prostate. The influence of preoperative and pathologic findings on biochemical disease-free outcome. *Urology* 1994;43:828–833.
13. D'Amico AV, Whittington R, Malkowicz SB, et al. PSA failure despite pathologically organ confined and margin negative disease: the basis for an adjuvant therapy trial. *J Clin Oncol* 1997;15:1465–1469.
14. D'Amico AV, Whittington R, Malkowicz SB, et al. Outcome based staging for clinically localized adenocarcinoma of the prostate. *J Urol* 1997;158:1422–1426.
15. Ragde H, Blasko JC, Grimm PD, et al. Interstitial iodine-125 radiation without adjuvant therapy in the treatment of clinically localized prostate carcinoma. *Cancer* 1997;80:442–453.
16. Blasko JC, Wallner K, Grimm PD, et al. Prostate specific antigen based disease control following ultrasound guided I 125 implantation for stage T1/T2 prostatic carcinoma. *J Urol* 1995;154:1096–1099.
17. Wallner K, Roy J, Harrison L. Tumor control and morbidity following transperineal Iodine 125 implantation for stage T1/T2 prostatic carcinoma. *J Clin Oncol* 1996;14:449–453.
18. Shipley WU, Thames HD, Sandler HM, et al. Radiation therapy for clinically localized prostate cancer: a multi-institutional pooled analysis. *JAMA* 1999;281:1598–1604.
19. Terris MK, Haney DJ, Johnstone IM, et al. Prediction of prostate cancer volume using prostate-specific antigen levels, transrectal ultrasound, and systematic sextant biopsies. *Urology* 1995;45:75–80.

20. Borirakchanyavat S, Bhargava V, Shinohara K, et al. Systematic sextant biopsies in the prediction of extracapsular extension at radical prostatectomy. *Urology* 1997;50:373–378.
21. Badalment RA, Miller MC, Peller PA, et al. An algorithm for predicting non-organ confined prostate cancer using the results obtained from sextant core biopsies with prostate specific antigen level. *J Urol* 1996;156:1375–1380.
22. D'Amico AV, Whittington R, Malkowicz SB, et al. A multivariable analysis evaluating the role of the percent positive biopsies and endorectal coil MRI in predicting extraprostatic disease and time to postoperative PSA failure in intermediate risk prostate cancer patients. *Cancer J* 1996;2:343–350.
23. Conrad S, Graefen M, Pichlmeier U, et al. Systematic sextant biopsies improve preoperative prediction of pelvic lymph node metastases in patients with clinically localized prostate carcinoma. *J Urol* 1998;159:2023–2029.
24. Epstein JI, Walsh PC, Carmichael M, et al. Pathologic and clinical findings to predict tumor extent of nonpalpable (stage T1c) prostate cancer. *JAMA* 1994;271:368–374.
25. Presti JC Jr., Shinohara K, Bacchetti P, et al. Positive fraction of systematic biopsies predicts risk of relapse after radical prostatectomy. *Urology* 1998;52:1079–1084.
26. Huland H, Graefen M, Hammerer P, et al. Multivariate analysis of preoperative parameters for prediction of early PSA relapse after radical prostatectomy. Proceedings of the 74th Annual Meeting of the American Urological Association. *J Urol* 1999;161:334(abst).
27. D'Amico AV, Whittington R, Malkowicz SB, et al. Clinical utility of the percent of positive prostate biopsies in defining biochemical outcome following radical prostatectomy for patients with clinically localized prostate cancer. *J Clin Oncol* 2000;18:1164–1172.
28. D'Amico AV, Schultz D, Schneider L, et al. The clinical utility of the percent of positive prostate biopsies in defining biochemical outcome following external beam radiation therapy for patients with clinically localized prostate cancer. *Int J Radiat Oncol Biol Phys* 2001;49:679–684.
29. Tempany CM, Zhou X, Zerhouni EA, et al. Staging of prostate cancer: results of the Radiology Diagnostic Oncology Group project comparison of three MR imaging techniques. *Radiology* 1994;192:47–54.
30. Perrotti M, Kaufman RP Jr., Jennings TA, et al. Endorectal coil magnetic resonance imaging in prostate cancer: Is it accurate? *J Urol* 1996;156:106–109.
31. D'Amico AV, Whittington R, Malkowicz SB, et al. A multivariable analysis evaluating the role of the percent positive biopsies and endorectal coil MRI in predicting extraprostatic disease and time to postoperative PSA failure in intermediate risk prostate cancer patients. *Cancer J* 1996;2:343–350.
32. D'Amico AV, Whittington R, Malkowicz SB, et al. Endorectal magnetic resonance imaging as a predictor of biochemical outcome following radical prostatectomy for men with clinically localized prostate cancer. *J Urol* 2000;164:759–763.
33. Kattan MW, Easthan JA, Stapleton AMF, et al. A preoperative nomogram for disease recurrence following radical prostatectomy for prostate cancer. *J Natl Cancer Inst* 1998;90:766–771.
34. D'Amico AV, Whittington R, Malcowicz SB, et al. A pre-treatment nomogram for prostate specific antigen recurrence following radical prostatectomy or external beam radiation therapy for clinically localized prostate cancer. *J Clin Oncol* 1999;17:168–172.
35. Pound CR, Partin AW, Eisenberger MA, et al. Natural history of progression after PSA elevation following radical prostatectomy. *JAMA* 1999;281:1591–1597.
36. Smith LG, Pollack A, Zagars GK. Predictor of distant metastasis 7 years after a rising PSA in prostate cancer patients treated with external beam radiotherapy. *Int J Radiat Oncol Biol Phys* 1999;45:218–224.
37. Beahrs OH, Henson DE, Hutter RVP, et al. *Manual for staging cancer*, 4th ed. American Joint Committee on Cancer Staging. Philadelphia: J.B. Lippincott Co, 1992.
38. Zagars GK, Pollack A, Kavadi VS, et al. Prostate specific antigen and radiation therapy for clinically localized prostate cancer. *Int J Radiat Oncol Biol Phys* 1995;32:293–306.
39. Pisansky TM, Kahn MJ, Rasp GM, et al. A multiple prognostic index predictive of disease outcome after irradiation for localized prostate cancer. *Cancer* 1997;79:337–344.
40. Leibel SA, Zelefsky MJ, Kutcher GJ, et al. The biologic basis and clinical application of three-dimensional conformal external beam radiation therapy in carcinoma of the prostate. *Semin Oncol* 1994;21:580–597.
41. Movsas B, Hanlon A, Teshima T, et al. Analyzing predictive models following definitive radiotherapy for prostate cancer. *Cancer* 1997;80:1093–2102.
42. D'Amico AV, Desjardin A, Chung A, et al. Assessment of outcome prediction models for patients with localized prostate carcinoma managed with radical prostatectomy or external beam radiation therapy. *Cancer* 1998;82:1887–1896.
43. Cox DR. Regression models and life tables. *J R Stat Soc B* 1972;34:187–199.
44. Akaike H. Factor analysis and AIC. *Psychometrika* 1987;52:317–332.
45. Schwartz G. Estimating the dimension of a model. *Ann Stat* 1978;6:461–464.
46. Efron R, Tibsherani R. *Introduction to the bootstrap*. New York: Chapman and Hall, 1993.
47. Lankford S, Pollack A, Zagars GK. Prostate-specific antigen cancer volume: a significant prognostic factor in prostate cancer patients at intermediate risk of failing radiotherapy. *Int J Radiat Oncol Biol Phys* 1997;38:327–333.
48. Kupelian P, Katcher J, Levin HS, et al. Stage T1-2 prostate cancer: a multivariate analysis of factors affecting biochemical and clinical failures after radical prostatectomy. *Int J Radiat Oncol Biol Phys* 1997;37:1043–1052.
49. D'Amico AV, Whittington R, Kaplan I, et al. Equivalent biochemical failure free survival after external beam radiation therapy or radical prostatectomy in patients with a pretreatment prostate specific antigen of >4–20 ng/mL. *Int J Radiat Oncol Biol Phys* 1997;37:1053–1058.
50. Kaplan EL, Meier P. Non-parametric estimation from incomplete observations. *J Amer Stat Assoc* 1958;53:457–500.
51. D'Amico AV, Whittington R, Malkowicz SB, et al. The combination of preoperative prostate specific antigen and postoperative pathological findings to predict prostate specific antigen outcome in clinically localized prostate cancer. *J Urol* 1998;160:2096–2101.
52. Cadeddu JA, Partin AW, Deweese TL, et al. Long-term results of radiation therapy for prostate cancer recurrence following radical prostatectomy. *J Urol* 1998;159:173–178.
53. Kattan MW, Wheeler TM, Scardio PT. Postoperative nomogram for disease recurrence after radical prostatectomy. *J Clin Oncol* 1999;17:1499–1507.

19

IMAGING AND STAGING OF PROSTATE CANCER

ANTJE E. WEFER
HEDVIG HRICAK

There has been a dramatic rise in the incidence of prostate cancer over the past decade, making it the most common malignancy, with the exception of skin cancers, in American men. Although an increased understanding of the underlying pathophysiology has made it possible to make significant advances in the diagnosis, pretreatment evaluation, and treatment of this disease, significant gaps in knowledge remain. As a result, clinical management of prostate cancer is one of the most controversial areas in modern medicine with uncertainty regarding the feasibility of cancer screening, choice of diagnostic tests for pretreatment evaluation, and appropriateness of treatment selection. Efforts to reduce treatment morbidity have led to a heightened demand for patient-specific and disease-targeted therapy. Achievement of this goal depends not only on clinical and laboratory information, but also on knowledge of cancer prognostic parameters, such as tumor location, volume, extent, and biologic behavior (aggressiveness).

At present, there are several major obstacles to optimal clinical management of prostate cancer. The first is related to cancer detection, location, and estimate of volume. In addition, there is a lack of reliable noninvasive tests to assess local and metastatic tumor extent. The stage of the disease at the time of diagnosis is an objective measure of tumor extent and an important consideration as a treatment and prognostic factor. Third, it is not now possible to differentiate indolent from aggressive disease. A unique and one of the most important characteristics of prostate cancer is its variability in biologic aggressiveness. Although a number of clinical tumor prognostic factors [e.g., patient age, prostate-specific antigen (PSA) level, and tumor grade and stage] can generally be used to predict disease at either end of the spectrum, most cancers fall into an intermediate range, in which it is difficult to distinguish with certainty those cancers likely to progress from those with a more indolent course (1,2). Therefore, there continues to be an intense debate about the ability to accurately assign patients to appropriate risk and treatment categories using currently available diagnostic methods (3). With diagnostic imaging, it is possible to assess tumor location and extent, important information in patient management. Although much progress in imaging has been made in the last decade, and imaging guidelines for the use of computed tomography (CT) and bone scanning have been developed, the use of imaging has been random and both over- and underused (4). Whether this is due to lack of communication among specialists, slow dissemination of knowledge, or difficulty in changing the old habits is not clear.

One of the most pressing needs in advancing the treatment of prostate cancer is the development of new and more powerful tumor prognostic factors, as well as a better understanding of how to use them and how to incorporate already available diagnostic imaging tests.

CLASSIFICATION AND STAGING

Two classification systems, the tumor-node-metastasis (TNM) and the Jewett-Whitmore systems, have been used to evaluate local and distant extent of disease for the staging of prostate cancer (5,6) (Table 19-1). For local staging, diagnostic tests must differentiate between disease confined to the prostate (stages T-T2) from locally invasive disease extending beyond the prostatic capsule (stage T3) (Table 19-2). Additional tests may be necessary to detect metastatic disease to lymph nodes (stages N1-3) or distant organs (stage M1). Identification of metastasis is important, because the prognosis for patients with metastatic disease is not good. Data from one study indicate that approximately 46% of patients with metastatic disease died within 22 months of diagnosis, whereas disease progression occurred in only 10% of patients who did not have lymph node metastases (7). Even in the absence of identifiable metastatic disease, extraprostatic spread of cancer [extracapsular extension (ECE) or seminal vesicle invasion (SVI)] is a poor prognostic indicator, owing to the increased likelihood of

TABLE 19-1. ADENOCARCINOMA OF THE PROSTATE: JEWETT-WHITMORE AND TUMOR-NODE-METASTASIS (TNM) STAGING SYSTEMS

Jewett-Whitmore	TNM	Extent of cancer
A	T1	Clinically localized: tumor not palpable on digital rectal examination
A1	T1a	Focal tumor (<5% of resected tissue on TURP) and low grade
A2	T1b	Diffuse tumor (>5% of resected tissue on TURP) or high grade
B	T2	Clinically localized: tumor palpable
B1	T2a	Tumor involves <1/2 lobe
B2	T2b	Tumor involves >1/2 lobe
B2	T2c	Tumor involves both lobes
C	T3	Locally invasive beyond prostatic capsule: tumor palpable
C1	T3a	Unilateral extracapsular extension
C1	T3b	Bilateral extracapsular extension
C1	T3c	Seminal vesicle invasion
C2	T4	Invades adjacent tissues (e.g., bladder, rectum, levator ani muscles)
D	N/M	Metastatic disease
D1	N1	Microscopic pelvic lymph node metastasis
D1	N2	Gross pelvic lymph node metastasis
D1	N3	Extrapelvic lymph node metastasis
D2	M	Distant metastases (e.g., bones, lung, liver, brain)

TURP, transurethral resection of the prostate.

occult metastases. It is well documented that lymph node metastases occur more frequently with increasing local stage and decreasing tumor differentiation (8,9).

Clinically localized prostate cancer is confined by the prostatic capsule, whereas locally invasive disease extends beyond the prostatic capsule into the periprostatic fat, lymphatics, and vessels. Involvement of organs other than the prostate may occur by three different routes: direct extension, lymphatic spread, or hematogenous dissemination. Owing to the proximity of the prostate to the seminal vesicles and bladder base, direct extension to these organs is not uncommon. Caudally, the tumor rarely extends below the membranous urethra. Although direct invasion of the rectum may occasionally occur, rectal involvement is rare, and it appears that Denonvillier's fascia, which separates the posterior aspect of the prostate from the anterior rectal wall, serves as a barrier. The most frequent sites of lymphatic spread are the obturator nodes; posterior and medial chains of the external nodes; and presacral, internal iliac and common iliac nodes (7,10). When paraaortic nodal disease is present, it is always associated with pelvic lymph node involvement. It is currently thought that lymphatic and hematogenous dissemination occur independently. Hematogenous spread of prostate cancer usually causes osseous metastases, which most commonly involve the lumbar spine, pelvic bones, femur, thoracic spine, and ribs (in decreasing order of frequency). Occasionally, extradural metastases cause spinal cord compression. Less commonly, hematogenous spread causes visceral metastases involving the lungs, liver, and adrenal glands. Pulmonary and pleural metastases may also occur via lymphatic spread. Visceral metastases are rarely seen in patients with newly diagnosed prostate cancer and are uncommon, even in patients dying of the disease. Liver metastases, for example, are found in only approximately 20% of patients dying of disseminated prostate cancer, and lymphangitic spread to the lungs is seen in only approximately 25% of these patients.

IMAGING STRATEGIES FOR DETECTION, DIAGNOSIS, AND STAGING

Prostate cancer screening is presently performed using digital rectal examination (DRE) and serum PSA testing. Although imaging studies do not now have a place in the early detection of prostate cancer, imaging does play a role in the diagnosis and evaluation of the disease. Transrectal ultrasound (TRUS) is used to guide biopsies of the prostate gland in patients with an abnormal DRE or elevated serum PSA level. Magnetic resonance imaging (MRI) and, particularly, combined MRI and three-dimensional 1H-MR spectroscopic imaging (proton 3D-1H-MRSI) can be used for patient stratification and targeted biopsies in patients with previously negative biopsy findings. Patients with negative biopsy findings may also be evaluated with endorectal MRI (eMRI) for classification into low-, moderate-, or high-risk groups for harboring cancer. In a study by Terratti and colleagues, MRI was found to have an overall accuracy of 70% and a negative predictive value (low suspicion for cancer) of 94.4% (11). Combining 3D-MRSI with eMRI further improves the ability to noninvasively identify cancer in a sextant location (12). Such information can be included in patient nomograms to help design patient-specific treatment protocols. For staging prostate cancer, MRI and MRI combined with MRSI are preferred for assessment of local disease extent, and CT and bone scintigraphy are valuable techniques for depicting distant spread of disease.

Technologic advances in imaging hardware and software continue at a rapid rate. Further improvements in imaging modalities currently used to image the prostate can be anticipated, with the promise of even greater diagnostic achievements. The development of new contrast media for ultrasound and MRI, the use of improved monoclonal antibodies specific for prostatic tissue, and metabolic imaging by magnetic resonance spectroscopy and positron emission tomography (PET) hold the promise of even greater diagnostic accuracy in the evaluation of prostate cancer.

ANATOMY OF THE PROSTATE GLAND

The anatomy of the prostate gland is well displayed on high-resolution cross-sectional imaging—TRUS, CT, and

TABLE 19-2. TRANSRECTAL ULTRASONOGRAPHY (TRUS), MAGNETIC RESONANCE IMAGING (MRI), AND COMPUTED TOMOGRAPHY (CT) STAGING CRITERIA AFTER THE JEWETT-WHITMORE (J-W) AND TUMOR-NODE-METASTASIS (TNM) CLASSIFICATIONS OF PROSTATE CANCER

J-W	TNM	Extent of cancer	TRUS	MRI	CT
A	T1	Tumor localized: nonpalpable	Normal peripheral zone or inhomogeneous echotexture	NA	NA
B	T2	Tumor localized: palpable	Lesion confined by prostatic capsule	Lesion confined by prostatic capsule	Periprostatic fat normal
B1,2	T2a,b	Single lobe involved	Normal peripheral zone or localized hypoechoic lesion	Normal peripheral zone or localized low signal intensity lesion on T2WI	Normal or enlarged prostate
B3	T2c	Both lobes involved	Large or multifocal hypoechoic lesions in peripheral zone	Large or multifocal low intensity lesions on T2WI	Normal or enlarged prostate
C	T3	Locally invasive tumor beyond prostatic capsule	Localized interruption or irregularity of prostatic capsule	Localized interruption or irregularity of prostatic capsule	Periprostatic fat abnormal
C1	T3a-b	Extracapsular extension (ECE) into periprostatic fat	Irregular bulge or disruption of prostatic capsule and tumor extension to periprostatic fat (hypoechoic strands extending from prostate into periprostatic fat)	Irregular bulge or disruption of prostatic capsule and tumor extension to periprostatic fat (obliteration of rectoprostatic angle, asymmetry of neurovascular bundles)	Soft tissue strands extending from prostate into periprostatic fat
C2	T3c	Seminal vesicle invasion	Seminal vesicle enlarged with soft tissue echogenicity, loss of the normal seminal vesicle "beak" at base of prostate on sagittal scan	Seminal vesicle enlarged with abnormal low intensity on T2WI, obliteration of the normal fat plane between seminal vesicle and base of prostate	Seminal vesicle enlarged, obliteration of the normal fat plane between seminal vesicle and base of prostate

NA, not applicable; T1WI, T1-weighted image; T2WI, T2-weighted image.

MRI. The display of the old anatomic descriptions of the lobar concept of the prostate gland division of the gland in five lobes can be referred to (13). More commonly used is the contemporary description, using the concept of *zonal anatomy* (14).

After the description of the zonal anatomy, three glandular regions of the prostate can be distinguished: *central, peripheral,* and *transition zones.* In young men, the peripheral zone occupies nearly 75% of the total volume of the prostatic gland, the central zone 25%, and the transition zone 5% (14). The relationships among the different zones change with age. The volume of the central zone is greatest in young men, but, with advancing age, there is progressive atrophy of this zone, sometimes leading to reduction of the total mass. In most men, however, there is an overall increase in gland size due to benign prostatic hypertrophy involving the transition zone. Differentiation of zonal anatomy is clinically important, because the peripheral zone is the site of origin of most carcinomas, and the transition zone is the site of origin of benign nodular hyperplasia.

From a radiologic viewpoint, most commonly used subdivisions of the glandular prostate are the peripheral zone and the central gland (15), in which the term *central gland* is used to refer collectively to the periurethral, transitional, and central zones. Using this terminology, the central gland contains the central and transition zones that are in variable proportion, depending on the degree of benign prostatic hyperplasia. It should be noted that the term *central* or *inner* gland is often used in the histologic and urologic literature, in which it refers to the combination of the central and peripheral zones. This latter approach was designed to separate those parts of the prostate that are susceptible to benign prostatic hyperplasia (the transition zone) from those parts susceptible to carcinoma (mainly the peripheral zone).

A final refinement to the anatomic divisions of the prostate is the concept of *sextants.* Systematic biopsy of six parts of the prostate was initially described in 1989 (16), and the associated sextant description of the prostate is frequently used in clinical practice. The sextants consist of base, midgland, and apex bilaterally. The sextants are not rigidly defined in the original description. On imaging, the arbitrary division is as follows: In the transverse plane of section, the base of the prostate extends from the bladder floor and seminal vesicle or ejaculatory duct junctions to the level with the largest transverse diameter of the gland. The prostatic midgland extends from the section with the largest transverse diameter to the level of the verumontanum. The prostatic apex extends from the level below the verumontanum to the external urethral sphincter or membranous urethra. The peripheral zone is defined as the part of the prostate between the true prostatic capsule and the surgical pseudocapsule. Both confines are characterized as low-signal intensity bands, the former separating the prostate from the surrounding periprostatic tissue, the latter separating the more homogenous, higher–signal intensity peripheral zone from the heterogenous, lower–signal intensity central gland.

The terminology is useful shorthand for describing the location of prostatic abnormalities, but the lack of well-defined anatomic landmarks for sextant definition should be remembered when interpreting prostatic imaging and attempting to correlate biopsy results with imaging.

Ultrasound

The prostate can be visualized with transabdominal transducers, but detailed assessment of the zonal anatomy is performed using a transrectal approach (15). In healthy young men, the zones of the prostate are not sonographically evident. With the development of benign prostatic hyperplasia, the transition zone becomes distinguishable as a well-demarcated area of heterogeneity, separable from a uniform, medium echogenicity peripheral zone. The transition zone and the central zone are typically referred as central gland. The peripheral zone forms an area of uniform echogenicity surrounding the central gland. The surgical or pseudocapsule may be evident as a discrete change in echogenicity or a hypoechoic rim. The anterior fibromuscular stroma forms a less echogenic band at the anterior aspect of the prostate. The seminal vesicles can be seen superolaterally, encased in hyperechoic fat that is continuous with the fat surrounding the prostate. The appearance of the seminal vesicles varies with the volume of contained fluid.

Computed Tomography

On CT, the prostate gland most commonly appears as a soft tissue structure of uniformly homogeneous attenuation and may be difficult to distinguish from surrounding muscles, vessels, and perineal structures. Spiral CT with thin sections and multiplanar reformations may partially overcome these problems. Nonetheless, CT of the prostate is generally limited to assessment of overall gland size. With the development of benign prostatic hyperplasia in the aging prostate, the central gland becomes heterogeneous and of higher attenuation relative to the peripheral zone on contrast-enhanced CT studies. This can allow distinction of the peripheral and central gland by CT. The clinical relevance, if any, of this finding is unknown.

Magnetic Resonance Imaging

Appearance of the prostate gland and depiction of zonal anatomy depend on the MR technique used. On T1-weighted images, the prostate demonstrates homogeneous intermediate signal intensity, and the zonal anatomy cannot be appreciated. Zonal anatomy is well depicted on T2-weighted images. The peripheral zone is of high T2 signal intensity, similar to or greater than the signal of adjacent periprostatic fat. It is surrounded by a thin rim of low T2 signal intensity that represents the anatomic or true capsule. The central and transition zones are both of lower T2 signal intensity than is the peripheral zone, possibly because of more compact smooth muscle and sparser glandular elements. Because the central and transition zones are of similar T2 signal intensity, their differentiation is based on their respective anatomic locations. Furthermore, benign prostatic hyperplasia develops in the transition zone and gradually compresses the central zone and may, ultimately, compress the peripheral zone as well. The typical changes of benign prostatic hyperplasia often facilitate identification of the transition zone in older men. The anterior fibromuscular stroma demonstrates low signal intensity on T1- and T2-weighted images.

The proximal urethra is rarely identifiable, unless a Foley catheter is present or a transurethral resection has been performed. The verumontanum can be visualized as a high T2 signal intensity structure. The distal prostatic urethra can be seen as a low T2 signal intensity ring in the apical region of the prostate. The vas deferens and seminal vesicles are particularly well seen on axial and coronal images, whereas the neurovascular bundles (NVB) can be seen best on axial images. The penile root can be seen inferiorly, separated from the prostatic apex by the urogenital membrane.

Prostate Cancer

Tumor Localization

Treatment innovations are aimed at maximizing cancer control while minimizing morbidity, making tumor detection and localization vitally important for optimal treatment planning. To date, transrectal TRUS-guided prostate biopsy has been considered the standard of reference for tumor localization. However, recent reports of biopsy sampling errors and inaccuracies are troubling (17,18). Furthermore, because prostate cancer is a multifocal and histologically heterogeneous disease, biopsy is limited in determining all cancer sites and grades. In fact, when biopsy results were compared with radical prostatectomy for sextant tumor localization, the positive predictive value (PPV) of biopsy was found to be 83.3%, and the negative predictive value was found to be 36.4% (18), limiting the value of biopsy results in risk stratification.

Transrectal Ultrasonography

Only prostate cancers located in the peripheral zone can be reliably detected by sonography. On TRUS scans, prostate cancer most commonly (60% to 70% of cases) appears hypoechoic, compared to the normal peripheral zone (Fig. 19-1). Up to 40% of lesions, however, are isoechoic and therefore are not detected by sonography (19,20). Rarely (1% to 5% of cases), even hyperechoic lesions can be seen. Except for ease of detection, there are

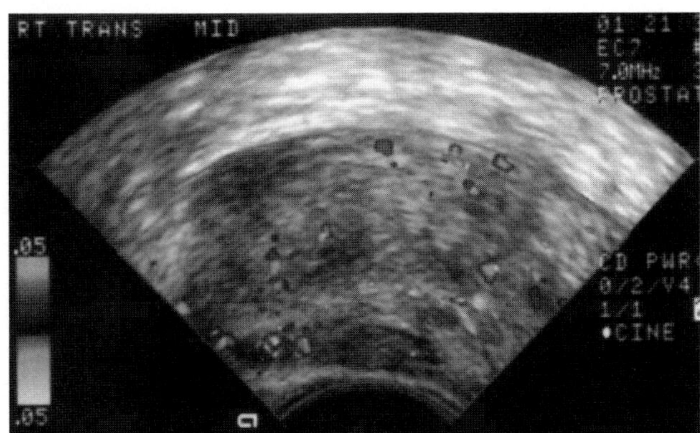

FIGURE 19-1. Transrectal ultrasound (TRUS). Transverse image of TRUS demonstrates abnormal echogenicity areas in the peripheral zone of the right midgland as highly suspicious for neoplasm.

no known differences among hypoechoic, isoechoic, and hyperechoic lesions. Their biologic behavior seems to be essentially the same (21).

The finding of a hypoechoic lesion on TRUS is not specific for carcinoma, and benign processes, such as prostatitis, frequently present as hypoechoic lesions. The low PPV of TRUS (18% to 52%) for the diagnosis of prostate cancer makes it inappropriate as a screening tool at the present time (22,23). However, color and power Doppler sonography are being investigated for their ability to increase the sensitivity and specificity of prostate cancer detection (24). Early reports on color Doppler sonography suggest that the combined use of gray-scale and color Doppler sonography results in improved cancer detection, with the PPV as high as 77%. There is, however, a corresponding decrease in sensitivity (24). Another emerging ultrasound technology is TRUS-sonoelasticity imaging. In comparison with gray-scale sonography, preliminary results for *in vitro* sonoelasticity imaging of prostatectomy specimens suggest greater sensitivity and accuracy in the detection and localization of prostate cancer by this technique (25).

Computed Tomography

CT lacks the soft tissue contrast resolution needed for the detection of intraprostatic cancer and offers no advantages over TRUS in biopsy guidance. The primary role of CT in prostate cancer is in the evaluation of distant spread of disease, mainly detection and biopsy of lymph nodes and distant organ parenchymal metastases.

Magnetic Resonance Imaging

Although MRI is the best imaging modality for demonstrating the normal zonal anatomy of the prostate (Fig. 19-2), at the present time it, like TRUS, has no established role in prostate cancer detection (26,27). This lack of a sufficiently high PPV for cancer detection, combined with its high cost, makes MRI inappropriate for cancer screening. Prostate cancer usually appears as an area of abnormal low signal intensity against the normal homogeneous high signal intensity background of the peripheral zone (Fig. 19-3) (28). Low signal intensity lesions in the peripheral zone represent a sensitive but not specific finding for cancer. Benign conditions, such as prostatitis, hemorrhage, or dystrophic changes related to radiation or androgen-deprivation therapy, can mimic cancer. In particular, prostatic biopsies may cause bleeding and abnormalities in signal intensity that lead to false-positive and false-negative results (29) (Fig. 19-4). To minimize this problem, MRI should be delayed for at least 3 weeks after biopsy (29). It should also be noted that a normal-appearing peripheral zone does not exclude the presence of cancer. Although detection rates as high as 95% have been reported, the results of large multicenter studies are disappointingly low, with only 60% of lesions larger than 5 mm being detected on MRI (30,31). Attempts to measure tumor volume by MRI have had somewhat more promising results than for TRUS. However, the use of MRI in the measurement of tumor volume remains unproven at the current time (31).

Three-Dimensional 1H–Magnetic Resonance Spectroscopic Imaging

Proton 3D-MRSI, a recently developed technique that provides metabolic information about the prostate, is a part of a complete eMRI examination. It is an added sequence that uses the same 1.5T magnet and hardware used for the eMRI study. In the last few years, significant progress has been made in the development of 3D-MRSI as a clinically useful tool. Technical developments have resulted in improved spatial resolution (from 0.7 cm^3 to 0.24 cm^3), an increase in gland coverage (from 30% to 50% to 80% to 100%), and a reduction in total examination time (for both MRI and 3D-MRSI).

In MRSI, metabolic information about the prostate gland is obtained by assessing the prostatic metabolites choline and citrate. In areas of cancer, there are significantly higher choline and significantly lower citrate levels than in the normal peripheral zone. In addition, the ratio of choline plus creatine to citrate in areas of cancer is more than three standard deviations (SD) higher than it is in the normal peripheral zone (32). When the metabolic data from 3D-MRSI is combined with the morphologic data from the MRI, it is possible to make a more specific diagnosis and to better localize prostate cancer than with the data from the MRI alone (33). Furthermore, in the presence of postbiopsy hemorrhage, the addition of 3D-MRSI findings significantly improves the specificity of cancer detection and localization (Fig. 19-5) (32,34).

A combined positive result from the MRI and 3D-MRSI (greater than three SD) indicates the presence of tumors with high probability (PPV, 88% to 92%). A combined negative result from both MRI and 3D-MRSI (greater than two SD) excludes the presence of cancer with high probability (NPV, 80%). Whether MRSI can increase

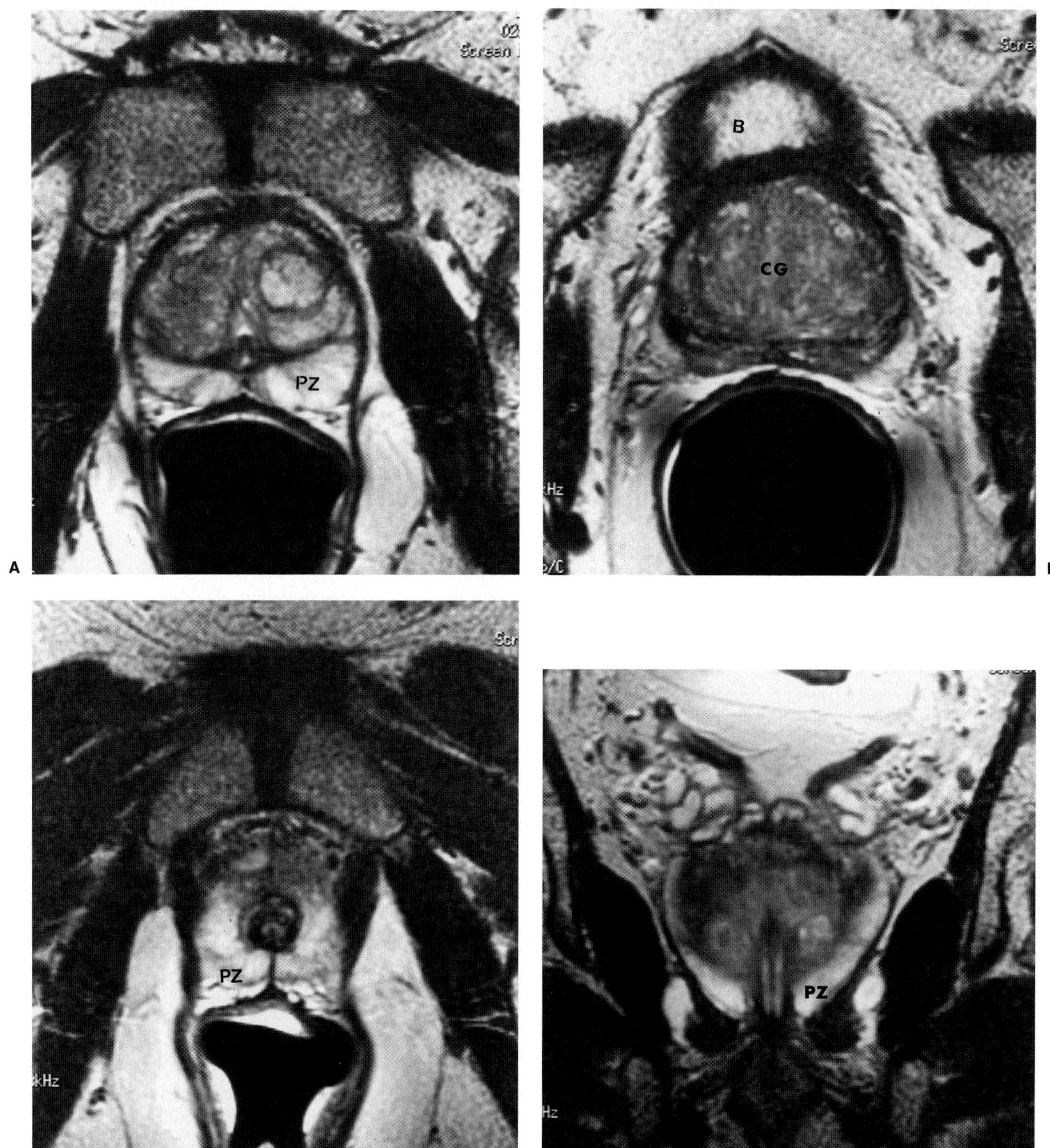

FIGURE 19-2. Magnetic resonance imaging anatomy of the prostate gland. The axial T2-weighted fast spin-echo (FSE) image **(A)** of a prostate demonstrates the zonal anatomy at the midgland. The peripheral zone (PZ) is of high signal intensity. The axial T2-weighted FSE image at the base shows that no PZ is present at this level of the gland close to the bladder (B). The central gland (CG) is large at this level **(B)**. At the apex, the axial T2-weighted FSE image **(C)** demonstrates the zonal anatomy, with PZ seen as a high signal intensity region. On the coronal T2-weighted FSE image, the PZ is demonstrated as a high signal intensity zone around the central gland **(D)**.

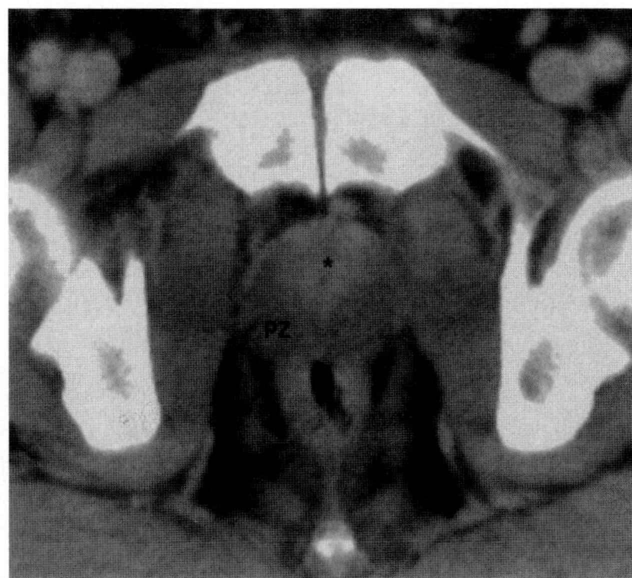

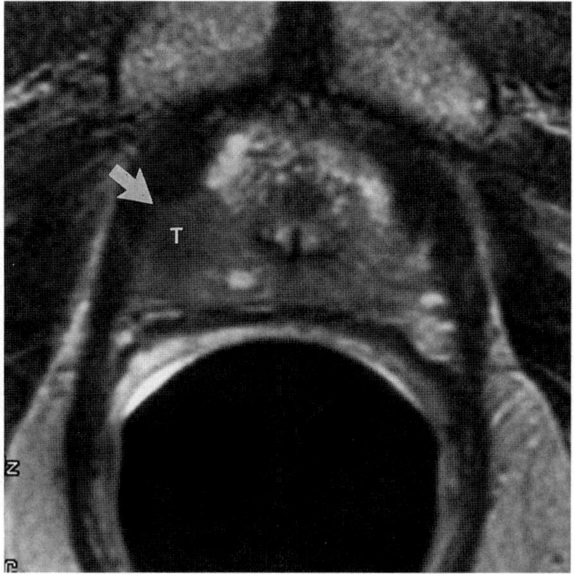

FIGURE 19-3. Magnetic resonance imaging: prostate cancer with extracapsular extension. This axial T2-weighted fast spin-echo image demonstrates prostate cancer on the right side in the peripheral zone toward the apex **(A)**. The tumor (T) is of low signal intensity and has contact to the right capsule (*arrow*) **(B)**. The capsule is not clearly separated from the tumor in this region. This finding is highly suspicious of extracapsular extension.

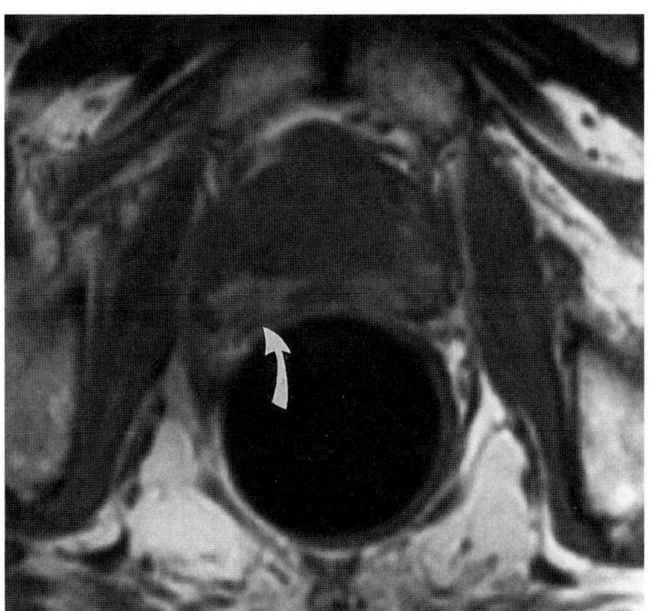

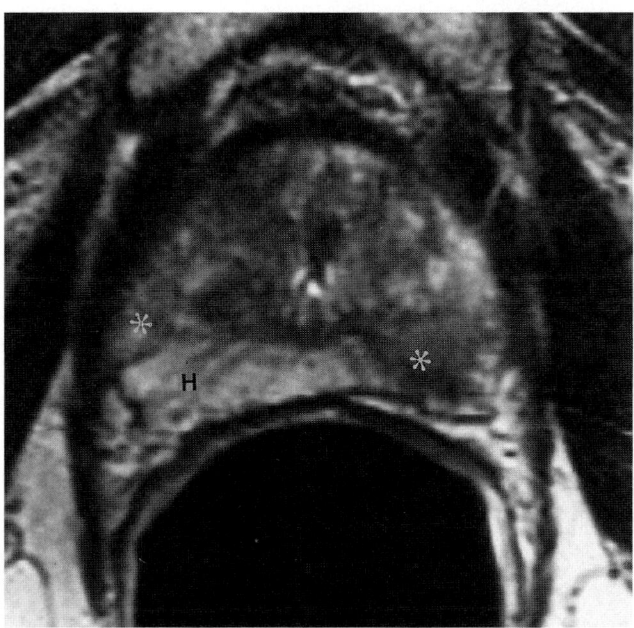

FIGURE 19-4. Postbiopsy hemorrhage (H). Extensive postbiopsy hemorrhage in the right peripheral zone (*arrow*) is seen on the T1-weighted axial image **(A)**. The T2-weighted axial image of the same level of the gland demonstrates a high signal intensity area, representing hemorrhage with relatively sharp delineation to the tumor in the anterior region of the right midgland (*asterisk*) **(B)**. The prostate cancer is multifocal. Another tumor is located on the left side in the peripheral zone (*asterisk*). Both tumors are seen as low signal intensity areas. Postbiopsy hemorrhage mostly demonstrates as low signal intensity regions but can present as high signal intensity as well, as demonstrated in this patient.

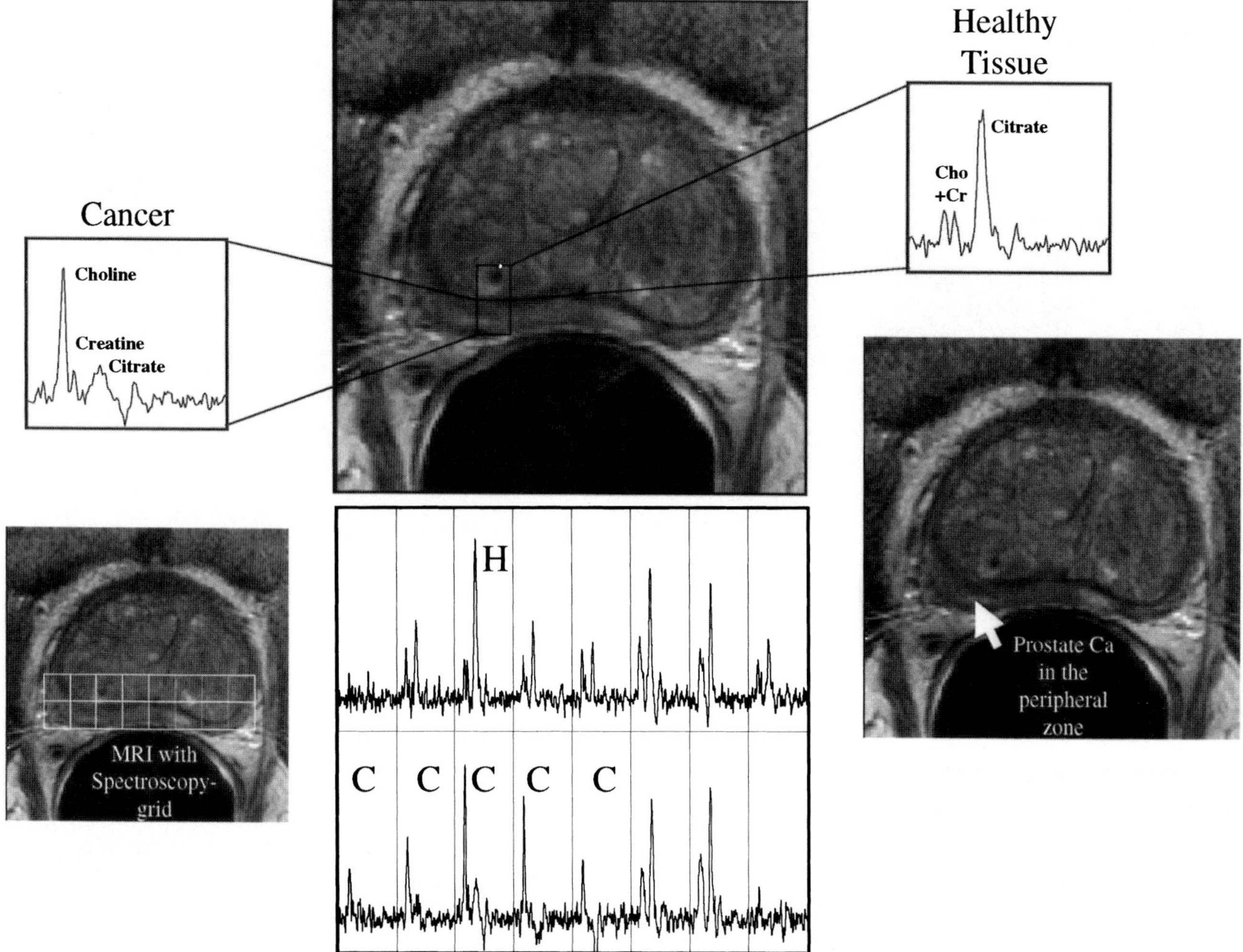

FIGURE 19-5. Three-dimensional 1H magnetic resonance spectroscopic imaging (3D-1H-MRSI). Images of a combined endorectal magnetic resonance imaging (eMRI) and 3D-1H-MRSI in a patient with prostate cancer. C, cancerous; Ca, cancer; Cho, choline; +Cr, creatine; H, healthy.

the specificity of MRI for cancer detection without compromising sensitivity is presently being investigated.

Evaluation of Tumor Aggressiveness

Attempts to evaluate tumor aggressiveness and add one more parameter to biologic tumor assessment have resulted in new developments in Doppler-ultrasound, TRUS, 3D-MRSI, and PET scanning.

The degree of tumor angiogenesis has been shown to correlate with the likelihood of metastatic disease in patients with prostate cancer (35) and may, therefore, represent an important prognostic factor. Recent advances, such as power Doppler sonography, with the capability to estimate tissue perfusion open up the possibility of using TRUS to image tumor angiogenesis (36), noninvasively providing information that may be useful in the management of patients with prostate cancer.

Early data also indicate that proton 3D-MRSI allows assessment of tumor aggressiveness by quantifying the assessment of two metabolites, citrate and choline. Choline to citrate ratios for cancer, benign prostatic lesions, and normal peripheral zones are reported to be 2.1 ± 1.3, 0.61 ± 0.21, and 0.45 ± 0.12, respectively (34,37). Overlap of this ratio between normal prostatic tissue and prostate cancer is minimal—98% of cancers have a choline to citrate ratio greater than three SD above normal values. A preliminary MRI/MRSI study of 26 biopsy-proven prostate cancer patients before radical prostatectomy and step-section pathologic examination has demonstrated a strong linear correlation between cancer aggressiveness and a decrease in citrate and elevation in choline levels (Gleason grade) (38). When comparing cancer patients with a high Gleason score (7 + 8) to those with a low score (5 + 6), a statistically significant ($p < .0001$) difference in cancer choline to normal choline ratios was observed (38).

Preliminary data on PET also show promise, as the level of uptake correlates with Gleason score and disease-free survival. However, results of Doppler sonography, 3D-MRSI, 18-fluoro-2-deoxyglucose (FDG)–PET, and use of new contrast media or tracers are preliminary and more data are needed.

Local Staging

The primary goal of local staging is to assist in treatment planning by differentiating between patients with organ-confined disease (stage T1-2) and those with extracapsular or SVI (stage T3). Although the simplest and most universally available method of local staging is derived from clinical parameters (e.g., DRE, serum PSA measurements, and biopsy tumor grade), clinical staging alone is not sufficiently accurate to be consistently useful in making treatment decisions. Clinical understaging has been reported in up to 30% to 60% of patients (39,40). Despite its inaccuracy, clinical staging remains in use because it is inexpensive and fairly specific for advanced (stage T3-4) disease (39,40). Although only a few patients with organ-confined disease are inappropriately excluded from surgery, patients with advanced disease who are clinically understaged are more likely to undergo surgery unnecessarily. Because of the limitations inherent in clinical staging, a variety of imaging techniques have been evaluated for their ability to improve staging accuracy. Of the currently available imaging techniques, eMRI shows the most promise for accurate local staging. The strengths and limitations of currently available imaging techniques are discussed separately for each technique.

Transrectal Ultrasonography

The role of TRUS in the local staging of prostate cancer remains controversial. Initial enthusiasm for the technique has been tempered by reports of widely varying results for the diagnosis of ECE, with sensitivity ranging from 50% to 92%, specificity from 46% to 91%, and accuracy from 58% to 86% (41–43). Relatively little progress has been made in improving TRUS staging accuracy, and the results from two large prospective multicenter studies suggest that TRUS is no better than DRE in the prediction of ECE (42,43). Drawbacks of TRUS in local staging include difficulty in diagnosing early ECE and high operator dependence, which limits the reproducibility of the results. Signs of early ECE include an irregular capsular bulge or obliteration of the rectoprostatic angle (RPA). Gross ECE is indicated by identification of strands of direct tumor extension into the periprostatic fat. Early SVI is suggested by fullness and loss of the normal tapering of the seminal vesicles near the prostatic base. Gross SVI is indicated by superior extension of the tumor from the prostatic base into the seminal vesicles. Sensitivity for the detection of SVI is reported to range from 22% to 60%, with specificity of approximately 88% and accuracy of approximately 78% (42,44). Because of the low sensitivity, TRUS-guided biopsy has been recommended in patients at increased risk for SVI (PSA greater than 20 ng per mL or Gleason score greater than 7) (45,46).

The use of 3D TRUS may improve the accuracy of TRUS staging of prostate cancer. Although data from a pilot study showed that 3D reconstruction of conventional TRUS imaging is superior to 2D imaging (47), 3D reconstruction presently relies on initial demonstration of the cancer by conventional ultrasonography, a potentially significant drawback. Further studies of this methodology are needed to fully explore its potential. Development of ultrasound contrast media may change the role of ultrasound in staging prostate cancer in the near future.

Computed Tomography

CT, once considered the mainstay of the imaging armamentarium for prostate cancer, is no longer routinely requested. A better understanding of how to use clinical tumor prognostic factors, such as PSA level, preoperative Gleason score, and clinical stage, to estimate the probability of advanced disease and lymph node involvement has limited the use of CT. Nomograms developed by Partin and colleagues that combine data from serum PSA levels, Gleason scores, and clinical stage provide probability estimates for lymph node involvement that can be used to determine the need for CT study or pelvic lymph node dissection (48).

In addition, CT is not recommended for local staging because of its low accuracy in the detection of extraprostatic disease (24% for ECE and 69% for SVI) (49). Although prostatic enlargement is well displayed on CT studies, it is a nonspecific finding that may be due to cancer or benign prostatic hyperplasia. Furthermore, a smooth outer prostatic margin does not exclude the presence of cancer within the gland, nor does an irregular margin accurately predict the presence of ECE. Even though the recent development of helical CT represents a significant advance in CT technology, no studies have been published that evaluate the accuracy of helical CT for local staging of prostate cancer. It is unlikely that the inherent limitation of low soft tissue contrast can be sufficiently overcome to significantly improve staging accuracy.

The accepted role of CT is in the evaluation of patients suspected of having advanced disease, including identification of extraprostatic spread of tumor into adjacent tissues, detection of lymph node metastasis, and planning radiation therapy. Gross ECE can be diagnosed when there is significant soft tissue extension into the periprostatic fat (Fig. 19-6). Unilateral enlargement of a seminal vesicle with obliteration of the fat plane between the seminal vesicle and prostatic base is suggestive of SVI, although images limited to the transaxial plane of section may create a false impression of unilateral enlargement when there is anatomic distortion from a distended rectum or bladder. Invasion of the bladder wall and rectum does not occur as frequently as SVI, which is seen in approximately 17% of patients with

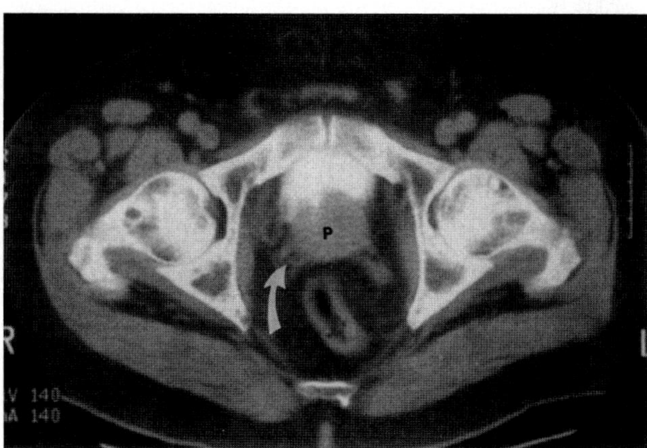

FIGURE 19-6. Pelvic computed tomography (CT): prostate gland with extracapsular extension (ECE). This contrast-enhanced delayed pelvic CT image of a patient with prostate cancer demonstrates an irregularity of the prostate gland (P). Strands from the gland into the periprostatic tissues are depicted (*arrow*). This is highly suspicious of ECE.

newly diagnosed prostate cancer (50). Because CT is limited to the transaxial plane, tumor invasion of the bladder base cannot be detected reliably. In the evaluation of lymph node invasion, CT, like MRI, relies on nodal size. The recommended size threshold for diagnosing lymph node metastases in patients with prostate cancer is a short axis diameter of greater than 1 cm.

Magnetic Resonance Imaging

The role of MRI in staging newly diagnosed prostate cancer remains controversial. The technology of MRI has undergone a marked evolution in the last decade, and the development of fast spin-echo T2-weighted imaging, surface coils, phased array coils, and subsequently endorectal coils has resulted in an incremental improvement in the efficacy of MRI staging. Its primary value appears to be in the local staging of patients with clinically localized prostate cancer.

MRI guidelines for staging prostate cancer follow the TNM staging criteria. TNM stage T1a tumors are not detectable by MRI. Most of these T1a tumors, incidentally, noted early-stage cancers are located within the transition zone, an area in which disease cannot reliably be detected with MRI. Clinical stage T2 tumors (i.e., palpable tumors confined to the prostate gland) are seen as areas of low signal intensity within the peripheral zone. Disease confined to the prostate can be diagnosed if the prostatic capsule appears intact (Fig. 19-7), even if there is broad contact between tumor and prostatic capsule or if a smooth capsular bulge is present (51,52). It is important to note that, although the prostatic margin may bulge, the bulge is usually smooth in contour. The ability to directly visualize the prostatic capsule increases the confidence level in diagnosis of these organ-confined stage T2 lesions.

Although tumor extension into periprostatic fat or seminal vesicles can be used to reliably diagnose gross extraprostatic disease, the diagnosis of early extraprostatic disease (stage T3) is necessary to ensure that as few patients as possible are deprived of potentially curative surgery owing to false-positive test findings (53). In stage T3 disease, the findings of importance are ECE and SVI. eMRI findings of extracapsular invasion include (a) an irregular bulge, (b) a step-off—angulated appearance—of the prostatic margin, (c) obliteration of the periprostatic fat in the RPA, (d) asymmetry of the NVB that indicates tumor extension through the prostatic capsule along the branches of the NVB, (e) breech of the capsule with direct tumor extension into the periprostatic fat, and (f) focal thickening or irregular bulging of the prostatic capsule. Using the findings of obliteration of the RPA and asymmetry of the NVB, a specificity of up to 95% can be achieved for the diagnosis of ECE, albeit with low sensitivity (less than 50%) (52).

SVI is indicated by (a) direct extension of tumor from the prostatic base into and around the seminal vesicles with loss of the normal fat plane separating the base of the prostate from the undersurface of the seminal vesicles, (b) the presence of asymmetric low signal intensity at the junction of the seminal vesicles and the base of the prostate, and (c) low signal intensity within the ejaculatory duct with direct extension into seminal vesicles (Fig. 19-7). High specificity (88%) and low sensitivity (22%) have been reported for diagnosis of SVI on MRI (42). Although transaxial plane images are essential in the evaluation of extracapsular invasion, detection of SVI is facilitated by using sagittal or coronal planes of section.

Gross extraprostatic extension of tumor can involve adjacent organs (stage T4 disease). Loss of the normal fat plane between the base of the prostate and bladder and interruption of the normal low signal intensity muscular bladder wall are findings indicative of bladder invasion. Similar diagnostic criteria can be used for the diagnosis of rectal invasion.

The recent literature has shown a trend toward improvement in results for local staging of prostate cancer by eMRI (54–57). MRI has been shown to be more accurate than DRE in local staging, and when MRI and TRUS are compared in the same patient population, there is a trend toward better performance with MRI (42,54,56,57). MRI and TRUS are more accurate than DRE in local staging (56), and MRI and CT are approximately equally accurate in the evaluation of lymph node metastases.

MRI is probably not suitable for local staging in all patients with newly diagnosed prostate cancer, although the precise indications for when to perform MR staging have yet to be defined. The patients in whom MRI is likely to be cost effective are those who are at intermediate risk for advanced disease as defined by DRE, preoperative PSA, and biopsy Gleason score. In one group of patients at intermediate risk for advanced disease, D'Amico and co-workers are able to demonstrate a significant correlation between

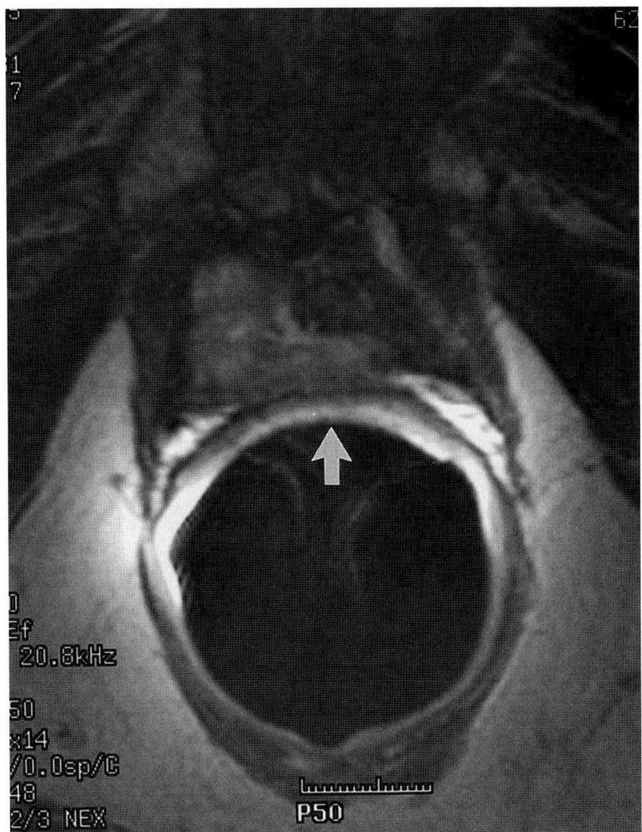

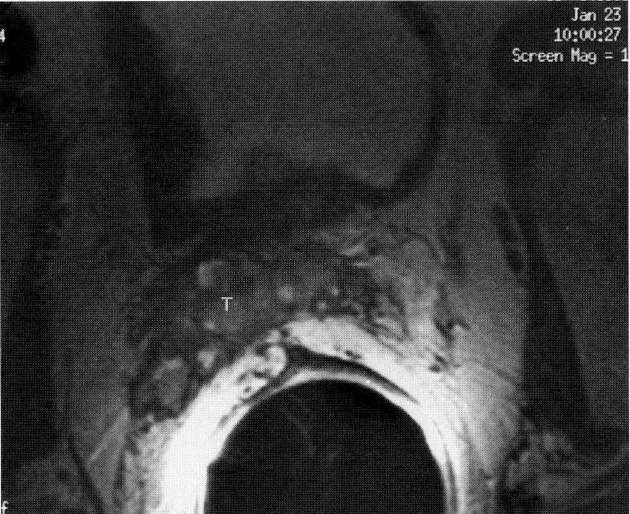

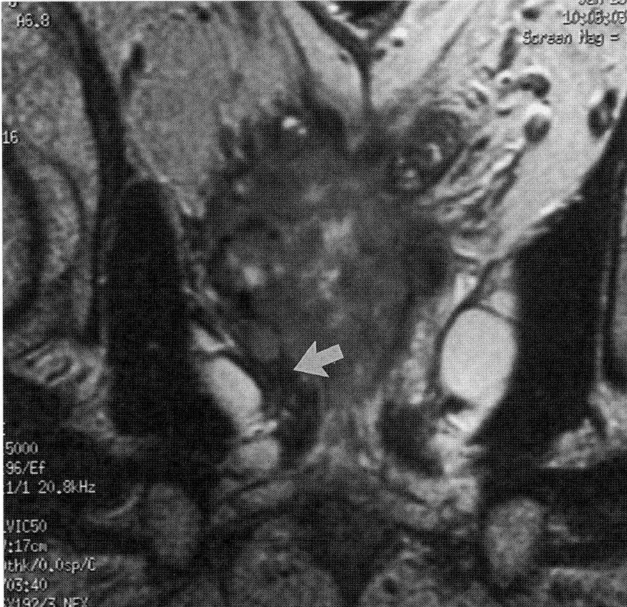

FIGURE 19-7. Magnetic resonance imaging: extracapsular extension and seminal vesicle invasion. These T2-weighted fast spin-echo images of a 66-year-old patient demonstrate extensive exophytic disease. The prostate cancer is invading the rectal mucosa (*arrow*) **(A)** and the seminal vesicles **(B)**, as demonstrated on the axial images [tumor (T)]. Normally, the seminal vesicles are of high signal intensity. On this image, they are infiltrated by a low-intensity T. The right levator ani muscle is also invaded, as demonstrated on the coronal image (*arrow*) **(C)**.

recurrence-free survival rates after radical prostatectomy and patient classification by MRI (58).

Although MRI offers great promise for the accurate local staging of prostate cancer, problems of reproducible image quality, interobserver variability, and higher examination cost must be resolved before it can be recommended for general clinical use. In addition, there is considerable concern about reports that indicate that the staging accuracy for eMRI spans a relatively wide range (30,31). Accuracy has been reported to be as low as 54% in one large multicenter trial (59) and as high as 82% to 88% in two other recently conducted studies (49,50). Sensitivity and specificity have been reported to range from 51% to 89% and 67% to 87%, respectively. In the Radiologic Diagnostic Oncology Group multicenter study, marked interobserver variability and the significance of reader experience in interpretation of endorectal images of the prostate became apparent. In this study, the staging accuracy for the same patient population varied from 50% to 79%, depending on the level of experience of the readers (59). These results suggest that development of standardized diagnostic criteria and more extensive training in interpreting eMRIs are required before interobserver variability can be reduced and MRI can be widely accepted.

Continued technologic advances in MR imaging and the development of new technologies, such as MRSI, provide hope for further improvement in the diagnostic performance of this technique in the local staging of prostate cancer. The use of the endorectal coil for prostate MRI allows not only higher-resolution anatomic images, but also the acquisition of metabolic information by MR spectroscopy. The development of analytic image correction may also help in establishing a reproducibly accurate approach to MR local staging.

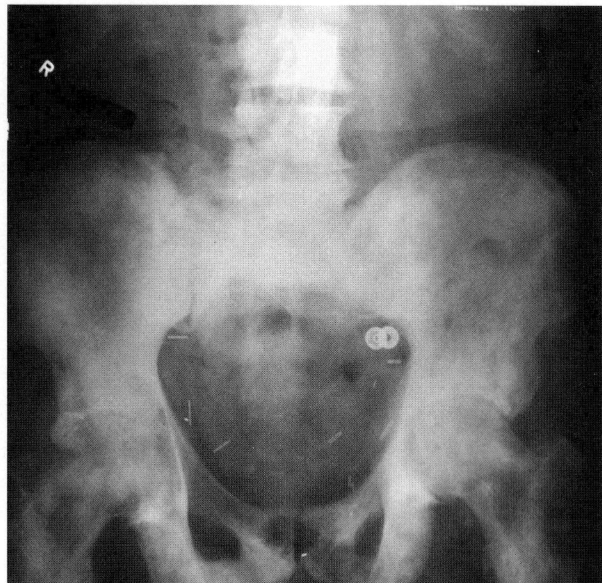

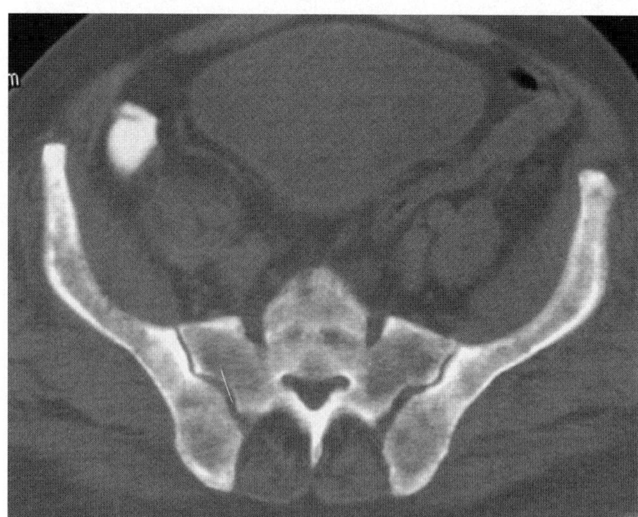

FIGURE 19-8. Conventional pelvic radiograph and pelvic computed tomography (CT). This pelvic radiography demonstrates extensive osteoblastic disease in a patient with prostate cancer **(A)**. The pelvic unenhanced helical CT demonstrates diffuse sclerosis of the bone consistent with osteoblastic bone metastasis **(B)**.

Three-Dimensional Magnetic Resonance Spectroscopic Imaging

As discussed earlier, spectroscopic imaging uses the same equipment as the MRI and is easily added to an MRI staging examination. When MRI and MRSI are performed as part of the same examination, the metabolic data can be correlated directly with the corresponding prostatic anatomy and pathology (Fig. 19-5). As is the case with tumor detection, the addition of 3D-MRSI to MRI in staging may improve accuracy and decrease interobserver variability (60). In one study, it was found that the strict application of specific MRI criteria for the diagnosis of ECE allowed reproducible high specificity to be achieved by readers of varying experience (93% for senior reader, 94% for junior reader). Variable sensitivity (50% for senior reader, 14% for junior reader), however, remained a problem for MRI alone. When MRSI data are added to the MRI data, there is a significant increase in sensitivity for the less experienced reader (from 14% to 39%) to a level approaching that of the more experienced reader (50%). These findings suggest that the addition of MRSI to MRI decreases interobserver variability and improves the accuracy of diagnosis of ECE in patients with clinically localized prostate cancer.

Evaluation of Distant Spread of Prostate Carcinoma

Bone Metastases

The skeleton is the most common site of hematogenous metastases from prostate cancer, and bone metastases can be found in 85% of patients dying of the disease (5). Plain films are not very sensitive for detecting bone metastases, because there must be a change in bone density of at least 50% before metastases can be seen radiographically (61). Radionuclide bone scintigraphy is very sensitive, however, and bone scans have replaced the skeletal survey in evaluating patients for osteoblastic bone metastases (Figs. 19-8 and 19-9). Reports from one study indicate that, with scintigraphy, bone metastases can be detected in 23% of patients with normal skeletal surveys. In addition, with information from bone scans, 16% of patients initially thought to have stage T1-3M0 disease are upstaged to T1-3M1 (62). Occasionally, a false-negative bone scan may occur. In these cases, a serum PSA greater than 50 ng per mL is suggestive of occult bone metastases. The use of serum PSA data can help to reduce the cost of pretreatment evaluation in patients with newly diagnosed prostate cancer by excluding patients who do not need a bone scan due to a low probability of bone metastases (63). It has been shown that if bone scans are performed only in asymptomatic patients with serum PSA levels greater than 10 ng per mL, then less than 1% of bone metastases will go undetected (63,64). In patients with stage T3 disease or poorly differentiated tumor on biopsy, however, a bone scan may be warranted regardless of PSA level (64). It should be noted that the high sensitivity of radionuclide scintigraphy is accompanied by low specificity. To increase diagnostic certainty, therefore, positive findings should be correlated with radiographs of the abnormal areas whenever necessary.

Conventional radiographs of selected bones are useful for evaluating inconclusive findings on bone scan and for evaluating specific sites of pain for impending pathologic fracture. Osteoblastic changes (80%), osteolytic changes (5%), or mixed osteoblastic-osteolytic changes (10% to

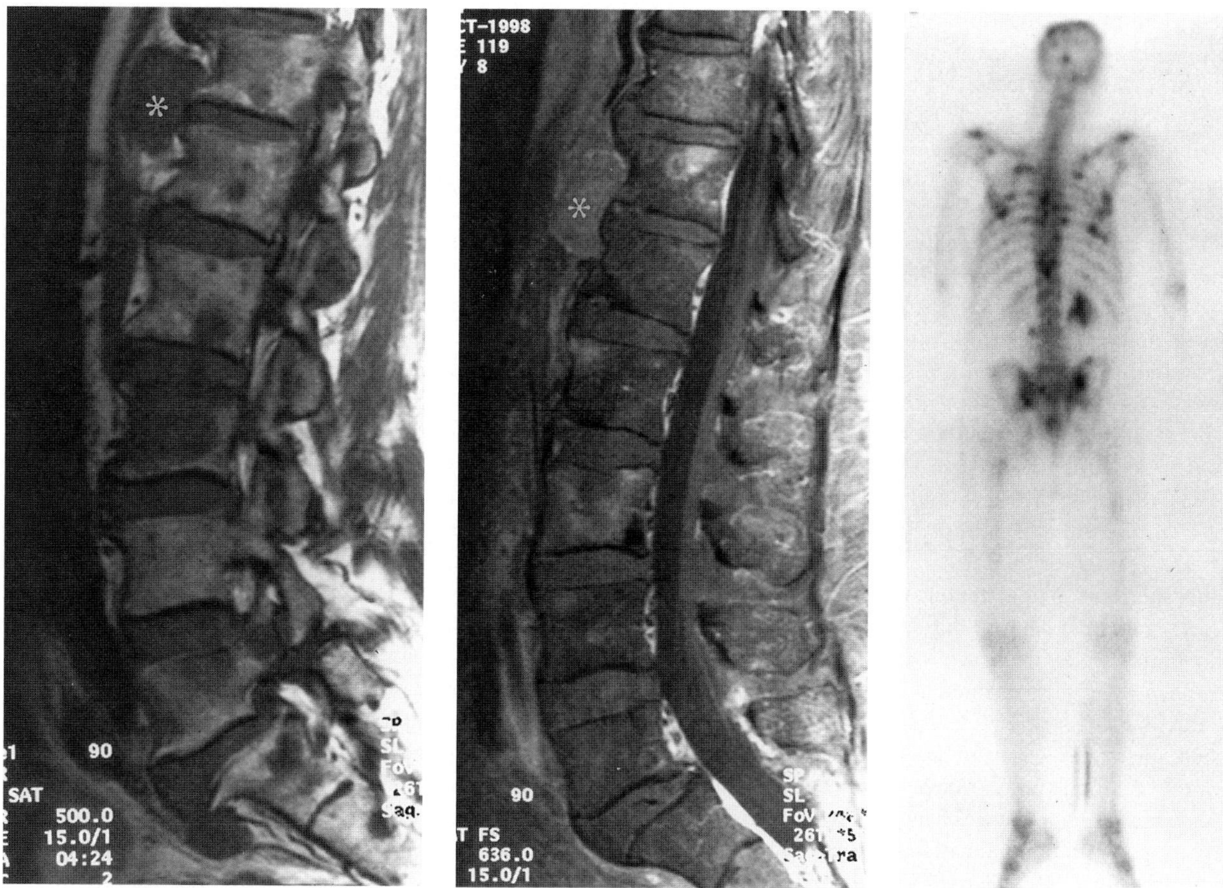

FIGURE 19-9. Bone metastasis on magnetic resonance imaging with bone scintigraphy. Images of a 64-year-old patient with prostate cancer. The sagittal T1-weighted spin-echo image **(A)** and the T2-weighted image with fat saturation **(B)** of the lumbar spine show numerous hypointense lesions on T1 consistent with bone metastases. An oval-shaped soft tissue mass (*asterisk*) ventral to the spinal segment T_{11} 12-L1 represents retrocrural adenopathy. The bone scintigraphy of the same patient **(C)** demonstrates multiple spots of enhancement throughout the whole skeleton, representing extensive metastatic disease.

15%) can be seen in the pelvis and lumbar spine of patients with bone metastases from prostate cancer (Fig. 19-8) (65). Early bone changes may present as focal areas of increased density that must be distinguished from benign bone islands. More commonly, large areas of bone are replaced by irregular dense deposits, leaving little question of the diagnosis (Fig. 19-8). Abnormal findings may be seen in only one bone, such as a lumbar vertebra, or may be extensive (Fig. 19-8). Bone findings may be completely reversed after endocrine therapy, although a paradoxic, transient increase in skeletal osteoblastic activity (the *flare* effect) may occur after orchiectomy or androgen blockade, even in the face of obvious clinical improvement.

Although CT is excellent for demonstrating osteoblastic, osteolytic, and mixed bony metastases from prostate cancer, it should not be used to screen for bone metastases (66). Radionuclide bone scintigraphy is preferred because it evaluates the entire skeleton and is more accurate in detecting small or early metastatic lesions. For similar reasons, scintigraphy is preferred over MRI. Because bone metastases are most commonly osteoblastic, they may appear hypointense compared to normal fatty marrow on T1- and T2-weighted MRI (67). The MRI may have a problem-solving role in the evaluation of patients with suspected bone metastases when other diagnostic studies are inconclusive or when spinal cord compression is suspected (67) (Fig. 19-9).

Lymph Node Metastases

Before the development of cross-sectional imaging techniques, such as CT and MRI, lymphangiography was used to evaluate patients with suspected lymph node metastases. *Lymphangiography* identifies lymph node metastases by finding intranodal filling defects. The ability to detect metastatic deposits as small as 5 mm in diameter is purported to be a unique advantage of lymphangiography. However, false-negative findings (nonvisualization of the node) may occur because of failure to fill the hypogastric and presacral lymphatics or because the entire node has been replaced by metastatic disease (68). In addition, an intranodal filling defect may be caused by inflammatory or other benign processes, and fine-needle aspiration biopsy may be required to confirm the diagnosis of metastatic disease (69). Enthusiasm for this technique has, therefore, declined, and lymphangiography is not currently recommended for lymph node staging in patients with prostate cancer. Not only is the procedure invasive and time consuming, but it also has not been found to be superior to CT or MRI.

CT is an excellent modality for the detection of lymph node metastases in patients with prostate cancer. In fact, it is the primary use of CT in these patients. Serum PSA data can be used to reduce the costs of pretreatment evaluation by excluding those patients who have a low probability of having an abnormal CT scan (63). In asymptomatic patients with serum PSA less than 20 ng per mL, fewer than 1% of patients will have a positive CT study (70).

The diagnosis of lymph node metastases by CT is based solely on size. All nodes larger than 1 cm in short axis diameter are considered abnormal. Dynamic scanning during bolus injection of intravenous contrast maximizes vascular opacification and helps to differentiate between blood vessels and lymph nodes in the pelvis and retroperitoneum. Unlike lymphangiography, the internal architecture of lymph nodes is not evaluated with CT. False-negative diagnoses result when metastases occur in normal-sized nodes, and false-positive diagnoses result when lymph node enlargement is due to benign hyperplastic changes. The sensitivity of CT for detecting lymph node metastases ranges from 30% to 78%, with a specificity of 77% to 97% and an accuracy of 70% to 94% (71–73). Although lowering the size threshold for the diagnosis of lymph node metastasis decreases the false-negative rate, it also increases the false-positive rate. Because a false-positive diagnosis denies potentially curative therapy to the patient, all enlarged lymph nodes should be biopsied to confirm the diagnosis. Combined CT and CT-guided fine-needle aspiration biopsy provide high specificity (up to 100%) for the diagnosis of lymph node metastases and may be considered an alternative to surgical or laparoscopic lymphadenectomy in some patients (71).

It is not necessary to include the retroperitoneum in pretreatment CT staging studies if there is no lymphadenopathy below the aortic bifurcation, because retroperitoneal lymphadenopathy does not occur in the absence of pelvic lymphadenopathy (74). Evaluation of suspected recurrent disease, however, requires examination of the abdomen and pelvis, owing to the higher prevalence of retroperitoneal lymphadenopathy (75).

The MRI can also be used to diagnose metastatic disease to lymph nodes. As with CT, the diagnosis of lymph node metastasis is based on the finding of lymph nodes larger than 1 cm in short axis diameter. On T1- and T2-weighted images, lymph nodes demonstrate intermediate signal intensity, as opposed to the low signal intensity flow voids usually seen in blood vessels. If necessary, gradient echo images may be obtained to help differentiate between lymph nodes and adjacent vessels.

Visceral Metastases

Distant metastases to liver, lung, and other viscera are readily detected by CT in symptomatic patients. The sensitivity of CT is maximized by dynamic scanning during bolus injection of intravenous contrast. Although the role of CT in patients with suspected distant spread of prostate cancer (PSA greater than 20 ng per mL) is well established, its use in screening for co-morbid disease that would affect treatment has not been found to be cost effective (70,76). Visceral metastases can also be identified with MR scanning, but because the MRI is obtained primarily for local staging, images above the aortic bifurcation are not usually obtained. Distant metastases occurring outside of the pelvis, therefore, are not detected.

In the search for lung metastases, the chest radiograph is still obtained routinely, even though its cost effectiveness as a routine study in evaluating all patients with prostate cancer is unproven (77). The case for routine examination is supported by the fact that in 10% to 15% of patients in the prostate cancer age group, a chest film will show evidence of significant nonneoplastic diseases, such as tuberculosis, cardiovascular disease, and pulmonary fibrosis (77,78). The chest radiograph also provides a simple and effective means of monitoring treatment in a patient with pulmonary metastases. Approximately 6% of all patients with newly diagnosed prostate cancer have intrathoracic metastases when first seen, and 25% of patients with documented distant spread of disease have chest involvement (78,79). Because some of these patients may demonstrate no other sites of distant spread, the true stage of disease may be underestimated if a chest radiograph is not obtained. Lymphangitic spread is a more typical presentation of metastatic disease than discrete pulmonary nodules. Thin-section CT of the chest can be used to detect early lymphangitic spread.

Radioimmunoscintigraphy and Positron Emission Tomography Scanning

Recent advances in metabolic imaging using radioimmunoscintigraphy [e.g., capromab pendetide (ProstaScint)] and PET may lead to improved detection of distant metastases from prostate cancer and provide an effective means of monitoring response to treatment and disease recurrence or progression (Fig. 19-10) (80–83). These new techniques may prove particularly useful in patients who are at high risk for having metastatic disease but do not demonstrate evidence of distant spread with conventional diagnostic imaging tests (83). Improved accuracy, particularly in the noninvasive evaluation of lymph node metastases, would represent a much-needed advance in the evaluation of patients with prostate cancer.

Radioimmunoscintigraphy

Radiolabeled monoclonal antibodies directed against prostate cancer–specific antigens are being developed to improve the diagnosis of metastatic disease to bone, lymph

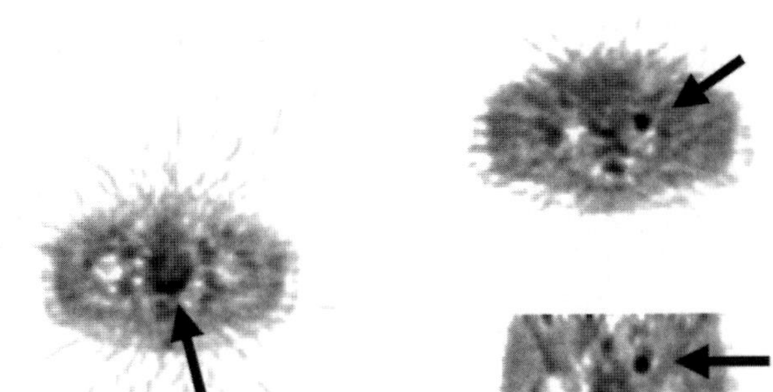

FIGURE 19-10. Radioimmunoscintigraphy and positron emission tomography. Arrows show increased activity in the region of lymph node metastasis.

nodes, and viscera. Research is under way to develop radiolabeled monoclonal antibodies that are highly specific for prostate cancer cell surface antigens (84). In the future, the large number of potential monoclonal antibodies may represent an advantage of radioimmunoscintigraphy over cross-sectional imaging techniques (85).

The best known of the monoclonal antibodies that have been developed is ProstaScint (81,86). ProstaScint, which recently received U.S. Food and Drug Administration approval, is a murine monoclonal antibody (CYT-356 or capromab pendetide) labeled with indium-111, which is directed against a glycoprotein expressed by prostate epithelium known as *prostate-specific membrane antigen.* It has shown efficacy in detecting lymph node and other metastases from prostate cancer with nuclear medicine single photon emission computed tomography (SPECT) and planar imaging techniques (87). Because of the kinetics of antibody binding, imaging is best performed approximately 72 to 120 hours after administration of the agent. The 2.8-day half-life of indium-111 facilitates timing of this imaging interval (81,84).

The greatest potential for ProstaScint radioimmunoscintigraphy is in selected patients with newly diagnosed prostate cancer, in patients who are suspected to have metastatic disease because of a rising serum PSA after definitive local therapy, and in high-risk patients in whom other diagnostic imaging tests have failed to demonstrate evidence of metastatic disease. Preliminary results from the ProstaScint Study Group suggest that ProstaScint imaging may help in differentiating between local and distant recurrence in patients in whom the only evidence of disease after radical prostatectomy is a detectable PSA level (88). Preliminary results also suggest that ProstaScint imaging can be used to differentiate between patients who will or will not respond to salvage radiation therapy after failed surgical therapy (89,90). In the identification of lymph node metastases, the detection threshold of ProstaScint imaging appears to be metastatic foci 5 mm or larger in size (91). Owing to the accumulation of radiolabel in the bladder, ProstaScint is of limited use in the prostate bed region, although it has been suggested that imaging can be performed during constant bladder irrigation.

Positron Emission Tomography

PET offers the capability of imaging biochemical processes *in vivo* and provides significantly better spatial resolution and image quality than standard nuclear medicine planar and SPECT imaging methods (82). Both PET and SPECT images can be co-registered to CT or other cross-sectional images, and such image fusion methods promise to become more clinically useful in the future, when standard image format protocols such as Dicom3 become implemented on imaging work and display stations. Another development in PET scanning is detection of abnormal uptake of the radiotracer FDG as a highly specific indicator for foci of metastatic disease in patients with prostate cancer (92). The relatively low metabolic activity of prostate cancer, however, may represent a potential limitation for FDG-PET (82). Preliminary studies suggest that PET cannot reliably differentiate between primary prostate cancer and benign prostatic hyperplasia. In addition, PET is not as sensitive as bone scintigraphy for the detection of bone metastases (93,94). Nonetheless, PET may have a role in the detection of lymph node metastases and may in the future prove to be a necessary staging modality in patients with prostate cancer.

REFERENCES

1. Stamey TA, Freiha FS, McNeal JE, et al. Localized prostate cancer. Relationship of tumor volume to clinical significance for treatment of prostate cancer. *Cancer* 1993;71[3 Suppl]:933–938.
2. Ohori M, Wheeler TM, Scardino PT. The New American Joint Committee on Cancer and International Union Against Cancer TNM classification of prostate cancer. Clinicopathologic correlations. *Cancer* 1994;74:104–114.
3. Slawin KM, Ohori M, Dillioglugil O, et al. Screening for prostate cancer: an analysis of the early experience. *CA Cancer J Clin* 1995;45:134–147.
4. Kindrick AV, Grossfeld GD, Stier DM, et al. Use of imaging tests for staging newly diagnosed prostate cancer: trends from the CaPSURE database. *J Urol* 1998;160:2102–2106.
5. Whitmore WJ Jr. Natural history and staging of prostate cancer. *Urol Clin North Am* 1984;11:209–220.
6. Schroder FH, Hermanek P, Denis L, et al. The TNM classification of prostate cancer. *Prostate Suppl* 1992;4:129–138.
7. Prout GR Jr., Heaney JA, Griffin PP, et al. Nodal involvement as a prognostic indicator in patients with prostatic carcinoma. *J Urol* 1980;124:226–231.
8. Epstein JI, Carmichael MJ, Pizov G, et al. Influence of capsular penetration on progression following radical prostatectomy. A study of 196 cases with long-term followup. *J Urol* 1993;150:135–141.
9. Ohori M, Scardino PT, Lapin SL, et al. The mechanisms and prognostic significance of seminal vesicle involvement by prostate cancer. *Am J Surg Pathol* 1993;17:1252–1261.
10. Morgan C, Calkins RF, Cavalcanti EJ. Computed tomography in the evaluation, staging, and therapy of carcinoma of the bladder and prostate. *Radiology* 1981;140:751–761.

11. Wefer AE, Hricak H, Vigneron DB, et al. Sextant localization of prostate cancer: comparison of sextant biopsy, magnetic resonance imaging and magnetic resonance spectroscopic imaging with step section histology. *J Urol* 2000;164:400–404.
12. Wefer AE, Hricak H, Vigneron DB, et al. Sextant localization of prostate cancer: comparison of sextant biopsy, magnetic resonance imaging and magnetic resonance spectroscopic imaging with step section histology. *J Urol* 2000;164:400–404.
13. Lowsley OS. The development of the human prostate gland with reference to the development of other structures at the neck of the urinary bladder. *Am J Anat* 1912;13:299–349.
14. McNeal JE. Normal and pathologic anatomy of the prostate. *Urology* 1981;17[Suppl]:11–16.
15. Older RA, Watson LR. Ultrasound anatomy of the normal male reproductive tract. *J Clin Ultrasound* 1996;24:389–404.
16. Hodge KK, McNeal JE, Terris MK, et al. Random systematic versus directed ultrasound guided transrectal core biopsies of the prostate. *J Urol* 1989;142:71–75.
17. Obek C, Louis P, Civantos F, et al. Comparison of digital rectal examination and biopsy results with the radical proctectomy specimen. *J Urol* 1999;161:494–498.
18. Salomon L, Colombel M, Patard JJ, et al. Value of ultrasound-guided systematic sextant biopsies in prostate tumor mapping. *Eur Urol* 1999;35:289–293.
19. Coffeld KS, Speights VO, Brawn PN, et al. Ultrasound detection of prostate cancer in postmortem specimens with histological correlation. *J Urol* 1992;147:822–826.
20. Shinohara K, Wheeler TM, Scardino PT. The appearance of prostate cancer on transrectal ultrasonography: correlation of imaging and pathological examinations. *J Urol* 1989; 142:76–82.
21. Ellis WJ, Brawer MK. The significance of isoechoic prostatic carcinoma. *J Urol* 1994;152:2304–2307.
22. Rifkin MD, Dahnert W, Kurtz AB. State of the art: endorectal sonography of the prostate gland. *AJR Am J Roentgenol* 1990;154:691–700.
23. Gustafsson O, Carlsson P, Norming U, et al. Cost-effectiveness analysis in early detection of prostate cancer: an evaluation of six screening strategies in a randomly selected population of 2,400 men. *Prostate* 1995;26:299–309.
24. Kelly IM, Lees WR, Rickards D. Prostate cancer and the role of color Doppler US. *Radiology* 1993;189:153–156.
25. Rubens DJ, Hadley MA, Alam SK, et al. Sonoelasticity imaging of prostate cancer: in vitro results. *Radiology* 1995; 195:379–383.
26. Hricak H, Dooms GC, McNeal JE, et al. MR imaging of the prostate gland. Normal anatomy. *AJR Am J Roentgenol* 1987;148:51–55.
27. Hricak H, White S, Vigneron D, et al. Carcinoma of the prostate gland: MR imaging with pelvic phased-array coils versus integrated endorectal—pelvic phased-array coils. *Radiology* 1994;193:703–709.
28. Schnall MD, Pollack HM. Magnetic resonance imaging of the prostate. *Urol Radiol* 1990;12:109–114.
29. White S, Hricak H, Forstner R, et al. Prostate cancer: effect of postbiopsy hemorrhage on interpretation of MR images. *Radiology* 1995;195:385–390.
30. Ohori M, Wheeler TM, Dunn JK, et al. The pathological features and prognosis of prostate cancer detectable with current diagnostic tests. *J Urol* 1994;152:1714–1720.
31. Waterbor JW, Bueschen AJ. Prostate cancer screening (United States). *Cancer Causes Control* 1995;6:267–274.
32. Kurhanewicz J, Vigneron DB, Nelson SJ, et al. Citrate as an in vivo marker to discriminate prostate cancer from benign prostatic hyperplasia and normal prostate peripheral zone: detection via localized proton spectroscopy. *Urology* 1995; 45:459–466.
33. Scheidler J, Hricak H, Vigneron DB, et al. Prostate cancer: localization with three-dimensional proton MR spectroscopic imaging—clinicopathologic study. *Radiology* 1999; 213:473–480.
34. Kurhanewicz J, Hricak H, Vigneron DB, et al. Prostate cancer: metabolic response to cryosurgery as detected with 3D H-1 MR spectroscopic imaging. *Radiology* 1996;200:489–496.
35. Weidner N, Carroll PR, Flax J, et al. Tumor angiogenesis correlates with metastasis in invasive prostate carcinoma. *Am J Pathol* 1993;143:401–409.
36. Rubin JM, Adler RS, Fowlkes JB, et al. Fractional moving blood volume: estimation with power Doppler US. *Radiology* 1995;197:183–190.
37. Kurhanewicz J, Vigneron DB, Hricak H, et al. Three-dimensional H-1 MR spectroscopic imaging of the in situ human prostate with high (0.24–0.7 cm^3) spatial resolution. *Radiology* 1996;198:795–805.
38. Vigneron D, Males R, Hricak H, et al. Prostate cancer: correlation of 3D MRSI metabolite levels with histologic grade. Abstract presented at the Radiological Society of North America. *Radiology* 1998;209:181.
39. Mukamel E, Hanna J, deKernion JB. Pitfalls in preoperative staging in prostate cancer. *Urology* 1987;30:318–321.
40. D'Amico A, Whittington R, Schnall M, et al. The impact of the inclusion of endorectal coil magnetic resonance imaging in a multivariate analysis to predict clinically unsuspected extraprostatic cancer. *Cancer* 1995;75:2368–2372.
41. Lorentzen T, Nerstrom H, Iversen P, et al. Local staging of prostate cancer with transrectal ultrasound: a literature review. *Prostate Suppl* 1992;4:11–16.
42. Rifkin MD, Zerhouni EA, Gatsonis CA, et al. Comparison of magnetic resonance imaging and ultrasonography in staging early prostate cancer—results of a multi-institutional cooperative trial. *N Engl J Med* 1990;323:621–626.
43. Smith JA, Scardino PT, Resnick MI, et al. Transrectal ultrasound versus digital rectal examination for the staging of carcinoma of the prostate: results of a prospective, multi-institutional trial. *J Urol* 1997;157:902–906.
44. Hardeman SW, Causey JQ, Hickey DP, et al. Transrectal ultrasound for staging prior to radical prostatectomy. *Urology* 1989;34:175–180.
45. Allepuz Losa CA, Sanz Velez JI, Gil Sanz MJ, et al. Seminal vesicle biopsy in prostate cancer staging. *J Urol* 1995;154: 1407–1411.
46. Pandey P, Fowler JE Jr., Seaver LE, et al. Ultrasound guided seminal vesicle biopsies in men with suspected prostate cancer. *J Urol* 1995;154:1798–1801.
47. Garg MK, Tekyi-Mensah S, Bolton S, et al. Impact of prostatectomy prostate-specific antigen nadir on outcomes following salvage radiotherapy. *Urology* 1998,51:998–1002.
48. Partin AW, Kattan MW, Subong EN, et al. Combination of prostate-specific antigen, clinical stage, and Gleason score to predict pathological stage of localized prostate cancer. A multi-institutional update. *JAMA* 1997;277:1445–1451.

49. Engeler CE, Wasserman NF, Zhang G. Preoperative assessment of prostatic carcinoma by computerized tomography. Weaknesses and new perspectives. *Urology* 1992;40:346–350.
50. Hricak H, Dooms GC, Jeffrey RB, et al. Prostatic carcinoma: staging by clinical assessment, CT, and MR imaging. *Radiology* 1987;162:331–336.
51. Outwater EK, Petersen RO, Siegelman ES, et al. Prostate carcinoma: assessment of diagnostic criteria for capsular penetration on endorectal coil MR images. *Radiology* 1994; 193:333–339.
52. Yu KK, Hricak H, Alagappan R, et al. Detection of extracapsular extension of prostate carcinoma with endorectal and phased-array coil MR imaging: multivariate feature analysis. *Radiology* 1997;202:697–702.
53. Langlotz C, Schnall M, Pollack H. Staging of prostatic cancer: accuracy of MR imaging. *Radiology* 1995;194:645–646.
54. Huch Boni RA, Boner JA, Debatin JF, et al. Optimization of prostate carcinoma staging: comparison of imaging and clinical methods. *Clin Radiol* 1995;50:593–600.
55. Bartolozzi C, Menchi L, Lencioni R, et al. Local staging of prostate carcinoma with endorectal coil MRI: correlation with whole-mount radical prostatectomy specimens. *Eur Radiol* 1996;6:339–345.
56. Vapnek JM, Hricak H, Shinohara K, et al. Staging accuracy of magnetic resonance imaging versus transrectal ultrasound in stages A and B prostatic cancer. *Urol Int* 1994;53:191–195.
57. Presti JC Jr., Hricak H, Narayan PA, et al. Local staging of prostatic carcinoma: comparison of transrectal sonography and endorectal MR imaging. *AJR Am J Roentgenol* 1996; 166:103–108.
58. D'Amico AV, Whittington R, Malkowicz SB, et al. Critical analysis of the ability of the endorectal coil magnetic resonance imaging scan to predict pathologic stage, margin status, and postoperative prostate-specific antigen failure in patients with clinically organ-confined prostate cancer. *J Clin Oncol* 1996;14:1770–1777.
59. Tempany CM, Zhou X, Zerhouni EA, et al. Staging of prostate cancer: results of Radiology Diagnostic Oncology Group project comparison of three MR imaging techniques. *Radiology* 1994;192:47–54.
60. Yu KK, Scheidler J, Hricak H, et al. Prostate cancer: prediction of extracapsular extension with endorectal MR imaging and three-dimensional proton MR spectroscopic imaging. *Radiology* 1999;213:481–488.
61. Lentle BC, McGowan DG, Dierich H. Technetium-99m polyphosphate bone scanning in carcinoma of the prostate. *Br J Urol* 1974;46:543–548.
62. Paulson DF. The impact of current staging procedures in assessing disease extent of prostatic adenocarcinoma. *J Urol* 1979;121:300–302.
63. Oesterling JE, Martin SK, Bergstralh EJ, et al. The use of prostate-specific antigen in staging patients with newly diagnosed prostate cancer. *JAMA* 1993;269:57–60.
64. Gleave ME, Coupland D, Drachenberg D, et al. Ability of serum prostate-specific antigen levels to predict normal bone scans in patients with newly diagnosed prostate cancer. *Urology* 1996;47:708–712.
65. Pontes JE, Choe B, Rose N, et al. Reliability of bone marrow acid phosphatase as a parameter of metastatic prostatic cancer. *J Urol* 1979;122:178–179.
66. Yoshida K, Akimoto M. Computed tomographic evaluation of bone metastases in prostatic cancer patients. *Adv Exp Med Biol* 1992;324:197–204.
67. Fujii Y, Higashi Y, Owada F, et al. Magnetic resonance imaging for the diagnosis of prostate cancer metastatic to bone. *Br J Urol* 1995;75:54–58.
68. McLaughlin AP, Saltzstein SL, McCullough DL, et al. Prostatic carcinoma: incidence and location of unsuspected lymphatic metastases. *J Urol* 1976;115:89–94.
69. Gothlin JH, Hoiem L. Percutaneous fine needle biopsy of radiographically normal lymph nodes in the staging of prostatic cancer. *Radiology* 1981;141:351–353.
70. Huncharek M, Muscat J. Serum prostate-specific antigen as a predictor of staging abdominal/pelvic computed tomography in newly diagnosed prostate cancer. *Abdom Imaging* 1996;21:364–367.
71. Oyen RH, Van Poppel HP, Ameye FE, et al. Lymph node staging of localized prostatic carcinoma with CT and CT-guided fine-needle aspiration biopsy: prospective study of 285 patients. *Radiology* 1994;190:315–322.
72. Weinerman PM, Arger PH, Coleman BG, et al. Pelvic adenopathy from bladder and prostate carcinoma: detection by rapid sequence computed tomography. *AJR Am J Roentgenol* 1983;140:95–99.
73. Golimbu M, Morales P, Al-Askari S, et al. CAT scanning in staging of prostatic cancer. *Urology* 1981;18:305–308.
74. Spencer J, Golding S. CT evaluation of lymph node status at presentation of prostatic carcinoma. *Br J Radiol* 1992;65: 199–201.
75. Spencer JA, Golding SJ. Patterns of lymphatic metastases at recurrence of prostate cancer: CT findings. *Clin Radiol* 1994;49:404–407.
76. Forman HP, Heiken JP, Brink JA, et al. CT screening for comorbid disease in patients with prostatic carcinoma: Is it cost-effective? *AJR Am J Roentgenol* 1994;162:1125–1128.
77. Forman HP, Fox LA, Glazer HS, et al. Chest radiography in patients with early stage prostatic carcinoma. Effect on treatment planning and cost analysis. *Chest* 1994;106: 1036–1041.
78. Apple JS, Paulson DF, Baber C, et al. Advanced prostatic carcinoma: pulmonary manifestations. *Radiology* 1985;154: 601–603.
79. Lindell MM, Doubleday LC, von Eschenbach AC, et al. Mediastinal metastases from prostatic carcinoma. *J Urol* 1982;128:331–333.
80. Vasallo P, Matei C, Heston WD, et al. Characterization of reactive versus tumor-bearing lymph nodes with interstitial magnetic resonance lymphography in an animal model. *Invest Radiol* 1995;30:706–711.
81. Burgers JK, Hinkle GH, Haseman MK. Monoclonal antibody imaging of recurrent and metastatic prostate cancer. *Semin Urol* 1995;13:103–112.
82. Bender H, Schomburg A, Albers P, et al. Possible role of FDG-PET in the evaluation of urologic malignancies. *Anticancer Res* 1997;17:1655–1660.
83. Hinkle GH, Burgers JK, Neal CE, et al. Multicenter radioimmunoscintigraphic evaluation of patients with prostate carcinoma using indium-111 capromab pendetide. *Cancer* 1998;83(4):739–747.
84. Feneley MR, Chengazi VU, Kirby RS, et al. Prostatic radioimmunoscintigraphy: preliminary results using techne-

tium-labeled monoclonal antibody, CYT-35 1. *Br J Urol* 1996;77:373–381.
85. Hoh CK, Schiepers C, Seltzer MA, et al. PET in oncology: will it replace the other modalities? *Semin Nucl Med* 1997;27:94–106.
86. Sodee DB, Conant R, Chalfant M, et al. Preliminary imaging results using IN-111 labeled CYT-356 (Prostascint) in the detection of recurrent prostate cancer. *Clin Nucl Med* 1996;21:759–767.
87. Hinkle GH, Burgers JK, Olsen JO, et al. Prostate cancer abdominal metastases detected with indium-111 capromab pendetide. *J Nucl Med* 1998;39:650–652.
88. Kahn D, Williams RD, Manyak MJ, et al. 111-Indium-capromab pendetide in the evaluation of patients with residual or recurrent prostate cancer after radical prostatectomy. The ProstaScint Study Group. *J Urol* 1998;159: 2041–2046.
89. Kahn D, Williams RD, Haseman MK, et al. Radioimmunoscintigraphy with In111-labeled capromab pendetide predicts prostate cancer response to salvage radiotherapy after failed radical prostatectomy. *J Clin Oncol* 1998;16:284–289.
90. Levesque PE, Nieh PT, Zinman LN, et al. Radiolabeled monoclonal antibody indium 111-labeled CYT-356 localizes extraprostatic recurrent carcinoma after prostatectomy. *Urology* 1998;51:978–984.
91. Babaian RJ, Sayer J, Podoloff DA, et al. Radioimmunoscintigraphy of pelvic lymph nodes with 111 indium-labeled monoclonal antibody CYT-356. *J Urol* 1994;152:1952–1955.
92. Effert PJ, Bare R, Handt S, et al. Metabolic imaging of untreated prostate cancer by positron emission tomography with 18fluorine-labeled deoxyglucose. *J Urol* 1996;155: 994–998.
93. Hoh CK, Seltzer MA, Franklin J, et al. Positron emission tomography in urological oncology. *J Urol* 1998;159:347–356.
94. Shreve PD, Grossman HB, Gross MD, et al. Metastatic prostate cancer: initial findings of PET with 2-deoxy-2(F-18)fluoro-D-glucose. *Radiology* 1996;199:751–756.

20

MOLECULAR STAGING OF PROSTATE CANCER

GEORGE V. THOMAS
MASSIMO LODA

Once the diagnosis of prostate cancer has been made, the local and distant extent of the primary tumor must be defined, as anatomic and clinical staging remains the mainstay by which clinical decision making is directed. The most commonly used system, tumor-node-metastasis (TNM), stages tumors according to the size of the primary tumor and the presence or absence of either lymph node metastasis or distant metastatic disease.

Pathologic staging is a measure of extent of disease. At present, organ-confined tumors benefit most from surgical excision of the primary tumor. Current clinical staging systems are limited by a number of factors, such as clinical understaging with transurethral resection or digital rectal examination, as well as the limited ability of imaging studies to evaluate the presence and extent of prostatic adenocarcinoma (1). No single diagnostic test can distinguish accurately between organ-confined (surgically curable) and non–organ-confined disease.

The widespread use of serum prostate-specific antigen (PSA) measurement has led to a marked shift in the pattern of disease presentation. As a result of PSA screening, patients now present more often with organ-confined disease (2). It is generally easy to predict the biologic behavior of patients with early-state cancers. Similarly, patients with extensive disease (e.g., extraprostatic extension) generally do poorly. Because patients with organ-confined disease mostly have the same TNM staging, this limits the predictive value of staging. In addition, there are still major differences with respect to outcome within the category of organ-confined prostate cancer. Among all patients undergoing prostatectomy for organ-confined disease, more than one-third will relapse and require additional therapy (3–7).

An additional valuable prognostic parameter is the degree of differentiation of the tumor based on Gleason score. Men with tumors of low Gleason grades (i.e., grades 2 to 4) face minimal risk (4% to 7%) of dying from prostate cancer in 15 years, whereas men having tumors of grades 8 to 10 face a much higher risk (60% to 87%) (8).

Using the preoperative serum PSA level, tumor grade (Gleason score), and the stage of the local tumor, patients can be stratified into groups that differ with respect to relapse-free survival (9,10). However, once again we are limited by the fact that the majority of patients undergoing radical prostatectomy presents with Gleason 6 or 7 tumors and have a serum PSA between 4 and 10 ng per mL. Although the combination of Gleason score and preoperative PSA is a better predictor of prognosis, it still does not accurately predict tumor behavior.

Further improvements in staging beyond tumor size and state of cellular differentiation will require the identification of new predictors of tumor behavior. In certain instances, the presence within a tumor of a characteristic molecular signature has been proven to be remarkably accurate in predicting the biologic behavior of these tumors. For hematologic neoplasms, multiple studies have demonstrated that cytogenetics can contribute valuable prognostic information, independent of morphologic or immunophenotypic features. Chromosomal analysis of pediatric leukemias is now considered the standard of care in many centers. These data have allowed predictions of the long-term survival rates of patients based on tumor-specific chromosomal translocations. For example, acute lymphoblastic leukemia patients with the TEL-AML1 fusion have a favorable prognosis, whereas those with the E2A-PBX1 fusion require more intensive therapy to obtain a good outcome (11). Similarly, patients with acute promyelocytic leukemia who carry the PML-RAR-alpha fusion respond to all-*trans*-retinoic acid and have an excellent outcome after treatment with all-*trans*-retinoic acid in combination with anthracyclines (12). Chimeric tumor genes obtained by reverse transcriptase-polymerase chain reaction (RT-PCR) have also been shown to provide diagnostic and prognostic information in synovial sarcoma (13,14). Among epithelial tumors, colorectal adenocarcinoma has the most advanced molecular staging, in which inactivation of tumor suppressor genes and activation of oncogenes at different stages of tumorigenesis have been mapped out (15). The molecular oncology paradigm is based on the belief that the behavior of a tumor is ultimately dependent on certain key molecular characteristics. More specifically, knowing these key molecular characteristics might, in time, allow one to predict important aspects of tumor behavior and patient outcome. Several emerging and experimental approaches to predicting tumor behavior fall under the heading of molecular staging tools. They look at genetic alterations or at changes in protein structure or concentration that are more characteristic of metastatic prostate cancer than of localized tumors or normal prostate tissue.

The aims of this chapter are to provide an introduction to the currently available molecular staging modalities that may be used in the clinical setting. Specific genes that have been shown to have potential as molecular staging tools are discussed. Knowledge of the signaling pathways, in which these markers are involved, may also help in selecting potential therapeutic targets for the treatment of prostate cancer.

SERUM BIOMARKERS

Prostate-Specific Antigen

PSA is a serine protease that functions to liquefy seminal coagulum (16) and has a molecular weight of 34 kD (17). It consists of 237 amino acids and four carbohydrate side chains. The gene encoding PSA is localized to chromosome 19 (18). It is produced by the epithelial cells lining the acini and ducts of the prostate gland, and under normal conditions it is secreted into the lumina of prostatic ducts and can be detected in high concentrations in seminal plasma.

PSA expression, although highly restricted and confined mainly to benign and malignant prostatic luminal epithelial cells, has also been documented in bladder adenocarcinomas (19), salivary gland neoplasms (20), and breast cancers (21). PSA levels can also be elevated in prostatitis (22) and benign prostatic hyperplasia (BPH) (23,24), and after prostate manipulation (25), thus making this marker not absolutely cancer specific. In prostate cancer, levels are dependent on the volume of cancer present (26), and the histologic differentiation of the tumor (more poorly differentiated tumors produce less PSA on an individual cell basis, but these tumors have more cells per unit of tumor volume) (27). These factors have important implications in using PSA for diagnosis and staging.

Serum PSA is currently used as a tumor marker for prostate cancer and also for the early detection, staging, and posttreatment follow-up of patients. Pretreatment serum PSA is related to clinical stage, Gleason grade, tumor volume, and pathologic stage (28–33). PSA levels correlate with clinical stage, but there is considerable overlap among the clinical stages (30). However, by combining the PSA level with the clinical findings on digital rectal examination and histologic grade by biopsy, several groups have developed normograms based on multivariate analyses to construct probability plots validated by pathologic staging to predict the probability of capsular penetration, seminal vesicle involvement, and nodal involvement (5,32). Immunohistochemical (IHC) staining for PSA is useful in the identification of metastatic tumor of unknown origin as prostate carcinoma. In addition, Epstein and Eggleston have shown a statistically significant correlation between progression of disease and negative to weak staining for PSA (34), suggesting that tumor cells that lack sufficient differentiation to express immunologically recognizable antigens normally expressed by nontransformed cells behave more aggressively (Fig. 20-1).

More recently, several groups have attempted to develop a more sensitive, molecular-based assay for the detection of PSA using the PCR. This technique allows the detection of one PSA-expressing cell in a background of 10^6 to 10^7 cells (35). In addition, RT-PCR PSA assays can detect the presence of occult prostate cells in tissues or circulating prostate tumor cells through amplification of PSA messenger RNA (mRNA). Several groups have evaluated peripheral blood mononuclear cells, lymph nodes, and bone marrow specimens using the mRNA for PSA as a template (36,37). Some investigators have shown a correlation between RT-

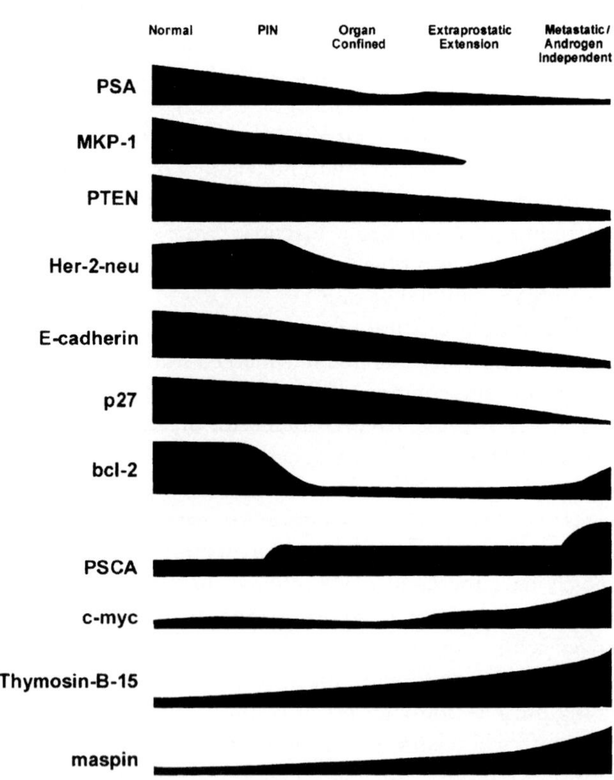

FIGURE 20-1. Immunohistochemical profile of tumor biomarkers at different stages of prostate cancer development and progression. MKP-1, MAP kinase phosphatase 1; PIN, prostatic intraepithelial neoplasia; PSA, prostate-specific antigen; PSCA, prostate stem cell antigen; PTEN, phosphatase and tensin homologue deleted on chromosome 10.

PCR results and clinical staging in prostate cancer. Olsson et al. evaluated a RT-PCR assay using nested primers and found that it correlated with positive surgical margins and extension into the seminal vesicles in 100 patients undergoing radical prostatectomy (38). The observed specificity and sensitivity for extraprostatic disease were 73% and 90%, respectively. They found the RT-PCR assay to be superior to Gleason score and serum PSA in predicting the presence of extraprostatic disease. On the other hand, they noted that the PSA RT-PCR test was a poor predictor of response to treatment. Ghossein et al. also found a correlation between positive peripheral blood RT-PCR results and clinical staging with 16% of men with apparent organ-confined disease, 30% with locally advanced or node-positive disease, and 35% with distant metastases (39). Jaakkola et al. found positive results in none of seven patients tested with clinically localized disease and 9 of 18 with metastatic disease (40). Others have reported a poor correlation between PSA RT-PCR results and pathologic or clinical stage (37,41,42). Limited cohorts of patients tested, technical variability in performance of the assays, and diverse populations tested may all contribute to the discordant results obtained by various groups.

Prostate-Specific Membrane Antigen

A novel marker with high specificity for prostate tissue is prostate-specific membrane antigen (PSMA) (43). PSMA is a membrane glycoprotein that is expressed in normal prostatic epithelial cells and elevated in prostate cancers, especially in poorly differentiated, metastatic, and hormone-refractory carcinomas (44,45). However, PSMA has been detected in nonprostatic tissue, namely salivary glands, brain, small intestine, cardiac muscle, skeletal muscle, and neoangiogenic endothelial cells (46–48). RT-PCR assays with primers specific for PSMA have been shown to be more effective than PSA-specific primers in detecting hematogenous circulating prostate cancer cells (49); however, no clear benefit in patient staging or use as a predictor of clinical outcome or response to treatment has been obtained using RT-PCR methods thus far (41,50).

Interestingly, Grasso et al. found that a combined nested RT-PCR assay for PSA and PSMA correlated with pathologic stage (51). In addition, PSA or PSMA RT-PCR was shown to be a better predictor of tumor extracapsular extension than initial serum PSA, clinical stage, and biopsy Gleason score.

The clinical applicability of PSA or PSMA RT-PCR assays is uncertain, because the detection of circulating prostate cancer cells in the peripheral blood or in tissues does not necessarily reflect the presence of metastatic disease. Large prospective studies will determine the clinical implications of such findings and the need, or lack thereof, for therapeutic intervention. The current predictive accuracy, however, does not permit basing treatment recommendations on the outcome of these tests.

Prostatic Acid Phosphatase

Prostatic acid phosphatase (PAP) was the biomarker most extensively used before the discovery of PSA for the diagnosis, staging, and monitoring of patients with prostate cancer. However, difficulties such as diurnal variation, cross-reactivity with serum acid phosphatases from other tissues, and elevations after digital rectal examination can alter the interpretation of the results and lead to false-negative and false-positive results (52). IHC staining for PAP (in combination with PSA) is useful in confirming metastatic prostate cancer (53).

TISSUE BIOMARKERS

p53

The *p53* gene, which is located on the short arm of chromosome 17, encodes for a nuclear transcription factor that functions in cell cycle control, DNA repair, and apoptosis (54–56). In response to DNA damage, wild-type *p53* arrests cells in the G_1 phase or can induce apoptosis (57,58). The *p21*^{cip1} gene plays a role in signaling cellular growth arrest, and, in response to DNA damage, p21 is induced by the *p53* gene, thereby playing a direct role in mediating *p53*-induced G_1 arrest (59). Loss of heterozygosity (LOH) on chromosome 17p occurs in 16% of prostate cancers with a range of 5% to 38% (60–63). LOH for *p53* in one allele can be coupled with a mutation in the other allele, most often occurring in exons 5 through 8, that can either result in no protein being produced or production of a dysfunctional protein. Cells having such *p53* mutations are genetically unstable and are prone to developing further mutations leading to tumor progression. Wild-type *p53* has a short half-life and is normally expressed at low levels in G_0 and G_1 phases. In contrast, most *p53* missense mutations result in a protein with a much longer half-life, facilitating detection by immunohistochemistry (64,65). It is important to bear in mind that IHC will not identify in-frame deletions, splicing errors, or nonsense mutations (66).

It has been shown that p53 protein expression is correlated with higher Gleason score, nuclear grade, pathologic stage, and proliferation in localized primary prostate carcinomas and that there is an increase in *p53* mutations in advanced prostate cancer, with the highest incidence occurring in androgen-independent tumors (67–69). Several studies have demonstrated that p53 protein expression serves as an adverse prognostic indicator and an independent prognostic marker for disease-free survival after radical prostatectomy (65,70–77). Stricker et al. compared p53, stage, age, race, Gleason score, and preoperative PSA by multivariate analysis to predict biochemical recurrence (76). They showed that p53, stage, and preoperative PSA levels were the best predictors of PSA recurrence. Bauer et al. have shown that the p53 status was positively associated with rising grade and stage and an independent predictor of disease-free survival (70). However, the major limitation of p53 in predicting behavior is the fact that its inactivation occurs primarily in advanced disease. In colorectal cancer, it has been recently shown that response to therapy aimed at inducing apoptosis was different according to p21 status in a background of p53 inactivation (78). This may have implications in prostate cancer as well.

Bcl-2

The *bcl-2* gene is the prototype of a newly described class of oncogenes that modulate apoptosis (79,80).

Subsequently, it has been demonstrated that the *bcl-2* gene is a member of a multigene family whose members function to inhibit or promote apoptosis (81). The regulation of cell death by members of this gene family may be achieved through competing dimerization of different family members (82–85). However, more recent evidence suggests that the individual *bcl-2* family members can independently regulate the susceptibility to undergo cell death and, thus, may not require heterodimerization (86).

Although initially discovered via the translocation in follicular lymphomas (t14,18), it has subsequently been found to be involved in the carcinogenesis of various epithelial tumors (87–90).

An increase in intracellular Ca^{2+} concentration has been implicated as an important signaling event associated with cell death in prostatic epithelial cells (91,92). *bcl-2* has been shown to inhibit the induction of cell death by thapsigargin, a selective inhibitor of the endoplasmic reticulum Ca^{2+} pump (93). Thapsigargin results in depletion of endoplasmic reticulum Ca^{2+} stores and subsequent capacitative influx of extracellular Ca^{2+}. Experimental evidence suggests that bcl-2 is able to inhibit the depletion of the endoplasmic reticulum Ca^{2+} pool and thereby inhibit capacitative Ca^{2+} entry. Of interest, thapsigargin can induce apoptosis in androgen-independent prostate cancer cells in a dose-dependent manner, and this effect is critically dependent on a sustained increase in intracellular Ca^{2+} (94), pointing to a novel therapeutic strategy.

bcl-2 is normally expressed in the basal cells of the prostate glandular epithelium, which is resistant to the effects of androgen withdrawal (95,96). In contrast, the bcl-2–negative secretory glandular epithelial cells undergo apoptotic cell death in response to androgen deprivation (95,97). High levels of bcl-2 expression are seen with greater frequency as prostate cancers progress from localized (7% of tumors overexpressing bcl-2) to metastasizing androgen-dependent (17%) to androgen-independent (67%) tumors (91,98). Several groups have shown that androgen-independent prostate cancers are typically immunoreactive for bcl-2 protein (95,97). Thus, it appears that bcl-2 may enable prostate cancer cells to remain viable despite castrate levels of androgen, and that hormone ablation therapy may be selecting for bcl-2–positive cells that fail to undergo apoptosis after hormone withdrawal (Fig. 20-1).

Expression of bcl-2 has been shown to correlate inversely with clinical outcome in patients undergoing radical prostatectomy for treatment of clinically localized prostate cancer (99). Expression of bcl-2 has also been shown to be an adverse prognostic indicator in patients with locally advanced or metastatic prostate cancer receiving hormonal therapy (97). Interestingly, expression of bcl-2 within prostate carcinoma cells is associated with resistance to cell death induction by various chemotherapeutic agents. A mechanism whereby bcl-2 induces its antiapoptotic effect may be via regulation of microtubule integrity (100). Anticancer drugs that inhibit microtubule function—for example, paclitaxel and vinblastine—also induce bcl-2 phosphorylation that leads to its inactivation and then apoptotic cell death. In contrast, drugs that damage deoxyribonucleic acid—for example, doxorubicin and cisplatin—do not induce bcl-2 phosphorylation or inhibit microtubule formation. The phosphorylation of bcl-2 involves the serine or threonine protein kinase c-Raf-1 (101). In contrast, the antiapoptotic function of bcl-2 may require phosphorylation of serine 70, one of several residues targeted by the c-jun-N-terminal kinase (102,103). Furthermore, it has been suggested that bcl-2 can target Raf-1 to mitochondrial membranes and that the localization of Raf-1 on the outer mitochondrial membrane protects cells from undergoing programmed cell death, resulting in the phosphorylation of the proapoptotic protein, Bad (104). Growth factor activation of phosphatidylinositol 3'-kinase (PI3K)/Akt signaling pathway (see section PTEN) also results in phosphorylation of Bad, thereby promoting cell survival (105,106).

The expression of the bcl-2 family members bcl-x_L and mcl-1 has also been assessed in prostate cancer using immunohistochemistry (107). Bcl-x_L expression was observed in all cases examined, with increasing intensity in higher-grade lesions. Similarly, the antiapoptotic mcl-1 protein was detected in 80% of tumors, and increased intensity was associated with higher tumor grade.

It may be anticipated that the inactivation of p53 and expression of bcl-2 may each confer a growth advantage to prostate cancer cells, as well as resistance to therapeutic cell death induction. Studies have shown that overexpression of bcl-2 and p53 in prostatectomy specimens independently predicts an aggressive clinical course (108,109). In addition, bcl-2 can function in p53-dependent and -independent pathways to apoptosis (110,111). The observations of an inverse correlation between p53 and bcl-2 expression in advanced, androgen-independent tumors, and the lack of genetic complementation between these two genes in animal models of multistep carcinogenesis, suggest an effector and repressor role, respectively, in a common cell death pathway (112).

The Cyclin-Dependent Kinase Inhibitor: p27

p27kip1 (p27) is a member of the universal cyclin-dependent kinase inhibitor family and is a putative tumor suppressor gene (113–115). The *p27* gene regulates progression of the cell cycle from G_1 to S phase by binding to and inhibiting the cyclinE-cdk2 complex (116,117). In the normal adult prostate, *p27* mRNA is localized in basal acinar cells (118,119). In contrast, p27 protein is present primarily in the terminally differentiated secretory cells. However, the normal basal cell compartment also shows selective p27 protein expression. Cells lacking p27 and expressing basal cell–specific cytokeratin are present between the basal and luminal cells and appear to be increased in prostate tissue previously subjected to androgen blockade and in BPH. The lack of nuclear p27 may, therefore, delineate a potential transiently proliferating subcompartment (119). Because reduced expression of p27 removes a cell-cycle block in human prostate epithelial cells, dysregulation of p27 expression may be a critical early event in the development of prostatic neoplasia. In fact, prostatic intraepithelial neoplasia, both in humans and in rats (M. Loda and I. Leav, *unpublished data*, 2000), shows low to absent p27 levels, suggesting that it may derive from (and persist as) the p27 negative-proliferating compartment of basal cells. Several groups observed that primary prostate carcinomas with lower levels of p27 protein were more biologically aggressive (118,120–123). In addition, Cordon-Cardo et al. observed that p27 protein and mRNA were almost undetectable in epithelial and stromal cells of BPH, supporting the hypothesis that lack of p27 is associated with proliferation (118).

In prostate cancer, p27 expression progressively decreases with increased tumor grade and stage in the majority of studies published to date (120–122,124,124a). In terms of predictive value, low p27 correlates with seminal vesicle involvement and positive surgical margins, whereas in poorly differentiated tumors, low p27 seems to predict a low likelihood of organ-confined disease (125). In several published series, loss of expression of p27 by immunohistochemistry has been shown to be a powerful indicator of poor prognosis, independent of the traditional predictive parameters, such as preoperative PSA levels and Gleason score, particularly in organ-confined disease. The prognostic value of p27 is particularly important in organ-confined disease, which has up to 20% PSA recurrence rate at 5 years. In a multivariate analysis, we found that loss of p27 confers a fivefold relative risk of recurrence independent of Gleason grade and preoperative PSA in patients with T2a-3b disease (122).

p27 expression in the prostate may also be regulated by androgens. Using the castrated-regenerating Noble rat prostate model, we found that reintroduction of testosterone-induced p27 levels to precastration levels with a notable (if transient) initial decrease in p27 due to an increase in its degradation (125a). Chen et al. also showed that p21 and p27 levels in the ventral prostate of the castrated rat increased after androgen treatment but diminished transiently at the peak of prostate epithelial proliferation and returned to high levels when the proliferation ceased (126). The androgen-dependent human prostate tumor cell line LNCaP can adapt to an androgen-depleted environment and give rise to androgen-independent cells. Growth in these cells has been shown to be paradoxically repressed by androgens through a mechanism involving p27 induction and accumulation. Taken together, these studies suggest the attractive hypothesis that p27, when expressed, may shift androgen action from a proliferative to a differentiating one. It is possible that androgens regulate p27 through a mechanism involving the protooncogene *c-myc*, which is amplified or overexpressed in late stages of prostate cancer (127,128) (see section c-myc and Prostate Stem Cell Antigen). Previous studies have shown that *c-myc* overexpression can block p27-induced cell cycle arrest and *c-myc* expression is repressed by androgen in LNCaP androgen-independent sublines (129,130). In untreated patients, low p27 predicts treatment failure. In addition, in patients treated with hormonal therapy, a low p27 level is a strong predictor of poor outcome (121). We have observed an increase in p27 staining after neoadjuvant hormonal therapy and suggest the possibility (supported by our studies in rats) that a block in p27 degradation is induced by this treatment modality (125a). In summary, p27 is arguably the best independent predictor of biologic behavior of prostate cancer, particularly in organ-confined disease, and may predict response to hormonal ablation therapy (Fig. 20-1).

E-Cadherin

The long arm of chromosome 16 (16q22.1) is deleted in 30% of primary and more than 70% of metastatic prostate cancer by LOH analysis (131). This region contains the *E-cadherin* gene. E-cadherin is a Ca^{2+}-dependent cell surface glycoprotein found on epithelial cells that functions as a Ca^{2+}-dependent epithelial cell adhesion molecule. Its intracellular domain binds directly to β-*catenin* that, along with α-*catenin*, links *E-cadherin* to the underlying actin cytoskeleton (132). In addition to its role in adhesion, β-*catenin* has been implicated in Wnt signal transduction and links the adenomatous polyposis coli (APC) tumor suppressor protein with transcription factors of the LEF/TCF family (133–136). Vogelstein et al. have shown that in colon cancers, inactivation of the APC tumor suppressor gene results in increased β-catenin accumulation and subsequent increased transcription of the *c-myc* oncogene (137).

In many carcinomas, cadherins or catenins are lost or down-regulated, resulting in a reduced level of intercellular adhesion. Loss of E-cadherin function may endow tumor cells with a relative growth advantage over normal contact-inhibited cells. Experimentally, expression of the E-cadherin protein suppresses, whereas loss of expression enhances, the invasiveness and motility of epithelial cells. Using immunohistochemistry, Umbas et al. were able to show a correlation between decreased E-cadherin expression and metastatic progression and show that loss of E-cadherin staining is a powerful predictor of poor outcome and overall survival (Fig. 20-1) (131). *E-cadherin* has been shown to mediate inhibition of invasion and proliferation via the induction of p27 in three-dimensional culture (138). These findings link extracellular stimuli to the cell-cycle machinery and suggest a role for *E-cadherin* and *p27* as both invasion and growth suppressors (139).

PTEN

*P*hosphatase and *ten*sin homologue deleted on chromosome ten (PTEN)/*m*utated in *m*ultiple *a*dvanced *c*ancers (MMAC)/transforming growth factor beta–regulated and epithelial cell–enriched phosphatase (TEP1) is a candidate tumor suppressor gene located at 10q2.3 (140–142). Homozygous inactivation of PTEN/MMAC/TEP1 (hereafter, PTEN) occurs in a large number of high-grade glioblastomas (143–146), melanomas (147), advanced prostate cancer (148,149), and endometrial cancers (150). Interestingly, PTEN appears to suppress cell growth by distinct mechanisms in different types of tumors, producing G_1 cell cycle arrest in glioblastoma cells but inducing apoptosis in carcinomas.

PTEN is able to dephosphorylate tyrosine and threonine residues and, in addition, can dephosphorylate a subset of inositol phospholipids, namely PI-3,4,5-trisphosphate (PI-3,4,5-P_3).

Tamura et al. reported that PTEN associated with and could dephosphorylate a phosphoprotein, focal adhesion kinase (FAK), suggesting a role for PTEN in regulation of focal adhesion structure, cell spreading, and mobility (151). However, extremely high (stoichiometric rather than catalytic) amounts of PTEN were required to dephosphorylate FAK. It is known that the biologically more relevant targets of PTEN are now phospholipids, namely PI-3,4,5-P_3 (152). The finding that PTEN dephosphorylates PI phosphates has led to a model of how PTEN acts as a tumor suppressor gene, a model linking PTEN to control of at least two known cellular protooncogenes, PI3K and Akt (153,154). PTEN inhibits PI3K-dependent activation of Akt (also called *protein kinase B*), a serine-threonine kinase. Deletion or inactivation of PTEN results in constitutive Akt activation. Activation of PI3K and Akt has been shown to provide a survival signal in response to nerve growth factor, insulinlike growth factor 1, platelet-derived growth factor, interleukin 3, and the extracellular matrix (155,156). Akt is likely to send survival signals by phosphorylating multiple targets, including the bcl-2 family member Bad and the cell death pathway enzyme caspase-9 (105,157).

In addition, PTEN-deficient cell lines show an accelerated entry into S phase, and this is accompanied by downregulation of p27 (158). These studies suggest that PTEN modulates two critical cellular processes, namely cell survival and cell-cycle progression. Furthermore, Gu et al. have also defined a role for PTEN in cellular signaling via the mitogen-activated protein kinase (MAPK) signaling pathways (159). They showed that PTEN dephosphorylates Shc and FAK, which is subsequently followed by inhibition of Ras activation, followed by further downstream effects targeting the extracellular signal-regulated kinases (Erk) pathway of MAPK signaling (see also section Mitogen-Activated Protein Kinase Phosphatase 1).

LOH at the PTEN locus has been observed in 29% to 42% of prostate tumors, and screening for homozygous deletions has identified a second mutational event in 43% of prostate tumors (148,160). LOH at 10q was found in 11 of 60 tumors (18%) that were localized to the prostate, but also in 12 of 20 pelvic metastases (60%). This observation suggested that PTEN may be an important tumor suppressor in a subset of prostate cancers and that inactivation of PTEN may be an important secondary genetic event that contributes to prostate cancer progression. We have found that 20% of primary prostate tumors lack detectable PTEN protein as assessed by IHC staining (161). In this series, PTEN loss was highly correlated with Gleason grade and advanced stage (Fig. 20-2). We and others have shown that cell lines and tumors in which PTEN is lost have elevated levels of Akt. Thus, loss of IHC detection of PTEN might predict for the presence of activated Akt and, in turn, might become useful as a factor predictive of success for therapies directed against this pathway. In general, the use of this type of predictive factor, such as the estrogen receptor in breast carcinoma, which can predict for the efficacy of a given therapy such as tamoxifen, has great clinical use as they directly impact treatment decisions.

Androgen Receptor and Her2/neu

Androgens are required for the development of the normal prostate and prostate cancer (162,163). Androgens act through the androgen receptor (AR), which belongs to the steroid receptor superfamily of ligand-dependent transcription factors (164,165). The AR has a central role in mediating the biologic effects of androgens to different downstream genes. After binding to the androgen, AR is phosphorylated, dimerized, and translocated to the cell nucleus, in which it binds to androgen-responsive elements (AREs) at the promoter region of target genes (166,167). New evidence suggests that AR can regulate genes that have and do not have AREs (168). Several candidate genes, which are androgen regulated, include cell cycle genes such as cyclins *A, D1-D3, E, cyclin-dependent kinases* (169–171); early response genes, such as *fos* and *jun* (172–174); signal transduction genes, such as *Ha-Ras* (175), *p21* (176–178), and *p27* (126); and peptide growth factors and their receptors (179–181).

The only effective treatment for metastatic prostate cancer is hormonal or androgen-ablative therapy (182). Although

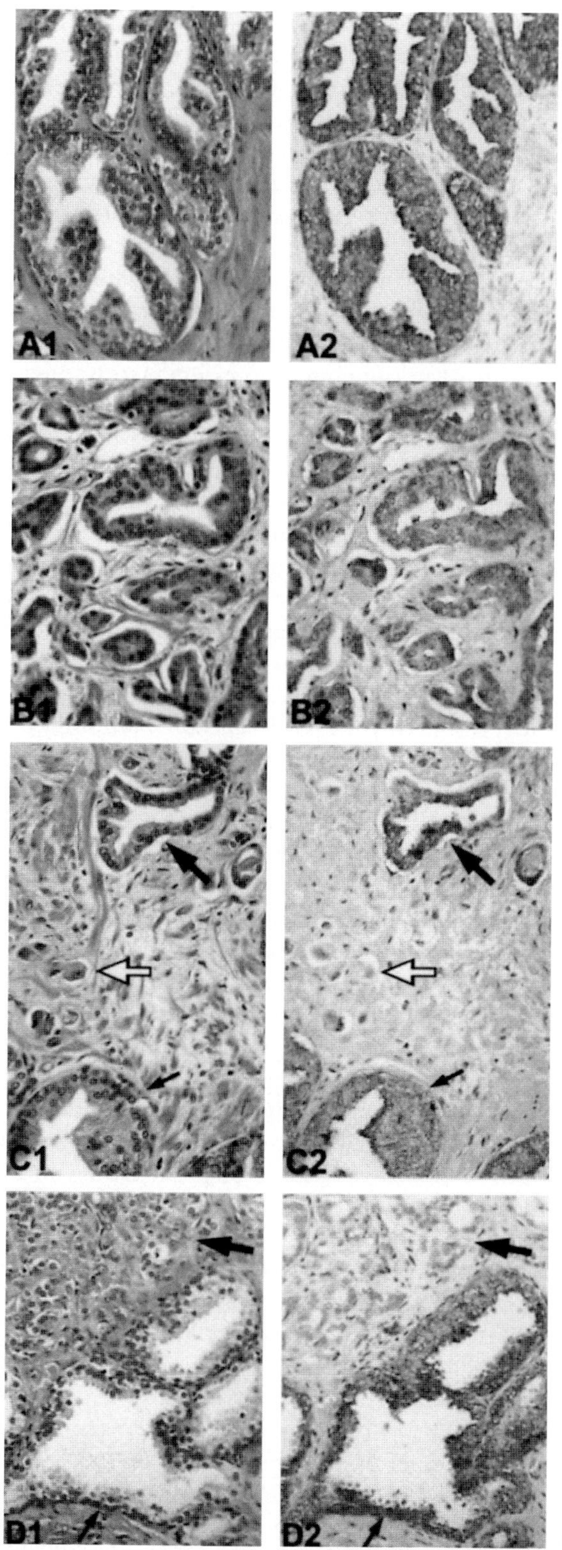

FIGURE 20-2. Gleason grades 3 and 5 prostate adenocarcinoma. **A:** Hematoxylin and eosin–stained section, the small arrow indicates a Gleason grade 3 tumor, and the large arrow indicates a Gleason grade 5 tumor. **B:** Positive staining for PTEN in Gleason grade 3 tumor (*small arrow*) and absence of staining for PTEN in Gleason grade 5 tumor (*large arrow*). (From McMenamin ME, Soung P, Perera S, et al. Loss of PTEN expression in paraffin-embedded primary prostate cancer correlates with high Gleason score and advanced stage. *Cancer Res* 1999;59:4291–4296.) (See also color Figure 20-2.)

an initial response to hormonal therapy is observed in 70% to 80% of patients with advanced disease, the duration of response is finite, lasting only 12 to 18 months (183,184).

Proposed mechanisms of progression to androgen-independent growth include loss of AR expression (185,186); amplification of the AR gene (187); mutations of the AR gene, including shortened numbers of CAG nucleotide repeat sequences; and recruitment of coactivators, such as ARA70 (188–190). In addition, Craft et al. have recently shown that the tyrosine kinase receptor *Her2/neu* can modulate responses in the setting of low androgen levels by restoring AR function, resulting in ligand-independent growth and, thus, clinical progression of the cancer (191). In addition, Yeh et al. have shown that *Her2/neu* can increase growth rate, PSA level, and AR transactivation in prostate cancer cells via the MAPK pathway (192).

IHC studies have demonstrated expression of AR in primary, advanced, and hormone-refractory prostate cancers, suggesting that disease progression is not necessarily associated with loss of AR expression (163). We and others report that there is also considerable heterogeneity of AR expression in specimens and among patients (193–198). Using computer-assisted image analysis, we have previously shown that the heterogeneity of AR expression increased with increasing Gleason grade (193). However, this method may not be practical for routine use. We have recently shown that Her2/neu protein expression increases progressively from untreated patients to those subjected preoperatively to androgen ablation to maximal levels in androgen-independent tumors (198a). These studies in human tumors strongly support the contention that Her2/neu overexpression can superactivate the existing AR pathway and substitute for it to confer androgen-independent tumor cell growth.

Mitogen-Activated Protein Kinase Phosphatase 1

In eukaryotic cells, activation of growth factor receptors activates the MAPK cascade, which is extensively used for transcytoplasmic signaling to the nucleus (199). After ligand growth factor receptor interaction, a number of molecules, including Ras and Raf, are recruited to the plasma membrane, in which they become sequentially activated (200–204). Ultimately, a family of enzymes, collectively known as *MAPKs*, are activated and transduce diverse cellular responses, such as cell growth, differentiation, and apoptosis (199). Recently, three structurally related MAPK subfamilies were identified: the Erks, the c-jun N-terminal kinases (JNKs)/stress-activated protein kinases (SAPKs), and the p38/reactivating kinase (RK) (205–208). JNK/SAPKs and p38/RK mediate signals in response to environmental stress, and cytokines transmit the effect of cellular insults or injury to the nucleus, mediating apoptosis (209–211). MAPK signaling is turned off in several cell systems by the action of a dual specific phosphatase MAPK phosphatase 1 (MKP-1) that hydrolyzes the phosphates on threonine and tyrosine residues (211–214).

In human prostate cancer, it has been shown that MKP-1 can differentially regulate the interaction or cross-talk between MAPK pathways and might be a key control point of their relative activities (215). Therefore, the balance between growth factor–activated Erk and stress-activated JNK/SAPK-p38/RK pathways selectively inhibited by MKP-1 may be essential in determining whether a prostate cancer cell survives or undergoes apoptosis. We have previously shown that MKP-1 is overexpressed in the early phases of prostate cancer, with progressive loss of expression with higher histologic grade and in advanced disease stage (216,217). In addition, MKP-1 expression was inversely correlated to JNK-1 but not to Erk-1 enzymatic activity (215). In the same series, we also showed that MKP-1 and bcl-2 were inversely related to apoptotic indices. This inverse correlation between MKP-1 and parameters of programmed cell death support the hypothesis that MKP-1 inhibits apoptosis in human prostate tumors via inhibition of stress-activated kinases. To support this hypothesis, current data from our laboratory also indicate that MKP-1 is able to block apoptosis induced by testosterone withdrawal in LNCaP cells via selective inhibition of the JNK/p38 pathways (G. Cangi, C. Magi-Galluzzi, and M. Loda, *unpublished data*, 2001). Assessment of MKP-1 and bcl-2 expression may, thus, be important in predicting response to therapy, particularly to hormonal ablation.

C-myc and Prostate Stem Cell Antigen

One of the most specific genetic changes detected by means of comparative genomic hybridization in hormone-refractory prostate cancer is the gain of 8q and especially the 8q-qter region (218–220). One possible target at the 8q24 region is the *myc* gene.

The *c-myc* gene is an immediate, early-response gene that is activated by mitogenic stimuli, resulting in proliferation (221). Recent studies have shown that *c-myc* activities are modulated by a network of nuclear basic region/helix-loop-helix/leucine zipper proteins (222). The Max protein is at the center of this network, in that it forms heterodimers with myc that result in transcriptional activation. Max also forms heterodimers with the Mad family of proteins, of which Mxi-1 is a member (223). Mad-Max complexes result in repression of transcription. Mad proteins, therefore, act as an antagonist of myc (224). Of note, Mxi-1 knockout mice demonstrate a cancer-prone phenotype with hyperplastic changes seen in the prostate (225).

Fluorescent *in situ* hybridization analysis has identified high-level amplification of *c-myc* in more than 20% of recurrent and metastatic prostate cancers (127,128). Amplification of c-myc correlates with high levels of c-myc protein expression (127). Furthermore, inhibition of c-myc expression by retrovirus encoding antisense c-myc can mediate tumor regression in a prostate cancer xenograft (226). *C-myc* can also cooperate with *Ras* to induce prostate cancer in various rat and murine model systems. Evaluation of case-matched prostate cancer biopsies from patients undergoing androgen ablation suggests that levels of c-myc expression increase after castration (227). Bubendorf et al., using fluorescent *in situ* hybridization analysis on tissue microarrays, showed high-level c-myc amplification in 11% of metastases from patients with hormone-refractory disease, suggesting a role for c-myc in metastatic progression (228). However, there may be other, currently unknown target genes at the distal 8q locus whose increased copy number is selected during cancer progression. One such candidate gene is the newly described prostate stem cell antigen (PSCA).

PSCA is a glycosyl PI (GPI)–anchored cell surface protein with predominant expression in the prostate (229). It shares a 30% nucleotide homology with stem cell antigen 2, a member of the Thy-1/Ly-6 superfamily of GPI-anchored cell surface antigens. The Ly-6 gene family is involved in signal transduction and cell-cell adhesion (230). Signaling through stem cell antigen 2 has been shown to prevent apoptosis in immature thymocytes (231). Thy-1 is involved in T-cell activation and transmits signals through srclike tyrosine kinases (232). Ly-6 genes have been implicated in tumorigenesis and homotypic cell adhesion (233–235). Although the biologic function of PSCA is not known at present, we hypothesize that it may play a role in stem cell or progenitor cell functions, such as self renewal (antiapoptosis) or proliferation, or both. PSCA maps distal to c-myc at the 8q24.2 locus. PSCA mRNA is expressed strongly in 80% of primary prostate cancers and is overexpressed in two prostate cancer xenografts (229). We have recently characterized PSCA protein expression using a panel of PSCA-specific monoclonal antibodies. These antibodies recognize PSCA on the cell surface of normal and malignant prostate cells. PSCA protein was overexpressed in cancer compared to normal in 36% of primary tumors and in 100% of bone metastases studied, suggesting that increased PSCA protein expression may correlate with prostate cancer progression and metastases to bone (235a). In addition, we have shown that PSCA is coamplified with *c-myc* (Fig. 20-3) and that PSCA amplification correlates with overexpression (236). As it localizes to the surface of prostate cancer cells and because of its almost exclusive expression in prostate, PSCA may also represent an important therapeutic target.

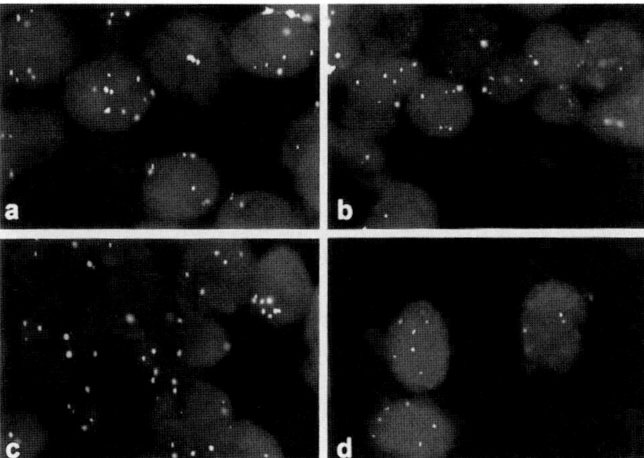

FIGURE 20-3. Fluorescent *in situ* hybridization analysis looking at *c-myc* and prostate stem cell antigen (PSCA) copy number in two patients with locally advanced prostate cancer. In **(A)** and **(C)**, for case No. 34 there is simple gain of chromosome 8 without any additional increase in *c-myc* or PSCA copy number. **A:** Most nuclei have three signals for both *c-myc* (red) and a probe for the centromere (green). A similar result is seen in **(C)**, with three signals for PSCA (red) and CEP-8 (green). In **(B)** and **(D)**, for case No. 75, there is additional increase in PSCA and *c-myc* copy number compared with the centromere, indicative of amplification of these two loci. **B:** There are, on average, five red signals (*c-myc*) and two green signals (CEP-8). Similarly, **(D)** there are five red signals (PSCA) and two green signals (CEP-8), again consistent with an additional increase of PSCA copy number. (See also color Figure 20-3.)

Thymosin β15

A well-characterized series of cell lines that show varying metastatic potential have been developed from the Dunning rat prostate carcinoma model (237). Thymosin β15 was cloned by differential mRNA display as a result of its overexpression in the highly motile and metastatic Dunning cancer cell line (238). Thymosin β15 binds monomeric actin and retards actin polymerization. Our studies revealed that thymosin β15 directly regulates cell motility in prostate cancer cell lines (239).

In situ hybridization for thymosin β15 in prostate carcinoma revealed the most extensive and intense staining in high-grade (Gleason scores 8 to 10) cancers, followed by moderately differentiated prostate cancers with Gleason scores of 6 to 7 (238). In addition, strong staining was seen in both lymph node and bone metastases. In contrast, all cases of BPH cases examined were negative. Thymosin β15 thus represents a powerful predictor of subsequent development of metastases when expressed in localized prostate cancer (Fig. 20-1).

Maspin

The novel tumor suppressor gene *maspin* was originally isolated from normal mammary epithelium by subtractive hybridization and differential display techniques and was shown to have tumor-suppressive activity, including inhibition of breast cancer tumor cell motility, invasion, and

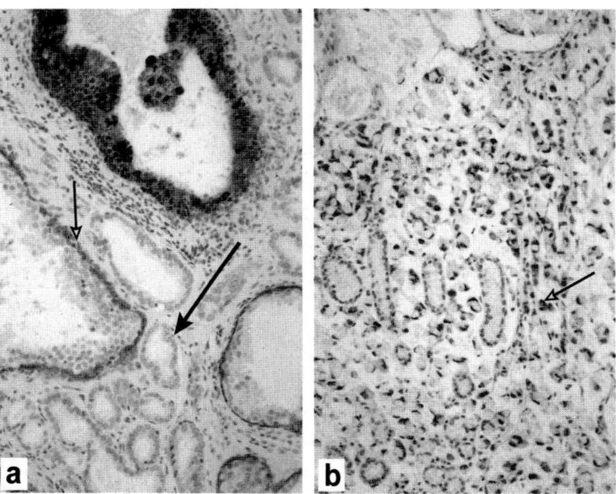

FIGURE 20-4. A: Positive staining for maspin localized to the basal cells and prostate intraepithelial neoplasia (*small arrow*) and absence of staining in Gleason grade 3 tumor (*large arrow*). **B:** Positive staining for maspin in androgen-independent tumor (*small arrow*). (See also color Figure 20-4.)

metastases (240–244). *Maspin* is located at chromosome 18q21.4 and contains sequence homology with several members of the serine protease inhibitor superfamily (serpins), including plasminogen activator inhibitor-1, -2, α-1 antitrypsin, as well as the noninhibitor serpin proteins, such as ovalbumin (245,246). The expression of maspin in prostate cell lines has been shown to be negatively regulated at the transcriptional level by a hormone-responsive site recognized by the AR. We investigated 207 prostate cancers by immunohistochemistry using a monoclonal maspin antibody.

Our results show that maspin is predominantly but not exclusively localized in basal cells of the prostate glands (Fig. 20-4). Although frequent loss of 18q has been demonstrated in prostate cancer (247–250), we found *maspin* expression in poorly differentiated tumors and in nonorgan-confined tumors (E. Macri and M. Loda, *unpublished data*, 2000). In addition, we found maspin expression in androgen-independent tumors, compared to androgen-dependent tumors, suggesting that *maspin* could be used as a predictor of cancer progression or androgen independence, or both.

CONCLUSION

Prostate cancer exhibits a wide range of biologic behavior. Preoperative serum PSA, Gleason tumor grade, and stage are the most widely used variables at present in predicting prognosis, relapse, and metastatic potential. As a result of screening, patients increasingly present with organ-confined disease. However, a significant percentage of these patients recur after prostatectomy. The goal of molecular staging of prostate cancer is to identify genes involved in pathways relevant to prostate cancer pathogenesis and to use them as prognostic or predictive markers, or both, in serum and tissue-based assays. In this chapter, we have discussed a variety of candidate markers that have been found to be relevant in the various stages of prostate cancer progression. Another emerging technology gaining widespread use is the complementary DNA (cDNA) arrays and oligonucleotide chips. cDNA microarrays consist of thousands of different cDNA clones spotted onto known locations on glass microscope slides, and these slides are then hybridized with differentially labeled cDNA populations made from the mRNAs of two different samples (251,252). The primary data obtained are the ratios of fluorescence intensity (red or green), representing the ratio of concentrations of mRNA molecules that hybridized to each of the cDNAs represented on the array. The oligonucleotide technology involves the hybridization of fluorescently labeled RNAs to oligonucleotides of known sequence that are photolithographically synthesized on a solid surface (253,254). Thousands of genes can be identified by these large-scale expression assays. To then confirm the prognostically meaningful genes that are involved in cancer progression, we need to examine large databases of tumor samples with clinical follow-up. This is best done by using the newly developed tissue microarray-based technology for high-throughput molecular analyses of tumor samples (255). This technique is based on arraying cylindric biopsy specimens from hundreds of different tumors into a single paraffin block. Consecutive sections of this tissue microarray block can then be used for analysis of multiple molecular alterations—for example, by *in situ* hybridization and immunohistochemistry. Both technologies complement each other and will undoubtedly be invaluable in identifying molecular signatures of tumors that may predict biologic behavior independent of or as an adjunct to morphologic classifications.

The challenge ahead is to conclusively determine the role some of these genes play as prognostic or predictive markers, or both, using large, retrospective, possibly multi-institutional databases with long-term follow-up. A difficult problem that needs to be overcome is the use of such markers as prognosticators in needle biopsies before any therapy. Unfortunately, the extreme heterogeneity of prostate cancer, in terms of cell by cell expression for a given marker, currently precludes their use as predictors in the initial assessment by needle biopsy. Potential therapeutic targets are also beginning to emerge. This will result in novel and more specific therapeutic modalities for a disease in which the mainstay of treatment, androgen ablation, is only temporarily effective.

SUPPORTING GRANTS AND ACKNOWLEDGMENTS

This work was supported by a CaPCURE award, National Cancer Institute Grant 5RO1CA-81755-03 and Department of Defense Grant PC 970273 to Massimo Loda.

We would like to thank Robert Reiter and Charles Sawyers for reviewing the chapter, Mairin McMenamin and John Hunt for organizational support, and Jane Hayward and Pam Godschal for photographic assistance.

REFERENCES

1. Bostwick DG, Foster CS. Examination of radical prostatectomy specimens: therapeutic and prognostic significance. In: Foster CS, Bostwick DG, eds. *Pathology of the prostate.* Philadelphia: WB Saunders, 1998:172–189.
2. Catalona WJ, Smith DS, Ratliff TL, et al. Measurement of prostate-specific antigen in serum as a screening test for prostate cancer. *N Engl J Med* 1991;324:1156–1161.
3. Catalona WJ, Smith DS. 5-year tumor recurrence rates after anatomical radical retropubic prostatectomy for prostate cancer. *J Urol* 1994;152:1837–1842.
4. Lu-Yao GL, Potosky AL, Albertsen PC, et al. Follow-up prostate cancer treatments after radical prostatectomy: a population-based study. *J Natl Cancer Inst* 1996;88:166–173.
5. Partin AW, Yoo J, Carter HB, et al. The use of prostate specific antigen, clinical stage and Gleason score to predict pathological stage in men with localized prostate cancer. *J Urol* 1993;150:110–114.
6. Partin AW, Pound CR, Clemens JQ, et al. Serum PSA after anatomic radical prostatectomy. The Johns Hopkins experience after 10 years. *Urol Clin North Am* 1993;20:713–725.
7. Pound CR, Partin AW, Epstein JI, et al. Prostate-specific antigen after anatomic radical retropubic prostatectomy. Patterns of recurrence and cancer control. *Urol Clin North Am* 1997;24:395–406.
8. Albertsen PC, Hanley JA, Gleason DF, et al. Competing risk analysis of men aged 55 to 74 years at diagnosis managed conservatively for clinically localized prostate cancer. *JAMA* 1998;280:975–980.
9. D'Amico AV, Desjardin A, Chung A, et al. Assessment of outcome prediction models for localized prostate cancer in patients managed with external beam radiation therapy. *Semin Urol Oncol* 1998;16:153–159.
10. Lerner SE, Blute ML, Bergstralh EJ, et al. Analysis of risk factors for progression in patients with pathologically confined prostate cancers after radical retropubic prostatectomy. *J Urol* 1996;156:137–143.
11. Rubnitz JE, Look AT. Molecular genetics of childhood leukemias. *J Pediatr Hematol Oncol* 1998;20:1–11.
12. Rubnitz JE, Pui CH. Molecular diagnostics in the treatment of leukemia. *Curr Opin Hematol* 1999;6:229–235.
13. Lu YJ, Birdsall S, Summersgill B, et al. Dual colour fluorescence in situ hybridization to paraffin-embedded samples to deduce the presence of the der(x)t(x;18)(p11.2;q11.2) and involvement of either the SSX1 or SSX2 gene: a diagnostic and prognostic aid for synovial sarcoma. *J Pathol* 1999; 187:490–496.
14. Nilsson G, Skytting B, Xie Y, et al. The SYT-SSX1 variant of synovial sarcoma is associated with a high rate of tumor cell proliferation and poor clinical outcome. *Cancer Res* 1999;59:3180–3184.

15. Fearon ER, Vogelstein B. A genetic model for colorectal tumorigenesis. *Cell* 1990;61:759–767.
16. Schellhammer PF, Wright GL Jr. Biomolecular and clinical characteristics of PSA and other candidate prostate tumor markers. *Urol Clin North Am* 1993;20:597–606.
17. Wang MC, Valenzuela LA, Murphy GP, et al. Purification of a human prostate specific antigen. *Invest Urol* 1979; 17:159–163.
18. Riegman PH, Vlietstra RJ, Klaassen P, et al. The prostate-specific antigen gene and the human glandular kallikrein-1 gene are tandemly located on chromosome 19. *FEBS Lett* 1989;247:123–126.
19. Epstein JI. PSA and PAP as immunohistochemical markers in prostate cancer. *Urol Clin North Am* 1993;20:757–770.
20. van Krieken JH. Prostate marker immunoreactivity in salivary gland neoplasms. A rare pitfall in immunohistochemistry. *Am J Surg Pathol* 1993;17:410–414.
21. Monne M, Croce CM, Yu H, et al. Molecular characterization of prostate-specific antigen messenger RNA expressed in breast tumors. *Cancer Res* 1994;54:6344–6347.
22. Neal DE Jr., Clejan S, Sarma D, et al. Prostate specific antigen and prostatitis. I. Effect of prostatitis on serum PSA in the human and nonhuman primate. *Prostate* 1992;20:105–111.
23. Oesterling JE. Prostate specific antigen: a critical assessment of the most useful tumor marker for adenocarcinoma of the prostate. *J Urol* 1991;145:907–923.
24. Partin AW, Carter HB, Chan DW, et al. Prostate specific antigen in the staging of localized prostate cancer: influence of tumor differentiation, tumor volume and benign hyperplasia. *J Urol* 1990;143:747–752.
25. Chybowski FM, Bergstralh EJ, Oesterling JE. The effect of digital rectal examination on the serum prostate specific antigen concentration: results of a randomized study. *J Urol* 1992;148:83–86.
26. Babaian RJ, Fritsche HA, Evans RB. Prostate-specific antigen and prostate gland volume: correlation and clinical application. *J Clin Lab Anal* 1990;4:135–137.
27. Aihara M, Lebovitz RM, Wheeler TM, et al. Prostate specific antigen and Gleason grade: an immunohistochemical study of prostate cancer. *J Urol* 1994;151:1558–1564.
28. Blackwell KL, Bostwick DG, Myers RP, et al. Combining prostate specific antigen with cancer and gland volume to predict more reliably pathological stage: the influence of prostate specific antigen cancer density. *J Urol* 1994;151: 1565–1570.
29. Frazier HA, Robertson JE, Humphrey PA, et al. Is prostate specific antigen of clinical importance in evaluating outcome after radical prostatectomy. *J Urol* 1993;149:516–518.
30. Hudson MA, Bahnson RR, Catalona WJ. Clinical use of prostate specific antigen in patients with prostate cancer. *J Urol* 1989;142:1011–1017.
31. Kleer E, Oesterling JE. PSA and staging of localized prostate cancer. *Urol Clin North Am* 1993;20:695–704.
32. Kleer E, Larson-Keller JJ, Zincke H, et al. Ability of preoperative serum prostate-specific antigen value to predict pathologic stage and DNA ploidy. Influence of clinical stage and tumor grade. *Urology* 1993;41:207–216.
33. Partin AW, Oesterling JE. The clinical usefulness of prostate specific antigen: update 1994. *J Urol* 1994;152:1358–1368.
34. Epstein JI, Eggleston JC. Immunohistochemical localization of prostate-specific acid phosphatase and prostate-specific antigen in stage A2 adenocarcinoma of the prostate: prognostic implications. *Hum Pathol* 1984;15:853–859.
35. Fey MF, Kulozik AE, Hansen-Hagge TE, et al. The polymerase chain reaction: a new tool for the detection of minimal residual disease in haematological malignancies. *Eur J Cancer* 1991;27:89–94.
36. Katz AE, Olsson CA, Raffo AJ, et al. Molecular staging of prostate cancer with the use of an enhanced reverse transcriptase-PCR assay. *Urology* 1994;43:765–775.
37. Seiden MV, Kantoff PW, Krithivas K, et al. Detection of circulating tumor cells in men with localized prostate cancer. *J Clin Oncol* 1994;12:2634–2639.
38. Olsson CA, de Vries GM, Raffo AJ, et al. Preoperative reverse transcriptase polymerase chain reaction for prostate specific antigen predicts treatment failure following radical prostatectomy. *J Urol* 1996;155:1557–1562.
39. Ghossein RA, Scher HI, Gerald WL, et al. Detection of circulating tumor cells in patients with localized and metastatic prostatic carcinoma: clinical implications. *J Clin Oncol* 1995;13:1195–1200.
40. Jaakkola S, Vornanen T, Leinonen J, et al. Detection of prostatic cells in peripheral blood: correlation with serum concentrations of prostate-specific antigen. *Clin Chem* 1995;41:182–186.
41. Sokoloff MH, Tso CL, Kaboo R, et al. Quantitative polymerase chain reaction does not improve preoperative prostate cancer staging: a clinicopathological molecular analysis of 121 patients. *J Urol* 1996;156:1560–1566.
42. Ignatoff JM, Oefelein MG, Watkin W, et al. Prostate specific antigen reverse transcriptase-polymerase chain reaction assay in preoperative staging of prostate cancer. *J Urol* 1997;158:1870–1874.
43. Horoszewicz JS, Kawinski E, Murphy GP. Monoclonal antibodies to a new antigenic marker in epithelial prostatic cells and serum of prostatic cancer patients. *Anticancer Res* 1987;7:927–935.
44. Gregorakis AK, Holmes EH, Murphy GP. Prostate-specific membrane antigen: current and future utility. *Semin Urol Oncol* 1998;16:2–12.
45. Murphy GP, Barren RJ, Erickson SJ, et al. Evaluation and comparison of two new prostate carcinoma markers. Free-prostate specific antigen and prostate specific membrane antigen. *Cancer* 1996;78:809–818.
46. Israeli RS, Grob M, Fair WR. Prostate-specific membrane antigen and other prostatic tumor markers on the horizon. *Urol Clin North Am* 1997;24:439–450.
47. Troyer JK, Beckett ML, Wright GL Jr. Location of prostate-specific membrane antigen in the LNCaP prostate carcinoma cell line. *Prostate* 1997;30:232–242.
48. Chang SS, Reuter VE, Heston WD, et al. Five different anti-prostate-specific membrane antigen (PSMA) antibodies confirm PSMA expression in tumor-associated neovasculature. *Cancer Res* 1999;59:3192–3198.
49. Okegawa T, Yoshioka J, Morita R, et al. Molecular staging of prostate cancer: comparison of nested reverse transcription polymerase chain reaction assay using prostate specific antigen versus prostate specific membrane antigen as primer. *Int J Urol* 1998;5:349–356.

50. Cama C, Olsson CA, Raffo AJ, et al. Molecular staging of prostate cancer. II. A comparison of the application of an enhanced reverse transcriptase polymerase chain reaction assay for prostate specific antigen versus prostate specific membrane antigen. *J Urol* 1995;153:1373–1378.
51. Grasso YZ, Gupta MK, Levin HS, et al. Combined nested RT-PCR assay for prostate-specific antigen and prostate-specific membrane antigen in prostate cancer patients: correlation with pathological stage. *Cancer Res* 1998;58:1456–1459.
52. Lowe FC, Trauzzi SJ. Prostatic acid phosphatase in 1993. Its limited clinical utility. *Urol Clin North Am* 1993;20:589–595.
53. Allsbrook WC Jr., Simms WW. Histochemistry of the prostate. *Hum Pathol* 1992;23:297–305.
54. Arrowsmith CH, Morin P. New insights into p53 function from structural studies. *Oncogene* 1996;12:1379–1385.
55. Kastan MB, Onyekwere O, Sidransky D, et al. Participation of p53 protein in the cellular response to DNA damage. *Cancer Res* 1991;51:6304–6311.
56. Soussi T, May P. Structural aspects of the p53 protein in relation to gene evolution: a second look. *J Mol Biol* 1996; 260:623–637.
57. Levine AJ, Momand J, Finlay CA. The p53 tumour suppressor gene. *Nature* 1991;351:453–456.
58. Vogelstein B, Kinzler KW. p53 function and dysfunction. *Cell* 1992;70:523–526.
59. Gartel AL, Serfas MS, Tyner AL. p21—negative regulator of the cell cycle. *Proc Soc Exp Biol Med* 1996;213:138–149.
60. Brewster SF, Browne S, Brown KW. Somatic allelic loss at the DCC, APC, nm23-H1 and p53 tumor suppressor gene loci in human prostatic carcinoma. *J Urol* 1994;151:1073–1077.
61. Cunningham JM, Shan A, Wick MJ, et al. Allelic imbalance and microsatellite instability in prostatic adenocarcinoma. *Cancer Res* 1996;56:4475–4482.
62. Ittmann MM. Loss of heterozygosity on chromosomes 10 and 17 in clinically localized prostate carcinoma. *Prostate* 1996;28:275–281.
63. Uchida T, Wada C, Wang C, et al. Microsatellite instability in prostate cancer. *Oncogene* 1995;10:1019–1022.
64. McDonnell TJ, Navone NM, Troncoso P, et al. Expression of bcl-2 oncoprotein and p53 protein accumulation in bone marrow metastases of androgen independent prostate cancer. *J Urol* 1997;157:569–574.
65. Navone NM, Troncoso P, Pisters LL, et al. p53 protein accumulation and gene mutation in the progression of human prostate carcinoma. *J Natl Cancer Inst* 1993;85: 1657–1669.
66. Bookstein R, MacGrogan D, Hilsenbeck SG, et al. p53 is mutated in a subset of advanced-stage prostate cancers. *Cancer Res* 1993;53:3369–3373.
67. Harris CC, Hollstein M. Clinical implications of the p53 tumor-suppressor gene. *N Engl J Med* 1993;329:1318–1327.
68. Heidenberg HB, Sesterhenn IA, Gaddipati JP, et al. Alteration of the tumor suppressor gene p53 in a high fraction of hormone refractory prostate cancer. *J Urol* 1995;154:414–421.
69. Yang G, Stapleton AM, Wheeler TM, et al. Clustered p53 immunostaining: a novel pattern associated with prostate cancer progression. *Clin Cancer Res* 1996;2:399–401.
70. Bauer JJ, Sesterhenn IA, Mostofi KF, et al. p53 nuclear protein expression is an independent prognostic marker in clinically localized prostate cancer patients undergoing radical prostatectomy. *Clin Cancer Res* 1995;1:1295–1300.
71. Berner A, Nesland JM, Waehre H, et al. Hormone resistant prostatic adenocarcinoma. An evaluation of prognostic factors in pre- and post-treatment specimens. *Br J Cancer* 1993;68:380–384.
72. Effert PJ, Neubauer A, Walther PJ, et al. Alterations of the P53 gene are associated with the progression of a human prostate carcinoma. *J Urol* 1992;147:789–793.
73. Myers RB, Oelschlager D, Srivastava S, et al. Accumulation of the p53 protein occurs more frequently in metastatic than in localized prostatic adenocarcinomas. *Prostate* 1994; 25:243–248.
74. Navone NM, Labate ME, Troncoso P, et al. p53 mutations in prostate cancer bone metastases suggest that selected p53 mutants in the primary site define foci with metastatic potential. *J Urol* 1999;161:304–308.
75. Shurbaji MS, Kalbfleisch JH, Thurmond TS. Immunohistochemical detection of p53 protein as a prognostic indicator in prostate cancer. *Hum Pathol* 1995;26:106–109.
76. Stricker HJ, Jay JK, Linden MD, et al. Determining prognosis of clinically localized prostate cancer by immunohistochemical detection of mutant p53. *Urology* 1996;47:366–369.
77. Thomas DJ, Robinson M, King P, et al. p53 expression and clinical outcome in prostate cancer. *Br J Urol* 1993;72:778–781.
78. Bunz F, Dutriaux A, Lengauer C, et al. Requirement for p53 and p21 to sustain G2 arrest after DNA damage. *Science* 1998;282:1497–1501.
79. Hockenbery D, Nunez G, Milliman C, et al. Bcl-2 is an inner mitochondrial membrane protein that blocks programmed cell death. *Nature* 1990;348:334–336.
80. Vaux DL, Cory S, Adams JM. Bcl-2 gene promotes haemopoietic cell survival and cooperates with c-myc to immortalize pre-B cells. *Nature* 1988;335:440–442.
81. Bruckheimer EM, Cho SH, Sarkiss M, et al. The Bcl-2 gene family and apoptosis. *Adv Biochem Eng Biotechnol* 1998;62: 75–105.
82. Hanada M, Aime-Sempe C, Sato T, et al. Structure-function analysis of Bcl-2 protein. Identification of conserved domains important for homodimerization with Bcl-2 and heterodimerization with Bax. *J Biol Chem* 1995;270: 11962–11969.
83. Sedlak TW, Oltvai ZN, Yang E, et al. Multiple Bcl-2 family members demonstrate selective dimerizations with Bax. *Proc Natl Acad Sci U S A* 1995;92:7834–7838.
84. Yang E, Zha J, Jockel J, et al. Bad, a heterodimeric partner for Bcl-XL and Bcl-2, displaces Bax and promotes cell death. *Cell* 1995;80:285–291.
85. Yin XM, Oltvai ZN, Korsmeyer SJ. BH1 and BH2 domains of Bcl-2 are required for inhibition of apoptosis and heterodimerization with Bax. *Nature* 1994;369:321–323.
86. Knudson CM, Korsmeyer SJ. Bcl-2 and Bax function independently to regulate cell death. *Nat Genet* 1997;16:358–363.
87. Bronner MP, Culin C, Reed JC, et al. The bcl-2 proto-oncogene and the gastrointestinal epithelial tumor progression model. *Am J Pathol* 1995;146:20–26.
88. Chandler D, el-Naggar AK, Brisbay S, et al. Apoptosis and expression of the bcl-2 proto-oncogene in the fetal and adult human kidney: evidence for the contribution of bcl-2

expression to renal carcinogenesis. *Hum Pathol* 1994;25:789–796.
89. Cleary ML, Sklar J. Nucleotide sequence of a t(14;18) chromosomal breakpoint in follicular lymphoma and demonstration of a breakpoint-cluster region near a transcriptionally active locus on chromosome 18. *Proc Natl Acad Sci U S A* 1985;82:7439–7443.
90. Moul JW, Bettencourt MC, Sesterhenn IA, et al. Protein expression of p53, bcl-2, and KI-67 (MIB-1) as prognostic biomarkers in patients with surgically treated, clinically localized prostate cancer. *Surgery* 1996;120:159–166.
91. Furuya Y, Krajewski S, Epstein JI, et al. Expression of bcl-2 and the progression of human and rodent prostatic cancers. *Clin Cancer Res* 1996;2:389–398.
92. Kyprianou N, English HF, Isaacs JT. Activation of a Ca2+-Mg2+-dependent endonuclease as an early event in castration-induced prostatic cell death. *Prostate* 1988;13:103–117.
93. Marin MC, Fernandez A, Bick RJ, et al. Apoptosis suppression by bcl-2 is correlated with the regulation of nuclear and cytosolic Ca2+. *Oncogene* 1996;12:2259–2266.
94. Furuya Y, Lundmo P, Short AD, et al. The role of calcium, pH, and cell proliferation in the programmed (apoptotic) death of androgen-independent prostatic cancer cells induced by thapsigargin. *Cancer Res* 1994;54:6167–6175.
95. Colombel M, Symmans F, Gil S, et al. Detection of the apoptosis-suppressing oncoprotein bc1-2 in hormone-refractory human prostate cancers. *Am J Pathol* 1993;143:390–400.
96. McDonnell TJ, Troncoso P, Brisbay SM, et al. Expression of the protooncogene bcl-2 in the prostate and its association with emergence of androgen-independent prostate cancer. *Cancer Res* 1992;52:6940–6944.
97. Apakama I, Robinson MC, Walter NM, et al. bcl-2 overexpression combined with p53 protein accumulation correlates with hormone-refractory prostate cancer. *Br J Cancer* 1996;74:1258–1262.
98. Oh WK, Kantoff PW. Management of hormone refractory prostate cancer: current standards and future prospects. *J Urol* 1998;160:1220–1229.
99. Herrmann JL, Bruckheimer E, McDonnell TJ. Cell death signal transduction and Bcl-2 function. *Biochem Soc Trans* 1996;24:1059–1065.
100. Haldar S, Basu A, Croce CM. Bcl2 is the guardian of microtubule integrity. *Cancer Res* 1997;57:229–233.
101. Blagosklonny MV, Schulte T, Nguyen P, et al. Taxol-induced apoptosis and phosphorylation of Bcl-2 protein involves c-Raf-1 and represents a novel c-Raf-1 signal transduction pathway. *Cancer Res* 1996;56:1851–1854.
102. Ito T, Deng X, Carr B, et al. Bcl-2 phosphorylation required for anti-apoptosis function. *J Biol Chem* 1997;272:11671–11673.
103. Maundrell K, Antonsson B, Magnenat E, et al. Bcl-2 undergoes phosphorylation by c-Jun N-terminal kinase/stress-activated protein kinases in the presence of the constitutively active GTP-binding protein Rac1. *J Biol Chem* 1997;272: 25238–25242.
104. Wang HG, Rapp UR, Reed JC. Bcl-2 targets the protein kinase Raf-1 to mitochondria. *Cell* 1996;87:629–638.
105. Datta SR, Dudek H, Tao X, et al. Akt phosphorylation of BAD couples survival signals to the cell-intrinsic death machinery. *Cell* 1997;91:231–241.
106. del Peso L, Gonzalez-Garcia M, Page C, et al. Interleukin-3-induced phosphorylation of BAD through the protein kinase Akt. *Science* 1997;278:687–689.
107. Krajewska M, Krajewski S, Epstein JI, et al. Immunohistochemical analysis of bcl-2, bax, bcl-X, and mcl-1 expression in prostate cancers. *Am J Pathol* 1996;148:1567–1576.
108. MacGrogan D, Bookstein R. Tumour suppressor genes in prostate cancer. *Semin Cancer Biol* 1997;8:11–19.
109. Theodorescu D, Broder SR, Boyd JC, et al. p53, bcl-2 and retinoblastoma proteins as long-term prognostic markers in localized carcinoma of the prostate. *J Urol* 1997;158:131–137.
110. Berges RR, Furuya Y, Remington L, et al. Cell proliferation, DNA repair, and p53 function are not required for programmed death of prostatic glandular cells induced by androgen ablation. *Proc Natl Acad Sci U S A* 1993;90:8910–8914.
111. Planchon SM, Wuerzberger S, Frydman B, et al. Beta-lapachone-mediated apoptosis in human promyelocytic leukemia (HL-60) and human prostate cancer cells: a p53-independent response. *Cancer Res* 1995;55:3706–3711.
112. Gjertsen BT, Logothetis CJ, McDonnell TJ. Molecular regulation of cell death and therapeutic strategies for cell death induction in prostate carcinoma. *Cancer Metastasis Rev* 1998;17:345–351.
113. Fero ML, Rivkin M, Tasch M, et al. A syndrome of multiorgan hyperplasia with features of gigantism, tumorigenesis, and female sterility in p27(Kip1)-deficient mice. *Cell* 1996; 85:733–744.
114. Kiyokawa H, Kineman RD, Manova-Todorova KO, et al. Enhanced growth of mice lacking the cyclin-dependent kinase inhibitor function of p27 (Kip1). *Cell* 1996;85:721–732.
115. Nakayama K, Ishida N, Shirane M, et al. Mice lacking p27(Kip1) display increased body size, multiple organ hyperplasia, retinal dysplasia, and pituitary tumors. *Cell* 1996;85:707–720.
116. Polyak K, Kato JY, Solomon MJ, et al. p27Kip1, a cyclin-Cdk inhibitor, links transforming growth factor-beta and contact inhibition to cell cycle arrest. *Genes Dev* 1994;8:9–22.
117. Slingerland JM, Hengst L, Pan CH, et al. A novel inhibitor of cyclin-Cdk activity detected in transforming growth factor beta-arrested epithelial cells. *Mol Cell Biol* 1994;14: 3683–3694.
118. Cordon-Cardo C, Koff A, Drobnjak M, et al. Distinct altered patterns of p27KIP1 gene expression in benign prostatic hyperplasia and prostatic carcinoma. *J Natl Cancer Inst* 1998;90:1284–1291.
119. De Marzo AM, Meeker AK, Epstein JI, et al. Prostate stem cell compartments: expression of the cell cycle inhibitor p27Kip1 in normal, hyperplastic, and neoplastic cells. *Am J Pathol* 1998;153:911–919.
120. Cote RJ, Shi Y, Groshen S, et al. Association of p27Kip1 levels with recurrence and survival in patients with stage C prostate carcinoma. *J Natl Cancer Inst* 1998;90:916–920.
121. Tsihlias J, Kapusta LR, DeBoer G, et al. Loss of cyclin-dependent kinase inhibitor p27Kip1 is a novel prognostic factor in localized human prostate adenocarcinoma. *Cancer Res* 1998;58:542–548.
122. Yang RM, Naitoh J, Murphy M, et al. Low p27 expression predicts poor disease-free survival in patients with prostate cancer. *J Urol* 1998;159:941–945.

123. Gao X, Porter AT, Grignon DJ, et al. Diagnostic and prognostic markers for human prostate cancer. *Prostate* 1997;31: 264–281.
124. Cheville JC, Lloyd RV, Sebo TJ, et al. Expression of p27kip1 in prostatic adenocarcinoma. *Mod Pathol* 1998;11: 324–328.
124a. Thomas GV, Schrage MI, Rosenfelt L, et al. Preoperative prostate needle biopsy correlates with subsequent radical prostatectomy p27, Gleason grade and pathological stage. *J Urol* 2000;164:1987–1991.
125. Guo Y, Sklar GN, Borkowski A, et al. Loss of the cyclin-dependent kinase inhibitor p27(Kip1) protein in human prostate cancer correlates with tumor grade. *Clin Cancer Res* 1997;3:2269–2274.
125a. Waltregny D, Leav I, Signoretti S, et al. Androgen-driven prostate epithelial cell proliferation and differentiation *in vivo* involve the regulation of 27. *Mol Endocrinol* 2001;15: 765–782.
126. Chen Y, Robles AI, Martinez LA, et al. Expression of G1 cyclins, cyclin-dependent kinases, and cyclin-dependent kinase inhibitors in androgen-induced prostate proliferation in castrated rats. *Cell Growth Differ* 1996;7:1571–1578.
127. Jenkins RB, Qian J, Lieber MM, et al. Detection of c-myc oncogene amplification and chromosomal anomalies in metastatic prostatic carcinoma by fluorescence in situ hybridization. *Cancer Res* 1997;57:524–531.
128. Nupponen NN, Kakkola L, Koivisto P, et al. Genetic alterations in hormone-refractory recurrent prostate carcinomas. *Am J Pathol* 1998;153:141–148.
129. Kokontis J, Takakura K, Hay N, et al. Increased androgen receptor activity and altered c-myc expression in prostate cancer cells after long-term androgen deprivation. *Cancer Res* 1994;54:1566–1573.
130. Vlach J, Hennecke S, Alevizopoulos K, et al. Growth arrest by the cyclin-dependent kinase inhibitor p27Kip1 is abrogated by c-Myc. *EMBO J* 1996;15:6595–6604.
131. Umbas R, Schalken JA, Aalders TW, et al. Expression of the cellular adhesion molecule E-cadherin is reduced or absent in high-grade prostate cancer. *Cancer Res* 1992;52:5104–5109.
132. Aberle H, Schwartz H, Kemler R. Cadherin-catenin complex: protein interactions and their implications for cadherin function. *J Cell Biochem* 1996;61:514–523.
133. Behrens J, von Kries JP, Kuhl M, et al. Functional interaction of beta-catenin with the transcription factor LEF-1. *Nature* 1996;382:638–642.
134. Huber O, Korn R, McLaughlin J, et al. Nuclear localization of beta-catenin by interaction with transcription factor LEF-1. *Mech Dev* 1996;59:3–10.
135. Rubinfeld B, Souza B, Albert I, et al. Association of the APC gene product with beta-catenin. *Science* 1993;262: 1731–1734.
136. Su LK, Vogelstein B, Kinzler KW. Association of the APC tumor suppressor protein with catenins. *Science* 1993;262: 1734–1737.
137. He TC, Sparks AB, Rago C, et al. Identification of c-MYC as a target of the APC pathway. *Science* 1998;281:1509–1512.
138. St. Croix B, Sheehan C, Rak JW, et al. E-Cadherin-dependent growth suppression is mediated by the cyclin-dependent kinase inhibitor p27(KIP1). *J Cell Biol* 1998;142:557–571.
139. Thomas GV, Szigeti K, Murphy M, et al. Down-regulation of p27 is associated with development of colorectal adenocarcinoma metastases. *Am J Pathol* 1998;153:681–687.
140. Li J, Yen C, Liaw D, et al. PTEN, a putative protein tyrosine phosphatase gene mutated in human brain, breast, and prostate cancer. *Science* 1997;275:1943–1947.
141. Li DM, Sun H. TEP1, encoded by a candidate tumor suppressor locus, is a novel protein tyrosine phosphatase regulated by transforming growth factor beta. *Cancer Res* 1997;57:2124–2129.
142. Steck PA, Pershouse MA, Jasser SA, et al. Identification of a candidate tumour suppressor gene, MMAC1, at chromosome 10q23.3 that is mutated in multiple advanced cancers. *Nat Genet* 1997;15:356–362.
143. Bostrom J, Cobbers JM, Wolter M, et al. Mutation of the PTEN (MMAC1) tumor suppressor gene in a subset of glioblastomas but not in meningiomas with loss of chromosome arm 10q. *Cancer Res* 1998;58:29–33.
144. Liu W, James CD, Frederick L, et al. PTEN/MMAC1 mutations and EGFR amplification in glioblastomas. *Cancer Res* 1997;57:5254–5257.
145. Rasheed BK, Stenzel TT, McLendon RE, et al. PTEN gene mutations are seen in high-grade but not in low-grade gliomas. *Cancer Res* 1997;57:4187–4190.
146. Wang SI, Puc J, Li J, et al. Somatic mutations of PTEN in glioblastoma multiforme. *Cancer Res* 1997;57:4183–4186.
147. Guldberg P, thor Straten P, Birck A, et al. Disruption of the MMAC1/PTEN gene by deletion or mutation is a frequent event in malignant melanoma. *Cancer Res* 1997;57:3660–3663.
148. Cairns P, Okami K, Halachmi S, et al. Frequent inactivation of PTEN/MMAC1 in primary prostate cancer. *Cancer Res* 1997;57:4997–5000.
149. Suzuki H, Freije D, Nusskern DR, et al. Interfocal heterogeneity of PTEN/MMAC1 gene alterations in multiple metastatic prostate cancer tissues. *Cancer Res* 1998;58:204–209.
150. Risinger JI, Hayes AK, Berchuck A, et al. PTEN/MMAC1 mutations in endometrial cancers. *Cancer Res* 1997;57: 4736–4738.
151. Tamura M, Gu J, Matsumoto K, et al. Inhibition of cell migration, spreading, and focal adhesions by tumor suppressor PTEN. *Science* 1998;280:1614–1617.
152. Maehama T, Dixon JE. The tumor suppressor, PTEN/MMAC1, dephosphorylates the lipid second messenger, phosphatidylinositol 3,4,5-trisphosphate. *J Biol Chem* 1998; 273:13375–13378.
153. Bellacosa A, Testa JR, Staal SP, et al. A retroviral oncogene, akt, encoding a serine-threonine kinase containing an SH2-like region. *Science* 1991;254:274–277.
154. Chang HW, Aoki M, Fruman D, et al. Transformation of chicken cells by the gene encoding the catalytic subunit of PI 3-kinase. *Science* 1997;276:1848–1850.
155. Downward J. Mechanisms and consequences of activation of protein kinase B/Akt. *Curr Opin Cell Biol* 1998;10:262–267.
156. Franke TF, Kaplan DR, Cantley LC. PI3K: downstream AKTion blocks apoptosis. *Cell* 1997;88:435–437.
157. Cardone MH, Roy N, Stennicke HR, et al. Regulation of cell death protease caspase-9 by phosphorylation. *Science* 1998;282:1318–1321.

158. Sun H, Lesche R, Li DM, et al. PTEN modulates cell cycle progression and cell survival by regulating phosphatidylinositol 3,4,5,-trisphosphate and Akt/protein kinase B signaling pathway. *Proc Natl Acad Sci U S A* 1999;96:6199–6204.
159. Gu J, Tamura M, Yamada KM. Tumor suppressor PTEN inhibits integrin- and growth factor-mediated mitogen-activated protein (MAP) kinase signaling pathways. *J Cell Biol* 1998;143:1375–1383.
160. Teng DH, Hu R, Lin H, et al. MMAC1/PTEN mutations in primary tumor specimens and tumor cell lines. *Cancer Res* 1997;57:5221–5225.
161. McMenamin ME, Soung P, Perera S, et al. Loss of PTEN expression in paraffin-embedded primary prostate cancer correlates with high Gleason score and advanced stage. *Cancer Res* 1999;59:4291–4296.
162. Trapman J, Brinkmann AO. The androgen receptor in prostate cancer. *Pathol Res Pract* 1996;192:752–760.
163. van der Kwast TH, Tetu B. Androgen receptors in untreated and treated prostatic intraepithelial neoplasia. *Eur Urol* 1996;30:265–268.
164. O'Malley B. The steroid receptor superfamily: more excitement predicted for the future. *Mol Endocrinol* 1990;4:363–369.
165. Tilley WD, Marcelli M, Wilson JD, et al. Characterization and expression of a cDNA encoding the human androgen receptor. *Proc Natl Acad Sci U S A* 1989;86:327–331.
166. Adler AJ, Danielsen M, Robins DM. Androgen-specific gene activation via a consensus glucocorticoid response element is determined by interaction with nonreceptor factors. *Proc Natl Acad Sci U S A* 1992;89:11660–11663.
167. Rennie PS, Bruchovsky N, Leco KJ, et al. Characterization of two cis-acting DNA elements involved in the androgen regulation of the probasin gene. *Mol Endocrinol* 1993;7:23–36.
168. Kallio PJ, Poukka H, Moilanen A, et al. Androgen receptor-mediated transcriptional regulation in the absence of direct interaction with a specific DNA element. *Mol Endocrinol* 1995;9:1017–1028.
169. Blanquet V, Wang JA, Chenivesse X, et al. Assignment of a human cyclin A gene to 4q26-q27. *Genomics* 1990;8:595–597.
170. Mashal RD, Lester S, Corless C, et al. Expression of cell cycle-regulated proteins in prostate cancer. *Cancer Res* 1996;56:4159–4163.
171. Xiong Y, Connolly T, Futcher B, et al. Human D-type cyclin. *Cell* 1991;65:691–699.
172. Bohmann D, Bos TJ, Admon A, et al. Human proto-oncogene c-jun encodes a DNA binding protein with structural and functional properties of transcription factor AP-1. *Science* 1987;238:1386–1392.
173. Bos TJ, Bohmann D, Tsuchie H, et al. v-jun encodes a nuclear protein with enhancer binding properties of AP-1. *Cell* 1988;52:705–712.
174. Saez E, Rutberg SE, Mueller E, et al. c-fos is required for malignant progression of skin tumors. *Cell* 1995;82:721–732.
175. Fujita J, Yoshida O, Yuasa Y, et al. Ha-ras oncogenes are activated by somatic alterations in human urinary tract tumours. *Nature* 1984;309:464–466.
176. Bushman EC, Nayak RN, Bushman W. Immunohistochemical staining of ras p21: staining in benign and malignant prostate tissue. *J Urol* 1995;153:233–237.
177. Viola MV, Fromowitz F, Oravez S, et al. Expression of ras oncogene p21 in prostate cancer. *N Engl J Med* 1986;314:133–137.
178. Yokota J, Tsunetsugu-Yokota Y, Battifora H, et al. Alterations of myc, myb, and rasHa proto-oncogenes in cancers are frequent and show clinical correlation. *Science* 1986; 231:261–265.
179. Culig Z, Hobisch A, Cronauer MV, et al. Regulation of prostatic growth and function by peptide growth factors. *Prostate* 1996;28:392–405.
180. Muir GH, Butta A, Shearer RJ, et al. Induction of transforming growth factor beta in hormonally treated human prostate cancer. *Br J Cancer* 1994;69:130–134.
181. Sherwood ER, Lee C. Epidermal growth factor-related peptides and the epidermal growth factor receptor in normal and malignant prostate. *World J Urol* 1995;13:290–296.
182. Gittes RF. Carcinoma of the prostate. *N Engl J Med* 1991;324:236–245.
183. Crawford ED, Eisenberger MA, McLeod DG, et al. A controlled trial of leuprolide with and without flutamide in prostatic carcinoma. *N Engl J Med* 1989;321:419–424.
184. Raghavan D. Non-hormone chemotherapy for prostate cancer: principles of treatment and application to the testing of new drugs. *Semin Oncol* 1988;15:371–389.
185. Quarmby VE, Beckman WC Jr., Cooke DB, et al. Expression and localization of androgen receptor in the R-3327 Dunning rat prostatic adenocarcinoma. *Cancer Res* 1990; 50:735–739.
186. Tilley WD, Wilson CM, Marcelli M, et al. Androgen receptor gene expression in human prostate carcinoma cell lines. *Cancer Res* 1990;50:5382–5386.
187. Visakorpi T, Hyytinen E, Koivisto P, et al. In vivo amplification of the androgen receptor gene and progression of human prostate cancer. *Nat Genet* 1995;9:401–406.
188. Giovannucci E, Stampfer MJ, Krithivas K, et al. The CAG repeat within the androgen receptor gene and its relationship to prostate cancer. *Proc Natl Acad Sci U S A* 1997;94:3320–3323.
189. Gottlieb B, Trifiro M, Lumbroso R, et al. The androgen receptor gene mutations database. *Nucleic Acids Res* 1996; 24:151–154.
190. Yeh S, Chang C. Cloning and characterization of a specific coactivator, ARA70, for the androgen receptor in human prostate cells. *Proc Natl Acad Sci U S A* 1996;93:5517–5521.
191. Craft N, Shostak Y, Carey M, et al. A mechanism for hormone-independent prostate cancer through modulation of androgen receptor signaling by the HER-2/neu tyrosine kinase. *Nat Med* 1999;5:280–285.
192. Yeh S, Lin HK, Kang HY, et al. From HER2/Neu signal cascade to androgen receptor and its coactivators: a novel pathway by induction of androgen target genes through MAP kinase in prostate cancer cells. *Proc Natl Acad Sci U S A* 1999;96:5458–5463.
193. Magi-Galluzzi C, Xu X, Hlatky L, et al. Heterogeneity of androgen receptor content in advanced prostate cancer. *Mod Pathol* 1997;10:839–845.
194. Miyamoto KK, McSherry SA, Dent GA, et al. Immunohistochemistry of the androgen receptor in human benign and malignant prostate tissue. *J Urol* 1993;149:1015–1019.
195. Sadi MV, Walsh PC, Barrack ER. Immunohistochemical study of androgen receptors in metastatic prostate cancer.

Comparison of receptor content and response to hormonal therapy. *Cancer* 1991;67:3057–3064.

196. Sadi MV, Barrack ER. Image analysis of androgen receptor immunostaining in metastatic prostate cancer. Heterogeneity as a predictor of response to hormonal therapy. *Cancer* 1993;71:2574–2580.
197. Takeda H, Akakura K, Masai M, et al. Androgen receptor content of prostate carcinoma cells estimated by immunohistochemistry is related to prognosis of patients with stage D2 prostate carcinoma. *Cancer* 1996;77:934–940.
198. van der Kwast TH, Schalken J, Ruizeveld de Winter JA, et al. Androgen receptors in endocrine-therapy-resistant human prostate cancer. *Int J Cancer* 1991;48:189–193.

198a. Signoretti S, Montironi R, Manola J, et al. Her-2-neu expression increase with progression towards androgen independence in human prostate cancer. *J Natl Cancer Inst* 2000;92:1918–1925.

199. Waskiewicz AJ, Cooper JA. Mitogen and stress response pathways: MAP kinase cascades and phosphatase regulation in mammals and yeast. *Curr Opin Cell Biol* 1995;7:798–805.
200. Bos JL. ras oncogenes in human cancer: a review. *Cancer Res* 1989;49:4682–4689.
201. Fanning P, Bulovas K, Saini KS, et al. Elevated expression of pp60c-src in low grade human bladder carcinoma. *Cancer Res* 1992;52:1457–1462.
202. Mizukami Y, Nonomura A, Noguchi M, et al. Immunohistochemical study of oncogene product ras p21, c-myc and growth factor EGF in breast carcinomas. *Anticancer Res* 1991;11:1485–1494.
203. Peehl DM. Oncogenes in prostate cancer. An update. *Cancer* 1993;71:1159–1164.
204. Slamon DJ, Clark GM, Wong SG, et al. Human breast cancer: correlation of relapse and survival with amplification of the HER-2/neu oncogene. *Science* 1987;235:177–182.
205. Chu Y, Solski PA, Khosravi-Far R, et al. The mitogen-activated protein kinase phosphatases PAC1, MKP-1, and MKP-2 have unique substrate specificities and reduced activity in vivo toward the ERK2 sevenmaker mutation. *J Biol Chem* 1996;271:6497–6501.
206. Gould GW, Cuenda A, Thomson FJ, et al. The activation of distinct mitogen-activated protein kinase cascades is required for the stimulation of 2-deoxyglucose uptake by interleukin-1 and insulin-like growth factor-1 in KB cells. *Biochem J* 1995;311:735–738.
207. Jiang Y, Chen C, Li Z, et al. Characterization of the structure and function of a new mitogen-activated protein kinase (p38beta). *J Biol Chem* 1996;271:17920–17926.
208. Marshall CJ. Specificity of receptor tyrosine kinase signaling: transient versus sustained extracellular signal-regulated kinase activation. *Cell* 1995;80:179–185.
209. Lee JC, Laydon JT, McDonnell PC, et al. A protein kinase involved in the regulation of inflammatory cytokine biosynthesis. *Nature* 1994;372:739–746.
210. Whitmarsh AJ, Shore P, Sharrocks AD, et al. Integration of MAP kinase signal transduction pathways at the serum response element. *Science* 1995;269:403–407.
211. Xia Z, Dickens M, Raingeaud J, et al. Opposing effects of ERK and JNK-p38 MAP kinases on apoptosis. *Science* 1995;270:1326–1331.
212. Alessi DR, Smythe C, Keyse SM. The human CL100 gene encodes a Tyr/Thr-protein phosphatase which potently and specifically inactivates MAP kinase and suppresses its activation by oncogenic ras in Xenopus oocyte extracts. *Oncogene* 1993;8:2015–2020.
213. Franklin CC, Kraft AS. Conditional expression of the mitogen-activated protein kinase (MAPK) phosphatase MKP-1 preferentially inhibits p38 MAPK and stress-activated protein kinase in U937 cells. *J Biol Chem* 1997;272:16917–16923.
214. Sun H, Charles CH, Lau LF, et al. MKP-1 (3CH134), an immediate early gene product, is a dual specificity phosphatase that dephosphorylates MAP kinase in vivo. *Cell* 1993;75:487–493.
215. Magi-Galluzzi C, Mishra R, Fiorentino M, et al. Mitogen-activated protein kinase phosphatase 1 is overexpressed in prostate cancers and is inversely related to apoptosis. *Lab Invest* 1997;76:37–51.
216. Loda M, Capodieci P, Mishra R, et al. Expression of mitogen-activated protein kinase phosphatase-1 in the early phases of human epithelial carcinogenesis. *Am J Pathol* 1996;149:1553–1564.
217. Magi-Galluzzi C, Montironi R, Cangi MG, et al. Mitogen-activated protein kinases and apoptosis in PIN. *Virchows Arch* 1998;432:407–413.
218. Cher ML, Bova GS, Moore DH, et al. Genetic alterations in untreated metastases and androgen-independent prostate cancer detected by comparative genomic hybridization and allelotyping. *Cancer Res* 1996;56:3091–3102.
219. Van Den Berg C, Guan XY, Von Hoff D, et al. DNA sequence amplification in human prostate cancer identified by chromosome microdissection: potential prognostic implications. *Clin Cancer Res* 1995;1:11–18.
220. Visakorpi T, Kallioniemi AH, Syvanen AC, et al. Genetic changes in primary and recurrent prostate cancer by comparative genomic hybridization. *Cancer Res* 1995;55:342–347.
221. Henriksson M, Luscher B. Proteins of the Myc network: essential regulators of cell growth and differentiation. *Adv Cancer Res* 1996;68:109–182.
222. Amati B, Dalton S, Brooks MW, et al. Transcriptional activation by the human c-Myc oncoprotein in yeast requires interaction with Max. *Nature* 1992;359:423–426.
223. Lee TC, Ziff EB. Mxi1 is a repressor of the c-Myc promoter and reverses activation by USF. *J Biol Chem* 1999;274:595–606.
224. Queva C, Hurlin PJ, Foley KP, et al. Sequential expression of the MAD family of transcriptional repressors during differentiation and development. *Oncogene* 1998;16:967–977.
225. Schreiber-Agus N, Meng Y, Hoang T, et al. Role of Mxi1 in ageing organ systems and the regulation of normal and neoplastic growth. *Nature* 1998;393:483–487.
226. Steiner MS, Anthony CT, Lu Y, et al. Antisense c-myc retroviral vector suppresses established human prostate cancer. *Hum Gene Ther* 1998;9:747–755.
227. Thompson TC, Southgate J, Kitchener G, et al. Multistage carcinogenesis induced by ras and myc oncogenes in a reconstituted organ. *Cell* 1989;56:917–930.
228. Bubendorf L, Kononen J, Koivisto P, et al. Survey of gene amplifications during prostate cancer progression by high-throughout fluorescence in situ hybridization on tissue microarrays. *Cancer Res* 1999;59:803–806.

229. Reiter RE, Gu Z, Watabe T, et al. Prostate stem cell antigen: a cell surface marker overexpressed in prostate cancer. *Proc Natl Acad Sci U S A* 1998;95:1735–1740.
230. Classon BJ, Boyd RL. Thymic-shared antigen-1 (TSA-1). A lymphostromal cell membrane Ly-6 superfamily molecule with a putative role in cellular adhesion. *Dev Immunol* 1998;6:149–156.
231. Noda S, Kosugi A, Saitoh S, et al. Protection from anti-TCR/CD3-induced apoptosis in immature thymocytes by a signal through thymic shared antigen-1/stem cell antigen-2. *J Exp Med* 1996;183:2355–2360.
232. Thomas PM, Samelson LE. The glycophosphatidylinositol-anchored Thy-1 molecule interacts with the p60fyn protein tyrosine kinase in T cells. *J Biol Chem* 1992;267:12317–12322.
233. Bamezai A, Rock KL. Overexpressed Ly-6A.2 mediates cell-cell adhesion by binding a ligand expressed on lymphoid cells. *Proc Natl Acad Sci U S A* 1995;92:4294–4298.
234. Brakenhoff RH, Gerretsen M, Knippels EM, et al. The human E48 antigen, highly homologous to the murine Ly-6 antigen ThB, is a GPI-anchored molecule apparently involved in keratinocyte cell-cell adhesion. *J Cell Biol* 1995;129:1677–1689.
235. Katz BZ, Eshel R, Sagi-Assif O, et al. An association between high Ly-6A/E expression on tumor cells and a highly malignant phenotype. *Int J Cancer* 1994;59:684–691.
235a. Thomas GV, Gu Z, Yamashiro J, et al. PSCA expression correlates with high Gleason Score, advanced stage, and bone metastases. *Oncogene* 2000;19:1288–1296.
236. Reiter RE, Watabe T, Thomas GV, et al. Co-amplification of PSCA and c-myc in locally advanced prostate cancer. *Genes and Dev* 2000;27:95–103.
237. Isaacs JT, Isaacs WB, Feitz WF, et al. Establishment and characterization of seven Dunning rat prostatic cancer cell lines and their use in developing methods for predicting metastatic abilities of prostatic cancers. *Prostate* 1986;9:261–281.
238. Bao L, Loda M, Janmey PA, et al. Thymosin beta 15: a novel regulator of tumor cell motility upregulated in metastatic prostate cancer. *Nat Med* 1996;2:1322–1328.
239. Bao L, Loda M, Zetter BR. Thymosin beta15 expression in tumor cell lines with varying metastatic potential. *Clin Exp Metastasis* 1998;16:227–233.
240. Sager R, Sheng S, Pemberton P, et al. Maspin: a tumor suppressing serpin. *Curr Top Microbiol Immunol* 1996;213:51–64.
241. Sager R, Sheng S, Pemberton P, et al. Maspin. A tumor suppressing serpin. *Adv Exp Med Biol* 1997;425:77–88.
242. Sheng S, Pemberton PA, Sager R. Production, purification, and characterization of recombinant maspin proteins. *J Biol Chem* 1994;269:30988–30993.
243. Sheng S, Carey J, Seftor EA, et al. Maspin acts at the cell membrane to inhibit invasion and motility of mammary and prostatic cancer cells. *Proc Natl Acad Sci U S A* 1996;93:11669–11674.
244. Zou Z, Anisowicz A, Hendrix MJ, et al. Maspin, a serpin with tumor-suppressing activity in human mammary epithelial cells. *Science* 1994;263:526–529.
245. Schneider SS, Schick C, Fish KE, et al. A serine proteinase inhibitor locus at 18q21.3 contains a tandem duplication of the human squamous cell carcinoma antigen gene. *Proc Natl Acad Sci U S A* 1995;92:3147–3151.
246. Sheng S, Truong B, Fredrickson D, et al. Tissue-type plasminogen activator is a target of the tumor suppressor gene maspin. *Proc Natl Acad Sci U S A* 1998;95:499–504.
247. Bergerheim US, Kunimi K, Collins VP, et al. Deletion mapping of chromosomes 8, 10, and 16 in human prostatic carcinoma. *Genes Chromosomes Cancer* 1991;3:215–220.
248. Bova GS, Carter BS, Bussemakers MJ, et al. Homozygous deletion and frequent allelic loss of chromosome 8p22 loci in human prostate cancer. *Cancer Res* 1993;53:3869–3873.
249. Bova GS, Isaacs WB. Review of allelic loss and gain in prostate cancer. *World J Urol* 1996;14:338–346.
250. Carter BS, Ewing CM, Ward WS, et al. Allelic loss of chromosomes 16q and 10q in human prostate cancer. *Proc Natl Acad Sci U S A* 1990;87:8751–8755.
251. Brown PO, Botstein D. Exploring the new world of the genome with DNA microarrays. *Nat Genet* 1999;21:33–37.
252. Eisen MB, Spellman PT, Brown PO, et al. Cluster analysis and display of genome-wide expression patterns. *Proc Natl Acad Sci U S A* 1998;95:14863–14868.
253. McGall G, Labadie J, Brock P, et al. Light-directed synthesis of high-density oligonucleotide arrays using semiconductor photoresists. *Proc Natl Acad Sci U S A* 1996;93:13555–13560.
254. Sapolsky RJ, Lipshutz RJ. Mapping genomic library clones using oligonucleotide arrays. *Genomics* 1996;33:445–456.
255. Kononen J, Bubendorf L, Kallioniemi A, et al. Tissue microarrays for high-throughput molecular profiling of tumor specimens. *Nat Med* 1998;4:844–847.

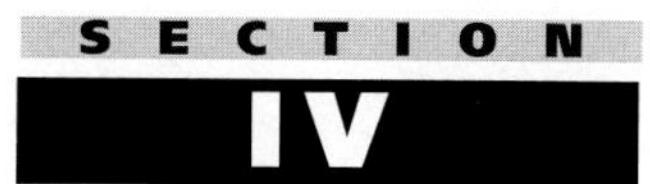

EARLY PROSTATE CANCER—SINGLE MODALITY TREATMENT

21

SURGICAL THERAPY OF CLINICALLY LOCALIZED PROSTATE CANCER: RATIONALE, PATIENT SELECTION, AND OUTCOMES

STEVEN R. POTTER
ALAN W. PARTIN

Prostate cancer is the most commonly diagnosed cancer and the second leading cause of cancer deaths in American men. More than 179,300 men will be diagnosed with prostate cancer in 1999, and an estimated 37,000 of them will die of their disease (1). Improvements in staging, primarily through the use of prostate-specific antigen (PSA) testing coupled with digital rectal examination (DRE), have revolutionized our ability to detect prostate cancer at an early, curable stage. Advances in surgical technique and perioperative care have revolutionized our ability to cure organ-confined prostate cancer with acceptable morbidity. This chapter focuses on the role of radical prostatectomy in the management of localized prostate cancer, including the rationale for surgical intervention, selection of patients, postoperative morbidity, and cancer control.

NATURAL HISTORY OF UNTREATED PROSTATE CANCER

Despite prostate cancer's epidemic proportions, it often has an indolent clinical course and characteristically afflicts older men. The histologic prevalence of occult prostate cancer greatly exceeds the clinical incidence of prostate cancer (2). Because of these issues, the role of definitive surgery in the management of prostate cancer has engendered enormous debate. Randomized and appropriately powered studies comparing active therapy with watchful waiting will not produce useful data for many years (3). Even when completed, these studies are unlikely, in isolation, to provide definitive answers regarding management of clinically localized prostate cancer. Men newly diagnosed with prostate cancer and their physicians require useful information now for making rational decisions regarding treatment. Insight for this decision process can be obtained by carefully studying the course of prostate cancer managed with deferred or ineffective therapies.

RESULTS OF DEFERRED THERAPY

Several investigators have evaluated the natural history of prostate cancer by studying patient cohorts receiving no therapy until progression. These studies, although often limited by selection bias, have been touted as evidence of the benignity of prostate cancer and used to support deferred therapy. Johansson and colleagues, in a widely quoted study, found 5- and 10-year progression-free survival rates of 68% and 53%, respectively (4). Whitmore and colleagues reported 100% and 84% cancer-specific survival in a group of men receiving deferred therapy at 5 and 10 years, respectively (5).

Although these progression-free survival rates are impressive, Whitmore and associates reported on a group of only 75 patients selected from a total of 4,000 men. Johansson reported on only 223 of 306 eligible patients. For the initial 24 months of patient accrual in the Johansson series, only men with well-differentiated (grade 1) tumors were enrolled. Men with moderately (grade 2) and poorly differentiated (grade 3) tumors were subsequently enrolled, but these men represented too small a fraction of the study population to allow valid comparison with men who are actually candidates for radical prostatectomy. During most of the studies' enrollment period, half of the men younger than 75 years of age received external beam radiotherapy, whereas all men older than 75 years were assigned to deferred therapy (observation). The patients in the Johansson series had predominantly low-grade disease, were significantly older (mean age, 72 years) than contemporary radical prostatectomy series, and had a mean follow-up of only 10 years. Many of these men were diagnosed with cytology performed on fine-needle biopsy specimens. This modality has been associated with an unacceptable level of false-positive results, making it possible that some of these men did not actually have prostate cancer (6). In fact, one patient reported to have expired free of progression was determined at autopsy to have died from prostate cancer, casting doubt on the rigor of follow-up. This study population cannot be considered typical of patients undergoing curative therapy in the United States. At 10-year follow-up, 47% of the men in this series had developed progression, and 84% of men progressing had received androgen ablation therapy. These results compare unfavorably with contemporary surgical series despite the much higher percentage of high-grade cancers in those series.

Fleming and associates attempted to assess the benefit of definitive therapy in comparison to deferred therapy using a decision analysis model, in which the likelihood of prostate cancer progression was estimated from review of the literature (7). The authors concluded that for patients with moderately or poorly differentiated prostate cancer, radical prostatectomy or radiotherapy provided approximately 3.5 additional years of "quality-adjusted life expectancy" and that these definitive therapies provided limited benefit relative to deferred therapy in men with well-differentiated tumors. The findings of this decision analysis model are critically dependent on the rates of progression to metastatic disease and the estimated morbidity of definitive therapy used to construct the model. Fleming and associates obtained estimated progression rates from five deferred therapy series, four of which contained only men with occult, incidentally discovered cancers (8–11). The fifth series used in this model was based on the cohort reported by Johansson et al. and was discussed earlier (12). These patients are not representative of candidates for radical prostatectomy. The progression rates found in these series were unrealistically low, minimizing any survival advantage found for definitive therapy.

In the Fleming model, any survival benefit from definitive therapy was arbitrarily reduced based on expected morbidity, and these expectations also played a critical role in determining any benefit found for definitive therapy. All men were assumed to be potent preoperatively, all men with focal extraprostatic extension of cancer were classified as not cured, and urinary incontinence and impotence were assigned more importance than death from metastatic prostate cancer. With these assumptions in place and with unrealistic rates of progression to metastatic disease, the results of this model must be viewed with skepticism.

In attempting to circumvent the problem of selection bias, Aus performed a retrospective analysis of all 536 patients dying of prostate cancer over a 2-year period in a single Swedish town (13). The intervals between diagnosis and death were as long as 25 years. In contrast to the findings of Johansson and Whitmore, approximately 63% of men surviving more than 10 years who were clinically metastasis free at diagnosis died of prostate cancer. When managed with noncurative intent, 75% of men younger than 65 years of age at diagnosis succumbed to prostate cancer. This study also demonstrates that, because of the prolonged natural history of prostate cancer, disease-specific mortality figures are only significant after approximately 15 years of follow-up. Certainly, prostate cancer death rates at 10 years reflect the number of men who presented with occult metastatic disease and were incurable at presentation.

Chodak and colleagues evaluated the natural history of prostate cancer by summarizing the results of six nonrandomized studies totaling more than 800 men treated with observation and delayed hormonal therapy for clinically localized prostate cancer (14). In these men, prostate cancer grade had a defining influence on outcome. Although 60% of the men in this study had grade 1 disease, overall metastatic rates at 10 and 15 years were substantial. At 15 years, 40% of grade 1 tumors had metastasized, as had 70% of grade 2 and 85% of grade 3 tumors (Fig. 21-1). Many men in this study received hormonal therapy at the time of biochemical (PSA) progression, actually delaying the appearance of metastatic disease.

Albertsen and colleagues used the Connecticut Tumor Registry to examine outcomes in 451 men with T1 and T2 tumors receiving either immediate or delayed hormonal therapy (15). Tumor grade had a dominant influence on long-term outcome, with 15-year cancer-specific mortality rates of 9% in men with Gleason sums 2 to 4 tumors, 28% in Gleason sums 5 to 7 tumors, and 51% in men with Gleason sums 8 to 10 tumors. Although the long-term survival of men with well-differentiated tumors was not significantly different from the general population, these low-grade tumors comprised only 10% of the study population. These low-grade tumors are rarely diagnosed on needle biopsy and are not representative of tumors removed at rad-

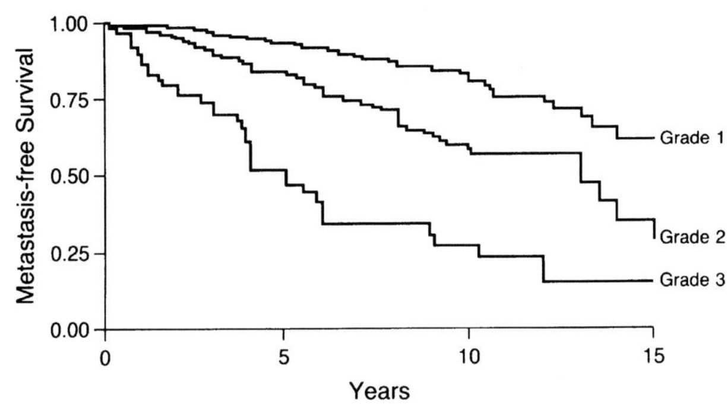

FIGURE 21-1. Metastasis-free survival among untreated patients with localized prostate cancer by tumor grade (1 to 3) illustrating the defining influence of grade on risk of prostate cancer progression. (From Chodak GW, Thisted RA, Gerber GS, et al. Results of conservative management of clinically localized prostate cancer. *N Engl J Med* 1994;330:242–248, with permission.)

ical prostatectomy. Albertsen and colleagues, again using the Connecticut Tumor Registry, reported that, depending on their age at diagnosis, men with Gleason sum 7 and Gleason sums 8 to 10 tumors had 42% to 70% and 60% to 87% cancer-specific death rates, respectively, when followed for 15 years (15,16).

RESULTS OF INEFFECTIVE THERAPIES

Most deferred therapy series are limited by the examination of men who are not comparable to patients undergoing radical prostatectomy and who would be unlikely surgical candidates. Series with younger patients and higher-grade cancers can be found if results from other treatment modalities are examined. Brachytherapy, as widely practiced 15 to 20 years ago, has proven ineffective in providing local control or stable biochemical (PSA) freedom from cancer progression. However, these men are more comparable to those in current surgical series in terms of clinical stage and grade. Indeed, additional staging information was provided for many of these men by staging lymphadenectomy performed before brachytherapy.

Fuks and associates reviewed a 15-year experience during which 679 men underwent iodine-125 brachytherapy for clinically localized prostate cancer (17). These men had a mean follow-up of 8 years and a mean age of 61 years. All patients included for analysis had negative lymph nodes at staging pelvic lymphadenectomy. Clinical stage at presentation was divided between T2 (87%) and T3 (13%) cancers. Histologic grade was low, moderate, and high in 37%, 53%, and 6% of these men, respectively. At 10 years, metastatic disease had developed in 30% of the patients with low-, 50% with moderate-, and 70% with high-grade disease. Overall, 5- and 10-year progression rates were 32% and 66%, respectively. Fuks and associates concluded that "early and complete eradication of the primary tumor is required if long-term cure is to be achieved." These patients are more representative of patients undergoing radical prostatectomy than are those in deferred therapy series. The devastating effect of cancer in these men and the favorable outcomes of surgery in relation to deferred or ineffective therapies lend support to the advocacy of radical prostatectomy in properly selected patients.

SELECTION OF PATIENTS FOR RADICAL PROSTATECTOMY

The ideal candidate for radical prostatectomy has early, curable disease, a biologically significant tumor, and a reasonable likelihood of living 10 to 20 years after surgery. Patients undergoing definitive surgery should ideally be free of serious co-morbidities. With conservative therapy of men with localized prostate cancer, 50% to 75% of tumors will have progressed at 10-year follow-up (16). Without treatment, some 13% to 20% of these men will die of prostate cancer during the decade after diagnosis.

Given that patients are healthy enough to be good surgical candidates and have a long enough life expectancy to benefit from surgery, the key becomes selecting candidates with curable disease. Men are increasingly being diagnosed with early-stage disease. In 1974, 43% of all staged patients were clinically T3 or T4, whereas by 1990, only 33% presented with T3 or T4 disease (18). The ubiquitous use of PSA as an intended or de facto screening tool has been largely responsible for current rates of organ confinement on the order of 65% to 75% in series of screen-detected cancers (19). When defined by strict histologic criteria, the vast majority of tumors detected in this fashion appears to be biologically significant (19–21).

The use of multivariate nomograms can increase the accuracy of preoperative staging. Probability models predicting capsular penetration, seminal vesicle involvement, and regional lymph node metastasis were introduced by Oesterling and colleagues, who constructed algorithms based on logistic regression analysis of 275 men with clinically localized prostate cancer undergoing radical prostatectomy (22). Using data from DRE, biopsy Gleason score, and serum PSA, Partin and associates developed a nomogram providing validated estimates of the likelihood of organ confinement and, thus, potential benefit from surgical intervention (23,24). For example, given a patient with clinical T2a disease, a PSA of 8 ng per mL, and a biopsy Gleason score of 6, the Partin nomogram predicts a 51% likelihood of organ-confined disease. The same patient has a 3% likelihood of seminal vesicle involvement and 2% likelihood of lymph node metastasis. Conversely, a man with a clinical T2c, biopsy Gleason score 8 tumor, and PSA level of 21 has only a 3% likelihood of organ confinement and a 35% probability of lymphatic metastasis. The role of imaging studies in selecting patients for radical prostatectomy has been an area of great controversy. The low sensitivity of computed tomography (CT) and magnetic resonance imaging (MRI) for the detection of local extension (CT, 55% to 75%; MRI, 20% to 70%) or lymph node metastases (CT, 25% to 45%; MRI, 0% to 15%) limits their usefulness in selecting patients for definitive surgical therapy (25–27).

The ideal candidates for radical prostatectomy present with a clinical stage T1c or T2 disease, a serum PSA less than 10 ng per mL, and a biopsy Gleason score less than 8. Patient age is also a strong predictor of curability, with the likelihood of findings at surgery consistent with curable disease declining with advancing age (28). Patients presenting with clinical T3 disease are not ideal candidates for surgical cure. However, those with low-grade disease and focal extracapsular extension may be curable. The surgeon must consider the likely pathologic stage and the age and health of the patient. In men with poor odds of favorable pathology, in whom surgery is unlikely to be curative, but without

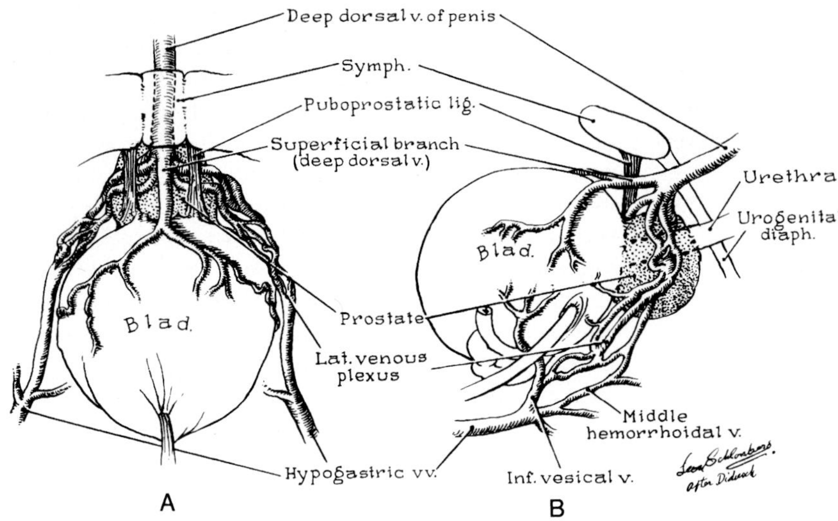

FIGURE 21-2. Santorini's venous plexus (dorsal vein complex). **A:** View of trifurcation of the dorsal vein of the penis. The relationship of venous branches to puboprostatic ligaments is depicted. **B:** Lateral view shows anatomic relationship at trifurcation. *In situ*, these structures are encased in the pelvic fascia. Blad, bladder; diaph, diaphragm; Inf, inferior; Lat, lateral; lig, ligament; symph, symphysis; v, vein. (From Reiner WG, Walsh PC. An anatomical approach to the surgical management of the dorsal vein and Santorini's plexus during radical retropubic surgery. *J Urol* 1979;121:198–200, with permission.)

evidence of systemic disease, three-dimensional conformal external beam radiotherapy is an excellent alternative and should be encouraged. Advances over the 1990s have dramatically reduced the morbidity of radical prostatectomy, and select patients can be offered a reasonable chance of surgical cure even with clinical parameters that suggest that organ-confinement is unlikely.

SURGICAL TECHNIQUE

The past two decades have seen a series of critical anatomic discoveries transform the surgeon's ability to cure localized prostate cancer while reducing attendant morbidity. Definition of the anatomy of the dorsal vein complex by Walsh and Reiner allowed radical prostatectomy to be performed in a controlled fashion and in a relatively bloodless field (29) (Fig. 21-2). Further anatomic studies led to delineation of the autonomic innervation to the corpora cavernosa, which runs outside the prostate and Denonvillier's fascia between the levator fascia and prostatic fascia (30) (Fig. 21-3).

The identification of these nerves and their relationship to the capsular vessels and investing layers of fascia made attainment of wider margins of resection possible (31) (Fig. 21-4). Preservation of the neurovascular bundles makes it

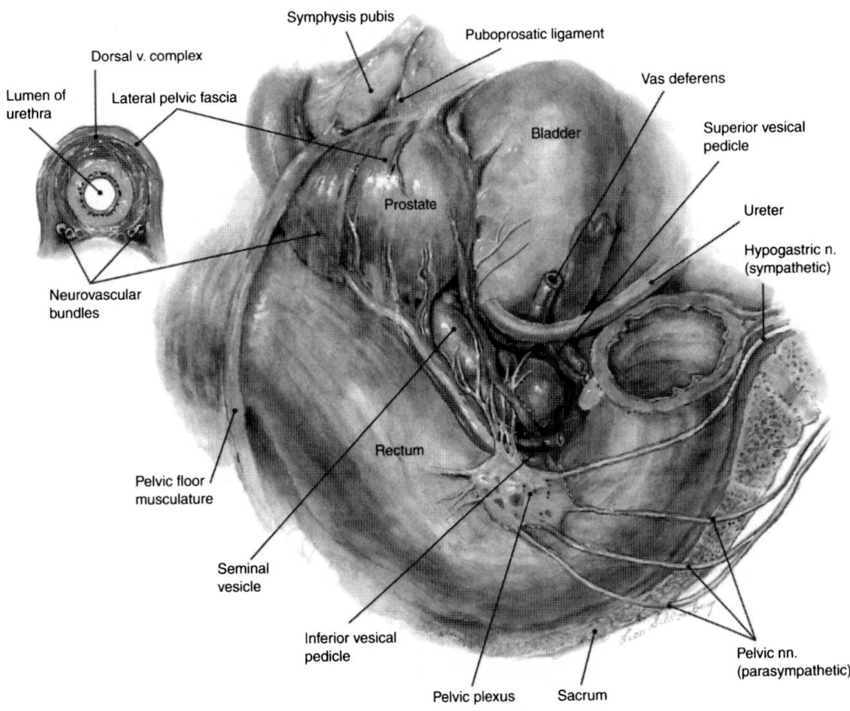

FIGURE 21-3. Anatomic relationship of the prostate to the pelvic fascia, the left pelvic plexus, and left neurovascular bundle. Inset: Cross section through the urethra just distal to the prostatic apex demonstrating the inner circular layer of smooth muscle, the outer striated urethral sphincter, and the perineal body (central tendon of the perineum). n, nerve; nn, nerves; v, vein.

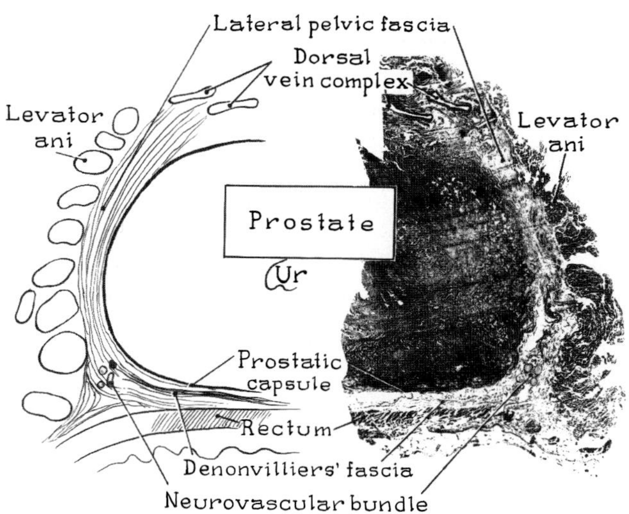

FIGURE 21-4. Cross section through the adult prostate demonstrating the anatomic relationships of the lateral pelvic fascia, Denonvillier's fascia, and neurovascular bundle (NVB). The NVB is sandwiched between the two layers of lateral pelvic fascia—the levator fascia and the prostatic fascia. Ur, urethra.

possible to preserve sexual function in many men (32). The techniques involved in delineation and preservation of these nerves have led to the somewhat inapt moniker of *nerve-sparing* radical prostatectomy. In fact, radical prostatectomy, as formerly practiced through either perineal or retropubic approaches, did not include excision of these nerves and their associated vasculature. Instead, the neurovascular bundles were cut and left in place (33). Recent modifications to the apical dissection and improved understanding of the striated urethral sphincter have altered the preparation of the vesicourethral anastomosis, resulting in improved rates of urinary continence (34,35). The evolution of the technique of radical retropubic prostatectomy has recently been elegantly summarized by Walsh (36).

INTRAOPERATIVE COMPLICATIONS AND POSTOPERATIVE MANAGEMENT

Hemorrhage has historically been the most frequent and troublesome intraoperative complication of radical prostatectomy. Refinements in technique have reduced blood loss substantially, and average blood loss of less than 1,000 cc has been reported in most recent series (37). With the use of careful technique and preoperatively donated autologous blood, transfusion of banked blood is necessary in only 2% of men (38).

Rectal injury is a rare intraoperative complication, occurring in 10 of 1,800 (0.5%) consecutive cases at our institution. These injuries typically occur while developing the plane between the rectum and Denonvillier's fascia. In the event of rectal injury, the prostatectomy is completed, the bladder neck is reconstructed, and hemostasis is obtained. The rectum is then primarily repaired in two layers with an omental pedicle placed between the repair and the vesicourethral anastomosis. The anal sphincter is widely dilated digitally and the patient placed on appropriate antibiotics. Using this technique, all patients recovered without need for colostomy and without developing a wound infection (39). Obturator nerve and ureteral injuries are exceedingly rare. Obturator nerve injuries are repaired by direct reanastomosis, whereas ureteral injuries occur at or near the trigone and are repaired by ureteroneocystostomy.

The vast majority of men undergoing radical retropubic prostatectomy has an uneventful postoperative course. Patients ambulate and start a clear liquid diet the morning after surgery and are typically discharged from the hospital on the morning of the third postoperative day with drains removed and urethral catheters to gravity drainage. The urethral catheter is removed within 2 to 3 weeks after surgery. Standardized radical prostatectomy care pathways provide significant reductions in hospitalization-related costs without increasing morbidity or decreasing patient satisfaction with their care (40,41). Standardized care pathways are used for all patients undergoing radical prostatectomy at our institution.

Operative mortality, defined as death within 30 days of surgery, has decreased substantially with improvements in patient selection, surgical technique, and perioperative care and is now exceedingly uncommon after radical prostatectomy. Operative mortality occurred in 11 (0.3%) of 3,834 men in a recent study pooling results from several institutions (42). Andriole and colleagues reported an operative mortality rate of 0.2% in a series of 1,342 men undergoing radical retropubic prostatectomy (43). The experience at The Johns Hopkins Hospital mirrors these results, with an operative mortality of 0.2% (38).

The majority of men undergoing radical prostatectomy does so uneventfully. Inpatient hospital stays have fallen dramatically, and the introduction of standardized postoperative care paths has streamlined patient care and helped decrease costs without increasing morbidity.

EARLY POSTOPERATIVE COMPLICATIONS

Postoperative complications include myocardial infarction, thromboembolic events, anastomotic stricture, and delayed bleeding. Postoperative myocardial infarction after radical prostatectomy occurred in 0.6% and 0.4% of men in a large series from Washington University and the Mayo Clinic, respectively (43,44). The frequency of cardiovascular events can be minimized by identification of patients with preexisting cardiac disease, judicious fluid management, and avoidance of postoperative anemia (45). Deep venous thrombosis (DVT) and pulmonary embolus occur in approximately 1.0% to 1.5% of patients. In our experience, thromboembolic events occurred in 1.5% of 1,300 consecutive patients, with associated deaths in two (0.15%) men (46). Sequential

TABLE 21-1. SUMMARY OF SEVERAL LARGE RADICAL RETROPUBIC PROSTATECTOMY SERIES

Series	Institution	n	Mean age (yr)	Mean follow-up (mo)	T2 lesions (%)	5-year PSA progression-free likelihood	10-year PSA progression-free likelihood
Partin et al.	Johns Hopkins	894	59	53	83	87	7
Pound et al.	Johns Hopkins	1,623	59	59	66	80	68
Catalona et al.	Washington University	925	63	63	79	78	65
Ohori et al.	Baylor University	500	63	36	78	76	73
Zincke et al.	Mayo Clinic	3,170	65	60	93	70	52

PSA, prostate-specific antigen.
Adapted from Pound CR, Partin AW, Epstein JI, et al. Prostate-specific antigen after anatomic radical retropubic prostatectomy: patterns of recurrence and cancer control. *Urol Clin North Am* 1997;24:395.

compression devices and surgical stockings are used routinely. The use of subcutaneous heparin is also efficacious in preventing DVT and pulmonary embolus (47). The use of heparin has been associated with increased lymphocele formation and bleeding and is used at our institution only in men with a history of prior DVT, pulmonary embolus, or thrombophlebitis (46). Avoidance of trauma to venous and lymphatic structures, postoperative dorsiflexion exercises, and early ambulation are important for DVT prophylaxis. Because most thromboembolic complications will occur after discharge from the hospital, thorough patient education and close follow-up are required.

Anastomotic stricture has been reported in 0.5% to 9% of men after radical retropubic prostatectomy (48). Precise construction of the vesicourethral anastomosis is critical in providing mucosal apposition and limiting the rate of bladder neck contracture (49). Most strictures are amenable to simple outpatient vesicourethral anastomotic dilation, although some strictures require cold knife incision under direct vision (50). Rare patients may require endoscopic reconstruction (51).

Postoperative bleeding requiring acute transfusion to maintain hemodynamic stability occurred in 7 (0.5%) of 1,300 consecutive men after radical prostatectomy at our institution (52). The undrained pelvic hematoma will eventually liquefy and drain through the vesicourethral anastomosis. Patients stabilized with transfusion and not returned to the operative theatre for exploration and drainage of their pelvic hematoma risk bladder neck contracture and are more likely to suffer imperfect urinary continence.

The vast majority of men has an uneventful postoperative course. Improvements in surgical technique and perioperative care have decreased complication rates dramatically, whereas experience has improved management of the few complications that do occur.

CANCER CONTROL AFTER RADICAL PROSTATECTOMY

The most important goal of radical prostatectomy is cure of cancer. Serum PSA is the most sensitive and specific marker available to monitor for progression of disease after definitive therapy of prostate cancer. Local or distant recurrence of prostate cancer after radical prostatectomy does not occur in the absence of a detectable serum PSA level. Pound et al. recently studied 1,900 consecutive men undergoing radical prostatectomy and followed them for more than 10,000 patient-years, finding that progression was accompanied in every instance by a detectable serum PSA (53). Evaluation of postoperative cancer control should, therefore, be based primarily on postoperative PSA monitoring. Biochemical (PSA) disease-free survival has been widely validated as a surrogate for cancer-specific survival and, thus, cancer control after radical prostatectomy.

Multiple institutions have reported on biochemical (PSA) disease progression rates in large radical prostatectomy series. Table 21-1 provides a summary of patient characteristics and outcomes in several of these series. Data from the The Johns Hopkins Hospital series by Walsh have recently been summarized (54). In a series of 1,623 men who underwent radical prostatectomy for clinically localized prostate cancer, recurrence occurred in 276 (13%) at a mean follow-up of 5 years. Overall, actuarial (Kaplan-Meier) biochemical progression-free rates at 5 and 10 years were 80% and 68%, respectively. These data are summarized in Figure 21-5.

Overall, actuarial cancer-specific survival rates were 99% and 93% at 5 and 10 years, respectively. Clinical stage, pretreatment PSA, and pathologic Gleason score were all independent predictors of progression after surgery. Patients with clinical stage T1c disease, who represented 21% of all men in this series, had an actuarial progression-free rate of 86% at 5 years. Preoperative PSA values were obtained in 1,354 (83%) men. When analyzed based on division of preoperative PSA values into groups of less than 4 ng per mL, 4 to 10 ng per mL, 10.1 to 20.0 ng per mL, and greater than 20 ng per mL, there was a statistically significant correlation between PSA and progression-free likelihood in all groups. Biochemical (PSA) progression rates rose with increasing Gleason score. No patient in this series developed a local or distant recurrence without concomitant PSA elevation.

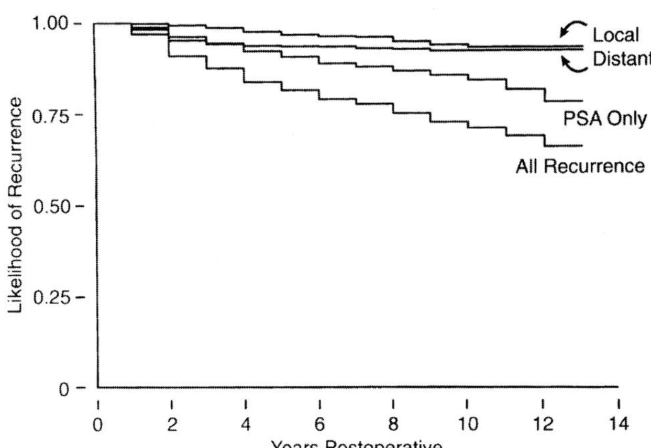

FIGURE 21-5. Kaplan-Meier actuarial progression-free likelihood for overall progression, isolated prostate-specific antigen (PSA) elevation only, local recurrence, and distant progression with or without local progression. One thousand six hundred and twenty-three men were included in the analysis. (From Pound CR, Partin AW, Epstein JI, et al. Prostate-specific antigen after anatomic radical retropubic prostatectomy: patterns of recurrence and cancer control. *Urol Clin North Am* 1997;24:395, with permission.)

Epstein and colleagues had previously reported that the probability of an undetectable PSA level 10 years after surgery was significantly higher with Gleason score 7 tumors in comparison to Gleason scores 8 to 10 tumors in this series (46% vs. 23%, $p < .00001$) (55). A combination of pathologic stage, Gleason score, and surgical margin status continued to be the best predictor of the probability of cancer recurrence (56). The results of several large radical prostatectomy series confirm those from The Johns Hopkins Hospital. In the Washington University series, actuarial progression-free probabilities of 78% and 65% were obtained at 5 and 10 years, respectively (57). The Baylor group demonstrated PSA progression-free rates of 76% at 5 years and 73% at 10 years (58).

These data indicate that radical prostatectomy is curative for most men presenting with organ-confined disease. A majority of men with well to moderately differentiated tumors with extraprostatic extension but otherwise negative margins can expect cure. In men with poorly differentiated tumors and focal extraprostatic extension, cure is less likely, whereas patients with lymph node involvement at the time of surgery are never free of progression with adequate follow-up.

URINARY CONTINENCE

Urinary incontinence has become less common but remains a potentially devastating sequela of radical prostatectomy. The rate and severity of incontinence are minimized through careful apical dissection, excellent visualization through control of hemorrhage, preservation of sphincteric innervation, and avoidance of injury to the smooth muscle of the urethral sphincter during construction of the vesicourethral anastomosis. Evaluation of 593 consecutive cases treated by Walsh at our institution revealed complete continence in 92%, with some degree of stress urinary incontinence in 8% (59). Of those with stress incontinence, 6% required zero or one pad per day, and no patients were totally incontinent. Ultimately, two men (0.3%) underwent artificial urinary sphincter placement. Continence was achieved in 94% of men with bilateral sparing of the neurovascular bundles, 92% of patients with excision of one bundle, and 81% of these with bilateral wide excision. Although these differences were not statistically significant, preserving autonomic innervation likely has subtle effects on urinary continence. Clearly, factors other than neurovascular bundle status are of primary importance in the maintenance of continence. There was no correlation between postoperative potency and continence. Similar results have been reported by other centers (60).

Although major centers consistently report urinary incontinence rates under 10%, with the majority of these men having mild stress incontinence easily managed with pads, survey studies of community hospital results throughout the United States show wide variation in radical prostatectomy outcomes. Murphy and colleagues surveyed 1,796 preoperatively continent men treated at 484 hospitals after undergoing radical prostatectomy. Postoperatively, 19% of these men required pads daily, whereas 3.6% were totally incontinent (61). Despite higher rates of incontinence in this and other broad-based population surveys, most men adapt well to pad use and report satisfaction with surgical outcomes. Quality-of-life studies, surprisingly, find that most men are minimally bothered by postoperative stress incontinence (62,63).

Improvement in continence may occur up to 2 years after surgery (64). During this time, patients need constant reinforcement and encouragement (65). Because improvement may continue long after radical retropubic prostatectomy, definitive incontinence surgery should be deferred at least a year after operation (37). When intervention is required, retrograde collagen injection has provided little durable benefit for men with mild stress incontinence (66,67). Men with persistent unexplained incontinence should be evaluated for the presence of anastomotic stricture, which characteristically produces a picture of overflow incontinence. Finally, a small minority of men will have primary detrusor dysfunction identified on urodynamics and may benefit from medical therapy (68,69).

PRESERVATION OF POTENCY

Before identification of the location of the autonomic branches of the pelvic plexus innervating the corpora cavernosa and development of techniques to preserve them, virtually all men were impotent after radical prostatectomy (36). The identification of these nerves by Walsh and Donker resulted in modification of the technique of radical prostatectomy, allowing preservation of potency (30). The initial experience with this procedure consisted of 600 consecutive men aged 34 to 72 years who underwent anatomic radical prostatectomy at The Johns Hopkins Hospital between 1982 and 1988. In the 503 of these men who were potent preoperatively and followed for a minimum of 18 months after surgery, 68% remained potent postoperatively (70). Preservation of potency was correlated with patient age, stage, and preservation or excision of the neurovascular bundles. Potency was preserved in 91% of men younger than 50 years of age, in 75% of men 50 to 60 years of age, in 58% of men 60 to 70 years old, and in 25% of men 70 years of age or older. Preservation of both rather than one neurovascular bundle assumed increasing importance with age, with young patients having similar potency rates with preservation of one or both neurovascular bundles. After controlling for age and neurovascular bundle status, the presence of extraprostatic extension or seminal vesicle invasion doubled the relative risk of postoperative impotence relative to men with organ-confined tumors. Similar results have been reported by a number of institutions (56,71–73). The preservation of potency does not result in decrease in biochemical disease-free survival (54,74).

Potency rates after radical prostatectomy have varied widely in some studies. Patient selection, co-morbidities, surgical technique, and the means of acquiring follow-up data (patient reported vs. physician acquired) have been cited as reasons for this variability and have contributed to the controversy surrounding postoperative potency rates. Walsh and associates prospectively studied 70 preoperatively potent patients undergoing radical prostatectomy for clinically localized disease. Physician-acquired potency rates were compared to patient-reported rates gathered via a validated, confidential questionnaire collected by a third party. One year after surgery, there was total consistency between physician and patient accounts of erectile function. The results offer evidence that, when asked in an informed and sensitive fashion, patients are forthcoming and honest in reporting postoperative potency rates to their physicians (75).

Zippe and associates have recently examined the role of sildenafil citrate (Viagra) in postprostatectomy erectile dysfunction. They found that 12 of 15 men who had undergone bilateral nerve-sparing procedures obtained erections sufficient for intercourse with sildenafil at standard dosages, whereas no men who had undergone excision or ligation of both neurovascular bundles had a positive response to this agent (76). This confirms the physiologic role of the autonomic innervation of the corpora first defined by Walsh and further strengthens the case for surgical intervention in appropriate patients.

CONCLUSION

Ideal candidates for radical prostatectomy are men in good health and with a life expectancy of more than 10 years who present with early curable prostate cancer. Largely owing to PSA testing coupled with DRE, men are presenting earlier and with lower-stage tumors. The vast majority of asymptomatic prostate cancers detected by isolated PSA elevations is clinically significant. Improvements in staging, largely owing to histologic grading of biopsy specimens and the development of predictive multivariate nomograms and neural networks, have helped to better select those patients with the highest chance of cure.

Since the 1980s, we have seen enormous advances in the treatment of localized prostate cancer through improvements in the technique of radical prostatectomy. The morbidity of surgery has been reduced dramatically, the length of hospital stays has fallen, and potency is preserved in many men. Younger men are more likely to remain potent after surgery as well as obtain the greatest benefit from cure of their cancer. The use of effective oral pharmacotherapy for erectile dysfunction restores potency in many men with at least one of their neurovascular bundles preserved.

Anatomic insight has also made the current practice of radical prostatectomy a better cancer operation than in the past. These improvements have made it possible to cure most men with organ-confined cancer. Most failures in these clinically low-stage tumors are due to distant metastases present at the time of surgery, and further improvements in cancer control will depend on earlier diagnosis, improvements in staging through the use of predictive neural networks and multivariate nomograms, and the development of effective systemic therapies.

REFERENCES

1. *Cancer facts & figures—1999.* American Cancer Society, 1999.
2. McNeal JE. Origin and development of carcinoma of the prostate. *Cancer* 1969;23:24–34.
3. Wilt TJ, Brawer MK. Prostate Cancer Intervention Versus Observation Trial: a randomized trial comparing radical prostatectomy versus expectant management for treatment of localized prostate cancer. *J Urol* 1994;152:1910–1914.
4. Johansson JE, Adami H-O, Andersson SO, et al. High 10-year survival rate in patients with early, untreated prostatic cancer. *JAMA* 1992;267:2191–2196.
5. Whitmore WF Jr., Warner JA, Thompson IM Jr. Expectant management of localized prostatic cancer. *Cancer* 1991;67: 1091–1096.
6. Servoll E, Halvorsen OJ, Haukaas S, et al. Radical retropubic prostatectomy: our experience with the first 54 patients. *Scand J Urol Nephrol* 1992;26:231–234.
7. Fleming C, Wasson JH, Albertsen PC, et al. A decision analysis of alternative treatment strategies for clinically localized prostate cancer. Prostate Patient Outcomes Research Team. *JAMA* 1993;269:2650–2658.
8. Zhang G, Wasserman NF, Sidi AA, et al. Long-term follow-up results after expectant management of stage A1 prostatic cancer. *J Urol* 1991;146:99–103.

9. Haapiainen R, Rannikko S, Makinen J, et al. T0 carcinoma of the prostate: influence of tumor extent and histologic grade on prognosis of untreated patients. *Eur Urol* 1986;12:16–20.
10. Blackard CE, Mellinger GY, Gleason DF. Treatment of stage 1 carcinoma of the prostate: a preliminary report. *J Urol* 1971;106:729–733.
11. Byar DP. Survival of patients with incidentally found microscopic cancer of the prostate: results of a clinical trial of conservative treatment. *J Urol* 1972;108:908–912.
12. Johansson JE, Adami HO, Andersson SO, et al. Natural history of localized prostatic cancer. A population-based study in 223 untreated patients. *Lancet* 1989;1:799–803.
13. Aus G. Prostate cancer: mortality and morbidity after noncurative treatment with aspects on diagnosis and treatment. *Scand J Urol Nephrol* 1994;167[Suppl]:1–41.
14. Chodak GW, Thisted RA, Gerber GS, et al. Results of conservative management of clinically localized prostate cancer. *N Engl J Med* 1994;330:242–248.
15. Albertsen PC, Fryback DG, Storer BE, et al. Long-term survival among men with conservatively treated localized prostate cancer. *JAMA* 1995;274:626–631.
16. Albertsen PC, Hanley JA, Gleason DF, et al. Competing risk analysis of men aged 55 to 74 years at diagnosis managed conservatively for clinically localized prostate cancer. *JAMA* 1998;280:975–980.
17. Fuks Z, Leibel SA, Wallner KE, et al. The effect of local control on metastatic dissemination in carcinoma of the prostate: long-term results in patients treated with ^{125}I implantation. *Int J Radiat Oncol Biol Phys* 1991;21:537–547.
18. Mettlin C, Jones GW, Murphy GP. Trends in prostate cancer care in the United States, 1974–1990: observations from the patient care evaluation studies of the American College of Surgeons Commission on Cancer. *Cancer J Clin* 1993;43: 83–91.
19. Catalona WJ, Smith DS, Ratliff TL, et al. Detection of organ-confined prostate cancer is increased through prostate-specific antigen based screening. *JAMA* 1993;270:948–954.
20. Epstein JI, Walsh PC, Carmichael M, et al. Pathologic and clinical findings to predict tumor extent of non-palpable (stage T1c) prostate cancer. *JAMA* 1994;271:368–374.
21. Stormont TJ, Farrow GM, Myers RP, et al. Clinical stage B0 or T1c prostate cancer: nonpalpable disease identified by elevated serum prostate-specific antigen concentration. *Urology* 1993;41:3–8.
22. Oesterling JE, Brendler CB, Epstein JI, et al. Correlation of clinical stage, serum prostatic acid phosphatase and preoperative Gleason grade with final pathological stage in 275 patients with clinically localized adenocarcinoma of the prostate. *J Urol* 1987;138:92–99.
23. Partin AW, Yoo J, Carter HB, et al. The use of prostate specific antigen, clinical stage and Gleason score to predict pathological stage in men with localized prostate cancer. *J Urol* 1993;150:110–114.
24. Partin AW, Kazan MW, Subong EN, et al. Combination of prostate specific antigen, clinical stage, and Gleason score to predict pathological stage of localized prostate cancer: a multi-institutional update. *JAMA* 1997;277:1445–1451.
25. Manyak MJ, Javitt MC. The role of computerized tomography, magnetic resonance imaging, bone scan, and monoclonal antibody nuclear scan for prognosis prediction in prostate cancer. *Semin Urol Oncol* 1998;16:145–152.
26. Ikonen S, Karkkainen P, Kivisaari L, et al. Magnetic resonance imaging of clinically localized prostatic cancer. *J Urol* 1998;159:915–919.
27. Huncharek M, Muscat J. Serum prostate-specific antigen as a predictor of staging abdominal/pelvic computed tomography in newly diagnosed prostate cancer. *Abdom Imaging* 1996;21:364–367.
28. Carter HB, Epstein JI, Partin AW. Influence of age and prostate-specific antigen on the chance of curable prostate cancer among men with nonpalpable disease. *Urology* 1999; 53:126–130.
29. Reiner WG, Walsh PC. An anatomical approach to the surgical management of the dorsal vein and Santorini's plexus during radical retropubic surgery. *J Urol* 1979;121:198–200.
30. Walsh PC, Donker PJ. Impotence following radical prostatectomy: insight into etiology and prevention. *J Urol* 1982;128:492–497.
31. Walsh PC, Lepor H, Eggleston JC. Radical prostatectomy with preservation of sexual function: anatomical and pathological considerations. *Prostate* 1983;4:473–485.
32. Walsh PC, Epstein JI, Lowe FC. Potency following radical prostatectomy with wide unilateral excision of the neurovascular bundle. *J Urol* 1983;138:823–827.
33. Walsh PC. Radical prostatectomy, preservation of sexual function, cancer control: the controversy. *Urol Clin North Am* 1987;14:663–673.
34. Walsh PC, Quinlan DM, Morton RA, et al. Radical retropubic prostatectomy: improved anastomosis and urinary continence. *Urol Clin North Am* 1990;17:679–684.
35. Walsh PC. Technique of vesicourethral anastomosis may influence recovery of sexual function following radical prostatectomy. *Atlas Urol Clin North Am* 1994;2:59–63.
36. Walsh PC. Anatomic radical prostatectomy: evolution of the surgical technique. *J Urol* 1998;160:2418–2424.
37. Eastham JA, Scardino PT. Radical prostatectomy. In: Walsh PC, Retik AB, Vaughn ED, et al., eds. *Campbell's urology*, 7th ed. Philadelphia: WB Saunders, 1998:2547–2564.
38. Walsh PC. Anatomic radical retropubic prostatectomy. In: Walsh PC, Retik AB, Vaughn ED, et al., eds. *Campbell's urology*, 7th ed. Philadelphia: WB Saunders, 1998:2565–2588.
39. Borland RN, Walsh PC. The management of rectal injury during radical retropubic prostatectomy. *J Urol* 1992;147: 905–907.
40. Litwin MS, Smith RB, Thind A, et al. Cost-efficient radical prostatectomy with a clinical care path. *J Urol* 1996;155: 989–993.
41. Litwin MS, Shpall AI, Dorey F. Patient satisfaction with short stays for radical prostatectomy. *Urology* 1997;49:898–905.
42. Dillioglugil O, Leibman BD, Leibman N, et al. Perioperative complications and morbidity of radical retropubic prostatectomy. *J Urol* 1997;157:1760–1767.
43. Andriole GL, Smith DS, Rao G, et al. Early complications of contemporary anatomic radical retropubic prostatectomy. *J Urol* 1994;152:1858–1860.
44. Zincke H, Oesterling JE, Blute ML, et al. Long-term (15 years) results after radical prostatectomy for clinically localized (stage T2c or lower) prostate cancer. *J Urol* 1994;152:1850–1857.

45. Hogue CW Jr., Goodnough LT, Monk TG. Perioperative myocardial ischemic episodes are related to hematocrit level in patients undergoing radical prostatectomy. *Transfusion* 1998;38:924–931.
46. Cisek LJ, Walsh PC. Thromboembolic complications following radical retropubic prostatectomy: influence of external pneumatic compression devices. *Urology* 1993;42:406–408.
47. Collins R, Scrimgeour A, Yusuf S, et al. Reduction in fatal pulmonary embolism and venous thrombosis by perioperative administration of subcutaneous heparin. Overview of results of randomized trials in general, orthopedic, and urological surgery. *N Engl J Med* 1988;318:1162–1173.
48. Schlossberg S, Jordan G, Schellhammer P. Repair of obliterative vesicourethral strictures after radical prostatectomy: a technique for preservation of continence. *Urology* 1995;45:510–513.
49. Goad JR, Scardino PT. Modifications in the technique of radical retropubic prostatectomy to minimize blood loss. *Atlas Urol Clin North Am* 1994;2:65–80.
50. Surya BV, Provet J, Johanson K-E, et al. Anastomotic strictures following radical prostatectomy: risk factors and management. *J Urol* 1990;143:755–758.
51. Potter SR, Marshall FF. Endoscopic reconstruction of vesicourethral obliteration after radical prostatectomy. *Urology* 1999;54:913–916.
52. Hedican SP, Walsh PC. Postoperative bleeding following radical retropubic prostatectomy. *J Urol* 1994;152:1181–1183.
53. Pound CR, Christens-Barry OW, Gurganus R, et al. Digital rectal examination and imaging studies are unnecessary in men with an undetectable PSA following radical prostatectomy. *J Urol* 1999;161:335(abst).
54. Pound CR, Partin AW, Epstein JI, et al. Prostate-specific antigen after anatomic radical retropubic prostatectomy: patterns of recurrence and cancer control. *Urol Clin North Am* 1997;24:395–406.
55. Epstein JI, Pizov G, Walsh PC. Correlation of pathologic findings with progression following radical retropubic prostatectomy. *Cancer* 1993;71:3582–3593.
56. Epstein JI, Partin AW, Sauvageot J, et al. Prediction of progression following radical prostatectomy: a multivariate analysis of 721 men with long-term follow-up. *Am J Surg Pathol* 1996;20:286–292.
57. Catalona WJ, Smith DJ. Five-year tumor recurrence rates after anatomic radical retropubic prostatectomy for prostate cancer. *J Urol* 1994;152:1837–1842.
58. Ohori M, Goad JR, Wheeler TM, et al. Can radical prostatectomy alter the progression of poorly differentiated prostate cancer? *J Urol* 1994;152:1843–1846.
59. Steiner MS, Morton RA, Walsh PC. Impact of anatomical radical prostatectomy on urinary continence. *J Urol* 1991;145:512–515.
60. Catalona WJ, Biggs SW. Nerve-sparing radical prostatectomy: evaluation of results after 250 patients. *J Urol* 1990; 143:538–543.
61. Murphy GP, Mettlin C, Menck H, et al. National patterns of prostate cancer treatment by radical prostatectomy: results of a survey by the American College of Surgeons Committee on Cancer. *J Urol* 1994;152:1817–1819.
62. Litwin MS, Hays RD, Fink A, et al. Quality-of-life outcomes in men treated for localized prostate cancer. *JAMA* 1995;273:129–135.
63. Arai Y, Okubo K, Aoki Y, et al. Patient-reported quality of life after radical prostatectomy for prostate cancer. *Int J Urol* 1999;6:78–86.
64. Eastham JA, Kattan MW, Rogers E, et al. Risk factors for urinary incontinence after radical retropubic prostatectomy. *J Urol* 1996;156:1707–1713.
65. Walsh PC, Worthington JF. Treating prostate cancer: radical prostatectomy. In: Walsh PC, Farrar J. *The prostate: a guide for men and the women who love them.* Baltimore: Johns Hopkins University Press, 1995:92–119.
66. Klutke JJ, Subir C, Andriole G, et al. Long-term results after antegrade collagen injection for stress urinary incontinence following radical retropubic prostatectomy. *Urology* 1999;53:974–977.
67. Smith DN, Appell RA, Rackley RR, et al. Collagen injection therapy for post-prostatectomy incontinence. *J Urol* 1998;160:364–367.
68. Foote J, Yun S, Leach GE. Postprostatectomy incontinence: pathophysiology, evaluation, and management. *Urol Clin North Am* 1991;18:229–241.
69. Goluboff ET, Chang DT, Olsson CA, et al. Urodynamics and the etiology of post-prostatectomy urinary incontinence: the initial Columbia experience. *J Urol* 1995;153: 1034–1037.
70. Quinlan DM, Epstein JI, Carter BS, et al. Sexual function following radical prostatectomy: influence of preservation of neurovascular bundles. *J Urol* 1991;145:998–1002.
71. Catalona WJ, Dresner ST. Nerve-sparing radical prostatectomy: extra-prostatic tumor extension and preservation of erectile function. *J Urol* 1985;134:1149–1151.
72. Leandri P, Rossignol G, Gautier J-R, et al. Radical retropubic prostatectomy: morbidity and quality of life. Experience with 620 consecutive cases. *J Urol* 1992;147:883–887.
73. Surya BV, Provet J, Dalbagni G, et al. Experience with potency preservation during radical prostatectomy. *Urology* 1988;32:498–501.
74. Eggleston JC, Walsh PC. Radical prostatectomy with preservation of sexual function: pathological findings in the first 100 cases. *J Urol* 1985;134:1146–1148.
75. Walsh PC, Marschke P, Ricker DD, et al. Potency and continence following anatomic radical prostatectomy: patient versus physician reported outcomes. *J Urol* 1999;161: 387(abst).
76. Zippe CD, Kedia AW, Kedia K, et al. Treatment of erectile dysfunction following radical prostatectomy with sildenafil citrate (Viagra). *Urology* 1998;52:963–966.

22

EXTERNAL BEAM RADIATION THERAPY: CONVENTIONAL AND CONFORMAL

JEFF M. MICHALSKI

Radiation therapy has been used in the treatment of prostate cancer for several decades. In the early part of the twentieth century, low-energy, poorly penetrating, orthovoltage x-ray machines limited the amount of radiation that could safely be delivered to the prostate and other deep target tissues, owing to the high surface dose these machines would deliver. The availability of high-energy megavoltage x-rays that deposit the maximum doses deep into the surface has reduced the risk of severe radiation sequelae, especially to skin and other superficial tissues. Modern linear accelerators facilitated the adoption of a variety of radiation techniques that could treat localized prostate cancer with acceptable morbidity. During the 1970s and through the early 1990s, the methods used to treat prostate cancer relied on broad anatomic and physical principles that were applied in a general fashion to all patients with presumed localized disease. During this era, radiation dose tolerance of normal organs was poorly understood and was based on limited information about whole-organ radiation distribution. Frequently, it would be assumed that the surrounding organs at risk, such as the bladder and the rectum, received nearly the same radiation dose as the target tissues, prostate, seminal vesicles (SVs), and pelvic lymph nodes. Treating large volumes of these normal organs to these high-radiation prescription doses was often unavoidable without the availability of modern imaging modalities, such as computed tomography (CT). Subsequently, the amount of radiation that could safely be administered to the prostate and adjacent targets was limited. As is discussed later, prostate cancer is a radiation-sensitive neoplasm that demonstrates a classic sigmoid dose response curve. The higher the radiation dose administered to a given volume of cancer, the more likely that the cancer will be permanently controlled.

The availability of cross-sectional imaging modalities (CT and magnetic resonance imaging) and computerized treatment planning with three-dimensional (3D) reconstructions, as well as a better understanding of the natural history of prostate cancer, has allowed radiation therapy to become a more effective and safer treatment option for men with localized prostate cancer. Community radiation oncology practices are rapidly adopting many of the new treatment methods previously developed and studied in academic medical centers. In this era of transition, it is appropriate to discuss traditional treatment methods and describe in detail the newer approaches to shaping radiation dose distributions using conformal radiation therapy (CRT).

BASIC RADIATION ONCOLOGY PHYSICS

Radiation can be emitted by the radioactive decay of nuclei of unstable isotopes or generated by the atomic collision interactions of fast electrons with dense elements such as tungsten. Photons generated by radioactive nuclear decay of unstable isotopes, such as cobalt 60 (^{60}Co), are referred to as *gamma rays*. Photons generated by the movement of atomic orbital electrons to new energy levels caused by atomic collision forces are referred to as *x-rays*. Most modern radiation therapy departments use linear accelerators to generate x-rays for cancer therapy. As the name implies, electrons are accelerated to near light speed through a linear vacuum tube and aimed at a tungsten target. The speed to which these electrons are accelerated will determine the energy of the x-rays emitted. The kinetic energy of these electrons is generally reported as the electronic potential difference between the two electrodes of the accelerator tube. The higher the potential difference, the faster the electrons, the higher the energy of x-rays produced, and the deeper the penetration of the x-ray energy in matter.

The radioactive decay of ^{60}Co results in an average radiation energy of 1.25 megavolts (MV). This megavoltage radiation source deposits its maximum energy 0.5 cm below the skin surface. When first introduced, ^{60}Co represented an improvement in existing methods that delivered maximum doses to the skin surface. No other isotope could generate sufficiently high-energy gamma rays at an acceptable dose rate for external beam radiation treatments. Eventually, ^{60}Co machines have been replaced by linear accelerators capable

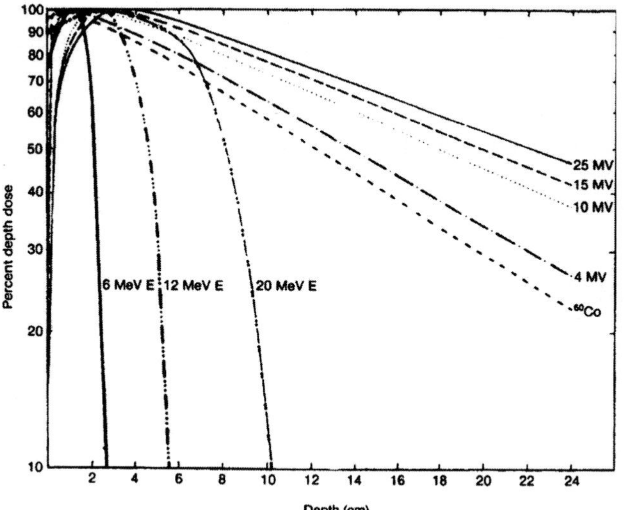

FIGURE 22-1. Examples of central axis percentage-depth dose for megavoltage x-ray beams and 6-MeV to 20-MeV electron beams. MeV and MV, megavolt. (From Purdy JA. The application of high energy x-rays and electron beams in radiotherapy in IEEE. *Trans Nucl Sci* 1979;26:1833, with permission.)

of producing higher-energy x-rays that deposit maximum energy 3 cm or more below the skin surface. Radioactive isotopes are still used in radiation oncology as brachytherapy sources. Brachytherapy (*brachy* means *short* in Greek) is the practice of placing radioactive sources in or around a malignant tumor to concentrate radiation dose. This subject is described in more detail in Chapters 23, 28, and 29.

Modern linear accelerators generate x-rays with energies ranging from 6 MV to 25 MV. Figure 22-1 illustrates the relationship between x-ray energy and the depth of penetration in tissue. With traditional radiation therapy techniques, patients would be treated with simple beam arrangements consisting of two or four fields. These techniques benefited from the use of the highest available energy to minimize radiation dose to superficial and intermediate-depth organs and tissues. Optimally, when traditional 2- or 4-field beam arrangements are used, an x-ray energy of 10 MV or greater should be used to treat deep pelvic tumors, such as prostate cancer. These higher energies will reduce the radiation dose to the femoral necks, bladder, and rectum and reduce the risk of late complications. With new multiple-field conformal methods, the advantage of the higher-energy x-rays may be less critical. In these circumstances, the additional radiation fields distribute their energy over a wider volume of normal tissues and organs, preventing them from receiving doses in excess of their tolerance.

Accelerated electrons can be used for therapy. More than 80% to 90% of the energy from electrons is deposited in the first few cm of tissue. The absorption properties of electrons in tissue make this modality ideal for treatment of superficial lesions. Generally, this low depth of penetration makes electrons a poor choice of treatment for early prostate cancers, but they can be used to treat superficial metastatic sites, such as groin lymph nodes or some bone lesions. The uses of other radiation particles (protons) are covered in Chapter 30.

Linear accelerators are configured with isocentric geometry (Fig. 22-2). The head of the accelerator houses the tungsten x-ray target mounted at a fixed distance from rotational isocenter, about which the gantry of the machine rotates. This same rotational center is used to define the treatment table motion. This geometry allows a tumor or treatment volume to be localized at the center of rotation of the accelerator and treatment couch in numerous directions. When isocentric gantry and treatment table rotations are used, the entrance directions of multiple x-ray beams can be changed to minimize radiation dose to surrounding tissues while keeping the cancer in the beam at all times.

As x-rays exit the head of a linear accelerator, the beam is shaped with collimators and customized apertures. The primary collimator jaws located closest to the x-ray target prevent leakage of x-rays in directions away from the patient. Secondary collimators are used to create a rectangular beam to minimize unintended radiation of the patient outside the treatment area. Finally, customized alloy blocks are used to shape the beam aperture to match the intended treatment volume within the patient. Lipowitz metal (Cerrobend) is the most commonly used alloy for blocks, consisting of 13% tin, 50% bismuth, 27% lead, and 10% cadmium. This metal alloy melts at a relatively low temperature and is easy to handle to create customized field shapes. Gradually, blocks fashioned with these metals are

A

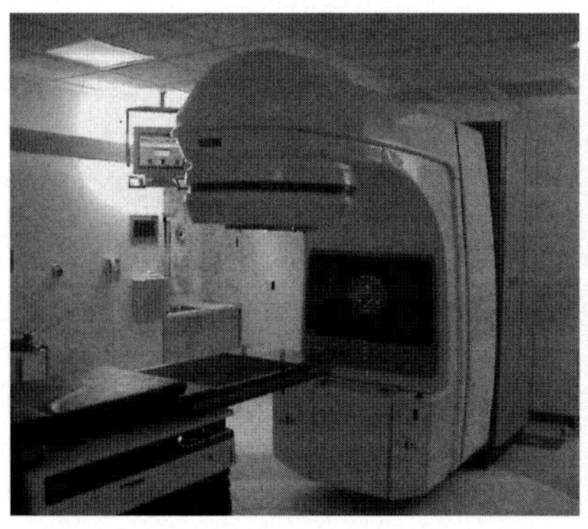

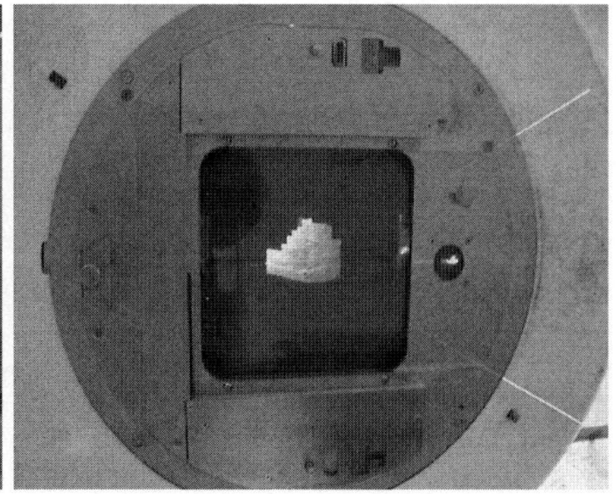

B

FIGURE 22-2. A: A modern dual-energy isocentric linear accelerator. **B:** A multileaf collimator mounted in head of linear accelerator. The 80 leaves (40 pair) move independently to shape the exiting radiation beam.

being replaced with tertiary collimator systems mounted permanently in the linear accelerator head. Multileaf collimators (MLCs) are computer-driven, dense metal leaves that can create custom-shaped beam apertures. MLCs minimize the handling time required for manual changing of blocks between treatment fields. They also allow for dynamic field shaping and intensity modulation.

BASIC RADIATION BIOLOGY

X-rays interact with matter in a myriad of ways. At energies used for radiation therapy, x-rays transfer their energy to the irradiated matter by interactions with orbital electrons. Photons may interact with water, the predominant molecule in cellular solutions, to produce free radicals. By direct interactions with DNA or indirectly by free radicals, the x-rays cause disruption of atomic or molecular bonds. Classic radiation biology teaching argued that injury to the cellular DNA by single- or double-strand breakage would result in the biologic end result of cellular dysfunction or death.

A double-strand DNA break is usually an irrevocably fatal injury. Single-strand DNA breaks, on the other hand, may undergo repair. Potentially lethal and sublethal damage occurs after radiation exposure. Elkind and Sutton (1) showed that repair of this damage occurs if the dose of radiation is divided into two fractions separated by a few hours. Therefore, two doses of radiation separated in time are less effective than the same total dose given as a single dose. The ability to correct this potentially lethal and sublethal damage varies among cell and tissue types. Compared with normally functioning human tissues, malignant tumors have a less effective repair mechanism. By fractionating a course of radiation therapy, radiation oncologists capitalize on these differences.

Many human cancers have a characteristic tumor control curve. If the dose of radiation is plotted against the likelihood for cure, then a sigmoid curve is generated. There is insufficient cell-kill to cause tumor cure at very low doses. As the dose is raised to approximately one lethal event per cell, the statistics of random cell-kill become important. The likelihood for cure rises rapidly with dose at the central part of the curve; it starts to plateau when the maximum effect is reached. The steepness of the curve in the effective range emphasizes the importance of small increases in dose. The shape and steepness of the sigmoid dose-response relationship for tumors can be affected by many factors. If the radiation survival curve is shallow for individual tumor cells (inherent radioresistance), then the dose-response curve for that tumor will also be shallow. Oxygen is an important modifier of the biologic effects of ionizing irradiation. The exact mechanism of the oxygen effect is unclear, but it is believed that oxygen affects the initial chemical products of the interactions of radiation with biologic material. Oxygen appears to favor the creation of free radicals or other highly reactive molecules.

Early in the history of the specialty of radiation oncology, it was recognized that fractionation affected cancerous and normal tissues in a variety of ways. Organs and tumors could be divided into acute and late-responding tissues. In general, acute effects are much more dependent on overall treatment time than late effects. Late effects are influenced primarily by the total dose and fraction size. Acute radiation effects occur largely in renewing tissues, such as skin, oropharyngeal mucosa, small intestine, rectum, and bladder mucosa. Acute effects are apparent during a course of radiation therapy and generally resolve within a few weeks or months. There is a balance between cell birth and cell death in these tissues. Late effects are most often the dose-limiting factor in radiation therapy. They are manifested months or years after completion of radiation therapy, and they are often irreversible. Late effects include necrosis, fibrosis, fistula formation, nonhealing ulceration, and damage to specific organs, such as spinal cord transection. Clinically, late effects appear to depend much more on the total dose of radiation and the radiation fraction size than on the duration of the radiation treatment course.

Tumor volume is an important factor in radiation therapy. The greater the tumor burden, the larger the radiation dose needed to eradicate it. Beyond the gross tumor periphery, the tumor cell density and burden decrease. Subclinical disease beyond the edge of gross tumor may respond more favorably to radiation because of the smaller number of malignant cells or improved oxygenation, or both, away from the central tumor. Radiation oncologists have adopted a shrinking-field technique, in which the volume of irradiation is decreased over the course of therapy. Modest doses of radiation are prescribed to larger volumes at risk of harboring subclinical disease, after which gross disease is boosted to a higher cumulative dose.

TRADITIONAL RADIATION SIMULATION AND TREATMENT PLANNING

Radiation therapy simulators were introduced in the 1970s to minimize the time required to set up patients for radiation therapy and to provide better diagnostic quality x-ray images on which the radiation oncologist could define the region to be treated. These simulators have identical isocentric gantry and table geometry as the treatment linear accelerators. Patient position is defined, and plain x-ray films of the treatment site are acquired. These films are then marked with wax or ink pens that indicate the treatment volume and shielding of normal structures. The films are then used to fabricate customized blocks that are to be mounted in the accelerator gantry at the time of treatment. At the time of simulation, indirect methods to identify the prostate gland on the simulation radiograph are used. Indwelling catheters or urethrograms with iodinated bladder contrast aid in defining the craniocaudal extent of the prostate. A rectal probe or radiopaque contrast assists in defining the posterior border. Anteriorly, the pubic bone limits the anterior extent of the gland.

Patient positioning is made reproducible with the aid of room setup lasers and immobilization devices. Skin markings or anatomic landmarks are aligned to laser lights that define the linear accelerator and treatment couch geometry. Occasionally, these skin marks are tattooed to ensure reproducibility. Foam or cast cradles can be used to conform to the shape of each patient while in the treatment position. These can then be used daily to duplicate body position on the treatment couch.

With traditional treatment planning, the geometry of the linear accelerator is generally limited to orthogonal (90-degree) angles. Anterior, posterior, and lateral radiation beam directions can be used to define treatment volumes based on clinical and radiographic landmarks. Although oblique treatment angles can be used, the possibility of geometric miss of the treatment target increases. Rotational methods with bilateral arcing gantry movements can be used for prostate irradiation to minimize treatment to the superficial tissues, but the field sizes need to be sufficient (10 cm × 10 cm to 12 cm × 12 cm) to ensure adequate target volume coverage. These arc or rotational methods can reduce bladder and rectal radiation doses when the prostate alone is being treated or boosted. If the pelvic lymph nodes are being electively irradiated, then orthogonal treatment geometry is preferred to encompass the internal and common iliac lymph nodes.

High-energy x-rays (greater than 10 MV) are preferred for patients treated with traditional radiation therapy planning for prostate cancer. The small number of radiation beam directions (two to four) concentrates radiation doses to subcutaneous tissues when low energies are used. High-energy x-rays avoid this superficial dose buildup that leads to subcutaneous fibrosis or other complications.

To verify that adequate radiation doses are being administered, a radiation treatment plan is created. The treatment plan reflects the radiation distribution in the patient from the shaped beams. Dosimetry information from the linear accelerator is used to indirectly compute the dose distribution of radiation to the target volume and surrounding critical structures. With traditional planning methods, the treatment will be represented on only one to three cross-sectional slices of a CT scan. Traditional treatment planning computers are unable to accommodate the full volumetric information on a complete CT data set. As a result, the limited information provided by the treatment plan may have missed undesirable dose distributions (hot or cold spots) outside of the plane of the calculated treatment plan.

Radiation therapy doses have been prescribed in a variety of ways that occasionally lead to confusion. Reporting a single dose parameter, such as central axis dose or the minimum dose delivered to a volume, may not fully describe the quality of the radiation distribution to a target or normal tissue. The International Commission on Radiation Units and Measurements (ICRU) (2) published guidelines for reporting, recording, and prescribing radiation doses. It is recommended that a dose to a central ICRU reference point (i.e., a point within the target volume, typically close to the isocenter of the radiation beams) be reported as well as the best estimates of maximum and minimum doses to the planned target volume and adjacent organs at risk.

Because of the heterogeneity of radiation distributions, the dose to the isocenter or ICRU reference can be 3% to 7% higher than the *minimum* dose to a target volume encompassing the prostate gland. This variation in dose reporting is critical, because the steep slope of the dose-response curve for prostate cancer is close to the tolerance doses of the bladder and rectum, the adjacent critical organs at risk.

CONFORMAL RADIATION THERAPY SIMULATION AND TREATMENT PLANNING

The availability of powerful computers and workstations has revolutionized the manner in which radiation therapy is delivered. CT has allowed capture of complete volumetric anatomic information on which a 3D-radiation therapy treatment plan can be developed. Unlike in traditional treatment planning, 3D CRT begins with the acquisition of a CT scan with the patient in the treatment position.

Patient Immobilization and Positioning

Patient immobilization devices are more frequently used in 3D CRT than in traditional treatment planning. Some investigators have reported improved treatment setup accuracy with these devices, whereas others have reported no significant advantage with their use (3,4). It is recommended that each treating physician study and review the treatment setup variations with either method and choose the one that gives the best reproducibility.

There is significant debate regarding the appropriate positioning for patients treated with localized prostate carcinoma. Some investigators advocate a prone position, which minimizes prostate positional uncertainty and the volume of rectum irradiated with CRT (5).

More recent data suggest that a prone position is associated with greater prostate motion accompanying normal ventilation. The increased intraabdominal pressure associated with breathing in a supine position results in significant movement of the prostate and SVs (6,7).

Target Volume Definition

To aid in the identification of the prostatic apex, a retrograde urethrogram can be performed. The prostatic apex is 3 mm to 13 mm above the most proximal aspect of the urogenital

TABLE 22-1. MARGINS NECESSARY TO ACCOUNT FOR UNCERTAINTY IN TREATMENT DELIVERY

					Total PTV margin		
Author	Position	Immobilization device	Organ	Margin SD[a] (CI%)	Anterior, posterior (mm)	Superior, inferior (mm)	Left, right (mm)
Rudat et al. (66)	Supine	None	P and SV	1 (68)	4.9	5.4[c]	3.5
Stroom et al. (67)	Supine prone	Knee foll	P and SV	$2\Sigma + 0.7\sigma^b$	8.3	8.2	4.0
		Belly board	P and SV		8.8	6.6	3.7
Tinger et al. (10)	Supine	Foam body cradle	P	2 (95)	8	8.8	6.4
			SV	2 (95)	9.6	8.2	7.0
Zelefsky et al. (68)	Prone	Thermoplastic body mask	P	1.5 (93)	3.6, 6.8	6.6, 6.7	5.0
			SV	1.5 (93)	5.8, 8.9	9.4, 8.0	7.2

Note: Data combine internal organ motion and setup error.
CI, confidence interval; P, prostate; PTV, planning target volume; SD, standard deviation; SV, seminal vesicles.
[a]Margins reported by authors correspond to variable probabilities of clinical target volume (CTV) coverage. Clinicians should adjust margin accordingly.
[b]$2\Sigma + 0.7\sigma$ corresponds to at least 95% dose covering (on average) 99% of the CTV.
[c]Margin reported for setup error only.

diaphragm, as defined by the urethrogram (8,9). Care should be taken not to overinflate the urethra with iodinated contrast, as this may distend or move the prostate from its relaxed position (7). A rubber catheter or hollow tube to deflate flatus in the rectum helps avoid the introduction of systematic errors in organ and target definition due to rectal distension (10). An enema before simulation will empty the rectum and allow the prostate to move to its most posterior position. This allows use of a tighter uncertainty margin posteriorly.

After the acquisition of the treatment planning CT scan, the image data need to be segmented for the treatment planning computer to render 3D images and compute dose to the various targets and normal organs. This target and normal organ definition can be done with a computer-pointing device, such as a mouse, and a drawing utility in the treatment-planning program. Organs with high contrast relative to adjacent tissues (skin, bone, and lung) can be segmented using automatic image-threshold identification utilities.

The critical element of 3D CRT is the identification of target volumes and normal organs at risk. The ICRU has encouraged the use of common terminology to describe the target volumes. The *gross tumor volume* (GTV) represents any disease that can be identified by imaging modalities or physical examination. Because prostate cancer is often found to be multifocal at the time of radical prostatectomy, the entire gland is considered the GTV for radiation treatment planning purposes. The *clinical target volume* (CTV) encompasses the GTV and adds margin for microscopic extension of disease. The CTV may expand the GTV to account for direct extension, or the CTV can be extended to encompass adjacent organs or regions of spread. In the case of prostate cancer, the CTV may encompass the SVs and, possibly, the regional pelvic lymph nodes. The *planning target volume* (PTV) envelops the CTV with a margin to account for uncertainties in treatment delivery. The uncertainties may be related to setup variations or internal organ motion. The magnitude of the PTV margin depends on several treatment-related factors. A technologist's inability to precisely reproduce a patient's position on a daily basis is one contributing factor. Some patients may move while on the treatment table because of fatigue or discomfort. Internal organs, including the prostate gland, can shift because of variable filling of the bladder and rectum. The shifts can be anisotropic, with most movement occurring in the anterior and posterior directions. Table 22-1 summarizes several studies of treatment uncertainty in prostate cancer patients. Each of these studies investigated internal organ motions and setup errors to determine an appropriate margin for the PTV. Increasing the size of the PTV margin increases the probability of encompassing the CTV by the prescribed isodose from a complete course of radiation therapy. To ensure that an adequate radiation dose is encompassing all areas at risk of harboring disease, the radiation oncologist needs to include an appropriate PTV margin. There is a trade-off between ensuring nearly 100% coverage during each treatment and that of the volume of adjacent organs irradiated unnecessarily. The PTV margin does not account for radiation beam penumbra. When beam aperture or field shape is defined, additional margin needs to be added to account for this dosimetric falloff near the edge of the beam.

Organs at risk need to be defined for the treatment planning process. In the treatment of prostate cancer, the organs at risk include the bladder, rectum, femoral heads, and, occasionally, the small bowel. There can be considerable variation in the definition of these organs from physician to physician. When dosimetric constraints and clinical outcomes from various series are compared, a consistent definition of these structures is important. The Radiation Therapy Oncology Group (RTOG) has described its method for normal organ definition (11). The femoral heads are contoured from the level of the ischial tuberosities to their proximal joint at the pelvis. The rectum and bladder are defined as solid organs. Inferiorly, the rectum is defined from the level of the ischial tuberosities; it extends superiorly until the colon moves anteriorly toward the sigmoid. The bladder is contoured inferiorly from the prostate base to the dome.

It has been argued that the bladder and rectum, being hollow organs, should have the inner contents subtracted from volumetric dose information. The remaining volume then represents the volume of the organ wall. Unfortunately, the calculation of wall volume is not a trivial task and requires either the added work of contouring the inner and outer rectal walls or additional software that is not available on many 3D CRT computer planning systems. As a result, most institutions and cooperative groups report dosimetry data to the whole organ volume. Early clinical outcomes suggest that wall volume may indeed be a more important parameter with respect to 3D dosimetry than the whole organ volume (12,13).

Beam Selection and Shaping

The process of beam selection and shaping with 3D CRT is analogous to the same process with conventional simulation. The 3D CRT planning systems display a "virtual patient" reconstructed from the CT image data and the segmented structures. Radiation beams can be added and displayed from the perspective of a subject in the treatment room (*room view* or *physician's eye view*) and from the perspective of the linear accelerator radiation source (*beam's eye view* or BEV). The BEV display allows a dosimetrist to set collimator positions and shape the field to encompass the projected PTV. The field shaping can be designated with free-hand shapes for Cerrobend blocks or with multileaf collimation (Fig. 22-3). The advantage that the BEV display offers over conventional simulation is the ability to actually see the spatial relationships of the target volume and organs at risk. The 3D renderings of the targets and adjacent organs can be adjusted with transparency or color controls to allow visualization of overlaps between them.

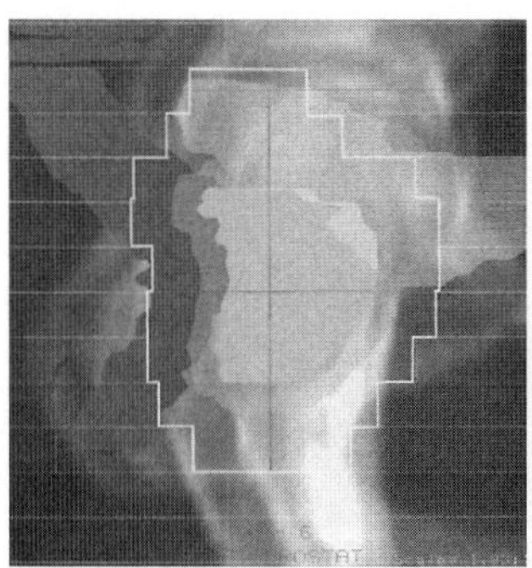

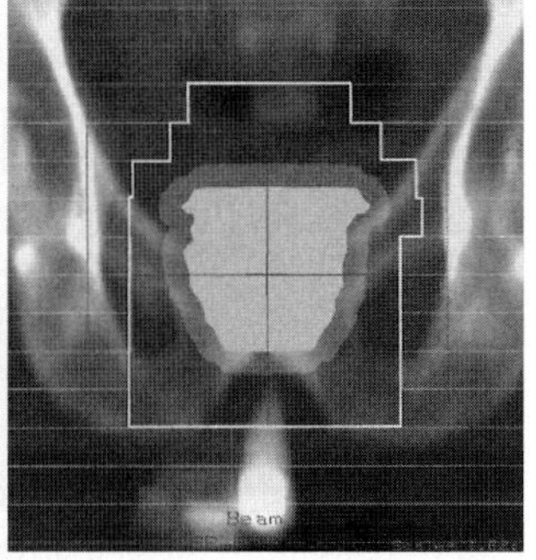

FIGURE 22-3. Beam's eye view displays of a right lateral prostate and anteroposterior fields. In addition to the gross tumor volume with planning target volume margin, the rectum and bladder contours are superimposed on the digitally reconstructed radiographs.

A critical enhancement of the BEV is the digitally reconstructed radiograph (DRR). The DRR is a projected plane x-ray image that is computed from the CT data. The DRR is helpful in the planning process and aids in treatment verification. In treatment planning, the DRR is used with the BEV to assist the physician or dosimetrist to define the treatment aperture. If all nearby anatomic structures have not been contoured, then the DRR helps to identify possible unintentional irradiation of those regions.

PLAN OPTIMIZATION AND REVIEW

After application of multiple radiation beams and shaping with BEV tools, the treatment planning computer will calculate the radiation distribution based on the characteristics of the treatment machine's x-ray output. The radiation dose distribution can be displayed on the segmented patient CT data with color-wash or wire-frame contours (Fig. 22-4). Room-view displays with interactive, real-time image manipulation tools help to review the adequacy of the dose distribution. Areas of radiation underdose to a target or overdose to an organ at risk can be identified.

Review of multiple dose levels is difficult with room-view displays because of overlap and crowding of objects on the computer screen. Planar two-dimensional (2D) displays of cross-sectional axial or reconstructed sagittal and coronal CT scans facilitate review of multiple dose levels.

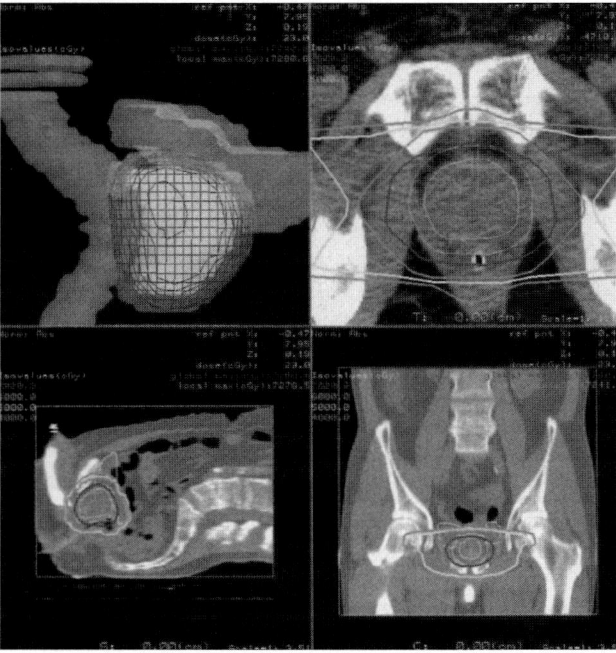

FIGURE 22-4. Isodose display in three-dimensional (3D) room view *(upper left)* and planar reconstructions. The 3D view displays the wire frame contour of the 70-Gy isodose volume. The axial, sagittal, and coronal views display the 70-, 60-, 50-, and 40-Gy isodose lines around the gross tumor volume and planning target volume.

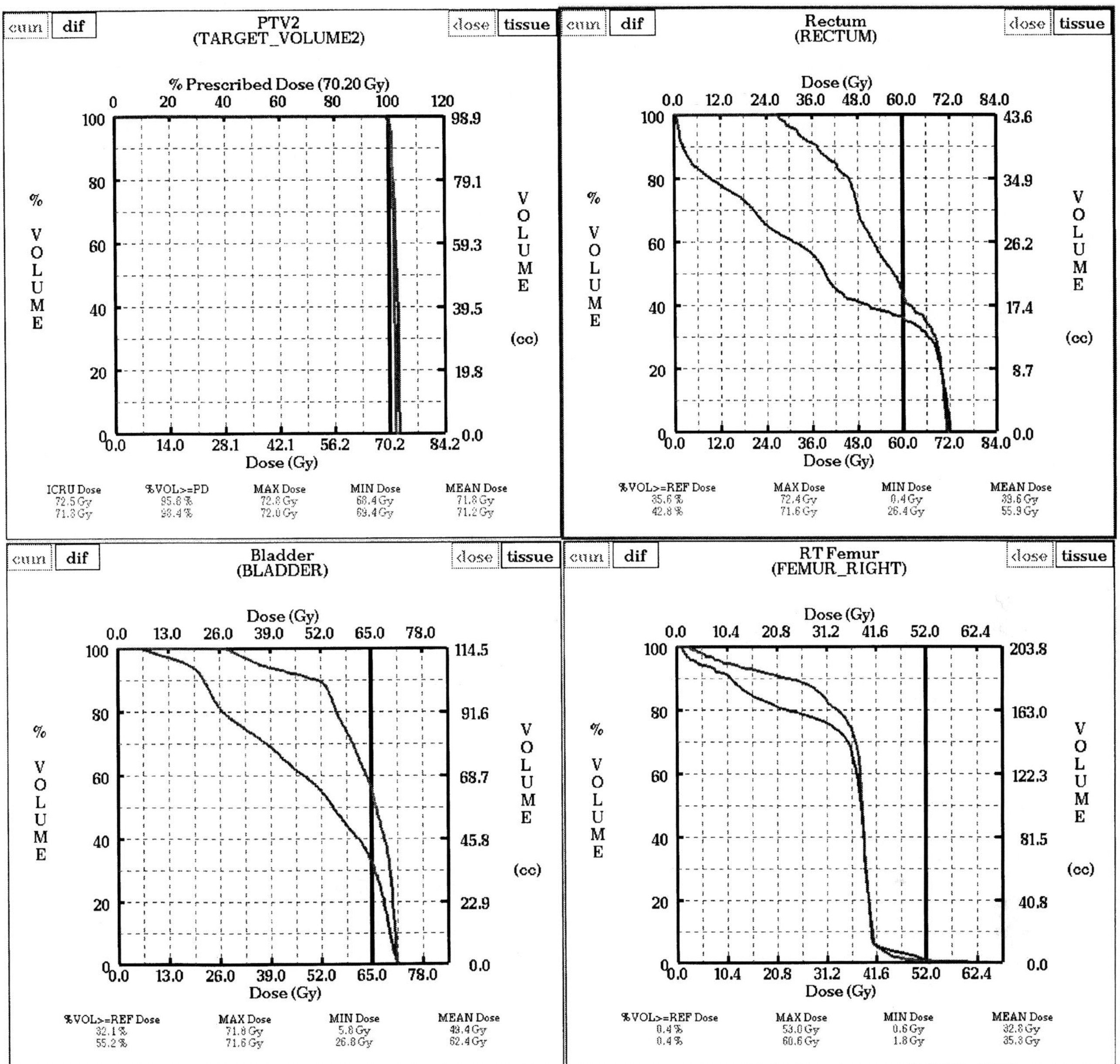

FIGURE 22-5. Cumulative dose-volume histograms of the planning target volume (PTV), bladder, rectum, and left femoral head. One plan represented includes nonconformal treatment to the whole pelvis (46 Gy) with a conformal prostate boost (70 Gy). The second plan represents conformal treatment to the prostate alone (70 Gy). Both plans deliver adequate dose to the PTV, but the boost-only plan treats substantially less rectum and bladder to high doses. cum, cumulative; dif, differential; ICRU, International Commission on Radiation Units and Measurements.

The room-view and 2D image reconstructions limit the radiation oncologist to a few dose levels reviewed at one time. To take advantage of the complete dosimetric data available for plan interpretation, dose-volume histograms (DVHs) are calculated. DVHs summarize the complete dose distribution to a target or organ at risk in a linear graph model. On the horizontal axis, the radiation dose can be represented in gray (Gy) or as a percent of the prescribed dose. The vertical axis represents the organ volume in cubic centimeters or as a percent of the whole organ. A differential DVH is a plot of equally spaced dose bins. A cumulative or integral DVH is a plot of the volume of a structure receiving more than a certain dose. The cumulative DVH is generally more helpful for plan interpretation and review (Fig. 22-5).

The DVH facilitates identification that an underdosed region of a target or an overdosed region of an organ at risk exists. The DVH can be displayed with dose statistics, such as minimum, maximum, or mean dose to the volume. The most significant shortcoming of the DVH is the lack of spatial information provided. The DVH may reveal that an unacceptable dose distribution is present, but it does not illustrate its location. For this reason, the DVH, room-view, and 2D reconstructions are complementary.

The radiation therapy planning process is iterative. The plan is created by a dosimetrist and then reviewed by the radiation oncologist and physicist. It is common for the plan to be redone with modifications in field shaping or with a change in the relative dose contribution per field to optimize the dose distribution.

RADIATION TREATMENT PRESCRIPTION

The radiation oncologist must decide the specific volumes requiring treatment and the radiation dose and fractionation schedule to be used. It is common to use variable dose levels depending on the likely volume of disease. Regions that are at risk of harboring microscopic or subclinical disease can be managed with radiation doses in the 45- to 50-Gy range. Gross disease requires radiation doses that approach or exceed 70 Gy. These different doses are accomplished by field or treatment volume reductions (shrinking-field technique) during the course of therapy. The pelvic lymph nodes can be treated with a large field to a dose of 45 Gy, followed by a boost to the prostate or prostate with SVs to a total exceeding 70 Gy.

TARGET VOLUME

Pelvic Lymph Nodes

Significant controversy exists as to whether there is any benefit to elective irradiation of the pelvic lymph nodes. The RTOG has conducted prospective clinical trials to address this issue. The RTOG 77-06 failed to show any difference in survival or patterns of failure in 445 patients with stage A2 and B tumors treated to the pelvis (45 Gy) and the prostate (additional 20 Gy) or the prostate only (65 Gy) (14). Leibel et al. (15) also reported in a series from Memorial Sloan-Kettering Cancer Center that pelvic lymph node irradiation offered no improvement in outcome over prostate irradiation alone in patients with lymph node metastases. Data published by Perez et al. (16) show a slightly lower incidence of pelvic failure in patients with poorly differentiated stage C cancers receiving greater than 50 Gy to the pelvis (23% vs. 46%, $p < .01$), but there were no survival or disease-free survival differences.

One of the important criticisms of these studies, prospective and retrospective alike, is that they may not have studied the patient population most likely to benefit. To show an advantage to pelvic irradiation, the patient population should be at high risk of having lymph node metastases without spread beyond. Furthermore, the effectiveness of the 65-Gy prescription for the primary tumor is doubtful. The RTOG completed accrual to another randomized study in the year 2000 that is expected to end the controversy. In the RTOG 94-13 study, patients at high risk of disease have been randomized to receive pelvic irradiation, 50.4 Gy plus a prostate boost (additional 19.8 Gy, 70.2 Gy total) versus prostate irradiation alone (70.2 Gy). A second randomization assigned patients to receive total androgen suppression therapy for 4 months versus no hormone therapy. High-risk disease is defined as having a lymph node metastasis rate of greater than 15%.

A preliminary analysis of these data from RTOG 94-13 suggests a significant advantage to whole pelvic irradiation when combined with neoadjuvant hormone therapy (M. Roach, *personal communication*, 2001). Partin et al. published tabulated data summarizing the risk of disease spread beyond the prostate gland in 4,133 men who underwent radical prostatectomy. The Partin (17) tables and other published nomograms have been helpful in estimating this risk. Roach et al. (18) described an equation that helps to estimate this risk:

$$\text{Risk of positive lymph node} = \tfrac{2}{3}\,\text{PSA} + [(\text{GS} - 6) \times 10]$$

The prostate-specific antigen (*PSA*) is the highest value before therapy, and *GS* is the biopsy Gleason score.

At the Mallinckrodt Institute of Radiology, we continue to electively irradiate the pelvis in patients with a high risk of lymph node metastases. This includes patients with Gleason scores greater than or equal to 8, initial PSA of greater than 20, or stage T3 disease. These patients will also receive neoadjuvant and adjuvant hormone therapy that may augment the oncolytic effects of radiation on prostate cancer (19–21).

Prostate and Seminal Vesicles

Given the multifocal nature of most prostate cancers, it is generally assumed that the entire prostate needs to be irradiated. Pickett et al. (22) have suggested that the dominant intraprostatic lesion, as defined by spectroscopic magnetic resonance imaging, could be boosted above the dose to the entire gland. This approach would require intensity-modulated radiation therapy (IMRT), a technique discussed later in this chapter.

The SVs are frequently invaded by cancer, even in patients without clinical evidence of tumor extension. This finding has led some physicians to recommend SV irradiation in all patients, disregarding the risk factors predictive of extension (23). Just as with lymph node metastases, data published by Partin et al. (17), Roach et al. (18), and others can help to identify patients who have a low risk of SV invasion. Diaz et al. (24) reported a significant reduction in the rectal dose if the SVs were excluded from the high-dose region; 20% of the rectal volume received on average above 86% of the total dose for five plans that included the SVs, compared to 68% for the five plans excluding the SVs. The doses to 40% of the rectal volume were 64% and 37% if the SVs were included and excluded, respectively.

The RTOG 94-06 dose-escalation study for CRT used target volumes that were based on the risk of SV invasion. For patients with clinical evidence of extraprostatic extension (T3), the prostate and SVs were considered the CTV for the entire prescribed study dose (group 3). Patients with T1-T2 cancers were irradiated to the SVs only if the calculated probability of invasion exceeded 15% (group 2). SV invasion risk was calculated using the formula (18)

$$\% \text{ SV risk} = \text{PSA} + ([\text{GS} - 6] \times 10).$$

The minimum dose to the PTV_1 (target encompassing prostate and SVs) was 55.8 Gy, after which the PTV_2 (target encompassing prostate only) was boosted to the study dose (range, 68.4 to 79.2 Gy). Patients with T1-T2 cancers with less than a 15% risk of SV invasion (group 1) were treated to the prostate only (11). All radiation doses were prescribed as a minimum to each PTV in that study.

DOSIMETRIC ADVANTAGES OF THREE-DIMENSIONAL CONFORMAL RADIATION THERAPY

Several studies have demonstrated a significant advantage in the use of 3D CRT over traditional treatment planning. Ten Haken et al. (25) showed that conventional radiation delivery methods using rotational arc techniques with field sizes ranging from 6 cm × 6 cm to 8 cm × 8 cm would be adequate only for small-stage T1 and T2a prostate cancers. An 8-cm × 8-cm field size is insufficient to cover large prostates or those with locally advanced disease. Larger field sizes also radiated more normal tissues than customized fields using BEV technology. Perez et al. (26) compared 174 patients planned with 3D CRT or standard radiation therapy and demonstrated that, when field sizes were adjusted to adequately encompass the PTV, there was a significant reduction in the volumes of bladder and rectum irradiated with the conformal technique. Table 22-2 summarizes these data.

TABLE 22-2. COMPARISON OF MEAN DOSIMETRIC PARAMETERS FOR THREE-DIMENSIONAL (3D) CONFORMAL OR STANDARD BILATERAL ARC ROTATION IN CARCINOMA OF THE PROSTATE

	Prostate irradiation only	
Parameter	3D conformal therapy	Standard therapy
Number of observations	87	87
Percent PTV receiving ≥ prescribed dose	92.9 ± 13.9	92.9 ± 10.8
ICRU dose (Gy)	69.1 ± 2.6	69.2 ± 2.6
Minimum tumor dose (Gy)	66.3 ± 5.3	63.5 ± 8.6
Mean tumor dose (Gy)	69.8 ± 2.6	69.7 ± 2.8
Maximum dose (Gy)	71.7 ± 2.4	71.3 ± 2.8
Percent volume rectum ≥65 Gy	33.7 ± 15	62.7 ± 21
Percent volume rectum ≥70 Gy	8.5 ± 11.8	28.8 ± 28.9
Percent volume bladder ≥65 Gy	22.3 ± 12.5	50.5 ± 22.8
Percent volume bladder ≥70 Gy	6.3 ± 8.4	19.4 ± 24.4

ICRU, International Commission on Radiation Units and Measurements; PTV, planning target volume.
From Perez CA, Michalski JM, Ballard S, et al. Cost benefit of emerging technology in localized carcinoma of the prostate. *Int J Radiat Oncol Biol Phys* 1997;39:875–883, with permission.

TREATMENT DELIVERY AND PATIENT MANAGEMENT

External beam radiation therapy is administered in once-daily fractions, 5 days per week over a period of 7 to 8 weeks. Each treatment session lasts approximately 10 to 20 minutes. On a weekly basis, the patients are seen by the radiation oncologist to assess tolerance to therapy and tumor response. Prostate cancer generally does not respond rapidly to radiation, so the prostate examination is unlikely to change.

Patients may report mild to moderate urinary and bowel symptoms. These may be more frequent and severe in patients receiving elective pelvic irradiation. The incidence of acute sequelae is equal or reduced in patients receiving CRT (27,28). Urinary symptoms may include dysuria, nocturia, and urinary urgency. It is occasionally necessary to rule out concomitant infection. These symptoms are managed with antispasmodics (e.g., hyoscyamine, oxybutynin, flavoxate, tolterodine) or phenazopyridine. Bowel symptoms include loose or more frequent bowel movements, tenesmus, or pain. Antiinflammatory suppositories containing hydrocortisone or mesalamine may reduce symptoms. A low-fiber diet can reduce the risk of diarrhea. Loperamide or diphenoxylate can control this symptom.

Treatment position is verified on a weekly basis by comparing the simulation radiograph or DRR to portal radiographs acquired on the linear accelerator during treatment (Fig. 22-6). These portal films are used to identify errors in patient setup and positioning. As 3D CRT is leading to dose escalation and shrinking margins for setup uncertainty, the frequency of checking portal films may need to be increased to twice weekly, especially for the first 2 weeks of therapy (29). Bel et al. (30) proposed an algorithm for digital portal imaging that reduces the magnitude of systematic error in setup over a course of radiation therapy.

RESULTS WITH EXTERNAL IRRADIATION

Prostate-Specific Antigen Outcome

PSA levels drawn during radiation therapy may show transient elevations that may be related to acinar cell death with release of PSA into the circulation (31). After radiation therapy, PSA levels decline gradually over the next 1 to 2 years. It is unclear whether the rate of fall carries any significant prognostic value. Hancock et al. (32) reported that patients who

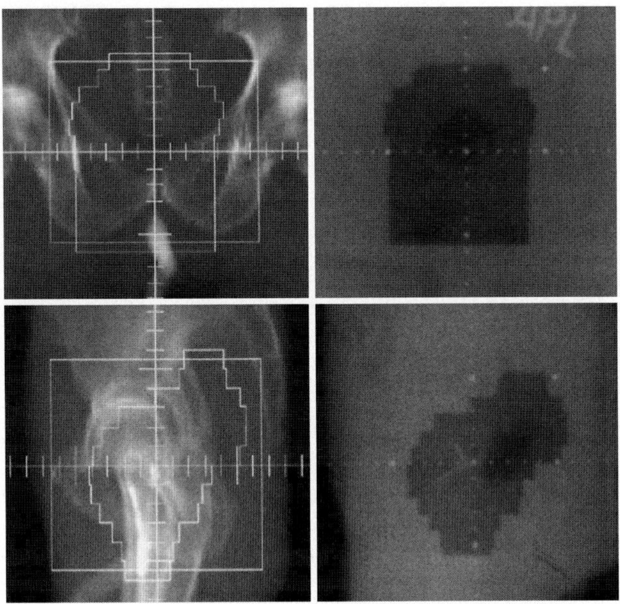

A,B

FIGURE 22-6. Digitally reconstructed radiograph **(A)** of an anteroposterior and left lateral prostate field and corresponding portal radiographs **(B)** used for treatment verification.

reached a postirradiotherapy PSA nadir more than 2 years after treatment had a risk of biochemical recurrence 18 times greater than patients who reached a nadir in less than 1 year.

Significant controversy exists regarding the appropriate nadir level that may correspond to long-term freedom from recurrence. Willett et al. (33) determined the PSA levels in 36 men who received pelvic irradiation (45 Gy to 65 Gy) for nonprostatic malignancies and compared them with those of 79 men of similar age without prostate cancer or pelvic irradiation. A group of 27 patients with prostate cancer who were treated with 68 Gy and who were disease-free were also evaluated. The median PSA level was 0.65 ng per mL in the patients receiving pelvic irradiation for nonprostatic malignancies, 1.1 ng per mL in the nonirradiated control group, and 0.5 ng per mL in patients previously treated for prostate cancer. These data suggest that patients whose PSA values do not reach less than 1 ng per mL after definitive irradiation for prostate cancer are unlikely to be long-term disease-free survivors. Kavadi et al. (34) demonstrated that a nadir of 1 ng per mL or less was an independent predictor of biochemical outcome. The 5-year biochemical relapse rate for patients who achieved nadir levels less than 1 ng per mL was 17%, compared to 70% with posttreatment nadir levels of greater than 1 ng per mL. A nadir level of less than or equal to 0.5 ng per mL does not predict for further improvement in outcome. Others have also demonstrated that PSA nadir values of less than 1 ng per mL are independent variables that predict for improved biochemical outcome (35,36).

In 1997, the American Society of Therapeutic Radiology and Oncology (37) gathered a panel of urologic radiation oncology experts to discuss the significance of postirradiation PSA values. This American Society of Therapeutic Radiology and Oncology consensus panel argued that postirradiation PSA nadir was an important prognostic variable, similar to pretreatment PSA value and Gleason score. The absolute PSA nadir value is not a surrogate or intermediate end point for defining treatment outcome. The panel established the definition of PSA relapse as three consecutive rises from a nadir level. For purposes of clinical trials or reports, the date of failure should be considered the midpoint between postirradiation nadir PSA and the first of three consecutive increases. It was recommended that series be presented for publication with a minimum observation of 24 months and that PSA determinations be obtained at 3- or 4-month intervals during the first 2 years after the completion of radiation therapy. Three consecutive rises were chosen to exclude the possibility of a benign PSA bounce (38).

PROSTATE BIOPSIES AFTER DEFINITIVE IRRADIATION

Microscopic disappearance of tumor, fibrosis, obliteration of glandular structure, and calcifications in the prostate have been reported after definitive radiation therapy. The number of positive biopsy specimens decreases with time; only those that show persistent tumors more than 18 months after radiation therapy may have clinical significance (39). Cell death after radiation therapy is a postmitotic event. In view of the long doubling time of many prostate tumors, cells that harbor biologically lethal damage but have not had an opportunity to morphologically express it may be misinterpreted as viable cancer. Patients with early positive biopsies after radiation therapy may convert to having a negative repeat biopsy with further follow-up. Cox and Kline (39,40) reported that the positive biopsy rate decreased from 19% at 24 months to 15% at 42 months in a series of 46 patients. Scardino (41) confirmed this observation, reporting that 32% of patients with a positive biopsy at 12 months had a negative pathologic specimen at 24 months.

Crook et al. (42) have studied a cohort of 498 men treated with conventional radiation therapy followed with systematic transrectal ultrasound-guided postirradiation prostate biopsies. The biopsies were started 12 to 18 months after receiving a radiation dose of 66 Gy. If there was residual tumor but further decline in the PSA, then biopsies were repeated every 6 to12 months. Patients with negative biopsies were rebiopsied at 36 months. At 5 years, freedom from clinical or histologic evidence of local recurrence was 83% for T1b, 88% for T1c, 72% for T2a, 66% for T2b and c, 58% for T3, and 0% for T4 tumors. The proportion of biopsies described as indeterminate decreased with time, being 33% for the first biopsy (median interval since radiation therapy, 13 months), 24% for the second biopsy (median interval since radiation therapy, 28 months), 18% for the third biopsy (median interval since radiation therapy, 36 months), and 7% for the fourth biopsy (median interval since irradiation, 44 months). They concluded that the timing of the biopsy is critical and seems to be the most predictive of outcome in the 24- to 36-month period after radiation therapy. By themselves, postirradiation prostate biopsies are not an indicator of treatment efficacy, but they are independent predictors of outcome.

Crook et al. (43) suggested that proliferating cell nuclear antigen (PCNA) staining might be useful to evaluate postirradiation prostate biopsies. Negative PCNA in a positive biopsy predicts for eventual resolution of tumor (83% to 97% of cases). On the other hand, positive PCNA correlates with local failure (49% to 79%) but, when present in an early biopsy (12 to 18 months), may eventually disappear.

CLINICAL OUTCOME WITH CONVENTIONAL AND THREE-DIMENSIONAL CONFORMAL RADIATION THERAPY

Zagars and Pollack (44) reported 5-year outcome after conventional external beam radiation therapy in 461 patients with stage T1-T2 disease. The 5-year biochemical disease-free survival rates for patients with pretreatment PSA levels of 0 to 4 ng per mL, greater than 4 to 10 ng per mL, greater than 10 to 20 ng per mL, and greater than 20 ng per mL were 91%, 69%, 62%, and 38%, respectively.

Shipley et al. (45) reported a multiinstitutional experience of 1,765 patients with T1 to T2 cancers treated with external beam radiation therapy. The PSA failure-free rates 5 and 7 years after treatment for patients presenting with a PSA of less than 10 ng per mL were 77.8% and 72.9%, respectively. Recursive partitioning analysis of initial PSA level, palpation stage, and the Gleason score groupings yielded four separate prognostic groups: group 1, patients with a PSA level of less than 9.2 ng per mL; group 2, PSA level greater than or equal to 9.2 to 19.7 ng per mL; group 3, PSA greater than or equal to 19.7 ng per mL and a Gleason score of 2 to 6; and group 4, PSA level greater than or equal to 19.7 ng per mL and a Gleason score of 7 to 10. The estimated rates of survival, free of biochemical failure at 5 years, were 81% for group 1, 69% for group 2, 47% for group 3, and 29% for group 4 (Fig. 22-7). Of the 302 patients followed up beyond 5 years who were free of biochemical disease, only 5% relapsed from the fifth to the eighth year.

Roach et al. (46) summarized results of 1,557 men treated with radiation therapy alone on four prospective clinical trials conducted by the RTOG between 1975 and 1992. Most of the patients had tumors clinically staged as T3 (59%), and 87 (36%) patients with clinical stage T1-T2 tumors had pathologically positive lymph nodes. The 10-year disease-specific survival for patients with a Gleason score of 2 to 5, 6 to 7, and 8 to 10 was 87%, 75%, and 44%, respectively. Gleason score was the single most important predictor of death.

The data from these large series demonstrate that conventional radiation therapy yields excellent long-term cancer-free survival for patients with favorable prognostic factors. Patients with unfavorable features, such as a high Gleason score or high initial PSA, require more aggressive treatment.

Dose Escalation

Prostate cancer has long been recognized as a dose-responsive neoplasm (47,48). Attempts at escalating the radiation dose beyond 70 Gy with standard 2D techniques have resulted in an unacceptable rate of rectal and other complications. Smit et al. (49) reported a dose-escalation study using conventional radiation therapy techniques. The 2-year rate of moderate to severe proctitis increased from 20% for patients receiving less than 75 Gy to 60% for those receiving higher dose levels.

The ability to reduce the volume of normal tissue that receives high radiation doses is central to the success of 3D CRT. Late effects of radiation therapy are related not only to the dose administered, but also to the volume of normal tissues that exceed that threshold. The availability of 3D CRT treatment-planning systems has prompted the initia-

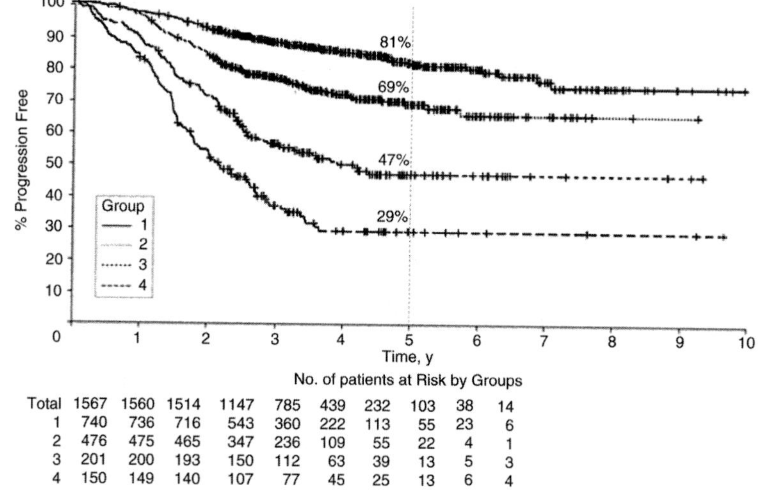

FIGURE 22-7. Estimated rates of no biochemical recurrence according to groupings by prognostic factor categories determined by recursive partitioning analysis. In group 1,116 of 740 patients were diagnosed as having an initial prostate-specific antigen (PSA) level of 9.2 ng per mL. In group 2, 130 of 476 patients were diagnosed as having an initial PSA level of 9.2 to less than 19.7 ng per mL. In group 3, 96 of 201 patients were diagnosed as having an initial PSA level of at least 19.7 ng per mL and a Gleason score from 2 to 6. In group 4, 97 of 150 patients were diagnosed as having an initial PSA level of at least 19.7 ng per mL and a Gleason score from 7 to 10. The *p* value is <.001 between all groups. (From Shipley WU, Thames HD, Sandler HM, et al. Radiation therapy for clinically localized prostate cancer: a multiinstitutional pooled analysis. *JAMA* 1999;17:1598–1604, with permission.)

TABLE 22-3. CARCINOMA OF THE PROSTATE: GRADES 2 TO 3 LATE SEQUELAE CORRELATED WITH TREATMENT GROUP

	3D conformal radiation therapy (n = 146)	Standard radiation therapy	
		Pelvic irradiation (n = 29)	Prostate and seminal vesicle irradiation (n = 102)
Proctitis	3 (1.7%)	2 (6.9%)	10 (9.8%)
Perianal abscess	—	—	1 (1%)
Fecal incontinence	—	—	1 (1%)
Small bowel obstruction	—	—	1 (1%)
Cystitis	1 (0.7%)	2 (6.9%)	1 (1%)
Urethral stricture	1 (0.7%)	—	1 (1%)

3D, three-dimensional.
From Perez CA, Michalski JM, Purdy JA, et al. Three-dimensional conformal therapy or standard irradiation in localized carcinoma of the prostate: preliminary results of a nonrandomized comparison. *Int J Radiat Oncol Biol Phys* 2000;47:629–637, with permission.

tion of several single and multiinstitutional prospective dose-escalation clinical trials.

At the Mallinckrodt Institute of Radiology, 6% to 9% of patients treated with standard radiation therapy reported moderately severe urinary symptoms compared with 2% to 5% of patients treated with 3D CRT. Moderate dysuria and nocturia were reported by 25% to 36% of patients in the standard treatment group compared with 27% to 33% of those treated with 3D CRT. The incidence of moderate diarrhea, usually after the fourth week of treatment, was 9% to 21% in the standard group and only 3% to 6% in the 3D CRT group. Chronic intestinal morbidity (proctitis, rectal bleeding) was very low (1.7%) in the 3D CRT group in contrast to the standard group (8%) (50) (Table 22-3). There was a significant improvement in biochemical disease-free survival in patients treated with 3D CRT. This improvement was seen even in patients treated with doses of less than or equal to 70 Gy, suggesting that 3D CRT by itself has improved tumor control by better targeting.

Decreased toxicity has been reported with 3D CRT, even when higher than standard irradiation doses are administered. Sandler et al. (51) reported the University of Michigan experience in 721 patients treated with 3D CRT. They described only 3% incidence of grade 3 or greater rectal morbidity. An update confirmed these findings (52). There were no grade 4 complications.

From the Fox Chase Cancer Center, Hanks et al. (53) reported 34% grade 2 toxicity in 247 patients treated with 3D CRT in comparison with 57% in 162 patients receiving standard irradiation. Only 12 gastrointestinal or genitourinary grade 3 complications were noted in the entire group of 409 patients. Patients in both the 3D CRT and standard radiation therapy groups receiving pelvic irradiation had a somewhat greater incidence of late treatment sequelae. Lee et al. (36) observed grade 2 to 3 rectal morbidity in 46 of 257 patients (18%) with 3D CRT; the majority of cases consisted of some rectal bleeding. The incidence of rectal morbidity was increased when higher doses of irradiation were delivered, particularly more than 76 Gy (actuarial rate of 23% at 18 months, compared with 7% to 16% with lower doses). However, when a rectal block on the lateral fields was interposed for the last 10 Gy of treatment, rectal morbidity was decreased to 10%.

Koper et al. (54) from Rotterdam reported a randomized trial of patients with T1-4N0M0 prostate cancer treated to 66 Gy (134 with conventional irradiation and 129 with 3D CRT). They observed reduced intestinal toxicity, primarily less anal toxicity in patients irradiated with 3D CRT. This was associated with a reduction in the anal volume irradiated (most distal 3 cm of the rectum).

Dearnaley et al. (55) updated results of a trial initially reported by Tait et al. (28) and reported that proctitis grade 1 or higher in severity occurred in 56% of patients receiving standard radiation, in contrast to 37% of those treated with 3D CRT ($p = .004$). Also, rectal bleeding occurred more frequently in the standard group (12%) than in the 3D CRT group (3%).

Zelefsky et al. (56) updated their experience with 743 patients with prostate cancer (stage T1c-T3) treated with 3D CRT to a target that always included the prostate and SVs; doses ranged from 64.8 to 81.0 Gy. With a median follow-up of 42 months, the 5-year actuarial incidence of grade 2 or 3 late gastrointestinal toxicity was 11.00% and 0.75%, respectively. The 5-year actuarial probability of developing grade 2 or 3 late genitourinary toxicity was 10% or 3%, respectively. On multivariate analysis, doses of 75.6 Gy or greater, history of diabetes mellitus, and the presence of acute gastrointestinal symptoms during treatment were independent predictors for grade 2 or 3 gastrointestinal toxicity. Among 544 patients who were potent before treatment, 211 (39%) became impotent after 3D CRT. Loss of erectile function was associated with doses of 75.6 Gy or higher and the use of neoadjuvant androgen deprivation. In a subsequent report on patients with stage T1c-T3 prostate cancer, 61 of whom were treated with 3D CRT and 171 with IMRT to doses of 81 Gy, the authors noted that the 2-year actuarial risk of grade 2 rectal bleeding was 10% for 3D CRT and only 2% for IMRT (57).

Michalski et al. (11) reported on the RTOG 94-06 prospective phase I dose-escalation study with 3D CRT for localized prostate cancer. Doses ranged from 68.4 Gy (level I) to 73.8 Gy (level II) and subsequently to 79.2 Gy (level III) with 1.8-Gy daily fractions. Data from RTOG 75-06 and 77-06 were used to calculate the expected probability of a greater than or equal to grade 3 late effect more than 120 days after the start of treatment. Group 1 and 2 cases (n = 288) were analyzed for toxicity. At dose level I, no grade 3 or worse late effects were observed when 9.1 and 4.8 complications were expected (p = .003 and p = .028), respectively, when compared to historical RTOG controls. At dose level II, there were no grade 3 or greater toxicities in group 1 patients and a single grade 3 toxicity in a group 2 patient when 12.1 and 13.0 complications were expected (p = .0005 and p = .0003), respectively.

Dose Response and Improved Tumor Control Probability

Fox Chase Cancer Center

Hanks et al. (58) conducted a dose-escalation study that began in 1989. Over the 1990s, they have implemented a program of image-guided radiation therapy simulation and treatment planning that has allowed them to gradually increase the irradiation dose to the ICRU reference from 6,260 cGy to 8,085 cGy in men with clinically localized prostate cancer. The results of this prospective clinical trial have recently been summarized. The 5-year biochemical disease-free survival was significantly improved for patients who had a pretreatment PSA greater than 10 and who received more than 76 Gy. Those patients with an initial PSA of 10.0 to 19.9 had a 5-year biochemical disease-free survival of 29%, 57%, and 73% if they received less than 71.5 Gy, 71.5 to 75.6 Gy, and greater than or equal to 75.6 Gy, respectively (p = .02). Patients with an initial PSA greater than 20 had a 5-year biochemical disease-free survival rate of 8%, 28%, and 30% if they received less than 71.5 Gy, 71.5 to 75.6 Gy, and greater than or equal to 75.6 Gy, respectively (p = .02). In that analysis, patients with an initial PSA less than 10 did not benefit from dose escalation (59). Subsequently, these investigators have divided their patient population into six subgroups. In addition to the three groups divided by initial PSA, they were grouped by favorable (T1,2a, Gleason score less than or equal to 6, and no perineural invasion) and unfavorable prognostic factors (one or more of T2b, T3, Gleason 7 to 10, perineural invasion) (58). Favorable patients with an initial PSA of less than 10 continued to show no improvement with dose escalation. Likewise, favorable patients with PSA of 10.0 to 19.9 also did not benefit from dose escalation. Unfavorable patients with an initial PSA of less than 10 and 10.0 to 19.9 demonstrated a 22% and 31% improvement in biochemical disease-free survival, respectively, if they received more than 77 Gy to the isocenter. Patients with an initial PSA of greater than 20 had a 40% improvement in biochemical disease-free survival if they received more than 77 Gy to the isocenter (p = .0029). Patients with favorable prognostic factors and a low initial PSA likely have small-volume disease that can be eradicated with doses between 70 and 75 Gy. Patients with unfavorable risk factors or high PSA may have improvement in local control with high irradiation doses. Patients with unfavorable risk factors and high PSA may have metastatic disease and, therefore, do not appear to benefit from the improvement in local control.

Memorial Sloan-Kettering Cancer Center

Radiation oncologists at Memorial Sloan-Kettering have been conducting a phase I dose escalation trial of 3D CRT for men with localized adenocarcinoma of the prostate. Zelefsky et al. (23) have summarized PSA relapse-free survival for 743 patients treated in this study. They divided patients into three prognostic groups by pretreatment PSA less than or equal to 10 ng per mL, stage T1-2 disease, and a Gleason score of less than or equal to 6. When all three indicators were present, the patient was classified in a favorable prognosis group. An increase in the value of any one of the indicators classified the patient in an intermediate group and two or more in an unfavorable prognosis group.

Patients in the favorable-risk group did not benefit from high-dose radiation therapy. The 5-year biochemical disease-free survival was excellent with any of the doses studied. Patients with intermediate- and high-risk disease who received a minimum PTV dose of greater than or equal to 75.6 Gy had a significant improvement in PSA-free survival (p = .04 and p = .03, respectively). In this trial, when patients were treated with doses in excess of 75.6 Gy, the investigators changed the treatment approach to IMRT. The topic of IMRT will be addressed later. Leibel et al. (60) reported the results of postirradiation biopsies performed more than 2.5 years after 3D CRT on 220 patients. Of patients who received 81 Gy, 30 of 33 (91%) patients had negative biopsies compared with 74 of 97 (76%) after 75.6 Gy, 44 of 67 (66%) after 70.2 Gy, and 11 of 23 (48%) after 64.8 Gy.

French Series

A multiinstitutional trial was initiated among five French hospitals in 1995 (61). The objective of the study was to test the feasibility and tolerance of increased doses from 66 to 80 Gy in patients with localized prostate cancer. In a preliminary analysis, patients were divided into a low-dose group (66 to 70 Gy) or a high-dose group (74 to 80 Gy). There was no difference between the two groups with respect to the incidence of late gastrointestinal and urinary toxicities. The probability of achieving a posttreatment PSA nadir of less than or equal to 1 ng per mL was significantly higher in the dose-escalation group and was directly related to the dose of irradiation given.

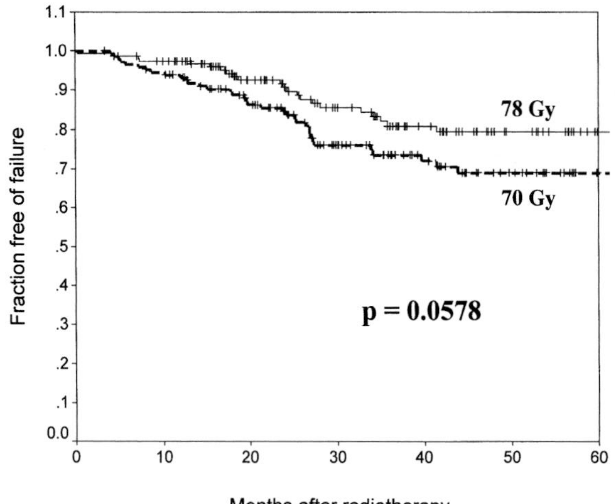

FIGURE 22-8. Kaplan-Meier fraction free-of-failure curves for all patients by dose randomization (70 vs. 78 Gy). The numbers of patients at risk at 10-month intervals are shown above the graph. (From Pollack A, Zagars GK, Smith LG, et al. Preliminary results of a randomized radiotherapy dose-escalation study comparing 70 Gy with 78 Gy for prostate cancer. *J Clin Oncol* 2000;18:3904–3911, with permission.)

M. D. Anderson Cancer Center

Pollack and Zagars (62) reviewed the clinical outcomes of 938 men consecutively treated between 1987 and 1995 at M. D. Anderson Cancer Center. Despite having more aggressive pretreatment prognostic features, men who received higher radiation doses had a better freedom-from-failure rate than men receiving lower doses. The only patients who did not appear to benefit from higher irradiation doses were those with a pretreatment PSA of less than 4 ng per mL. For all other pretreatment PSA groups, there was incremental increased freedom from failure with a dose of greater than 67 to 77 Gy or greater than 77 Gy. Pollack et al. (63) updated the M. D. Anderson Cancer Center experience with 1,127 consecutively treated patients in the PSA era. The analysis largely confirmed their initial findings of a dose response. The improved outcome with high doses led these investigators to initiate a randomized trial of CRT to a dose of 70 Gy versus CRT to a dose of 78 Gy with each treatment prescribed to the isocenter. In this study, all patients received 46 Gy to a small pelvic volume encompassing the prostate and SVs using a four-field box technique. Patients then received a 24-Gy conventional boost using four fields or a 32-Gy conformal boost using a six-field technique. The ICRU 50 PTV convention was not used, and doses were prescribed to the treatment isocenter. Fields were shaped with a BEV treatment planning utility.

One hundred fifty patients were randomized to the 70-Gy arm and 151 to the 78-Gy arm. The rates for freedom from biochemical or disease failure, or both, were 69% for the 70-Gy arm and 79% for the 78-Gy arm (p = .058) (Fig. 22-8). Patients with a pretreatment PSA level of greater than 10 ng per mL benefited the most from dose escalation with a 5-year freedom-from-failure rate of 48% versus 75% for the 70-Gy and 78-Gy arms, respectively (p = .011) (64). This group of

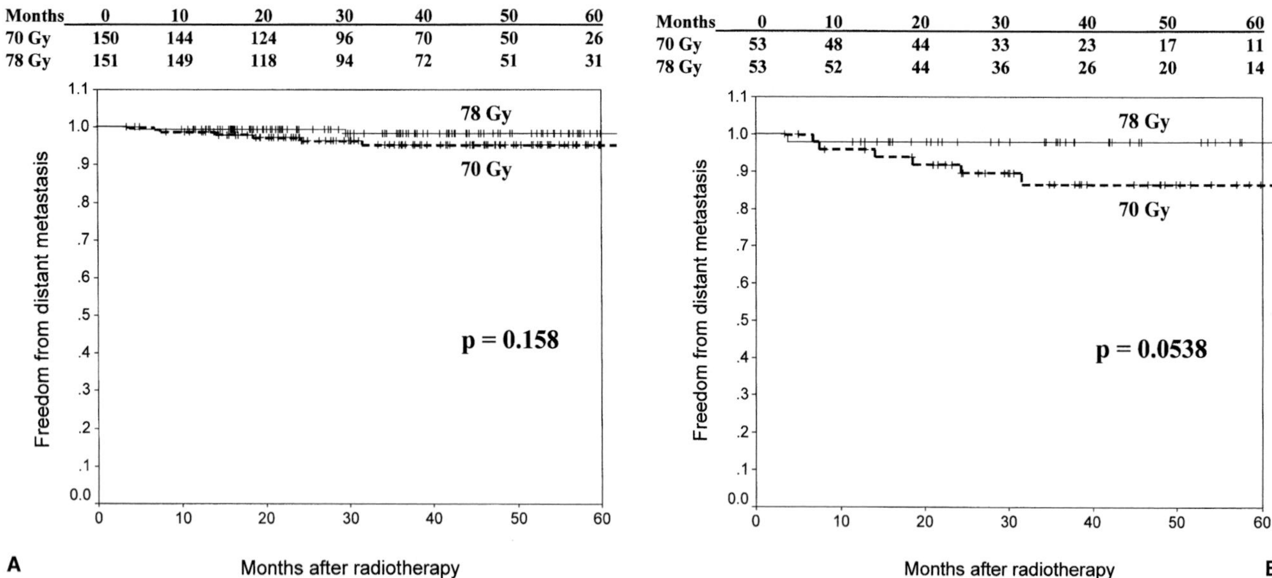

FIGURE 22-9. Kaplan-Meier freedom from distant metastasis for all patients **(A)** and those with prostate-specific antigen levels of greater than 10 ng per mL **(B)** by dose randomization (70 vs. 78 Gy). The numbers of patients at risk at 10-month intervals are shown above the graphs. (From Pollack A, Zagars GK, Smith LG, et al. Preliminary results of a randomized radiotherapy dose-escalation study comparing 70 Gy with 78 Gy for prostate cancer. *J Clin Oncol* 2000;18:3904–3911, with permission.)

patients with a PSA greater than 10 at diagnosis also had a better freedom-from–distant metastasis rate with 78 Gy than with 70 Gy (98% vs. 87%, respectively, $p = .054$) (Fig. 22-9). It is tempting to speculate that the reduction in distant metastasis seen in the higher-dose arm is related to improved eradication of local tumors, which would serve as a nidus for subsequent metastatic spread of disease.

INTENSITY-MODULATED RADIATION THERAPY VERSUS THREE-DIMENSIONAL CONFORMAL RADIATION THERAPY

3D CRT refers broadly to a variety of radiation therapy planning and delivery techniques designed to shape or conform a radiation dose distribution to the shape of a specific target volume. Likewise, 3D CRT may also allow conformal avoidance of radiation-sensitive structures. A specific and important subset of 3D CRT is IMRT. Conventional unmodulated radiation therapy beams achieve conformality by aperture or field shaping of uniform radiation output from a linear accelerator. The BEV tool, described earlier, is used to accomplish this field shaping. As the name implies, IMRT changes the fluence or intensity of the x-ray beam as it exits the linear accelerator. This modulation of radiation intensity adds another dimension of radiation dose shaping capabilities that allows more complex dose distributions than achievable with standard 3D CRT.

Differences in Planning

In traditional 3D CRT treatment planning, the dose distribution is computed only after radiation beams are applied. If the distribution is unacceptable, then the plan can be modified by reshaping the radiation fields or by changing the relative weight of the contributing radiation beams. IMRT introduces another level of complexity. Although the forward iterative or trial and error method of treatment plan optimization can be used with IMRT, most treatment planning systems incorporating IMRT use an inverse treatment planning approach.

Forward versus Inverse Planning

Forward treatment planning refers to the process of dose calculation after the radiation fields, and relative beam weights are chosen or designed by the treatment planner. The resultant computed dose distribution is then reviewed for plan quality, evaluating dose to targets and normal structures for clinical acceptability. *Inverse planning* refers to the process of determining a dose distribution or defining dose constraints that are used to determine the radiation beam shapes and intensity exiting the linear accelerator. These beam intensities are determined by "back projection" from the desired dose distribution. A radiation beam can be divided into multiple hypothetical beamlets. A large relative thickness or density of the target will increase the intensity of the beamlet intersecting with that portion of the target. Likewise, beamlets passing through normal radiosensitive structures will have a reduced intensity.

Implementation of inverse planning and IMRT places greater demand on the radiation oncologist to define target volumes and critical structures carefully. The intuitive input of forward planning is eliminated in the inverse planning process. If dose to adjacent tissues is an important clinical factor, then the DVH may not accurately represent this unless appropriate attention has been paid to anatomical segmentation or definition of that region. The treatment planning team, consisting of the radiation oncologist, physicist, and dosimetrist, needs to give considerable thought to the dose prescription and constraints. There is significant trade-off between coverage of a target, avoidance of adjacent critical structures, and the homogeneity of the distribution within the target. The radiation oncologist must apply various weights or levels of importance to his or her dosimetric goals. Even with IMRT, the "perfect" dose distribution that creates a complete homogeneous coverage of the target volume and zero or small dose to the adjacent radiation-sensitive structures may not be physically achievable. In many cases, compromises between target dose and normal tissue dose will need to be considered. Similarly, evaluation of the treatment plan requires careful review of DVHs and dose displays. The price that is paid by the increased conformality around the target is the possible increase in dose to adjacent tissues that, unless defined and constrained with dose limits *a priori*, may lead to their excessive irradiation.

Differences in Treatment Delivery

There are several ways in which radiation beam intensities can be modulated. One of the simplest methods used to modulate a radiation beam is the shrinking field technique. Similar to a boost in conventional radiation therapy, small subfields can supplement larger fields to bring regions within the field to a greater intensity. Because most IMRT plans have numerous levels of varying intensity, this method is most commonly accomplished using multiple static radiation fields shaped using the MLC. With an MLC, beam shaping can take place remotely and quickly by computer control. In our experience, as many as 30 segments can be used in each field when applying the segmental MLC method. When automatically driven by the MLC computer, the treatment time can be kept to a range similar to that used for standard 3D CRT. Figure 22-10 depicts a fluence map that could be derived from an inverse treatment plan. There is a corresponding portal radiograph exposed by the modulated x-ray beam.

A greater degree of conformality and treatment efficiency can be achieved with a dynamic MLC method of

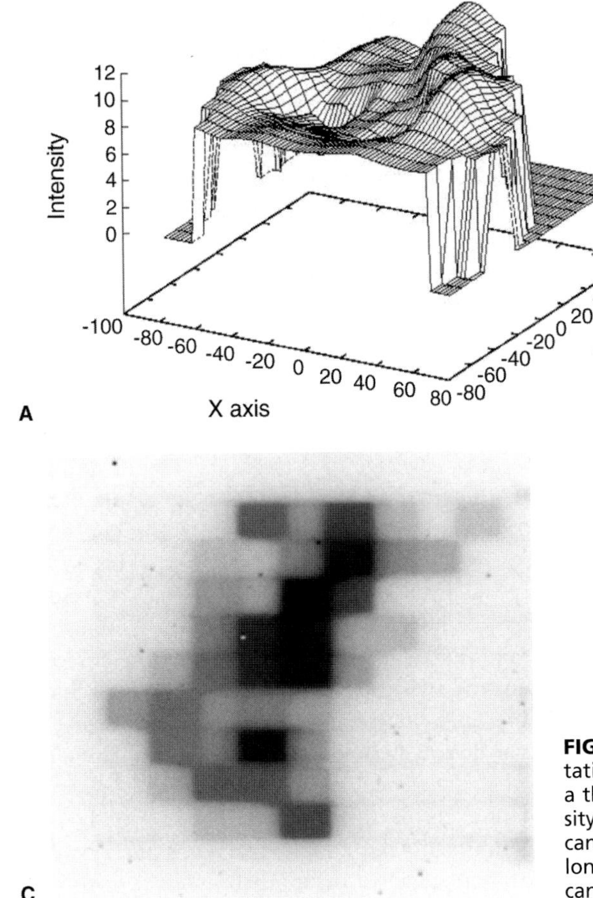

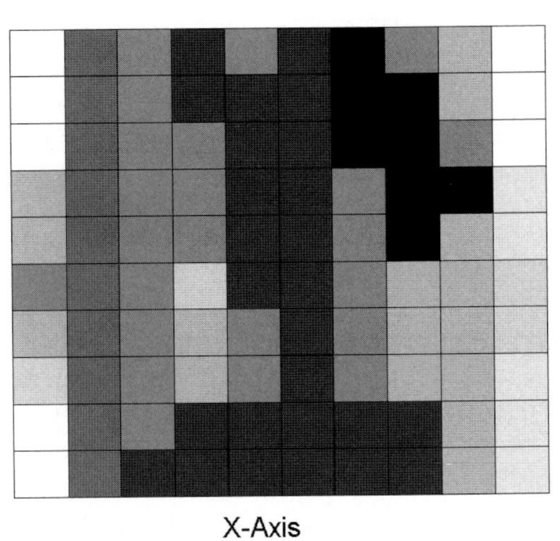

FIGURE 22-10. Intensity-modulated radiation therapy dose intensity representations. **A:** The relative fluence or intensity of the radiation beam is depicted in a three-dimensional map. **B:** The darker shades correspond to a greater intensity of radiation emitted to a region within the target. More intense radiation can be delivered to subfields by a multileaf collimator remaining open for longer exposures. **C:** As the radiation exits from the patient, a portal radiograph can demonstrate the variable intensities across the radiation field.

treatment delivery. With dynamic MLC, the independent leaf pairs of the MLC move continuously across the radiation field. The speed of the MLC motion and the relative separation between opposing leaf pairs determine the amount of radiation emitted in various regions of the field.

One of the first clinical methods of IMRT was delivered with a helical tomographic treatment device. The MIMiC (NOMOS Corporation, Sewickley, PA) is a tertiary collimator system that is inserted into the block tray of most linear accelerators. As the linear accelerator gantry rotates around the patient, the MIMiC modulates the beam continuously in a plane perpendicular to the treatment table. The MIMiC treats 1.6-cm slices of tissue in a manner inversely analogous to a diagnostic CT scan. Once a slice of tissue is irradiated, the table is moved 1.6 cm in a longitudinal direction to allow irradiation of another 1.6-cm slice. The treatment of a prostate patient generally takes five table positions or slices to complete treatment. Some institutions have used a wider treatment slice of 3.2 cm to make the delivery more efficient, albeit at the cost of diminished conformality (64a).

Engineers and physicists at the University of Wisconsin have proposed a novel linear accelerator design. In this system, a small linear accelerator is mounted on a ring gantry that can rotate beyond the 360-degree constraint on all other medical linear accelerators. The accelerator rotates around the patient in a spiral or corkscrew fashion with the beam intensity modulated by an internal MIMiC. This design potentially allows for megavoltage CT image acquisition that can be used to verify internal target position and treatment (64b).

Potential Clinical Advantages

As described earlier, the rate of rectal toxicity begins to rise substantially after a prescribed dose of 75 to 80 Gy with conventional fractionation using 3D CRT. To continue to safe escalation of radiation dose above 75 to 80 Gy, several institutions have moved to implementation of IMRT. Investigators at the Memorial Sloan-Kettering Cancer Center described an IMRT method that allowed a significantly improved conformality and increased dose homogeneity than the plan produced by a conventional 3D CRT technique. Subsequently, clinical results have been published describing a group of 171 prostate cancer patients treated to 81 Gy using IMRT. A dynamic MLC treatment delivery method was used. When compared to a group of 61 patients treated to 81 Gy delivered with a conventional 3D CRT approach, the IMRT technique resulted in a decrease in late grade 2 rectal toxicity. The 2-year actuarial risk of grade 2 bleeding was 2% for IMRT and 10% for conventional 3D CRT (p <.001) (57).

Teh et al. (64a) have described clinical IMRT results with a tomotherapy device in 100 patients treated to a prescribed dose of 70 Gy. To eliminate internal organ motion, an internal rectal balloon was used for daily prostate immobilization. Eighty-three percent of patients had no acute gastrointestinal complaints, and 27% had no acute genitourinary complaints. No patient in that series experienced any grade 3 or greater toxicity.

At the Cleveland Clinic, IMRT is being used to escalate the daily dose fraction size. Unlike the dose escalation trials previously described, this paradigm seeks to reduce the overall treatment time to 5 1/2 weeks by delivering 70 Gy in 28 2.5-Gy fractions. Without IMRT, the risk of late normal tissue toxicity rises significantly with this dose per fraction. By using IMRT, the dose per fraction to the adjacent normal structures, such as the rectum and bladder, can be maintained to conventional levels of 1.8 to 2.0 Gy or less. Preliminary results of this dose escalation scheme have demonstrated no increase in acute toxicity. It is too soon to know whether late effects, such as rectal bleeding, will be kept to acceptable levels (64c).

SUMMARY

External beam radiation therapy is a suitable alternative to radical prostatectomy and brachytherapy for men with localized prostate cancer. Advances in diagnostic imaging and radiation therapy planning and an improved understanding of the natural history of localized prostate cancer have resulted in improved outcomes for men choosing external beam radiation therapy for primary treatment. The reduction in late effects with 3D CRT by itself justifies the use of this modality in the majority of men receiving this treatment. The improvement in biochemical disease-free survival seen in the series from the Mallinckrodt Institute of Radiology (50) and the Fox Chase Cancer Center (53) argue that improved targeting has come about with 3D CRT. More important, the ability to safely escalate dose with the use of 3D CRT is yielding exciting results. The dose escalation series from the Fox Chase and Memorial Sloan-Kettering Cancer Centers (56–59) provide some evidence that higher doses will lead to more cures. Series such as these may suffer from selection or lead-time biases. The randomized study conducted at the M. D. Anderson Cancer Center provides strong evidence that a higher dose will indeed control more cancers. This study needs to be repeated on a larger scale before a prescription dose of 78 Gy becomes the community standard. The RTOG is currently planning this study.

REFERENCES

1. Elkind MM, Sutton H. Radiation response of mammalian cells grown in culture. Part 1. Repair of x-ray damage in surviving Chinese hamster cells. *Radiat Res* 1960;13:556.
2. International Commission on Radiation Units and Measurements. *Prescribing, recording, and reporting photon beam therapy.* Bethesda, MD: ICRU, 1993.
3. Nutting CM, Khoo VS, Walker V, et al. A randomized study of the use of a customized immobilization system in the treatment of prostate cancer with conformal radiotherapy. *Radiother Oncol* 2000;54:1–9.
4. Rosenthal SA, Roach M, Goldsmith BJ, et al. Immobilization improves the reproducibility of patient positioning during six-field conformal radiation therapy for prostate carcinoma. *Int J Radiat Oncol Biol Phys* 1993;27:921–926.
5. Zelefsky MJ, Aschkenasy E, Kelsen S, et al. Tolerance and early outcome results of postprostatectomy three-dimensional conformal radiotherapy. *Int J Radiat Oncol Biol Phys* 1997;39:327–333.
6. Dawson LA, Litzenberg DW, Brock KK, et al. A comparison of ventilatory prostate movement in four treatment positions. *Int J Radiat Oncol Biol Phys* 2000;48:319–323.
7. Malone S, Crook JM, Kendal WS, et al. Respiratory-induced prostate motion: quantification and characterization. *Int J Radiat Oncol Biol Phys* 2000;48:105–109.
8. Wilder RB, Fone PD, Rademacher DE, et al. Localization of the prostatic apex for radiotherapy treatment planning using urethroscopy. *Int J Radiat Oncol Biol Phys* 1997;38: 737–741.
9. Rasch C, Barillot I, Remeijer P, et al. Definition of the prostate in CT and MRI: a multi-observer study. *Int J Radiat Oncol Biol Phys* 1999;43:57–66.
10. Tinger A, Michalski JM, Cheng A, et al. A critical evaluation of the planning target volume for 3-D conformal radiotherapy of prostate cancer. *Int J Radiat Oncol Biol Phys* 1998;42:213–221.
11. Michalski JM, Purdy JA, Winter K, et al. Preliminary report of toxicity following 3D radiation therapy for prostate cancer on 3DOG/RTOG 9406. *Int J Radiat Oncol Biol Phys* 2000;46:391–402.
12. Boersma LJ, van den Brink M, Bruce AM, et al. Estimation of the incidence of late bladder and rectum complications after high-dose (70–80 Gy) conformal radiotherapy and prostate cancer, using dose-volume histograms. *Int J Radiat Oncol Biol Phys* 1998;41:83–92.
13. Skwarchuk MW, Jackson A, Zelefksy MJ. Late rectal toxicity after conformal radiotherapy of prostate cancer (I): multivariate analysis and dose-response. *Int J Radiat Oncol Biol Phys* 2000;47:103–113.
14. Asbell SO, Krall JM, Pilepich MV, et al. Elective pelvic irradiation in stage A2, B carcinoma of the prostate: analysis of RTOG 77-06. *Int J Radiat Oncol Biol Phys* 1988;15:1306–1316.
15. Leibel SA, Fuks Z, Zelefsky MJ, et al. Significance of normal serum prostate-specific antigen in the follow-up period after definitive radiation therapy for prostatic cancer. *Int J Radiat Oncol Biol Phys* 1994;28:7–16.
16. Perez CA, Michalski JM, Hanlon AL, et al. Nonrandomized evaluation of pelvic lymph node irradiation in localized carcinoma of the prostate. *Int J Radiat Oncol Biol Phys* 1996; 36:573–584.

17. Partin AW, Kattan MW, Subong EN, et al. Combination of prostate-specific antigen, clinical stage, and Gleason score to predict pathological stage of localized prostate cancer: a multi-institutional update. *JAMA* 1997;18:1445–1451.
18. Roach M, Pickett B, Rosenthal SA, et al. Defining treatment margins for six field conformal irradiation of localized prostate carcinoma. *Int J Radiat Oncol Biol Phys* 1994;28: 267–275.
19. Zietman AL, Prince EA, Nakfoor BM, et al. Androgen deprivation and radiation therapy: sequencing studies using the Shionogi in vivo tumor system. *Int J Radiat Oncol Biol Phys* 1997;38:1067–1070.
20. Granfors T, Modig H, Damber J-E, et al. Combined orchiectomy and external radiotherapy versus radiotherapy alone for nonmetastatic prostate cancer with or without pelvic lymph node involvement: a prospective randomized study. *J Urol* 1998;159:2030–2034.
21. Pilepich MV, Sause WT, Shipley WU, et al. Androgen deprivation with radiation therapy compared with radiation therapy alone for locally advanced prostatic carcinoma: a randomized comparative trial of the Radiation Therapy Oncology Group. *Urology* 1995;45:616–623.
22. Pickett B, Vigneault E, Kurhanewicz J, et al. Static field intensity modulation to treat a dominant intra-prostatic lesion to 90 Gy compared to seven field 3-dimensional radiotherapy. *Int J Radiat Oncol Biol Phys* 1999;43:921–929.
23. Zelefsky MJ, Leibel SA, Gaudin PB, et al. Dose escalation with three-dimensional conformal radiation therapy affects the outcome in prostate cancer. *Int J Radiat Oncol Biol Phys* 1998;41:491–500.
24. Diaz A, Roach M, Marquez C, et al. Indications for and the significance of seminal vesicle irradiation during 3D conformal radiotherapy for localized prostate cancer. *Int J Radiat Oncol Biol Phys* 1994;30:323–329.
25. Ten Haken RK, Perez-Tamayo C, Tersser RJ, et al. Boost treatment of the prostate using shaped, fixed fields. *Int J Radiat Oncol Biol Phys* 1989;16:193–200.
26. Perez CA, Michalski JM, Ballard S, et al. Cost benefit of emerging technology in localized carcinoma of the prostate. *Int J Radiat Oncol Biol Phys* 1997;39:875–883.
27. Nguyen LN, Pollack A, Zagars G. Late effects after radiotherapy for prostate cancer in a randomized dose-response study: results of a self-assessment questionnaire. *Urology* 1998;51:991–997.
28. Tait DM, Nahum AE, Meyer LC. Acute toxicity in pelvic radiotherapy: a randomized trial of conformal versus conventional treatment. *Radiother Oncol* 1997;42:121–136.
29. Denham JW, Dally MJ, Hunter K, et al. Objective decision-making following a portal film: the results of a pilot study. *Int J Radiat Oncol Biol Phys* 1993;26:869–876.
30. Bel A, Vos PH, Rodrigus PT, et al. High-precision prostate cancer irradiation by clinical application of an offline patient setup verification procedure, using portal imaging. *Int J Radiat Oncol Biol Phys* 1996;35:321–332.
31. Vijayakumar S, Quadri SF, Sen S, et al. Measurement of weekly prostate specific antigen levels in patients receiving pelvic radiotherapy for nonprostatic malignancies. *Int J Radiat Oncol Biol Phys* 1995;32:189–195.
32. Hancock SL, Cox RS, Bagshaw MA. Prostate specific antigen after radiotherapy for prostate cancer: a re-evaluation of long-term biochemical control and the kinetics of recurrence in patients treated at Stanford University. *J Urol* 1995;154:1412–1417.
33. Willett CG, Zietman AL, Shipley WU, et al. The effect of pelvic radiation therapy on serum levels of prostate specific antigen. *J Urol* 1995;154:1579–1581.
34. Kavadi VS, Zagars GK, Pollack A. Serum prostate specific antigen after radiation therapy for clinically localized prostate cancer: prognostic implications. *Int J Radiol Oncol Biol Phys* 1997;30:279–287.
35. Zelefsky MJ, Leibel SA, Wallner KE, et al. Significance of normal serum prostate-specific antigen in the follow-up period after definitive radiation therapy for prostate cancer. *J Clin Oncol* 1995;13:459–463.
36. Lee WR, Hanks GE, Hanlon AL. Lateral rectal shielding reduces late rectal morbidity following high dose three dimensional conformal radiation therapy for clinically localized prostate cancer: further evidence of significant dose effect. *Int J Radiat Oncol Biol Phys* 1996;35:251–257.
37. American Society for Therapeutic Radiology and Oncology Consensus Panel. Consensus statement: guidelines for PSA following radiation therapy. *Int J Radiat Oncol Biol Phys* 1997;37:1035–1041.
38. Critz FA, Williams WH, Benton JB, et al. Prostate specific antigen bounce after radioactive seed implantation followed by external beam radiation for prostate cancer. *J Urol* 2000;163:1085–1089.
39. Cox JD, Klein RW. Do prostatic biopsies 12 months or more after external irradiation for adenocarcinoma, stage III, predict long-term survival? *Int J Radiat Oncol Biol Phys* 1983;9:299–303.
40. Cox JD, Klein RW. The lack of prognostic significance of biopsies after radiotherapy for prostatic cancer. *Semin Urol* 1983;1:237–242.
41. Scardino PT. The prognostic significance of biopsies after radiotherapy for prostatic cancer. *Semin Urol* 1983;1:243–252.
42. Crook J, Malone S, Perry G, et al. Postradiotherapy prostate biopsies: What do they really mean? Results for 498 patients. *Int J Radiat Oncol Biol Phys* 2000;48:355–367.
43. Crook J, Robertson S, Esche B. Proliferative cell nuclear antigen in postradiotherapy prostate biopsy. *Int J Radiat Oncol Biol Phys* 1994;30:303–308.
44. Zagars GK, Pollack A. Radiation therapy for T1 and T2 prostate cancer: prostate specific antigen and disease outcome. *Urology* 1995;45:476–483.
45. Shipley WU, Thames HD, Sandler HM, et al. Radiation therapy for clinically localized prostate cancer: a multi-institutional pooled analysis. *JAMA* 1999;17:1598–1604.
46. Roach M, Lu J, Pilepich MV, et al. Long-term survival after radiotherapy alone: Radiation Therapy Oncology Group prostate cancer trials. *J Urol* 1999;161:864–868.
47. Perez CA, Pilepich MV, Zivnuska F. Tumor control in definitive irradiation of localized carcinoma of the prostate. *Int J Radiat Oncol Biol Phys* 1986;12:523–531.
48. Hanks GE, Martz KL, Diamond JJ. The effect of dose on local control of prostate cancer. *Int J Radiat Oncol Biol Phys* 1988;15:1299–1305.
49. Smit WG, Helle PA, van Putten WL, et al. Late radiation damage in prostate cancer patients treated by high dose

external radiotherapy in relation to rectal dose. *Int J Radiat Oncol Biol Phys* 1990;18:23–29.

50. Perez CA, Michalski JM, Purdy JA, et al. Three-dimensional conformal therapy or standard irradiation in localized carcinoma of the prostate: preliminary results of a nonrandomized comparison. *Int J Radiat Oncol Biol Phys* 2000;47:629–637.
51. Sandler HM, McLaughlin PW, Ten Haken RK. Three dimensional conformal radiotherapy for the treatment of prostate cancer: low risk of chronic rectal morbidity observed in a large series of patients. *Int J Radiat Oncol Biol Phys* 1995;33:797–802.
52. Fukunaga-Johnson N, Sandler HM, McLaughlin PW, et al. Results of 3D conformal radiotherapy in the treatment of localized prostate cancer. *Int J Radiat Oncol Biol Phys* 1997;38:311–317.
53. Hanks GE, Schultheiss GE, Hunt MA. Factors influencing incidence of acute grade 2 morbidity in conformal and standard radiation treatment of prostate cancer. *Int J Radiat Oncol Biol Phys* 1995;31:25–29.
54. Koper PCM, Stroom JC, van Putten WLJ, et al. Acute morbidity reduction using 3D CRT for prostate carcinoma: a randomized study. *Int J Radiat Oncol Biol Phys* 1999;43:727–734.
55. Dearnaley DP, Khoo VS, Norman AR, et al. Comparison of radiation side-effects of conformal and conventional radiotherapy in prostate cancer: a randomized trial. *Lancet* 1999;353:267–272.
56. Zelefsky MJ, Cowen D, Fuks Z, et al. Long-term tolerance of high dose three dimensional conformal radiotherapy in patients with localized prostate carcinoma. *Cancer* 1999;85:2460–2468.
57. Zelefsky MJ, Fuks Z, Happersett L, et al. Clinical experience with intensity modulated radiation therapy (IMRT) in prostate cancer. *Radiother Oncol* 2000;55:241–249.
58. Hanks GE, Hanlon AL, Pinover WH, et al. Dose selection for prostate cancer patients based on dose comparison and dose response studies. *Int J Radiat Oncol Biol Phys* 2000;46:823–832.
59. Hanks GE, Hanlon AL, Schultheiss TE, et al. Dose escalation with 3D conformal treatment: five year outcomes, treatment optimization, and future directions. *Int J Radiat Oncol Biol Phys* 1998;41:501–510.
60. Leibel SA, Fuks Z, Zelefsky MJ, et al. Prostate cancer: three dimensional conformal and intensity modulated radiation therapy. In: Rosenberg DH, ed. *PPO updates: principles & practice of oncology*, vol. 14. New York: Lippincott Williams & Wilkins, 2000.
61. Bey P, Carrie C, Beckendorf V, et al. Dose escalation with 3-D CRT in prostate cancer: French study of dose escalation with conformal 3-D radiotherapy and prostate cancer—preliminary results. *Int J Radiat Oncol Biol Phys* 2000;48:513–517.
62. Pollack A, Zagars GK. External beam radiotherapy dose response of prostate cancer. *Int J Radiat Oncol Biol Phys* 1997;39:1011–1108.
63. Pollack A, Smith LG, von Eschenbach AC. External beam radiotherapy dose response characteristics of 1127 men with prostate cancer treated in the PSA era. *Int J Radiat Oncol Biol Phys* 2000;48:507–512.
64. Pollack A, Zagars GK, Smith LG, et al. Preliminary results of a randomized radiotherapy dose-escalation study comparing 70 Gy with 78 Gy for prostate cancer. *J Clin Oncol* 2000;18:3904–3911.

64a. Teh BS, Mai WY, Uhl BM, et al. Intensity-modulated radiation therapy (IMRT) for prostate cancer with the use of a rectal balloon for prostate immobilization: acute toxicity and dose volume analysis. *Int J Radiat Biol Phys* 2001;49:705–712.

64b. Mackie TR, Balog J, Ruchala K, et al. Tomotherapy. *Semin Radiat Oncol* 1999;9:108–117.

64c. Mohan D, Kupelian PA, Willoughby TR. Short-course intensity modulated radiotherapy for localized prostate cancer with daily transabdominal ultrasound localization of the prostate gland. *Int J Radiat Biol Phys* 2000;46:575–580.

65. Purdy JA. The application of high energy x-rays and electron beams in radiotherapy in IEEE. *Trans Nucl Sci* 1979;26:1833.
66. Rudat V, Schraube P, Oetzel D, et al. Combined error of patient positioning variability and prostate motion uncertainty in 3D conformal radiotherapy of localized prostate cancer. *Int J Radiat Oncol Biol Phys* 1996;35:1027–1034.
67. Stroom JC, Koper PC, Korevaar GA, et al. Internal organ motion in prostate cancer patients treated in prone and supine treatment positions. *Radiother Oncol* 1999;51:237–248.
68. Zelefsky MJ, Crean D, Mageras GS, et al. Quantification and predictors of prostate position variability in 50 patients evaluated with multiple CT scans during conformal radiotherapy. *Radiother Oncol* 1999;50:225–234.

23

BRACHYTHERAPY AS MONOTHERAPY

JOHN E. SYLVESTER
JOHN C. BLASKO
PETER D. GRIMM

Prostate cancer is the most common cancer (other than skin cancer) and the second leading cause of cancer mortality in men. The incidence increased rapidly with the introduction of the prostate-specific antigen (PSA) blood test (1). Not only did the incidence of newly diagnosed cases increase, but also the percentage of patients diagnosed with early stage disease increased dramatically. It has been recently reported that 77% of newly diagnosed cases are early stage (T1 and T2) at the time of diagnosis, compared to 57% between 1975 and1979 (2).

The high incidence of early stage disease being diagnosed has resulted in an increased demand by patients for aggressive definitive treatment. The therapeutic options of radical prostatectomy and external beam radiation therapy are under more scrutiny (3–6). Talcott has discussed the toxicity of these treatment modalities by way of patient interviews and surveys (7). PSA testing in follow-up of patients treated with modern external beam radiation therapy or surgery has shown these modalities to be less effective at eradicating all the malignancy than we once thought they were (in the pre-PSA era). It has also shown that neither modality appears to be superior to the other in terms of biochemical control when the major pretreatment risk factors are taken into account (8–12).

Permanent, interstitial prostate brachytherapy is a form of radiation therapy in which radioactive sources are placed permanently, directly into the prostate. The primary goal of prostate brachytherapy is to deliver very high doses of radiation to the prostate and relatively low doses to the surrounding normal structures. Ultrasound- and template-guided permanent transperineal radioactive seed implantation is emerging as a reasonable treatment option for men with early-stage prostate cancer.

The demand for radioactive seed implantation has increased dramatically over the 1990s. This is a result of many factors, including improved outcomes with the modern seed implantation techniques, acceptably low rates of permanent complications in properly selected patients, and the conveyance of a single outpatient treatment (13).

PROSTATE BRACHYTHERAPY HISTORY

In 1903, Alexander Graham Bell postulated that an effective way to control tumors might be to insert radioactive sources directly into them. In 1911, Pasteur suggested treating prostate cancer by inserting radium into the prostate (14). In 1922, Denning reported a series of 100 patients with prostate cancer whom he treated with transurethral radium insertion (15). Compared to other methods of prostate cancer treatment in that era, the control rates he achieved were quite good. Complication rates were high, however, as there was no way to adequately measure the radiation dose delivered. Prostate brachytherapy fell into disuse with the advent of the radical prostatectomy and improved anesthetic and surgical techniques. With the development of megavoltage radiation therapy, external beam radiation therapy became a popular treatment for prostate cancer in the 1960s.

In the late 1960s, Scardino and Carlton reintroduced prostate cancer brachytherapy (16). They used a combination therapy approach of interstitial gold 198 implantation and external beam radiation therapy. In the early 1970s, Dr. Whitmore and his colleagues developed and reported on the use of permanent interstitial iodine 125 (^{125}I) seed implantation (17). This was at Memorial Sloan-Kettering Cancer Center (MSKCC) in New York City. They placed the seeds at the time of open laparotomy by way of a retropubic approach. This technique became quite popular throughout the United States. However, as more follow-up was obtained, it became apparent that the control rate, in general, achieved with open laparotomy retropubic interstitial seed implantation was inferior to the results of surgery and external beam radiation in that era. At open laparotomy, the brachytherapist was not able to clearly visualize the placement of the seeds into the prostate. It was common for these implants to have an inhomogeneous distribution of seeds, as identified on orthogonal films taken for postimplant dosimetry. In that era, they used a spacing nomogram to determine the number of seeds needed, because sophisticated computerized preplanning was not available. It was not known that patients with stage C disease or large transurethral resection of the prostate (TURP) defects were poor candidates for permanent seed implantation.

Historical Retropubic Results

The outcomes and results of the open retropubic approach have been thoroughly debated and reviewed in the literature (8,14,18). The end points available in the 1970s and early 1980s were survival and local control. For stage A and B disease, the survival rates with brachytherapy and external beam radiation therapy were similar in institutions that used both treatment modalities (19–24). This similarity in survival could be due to two incongruous hypotheses. First, each form of radiation therapy was equally effective at controlling disease. Second, neither form of therapy was particularly effective or ineffective. By its very nature, early-stage prostate cancer is often only slowly progressive; thus, similar survival rates could be expected in this older population, whether or not therapy was effective at totally eradicating the disease.

Local control became the benchmark by which effectiveness of local therapy was evaluated in the pre-PSA era. The interpretation of local control was problematic. Without PSA evaluations or the common use of posttreatment biopsies, local control was determined by relatively insensitive clinical criteria. Local failure was defined by a progressing palpable abnormality on serial digital rectal examinations (DREs) or by development of urinary obstructive symptoms. With these relatively crude end points and the absence of modern actuarial statistical models comparing the local control rates of brachytherapy, external beam ration therapy and surgery are challenging at best. In those few centers that have reported long-term results with both methods of radiation therapy (in early-stage low-grade disease), there does not appear to be a significant difference in local control for either treatment. However, as stage or grade progressed, external beam radiation produced better results (21,24,25).

The clinical data at that time suggested those patients with poorly differentiated lesions had high failure rates, but those with well to moderately differentiated lesions appeared to have reasonable control rates if adequate doses were obtained at implantation. In those patients with early-stage disease without large TURP defects, in whom postimplant dosimetry appeared good, excellent local control was obtained (19,20,23,26). The long-term results of retropubic implantation at MSKCC reveal a 60% local control rate if the matched peripheral dose (MPD) was greater than 140 Gy but only 20% if that MPD was not achieved (20). Hilaris et al. reported 15-year survivals of 70% in patients with stage B1 disease (27). These published reports suggest that successful outcomes are more dependent on patient selection and accurate placement of the radioactive isotopes than on some inherent radiobiologic resistance of prostate cancer to low-dose-rate brachytherapy. However, high-quality implantation was not achieved consistently with the open laparotomy technique. This, combined with suboptimal outcomes, led to the abandonment of prostate permanent seed implantation in the early 1980s.

It became clear that permanent radioactive seed implantation would not become an accepted treatment option until high-quality implants could be consistently obtained in properly selected patients. Technical advances needed to be made before this could become a reality.

TECHNICAL ADVANCES IN PROSTATE BRACHYTHERAPY

In the 1980s, several important advances were achieved and refined. At Long Beach Memorial Hospital, Puthawala and Syed pioneered a transperineal approach to prostate brachytherapy done at the time of open laparotomy (28). Martinez et al. treated locally advanced prostate cancer with the combination of external beam radiation therapy and a multiple site transperineal applicator (29).

Advances in transrectal ultrasonography led Dr. Holm to use this new technology to guide radioactive ^{125}I seeds into the prostate. This was done by inserting the ^{125}I radioactive seeds transperineally, while the ultrasound probe in the rectum visualized the precise location of the needles used to deposit the radioactive seeds. Even seed distribution was noted on orthogonal films. He published his technique in 1983 (30). This technology allowed the brachytherapist to image the prostate before implantation and develop a three-dimensional (3D) representation of that individual's prostate. From this, a conformal pretreatment plan could be rendered in which the precise location of each radioactive source "seed" could be determined. This preplan could then be carried out at the time of the implantation. Real-time transrectal ultrasound (TRUS) imaging allowed the brachytherapist to guide the placement of the needles carrying the radioactive seeds into their proper position.

In 1985, Dr. Blasko performed the first TRUS and template-guided closed transperineal ^{125}I permanent seed implantation of the prostate for early-stage prostate cancer in the United States, in Seattle. The Seattle team used TRUS preoperatively to map out the size and shape of the prostate from base to apex. This was used to develop a customized conformal preplan that identified the precise location (in x, y, and z coordinates) within the prostate for each radioactive seed to be used. The patient position and ultrasound measurements were then duplicated in the operating room (OR) a few weeks later, at which time the radioactive seeds were inserted under ultrasound guidance in accordance with that patient's individualized, conformal preplan (Fig. 23-1). Early on, fluoroscopy showed even seed distribution consistently in implants performed in Seattle and other centers that had passed the learning curve of modern brachytherapy (Fig. 23-2).

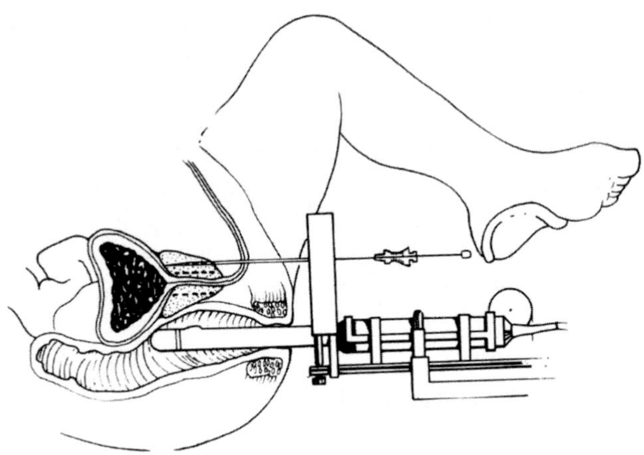

FIGURE 23-1. Schematic illustration of ultrasound-guided transperineal prostate brachytherapy.

In the late 1980s and 1990s, the widespread availability of sophisticated, computerized planning systems specifically developed for prostate brachytherapy made treatment planning quicker and more flexible. It allowed this technology to be moved out of specific institutions into the general community. Improvements in template design, stabilization equipment, and OR technique have further improved the accuracy and speed of the procedure. The addition of another low-dose-rate, low-energy radioisotope, palladium 103 (^{103}Pd), and the widespread availability of computed tomography (CT) have further increased the medical profession's interest in prostate brachytherapy. It is now performed as a closed, percutaneous 45-minute outpatient procedure in many centers. There are some who prefer to use the Mick applicator system, and others prefer the preloaded needles (31–34). Some prefer to use ^{125}I as loose seeds or stranded seeds, and others prefer ^{103}Pd. An advantage to stranded seeds [seeds embedded in Vicryl suture (RAPID Strand)] is the low rate of seed embolization, 0.7% for embedded seeds, versus 11% for loose seeds (35). A theoretic advantage for ^{103}Pd is that its lower energy may deliver a lesser dose to the rectum. Most use an ultrasound-planned and ultrasound-guided technique (30,36–38).

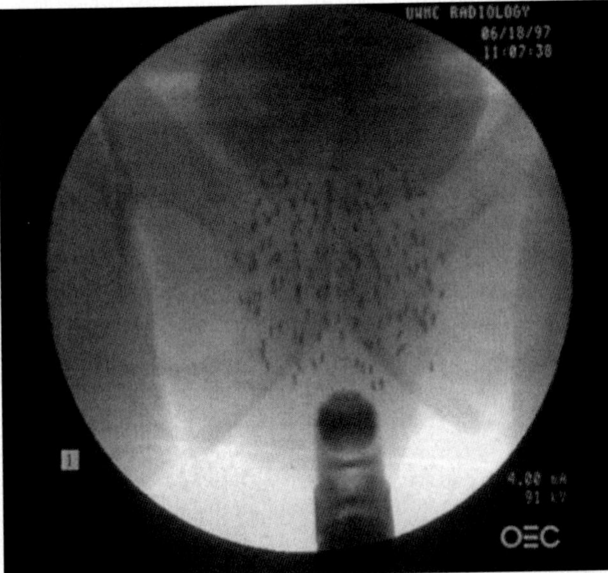

FIGURE 23-2. Fluoroscopic image showing even seed distribution after ultrasound-guided prostate brachytherapy.

However, there are proponents of CT-planned (39–42) and, recently, magnetic resonance imaging (MRI)–directed permanent interstitial seed implantation (43). Multiple institutions have published results demonstrating that the previously discussed advances in technology and patient selection have led to an improvement in the accuracy and consistency of permanent interstitial radioactive seed implantation (30,39,44,45). Differences in technique are prevalent. Individuals and institutions commonly attach a label to their own particular variation in methodology, such as "real-time," "CT scan based," or "interactive," so as to separate their methods from others. Most involve a closed transperineal percutaneous approach that is guided in real time by an imaging apparatus to guide seed placement in accordance with the conformal treatment preplan. Most agree that the important point is the end result: the postimplantation dosimetry. There are no studies that have compared the dosimetric outcomes of these various differences in technique. In the 1990s, it became apparent that postimplantation dosimetry needed to be CT or MRI based, or both (46). Postimplantation dosimetry based on orthogonal films is no longer acceptable (13,47,48).

In essence, modern transperineal permanent low-dose-rate prostate brachytherapy can be divided into four parts: (a) patient selection, (b) conformal preplanning, (c) the implant procedure, and (d) postimplantation dosimetric evaluation.

PATIENT SELECTION

Among brachytherapists, there is some variation in selection criteria. In general, patients who are candidates for seed implantation alone are often equally suitable candidates for other treatment options, such as external beam radiation therapy or radical prostatectomy. To be considered as candidates for monotherapy seed implantation, patients should meet certain technical and clinical conditions.

Technical factors deal with the ability to physically place the radioactive seeds in such a distribution that postimplantation dosimetry will be deemed adequate. A large gland (larger than 60 cc) will often be difficult to implant, owing to pubic arch interference. The seeds are typically placed by way of a transperineal template-guided approach. If the prostate is too large, then some of the gland (anterior and laterally) will be blocked to needle insertion by the pubic arch. If the prostate is smaller than 40 cc, then pubic arch interference is uncommon. In a 40- to 60-cc prostate pubic arch, interference occurs often enough to justify a pubic arch correlate CT scan. When more than 25% of the prostate appears to be blocked by the pubic arch on the CT correlate scan, implantation of the prostate in the OR will be difficult. Often, this problem can be overcome by downsizing the prostate with androgen ablation. Three months of total androgen ablation will downsize the prostate volume by an average of 45% (49). Even if the pubic arch were not a factor, many brachytherapists shy away from implanting very large prostates because of concerns over possible toxicities that might occur with irradiation of such a large volume to such a high dose, especially when other reasonable treatment options are usually available (46).

Patients with a history of a TURP need to be evaluated carefully. A large TURP defect can limit the number and distribution of seeds placed within the interior of the prostate and lead to underdosing problems. Patients with a history of a TURP, large or small, recent or remote, have been reported to experience more long-term urinary side effects (13,47,50). Thus, both technical and clinical factors come into play in TURP patients.

Patients with a large median lobe can be technically challenging. It is difficult to deliver prescription-level doses to the median lobe with seed monotherapy. Fortunately, this region seldom harbors malignant cells in early-stage disease, so it is not clear that full-prescription doses of radiation need to be delivered to the entire median lobe.

Clinical factors deal with the suitability of an individual patient based on how extensive the patient's disease is and how well the patient is expected to tolerate therapy. Local therapy, such as surgery or permanent seed implantation alone, is suitable for patients with a high chance of having organ-confined disease. For those patients considered to have a substantial risk of extensive extracapsular spread of disease beyond the confines of surgery or monotherapy seed implantation, external beam radiation with or without a seed implant boost is often reasonable. The challenge lies in identification of those patients with disease that is too advanced for seed monotherapy. Studies indicate that patients with clinically staged disease are often upstaged at time of radical prostatectomy (33,51–60).

Partin et al. established that pretreatment PSA, grade, and clinical stage (by DRE) are important clinical factors predicting for extraprostatic disease (61). The Partin tables divide the risk of extraprostatic extension of disease into the risk of lymph node (LN), seminal vesicle (SV), and established capsular penetration (ECP). The total ECP risk is the sum of the LN, SV, and ECP risks. The penetration through the prostate capsule (ECP) is often only a short distance (a few millimeters). When this is the case, ECP may be encompassed within a surgical and, therefore, an implant volume. Epstein et al. demonstrated that, for patients with pathologically determined ECP but negative LNs and negative SVs and a Gleason of 6 or less, the chance of failing radical prostatectomy was 25% at 7 years (54). An explanation for this relatively low failure rate in these ECP patients is that the ECP was such a short distance that it was all encompassed within the surgical margins in the failure-free patients (62,63). Conversely, the risk of failure was 50% if the Gleason score was 7 or greater in patients with ECP yet negative LNs and negative SVs (54). The approximate risk of failure with surgery (and presumably monotherapy seed implantation) might therefore be expressed as a percentage of the ECP added to the risk of LN and SV involvement. As illustrated in Table 23-1, by multiplying the risk of ECP by 25% or 50% (depending on Gleason score) and adding to that the risk of LN and SV involvement (as predicted by the Partin tables), the clinician can estimate the risk of disease beyond the confines of local therapy (surgery or monotherapy seed implantation) (64). When one plugs in the numbers to this equation, the predicted total risk of disease beyond the confines of local therapy comes quite close to the failure rates of the surgical and seed monotherapy results reported in the medical literature.

TABLE 23-1. RELATIONSHIP OF GLEASON SCORE TO THE RISK OF DISEASE BEYOND REACH OF LOCAL THERAPY

Gleason scores	Risk of disease beyond reach of local therapy
2–6	SV risk + LN risk + 0.25 ECP risk
7–10	SV risk + LN risk + 0.50 ECP risk

ECP, established capsular penetration; LN, lymph node; SV, seminal vesicle.

This calculation can be helpful when discussing with a potential brachytherapy candidate whether to treat with seed monotherapy or external beam radiation with a seed implant boost. Other factors that the clinician will wish to take into account are the number and percentage of positive biopsies and whether perineural invasion was noted in the biopsy specimens.

Using the Partin tables, number of positive biopsies, and recent clinical results with local therapy, patients usually can be divided into a low-risk group suitable for implant alone and a high-risk group more suitable for external beam radiation and an implant boost.

In general, low-risk patients (cT1 and cT2a disease, PSA less than or equal to 10 ng per mL, and Gleason score of 2 to 6) are reasonable candidates for implant alone. Although this stratification is helpful, other clinical factors may need to be considered. Perineural invasion and multiple positive sextant biopsies have been demonstrated risk factors for extracapsular extension of disease (52,54,58,65–67). These factors have been shown to increase the risk of extracapsular penetration, but how significant they are compared to Gleason score, stage, and PSA has yet to be determined. Further studies will need to be done to determine how critical these other factors are clinically in monotherapy seed implantation, independent of the already established Partin tables. The use of MRI in patient selection for seed implantation monotherapy is unresolved (68).

The use of combined external beam and seed implantation for all patients, as advocated by some practitioners, does not seem justified in the light of current data (13,47,69). One of the rationales for combining external beam radiation and implantation in all patients is the high risk of extracapsular spread in most patients. This philosophy fails to recognize that ECP in favorable low-risk patients is rarely beyond 1 to 5 mm, clearly within the confines of local treatment (62,63). Clinical results for these low-risk patients treated with implant alone have been excellent (70).

High-risk patients are those with two of three poor prognostic factors (cT2c, Gleason score of 7 or greater, PSA between 10.1 and 20) or PSA greater than 20. These patients are not generally considered suitable for seed monotherapy. They are usually treated by brachytherapists with a combination of external beam radiation and a permanent seed or temporary high-dose-rate (HDR) boost.

Patients in the intermediate-risk group are patients with one poor risk factor (Gleason score 7 or greater, stage cT2c, or PSA between 10 and 20). Results of monotherapy in this group are mixed. Some centers have presented excellent results with monotherapy in this risk cohort, others poor results (64,71–74). It is possible that the contrasting outcomes are a result of differences in implant quality due to the differences in technique and experience of the various brachytherapists. Other explanations could include hidden selection biases among the various patient populations that are impossible to control for when comparing reports of retrospective reviews between different institutions.

Certain patients are not considered suitable candidates for permanent transperineal seed implantation. Patients who are stage cT3 or higher or LN positive, and patients with metastatic disease are not expected to benefit from permanent seed brachytherapy. Age has not been demonstrated to be a selection factor. Relative contraindications include a history of even a small TURP. Patients with prior TURP, even in the remote past, have been reported to experience higher rates of incontinence and superficial urethral necrosis (47,75). Patients with significant obstructive voiding symptoms may be at risk for needing a TURP postimplantation and should be approached with caution. In these patients, it is prudent to perform uroflow voiding studies, check postvoid residuals, and consider cystoscopy before accepting the patient as a permanent seed implant candidate. In some of these patients, the obstructive voiding symptoms respond well to alpha blockers or androgen ablation, or both. If the symptoms do respond well, the patient would then be an appropriate candidate for seed implantation.

Patients who fall into a gray area, technically or clinically, might be best served by having a second opinion by a radiation oncologist who subspecializes in prostate cancer brachytherapy (46). This could include patients technically difficult to implant adequately, such as patients with a large median lobe, prior TURP, or large prostate volume. It could also include clinically challenging patients, such as those with a history of some prior pelvic radiation therapy, significant prior pelvic surgery, severe diabetes, and patients with moderate to severe obstructive urinary symptoms.

PREIMPLANT CONFORMAL DOSIMETRY

The goal of treatment is to deliver doses to the prostate higher than that which is achievable with external beam radiation therapy or temporary low-dose-rate or HDR brachytherapy. The assumption is that the higher the dose delivered, the higher the likelihood that all malignant clonogens will be destroyed. Despite the dose inhomogeneity seen and expected with permanent radioactive seed implantation, the total dose and the radiobiologic effective dose delivered to the prostate with this technique are significantly higher than standard external beam radiotherapy, 3D conformal, particle-beam, or HDR temporary brachytherapy can achieve (13,46,76).

Because radiation emanates from a single source or seed, dose inhomogeneity is inherent to any temporary or permanent brachytherapy implant. Therefore, to standardize the dose prescription, the prescribed dose was described in the past as the MPD. The MPD is the dose delivered to a volume equal to an ellipsoid volume with the same average dimension as the prostate gland. This definition is admittedly confusing. Most practitioners consider the prescription dose to be the dose encompassing the *target volume.* The target volume for prostate cancer is typically the entire prostate and a small amount of surrounding normal tissue. Using standard dose nomograms, as was done in the past with the open laparotomy retropubic implants, is reasonable if the prostate is relatively symmetric and ellipsoid in shape. However, using a target volume approach based on the individual patient's prostate volume and shape (as determined by ultrasound or MRI) is intuitively a more precise therapy. CT scans appear to overestimate the size of the prostate compared to pathologic specimens, whereas volumes from TRUS volume studies appear to match the pathologic prostatectomy volume well (77).

The MPD (implant prescription dose) only describes the dose at the periphery of the target volume. Dramatic differences in source distribution philosophy exist from one institution to another. Whereas the dose prescribed for an implant will be the same from one center to the next (as described by the MPD), the dose distribution within and adjacent to the gland can vary significantly due to differences in source distribution loading patterns. Actual doses to the central portion of the prostate and tumor are often considerably higher (200 to 400 Gy for ^{125}I implants) than the MPD. The central dose varies significantly, depending on the activity of the seed used and placement technique. The dose to the rectum can also vary from one center to the next, depending on source distribution and seed activity.

Uniform loading dictates that each seed is evenly spaced (1 cm from seed center to seed center) throughout the prostate gland. With this technique, a relatively large number of low-activity seeds are used. This has the theoretic advantage of relying less on the precise position of each individual seed. With this technique, if a few seeds migrate out of position during the implant, there will be little disturbance in the ultimate postimplantation dosimetry and, therefore, a low risk of local disease relapse. The potential disadvantage is that this technique delivers a very high dose to the center of the implant volume (the urethra), and it is a more expensive technique due to the higher number of seeds required.

The peripheral loading philosophy of seed distribution dictates placing the seeds just inside of the peripheral edge of the prostate. This relies on relatively few seeds of higher activity to achieve adequate dose to the center of the gland. The potential advantage of this technique is the avoidance of overdosing the central portion of the prostate. The theoretic disadvantage lies in the importance of the precisely accurate placement of each individual seed. Even a few seeds misaligned would be expected to result in a cold spot in the prostate and a hot spot outside the gland. This could be expected to result in overdosing structures outside the prostate (rectum and neurovascular bundle) and underdosing tissue inside the planned treatment volume (cancer).

Modified uniform loading is a fusion of the pure uniform seed spacing system and the pure peripheral seed spacing system. The theoretic advantage of the modified uniform loading technique is that the dose delivered to any specific point within the target volume is relatively independent of the precise position of a specific seed and therefore may be more forgiving of slight errors in seed placement than the peripheral technique. The modified uniform loading technique uses fewer seeds in the central aspect of the target volume than the pure uniform loading system and more than the pure peripheral loading system. It uses more seeds in the periphery of the target volume than the pure uniform loading system. Thus, the dose delivered centrally is less than that expected with the pure uniform technique, yet still greater than the dose delivered to the peripheral edge of the gland.

Clinical studies will have to be performed to determine whether one technique is truly superior in daily practice to another. Because these different planning techniques and implant philosophies have a potential impact on tumor control and treatment morbidity, physicians should be aware of the results of these various implant techniques when advising patients.

The primary dosimetry philosophies used today are modifications of the Manchester (peripheral loading) and Quimby (uniform loading) systems. In considering the merits and pitfalls of each of these systems, it is important to keep in mind the locations anatomically of the rectum, bladder, urethra, neurovascular bundle, and peripheral zone of the prostate. Most centers currently preplan the seed arrangement based on a preoperative TRUS volume study and use a fusion of the Manchester and Quimby loading systems to develop a modified uniform loading preplan for each individual patient (13,78,79). Depending on physician preference and logistics, this preplanning can be done in the clinic weeks before the implant or in the OR minutes before the implant.

The American Brachytherapy Society (ABS) recently recommended that all patients undergo dosimetric planning before the implant procedure itself (46). The initial TRUS volume study is a critical first step in the evaluation and treatment planning of patients who intend to undergo TRUS-guided seed implantation. It is used to develop a treatment plan that identifies the number and activity of the seeds and the precise 3D coordinate into which each seed will need to be placed within the prostate. Most centers perform the TRUS volume study and preimplantation dosimetry weeks before the actual implant, although some prefer to do this in the OR immediately before the procedure (32,45,80–83). It is important to perform this study before the initiation of external beam in those patients receiving combined treatment. It is common to find the TRUS prostate volume to be much larger than initially anticipated by DRE or at the time of ultrasound-guided biopsy. Once the external beam starts, the clock starts running.

The TRUS volume study should be performed with the patient in the same position he will be in at implantation, which is extended dorsal lithotomy. Serial transverse images are taken at 5-mm intervals from base to apex. It is important to take a sagittal image to verify that the sum of the transverse images adds up to the correct prostate length. The number of transverse images should be equal to two times the length of the prostate (in cm) plus one. During the TRUS volume study (and the implant itself), care should be taken to avoid compressing the gland with the ultrasound probe. The normal prostate does not wrap around the rectum in a dog-ear shape. Usually, the ideal megahertz frequency to use during the TRUS volume studies and for implantation is 5.0 to 6.5 MHz and not the 7.5 MHz frequency often used during a diagnostic scan. The ultrasonographer should outline the prostate with the white dotted cursor line (Fig. 23-3). After that, the radiation oncologist outlines the planned target volume. The target volume is usually larger than the prostate volume, especially at the base and apex of the gland. From this, the preplan for a peripheral or modified uniform seed-loading pattern can be run. In the early 1990s, MSKCC used CT-planned implant dosimetry (but not CT or ultrasound guided) and has had success in patients with pretreatment PSA level less

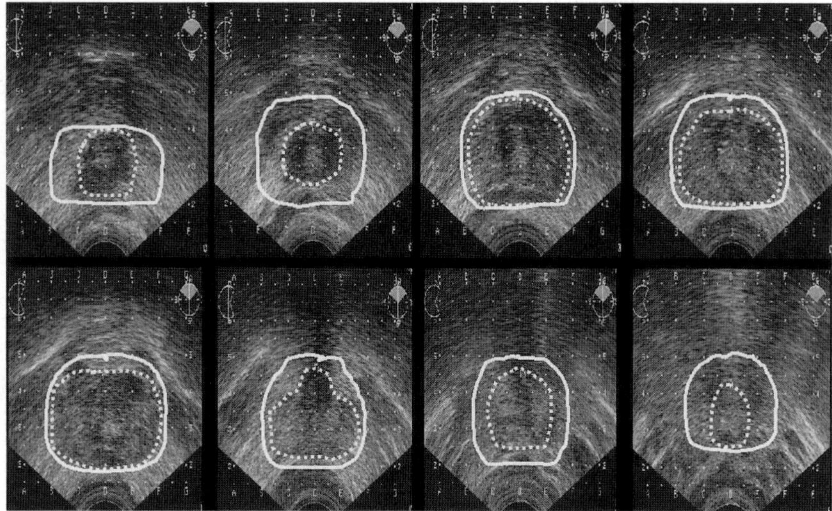

FIGURE 23-3. Transrectal ultrasound images with prostate volume (pv) (*dotted line*) and target volume (tv) (*solid line*) contours.

than or equal to 10 ng per mL but less favorable results in patients with higher pretreatment PSA levels (39,84,85).

DOSE

The exact dose needed to sterilize early stage prostate cancer when treated by brachytherapy is not fully established. Moreover, most studies to date have reported the planned prescription dose for the prostate, not the dose actually achieved at time of implantation.

Current prescription doses have evolved from the old retropubic data from MSKCC and the modern ultrasound-guided technique pioneered by the Seattle team. The retropubic implant MSKCC results reported by Fuks et al. revealed a 60% 10-year local control rate (by DRE) in patients achieving an MDP of 140 Gy or greater but only a 20% local control in those with a dose less than 140 Gy (20). The Seattle team used a prescribed dose of 160 MPD [144-Gy task group (TG)-43] and achieved local control rates in excess of 93% using DRE and biopsy to evaluate local control (13,47,64). A recent report from Stock et al. suggests superior PSA progression-free survival in patients achieving a dose in which 90% of prostate receives (D90) greater than 140 Gy (TG-43) in patients treated with ^{125}I monotherapy (81).

In modern practice, the dose prescribed depends on whether the isotope being used is ^{103}Pd or ^{125}I. Only a few centers worldwide still use gold seeds. For monotherapy with ^{103}Pd, the ABS recommends a prescribed MPD of 115 to 120 Gy and 144 Gy for ^{125}I (45,46,82,86). The doses prescribed for ^{103}Pd and ^{125}I monotherapy are different because the dose rates are different. ^{103}Pd has a half-life of 17 days and a dose rate of 18 to 20 cGy per hour. ^{125}I has a half-life of approximately 59.4 days and a dose rate of 7 cGy per hour (50). ^{125}I has a photon energy of 28 kev and was introduced into clinical practice in 1965. ^{103}Pd has a photon energy of 21 keV and was introduced in 1986. The clinical significance of these differences are controversial. Mathematical models described by Ling et al. suggest that ^{125}I may be more appropriate in slower-growing tumors and ^{103}Pd more effective in faster-growing tumors (87,88). Because of these models, some investigators use ^{125}I for lower Gleason score tumors and ^{103}Pd for higher-grade lesions (79). However, a recent study by Haustermans et al. showed no correlation between cell kinetics and histology in human prostate biopsies (89). Retrospective clinical reviews have not shown a difference in the effectiveness of either isotope for any Gleason score. A randomized trial involving intermediate Gleason score tumors is currently under way at the University of Washington to try to shed some light on this issue. At the present time, the ABS does not recommend one isotope over the other for any Gleason score (46).

Due to the differences in dose rate and half-life, different prescription doses are used for ^{103}Pd and ^{125}I in an attempt to achieve the same radiobiologic effect (45). The MPD of 145 Gy for ^{125}I is believed to be radiobiologically equivalent to the MPD of 115 Gy for ^{103}Pd.

In 1995, the American Association of Physicists in Medicine issued its TG-43 report on interstitial brachytherapy dosimetry. The TG-43 report included a new, single-source dose calculation formalism and recommended dosimetry constraints for ^{125}I sources. The dose rates are predicted to be 10% to 18% less than the pre–TG-43 dose rates. In the end, the prescribed MPD (done with post–TG-43 calculations) would translate into a 10% to 18% higher dose delivered. As a result, to achieve the same biologic effect as 160 Gy MPD pre–TG-43, institutions should now prescribe 144-Gy MPD post–TG-43 (90). The V150 is the volume of prostate that receives 150% or greater of the prescription dose. Most experienced brachytherapists preplan the V150 to be less than 50% of the MPD (79).

The dose delivered to the peripheral edge of the prostate with monotherapy seed implantation is dramatically higher than can be attempted with even 3D conformal external beam radiation therapy or HDR temporary brachytherapy. For a patient to receive the radiobiologic-equivalent dose of a 144-Gy ^{125}I MPD implant, the patient would need to undergo approximately 120 Gy (12,000 cGy) of external beam therapy (87,88). That is just the dose to the outside edge of the prostate. A 144-Gy MDP ^{125}I implant often delivers greater than 20,000 cGy to the peripheral zone of the prostate. The ^{125}I source strength used is usually 0.25 to 0.37 mCi per seed, although some prefer to use higher-strength sources of 0.4 to 0.6 mCi per seed (85,91). In general, peripheral loading philosophies use fewer seeds of higher activity placed more along the periphery of the prostate, whereas modified uniform loading enthusiasts use a higher number of low-strength seeds scattered more evenly throughout the prostate. The use of significantly different seed activities requires different source distribution patterns. These differences should be kept in mind when comparing the results from institutions that use these different seed activities and source loading patterns. The clinical results of one permanent seed implantation technique and loading philosophy may not be the same as a different technique or a different seed-spacing philosophy.

IMPLANT PROCEDURE

The implant procedure can be performed by a radiation oncologist alone or working with a urologist as a team. In most centers, the urologist and radiation oncologist work closely together as a team. The team approach is recommended by most experienced centers, as well as most training courses. The implant usually takes approximately 1 hour to perform. It is typically done under spinal anesthesia and as a clean procedure.

Operating Room Set-Up

Intraoperatively, most centers treat patients with intravenous broad-spectrum antibiotics. The equipment required in the OR includes the ultrasound machine with rectal probe, preferably with multiple MHz frequency options and transverse and sagittal imaging capability. Few centers perform seed implantation under CT guidance. Also needed are the stabilization apparatus (preferably with fine-tuning x-, y-, and z-axis control knobs), needle guidance template, stepper unit to hold the ultrasound probe to the stabilization apparatus, and needles (or Mick apparatus) to place the seeds. Periodically, the apparatus consisting of the stepper, template, and ultrasound system needs to undergo needle-path verification calibrations.

The implant is performed with the patient in dorsal lithotomy position. It is important that the patient be centered symmetrically on the table. The femurs should be perpendicular to the floor. A standard povidone-iodine, 7.5% (Betadine) perineal prep is done, then a KY Jelly infusion aerated urethrogram is performed. The aerated KY Jelly urethral infusion allows visualization of the urethra without distortion of the prostate gland (92). Some centers use a Foley catheter to visualize the urethra. However, a Foley catheter can obstruct visualization of the prostate anterior to the urethra, and it does not allow for visualization of the sulci on either side of the verumontanum, and the balloon can compress the base of the prostate.

After this, the stabilization apparatus, stepper, needle guide spacing template, and ultrasound equipment are set up. The stabilization apparatus anchors the stepping unit to the OR table. The ultrasound probe fits into the stepping unit, and the template is positioned close to the perineum (Fig. 23-4). The physician then centers and aligns the ultrasound probe in the patient's rectum, such that the ultrasound images obtained correlate well with those obtained at the TRUS volume study. The base plane (prostate-bladder interface plane) is established as the 0.0 plane. The other planes are described in relation to the base plane (0.5, 1.0, 1.5, and others from the base plane). The gland is scanned from base to apex to ensure that the probe is properly aligned. The aerated KY Jelly urethral infusion can aid in this regard as well. It is critical that the radiation oncologist double checks the pretreatment plan and the seed strength and isotope that have been brought into the OR to make sure that they match with that particular patient. If multiple cases are done in a single day, then the OR staff might accidentally bring the wrong patient's seeds into the OR.

The physician then begins needle insertion to deposit the radioactive ^{125}I or ^{103}Pd seeds. Some centers use the Mick apparatus to guide seed placement; others prefer preloaded disposable needles (18,86,93). Some prefer to use loose seeds; others prefer seeds within an absorbable Vicryl suture. It typically takes 30 to 60 minutes to deposit the seeds in accordance with the pretreatment plan (whether the plan was done weeks before the implant or in the OR just minutes before). Many have published their own implant techniques (32,45,71,84,94).

Regardless of the particular technical variation used, certain aspects of the transperineal ultrasound-guided permanent implant are universal. During the implant procedure, both physicians need to constantly review prostate and ultrasound probe alignment. Prostate movement can be dramatic as one inserts and withdraws each needle. This is why it is critically important to visualize the prostate while performing the implant procedure. Prostate movement during implantation may help explain the relatively poor results achieved in patients with pretreatment PSA of 10 or greater that underwent CT-planned (but not CT- or ultrasound-guided) monotherapy (41,85). The prostate will distort with each needle insertion. As the needle is inserted, the prostate moves (tents) in a cephalad direction. If the first seed is deposited without correcting this tenting distortion of the prostate, then the seed will be pushed away from its planned position and end up nearer the prostate apex than planned. During the procedure, some bleeding will occur in the perineum; this, combined with swelling of the prostate itself

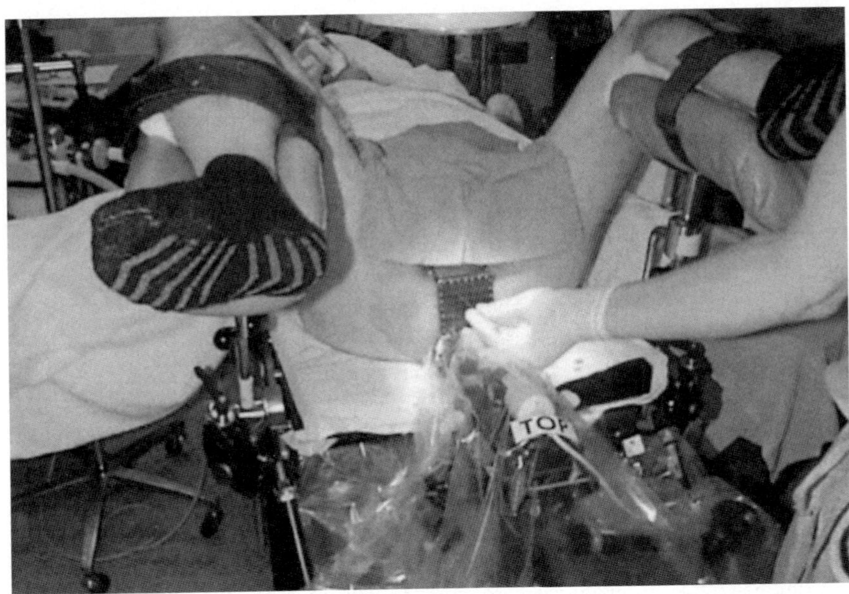

FIGURE 23-4. Photograph showing prostate brachytherapy procedure in process.

during the procedure, will cause the base of the gland to move away from the perineum in a cephalad direction. The combined effects of prostate tenting and cephalad movement explain why so many brachytherapists fail to achieve adequate dose coverage of the base of the prostate during their initial cases (46,95,96). The most common technique used to overcome this problem is to constantly monitor the base position and readjust the base position throughout the case. The base moves in a cephalad direction an average of 1.2 cm per case (64). Overinsert each needle 1 to 2 cm, then slightly overretract, then reinsert each needle until the tip is just barely visible in the ultrasound plan it is planned for. Verify that the base has not moved. Be sure that the needle is not under tension (it does not move in or out when you release your grip on it). All of the above aid in proper positioning of each needle and seed. The prostate also deviates laterally with each needle insertion, especially with the more peripheral needles. To overcome this, target the peripheral-most needles 1 to 2 mm medial of their planned target coordinate. Stabilization needles can help to reduce prostate motion but will not completely eliminate it. Needle depth confirmation can be accomplished by measuring the distance from the needle hub to the template and verifying that the distance is consistent for each needle tip (or seed) placed at that particular transverse image plane. Sagittal view imaging is also helpful in this regard, especially for needles delivering seeds to the base plane.

Pubic Arch Interference

Occasionally, pubic arch interference will be encountered during the procedure despite meticulous preplanning, which includes pubic arch CT scan evaluation. If this occurs, it is in the anterior and lateral needle grid coordinates. This interference can usually be overcome by placing the needle into the coordinate in the template that is 0.5 cm posterior and 0.5 mm medial of the planned template coordinate. Then, the needle can be angled up and out into the proper preplanned coordinate within the prostate with the aid of the needle bevel angle. If that is not enough, then gentle pressure with the physician's finger on the needle between the template and the perineum can guide the needle into the proper position within the prostate. If there is still too much pubic arch interference, put the needle(s) back into the needle holding box and come back to the coordinate(s) at the end of the implant. After placing the seeds that are designated for coordinates that are not obstructed by the pubic arch, change the position of the ultrasound probe so it angles up instead of down. This will usually enable the needle(s) previously obstructed by the pubic arch to get under the pubic arch and into a position very close to its original preplanned position.

Postoperative Procedures

Exposure measurements are taken in the OR or recovery room. These readings in radiation exposure measurements are taken at the patient's surface and at 1 m from the patient. Standard radiation safety procedures are followed with room surveys and Foley bag and catheter and bedding radiation surveys. Many centers recommend placing an ice pack on the patient's perineum while the patient is in the recovery room. The Foley catheter is usually removed when the anesthesia wears off. Postoperative discharge medications typically include an alpha blocker, doxazosin mesylate or tamsulosin hydrochloride (Cardura or Flomax, respectively); acetaminophen with codeine; and an oral antibiotic (trimethoprim-sulfa or ciprofloxacin, 250 mg twice a day). Few centers routinely prescribe a methylprednisolone (Medrol) dose pack.

The radiation oncologist reminds the patient not to have close contact with children younger than 18 years and pregnant women. These restrictions are 1 month for ^{103}Pd implants and 2 months for ^{125}I implants. In general, the previously mentioned guidelines exceed nuclear regulatory commission guidelines.

POSTOPERATIVE DOSIMETRIC EVALUATION

In the past, orthogonal anteroposterior and lateral x-rays were used to develop isodose curves for postoperative dosimetric purposes. Unfortunately, isodose curves based on orthogonal films do not always correlate with the dose the prostate received, because the prostate is not visualized on plain x-rays. Thus, orthogonal film has been for the most part replaced by CT-based dosimetry (Fig. 23-5).

However, CT dosimetry is not without problems. The CT scan has difficulty in delineating the prostate capsule from the periprostatic vasculature. CT scans are not good at identifying the apex of the gland. Image degradation occurs owing to artifacts created by the metallic seeds themselves. This results in CT scans' overestimating the size of the prostate compared to MRI, TRUS, and intraoperative measurements (97–100). This makes it difficult to outline the appropriate prostate area on transverse CT images that are used to develop postimplant dosimetric isodose curves and dose-volume histograms. Furthermore, considerable postimplantation swelling occurs with the procedure. Prestige et al. demonstrated that the CT prostate volume was 41% larger than the preoperative TRUS-planning prostate volume. The prostate volume was found to progressively decrease as CT scans were taken further out from the date of implantation. Thus, even if one reproducibly and accurately outlines the prostate contours on CT scan, significant differences in perceived implant quality occur depending on how many days postoperatively the CT scan is done (101,102). Waiting 3 to 4 weeks before performing the postimplant CT scan allows most of the swelling to resolve. It is important to keep in mind on which postoperative day the CT scan was done when comparing the dosimetric results of one institution with another. Because of prostate swelling, postimplantation dosimetry derived from CT scans performed on day 1 postimplantation will result in lower volume of prostates receiving 100% of prescription dose (V100s), D90s, et cetera, than those run from CT scans performed 3 to 4 weeks postimplantation. Some recent reports indicate that 4 weeks postimplantation may be the best time for posttreatment CT dosimetry scanning (102,103).

Some centers use the preoperative TRUS study to aid in outlining the prostate contours on the postoperative CT scan, and others use a free-hand approach (90).

Most studies to date have claimed to have achieved superior dosimetric results with modern brachytherapy techniques but have evaluated implants qualitatively (not quantitatively with CT dosimetry) (18,30,32,36,38,39,45,94,104). A few reports have been published that quantify the implant quality (41,80,81).

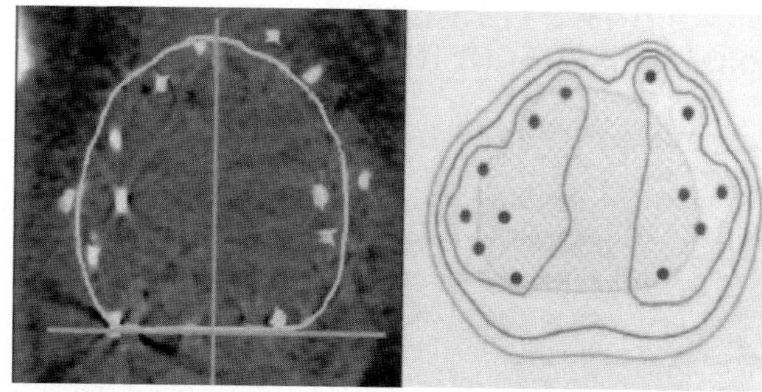

FIGURE 23-5. Illustration showing postimplant computed tomography dosimetry results.

Moreover, at least one paper has correlated an improvement in PSA progression-free survival with improved postimplant dosimetry. Stock and Stone have shown that the patients whom they treated who achieved a D90 of 140 Gy or greater with ^{125}I had superior PSA progression-free survival rates than those who achieved a D90 of less than 140 Gy (81). This is consistent with the historical results reported by MSKCC with the open retropubic technique, although follow-up on the patients with postimplantation D90s greater than 140 Gy was significantly shorter than on those with D90s less than 140 Gy. If the initial implant achieves a D90 or V100 significantly less than planned, then the patient may be a candidate for further therapy, such as external beam irradiation or a second brachytherapy procedure.

At this time, the ABS is recommending postimplantation CT-based dosimetry on patients receiving permanent seed implantation (46). It is important that this be done consistently to document the dose the patient actually received. It also provides feedback to the brachytherapist on the quality of the implants being performed and which regions of the gland are consistently being under- or overdosed. By evaluating implant quality case by case, improvements can be made by altering technique in subsequent implants. The learning curve for this procedure is significant. Postimplant CT dosimetry is the key measuring stick by which the brachytherapy team can be evaluated (46,76,80). The ABS also recommends that implant quality be reported when brachytherapy results are published. The postoperative evaluation should include the D90, V100, and V150. Without quantitative uniform measurements of implant quality, it will be difficult to compare the quality of the implants from one center to the next. If implant quality cannot be compared, then it will not be possible to know if poor clinical outcomes reported at a particular institution are due to brachytherapy (as a treatment option) itself or poor-quality implants at a specific center.

MORBIDITY OF MODERN PROSTATE BRACHYTHERAPY

Intraoperative Morbidity

Intraoperative morbidity has been negligible for modern permanent transperineal ultrasound-guided prostate brachytherapy. Virtually no significant intraoperative complications have been published (28,105). The Seattle team has implanted more than 5,000 patients and has noted no postoperative or intraoperative deaths and no septic complications or other serious perioperative complications.

Early Postoperative Side Effects

The majority of patients can be expected to experience an increase in irritative and obstructive urinary symptoms. These are typically Radiation Therapy Oncology Group (RTOG) grades 1 to 2 urinary symptoms, such as increased frequency, urgency, nocturia, and variable degrees of bladder outlet obstruction (42,47,106). The symptoms are most noted during the first 2 to 6 weeks' status postimplantation, but they can often be bothersome for 2 to 6 months.

These symptoms are probably due to the continual emission of radiation during this time frame. Virtually all patients undergoing seed implantation are placed on alpha blockers, such as doxazosin mesylate or tamsulosin hydrochloride. These symptoms usually have only a minor impact on lifestyle. However, some patients have significant acute urinary retentive effects and temporarily require catheterization. When a catheter is needed, it is usually for a few days or a few weeks; this occurs in approximately 5% to 7% of patients (32,34,42,71,72,75). The incidence of prolonged catheterization (a few months) is approximately 2% to 3% (107). If the patient needs a catheter for longer than just a few weeks, he will usually undergo placement of a suprapubic catheter or be taught self-catheterization. In the very few who fail to have their retentive symptoms resolve, surgical intervention, such as a transurethral incision of the prostate or TURP, can be considered. It must be emphasized that surgical intervention should not be performed until the patient is at least 6 months, and preferably more than 9 months, postimplantation. The published literature indicates an increased incidence of incontinence in patients who undergo TURP before or after permanent seed implantation (18,75). The patient who presents with benign prostatic hypertrophy and a high urinary obstructive score is at highest risk for developing retention (47).

Occasionally, patients will develop proctitis symptoms expressed as increased bowel frequency or urgency, or both. Temporary hematuria and hematospermia are expected, as well as tenderness and bruising in the perineum. Approximately 50% of patients will experience some degree of pain or discomfort at time of orgasm during the first several months after seed implantation. Sexual intercourse may resume shortly after seed implantation. Only 3 of 5,000 patients treated by the Seattle team have reported ejaculation of a seed (P. G. Grimm, *personal communication*, 1999). A bloody ejaculation is expected the first few times. Seed implantation cannot be counted on as birth control. The prostatic fluid component of the ejaculate will decrease dramatically, but sperm in the ejaculate can remain viable. Whether the sperm has been damaged by radiation exposure or by changes in the composition of the ejaculate is not documented.

Long-Term Side Effects

The incidence of long-term side effects is what most patients are concerned about. Many patients chose permanent seed implantation, not only because the tumor control rates appear equivalent to other treatment options, but also because the risk of permanent side effects appears to be relatively low (Table 23-2). There are no RTOG grade 5 complications, only 1% grade 4 and 7% grade 3 permanent urinary effects with modern permanent seed implantation (18,42,44,69,72,85,105,108,109).

TABLE 23-2. TRANSPERINEAL PERMANENT INTERSTITIAL BRACHYTHERAPY: COMPLICATIONS

Series	Tx	Retention (%)	Incontinence (%)	Cystitis (%)	Proctitis (%)	Impotency (%)
Beyer et al. (44)	^{125}I	—	1	4	1	—
Blasko et al. (47)	^{125}I	7	6[a]	7	2	15–50[e]
Stock et al. (32)	^{125}I/^{103}Pd	6	0	3	1.7	6
Wallner et al. (39)	^{125}I	0	0	—	12[d]	19
Blasko et al. (47)	^{125}I + EBRT	4	4[b]	1	6	15–50[e]
Datolli (148)	^{103}Pd + EBRT	7	1	—	—	23
Kaye et al. (38)	^{125}I + EBRT	5	4[c]	4	6	25

EBRT, external beam radiation therapy; ^{125}I, iodine 125; ^{103}Pd, palladium 103; Tx, treatment.
[a]Transurethral resection of the prostate (TURP) patients,17%; non-TURP patients, 0%.
[b]TURP patients, 11%; non-TURP patients, 0%.
[c]TURP patients, 11%; non-TURP patients, 1%.
[d]Computed tomography–planned peripheral loading technique.
[e]Patients <70 years old, 15%; >70 years old, 50%.

Late urinary complications are usually manifested as chronic radiation cystitis, incontinence, or urethral stricture. The bladder neck and the urethra are located in the central high-dose region of the implant and are subject to substantial doses of radiation. Depending on the size of the prostate, the philosophy of seed distribution, and the presence of risk factors, such as a previous TURP, urinary complications have been variable. In patients with a modest-size prostate and no history of a TURP, the incidence of urinary incontinence and chronic cystitis is less than 3% (18,105). In the Seattle series (modified uniform loading technique), the presence of a TURP posed a risk of incontinence of 17% with short follow-up and 32% with 6 years' actuarial follow-up. In patients without a TURP history, the Seattle group found only a 0.4% risk of permanent incontinence (stress or gravity incontinence) (47). The MSKCC series found TURP patients to be only at a slightly higher risk (6%) for incontinence than non-TURP patients (42,72). Whether this lower incidence was due to the use of the peripheral loading technique or because of shorter follow-up (or a combination of the two) is subject to debate. In the Seattle series, urinary complications for seed implantation alone are similar to combined external beam radiation therapy (45 Gy) with a seed boost (110 Gy ^{125}I or 90 Gy ^{103}Pd). From a urinary toxicity view point, the ideal patient for permanent interstitial seed implantation monotherapy is a patient with an intact prostate, only mild to moderate obstructive symptoms, and a gland with a volume of less than 50 to 60 cc.

Rectal complications are noted in 2% to 12% of patients. These are usually self-limited RTOG grades 1 to 2 symptoms in series that adhere to standard dose prescriptions (34,42,69,72,73,75,85). Rectal fistula is quite rare at institutions that use modified uniform seed spacing (18,105). In those patients who undergo external beam radiation with a permanent seed boost, the rectal complication incidence appears to be higher if the external beam portion of therapy is given first. In the initial Danish experience, a 42% incidence of severe rectal complications was reported. In this series, the patients received a 160-Gy (pre–TG-43) ^{125}I implant followed immediately by 47.4-Gy external beam at a high dose per fraction (110); Critz et al. were much more conservative. They delivered only 80 Gy with an ^{125}I implant followed by external beam at 1.5 Gy per fraction to 45 Gy. He reported a 15% incidence of proctitis, despite using relatively low doses at a low dose per fraction (111).

Although the incidence of incontinence and proctitis is low, these toxicities help to fuel the debate over modified uniform versus peripheral source spacing philosophies. As previously mentioned, the modified uniform spacing philosophy delivers higher doses to the center of the target (urethra) than are expected with the peripheral loading technique. This could be expected to lead to a higher risk of late urethral damage and incontinence (112). The peripheral loading philosophy requires distributing higher-activity seeds just inside the periphery of the prostate (close to the rectum). This would be expected to deliver higher doses to the rectum and, thus, a higher incidence of proctitis. The results reported to date do not prove or disprove these points (Table 23-2). The incidence of proctitis was 1% to 2% in the Seattle- and Beyer-modified uniform loading series in patients treated with ^{125}I monotherapy. The two series that used peripheral loading (Stock and Wallner) reported a 2% to 12% rate of proctitis (31,47,71,80,84). The rate of incontinence was 1% to 6% in the modified uniform loading series and 0% in the peripheral loading series. On the surface, this seems to substantiate the theoretic advantages and disadvantages of the two different loading philosophies. However, the risk of incontinence in the modified uniform loading series reported by Beyer, Kaye, and Seattle was only 0% to 1% in patients without a TURP before or after implantation. Moreover, the median follow-up was an average of 35.5 months in the Seattle and Beyer series, but only 18.5 months in the Wallner and Stock series (31,47,71,73,80,84). Longer follow-up is needed in the peripheral loading series to prove a lower incidence of incontinence in the TURP patients treated with this technique.

The patient with an intact urethra can tolerate very high central doses, whereas a patient with a history of urethral surgery is more sensitive to permanent radioactive seed implantation doses. At this time, it is unclear what the long-term risk of incontinence is in the patient with a history of prior urethral surgery. Thus, for the time being, it is reasonable to avoid permanent seed implantation in these patients or use a more peripheral loading approach and explain to the patient that this issue is unresolved.

Impotency data are not yet widely available for brachytherapy. Potency status after definitive prostate cancer treatment is confounded by the fact that different treatment series define potency differently, and patients have different potency rates (related to age and general medical condition) before undergoing treatment. Impotency can also occur later than other complications; thus, series with short follow-up and younger-aged patients would be expected to report superior potency rates.

Preliminary data on a group of 38 patients reported by Wallner et al. suggest that potency can be maintained in 81% of patients at 3 years (85). In the Seattle series, 69% of patients who received combined external beam radiation and seed implantation maintained potency (90). The Seattle group reported a 20% to 30% risk of complete impotency in patients treated with monotherapy and combination therapy, respectively (64,69) (Table 23-2). Approximately 30% to 40% noted a partial loss of erection ability. Kaye reported a 75% potency rate in 44 patients at 1 year (73). Potency data presented in Table 23-2 are not stratified by patient age or preexisting medical conditions. A permanent decrease in the volume of ejaculate is expected after implantation.

RESULTS

Despite the growing level and quality of research on prostate cancer, there is no agreement as to the clinical end points to be used in evaluating the efficacy of the various treatment modalities currently available. In addition, comparisons between surgery and radiation therapy series have been hampered by inadequate staging systems, lack of randomized trials, and the long, natural history of the disease itself. Many surgical series, for example, report results based on pathologic postoperative staging (113). Under these circumstances, meaningful comparison between surgical and radiation series is nearly impossible, even for similarly staged patients, because, in the radiation series, there is not the opportunity to remove patients with positive LNs or extraprostatic disease. Another difficulty is that patients in the radiation series often have higher pretreatment PSA levels than do patients in the surgical series (9,114). In the radiation series, there is still debate as to how biochemical PSA disease-free survival should be defined. What is clear is that it will take improvements in study design, patient groupings, and standards of evaluation for there to be greater confidence in judging the therapeutic impact of individual treatment modalities with one another. Regardless of the method of treatment, it is important for clinicians to recognize that failures will continue to occur at 10 years and beyond (10,115).

Pretreatment Prognostic Factors

Stage has historically been reported as the most important pretreatment prognostic factor for predicting outcome of treatment. However, directly comparing surgery and radiation outcomes on the basis of stage alone is extremely naïve. Patients in the radiation series usually have higher PSAs and grades (9). Comparing radiation series to pathologically staged surgical series is pointless.

Gleason score is clearly another important prognostic factor to take into account when comparing results of various treatment modalities (11,116–118). Zietman et al. demonstrated on a recent analysis that a high PSA (greater than 15) or high grade predicted for a high probability of failure after external beam radiation (9).

PSA has also been demonstrated to be an important independent pretreatment prognostic factor (11,12,118,119). Comparison of pre–PSA era cases and post–PSA era cases in the study by Zagars et al. demonstrated that pretreatment PSA is a useful prognosticator for local control with external beam radiation therapy (12).

Stage and grade, although perhaps only weak prognosticators of local control, are major determinants of metastatic disease (11). Because stage, grade, and PSA influence the risk of extraprostatic disease and treatment outcome, stratification of patients by stage, grade, and PSA will be important to evaluate various treatment modalities adequately. Comparison of treatment results is further complicated by other prognostic factors. Perineural invasion has been shown to increase the risk of extracapsular extension (52). This is especially true for tumors located at the base near the neurovascular bundle (54,58,120). The risk of ECP is increased in patients with four or more positive biopsies (65,66). The risk of ECP may be decreased when the tumor is found to be located in the transitional zone (56,121). Expression of specific genes, such as *bcl-2* and *p53*, may predict for increased risk of external beam radiation failure (122).

Thus, it is difficult to adequately compare treatment results from different centers and between different modalities in the absence of randomized trials. In the meantime, whether treatment is with external beam radiation, radioactive seed implantation, or surgery, it seems prudent to report pretreatment clinical stage, PSA, and Gleason score when evaluating and publishing treatment results in prostate cancer. It would be helpful to stratify results by grouping patients by risk groups. Some centers, such as the Seattle Prostate Institute, and some individuals, such as D'Amico, are presenting PSA outcomes stratified by patient risk groups (64,74). Low or favorable risk groups are patients with pretreatment PSA less than 10 ng per mL, Gleason sum scores 2 to 6, and stage cT1-cT2. High-risk or unfavorable patients in general have two of the three prognostic factors not favorable or a PSA greater than 20 ng per mL. Intermediate-risk patients have one prognostic factor not favorable (e.g., PSA 10 to 20, or Gleason score of 7 or greater, or stage cT3 or greater) (64,74). As can be seen in Figure 23-6, in the Seattle experience, intermediate-risk patients appear to have done well with monotherapy treatment.

Treatment End Point: Local Control

Local control historically was based on the DRE. A suspicious or progressing palpable abnormality on follow-up serial DRE

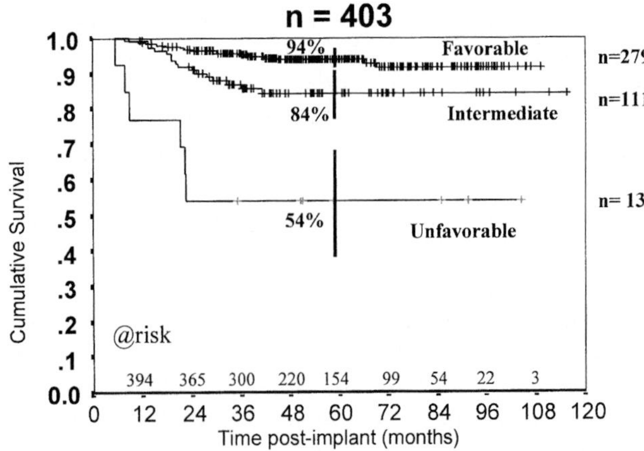

FIGURE 23-6. Iodine 125/palladium 103 monotherapy prostate-specific antigen progression-free survival by risk group. (From Grim P. Clinical results of prostate brachytherapy. Radiological Society of North America Annual Meeting. Chicago, 1998, with permission.)

was considered a local failure. However, because DRE evidence of local failure can take a decade or more to manifest, more sensitive outcome parameters—that is, biopsy, absolute PSA, and, more recently, PSA-free progression—are now used to evaluate local control (9,11,18,23,26,119,123,124).

The significance of biopsy data after external beam radiation or brachytherapy is controversial. The incidence of residual cancer (positive biopsy) after external beam radiation therapy has been reported to range from 25% to 90% (123,125–127). After external beam radiation alone, clinical progression after a positive biopsy has been reported to be 14% to 80% (127,128). In contrast, for external beam radiation followed by ^{125}I seed implantation, Abadir et al. found no prognostic significance for positive biopsy posttreatment (129). This wide range of positive biopsies after external beam radiation and their prognostic significance suggest an inherent problem in pathologic interpretation. This may have been further complicated by patient selection for biopsy and timing of biopsies (130). As radiation can distort the architecture of normal cells, interpretation of postradiation biopsies can be difficult. Often, nonreproductive and nonviable cells can be confused with persistent carcinoma. In addition, malignant cell mortally wounded by radiation and destined for reproductive death may appear undamaged for many months. Thus, positive biopsies can convert to negative even beyond 2 years posttherapy (131,132).

Some pathologists recognize the difficulty in interpretation and have established a separate, "indeterminate" category (131). However, many series do not recognize this indeterminate group or, if so, it is placed in the positive category (127,133–134). The prognostic significance of this indeterminate group is not fully established; however, the Seattle group demonstrated that 85% of the indeterminate biopsies in seed implant patients convert to negative with further follow-up biopsies (131). The lack of consensus in pathology interpretation and the arbitrary placement of the indeterminate biopsies into the positive category make comparisons of treatment outcome by biopsy criteria difficult. This is demonstrated in Table 23-3.

The largest prospective external beam radiation–posttreatment biopsy series is 100 patients with cT1-cT3 disease treated in Ottawa. In this study, 38% of the patients received androgen ablation, whereas none of the patients in the Seattle brachytherapy series did. The Seattle series defined indeterminate and positive categories separately, whereas the Ottawa series did not. Of the 201 patients in the Seattle brachytherapy series who agreed to posttreatment biopsy, six (3%) were positive, and 34 (17%) were called indeterminate. Not all patients in the Seattle series agreed to posttreatment biopsies. However, the patients with higher pretreatment stage and posttreatment PSA were biopsied more than the lower-risk patients. If the positive and indeterminate biopsies in the Seattle series are lumped together (as they are in the Ottawa series), the biopsy positive rates are relatively comparable stage for stage to the Ottawa series. Otherwise, the Seattle series' lower rate of true positive biopsies would appear superior.

What is the significance of a positive biopsy after brachytherapy or external beam radiation? Using a strict definition for positive biopsy, five of six (83%) patients with a positive biopsy in the Seattle series have clinically evident local or distant failure. In the Ottawa series, in which the indeterminate group was included as positive, only 8 of 26 (26%) have evidence of biochemical or clinical failure. The interpretation of and distinction between indeterminate and positive biopsies may therefore be very important. In the Seattle series, 33 patients had an initial biopsy interpreted as indeterminate. In this group, 28 of 33 (85%) subsequently converted to negative on later biopsies (135). Moreover, the median PSA levels in the patients with negative biopsies and in the patients with indeterminate biopsies were both less than 1 ng per mL, whereas in the positive biopsy cohort, the median PSA was greater than 6.9 ng per mL. The Seattle and Ottawa studies suggest that the indeterminate group is more likely to convert to negative or behave clinically similarly to the negative biopsy group, or both. Inclusion of this indeterminate group in the positive posttreatment biopsy group will overestimate the ultimate clinical failure rate (131,132,135).

As a treatment end point, biopsy data have significant limitations. For individual patient care, however, proliferative nuclear cell antigen staining of the biopsy specimens does hold some promise in helping to segregate the truly positive biopsies from the rest (134,136,137). Before making a clinical decision, a positive biopsy specimen after seed implantation should be reviewed by a pathologist experienced in reading postradiation biopsies.

TABLE 23-3. CONVENTIONAL EXTERNAL BEAM RADIATION THERAPY VERSUS BRACHYTHERAPY: BIOPSY RESULTS BY STAGE

	Brachytherapy (Seattle) (64)		External beam (Ottawa) (132)
Stage	Positive	Positive and intermediate	Positive and intermediate
T1b	0%, 0/6	0%, 0/6	0%
T1b/T1c	2%, 1/45	26%, 12/45	21%, 4/19
T2a	2%, 3/125	20%, 26/125	29%, 7/24
T2b	10%, 2/22	10%, 2/22	28%, 10/36
Total	3%, 6/198	21%, 40/192	34%, 21/61

Prostate-Specific Antigen Biochemical Control

Most recent radical prostatectomy and radiation therapy series support posttreatment PSA biochemical failure as the earliest and most sensitive determinate of control and the most significant predictor of clinical failure (114,118,119,130,138). After surgery, an absolute PSA value should approach 0; however,

TABLE 23-4. BRACHYTHERAPY: EARLY PROSTATE-SPECIFIC ANTIGEN (PSA) RESULTS

Series	n	Stages	Tx	PSA control (%)	Follow-up (yr)
Wallner (85)	62	T1, T2	^{125}I	83[a]	3
Kaye et al. (73)	45	T2a	^{125}I	98[b]	2
Beyer et al. (71)	465	T1, T2	^{125}I/^{103}Pd	67[b]	3
Grado et al. (141)	241	T2	^{125}I/^{103}Pd	87[a]	3
Kaye et al. (73)	31	T2b+	EBRT + ^{125}I	95[b]	2
Dattoli et al. (148)	72	T2, T3	EBRT + ^{103}Pd	78[c]	3

EBRT, external beam radiation therapy; ^{125}I, iodine 125; ^{103}Pd, palladium 103; Tx, treatment.
[a]Progression free.
[b]<4.0.
[c]<1.0.

most surgical series use cut-off points of 0.3 to 0.6 ng per mL (10,124,130,139). Some radiation therapy series have used an absolute PSA level as well. These have arbitrarily defined control as PSA less than 4.0, 1.5, 1.0, or 0.5 ng per mL (18,31,101,118,140). One limitation of using an absolute PSA level in radiation series is that in some patients, it takes a long time for the PSA to nadir posttreatment. These patients are censored as failure by absolute PSA criteria, even when their PSA levels are continuing to fall, if they are evaluated when their PSA is still above the absolute PSA value chosen for that particular study or comparison. This would overestimate the failure rate.

A PSA nadir less than 1 ng per mL after external beam radiation is an important predictor of control (11,18,31,101,118,140). A low PSA nadir of less than 0.5 ng per mL has been associated with improved disease-free survival after permanent radioactive seed implantation (141,142). However, absolute PSA values above 0.5, 1.0, and 4.0 have been associated with a disease-free clinical state as well (141–143). The usefulness of choosing an absolute PSA level in selecting and evaluating the ultimate effectiveness of various treatment options or techniques is unresolved.

PSA progression-free survival has recently become a more popular method of evaluating outcomes after radiation therapy (external beam or seed implantation, or both). The American Society of Therapeutic Radiation Oncology consensus conference in 1996 defined *biochemical control* of prostate cancer after radiation therapy as a nonrising PSA or PSA progression-free survival. A patient with three consecutive PSA rises in follow-up is considered to have failed biochemically. The date of that failure is halfway between the PSA nadir and the first PSA rise (114,144). Although this appears to be a sensible definition, it may underestimate failure rates in those series with relatively short follow-up, as the patients may not have been followed long enough to experience the third PSA rise.

Modern Permanent Seed Implantation Results

Modern ultrasound-guided transperineal permanent seed prostate brachytherapy is still relatively new, and, therefore, with the exception of Seattle, most of the available series report short follow-up (18,31,34,73) (Table 23-4). The Seattle results have been presented as absolute PSA levels and as PSA progression-free survival using the American Society of Therapeutic Radiation Oncology consensus conference definition (64).

There are a limited number of surgery and brachytherapy series evaluating absolute PSA results (10,18,47,73,124,139). Figure 23-7 shows a comparison of two recent, large, retrospective surgical series of consecutively treated patients at Washington University, St. Louis, and The Johns Hopkins University to the Seattle brachytherapy series of consecutively treated patients (125,139,145). Using absolute PSA criteria of less than 0.5 ng per mL for surgery and less than 1 ng per mL for permanent seed implantation, the results of brachytherapy are at least as good as surgery at 10 years. Although it is impossible to control for all prognostic factors when comparing the results of retrospective reviews, the generally accepted three most important prognostic factors are listed by series here. The brachytherapy series does not appear to contain patients with more favorable prognostic factors than the surgical series.

A comparison of the major treatment modalities on a basis of PSA progression-free survival at 5 years is noted and shown in Table 23-5. It appears that PSA progression-

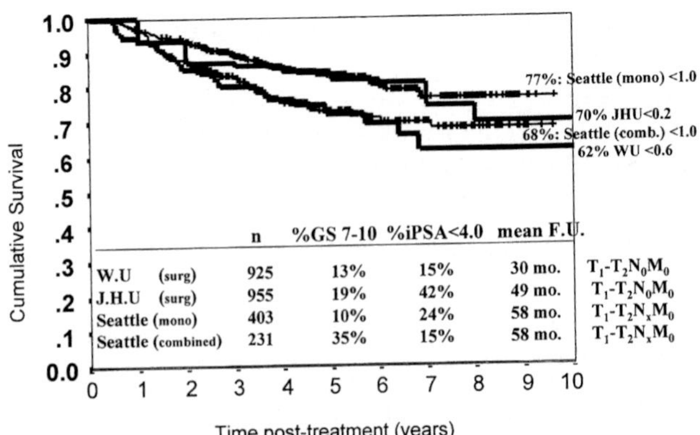

FIGURE 23-7. Surgery versus seeds: biochemical relapse-free survival cT1-T2. FU, follow-up; GS, Gleason score; JHU, The Johns Hopkins University; WU, Washington University.

TABLE 23-5. INTERMEDIATE RISK PATIENTS: T1C-T2/GLEASON SCORE 2–6/iPROSTATE-SPECIFIC ANTIGEN (iPSA) 10–20: FIVE-YEAR PSA-BASED OUTCOMES

Tx	Series	n	Fail definition	Follow-up (yr)	bNED (%)
EBRT	Zagars et al. (12)	140	2 rises	4	45
Surgery	Catalona et al. (139)	253	>0.6 ng/mL	5	70
	Kupelian (155)	73	>0.2 ng/mL	5	56
	Partin (124)	105	>0.2 ng/mL	5	56
Seeds	Beyer et al. (71)	—	>4 ng/mL	5	45
	Wallner et al. (72)	29	>1 ng/mL	4	45
	Blasko et al. (8)	77	>1 ng/mL	5	78
EBRT + seeds	Blasko et al. (8)	71	>1 ng/mL	5	75
	Dattoli et al. (148)	21	>1 ng/mL	5	82

bNED, biochemical no evidence of disease; EBRT, external beam radiation therapy; Tx, treatment.

free survival rates in the brachytherapy series are on a par with the external beam radiotherapy and surgical results across all pretreatment PSA risk cohorts.

In the Seattle series, patients with pretreatment PSAs in the 10 to 20 ng per mL range faired well with seed implantation alone (Fig. 23-8). This was not the case in the series reported by Beyer et al. or in the MSKCC series reported by Wallner et al. (Table 23-5). Whether this difference is due to hidden selection bias or to technique of implantation is unclear. If due to *cold spots* within the implant volume, then one could envision that 45-Gy external beam radiation would "fill in" these underdosed areas. The use of external beam radiation for this purpose has been dubbed *radiation spackle* by Zietman (146). In low-risk patients, a few cold spots might not place the patient at significant risk of subsequent PSA relapse; thus, relatively good results may be seen in the low-risk patient with seed monotherapy in centers that perform excellent-quality implants and in those centers that do not. In the intermediate-risk patient, one would expect a higher volume or density of disease. In these patients, implant quality may be especially important. If this is true, it could explain the variable results reported in the intermediate-risk patients implanted at different institutions. These institutions have variable levels of experience and use different techniques. Patients treated with external beam radiation therapy and a seed implant boost did well in the Seattle series and in Dattoli's series (148).

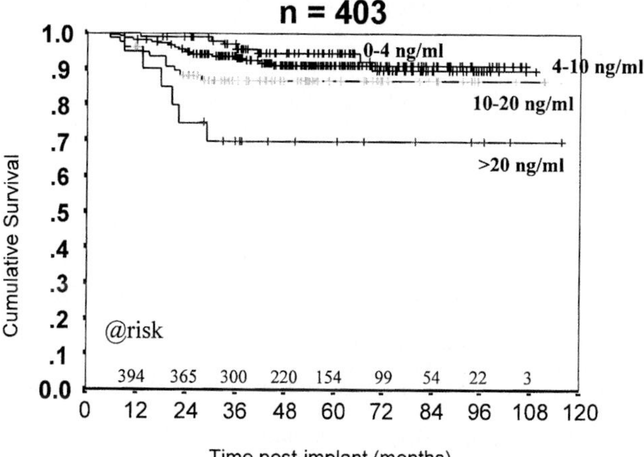

FIGURE 23-8. Iodine 125/palladium 103 monotherapy prostate-specific antigen (PSA) progression-free survival by iPSA.

CONCLUSION

What is the role of brachytherapy in the treatment of prostate cancer? The goal is to deliver a highly conformal dose of radiation to the prostate while relatively sparing normal surrounding tissues. Compared to external beam radiation (standard, 3D conformal, or particle beam), modern transperineal permanent seed implantation is capable of delivering one and a half to two times the radiobiologically equivalent dose of radiation to the prostate. If one believes dose escalation is important to maximize the chance of tumor eradication, then it is apparent that no other radiation modality can compete with brachytherapy in this regard.

Prostate brachytherapy has a long history. The retropubic approach was inconsistent in its effectiveness, owing to limitations in experience, technology, and patient selection in that era. Improvements in patient selection and the development of PSA screening have allowed more men to become appropriate candidates for permanent seed implantation. Advances in technology, such as transrectal ultrasonography, CT scans, sophisticated computerized dosimetry, and the transperineal template-guided approach, have improved the consistency and quality of permanent seed implantation (13,35,46–50). As an outpatient, one-time nonsurgical therapy with minimal long-term morbidity (in non-TURP patients), permanent radioactive seed implantation is becoming a very attractive alternative to radical prostatectomy and daily external beam radiation therapy to a rapidly increasing percentage of men with early-stage prostate cancer (8,18,70,72,73,86,111,147–151).

Accurate comparisons of the efficacy of brachytherapy to surgery and external beam radiation require a randomized study. Comparisons of current retrospective studies are hindered by imbalances in stage, grade, initial PSA, extraprostatic disease, LN status, and other prognostic factors. Most of the long-term data for permanent seed implantation are the result of the work of the Seattle group using a modified uniform seed-spacing preplanned dosimetric philosophy and a transperineal ultrasound- and template-guided approach. These results will need to be repeated by other centers that manage patients with the same planning philosophy and implantation techniques (45). As planning philosophy and implantation techniques may vary from center to center, permanent implant results will also need to be evaluated for technique along with pretreatment prognostic factors.

Selection of patients for seed implantation alone versus combined external beam radiation and seed implant boost is difficult in the intermediate-risk cohort. The results of seed implantation alone in the low-risk patient cohort have been so favorable that it appears adding external beam will not significantly improve results (Fig. 23-6). However, in the intermediate-risk group (initial PSA 10 to 20 ng per mL or Gleason score 7 or greater), results have varied greatly from center to center with seed implantation alone (Table 23-5). Whether this is due to differences in treatment planning and technique, experience, or hidden selection biases remains to be seen. In the high-risk patient, with his substantial risk of ECP, it is difficult not to include an external beam component to the overall treatment plan. In fact, those patients with a pretreatment PSA greater than 20 ng per mL or greater than 15 ng per mL with a Gleason score of 7 or greater have a high risk of PSA progression and failure with any treatment modality (105). In these poor-prognosis patients, the combination of androgen ablation, external beam radiation (45 Gy), and seed implantation may improve the results of seed implantation or external beam irradiation, or both (12,91,152).

Using only PSA data to define risk of relapse is problematic, as it ignores the prognostic impact of Gleason score and stage. Reporting results based on risk cohorts that include PSA, Gleason score, and stage should help us to compare results between various institutions more accurately. Although there is some variation in the definitions of the intermediate- and high-risk cohorts, these are relatively minor. The results of seed implantation, radical prostatectomy, and high-dose 3D conformal radiation therapy have recently been reported by a few centers by risk cohort analysis (Table 23-6).

Currently, the Prostate Brachytherapy Research Group is running a randomized trial to look at whether 6 months of total androgen ablation will improve on the results of 45-Gy external beam radiation with a ^{103}Pd or ^{125}I seed boost in the intermediate- and high-risk cohorts. To date, there is no reported good-quality brachytherapy series with adequate follow-up that demonstrates that adjuvant androgen ablation improves the results of seed implantation monotherapy. Most reports that have included androgen ablation thus far have had poor results in the seed implant–alone arm or have such short follow-up that the androgen ablation may be masking PSA failure in the combination arm (74,153,154).

As mentioned earlier, posttreatment prostate biopsy interpretation is difficult, as indeterminate biopsies may convert to negative at a later date, different pathologists have various levels of expertise in postimplant biopsy interpretation, and, at some centers, a "positive" posttreatment biopsy does not correlate well with clinical outcome. Most authors agree that PSA progression-free survival (rather than an absolute PSA level) is the most reasonable measurement of treatment effectiveness in patients who receive radiation therapy. Few studies to date have 5-year follow-up evaluated by PSA progression-free survival. However, the

TABLE 23-6. FIVE-YEAR BIOCHEMICAL PROSTATE-SPECIFIC ANTIGEN NO EVIDENCE OF DISEASE

	Radical retropubic prostatectomy (%)		3D CRT (%)	Seeds (%)	
Risk group	D'Amico[a] (HUP)	D'Amico[a] (B and W)	Zelefsky[b] (4-yr follow-up)	Blasko[c] (Mono)	Sylvester[d] ± EBRT/TAB
Low	85	83	95	94	94
Intermediate	65	50	79	82	84
High	32	28	60	65	69 77[e]

3D CRT, three-dimensional conformal radiation therapy; B and W, Brigham and Women's Hospital; EBRT, external beam radiation therapy; HUP, Hospital of the University of Pennsylvania; TAB, total androgen blockade.
[a]D'Amico A, Whittington R, Malkowicz S, et al. Clinical utility of the percentage of positive prostate biopsies in defining biochemical outcome after radical prostatectomy for patients with clinically localized prostate cancer [see comments]. *J Clin Oncol* 2000;18:1164–1172.
[b]Zelefsky M, Leibel S, Gaudin P, et al. Dose escalation with three-dimensional conformal radiation therapy affects the outcome in prostate cancer. *Int J Radiat Oncol Biol Phy* 1998;41:491–500.
[c]Blasko J, Grimm P, Sylvester J. Palladium-103 brachytherapy for prostate carcinoma. *Int J Radiat Oncol Biol Phy* 2000;46:839–850.
[d]Sylvester J, Blasko J, Grimm P, et al. Neoadjuvant androgen ablation combined with external-beam radiation therapy and permanent interstitial brachytherapy boost in localized prostate cancer. *Mol Urol* 1999;3:231–236.
[e]Sylvester J, Blasko J, Grimm P, et al. Short-course androgen ablation combined with external-beam radiation therapy and low-dose rate permanent brachytherapy in early-stage prostate cancer: a matched subset analysis. *Mol Urol* 2000;4:155–161.

TABLE 23-7. PROSTATE-SPECIFIC ANTIGEN (PSA) OUTCOMES BY iPSA

iPSA	EBRT[a] (%)	3D CRT[b] (%)	Seeds[c] (%)	Surgery[d] (%)
0–4	69–93	90–97	94–100	92–95
4–10	44–84	83–85	70–90	83–93
10–20	27–72	56–83	47–89	56–71
20+	14–38	20–56	38–80	45

3D CRT, three-dimensional conformal radiation therapy; EBRT, external beam radiation therapy.
[a]8 series (9,11,118,133,138,156–158).
[b]3 series (158–161).
[c]6 series (8,44,73,80,85,148).
[d]2 series (124,162).

few studies available with 5-year follow-up suggest that brachytherapy may be superior to external beam radiation therapy and equal to surgery in the patients who present with a low PSA level. As the presenting PSA level rises, brachytherapy (with or without external beam) becomes an even more attractive option (Table 23-7).

For the patient, brachytherapy is an attractive alternative to surgery and external beam irradiation. In most cases, treatment can be delivered in a single outpatient visit, and patients return to normal activities within a few days. The risk of permanent incontinence is extremely low in the non-TURP patient. The potency preservation rate appears to be relatively good compared to other treatment options. For the radiation oncologist, permanent radioactive seed implantation allows the delivery of radiation doses to the prostate that far surpass conformal external beam radiotherapy, particle beam (proton and neutron) therapy, and HDR temporary brachytherapy. For the urologist, brachytherapy appears to produce tumor control equivalent to radical prostatectomy, yet is a 1-hour outpatient treatment and is suitable not only for patients who are radical prostatectomy candidates, but also for those patients unwilling to have or unsuitable for surgery.

ACKNOWLEDGMENTS

The authors wish to thank William Cavanagh and Charles Heaney for their valuable assistance in the research and editorial preparation of this chapter.

REFERENCES

1. Garfinkel L, Mushinski M. Cancer incidence, mortality, and survival: trends in four leading sites. *Stat Bull Metrop Insur Co* 1994;75:19–27.
2. Mettlin C, Jones GW, Murphy GP. Trends in prostate cancer care in the United States, 1974–1990: observations from the patient care evaluation studies of the American College of Surgeons Commission on Cancer. *CA Cancer J Clin* 1993;43:83–91.
3. Fleming C, Wasson JH, Albertsen PC, et al. A decision analysis of alternative treatment strategies for clinically localized prostate cancer. *JAMA* 1993;269:2650–2658.
4. Talcott JA, Rieker P, Propert K, et al. Complications of treatment for early prostate cancer: a prospective, multi-institutional outcomes study. *Proc Am Soc Clin Oncol* 1994; 13:711(abst).
5. Litwin MS. Health-related quality of life after treatment for localized prostate cancer. *Cancer* 1995;75:2000–2003.
6. Johansson JE, Adami HO, Andersson SO, et al. High 10-year survival rate in patients with early, untreated prostatic cancer [see comments]. *JAMA* 1992;267:2191–2196.
7. Talcott JA, Rieker P, Clark JA, et al. Patient-reported symptoms after primary therapy for early prostate cancer: results of a prospective cohort study. *J Clin Oncol* 1998;16:275–283.
8. Blasko JC, Wallner K, Grimm PD, et al. Prostate specific antigen based disease control following ultrasound guided 125iodine implantation for stage T1/T2 prostatic carcinoma. *J Urol* 1995;154:1096–1099.
9. Zietman AL, Coen JJ, Shipley WU, et al. Radical radiation therapy in the management of prostatic adenocarcinoma: the initial prostate specific antigen value as a predictor of treatment outcome. *J Urol* 1994;151:640–645.
10. Trapasso JG, deKernion JB, Smith RB, et al. The incidence and significance of detectable levels of serum prostate specific antigen after radical prostatectomy [see comments]. *J Urol* 1994;152:1821–1825.
11. Zagars GK, Pollack A, Kavadi VS, et al. Prostate-specific antigen and radiation therapy for clinically localized prostate cancer. *Int J Radiat Oncol Biol Phys* 1995;32:293–306.
12. Zagars GK. Prostate-specific antigen as a prognostic factor for prostate cancer treated by external beam radiotherapy. *Int J Radiat Oncol Biol Phys* 1992;23:47–53.
13. Sylvester J, Blasko JC, Grimm P, et al. Interstitial implantation techniques in prostate cancer. *J Surg Oncol* 1997; 66:65–75.
14. Porter AT, Blasko JC, Grimm PD, et al. Brachytherapy for prostate cancer. *CA Cancer J Clin* 1995;45:165–178.
15. Denning CL. Carcinoma of the prostate seminal vesicles treated with radium. *Surg Gynecol Obstet* 1922;34:99–118.
16. Scardino P, Carlton C. Combined interstitial and external irradiation for prostatic cancer. In: Javadpour N, ed. *Principles and management of urologic cancer.* Baltimore: Williams & Wilkins, 1983:392–408.
17. Whitmore WF Jr., Hilaris B, Grabstald H. Retropubic implantation to iodine 125 in the treatment of prostatic cancer. *J Urol* 1972;108:918–920.
18. Blasko JC, Grimm PD, Ragde H. Brachytherapy and organ preservation in the management of carcinoma of the prostate. *Semin Radiat Oncol* 1993;3:240–249.
19. DeLaney TF, Shipley WU, O'Leary MP, et al. Preoperative irradiation, lymphadenectomy, and 125iodine implantation for patients with localized carcinoma of the prostate. *Int J Radiat Oncol Biol Phys* 1986;12:1779–1785.
20. Fuks Z, Leibel SA, Wallner KE, et al. The effect of local control on metastatic dissemination in carcinoma of the prostate: long-term results in patients treated with 125I implantation. *Int J Radiat Oncol Biol Phys* 1991;21:537–547.
21. Giles GM, Brady LW. 125-Iodine implantation after lymphadenectomy in early carcinoma of the prostate. *Int J Radiat Oncol Biol Phys* 1986;12:2117–2125.

22. Kuban DA, el-Mahdi AM, Schellhammer PF. I-125 interstitial implantation for prostate cancer. What have we learned 10 years later? *Cancer* 1989;63:2415–2420.
23. Morton JD, Peschel RE. Iodine-125 implants versus external beam therapy for stages A2, B, and C prostate cancer. *Int J Radiat Oncol Biol Phys* 1988;14:1153–1157.
24. Schellhammer PF, Whitmore WF, Kuban DA, et al. Morbidity and mortality of local failure after definitive therapy for prostate cancer. *J Urol* 1989;141:567–571.
25. Morton JD, Harrison LB, Peschel RE. Prostatic cancer therapy: comparison of external-beam radiation and I-125 seed implantation treatment of stages B and C neoplasms. *Radiology* 1986;159:249–252.
26. Koprowski CD, Berkenstock KG, Borofski AM, et al. External beam irradiation versus 125 iodine implant in the definitive treatment of prostate carcinoma [see comments]. *Int J Radiat Oncol Biol Phys* 1991;21:955–960.
27. Hilaris B, Fuks Z, Nori D, et al. Interstitial irradiation in prostatic cancer: report of 10-year results. In: Rolf, ed. *Interventional radiation therapy techniques/brachytherapy.* Berlin: Springer-Verlag, 1991:235.
28. Puthawala A, Syed A, Tansey L. Temporary iridium implant in the management of carcinoma of the prostate. *Endocurie Hyper Oncol* 1985;1:25–33.
29. Martinez A, Edmundson GK, Cox RS, et al. Combination of external beam irradiation and multiple-site perineal applicator (MUPIT) for treatment of locally advanced or recurrent prostatic, anorectal, and gynecologic malignancies. *Int J Radiat Oncol Biol Phys* 1985;11:391–398.
30. Holm HH, Juul N, Pedersen JF, et al. Transperineal 125-iodine seed implantation in prostatic cancer guided by transrectal ultrasonography. *J Urol* 1983;130:283–286.
31. Priestly JB Jr., Beyer DC. Guided brachytherapy for treatment of confined prostate cancer. *Urology* 1992;40:27–32.
32. Stock RG, Stone NN, Wesson MF, et al. A modified technique allowing interactive ultrasound-guided three-dimensional transperineal prostate implantation. *Int J Radiat Oncol Biol Phys* 1995;32:219–225.
33. D'Amico AV, Coleman CN. Role of interstitial radiotherapy in the management of clinically organ-confined prostate cancer: the jury is still out [see comments]. *J Clin Oncol* 1996;14:304–315.
34. Dattoli MJ, Wasserman SG, Koval JM, et al. Conformal brachytherapy boost to external beam irradiation for localized high risk prostate cancer. *Int J Radiat Oncol Biol Phys* 1995;32[Suppl]:251(abst).
35. Tapen EM, Blasko JC, Grimm PD, et al. Reduction of radioactive seed embolization to the lung following prostate brachytherapy. *Int J Radiat Oncol Biol Phys* 1998;42:1063–1067.
36. Blasko JC, Radge H, Schumacher D. Transperineal percutaneous iodine-125 implantation for prostatic carcinoma using transrectal ultrasound and template guidance. *Endocurie Hyper Oncol* 1987;3:131–139.
37. Grado GL, Larson TR, Collins JM, et al. Fluoroscopic and ultrasound guided prostate implant: technique and experience at Mayo clinic Scottsdale. *American Brachytherapy Society, 18th Annual Meeting* 1995:10(abst).
38. Kaye KW, Olson DJ, Lightner DJ, et al. Improved technique for prostate seed implantation: combined ultrasound and fluoroscopic guidance. *J Endourol* 1992;6:61–66.
39. Wallner K, Chiu-Tsao ST, Roy J, et al. An improved method for computerized tomography-planned transperineal 125iodine prostate implants. *J Urol* 1991;146:90–95.
40. Roy JN, Wallner KE, Chiu-Tsao ST, et al. CT-based optimized planning for transperineal prostate implant with customized template. *Int J Radiat Oncol Biol Phys* 1991;21:483–489.
41. Willins J, Wallner K. CT-based dosimetry for transperineal I-125 prostate brachytherapy. *Int J Radiat Oncol Biol Phys* 1997;39:347–353.
42. Arterbery VE, Wallner K, Roy J, et al. Short-term morbidity from CT-planned transperineal I-125 prostate implants. *Int J Radiat Oncol Biol Phys* 1993;25:661–667.
43. D'Amico AV. MRI-guided Seeds Second Annual Advanced Prostate Brachytherapy Conference. Seattle, WA: Seattle Prostate Institute, 1999.
44. Beyer DC, Priestley JB Jr. Biochemical disease-free survival following 125I prostate implantation. *Int J Radiat Oncol Biol Phys* 1997;37:559–563.
45. Grimm PD, Blasko JC, Ragde H. Ultrasound-guided transperineal implantation of Iodine-125 and Palladium-103 for the treatment of early-stage prostate cancer: technical concepts in planning, operative technique, and evaluation. In: Schellhammer PF, ed. *New techniques in prostate surgery.* Philadelphia: WB Saunders, 1994:113–126.
46. Nag S, Beyer D, Friedland J, et al. American Brachytherapy Society (ABS) recommendations for transperineal permanent brachytherapy of prostate cancer. *Int J Radiat Oncol Biol Phys* 1999;44:789–799.
47. Blasko JC, Ragde H, Luse RW, et al. Should brachytherapy be considered a therapeutic option in localized prostate cancer? *Urol Clin North Am* 1996;23:633–649.
48. Wallner K, Blasko J, Dattoli M. *Prostate brachytherapy made complicated.* Seattle: Smart Medicine Press, 1997.
49. Blasko JC, Ragde H, Grimm PD, et al. Potential for neoadjuvant hormonal therapy with brachytherapy for prostate cancer. *Mol Urol* 1997;1:207–214.
50. Grimm PD, Blasko JC, Ragde H, et al. Does brachytherapy have a role in the treatment of prostate cancer? *Hematol Oncol Clin North Am* 1996;10:653–673.
51. Ackerman DA, Barry JM, Wicklund RA, et al. Analysis of risk factors associated with prostate cancer extension to the surgical margin and pelvic node metastasis at radical prostatectomy. *J Urol* 1993;150:1845–1850.
52. Bastacky SI, Walsh PC, Epstein JI. Relationship between perineural tumor invasion on needle biopsy and radical prostatectomy capsular penetration in clinical stage B adenocarcinoma of the prostate. *Am J Surg Pathol* 1993;17:336–341.
53. Epstein JI, Walsh PC, Carmichael M, et al. Pathologic and clinical findings to predict tumor extent of nonpalpable (stage T1C) prostate cancer. *JAMA* 1994;271:368–374.
54. Epstein JI, Carmichael MJ, Pizov G, et al. Influence of capsular penetration on progression following radical prostatectomy: a study of 196 cases with long-term followup. *J Urol* 1993;150:135–141.
55. Epstein JI, Pizov G, Walsh PC. Correlation of pathologic findings with progression after radical retropubic prostatectomy. *Cancer* 1993;71:3582–3593.
56. McNeal JE. Cancer volume and site of origin of adenocarcinoma in the prostate: relationship to local and distant spread. *Hum Pathol* 1992;23:258–266.

57. Partin AW, Carter HB, Chan DW, et al. Prostate specific antigen in the staging of localized prostate cancer: influence of tumor differentiation, tumor volume and benign hyperplasia. *J Urol* 1990;143:747–752.
58. Partin AW, Yoo J, Carter HB, et al. The use of prostate specific antigen, clinical stage and Gleason score to predict pathological stage in men with localized prostate cancer [see comments]. *J Urol* 1993;150:110–114.
59. Partin AW, Kattan MW, Subong EN, et al. Combination of prostate-specific antigen, clinical stage, and Gleason score to predict pathological stage of localized prostate cancer. A multi-institutional update [see comments] [published erratum appears in *JAMA* 1997;278:118]. *JAMA* 1997;277: 1445–1451.
60. Rosen MA, Goldstone L, Lapin S, et al. Frequency and location of extracapsular extension and positive surgical margins in radical prostatectomy specimens. *J Urol* 1992; 148:331–337.
61. Partin AW, Pearson JD, Landis PK, et al. Evaluation of serum prostate-specific antigen velocity after radical prostatectomy to distinguish local recurrence from distant metastases. *Urology* 1994;43:649–659.
62. Davis BJ, Pisansky TM, Wilson TM, et al. The radial distance of extraprostatic extension of prostate carcinoma: implications for prostate brachytherapy. *Cancer* 1999;85: 2630–2637.
63. Sohayda C, Kupelian PA, Ciezki J, et al. Extent of extracapsular extension: implications for planning for conformal radiotherapy and brachytherapy. *Int J Radiat Oncol Phys* 1998;42[Suppl]:132(abst).
64. Grimm P. Clinical results of prostate brachytherapy. Radiological Society of North America Annual Meeting. Chicago, 1998.
65. Daniels GF Jr., McNeal JE, Stamey TA. Predictive value of contralateral biopsies in unilaterally palpable prostate cancer. *J Urol* 1992;147:870–874.
66. Peller PA, Young DC, Marmaduke DP, et al. Sextant prostate biopsies. A histopathologic correlation with radical prostatectomy specimens. *Cancer* 1995;75:530–538.
67. Stamey TA, McNeal JE, Freiha FS, et al. Morphometric and clinical studies on 68 consecutive radical prostatectomies. *J Urol* 1988;139:1235–1241.
68. Chelsky MJ, Schnall MD, Seidmon EJ, et al. Use of endorectal surface coil magnetic resonance imaging for local staging of prostate cancer. *J Urol* 1993;150:391–395.
69. Ragde H, Blasko JC, Grimm PD. *Complications of permanent seed implantation transperineal brachytherapy: into the mainstream*. Seattle: Pacific NW Cancer Foundation, 1995.
70. Grimm PD, Blasko JC, Ragde H, et al. Transperineal ultrasound guided I-125/PD-103 brachytherapy for early stage prostate cancer: update on clinical experience at seven years. *Int J Radiat Oncol Biol Phys* 1997;39[Suppl]:219(abst).
71. Beyer DC, Priestley JB. Biochemical disease-free survival following I-125 prostate implantation. *Int J Radiat Oncol Biol Phys* 1995;32[Suppl]:254(abst).
72. Wallner K, Roy J, Zelefsky M, et al. Short-term freedom from disease progression after I-125 prostate implantation. *Int J Radiat Oncol Biol Phys* 1994;30:405–409.
73. Kaye KW, Olson DJ, Payne JT. Detailed preliminary analysis of 125iodine implantation for localized prostate cancer using percutaneous approach. *J Urol* 1995;153:1020–1025.
74. D'Amico AV, Whittington R, Malkowicz SB, et al. Biochemical outcome after radical prostatectomy, external beam radiation therapy, or interstitial radiation therapy for clinically localized prostate cancer [see comments]. *JAMA* 1998;280:969–974.
75. Blasko JC, Ragde H, Grimm PD. Transperineal ultrasound-guided implantation of the prostate: morbidity and complications. *Scand J Urol Nephrol Suppl* 1991;137:113–118.
76. Prestidge BR, Bice WS, Prete JJ, et al. A dose-volume analysis of permanent transperineal prostate brachytherapy. *Int J Radiat Oncol Biol Phys* 1997;39[Suppl]:289.
77. Hastak SM, Gammelgaard J, Holm HH. Transrectal ultrasonic volume determination of the prostate—a preoperative and postoperative study. *J Urol* 1982;127:1115–1118.
78. Paulson DF. Impact of radical prostatectomy in the management of clinically localized disease. *J Urol* 1994;152:1826–1830.
79. Prestidge BR, Prete JJ, Buchholz TA, et al. A survey of current clinical practice of permanent prostate brachytherapy in the United States. *Int J Radiat Oncol Biol Phys* 1998; 40:461–465.
80. Stock RG, Stone NN, DeWyngaert JK, et al. Prostate specific antigen findings and biopsy results following interactive ultrasound guided transperineal brachytherapy for early stage prostate carcinoma. *Cancer* 1996;77:2386–2392.
81. Stock RG, Stone NN, Tabert A, et al. A dose-response study for I-125 prostate implants. *Int J Radiat Oncol Biol Phys* 1998;41:101–108.
82. Nag S, Scaperoth DD, Badalament R, et al. Transperineal palladium 103 prostate brachytherapy: analysis of morbidity and seed migration. *Urology* 1995;45:87–92.
83. Nag S. Transperineal iodine-125 implantation of the prostate under transrectal ultrasound and fluoroscopic control. *Endocuriether Hypertherm* 1985;1:207–211.
84. Wallner K. I-125 brachytherapy for early stage prostate cancer: new techniques may achieve better results. *Oncology* 1991;5:115–126.
85. Wallner K, Roy J, Harrison L. Tumor control and morbidity following transperineal iodine 125 implantation for stage T1/T2 prostatic carcinoma. *J Clin Oncol* 1996;14:449–453.
86. Nag S, Pak V, Blasko J, et al. Prostate brachytherapy. In: Nag S, ed. *Principles and practices of brachytherapy*. Armonk, NY: Futura Publishing, 1997:421–440.
87. Ling CC. Permanent implants using Au-198, Pd-103 and I-125: radiobiological considerations based on the linear quadratic model. *Int J Radiat Oncol Biol Phys* 1992;23:81–87.
88. Ling CC, Li WX, Anderson LL. The relative biological effectiveness of I-125 and Pd-103. *Int J Radiat Oncol Biol Phys* 1995;32:373–378.
89. Haustermans KM, Hofland I, Van Poppel H, et al. Cell kinetic measurements in prostate cancer. *Int J Radiat Oncol Biol Phys* 1997;37:1067–1070.
90. *First Advanced Prostate Brachytherapy Workshop*. Seattle: Seattle Prostate Institute, 1998.
91. Stone NN, Stock RG. Brachytherapy for prostate cancer: real-time three-dimensional interactive seed implantation. *Tech Urol* 1995;1:72–80.
92. Sylvester JE, Grimm PD, Blasko JC. Urethral visualization during transrectal ultrasound guided interstitial implantation for early stage prostate cancer. *Annual Meeting of the Radiological Society of North America*. Chicago, IL, 1998.
93. Butler WM. I-125 rapid strand loading technique. *Radiat Oncol Invest* 1996;4:48–49.
94. Wallner K, Roy J, Zelefsky M, et al. Fluoroscopic visualization of the prostatic urethra to guide transperineal prostate implantation. *Int J Radiat Oncol Biol Phys* 1994;29:863–867.

95. Dattoli M, Waller K. A simple method to stabilize the prostate during transperineal prostate brachytherapy. *Int J Radiat Oncol Biol Phys* 1997;38:341–342.
96. Feygelman V, Friedland JL, Sanders RM, et al. Improvement in dosimetry of ultrasound-guided prostate implants with the use of multiple stabilization needles. *Med Dosim* 1996;21:109–112.
97. Gomella LG, Lotfi MA, Reagan GN. Laboratory parameters following contact laser ablation of the prostate for benign prostatic hypertrophy. *Tech Urol* 1995;1:168–171.
98. Hastak SM, Gammelgaard J, Holm HH. Transrectal ultrasonic volume determination of the prostate—a preoperative and postoperative study. *J Urol* 1982;127:1115–1118.
99. Sandler HM, Bree RL, McLaughlin PW, et al. Localization of the prostatic apex for radiation therapy using implanted markers. *Int J Radiat Oncol Biol Phys* 1993;27:915–919.
100. Hricak H, Jeffrey RB, Dooms GC, et al. Evaluation of prostate size: a comparison of ultrasound and magnetic resonance imaging. *Urol Radiol* 1987;9:1–8.
101. Corn BW, Hanks GE, Schultheiss TE, et al. Conformal treatment of prostate cancer with improved targeting: superior prostate-specific antigen response compared to standard treatment [see comments]. *Int J Radiat Oncol Biol Phys* 1995;32:325–330.
102. Waterman FM, Yue N, Reisinger S, et al. Effect of edema on the post-implant dosimetry of an I-125 prostate implant: a case study. *Int J Radiat Oncol Biol Phys* 1997;38:335–339.
103. Prestidge BR, Bice WS, Kiefer EJ, et al. Timing of computed tomography-based postimplant assessment following permanent transperineal prostate brachytherapy [see comments]. *Int J Radiat Oncol Biol Phys* 1998;40:1111–1115.
104. Ragde H, Blasko JC, Schumacher D, et al. Use of transrectal ultrasound in transperineal Iodine-125 seeding for prostate cancer: methodology. *J Endourol* 1989;3:209–218.
105. Blasko JC, Grimm PD, Ragde H. *6 and 7 year results of permanent seed implantation transperineal brachytherapy: into the mainstream.* Seattle: Pacific NW Cancer Foundation, 1995.
106. Blasko JC, Grimm PD, Ragde H. External beam irradiation with palladium-103 implantation for prostate carcinoma. *Int J Radiat Oncol Biol Phys* 1994;30:219.
107. Meier R. *Second advanced prostate brachytherapy workshop.* Seattle: Seattle Prostate Institute, 1999.
108. Stock RG, Stone NN, DeWyngaert JK. PSA findings and biopsy results following interactive ultrasound guided transperineal brachytherapy for early stage prostate cancer. *Proceedings of the American Radium Society 78th Annual Meeting*. Paris, 1995:58.
109. Wallner K, Lee H, Wasserman S, et al. Low risk of urinary incontinence following prostate brachytherapy in patients with a prior transurethral prostate resection. *Int J Radiat Oncol Biol Phys* 1997;37:565–569.
110. Iversen P, Bak M, Juul N, et al. Ultrasonically guided 125iodine seed implantation with external radiation in management of localized prostatic carcinoma. *Urology* 1989; 34:181–186.
111. Critz FA, Tarlton RS, Holladay DA. Prostate specific antigen-monitored combination radiotherapy for patients with prostate cancer. *Cancer* 1995;75:2383–2391.
112. Roy JN, Ling CC, Wallner KE, et al. Determining source strength and source distribution for a transperineal prostate implant. *Endocurie Hyperthermia Oncology* 1996;12:35–41.
113. Stein A, deKernion JB, Smith RB, et al. Prostate specific antigen levels after radical prostatectomy in patients with organ confined and locally extensive prostate cancer. *J Urol* 1992;147:942–946.
114. Pollack A, Zagars GK, Kavadi VS. Prostate specific antigen doubling time and disease relapse after radiotherapy for prostate cancer. *Cancer* 1994;74:670–678.
115. Zincke H, Oesterling JE, Blute ML, et al. Long-term (15 years) results after radical prostatectomy for clinically localized (stage T2c or lower) prostate cancer [see comments]. *J Urol* 1994;152:1850–1857.
116. Stamey TA, Yang N, Hay AR, et al. Prostate-specific antigen as a serum marker for adenocarcinoma of the prostate. *N Engl J Med* 1987;317:909–916.
117. Bova GS, Partin AW, Isaacs SD, et al. Biological aggressiveness of hereditary prostate cancer: long-term evaluation following radical prostatectomy. *J Urol* 1998;160:660–663.
118. Pisansky TM, Cha SS, Earle JD, et al. Prostate-specific antigen as a pretherapy prognostic factor in patients treated with radiation therapy for clinically localized prostate cancer. *J Clin Oncol* 1993;11:2158–2166.
119. Ritter MA, Messing EM, Shanahan TG, et al. Prostate-specific antigen as a predictor of radiotherapy response and patterns of failure in localized prostate cancer [see comments]. *J Clin Oncol* 1992;10:1208–1217.
120. Villers A, McNeal JE, Redwine EA, et al. The role of perineural space invasion in the local spread of prostatic adenocarcinoma. *J Urol* 1989;142:763–768.
121. Stamey TA, Dietrick DD, Issa MM. Large, organ confined, impalpable transition zone prostate cancer: association with metastatic levels of prostate specific antigen. *J Urol* 1993; 149:510–515.
122. Scherr DS, Vaughan ED Jr., Wei J, et al. BCL-2 and p53 expression in clinically localized prostate cancer predicts response to external beam radiotherapy. *J Urol* 1999;162:12–16.
123. Kuban DA, el-Mahdi AM, Schellhammer P. The significance of post-irradiation prostate biopsy with long-term follow-up. *Int J Radiat Oncol Biol Phys* 1992;24:409–414.
124. Partin AW, Pound CR, Clemons JQ, et al. Serum PSA after anatomic radical prostatectomy. The Johns Hopkins experience after 10 years. *Urol Clin North Am* 1993;20:713–725.
125. Dugan TC, Shipley WU, Young RH, et al. Biopsy after external beam radiation therapy for adenocarcinoma of the prostate: correlation with original histological grade and current prostate specific antigen levels [see comments]. *J Urol* 1991;146:1313–1316.
126. Kabalin JN, Hodge KK, McNeal JE, et al. Identification of residual cancer in the prostate following radiation therapy: role of transrectal ultrasound guided biopsy and prostate specific antigen. *J Urol* 1989;142:326–331.
127. Scardino PT, Frankel JM, Wheeler TM, et al. The prognostic significance of post-irradiation biopsy results in patients with prostatic cancer. *J Urol* 1986;135:510–516.
128. Kuban DA, el-Mahdi AM, Schellhammer PF. Prognostic significance of post-irradiation prostate biopsies. *Oncology (Huntingt)* 1993;7:29–38.
129. Abadir R, Ross G Jr., Weinstein SH. Carcinoma of the prostate irradiated by combined I125 and external irradiation. Analysis of failure and significance of positive biopsy one year or more after therapy. *Int J Radiat Oncol Biol Phys* 1983;9:305–309.

130. Zietman AL, Shipley WU, Coen JJ. Radical prostatectomy and radical radiation therapy for clinical stages T1 to 2 adenocarcinoma of the prostate: new insights into outcome from repeat biopsy and prostate specific antigen followup [see comments]. *J Urol* 1994;152:1806–1812.
131. Prestidge BR, Hoak DC, Grimm PD, et al. Post-treatment biopsy results following interstitial brachytherapy in early stage prostate cancer. *Int J Radiat Oncol Biol Phys* 1995; 32[Suppl]:144(abst).
132. Crook J, Robertson S, Collin G, et al. Clinical relevance of trans-rectal ultrasound, biopsy, and serum prostate-specific antigen following external beam radiotherapy for carcinoma of the prostate. *Int J Radiat Oncol Biol Phys* 1993;27:31–37.
133. Kuban DA, el-Mahdi AM, Schellhammer PF. Prostate-specific antigen for pretreatment prediction and posttreatment evaluation of outcome after definitive irradiation for prostate cancer [see comments]. *Int J Radiat Oncol Biol Phys* 1995;32:307–316.
134. Schellhammer PF, Ladaga LE, El-Mahdi A. Histological characteristics of prostatic biopsies after 125iodine implantation. *J Urol* 1980;123:700–705.
135. Prestidge BR, Hoak DC, Grimm PD, et al. Posttreatment biopsy results following interstitial brachytherapy in early-stage prostate cancer. *Int J Radiat Oncol Biol Phys* 1997;37:31–39.
136. Crook J, Robertson S, Esche B. Proliferative cell nuclear antigen in postradiotherapy prostate biopsies. *Int J Radiat Oncol Biol Phys* 1994;30:303–308.
137. Crook JM, Bahadur YA, Bociek RG, et al. Radiotherapy for localized prostate carcinoma. The correlation of pretreatment prostate specific antigen and nadir prostate specific antigen with outcome as assessed by systematic biopsy and serum prostate specific antigen. *Cancer* 1997;79:328–336.
138. Kaplan ID, Cox RS, Bagshaw MA. Prostate specific antigen after external beam radiotherapy for prostatic cancer: followup. *J Urol* 1993;149:519–522.
139. Catalona WJ, Smith DS. 5-year tumor recurrence rates after anatomical radical retropubic prostatectomy for prostate cancer [see comments]. *J Urol* 1994;152:1837–1842.
140. Russell KJ, Dunatov C, Hafermann MD, et al. Prostate specific antigen in the management of patients with localized adenocarcinoma of the prostate treated with primary radiation therapy. *J Urol* 1991;146:1046–1052.
141. Grado GL, Larson TR, Balch CS, et al. Actuarial disease-free survival after prostate cancer brachytherapy using interactive techniques with biplane ultrasound and fluoroscopic guidance. *Int J Radiat Oncol Biol Phys* 1998;42:289–298.
142. Critz FA, Levinson AK, Williams WH, et al. The PSA nadir that indicates potential cure after radiotherapy for prostate cancer. *Urology* 1997;49:322–326.
143. Zietman AL, Tibbs MK, Dallow KC, et al. Use of PSA nadir to predict subsequent biochemical outcome following external beam radiation therapy for T1-2 adenocarcinoma of the prostate. *Radiother Oncol* 1996;40:159–162.
144. Horwitz EM, Hanlon AL, Pinover WH, et al. The treatment of nonpalpable PSA-detected adenocarcinoma of the prostate with 3-dimensional conformal radiation therapy. *Int J Radiat Oncol Biol Phys* 1998;41:519–523.
145. Blasko JC. *Localized prostate cancer: external beam vs. brachytherapy: American Urological Association Annual Meeting.* Dallas: American Urological Association, 1999.
146. Zietman A. Role of external beam radiation. *First Advanced Prostate Brachytherapy Workshop.* Seattle: Seattle Prostate Institute, 1998.
147. Blasko JC, Ragde H, Grimm PD, et al. Transperineal ultrasound-guided brachytherapy with I-125 or Pd-103 for prostate cancer: the Seattle experience in 508 patients. *37th Annual Meeting of the American Society for Therapeutic Radiology and Oncology*, October Miami Beach, FL, 1995.
148. Dattoli M, Wallner K, Sorace R, et al. 103Pd brachytherapy and external beam irradiation for clinically localized, high-risk prostatic carcinoma [see comments]. *Int J Radiat Oncol Biol Phys* 1996;35:875–879.
149. Prestige BR. Radioisotopic implantation for carcinoma of the prostate. *Semin Radiat Oncol* 1998;8:124–131.
150. Stokes SH, Real JD, Adams PW, et al. Transperineal ultrasound-guided radioactive seed implantation for organ-confined carcinoma of the prostate. *Int J Radiat Oncol Biol Phys* 1997;37:337–341.
151. Stock RG, Stone NN, Iannuzzi C. Sexual potency following interactive ultrasound-guided brachytherapy for prostate cancer. *Int J Radiat Oncol Biol Phys* 1996;35:267–272.
152. Sylvester J, Blasko JC, Grimm PD, et al. Neoadjuvant androgen ablation combined with external beam radiation therapy and permanent interstitial brachytherapy boost in localized prostate cancer. *Mol Urol* 1999;3:231–236.
153. Sharkey J, Chovnick SD, Behar RJ, et al. Outpatient ultrasound-guided palladium 103 brachytherapy for localized adenocarcinoma of the prostate: a preliminary report of 434 patients. *Urology* 1998;51:796–803.
154. Stone NN, Stock RG. Prostate brachytherapy: treatment strategies. *J Urol* 1999;162:421–426.
155. Kupelian P, Katcher J, Levin H, et al. Correlation of clinical and pathological factors with rising prostate-specific antigen profiles after radical prostatectomy alone for clinically localized prostate cancer. *Urology* 1996;48:249–260.
156. Lee WR, Hanks GE, Schultheiss TE, et al. Localized prostate cancer treated by external-beam ratiotherapy alone: serum prostate-specific antigen–driven outcome analysis. *J Clin Oncol* 1995;13:464–469.
157. Horwitz EM, Vincini FA, Ziaja EL, et al. Assessing the variability of outcome for patients treated with localized prostate irradiation using different definitions of biochemical control [see comments]. *Int J Radiat Oncol Biol Phys* 1996;36:565–571.
158. Schneider SB, Schweitzer VG, Parker RG, et al. The prognostic value of PSA levels in radiation therapy of patients with carcinoma of the prostate: the UCLA experience, 1988–1992. *Am J Clin Oncol* 1996;19:65–72.
159. Zelefsky MJ, Leibel SA, Kutcher GJ, et al. The feasibility of dose escalation with three-dimensional conformal radiotherapy in patients with prostatic carcinoma escalation. *Cancer J Sci Am* 1995;1:142.
160. Hanks GE, Schultheiss TE, Hanlon AL, et al. Optimization of conformal radiation treatment of prostate cancer: report of a dose escalation study. *Int J Radiat Oncol Biol Phys* 1997;37:543–550.
161. Hanks GE, Lee WR, Hanlon AL, et al. Conformal technique dose escalation for prostate cancer: biochemical evidence of improved cancer [see comments]. *Int J Radiat Oncol Biol Phys* 1996;35:861–868.

24

NEW METHODS OF FOCAL ABLATION OF THE PROSTATE

JOHN P. LONG

When faced with a new diagnosis, the task of determining the ideal therapy with which to treat clinically localized prostate cancer (CaP) continues to be a challenging one for both physician and patient. Currently, the two most common therapies used in the United States to treat CaP remain radical prostatectomy and external beam radiotherapy, together accounting for nearly 80% of initial treatments administered to patients with CaP in the United States (1).

The purpose of this chapter is to summarize the current experience with newer focal therapy modalities that do not involve radiotherapy or surgery. These consist of cryoablation techniques and heat energy–based treatments [high intensity focused ultrasound (HIFU), radiofrequency interstitial tumor ablation (RITA), and thermal brachytherapy]. The current clinical experience with these approaches is examined, and any potential role in managing CaP is assessed for each in turn.

FOCAL ABLATION OF THE PROSTATE: IS IT EVEN POSSIBLE?

Focal ablation refers to treatment modalities that are designed to arrest the growth of or destroy all foci of CaP in a given gland *in situ* without the use of radiation or surgical extirpation. Unlike radiation (mitotic arrest) or androgen deprivation (apoptosis), the mechanism of cytotoxicity, by way of which cryo- and heat-based focal therapies work, is the creation of areas of coagulative necrosis in a designated target area. To be a legitimate therapeutic option for patients, any potential focal ablation modality needs to meet several essential criteria.

CaP poses a particular challenge to focal ablation in that it is difficult to reliably define the location or extent of local tumor burden in the prostate. For example, it has been shown that CaPs are usually multifocal, typically consisting of two to five tumors per gland (2). Unfortunately, there is still no radiographic modality that can identify, with satisfactory degrees of resolution, the intraprostatic tumor volume distribution to any degree of reliability. Thus, until such time that clinically significant foci (greater than 0.5 cm^3) of CaP can be reliably identified preoperatively, the application of focal ablation modalities for treating patients with CaP must be directed toward treating the *entire prostate gland* as the ideal means of eradicating the disease.

Because all current focal ablation modalities rely on temperature changes to produce the desired treatment effect, the temperature thresholds necessary to produce a *reliable correlation between treatment parameters and histopathology* (i.e., coagulative necrosis in the target area) need to be defined for any particular treatment modality. For human prostate tissue, these targets currently appear to be less than –40° to –50°C for cryoablation and greater than 55° to 60°C for heat-based ablation techniques. One of the best ways to demonstrate that necrosis is being generated in the targeted area is by using temperature monitoring in real time during a given focal ablation procedure. It is conceivable that models could be constructed to predict reliably the three-dimensional areas of coagulative necrosis that will be created in the prostate by a given set of treatment variables (wattage, time, duration of freeze, and others). Yet, such *operator-independent* models that are sufficiently reliable are lacking. At the moment, the only reliable means of real-time temperature monitoring during focal ablation requires the interstitial placement of multiple thermocouples in strategic locations in and around the targeted treatment area.

Because the use of focal ablation modalities in the prostate gland involves fairly narrow margins of error in destroying cancerous tissue, while avoiding damage to closely proximate structures, such as the bladder neck, rectum, and periurethral tissue, any successful modality must have a very *sharp demarcation between treatment effect and normal tissue.* Treatments that involve greater than 1- to 2-mm *buffer zones* of variable tissue changes around cores of coagulative necrosis are problematic, because these may amount to an inadequate degree of cell kill for any tumor cells in this area or an excessive amount of tissue damage to surrounding structures with resultant unnecessary morbidity.

It seems fairly evident that to have any potential role in treating patients with CaP, focal ablation modalities must be genuinely *minimally invasive* with lower morbidity rates than established treatments or shorter hospitalizations, or both. Based on current experience, it appears that these goals can be best achieved if a fair degree of control exists in directing the ablation energy source to avoid damage to the bladder neck, prostatic urethral musculature, rectum, voluntary sphincter complex, pudendal vasculature, and neurovascular bundles.

CRYOABLATION OF THE PROSTATE

The first report of cryoablation of the human prostate was in 1966, when Gonder and Soanes published the results of using a transurethral, single cryoprobe in ablating periurethral adenomatous tissue in patients with outlet obstructive symptoms (3). Over the next 15 years, transurethral and transperineal approaches for treating patients with various clinical stages of CaP were used with mixed results (4–6). Fundamentally, these procedures suffered from the inability to monitor the cryodestruction in real time, and, ultimately, cryoablation was generally abandoned owing to modest rates of local recurrence along with frequent morbidities (7).

With the development of transrectal ultrasonographic imaging, interest in percutaneous cryoablation of the prostate was renewed in the late 1980s. Three critical modifications to the older techniques were made. The first was the use of real-time transrectal ultrasonographic monitoring of the cryoprobe placement as well as the propagation of the advancing ice. The second was the development of 3-mm cryoprobes that could be placed transperineally into targeted areas of the prostate. Last, a urethral warming system was devised to maintain sufficient viability of the periurethral tissues to lower tissue sloughing rates relative to the older approaches (Fig. 24-1).

Using these components and based on somewhat limited animal testing (8,9), the first clinical experience in humans with percutaneous cryoablation was published in 1993, when Onik reported early results after treatment of 63 patients with localized CaP (10). Given that this was the first focal ablative therapy introduced for treating CaP and that it may have been marketed prematurely, it is fair to say that since that time, cryoablation has been a work in evolution. Perhaps not surprisingly, a number of technical variations have been proposed since the initial report, and the absence of a validated treatment protocol before marketing is probably the reason why the clinical results presented in more than 40 peer-reviewed reports since then have been somewhat mixed. These technical modifications are reviewed in the next section.

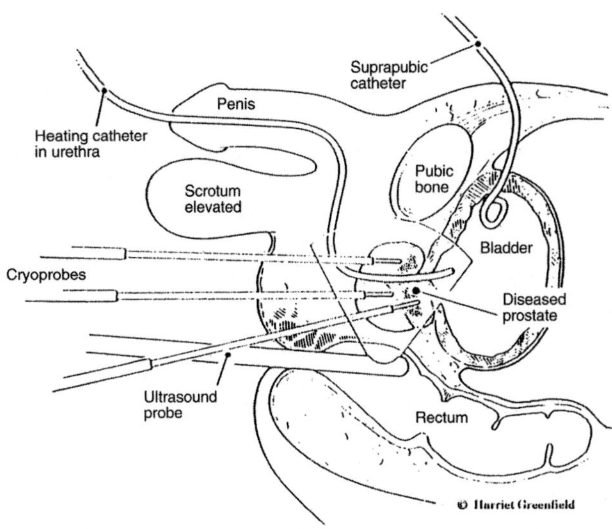

FIGURE 24-1. Graphic illustration of transperineal cryoablation of the prostate. Posttreatment urinary drainage can be either with a suprapubic tube, as here, or with urethral catheters.

CRYOABLATION TECHNICAL VARIATIONS

Multiple Freeze-Thaw Cycles

It has been demonstrated that cellular destruction occurs during the freeze and the thaw (rapid freeze, slow thaw) portions of a cryoablation cycle (11). Two freeze-thaw cycles have been shown to produce more efficient cell kill when compared to single cycles in both human prostate monolayers *in vitro* (12), although this may not be as important as reaching –40°C in human prostate models *in vivo* (13). Furthermore, two freeze-thaw cycles during prostate cryoablation in humans have been associated with lower positive biopsy rates as well as improved prostate-specific antigen (PSA) results when compared to single freeze cycles without any apparent increase in developing cryo-related morbidities (14–16). Finally, in single-probe temperature mapping experiments performed on patients before radical prostatectomy, two consecutive 10-minute freeze cycles produced a larger area of coagulative necrosis than a single 20-minute freeze (16a). Thus, the available literature supports the use of a minimum of two freeze-thaw cycles, although whether there is any additional benefit to more than two cycles is not known.

Urethral Warming

The primary objective of the use of urethral warming catheter systems during cryoablation is to minimize urethral sloughing. The first urethral warming system was marketed as a nonsignificant risk device until approximately July 1994. Initial experiences with this system were notable for fairly low rates of urethral sloughing, ranging from 4% to 10% (10,18,19). Due, apparently, to concerns submitted to the U.S. Food and Drug Administration surrounding the safety of this particular device, it was taken off the market in mid 1994 for approximately 18 months while it underwent regulatory review. During this time period, numerous authors reported a sharp increase in post–cryo transurethral resection (TUR) rates and overall urethral sloughing rates due to varying operator experience as well as to the use of alternate warmers that did not have many of the features of the original one, which has since been made available (14–16,20,21). Currently, although the precise features of urethral warming, which ensure the most protective heat transfer during cryoablation, are still being evaluated, it is clear that the warming system as originally designed was effective in reducing slough-related morbidities. Currently, post-cryo sloughing rates lie between 3% and 9% (22,23), provided that the appropriate warming catheters are used and patients have not been radiated. With increased attention to corroborating better catheter design, it is entirely possible that these slough rates will decline further.

Thermocouple Monitoring

Early in the experience with performing cryoablation of the prostate, several authors in particular noted that real-time interpretation of the leading edge of the ice ball on sonographic imaging underestimated the actual extent of cellular destruction (15,24,25). In addition, a number of reports in the cryobiologic literature had documented in several human tissues fairly reliable coagulative necrosis when temperatures of –40° to –50°C were achieved in the target areas (11). As a result, some programs began to place thermocouples at the margins of the targeted treatment zones (e.g., neurovascular bundles, apex) to ensure that these cytotoxic temperatures were achieved during freezing. Wong and Bahn were among the first to relate improved PSA rates and post-cryo biopsy results with thermocouple monitoring when compared to patients in whom this had not been used (15,26,27). Currently, it is evident that transrectal ultrasonography alone is inadequate for monitoring and planning a successful cryoablation. Although the precise number of thermocouples that constitute a satisfactory number of data points to ensure an adequate freeze is still being evaluated, a minimum of four to perhaps five thermocouple positions around the periphery of the prostate, as well as at the apex of the prostate, is recommended.

Probe Number and Probe Distribution

The device first used to perform percutaneous cryoablation in patients with CaP was manufactured with exit ports for five cryoprobes (28). Not surprisingly, the initial report on this procedure described a technique involving the placement of five cryoprobes radially around the urethra. To what degree this probe distribution effectively produced reliably confluent areas of coagulative necrosis around the urethra had not been confirmed in human prostate settings and was based to some extent on patterns of ice propagation using five cryoprobes in agar phantoms.

Recently, temperature mapping studies done in patients with localized CaP who agreed to undergo focal cryoablation of the prostate before undergoing a radical prostatectomy have begun to define the mechanics of freezing in human prostate tissue more clearly (17). These studies found that, for single probes engaged in two consecutive 10-minute freeze-thaw cycles, a radius of approximately 7 to 8 mm from the cryoprobe correlated consistently with a –40° to –50°C isotherm. Subsequent histopathologic evaluation of the surgical specimens after 3-mm step sectioning indicated that this isotherm also consistently correlated with zones of complete coagulative necrosis. Temperatures ranging from –20° to –40°C (i.e., 8- to 10-mm radii) correlated with a zone of histopathologic changes that was characterized by viable cells' exhibiting signs of cellular injury, the significance of which is difficult to discern from the preliminary studies. Follow-up temperature mapping studies in patients undergoing full-gland (i.e., six probes) cryoablation demonstrated that the effect of multiple probe placement produces a larger effective freezing zone than that predicted by simply adding single probe properties. The arcuate, peripheral placement of cryoprobes 1.2 to 1.4 cm apart consistently produced temperatures lower than –100°C at points 8 to 10 mm medial to the probe arc. Interestingly, temperatures measured at 7 to 8 mm peripheral to the arc rarely were lower than the targeted threshold of –50°C, presumably because no additive effect was being produced.

These preliminary data strongly indicate that for many patients (especially those with larger glands), the originally suggested five-probe distribution may have been inadequate to reliably produce an area of coagulative necrosis that was large enough to cover all viable tissue in the prostate. Moreover, these data begin to define critical elements of probe placement for individual glands. These features may include keeping probes within 7 to 8 mm of the capsule, placing probes no less than 1.2 to 1.4 mm apart (i.e., 6- to 7-mm radii) around the gland, and using as many probes within these guidelines as the volume or shape of the prostate requires. Whether such a treatment design will produce reliable targeted ablation in all patients requires additional study, but it is interesting that Lee has demonstrated a clear clinical improvement in results with six versus five cryoprobes (50).

Thus, although there has been significant technical variation in published reports on cryoablation of the prostate, the essential elements of an effective treatment are starting to emerge (Fig. 24-2). Ideally, candidate prostate glands should be between 40 and 55 cc. The targeted temperatures are –40° to –50°C at the periphery of the prostate with a minimum of six peripherally loaded cryoprobes. Urethral warming using approved devices has to be used to ensure a minimized TUR slough rate. A minimum of two freezes

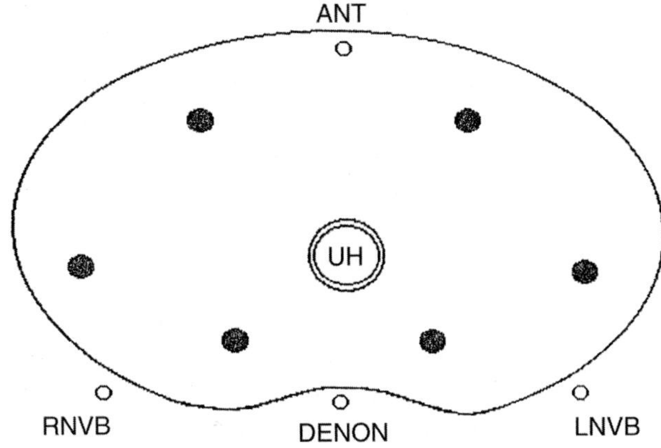

FIGURE 24-2. Graphic illustration of current cryoablation technique. Filled circles represent standard 6-probe distribution; more can be added for selected glands. Open circles represent thermocouple positions for monitoring. Occasionally, a fifth is placed at the apical level. ANT, anterior (and just subcapsular); DENON, Denonvilliers' layer in the midline; R/LNVB, right and left neurovascular bundles (just extracapsular at levels of NVBs); UH, urethral heater.

should be used, and the entire procedure should be done under real-time temperature monitoring to maximize the likelihood of achieving large areas of coagulative necrosis throughout the prostate.

CRYOABLATION CLINICAL RESULTS

Because the first reported results with contemporary cryoablation of the prostate were published in 1993, standard criteria for treatment efficacy, such as 10- to 15-year cause-specific survival data, are lacking for this procedure. However, surrogate outcomes that are increasingly being used to assess treatment efficiency are available from many centers using this modality. The three primary surrogate outcomes in this regard are posttreatment PSA results, posttreatment biopsy results (occult local control), and posttreatment morbidities. These are briefly summarized below.

Prostate-Specific Antigen Results

The post-cryo PSA results that have appeared in the literature have been reported variably. Very few programs have follow-ups that are sufficient with an adequate number of patients treated to determine actuarial projections for 5-year biochemical-free survival at any PSA threshold definition. A number of early studies tend to document post-cryo PSA outcomes by reporting crude PSA rates at fixed postoperative time points; for example, post-cryo PSA values of less than 0.5 ng per mL ranged from 41% to 74% (14,18,30). Longer projections of PSA-based disease-free survivals from single institutions, postcryo, are few. Long reported an overall actuarial biochemical progression-free rate at 5 years of 56% (22). Cohen recently reported 5-year biochemical-free survivals of 42% for PSA less than 0.4 ng per mL and 58% for PSA less than 1 ng per mL among patients with Gleason grade 7 or higher CaP or PSA greater than 10 ng per mL who undergo cryoablation (31).

More recently, a retrospective multiinstitutional database designed to stratify patients and outcomes to minimize selection bias inherent in single institutional reporting was constructed. In this study, 975 patients were found among five institutions performing cryoablation over the course of five years. For these patients, the overall 5-year actuarial biochemical-free survival postcryo was 51% and 63% for PSA less than 0.5 ng per mL and PSA less than 1 ng per mL, respectively (32). When patients were stratified by factors predicting higher risks of progression, the 5-year biochemical-free survival rates, not surprisingly, declined according to increasing risk (Table 24-1). A brief synopsis of contemporary radiotherapeutic techniques, including three-dimensional conformal modifications as well as interstitial brachytherapy results reported in the last three years, suggests that these results are fairly comparable to what has been reported by other institutions (37–46). This is despite the fact that these cryo data likely reflect a "least common denominator" effect among the institutions studied, because no attempt to segregate patients based on the actual technique used during the procedure for each patient in the database was made.

Postcryoablation Biopsy Results

The value of posttreatment biopsy results continues to be a subject of some debate (33). What is clear is that with any type of ablative approach to the prostate, there still remains a sonographically evident residuum of tissue in which persistent or resistant foci of carcinoma have an opportunity to progress. Usually, radiographic evaluations such as transrectal ultrasound are not helpful in demonstrating the presence or absence of residual disease, although spectroscopically enhanced magnetic resonance imaging may have some

TABLE 24-1. FIVE-YEAR ACTUARIAL BIOCHEMICAL SUCCESS RATE POSTCRYO STRATIFIED BY RISK CATEGORY

		PSA <0.5		PSA <1	
	n	% Rate (SE)	% 5 yr at risk	% Rate (SE)	% 5 yr at risk
Overall	975	51.1 (2.7)	67	63 (2.7)	81.5
Low risk[a]	238	59.5 (4.7)[b]	26	76 (4.2)	34
Medium risk[c]	321	61 (4.3)	23	71 (4.3)	25.5
High risk[d]	385	36 (5)	16.5	45 (5.2)	20.5

PSA, prostate-specific antigen; SE, standard error.
[a]PSA <10, Gleason grade (GG) <7, and stage <cT2b.
[b]p <.05 across groups, logrank.
[c]Any one of the following: PSA >10, GG >6, or stage >cT2a.
[d]Two or more of the following: PSA >10, GG >6, or stage >cT2a.

TABLE 24-2. POSTCRYO POSITIVE BIOPSY RATES (OF PATIENTS BIOPSIED) STRATIFIED BY RISK CATEGORY

	n	%
Overall	141/779	18
Low risk[a]	25/198	12
Medium risk[b]	31/255	12
High risk[c]	82/305	27

[a]Prostate-specific antigen (PSA) <10, Gleason grade (GG) <7, and stage <cT2b.
[b]Any one of the following: PSA >10, GG >6, or stage >cT2a.
[c]Two or more of the following: PSA >10, GG >6, or stage >cT2a.

value (34,35). In this context, the value of random biopsies after these treatments, particularly for patients who have a rising PSA, seems obvious.

Numerous authors have reported fairly low positive biopsy rates after cryoablation, ranging from 8% to 35%, with rates dependent on operator experience, patient selection factors, and duration of follow-up (14,15,18,22,26,29–31,36). Biopsies have been done at predetermined time points posttreatment or in response to unfavorable clinical developments, such as a rising PSA, and usually 6 to 12 core techniques have been cited. In the retrospective multiinstitutional study noted previously, the overall positive biopsy rate was only 18% (Table 24-2). Among patients at low risk for progression, the positive biopsy rate was even lower at 10%. These results are very comparable, if not superior, to positive biopsy rates after external beam radiotherapy and brachytherapy (37–42). Thus, it would appear that these data suggest that, at least insofar as posttreatment biopsy sampling can indicate, cryoablation can produce fairly impressive degrees of local control with a very small risk of harboring occult persistent disease in the residuum.

PostCryo Morbidities

As with cancer-related outcomes, morbidities postcryo are also variably reported (Table 24-3). Prior radiation appears to be a significant risk factor for postcryoablation-related side effects, and this is discussed separately. The rates of rectourethral fistulae have been fairly low, ranging from 0% to 3% (14,15,18–22). Urethral drainage alone will resolve most of these fistulae, although colonic diversion and primary repair may be needed in rare instances. Reported rates of urethral sloughing in reports cited earlier range from 4% to 38%. As noted earlier, alternate urethral warming is clearly the chief risk factor among these studies for developing posttreatment sloughing. For patients with no prior therapies undergoing cryoablation with standard warming catheters, the slough rate can be as low as 4% to 8% (19,22). Typically, sloughing is best managed with a TUR of the prostate (TURP) limited only to the removal of obviously necrotic material, as extensive resections may decrease ultimate continence (15,26). Overall, the reported rates of incontinence in nonradiated patients after cryoablation range widely from 3% to 27% (14,15,18–22). Again, as with urethral sloughing, factors that contribute to incontinence postcryo include operator inexperience and inadequate urethral warming. In fact, it is probably accurate to note that in the absence of tissue sloughing or prior radiation treatment, pad-dependent incontinence postcryo occurs in fewer than 3% of cases (22,23,26).

Currently, reported rates of potency after cryoablation are generally low, ranging from 0% to 20% (14,15,19,22,23). As with other therapies for managing CaP, it is difficult to provide objective determinations of erectile function postcryo, yet these low potency rates have been noted in physician-based as well as patient-based outcome assessment studies (23). The etiology of erectile dysfunction after cryoablation is poorly understood. One recent report suggests that it is likely due to vasculogenic rather than exclusively neurogenic changes after the procedure, although this needs further study to be corroborated (51). At the moment, there are few data documenting the effectiveness of different treatment strategies for postcryo erectile dysfunction, although anecdotal experience suggests that intracavernous injection can be effective for most patients in this setting.

Overall, the rates of developing lower urinary tract infections postcryo range from 4% to 9% (14,20,22,29). These are invariably easily managed with antibiotics. Other, rarer potential complications after cryo that have been reported include sepsis, venous thrombosis, ureteral obstruction, ureteral hydronephrosis, and chronic penile pain. In the aggregate, these more serious problems have typically occurred in fewer than 10% of cases and are noted to occur infrequently in institutions with many experiences performing this procedure.

Thus, based on the clinical evidence available from the literature presented earlier, cryoablation seems to be a potentially effective treatment option for patients with new diagnoses of CaP. Unfortunately, the technical features that comprise a reliably effective treatment for individual patients have been evolving since its reintroduction in 1992. This lack of a genuinely validated method of applying cryoablation technology to adequately treat CaP has probably been the main reason hindering a broader acceptance of this procedure, as unfavorable outcomes after cryo were noted after the initial experiences of a number of urologists with cryo (20,21,52). However, the currently recommended method is considerably different from that used during the initial marketing of this technique and is based on carefully controlled clinical studies in humans. It seems reasonable to conclude that using six or more cryoprobes, standard urethral warming, multiple freeze-thaw cycles, and thermocouple monitoring cryo will produce clinical outcomes that are comparable to those reported for other nonsurgical therapies, such as external beam radiation or brachytherapy.

TABLE 24-3. REPORTED MORBIDITY RATES AFTER CRYOABLATION OF THE PROSTATE

	Nonradiated/previously radiated, where reported									Previously radiated only		
	Shinohara et al. (14)	**Lee et al. (26)**	**Cox et al. (20)**	**Long et al. (22)**	**Wong et al. (15)**	**Cohen et al. (29)**	**Sosa et al. (21)**	**Coogan et al. (18)**	**Weider et al. (19)**	**Miller et al. (47)**	**Bales et al. (48)**	**Pisters et al. (16)**
No. of patients	92/10	301/46	51/12	127/18	83/7	239	1,467	95	83	33	23	150
Complications (%)												
Rectourethral fistula	0/10	0.33/8.7	3	0/17	0	0.4	1.4	1	0	0	0	1.5
Slough requiring TURP	23	NR	19	3/50	19	9.8	9.9/38.0[a]	10	3.8	15	52	17
Bladder outlet obstruction	NR	3.2	29	17.2	NR	3	6.8	6	13	18	41	44
Incontinence	15	0.3/8.7	27	2/83	6	4	11	3.5	2.5	10	95	73
Impotence	86	92	NR	88	94	NR	100	47	80	NR	100	72
Urethral stricture/BNC	NR	NR	3	3.4	11	2.2	5	1	3.8	5	14	NR
UTI/epididymitis	4	NR	NR	3/40	NR	4	9.1	4	9	NR	59	NR
Perineal pain	3	NR	11	2/37	NR	0.4	9.4	1	NR	NR	37	8
Sepsis	3	NR	3	1	NR	0.7	2.3	0	NR	0	9	NR
Other (hematoma, bladder injury, ureteral obstruction, and others)	4	NR	13	5	1	2	NR	2	2.6	2	13	4
Total complications	NR	NR	46/82	17/89	NR	NR	NR	NR	NR	NR	NR	NR

BNC, bladder neck contracture; NR, not reported; TURP, transurethral resection of the prostate; UTI, urinary tract infection.
[a]Approved or nonapproved warmer.

SALVAGE CRYOABLATION RADIATION FAILURES

On its introduction in 1993, there was a fair degree of enthusiasm for cryoablation as a salvage option for patients who had failed radiotherapy. However, clinical outcomes from several programs examining this select patient group have been suboptimal. Using older prostate cryoablation techniques (e.g., less than six probes, no thermocouple monitoring, nonstandard urethra; warming catheters), the rates of attaining undetectable PSA nadirs postcryo in these patients range from 36% to 38%, but the likelihood of maintaining an undetectable PSA 12 to 18 months posttreatment drops to between 11% and 28% (16,47,48). Postcryo positive biopsy results for these patients have been a bit more encouraging, ranging between 14% and 27%, with lower rates noted in patients receiving more than one freeze-thaw cycle (16). Yet in most of these studies, the biopsies were done fairly early (i.e., less than 1 year) after the treatment. Longer follow-ups demonstrating the rate of maintaining a negative biopsy status in this group are lacking. Regardless of the mixed cancer-related outcomes, the primary concern with using cryoablation in managing these difficult patients has to do with the attendant morbidities. Again, in reports using older cryoablation techniques, the side effect profile for patients undergoing cryoablation after radiotherapy clearly appears to be higher than that seen in patients without prior radiation (Table 24-3). Incontinence rates range anywhere from 10% to 95% (16,21,22,47–49), with all but one study noting very high rates of poor urinary control. Rectourethral fistula rates ranged between 0% and 17%, and tissue sloughing has been noted in between 15% and 52% of cases, with lower rates for approved urethral warmer use (49). More severe side effects, such as chronic and unrelenting pelvic pain (16,21,22) and osteitis pubis (53), may be specific to prior radiation patients, as these outcomes are much less common after cryoablation used as primary therapy.

However, one recent report using contemporary thermocouple-controlled technique with a modified urethral warning system noted a significantly lower morbidity profile than in these initial studies (53a). In this report, PSA nadirs of less than 0.1 were reached in 60% of patients, and the 12-month actuarial PSA-free survival of those patients with nadirs of less than 0.1 was 73%. Side effects in this study were significantly lower than those reported in prior prostate cryoablation studies mentioned earlier and included transient rectal pain in 26% of patients, urinary tract infection in 9%, incontinence in 9%, outlet obstruction in 5%, and urethral structure in 5%. A recent update of this series suggests that the incontinence rates may be even lower with less than 3% of current patients experiencing slough.

Given that nearly all of the initial studies did not employ the elements of technique used in this more recent trial, these data are very encouraging. In fact, based chiefly on the updated experience from this group using more recent elements of technique (i.e., thermocouple monitoring, seminal vesicle biopsies, approved urethral warming extended for 2 hours in the recovery room post cryoablation, six cryoprobes), the Health Care Financing Administration has recently reversed its previous position and approved coverage for the use of prostate cryoablation as salvage therapy for patients with Gleason grade less than 9, PSA less than 8, and tumor stage less than 2c post CaP radiation therapy (53b). These developments may reestablish a role for prostate cryoablation in treating these difficult management problems. Additional studies are needed to determine whether the use of contemporary technique in previously radiated patients can continue to produce fewer morbidities than initially found.

HIGH INTENSITY WITH FOCUSED ULTRASOUND

HIFU was first demonstrated to produce clinically significant areas of focal tissue ablation in 1955 in the central nervous system (54). A number of centers, chiefly located in Europe, since 1990 have been examining the potential feasibility of HIFU in treating various forms of prostate disease, including and in particular CaP.

HIFU treatment of human CaP consists of several features (55). First, a piezoelectric transducer placed transrectally emits a highly focused convergent ultrasound beam in pulses lasting 3 to 5 seconds. These pulses produce areas of ablation that are ellipsoid in shape and typically measure approximately 2 cm in height by 2 mm in diameter. Temperatures in the target area range between 85° and 100°C, clearly high enough to produce discrete areas of coagulative necrosis. The transducer is then moved sequentially (usually under computer-assisted control) through various areas of the prostate to produce large areas of focal ablation. The transducer is positioned in the rectum with a latex balloon that is filled with noncavitation coupling fluid. Recent modifications involve a system of continuous cooling for the rectal wall and software that monitors the distance from the transducer to the rectal wall continuously in real time to assist planning for each sequential pulse to minimize damage to the rectal wall (56).

As a general rule, each procedure takes between 2 and 3 hours to complete, involving between 700 and 1,500 firings per session. To date, several studies investigating its use in patients with CaP have used anywhere from one to four total sessions, usually treating no more than one lobe of the prostate per session (55). The procedures have been predominantly done under a spinal anesthetic, although a general anesthetic can be used as well. Urinary drainage posttreatment is typically maintained with suprapubic tube catheters that are removed when spontaneous voiding resumes; this can take from 2 to 3 weeks.

Preliminary results with this technique in patients with clinically localized CaP (i.e., clinical stage T1 to T2) who are poor candidates for radical prostatectomy have been recently presented (56–58). Overall, positive biopsies at 3 months after treatment have ranged between 27% and 28% of patients. PSA nadirs of less than 1 within 3 months of the procedure have ranged between 35% and 77% of patients, depending on the technique and operator experience (57). In one study, PSA nadirs of less than 0.5 were achieved in approximately 49% of patients (58). The clinical experience so far is not of sufficient duration to project biochemical-free survivals over even short-term periods of time. Morbidities after the procedure include rectourethral fistulae in 1% to 2% of treated patients, post-HIFU TURP rates of 20%, incontinence rates of 9%, and impotence rates of greater than 50% (56). One group reported that the risk of treatment-related morbidities might escalate with additional follow-up treatments (58). Most investigators engaged in HIFU were cautiously enthusiastic about its use as a possible therapeutic alternative that is minimally invasive to the standard therapies.

Considering its potential as a treatment option for patients with localized CaP, HIFU has some promise, although 5-year outcome data are lacking. Potential advantages of HIFU include that it appears to be able to be repeated; however, further study will be need to corroborate whether repeat treatments do in fact increase morbidity risk. It does appear to be able to be offered in patients who have undergone previous TURP, and it may be an effective salvage option for patients who have failed radiotherapy, although an inadequate number of patients have been treated to draw any conclusions.

One of the more obvious problems with HIFU is the absence of any real-time temperature monitoring system on which to base the end points of a given treatment. Furthermore, the fact that many patients may not have their entire prostate treated at one sitting is at best very inconvenient. At the moment, durable post-HIFU PSA data are lacking and prevent any valid comparisons with other therapies. Post-HIFU–positive biopsy rates have been encouraging, but follow-up is short. Post-HIFU morbidities may be comparable to other *in situ* therapies (e.g., cryoablation or brachytherapy), yet the potential risk of higher side effects with multiple treatments is a matter of concern in this regard. Last, the fact that what clinical data do exist after the use of HIFU for patients with CaP pertains only to patients with stage T1-2 disease limits comparisons with other therapies (e.g., cryo- or radiation-based therapies) that have been used to treat broader ranges of clinical presentations. This selection bias also precludes any assessment of the potential value of HIFU as a local control option for patients with more locally advanced disease. Certainly, further study with this interesting technology in treating patients with CaP is warranted, and it is hoped that such studies will continue in the future.

OTHER HEAT-BASED ABLATIVE SYSTEMS

Two other heat-based focal ablation modalities have been proposed as potential treatment options for patients with CaP. The first is transperineal, ultrasound-guided RITA. In this procedure, radio frequency electrodes are placed under sonographic guidance transperineally into target areas of the prostate, and large spherical areas of coagulative necrosis can be produced (59). Treatment times are fairly short (i.e., 8 to 12 minutes), and, depending on the time of treatment and the power setting chosen, various-sized lesions can be generated. This technology has been demonstrated to produce moderately predictable lesion areas in the prostate in patients undergoing RITA before radical prostatectomy, with subsequent subsectioning of the specimens. The total number of patients who were pathologically free of carcinoma, however, was not stated (59).

The second modality involves interstitial thermal ablation using self-regulating seed implants. In this procedure, specially derived cobalt-palladium alloy seeds are placed in the targeted area (i.e., the prostate) under transrectal sonographic guidance in a manner similar to that being used for high-dose interstitial brachytherapy. The seeds are 1 mm in diameter by 14 mm in length and will self regulate to desired temperatures (usually 55°C) when placed in a magnetic field. At the moment, only very preliminary clinical work exists with this technology, and studies are ongoing to determine its effectiveness as primary therapy in patients with CaP (60). One potential advantage of this therapy is that it appears to be among the most easily repeatable of proposed ablative technologies, in that patients with the implants in place need only to sit within a magnetic field to have a thermal treatment of the prostate. However, there are no morbidity or clinical outcome data available in the literature on this technology at the present time.

Neither of these two interesting approaches has generated enough peer-reviewed clinical information as treatment options for patients with CaP to assess their efficacy or compare them to other treatment options. However, the prospect of simplicity of design (RITA) and safe repeatability (self-regulating thermal seeds) certainly merits continued investigation.

CONCLUSION

Although the current results with focal ablative therapies for managing patients with localized CaP presented in this chapter are promising, they are nonetheless somewhat preliminary. It has been only since January 2000 that a consensus on technique has begun to be established for cryoablation, and whether the encouraging results seen in several institutions skilled in this procedure can be successfully transferred to other programs requires further study. Similarly, the initial users of HIFU have modified the technique several times in an effort to minimize morbidity, yet whether their encouraging initial results can be translated to wider patient selection remains unknown. In the absence of randomized prospective comparisons, it is particularly difficult to determine clear indications for when focal ablative modalities would be better than more established therapies. An ongoing prospective comparison between cryoablation and external beam radiotherapy for patients with localized CaP being conducted by the Canadian National Cancer Institute should provide very useful information in this regard over the next 5 years. In the meantime, data in the literature support the use of focal ablation and, in particular, cryoablation as reasonable therapeutic alternatives in select institutions for managing patients with new diagnoses of localized CaP.

REFERENCES

1. Mettlin C. The American Cancer Society National Prostate Cancer Detection Project and national patterns of prostate cancer detection and treatment. *CA Cancer J Clin* 1997;47: 265–267.
2. Miller GJ, Cygan JM. Morphology of prostate cancer: the effects of multifocality on histological grade, tumor volume, and capsular penetration. *J Urol* 1994;152:1709–1713.
3. Gonder MJ, Soanes WA, Shulman S. Cryosurgical treatment of the prostate. *Invest Urol* 1966;3:372–378.
4. Soanes WA, Gonder MJ. Use of cryosurgery in prostatic cancer. *J Urol* 1968;99:793–797.
5. Flocks RH, Nelson CM, Boatman DL. Perineal cryosurgery for prostatic carcinoma. *J Urol* 1972;108:933–935.
6. Bonney WW, Fallon B, Gerber WL, et al. Cryosurgery in prostatic carcinoma: survival. *Urology* 1982;19:37–42.
7. Bonney WW, Fallon B, Gerber WL, et al. Cryosurgery in prostatic carcinoma: elimination of local lesion. *Urology* 1983;22:8–15.
8. Onik G, Cobb C, Cohen JK, et al. US characteristics of frozen prostate. *Radiology* 1988;168:629–631.
9. Onik G, Porterfield B, Rubinsky B, et al. Percutaneous transperineal prostate cryosurgery using transrectal ultrasound guidance: animal model. *Urology* 1991;37:277–281.
10. Onik GM, Cohen JK, Reyes GD, et al. Transrectal ultrasound guided percutaneous radical cryosurgical ablation of the prostate. *Cancer* 1993;72:1291–1299.
11. Gage AA, Baust J. Mechanisms of tissue injury in cryosurgery. *Cryobiology* 1998;37:171–186.
12. Tatsutani K, Rubinsky B, Onik G, et al. Effect of thermal variables on frozen human primary prostatic adenocarcinoma cells. *Urology* 1996;48:441–447.
13. Turk TM, Ries MA, Pietrow P, et al. Determination of optimal freezing parameters of human prostate cancer in a nude mouse model. *Prostate* 1999;38:137–143.
14. Shinohara K, Connolly JA, Presti JC Jr., et al. Cryosurgical treatment of localized prostate cancer (stages T1 to T4): preliminary results. *J Urol* 1996;156:115–121.
15. Wong WS, Chinn DO, Chinn M, et al. Cryosurgery as a treatment of prostate carcinoma: results and complications. *Cancer* 1997;79:963–974.
16. Pisters LL, von Eschenbach AC, Scott SM, et al. The efficacy and complications of salvage cryotherapy of the prostate. *J Urol* 1997;157:921–925.

16a. Larson TR, Robertson DW, Corica AP, et al. In vivo interstitial temperature mapping of the human prostate during cryosurgery with correlation to histopathologic outcomes. *Urology* 2000;55:547–552.

17. Larson TR, Corica AP, Robertson DW. What cryotherapy temperature really kills tissue: in vivo temperature mapping correlated to pathological changes in human prostates. *J Endourol* 1998;12:87,BS3–3A.
18. Coogan CL, McKiel CF. Percutaneous cryoablation of the prostate: preliminary results after 95 procedures. *J Urol* 1995;154:1813–1817.
19. Wieder J, Schmidt JD, Casola G, et al. Transrectal ultrasound-guided transperineal cryoablation in the treatment of prostate carcinoma: preliminary results. *J Urol* 1995;154: 435–441.
20. Cox RL, Crawford ED. Complications of cryosurgical ablation of the prostate to treat localized adenocarcinoma of the prostate. *Urology* 1995;45:932–935.
21. Sosa RE, Martin T, Lynn K. Cryosurgical treatment of prostate cancer: a multicenter review of complications. *J Urol* 1996;155:361.
22. Long JP, Fallick ML, LaRock DR, et al. Preliminary outcomes following cryosurgical ablation of the prostate in patients with clinically localized prostate carcinoma. *J Urol* 1998;159:477–484.
23. Badalament RA, Balm DK, Kim H, et al. Patient-reported complications after cryoablation therapy for prostate cancer. *Urology* 1999;54:295–300.
24. Grampsas SA, Miller GJ, Crawford ED. Salvage radical prostatectomy after failed transperineal cryotherapy: histologic findings from prostate whole-mount specimens correlated with intraoperative transrectal ultrasound images. *Urology* 1995;45:936–941.
25. Steed J, Saliken JC, Donnelly BJ, et al. Correlation between thermosensor temperature and transrectal ultrasonography during prostate cryoablation. *Can Assoc Radiol J* 1997;48: 186–190.
26. Lee F, Bahin DK, McHugh TA, et al. Cryosurgery of prostate cancer. Use of adjuvant hormonal therapy and temperature monitoring—a one year follow-up. *Anticancer Res* 1997;17:1511–1515.
27. Lee F, Bahn DK, McHugh TA, et al. US-guided percutaneous cryoablation of prostate cancer. *Radiology* 1994;192:770.
28. Chang Z, Finkelstein JJ, Ma H, et al. Development of a high-performance multiprobe cryosurgical device. *Biomed Instr Tech* 1994;28:383–390.
29. Cohen JK, Miller RJ, Rooker GM, et al. Cryosurgical ablation of the prostate: two-year prostate-specific antigen and biopsy results. *Urology* 1996;47:395–401.
30. Wake RW, Hollabaugh RS, Bond KH. Cryosurgical ablation of the prostate for localized adenocarcinoma: a preliminary experience. *J Urol* 1996;155:1663.
31. Cohen JK, Miller RJ, Benoit RM, et al. Cryosurgical ablation of the prostate in men with an unfavorable presentation of clinically localized prostate cancer. *J Urol* 1999; 161:1378A.
32. Long JP, Balm DK, Lee F, et al. Five-year retrospective, multi-institutional pooled analysis of cancer-related outcomes following cryosurgical ablation of the prostate. *Urology* 2001;57:518–523.

33. Zietman AL, Shipley WU, Willett CG. Residual disease after radical surgery or radiation therapy for prostate cancer. *Cancer* 1993;71[3 Suppl]:959–969.
34. Parivar F, Hricak H, Shinohara K, et al. Detection of locally recurrent prostate cancer after cryosurgery: evaluation by transrectal ultrasound, magnetic resonance imaging, and 3-dimensional proton magnetic resonance spectroscopy. *Urology* 1996;48:594–599.
35. Salomon CG, Kalbhen CL, Dudiak CM, et al. Prostate carcinoma: transrectal US after cryosurgical ablation. *Radiology* 1998;206:533–538.
36. Cohen JK, Miller RJ, Benoit R, et al. Five-year outcomes of PSA and biopsy following cryosurgery as primary treatment for localized prostate cancer. *J Urol* 1998;159:976A.
37. Ragde H, Elgamal AA, Snow PB, et al. Ten-year disease-free survival after transperineal sonography-guided inodine-125 brachytherapy with or without 45-gray external beam irradiation in the treatment of patients with clinically localized, low to high Gleason grade prostate carcinoma. *Cancer* 1998; 83:989–1001.
38. Stock RG, Stone NN, Tabert A, et al. A dose-response study for I-125 prostate implants. *Int J Radiat Oncol Biol Phys* 1998;41:101–108.
39. Zelefsky MI, Leibel SA, Gaudin PB, et al. Dose escalation with three-dimensional conformal radiation therapy affects the outcome in prostate cancer. *Int J Radiat Oncol Biol Phys* 1998;41:491–500.
40. Scardino PT, Wheeler TM. Local control of prostate cancer with radiotherapy: frequency and prognostic significance of positive results of postirradiation prostate biopsy. *NCI Monogr* 1988;7:95–103.
41. Laverdiere J, Gomez JL, Cusan L, et al. Beneficial effect of combination hormonal therapy administered prior and following external beam radiation therapy in localized prostate cancer. *Int J Radiat Oncol Biol Phys* 1997;37:247–252.
42. Crook JM, Bahadur YA, Bociek RG, et al. Radiotherapy for localized prostate carcinoma. The correlation of pretreatment prostate specific antigen and nadir prostate specific antigen with outcome as assessed by systematic biopsy and serum prostate specific antigen. *Cancer* 1997;79:328–336.
43. D'Amico AV, Whittington R, Malkowicz SB, et al. Biochemical outcome after radical prostatectomy, external beam radiation therapy or interstitial radiation therapy for clinically localized prostate cancer. *JAMA* 1998;280:969–974.
44. Beyer DC, Priestly JB Jr. Biochemical disease-free survival following I125 prostate implantation. *Int J Radiat Oncol Biol Phys* 1997;37:559–563.
45. Fukunaga-Johnson N, Sanadler HM, McLaughlin PW, et al. Results of 3D conformal radiotherapy in the treatment of localized prostate cancer. *Int J Radiat Oncol Biol Phys* 1997;38:311–317.
46. Corn BW, Valicenti RK, Mulholland SG, et al. Stage T3 prostate cancer: a nonrandomized comparison between definitive irradiation and induction hormonal manipulation plus prostatectomy. *Urology* 1998;51:782–787.
47. Miller RJ, Cohen JK, Shuman B, et al. Percutaneous, transperineal cryosurgery of the prostate as salvage therapy for post-radiation recurrence of adenocarcinoma. *Cancer* 1996;77: 1510–1514.
48. Bales GT, Williams MI, Simmer M, et al. Short-term outcomes after cryosurgical ablation of the prostate in men with recurrent prostate carcinoma following radiation therapy. *Urology* 1995;46:676–680.
49. Cespedes RD, Pisters LL, von Eschenbach AC, et al. Long-term followup of incontinence and obstruction after salvage cryosurgical ablation of the prostate: results in 143 patients. *J Urol* 1997;157:237–240.
50. Lee F, Bahn DK, Badalament RA, et al. Cryosurgery for prostate cancer: improved glandualr ablation by use of 6 to 8 cryoprobes. *Urology* 1999;54:135–140.
51. Aboseif S, Shinohara K, Borirakchanyavant S, et al. The effect of cryosurgical ablation of the prostate on erectile function. *Br J Urol* 1997;80:918–922.
52. Cox RL, Crawford ED. Cryosurgical ablation of the prostate: the con side in 1996. *Urology* 1996;48:181–183.
53. Seigne JD, Pisters LL, von Eschenbach AC. Osteitis pubis as a complication of prostate cryotherapy. *J Urol* 1996;156:182.

53a. de la Taille A, Hayek O, Benson MC, et al. Salvage cryotherapy for recurrent prostate cancer after radiation therapy: the Columbia experience. *Urology* 2000;55:79–84.

53b. Medicare Intermediary Manual. Transmittal 1835, chap. VII, sec. 3617, p. 6–136. 11 June 2001.

54. Fry WJ, Barnard JW, Fry FJ, et al. Ultrasonic lesions in mammalian central nervous system. *Science* 1955;122:517–521.
55. Gelet A, Chapelon JY, Bouvier R, et al. Local control of prostate cancer by transrectal high intensity focused ultrasound therapy: preliminary results. *J Urol* 1999;161:156–162.
56. Gelet A, Chapelon JY, Bouvier R, et al. Treatment of localized prostate cancer by transrectal high intensity focused ultrasound therapy (HIFU). *J Urol* 1999;161:1301A.
57. Vallancien G, Guillonneau B, Desgrandchamps F, et al. Local control of prostate cancer with HIFU: preliminary results of European study. *J Urol* 1999;161:1274A.
58. Chaussy C, Thuroff S, Zimmermann R. Localized prostate cancer treated by transrectal high intensive ultrasound (HIFU) outcome of 150 patients after 3 years. *J Urol* 1999;161:1279A.
59. Djavan B, Susani M, Sharait S, et al. Transperineal radiofrequency interstitial tumor ablation (RITA) of the prostate. *Tech Urol* 1998;4:103–109.
60. Paulus JA, Tucker RD, Loening SA, et al. Thermal ablation of canine prostate using interstitial temperature self-regulating seeds: new treatment for prostate cancer. *J Endourol* 1997;11:295–300.

25

QUALITY OF LIFE IN PROSTATE CANCER

JAMES A. TALCOTT
MARK S. LITWIN

WHY DOES QUALITY OF LIFE MATTER IN PROSTATE CANCER?

It is reasonable to ask why we choose to discuss quality of life in a book about a cancer that kills more American men than any other cancer except lung cancer. For patients with many cancers, especially those that are rapidly lethal and may be cured, health-related quality of life (HRQL) is almost irrelevant to choosing a treatment. Although these patients must understand the potential complications of their treatment accurately enough to give informed consent to it, the required recitation of the known side effects has little impact on whether or which treatment will start. The most efficacious treatment, once identified, will be chosen. The information about toxicity simply increases the anxiety of a patient who realistically believes himself to be without meaningful alternatives. For the patient with prostate cancer, however, particularly those with early (nonmetastatic) disease, the scenario can be very different. All of the established treatments can cause serious and long-lasting complications, whereas little definitive evidence supports the belief that they differ importantly in efficacy for most patients. Thus, for clinically localized prostate cancer, it is difficult to avoid concluding that quality of life matters, at least to some patients.

Radical prostatectomy and radical external beam radiotherapy are well-established alternative treatments, and additional options, such as brachytherapy and cryotherapy, have become widely available to patients in the 1990s. Chemical castration of varying duration using luteinizing hormone releasing hormone (LHRH) agonists or antiandrogens, or both, has been added to potentiate these local treatments and perhaps delay progression of micrometastatic cancer. Furthermore, patients and clinicians now commonly discuss the active choice to defer initial local treatment, sometimes called *watchful waiting*. Long an option for older patients and those with other life-threatening illnesses, observation has been considered in wider contexts based on recent published reports. Natural history studies have documented favorable outcomes for carefully selected observed patients, especially those with low Gleason scores (1–4), and a decision analytic model found little average survival benefit of active treatment for older patients and those with well-differentiated tumors (5). Each of these treatment alternatives has a distinctive pattern of potential complications, both short and long term. For watchful waiting, the potential complications come, of course, not from the treatment itself, but from the fear, risk, and occurrence of future progression of initially untreated cancer.

Although patients need accurate information about the likely complications of treatment to give ethically and legally acceptable informed consent, the knowledge may be beneficial *per se*: Patients provided with accurate information about likely complications can anticipate, prepare for, and, when they occur, adapt to them more easily. When a treatment-related complication occurs, a patient accurately forewarned of the risk feels unlucky, whereas a patient falsely reassured that it is unlikely feels injured and misused. Toxicity from cancer treatment is certainly not confined to surgery and radiation for prostate cancer. Side effects of cytotoxic cancer chemotherapy may be extraordinarily unpleasant, and some are life threatening. Yet patients receiving, say, bone marrow transplantation rarely blame their medical oncologists for complications they were warned about, even when toxicity is severe and the indication for initiating treatment uncertain. Although it may be tempting to providers to spare patients unnecessary anxiety by minimizing potential complications, particularly when they lack realistic alternatives, accurate information, even if unpleasant to contemplate, is what they need and usually know they need to get through treatment.

Because of prostate cancer's long natural history, the need for information about treatment-related quality of life factors is greater than for most other cancers. Prostate cancer progresses slowly, compared to quick killers like lung cancer, acute leukemia, and high-grade lymphoma. For prostate cancer to kill within 5 years is uncommon; for many other cancers, 5-year survival is an infrequently accomplished harbinger of cure. Furthermore, prostate cancer *usually* occurs in older men during a time in their lives when other potentially lethal illnesses are increasingly likely to arise. Presumably because of screening with the prostate-specific antigen (PSA) test (6,7), the average age at diagnosis has fallen rapidly to below 70 years, and the number of patients diagnosed spectacularly increased before falling almost as rapidly beginning in 1992 (8–10). There is no reason to think that the natural history of prostate cancer, which most men die with and not of, has changed since screening emerged. Rather, cancers are simply being discovered sooner, possibly allowing more patients to receive curative therapy but certainly forcing many more men to face choosing a cancer therapy years earlier than men used to do. Thus, a man destined to die of prostate cancer at age 80 years may now be diagnosed at age 65 years because of an abnormal PSA, rather than at age 70 years because of an abnormal digital rectal examination. This hypothetical 5-year interval between diagnosis from PSA screening and that from earlier techniques used in the past is not arbitrary. A retrospective analysis of blood specimens taken from the Physicians Health Study, a randomized cancer and coronary artery disease prevention trial, found an average delay of more than 5 years between an abnormal PSA and the later diagnosis (in the pre-PSA era) of prostate cancer (11). This lead time bias, or apparently prolonged cancer survival because of earlier diagnosis, is one of two analytic problems that make the prognosis of screening-diagnosed cancers appear better than those diagnosed because of symptoms. The other length bias may be as important but is much harder to estimate. It arises because slow-growing tumors spend more time at the stage when they can be detected by screening but do not yet cause symptoms. These more indolent tumors, slower to metastasize and kill, are more likely to be diagnosed by screening than rapidly growing tumors. Because of both effects of screening, men diagnosed with prostate cancer now are likely to live significantly longer without harm from their cancers after diagnosis than are men diagnosed in previous generations. As a result, the average time between the diagnosis and treatment of prostate cancer and symptoms of metastatic cancer has lengthened.

The goal of local treatment of prostate cancer is to prevent the first metastasis, because metastatic cancer, not local disease, causes death. Therefore, local therapy will provide no survival benefit at all for the patient who already has metastatic spread, even if the metastases remain microscopic and undetectable for years. After metastatic seeds are planted in the patient's bones, only the race between his cancer and any other potentially lethal diseases he might develop will determine whether he will die of prostate cancer. The patient without micrometastasis will not necessarily benefit from therapy either: If the prostate cancer progresses more slowly than competing coexisting diseases, then treatment would be unneeded and again without benefit. Thus, for many, if not for most, therapy may provide no benefit in terms of prolonged life. When local therapy does prevent clinically important metastatic disease, the benefit of treatment is not realized until micrometastases have grown to a size that causes symptoms, a period likely to be a decade or more for most patients. As a result, even successful treatment of the prostate provides no tangible benefit for years. However, whereas the intended benefit of treatment is in the future, the complications of treatment may be immediate and enduring. Permanent effects of prostate cancer therapy on sexual potency, urinary incontinence, and bowel function may begin immediately after radical prostatectomy and within the first year or two after radiation therapy. Because of prostate cancer's long natural history, men with complications will survive to experience them for years.

Paradoxically, the complications of treatment matter particularly to prostate cancer patients, because, regardless of whether treatment is successful, their prognosis is so good relative to other cancer patients. However, the recent publicity given to studies documenting good results for some men after observation (2,3,5) has not apparently led large numbers of men to reject local therapy. For most patients in the United States, to knowingly allow a cancer to go untreated is intuitively wrong, even if some evidence suggests that the tradeoff of treatment complications for protection against future metastatic cancer may benefit only a minority of patients. But these results have made men increasingly aware that their treatment choices may well contribute importantly to the quality of the final decade or more of their lives. To a young person, prolonging life may mean the opportunity to accomplish significant life goals, such as starting and raising a family, building a career, and cultivating avocations and friendships. For an older man, many of those goals have been accomplished, and most men have seen in the lives of their friends, family, and acquaintances that death cannot be postponed indefinitely. In this latter setting, in which other infirmities of advancing age may have become manifest, men may be more cautious about accepting the chance of significant new iatrogenic ones.

Although the harms of treatment are increasingly well established and well known, the benefits of active treatment remain controversial. Randomized trials of treatments for early prostate cancer are few and inadequate. Small trials of radical prostatectomy against radiation therapy and observation were completed many years ago, when the close attention to study design issues now practiced was not routine and provided inconclusive results (12,13). Although the need for randomized trials saturates thoughtful discussions of early prostate cancer treatments, few have been initiated and none completed in the last decade. The remarkable, although still slow, accrual to the most ambitious such trial, the Prostate Intervention versus Observation Trial, will not yield its results soon. The first analysis is planned after 10 years of follow-up (14). Whereas progress documenting the benefits of treatment has been slow, several important studies have documented the substantial likelihood of treatment-related complications. By asking patients directly about their symptoms and other measures of the quality of life rather than relying on their treating physicians to observe and report them, these studies have documented that erectile dysfunction (ED) after treatment is more probable than not, whereas other important symptoms, such as urinary incontinence after radical prostatectomy and radiation proctitis, are more frequent than previously thought (15–20). The combination of poorly defined benefit and increasingly evident complications of treatment has made the discussion of treatment complications an essential part of treatment discussions and, by extension, of this book.

Despite this murky picture, the overwhelming majority of men with localized prostate cancer does choose to be treated, typically with prostatectomy or pelvic irradiation. Although the risks of sexual, urinary, and bowel impairment are well established, individual patients often find it difficult to base their decisions on population statistics. Rather, they make implicit judgments about the relative value of maintaining their quality of life versus maximizing their survival. Although the chance of dying from prostate cancer is low for men with well- to moderately differentiated tumors, for most American men the idea of not treating a malignancy is so foreign that they cannot conceive of choosing observation. Hence, they choose to expose themselves to the risks of impotence, incontinence, and proctitis without a clear survival advantage. Nevertheless, this choice is not simply suppression of cognitive dissonance. Indeed, for many men, the decline of their PSA to undetectable levels provides crucial reassurance and relief of the anxiety their cancer diagnosis has caused. Although their risk of terminal prostate cancer may be low, the inherent benefit of feeling "cured," which an undetectable PSA produces, may powerfully benefit their quality of life. Whereas we lack solid evidence that early intervention meaningfully prolongs life for men with localized prostate cancer, we also lack solid evidence that it does not. The choice to accept known risks for an unknown, deferred benefit usually implies neither ignorance nor indifference but determination married to necessity. Having given them what we think they need to make an informed decision, our job as physicians is to support their decision and life in the shadow of cancer.

However, for prostate cancer, as for all cancers, the event (after the cancer's diagnosis) that erodes quality of life most dramatically for patients and their spouses is evidence that it has become metastatic and thus incurable (21). By using PSA to monitor the course of treated patients, we have accelerated our discovery of each patient's treatment failure. PSA levels first rise long before bone metastases cause symptoms. A recent review of surgically treated patients found a median delay of 8 years between the rise of PSA and the detection of metastases (22). These facts led to the awkward conclusion that to optimize the quality of life in men with prostate cancer requires either that a lab value or PSA remain low or that it not be measured. Because most men with prostate cancer are unable to suppress their interest in the one reliable indicator of the status of their cancer, patients usually rule out not measuring PSA. Therefore, clinicians confronted with their patient's anguish at a rising PSA may feel compelled to suppress it to improve their patient's quality of life. This motive may partially account for a puzzling trend—that is, physicians' increasing use of hormonal ablation for patients with rising PSA alone without other evidence of metastatic prostate cancer. Surgical or chemical castration provides reliable temporary suppression of PSA levels but without proven survival benefit and a growing body of evidence that documents the treatment's side effects. The use of quality of life to justify an unproved treatment with known side effects shows that, even in the setting of metastatic prostate cancer, quality of life aspects of treatment deserve thoughtful discussion.

Yet, compared to the treatments given for other advanced cancers, hormone ablation is benign. By some measures, patients in remission receiving an LHRH agonist and flutamide have a quality of life that is indistinguishable from a matched male population without prostate cancer and a quality of life significantly better than that of men with androgen-resistant disease. Among patients who respond to total androgen ablation, flutamide and an LHRH agonist provide significant, measurable benefits to recipients independent of improvement in longevity as yet unproven (23). However, the tumor invariably becomes refractory to this therapy. As metastatic prostate cancer progresses, quality of life not only qualifies survival, but it also predicts it (24). During the stage of advanced prostate cancer, the importance of spousal support apparent from the time of diagnosis becomes even more evident. Krongrad and colleagues have documented that survival is better among married men (25,26). As the various factors contributing to quality of life become better understood, interventions to assist patients may become an increasing part of our treatment of men with prostate cancer, particularly when advanced.

METHODOLOGIC ISSUES IN QUALITY OF LIFE MEASUREMENT

Although duration of survival is relatively easy to quantify, the measurement of quality of life is more difficult, primarily because the process is less familiar to physicians. In quality of life research, data are collected with HRQL surveys called *instruments* that contain questions or items organized into scales. Each scale measures an aspect or domain of HRQL. For example, items of a particular instrument may address a patient's ability to have an erection and his satisfaction with ejaculation, both of which might be included in a sexual domain. Some scales include several items, whereas others may include only one or two. Each item contains a stem, which may be a question or a statement, and a response set.

Because HRQL assessment must involve individuals' own perceptions of health and ability to function, instruments are best when they are self-administered by the patient. Physicians typically underestimate the symptom burden experienced by prostate cancer patients, either because their queries are not sensitive enough or patients tend to understate their problems when responding directly to their primary caregiver (27–29). HRQL measurement must adhere to a rigorous discipline known as *psychometric test theory*, which seeks to optimize the attributes of reliability, validity, and responsiveness.

Reliability refers to how reproducible an instrument or scale is. *Test-retest reliability* is a measure of response stability over time. It is assessed by administering scales to subjects at two time points, with the time interval short enough to preclude the possibility that the domains being assessed will have been affected by the disease or its treatment during the intervening period. Correlation coefficients between the two scores reflect the stability of responses. *Internal consistency reliability* measures the similarity of an individual's responses across several items, indicating the homogeneity of a scale. The statistic used to quantify the internal consistency or unidimensionality of a scale is called *Cronbach's coefficient alpha* (30). Generally accepted standards dictate that, for group comparisons, reliability statistics measured by these two methods should exceed 0.7 (31). When used at the level of individual patients (e.g., monitoring HRQL over time), a reliability coefficient of at least 0.9 is preferred. Although some scales may function well as single-item measures, in general a health concept is better measured by a set of questions than by a single question. Multi-item measures are thus more reliable.

Validity refers to how well the scale or instrument measures the attribute it is intended to measure. *Content validity*, sometimes referred to as *face validity*, involves qualitative assessments of the scope, completeness, and relevance of a proposed scale (32). *Criterion validity* is a more quantitative approach to assessing the performance of scales and instruments. It requires the correlation of a scale's score with other measurable health outcomes (predictive validity) and with results from established tests (concurrent validity). Generally accepted standards also dictate that validity statistics should exceed 0.7. *Construct validity*, perhaps the most valuable assessment of a survey instrument, is a measure of how meaningful the scale or survey instrument performs in a multitude of settings and populations over a number of years. Construct validity comprises two other forms of validity: convergent and divergent. *Convergent validity* implies that several different methods for obtaining the same information about a given trait or concept produce similar results. *Divergent validity* means that the scale does not correlate too closely with similar but distinct concepts or traits. Because instruments are not simply valid or invalid, the task of validating them is always ongoing.

Responsiveness of an HRQL instrument refers to how sensitive the scales are to change over time. That is, a survey may be reliable and valid when used at a single point in time, but in some circumstances it must also be able to detect meaningful improvements or decrements in quality of life during longitudinal studies. The instrument must "react" in a time frame that is relevant for patients over time. Because HRQL may change over time, longitudinal measurement of these outcomes is important (33,34). Different domains may become more or less prominent over time as the course of disease and recovery evolves. Although their perception of cure waxes and wanes with time since treatment or the latest PSA level, patients may feel more or less impacted by their HRQL impairments. In addition, patients may experience a "response shift" as they learn to adapt to the chronicity of HRQL alterations (35).

Prospective, longitudinal data collection is always best, because this approach may reveal time-dependent evolution of HRQL domains (36,37). Patients may then serve as their own controls. Assessing HRQL at baseline before treatment allows for the inclusion of baseline age-related changes that should not be attributed to treatments. Because prostate cancer is largely a disease of older men, many of them may already be troubled by sexual, urinary, or bowel dysfunction. If they are surveyed cross sectionally after surgery or radiation, then it is impossible to determine whether any quality of life impairments have occurred as a result of the treatment or whether they were already present. Studies that use longitudinal methods can determine how long it takes for patients to return to their own individual baseline status in the various quality of life domains.

However, investigators often use methodologies in which HRQL is assessed cross sectionally rather than longitudinally. In cross-sectional surveys, patients cannot serve as their own temporal controls, because it is well established that patients' recall of pretreatment HRQL is inaccurate (38–41). Hence, studies must rely on appropriate comparison groups. Selecting the best normal comparison group is a critical step in conducting a meaningful analysis of HRQL outcomes. If normal is defined as the absence of any dysfunction, then prostate cancer treatment groups may be held to too high a standard. If normal is determined by assessing older men without prostate cancer (or, even better, prostate cancer patients on watchful waiting), then HRQL outcomes after prostate cancer treatment may be interpreted in a more valid context (42).

Investigators must be parsimonious when selecting HRQL instruments. Although longer instruments may provide richer databases, researchers must recognize that fatigue may limit the ability of patients to provide useful information. This phenomenon, known as *response burden*, must be considered when assessing HRQL in clinical or research settings.

Cultural issues must also be taken into account. Although an instrument may have been translated into a new language, it may not have the same meaning in that culture. This is particularly relevant when studying quality of life, social attitudes, and health behaviors in different countries or cultures. Different nations and cultures may have very different concepts of health, well being, illness, and disease. Therefore, a well-developed concept in one group of people may not even exist in another. Even with an instrument that is well validated in English, various English-speaking populations across the world may not approach the concept with the same ideas (43–45). Failing to be attentive to multicultural issues may result in significant bias when collecting and interpreting data. New instrument development should always be undertaken with an eye toward eventual international translation and cultural adaptation.

General and Disease-Specific Quality of Life Assessment

HRQL instruments may be general or disease-specific. General HRQL domains address the components of overall well being, whereas disease-specific domains focus on the impact of particular organic dysfunctions that affect HRQL (46). General HRQL instruments typically address general health perceptions, a sense of overall well being, and function in the physical, emotional, and social domains. Disease-specific HRQL instruments focus on more directly relevant domains, such as anxiety about cancer recurrence, urinary, sexual, and bowel impairment, and any bother caused by these dysfunctions. Disease-specific and general HRQL domains often impact each other, leading to important interactions that must be considered in the interpretation of HRQL data. In early-stage prostate cancer, the treatments alter intimate bodily functions that may not be fully appreciated by assessing only the broader domains of general HRQL. Conversely, in patients with advanced prostate cancer, HRQL may be affected predominantly by pain, fatigue, and other constitutional symptoms that are well captured by general HRQL instruments.

General Quality of Life Instruments

General HRQL instruments have been extensively studied and validated in many types of patients, sick and well. Examples include the RAND Medical Outcomes Study 36-Item Health Survey (also known as the SF-36) (47,48), the Quality of Well-Being scale (QWB) (49,50), the Sickness Impact Profile (51,52), and the Nottingham Health Profile (53,54). Each assesses various components of HRQL, including physical and emotional functioning, social functioning, and symptoms. Each has been thoroughly validated and tested.

The SF-36 is one of the most commonly used instruments and is regarded by some as a gold-standard measure of general HRQL. It is a 36-item, self-administered instrument that takes fewer than 10 minutes to complete and quantifies HRQL in multi-item scales that address eight different health concepts—physical function, role limitation due to physical problems, bodily pain, general health perceptions, social function, emotional well being, role limitation due to emotional problems, and energy and fatigue. The SF-36 may also be scored in two summary domains: physical and mental. Recently, a shorter 12-item version, the SF-12, has been developed for use in studies requiring greater efficiency. It provides a somewhat narrower view of overall health status and is scored only in the two summary domains (55,56).

The QWB summarizes three aspects of health status—mobility, physical activity, and social activity—in terms of quality-adjusted life years, quantifying HRQL as a single number that may range from death to complete well being. The original QWB contains only 18 items, but it requires a trained interviewer. A newer self-administered version of the QWB is now available and has been shown to produce scores that are equivalent to the interviewer-administered version and stable over time (57).

The Sickness Impact Profile measures health status by assessing the impact of sickness on changing daily activities and behavior. It is self-administered but contains 136 items and can take 30 minutes or longer to complete. Test-retest reliability is consistently high (0.88 to 0.92) in validation populations.

The Nottingham Health Profile covers six types of experiences that may be affected by illness, pain, physical mobility, sleep, emotional reactions, energy, and social isolation by using a series of weighted yes or no items. It contains 38 self-administered items and can be completed fairly quickly.

Cancer-Specific Quality of Life Instruments

Because of the well-documented impact of malignancies and their treatment on HRQL, cancer-specific quality of life also has been investigated extensively. Various instruments have been developed and tested that measure the special impact of cancer in general on patients' daily activities. Examples include the European Organization for the Research and Treatment of Cancer Quality of Life Questionnaire C30 (EORTC QLQ-C30) (58,59), the Functional Assessment of Cancer Therapy (FACT) (60), and the Cancer Rehabilitation Evaluation System Short Form (CARES-SF) (61,62). Each has been validated and tested in patients with various types of cancer. Readers are also directed to a comprehensive website (http://www.qlmed.org/) developed by Tamburini. It is an invaluable resource in the selection of quality of life instruments for studies in prostate cancer, other malignancies, and a variety of acute and chronic benign conditions. It contains up-to-date psychometric data, bibliographies, and easily downloadable copies of dozens of HRQL instruments.

The EORTC QLQ-C30 was designed to measure cancer-specific HRQL in patients with a variety of malignancies. Its 30 items address domains that are common to all cancer patients. The questionnaire includes five functional scales (physical, role, emotional, cognitive, and social functioning); a global health scale; three symptom scales (fatigue, nausea/vomiting, and pain); and six single items concerning dyspnea, insomnia, appetite loss, constipation, diarrhea, and financial difficulties due to disease. The EORTC QLQ-C30 does not include items specific to prostate cancer, but it has performed well in this population (63). Other disease-specific modules for prostate cancer (see later) are presently under development.

The FACT is usually applied as a two-part instrument that includes a general item set pertaining to all cancer patients [FACT-general (G)] and one of several item sets containing special questions for patients with specific tumors (see later). Each item is a statement that a patient may agree or disagree with across a 5-point range. The FACT-G domains include well being in five main areas: physical, social/family, relationship with doctor, emotional, and functional. The FACT-G includes 28 items and is easily self-administered.

The CARES-SF is a 59-item, self-administered instrument that measures cancer-related quality of life with five multi-item scales: physical, psychosocial, medical interaction, marital interaction, and sexual function. A large and valuable database of patients with many different tumors, including urologic tumors, has been collected by the instrument's authors (64). These data are helpful when comparing the experience of prostate cancer patients with that of patients with other types of cancer.

The Rotterdam Symptom Checklist contains 27 items that are scored in two domains (psychosocial and physical distress), as well as several miscellaneous items relevant to cancer patients. Its two dimensions are reliable across populations (65).

Prostate Cancer–Specific Quality of Life Instruments

The University of California, Los Angeles Prostate Cancer Index (PCI) has been popularized as a reliable, valid instrument to measure disease-targeted HRQL in men treated for early-stage prostate cancer (17,66). The PCI is a self-administered, 20-item questionnaire that quantifies prostate cancer–specific HRQL in six separate domains: urinary function, urinary bother, sexual function, sexual bother, bowel function, and bowel bother. The six scales are scored from 0 to 100, with higher scores representing better outcomes. The PCI has been shown to be reliable and valid, with test-retest reliability coefficients of 0.77 in five of six scales and internal consistency alpha coefficients of 0.65 to 0.93 in populations of older men with and without prostate cancer. A cross-cultural Spanish translation of the PCI is available for Spanish-speaking men living in the United States (67).

The FACT-Prostate (FACT-P) is a supplemental prostate-targeted module that is used with the FACT-G. It is a 12-item scale that addresses weight loss, appetite, and urinary and erectile difficulties (68). Its internal consistencies range from 0.65 to 0.69 in populations of men with prostate cancer, and it is responsive to changes in performance status and PSA over time. Although it has been used in patients with localized or advanced disease, its items focus primarily on the symptoms of metastatic prostate cancer.

The Prostate Cancer Treatment Outcome Questionnaire (PCTOQ) (69) was also designed as a supplement to the FACT-G. Its self-administered 41 items probe domains relevant to prostate cancer patients. The PCTOQ provides scores in the sexual, urinary, and bowel domains, but it is much longer than the FACT-P. A newer version of the PCTOQ based on further analysis includes 29 items in the three domains of sexual, urinary, and bowel dysfunction. Both the PCTOQ and the FACT-P are relatively new, so additional research is needed to determine their usefulness.

The Radiumhemmets Scale of Sexual Function, another disease-specific instrument (70), was initially developed to address sexual dysfunction in the setting of treatment for prostate cancer. An expanded version of this questionnaire, available from its authors, also addresses micturition and continence (incorporating the International Prostate Symptom Score), as well as bowel function, co-morbidity, overall health status, and demographics. This instrument has been used in a number of Swedish prostate cancer health-related quality of life studies, although published data on its reliability and validity are limited (71,72).

Another HRQL disease-specific instrument presently under investigation and soon to be published is the prostate cancer module of the EORTC QLQ-PR25. Researchers are developing this module to be used in conjunction with the EORTC QLQ-C30 as a measure of disease-specific HRQL in prostate cancer. Its 25 items include bowel, urinary, and sexuality symptom scales and are reliable and valid in men with localized and metastatic prostate cancer. Its transformed scales are scored from 0 to 100, with higher scores representing worse outcomes in functional status domains.

Some investigators believe that comparisons of various quality of life studies will only be possible if the research community establishes a single instrument to be used throughout the world. Others contend that patients' life experiences and values vary so widely across cultures that conforming to one unified instrument would be neither possible nor desirable. Clearly, the existing general and disease-specific quality of life instruments adequately address the domains of importance to men with early and late-stage prostate cancer. Although it might be useful to develop a core set of items to use in international studies, the literature is enriched with data from a variety of validated quality of life measures.

As useful as multi-item scales are, particularly for comparing the outcomes of groups of patients, combining several items into a domain and several domains into a summary score for HRQL to some extent substitutes mathematical confidence for interpretability, particularly at the individual level. Summary scores are essential to obtain a single number for a complex outcome but, like any aggregation, may conceal particular outcomes of interest. For example, a patient trying to choose a treatment may care less that patients receiving radiation therapy have on average lower urinary dysfunction scores than surgery patients than the actual frequency of developing urinary incontinence of a particular severity after each treatment. It is important that studies of quality of life keep in mind health policy makers and individual patients and reporting results, including specific outcomes of interest in addition to scores.

LESSONS FROM THE QUALITY OF LIFE LITERATURE

The literature on quality of life in men treated for early and late-stage prostate cancer expanded rapidly during the 1990s. Despite the absence of randomized controlled trials, a variety of well-conducted studies have used cross-sectional and longitudinal designs to reveal several important lessons. The best studies have relied on validated instruments. The central findings reported in the literature include the following. First, the domains of general quality of life, such as physical, emotional, and social functioning, do not differ substantially across treatment groups. This suggests that patients undergoing surgery or radiation appear to adjust equally well to any changes that prostate cancer or its treatments may cause. Second, the domains of disease-specific quality of life, such as sexual, urinary, and bowel dysfunction, vary markedly, qualitatively, and quantitatively across treatment groups. Third, over time, patients accommodate at least partially to any dysfunction they may experience. Fourth, some differences in disease-specific quality of life between groups undergoing surgery or radiation diminish significantly over time. For example, the effects of radical prostatectomy on potency (and continence) occur acutely after treatment. However, after approximately 2 years, the continuing progression of ED after pelvic irradiation results in approximately similar levels of impairment. Fifth, when performing group comparisons of quality of life in prostate cancer patients, it is important to use them to age-matched controls, as older men may develop sexual, urinary, or bowel dysfunction independent of prostate cancer treatment. Furthermore, documentation of pretreatment function, possible in prospective cohort studies and, still better, randomized trials, but not cross-sectional surveys, allows the distinction to be made between preexisting impairments and those arising after and potentially because of treatment. Sixth, it is important to adhere to rigorous methodologic guidelines when measuring quality of life, as these issues can profoundly impact study results. For example, quality of life is best measured by patient self report, as physicians have been shown to underestimate the effects of treatment.

Treatment-Related Symptoms

Treatments for early prostate cancer differ in their expected side effects. Because the prostate is anatomically central to sexual functioning adjacent to the neurovascular bundles implicated in initiating erections (73) and the corpora cavernosa, whose engorgement with arteriolar blood provides mechanical support, all active treatments may cause ED. Radical prostatectomy invariably resulted in impotence before the importance of the neurovascular bundles was appreciated. New "nerve-sparing" surgical techniques to preserve these structures developed by Walsh and colleagues had little impact on the nearly universal impotence experienced immediately after surgery but made recovery within a year or two to full erectile function possible for some men (74). Because prostate cancer is often multifocal in the prostate and the neurovascular bundles lie immediately adjacent to it, nerve preservation theoretically risks compromising the primary surgical goal of excising all tumors. Therefore, most urologists are reluctant to preserve bundles on the same side of the prostate as the evident tumor, leaving many men who desired nerve preservation, particularly if their cancers are palpable, with only unilateral preservation or without it. Unilateral nerve preservation is much less successful than bilateral preservation in preserving potency (19,75). The likelihood of erectile function varies with the definition of potency; patient's age and other comorbid conditions; stage of the cancer; and, probably, surgeon and institution-specific characteristics, such as frequency of surgery. The most commonly cited outcomes arise from specialized referral centers with selected patients, although most procedures are performed in community settings where outcomes are usually not measured or published. The contrast between the results at centers and more representative patient samples can be striking (15).

External beam radiation therapy also causes ED, although the time course is slower than for surgery, and the etiology is complex (17,76–78). Little evidence of ED is evident until a year after treatment (18,20), but impotence continues to progress for at least another year (79). The quality of ED after radiation therapy may also differ; many, if not most, men with ED report erections that are not firm enough for intercourse. The significance of the differences between radical prostatectomy and external beam radiation therapy is not understood. Some have argued that erections of inadequate firmness may be caused by leakage of blood from the corpora due to radiation-induced damage, but little data exist to support this mechanism.

Brachytherapy also likely causes ED, but it has been less well studied than more common modalities. ED after brachytherapy is likely to follow a similar slow time course like that after external beam radiation therapy, because radiation-induced fibrosis is likely a common mechanism. These techniques may differ in the dose to the neurovascular bundles and corpora.

The use of neoadjuvant or adjuvant androgen ablation with these primary local treatments may have an important impact on erectile function. The duration of treatment is increasing. Earlier trials used hormonal ablation for 2 or 3 months. Because the PSA nadir may be found 8 to 12 months after treatment begins, longer periods are now used. In the sole adjuvant trial in which a survival advantage was found, hormonal treatment was extended for 3 years (80). Prolonged hormonal ablation may significantly delay recovery of endogenous androgen production.

Localized Prostate Cancer

Prostate-specific HRQL in the sexual, urinary, and bowel domains has been studied in a cross-sectional survey using the University of California, Los Angeles PCI (17). In a study of 528 men in a managed care population, general HRQL was similar when comparing patients who had undergone surgery, radiation, or observation alone for clinically localized prostate cancer or when comparing them to a group of age-matched control subjects without prostate cancer. Among the subjects, significant treatment group differences in HRQL were identified in the prostate-specific sexual, urinary, and bowel domains. Patients who had undergone radical prostatectomy had worse sexual and urinary function, but they were no more bothered than patients who had received radiation. Radiated patients had worse bowel function, but they were no more bothered than those undergoing surgery. Function and bother were clearly shown to be independent HRQL domains. Interestingly, the prostate-specific HRQL decrements did not translate into differences in general HRQL.

In a longitudinal prospective study of 260 newly diagnosed patients with early prostate cancer who later chose radical prostatectomy or external beam radiation therapy, Talcott and colleagues were able to compare the treatment groups' pretreatment status and subsequent changes (18–20,81). ED, but not bowel symptoms or urinary incontinence, was prevalent pretreatment, particularly among radiation therapy patients. Radiation patients averaged 6 years older than the surgery patients, which was an expected difference given the commonly preferred recommendation of surgery for younger, healthier men. At 3 months after treatment, nearly all surgery patients reported ED, more than half wore absorptive pads for urinary incontinence, and 16% of radiation therapy patients reported several episodes of diarrhea and at least mild rectal urgency in the last week. Despite subsequent improvement in the first year, at 12 months, 69% of surgery patients with erections pretreatment reported complete impotence in the last month, and 91% reported erections inadequate for intercourse. In addition, 11% reported "a lot" of urinary incontinence, and 35% reported wearing pads within the last week. Although diarrhea and rectal urgency improved, ED increased among radiation patients after 3 months. At 12 months after radiotherapy, 24% of men with erections pretreatment had none, 61% had erections inadequate for intercourse (20), and ED increased further the following year, the proportion with inadequate erections approaching that of surgery patients (79).

Others have documented the evolution of HRQL over time. In men treated with radical prostatectomy for early-stage disease, Pedersen and colleagues (56) carried out a longitudinal study of quality of life changes for 18 months after surgery. The initial distress associated with diagnosis of cancer improved over time, although bother from ED persisted. Overall well being was minimally affected. In the initial 12 months after initial therapy for early prostate cancer, Clark and colleagues found sluggish responsiveness of only three SF-36 domains (global health perception, vitality, and social function). Even these changes showed a modest association with symptoms and responded little to the development of new symptoms (81). Litwin and colleagues found similarly poor correlation between global measures of HRQL symptoms. These global measures were more responsive to anxiety over cancer than to treatment-related symptoms. In a prospective study of patients in the year after radical prostatectomy for early-stage prostate cancer, patients experienced steady improvement in their quality of life. By 3 months postoperatively, 30% to 40% of patients had already recovered their baseline levels of physical, mental, and social functioning, by 6 months more than 70%, and by 12 months after surgery, 86% to 97% of patients had returned to baseline levels in each domain (82). Similar results were found in patients included in the Cancer of the Prostate Strategic Urology Research Endeavor (CaPSURE) database. After initial decreases after prostatectomy, patients reported an improvement in general and disease-specific HRQL within 9 months of their initial diagnosis with prostate cancer. Being married was associated with better HRQL, whereas advancing age was associated with steeper HRQL declines over time (83).

Talcott et al. (19) compared erectile function of men who underwent nerve-sparing radical prostatectomy and non-nerve-sparing surgery. Using a newly validated HRQL instrument, they found that the surgical procedure patients received was correlated with pretreatment erectile function and cancer prognostic factors: non-nerve-sparing, unilateral nerve-sparing (one neurovascular bundle preserved), and bilateral nerve-sparing patient groups had progressively better erectile function, a younger age, and better PSA, Gleason scores, and tumor stage. At 12 months after surgery, there was no difference in erectile function between non-nerve-sparing and unilateral nerve-sparing patients, and only 21% of patients who had bilateral nerve-sparing surgery reported erections usually adequate for intercourse. This study did not examine the degree to which sexual dysfunction bothered patients, nor did it examine general HRQL in these patients.

Fortunately, a variety of treatments are available for men with impotence. One study found that when postprostatectomy patients use erectile aids, their HRQL in the sexual domains is returned to levels similar to men awaiting surgery (84). However, another longitudinal study of outcomes 18 months after surgery found that whereas the initial distress associated with diagnosis of cancer improved over time, bother from ED persisted. Overall well being was minimally affected (85). Lim and colleagues (86) surveyed HRQL in 136 men who had undergone radical retropubic prostatectomy and 60 men who had received external beam irradiation for clinically localized prostate cancer. Although the prostatectomy group initially had more impotence and incontinence, the radiation group had worse bowel function. Radiated patients who were incontinent perceived this as a greater problem than did incontinent patients in the prostatectomy group. The study also showed that sexual function correlated positively with physical vigor and negatively with incontinence and depression, implying that impotence may affect general HRQL. Approximately 90% of each group stated that they would choose the same treatment again.

Brasilis et al. (87) studied 79 men who had undergone prostatectomy and found that although impotence had little effect on most domains of general HRQL, patients with better sexual function tended to have better scores in the physical vigor domain. Rossetti and Terrone (88) also found that ED in 161 men after radical prostatectomy did not correlate strongly with general HRQL. Shrader-Bogen et al. (69) compared men who had undergone prostatectomy or radiation therapy and also found that whereas sexual function was worse among the surgery patients, general HRQL was similar between the two groups.

Fowler and colleagues on the Prostate Patient Outcomes Research Team (89,90) studied a large national sample of Medicare beneficiaries who had undergone radical prostatectomy. They documented that although sexual and urinary dysfunction are much more common after surgery than previously reported, general HRQL domains, such as physical and mental health, do not correlate well with decrements in prostate-specific HRQL.

Incontinence after prostate cancer treatment appears to have a greater impact than ED on general HRQL. Herr (91) demonstrated that among men who were incontinent after radical prostatectomy, 26% reported limitations in their usual physical activity, and more than half experienced moderate to severe emotional distress. Interestingly, 79% of those evaluated fewer than 5 years after surgery said they would choose surgery again despite their leakage problems. Lim and colleagues (86) found that men who were incontinent after prostatectomy or radiation therapy were more likely to have emotional tension, physical fatigue, depression, low physical vigor, and poor social well being. In their study of men who underwent radical prostatectomy, Shrader-Bogen and colleagues (69) showed that 19% of subjects reported that their urinary problems affected their quality of life "quite a bit" or "very much." Fossa and colleagues (92) also found lower urinary tract symptoms after treatment to be an independent predictor of global HRQL in a logistic regression model. As continence improves during the months after prostatectomy, quality of life follows a similar course (93).

Borghede (94) used an early version of the EORTC prostate module to study a population of men with localized prostate cancer who had undergone external beam radiation therapy. Patients had significant decreases in the sexual domain but relatively good general HRQL. HRQL scores on the sexuality and general scales did not correlate well with each other, again suggesting that general HRQL tends to be well preserved, even in the setting of specific pelvic dysfunction. In a prospective cohort study, Beard et al. (95) used the SF-36 to demonstrate that general HRQL did not change significantly in men receiving external beam radiation for prostate cancer. Bowel symptoms were common during the initial 3 months after therapy but improved at 6 months. Those receiving whole-pelvis treatment fared worse than those receiving conformal therapy. Likewise, Caffo et al. (96) showed that although 44% of men had significant decreases in the sexual domain after radiation therapy, physical, psychologic and relational well being remained high.

Fowler et al. (16) studied HRQL in 621 men who had undergone pelvic irradiation for prostate cancer. Patients were identified through the National Institutes of Health's Surveillance, Epidemiology, and End Results program in three regions of the United States. Compared to those who had received radical prostatectomy, radiated patients had significantly less incontinence (7% vs. 32%) and ED (23% vs. 56%) but significantly more bowel dysfunction (10% vs. 4%). Radiated patients also worried more about cancer recurrence than did those treated with surgery. In a comprehensive study of sexual function in 199 men who had undergone pelvic irradiation compared to 200 age-matched controls, Fransson and Widmark (97) showed that radiated patients were more than four times more likely to be impotent, except in those younger than 70 years, in whom the frequency of sexual activity was almost equal to the control population without prostate cancer.

Other investigators examining the effect of ED on HRQL after radiation have shown differences in general HRQL. Helgason et al. (70) used the Radiumhemmets Scale of Sexual Functioning, which includes an item that addresses global quality of life, to determine the effect of decreased sexual capacity on HRQL in this patient population. They showed that sexual desire diminished 77% after treatment and that although 66% of men still had an erection sufficient for intercourse, 77% of men reported some loss of stiffness. More important, half of men reported that their overall quality of life had decreased much or very much as a direct result of their decrease in erectile function. Roach et al. (98) noted similar outcomes.

Although patients undergoing radiation therapy tend to score better in the urinary domains than do those undergoing radical prostatectomy, these scores are still worse than in age-matched controls (99).

ISSUES FOR THE FUTURE

Although we have learned a great deal about quality of life in men with prostate cancer in the 1990s, more questions remain unanswered than resolved. These issues involve choosing methods for measuring and reporting quality of life, identifying situations in which quality of life matters most, and fitting quality of life into the question of treatment choice, in which the most important issue for most patients is preventing death from cancer.

We need to be consistent in how we measure and report quality of life. Even when the methodologic guidelines described previously are followed, methodologic issues remain. Even thoroughly validated instruments are not interchangeable. Although consistent results using different instruments in different populations reinforce one another, the reasons for conflicting results are less clear when instruments vary between studies. Converging on a single instrument may be premature and disadvantageous, however. Available instruments may not collect all we need to understand HRQL in prostate cancer. For example, the limited and inconsistent correlation between ED and general HRQL appears to contradict the importance many men ascribe to sexual potency. To clarify this relationship, we may need to better understand men's concept of sexuality and its changing relationship to ED; cancer and other diseases; masculine self-identity; social support, especially from a sexual partner; regret over treatment decisions; and treatments for ED, to name a few. Flexibility and inventiveness in developing assessment tools will be necessary to clarify such complex relationships.

Almost all of the current reports on the effects of treatment are nonrandomized. As a result, reported results are confounded by the treatment patients receive. Men choose and are steered toward different treatments by their physicians based on factors that affect their prognosis: the extent of their prostate cancer, the number and seriousness of their coexisting diseases, their age, and, perhaps, other less directly relevant factors, such as their sociodemographic status or race. These factors also influence the likelihood of symptoms that may be caused by prostate cancer treatment, such as ED or urinary incontinence. Physicians, for example, more often recommend that older patients receive radiation therapy rather than radical prostatectomy. Because ED increases with age, radiation therapy patients are more often impotent before treatment than surgery patients (20). Radiation therapy patients thus go into treatment disadvantaged compared to surgery patients, making a comparison of their potency rates after treatment misleading, unless their pretreatment differences are accounted for. Similarly, the decision of whether to perform nerve-sparing radical prostatectomy depends on the patient's desire to preserve his potency and the urologist's belief that all prostate cancer can be safely removed if one or both neurovascular bundle(s) is spared excision. The patient's pretreatment erectile function, age, and the extent of his cancer all influence the choice of the surgical technique, and each may influence later potency independent of the treatment he receives. Men who are impotent before surgery are the least likely to be potent after surgery and to request potency-sparing surgery, whereas younger men with early prostate cancer and without ED are the most likely to request bilateral nerve-sparing surgery and to have it accomplished. Therefore, at least some of the apparent benefit of nerve-sparing surgery is confounded by the patient's pretreatment characteristics (19). Thus, without assurance that patients were similar before treatment or that differences were adjusted for, separating outcomes due to the particular treatment received and to other patient factors is impossible. The best assurance comes from random assignment of patients to treatment in controlled trials. The track record for completing randomized trials among men with prostate cancer, particularly early prostate cancer, is nothing short of scandalous.

Until we can complete and analyze randomized trials, we need to collect information consistently to make approximate comparisons of the primary treatments for early prostate cancer consistent with the principles described earlier. The patient is the best judge of his own quality of life and should be the direct source of information reported.

We need to study the quality of life impact of changes in our treatment approach, particularly when the changes lack a strong evidence-based rationale. For example, hormonal ablation is increasingly often used to increase the efficacy of external beam radiation therapy preceding definitive local therapy for short periods of 2 to 3 months but increasingly prolonged for as long as 12 months. Although large trials of the Radiation Therapy Oncology Group have found that neoadjuvant hormone ablation delays cancer progression, such a benefit would be expected based on the treatment's known antitumor effect, which control arm patients have not yet received. When control patients progress and receive hormonal ablation, the early advantage of the other group would be expected to be largely made up, whereas patients receiving hormonal therapy at progression would be expected to have a lesser benefit, because many cancer cells that are sensitive to hormonal ablation will have already died. Therefore, the only reliable end point to test this treatment is overall survival. The Radiation Therapy Oncology Group studies have found a survival benefit for only a single subset of one study, patients with centrally reviewed Gleason scores of 8 to 10 (100,101). The sole (unconfirmed) randomized trial that found an overall survival benefit for early hormonal ablation continued treatment for 3 years (80). Despite the incomplete evidence regarding this approach, many radiation oncologists consider neoadjuvant hormonal ablation a standard approach, especially for patients with adverse prognostic factors, such as high Gleason score, PSA greater than 10 ng per mL, or large palpable tumors. This gradual enlargement of the indications and duration of treatment have occurred with little study of the adverse side effects of treatment. For example, recovery of endogenous testosterone production is prolonged after androgen ablation of increasing lengths and may not recover for all men (102). The impact of these changes on erectile function may be important. Perhaps most striking is the increasingly common practice of instituting hormone ablation in response to the initial rise of PSA after primary treatment based on a single study of uncertain relevance to current standards of practice (103). These examples emphasize that measuring quality of life remains integral to improving our care of prostate cancer patients. We hope that when this text is revised, HRQL measurement will have become a useful, integrated aspect of management of men with prostate cancer.

REFERENCES

1. Albertsen PC, Hanley JA, Gleason DF, et al. Competing risk analysis of men aged 55 to 74 years at diagnosis managed conservatively for clinically localized prostate cancer. *JAMA* 1998;280:975–980.
2. Johansson JE, Adami HO, Andersson SO, et al. Natural history of localised prostatic cancer. A population-based study in 223 untreated patients. *Lancet* 1989;1:799–803.
3. Chodak GW, Thisted RA, Gerber GS, et al. Results of conservative management of clinically localized prostate cancer. *N Engl J Med* 1994;330:242–248.
4. Johansson JE, Holmberg L, Johansson S, et al. Fifteen-year survival in prostate cancer. A prospective, population-based study in Sweden [see comments] [published erratum appears in *JAMA* 1997;278:206]. *JAMA* 1997;277:467–471.
5. Fleming C, Wasson JH, Albertsen PC, et al. A decision analysis of alternative treatment strategies for clinically localized prostate cancer. *JAMA* 1993;269:2650–2658.
6. Potosky AL, Miller BA, Albertsen PC, et al. The role of increasing detection in the rising incidence of prostate cancer. *JAMA* 1995;273:548–552.
7. Jacobsen SJ, Katusic SK, Bergstralh EJ, et al. Incidence of prostate cancer diagnosis in the eras before and after serum prostate-specific antigen testing. *JAMA* 1995;274:1445–1449.
8. Etzioni R, Legler JM, Feuer EJ, et al. Cancer surveillance series: interpreting trends in prostate cancer—part III: quantifying the link between population prostate-specific antigen testing and recent declines in prostate cancer mortality. *J Natl Cancer Inst* 1999;91:1033–1039.
9. Feuer EJ, Merrill RM, Hankey BF. Cancer surveillance series: interpreting trends in prostate cancer—part II: cause of death misclassification and the recent rise and fall in prostate cancer mortality. *J Natl Cancer Inst* 1999;91:1025–1032.
10. Hankey BF, Feuer EJ, Clegg LX, et al. Cancer surveillance series: interpreting trends in prostate cancer—part I: evidence of the effects of screening in recent prostate cancer incidence, mortality, and survival rates. *J Natl Cancer Inst* 1999;91:1017–1024.
11. Gann PH, Hennekens CH, Stampfer MJ. A prospective evaluation of plasma prostate-specific antigen for detection of prostatic cancer. *JAMA* 1995;273:289–294.
12. Paulson DF, Lin GH, Hinshaw W, et al. Radical surgery versus radiotherapy for adenocarcinoma of the prostate. *J Urol* 1982;128:502–504.
13. Hanks GE. More on the Uro-Oncology Research Group report of radical surgery vs. radiotherapy for adenocarcinoma of the prostate [Letter]. *Int J Radiat Oncol Biol Phys* 1988;14:1053–1054.
14. Wilt TJ, Brawer MK. The Prostate Cancer Intervention Versus Observation Trial: a randomized trial comparing radical prostatectomy versus expectant management for the treatment of clinically localized prostate cancer. *J Urol* 1994;152:1910–1914.
15. Fowler F Jr., Barry MJ, Lu-Yao G, et al. Patient-reported complications and follow-up treatment after radical prostatectomy. The National Medicare Experience: 1988–1990 (updated June 1993). *Urology* 1993;42:622–629.
16. Fowler FJ Jr., Barry MJ, Lu-Yao G, et al. Outcomes of external-beam radiation therapy for prostate cancer: a study of Medicare beneficiaries in three Surveillance, Epidemiology, and End Results areas. *J Clin Oncol* 1996;14:2258–2265.
17. Litwin MS, Hays RD, Fink A, et al. Quality-of-life outcomes in men treated for localized prostate cancer. *JAMA* 1995;273:129–135.
18. Beard CJ, Propert KJ, Rieker PP, et al. Complications after treatment with external-beam irradiation in early-stage prostate cancer patients: a prospective multiinstitutional outcomes study. *J Clin Oncol* 1997;15:223–229.
19. Talcott JA, Rieker P, Propert KJ, et al. Patient-reported impotence and incontinence after nerve-sparing radical prostatectomy. *J Natl Cancer Inst* 1997;89:1117–1123.
20. Talcott JA, Rieker P, Clark JA, et al. Patient-reported symptoms after primary therapy for early prostate cancer: results of a prospective cohort study. *J Clin Oncol* 1998;16:275–283.
21. Kornblith AB, Herr HW, Ofman US, et al. Quality of life of patients with prostate cancer and their spouses. The value of a data base in clinical care. *Cancer* 1994;73:2791–2802.
22. Pound CR, Partin AW, Eisenberger MA, et al. Natural history of progression after PSA elevation following radical prostatectomy [see comments]. *JAMA* 1999;281:1591–1597.
23. Albertsen PC, Aaronson NK, Muller MJ, et al. Health-related quality of life among patients with metastatic prostate cancer. *Urology* 1997;49:207–216.
24. Ganz PA, Schag CA, Lee JJ, et al. The CARES: a generic measure of health-related quality of life for patients with cancer. *Qual Life Res* 1992;1:19–29.
25. Krongrad A, Lai H, Burke MA, et al. Marriage and mortality in prostate cancer. *J Urol* 1996;156:1696–1670.
26. Krongrad A, Lai H, Lai S. Variation in prostate cancer survival explained by significant prognostic factors. *J Urol* 1997;158:1487–1490.
27. Fossa SD, Aaronson NK, Newling D, et al. Quality of life and treatment of hormone resistant metastatic prostatic

cancer. The EORTC Genito-Urinary Group. *Eur J Cancer* 1990;26:1133–1136.

28. da Silva FC, Fossa SD, Aaronson NK, et al. The quality of life of patients with newly diagnosed M1 prostate cancer: experience with EORTC clinical trial 30853. *Eur J Cancer* 1996;32A:72–77.
29. Litwin MS, Lubeck DP, Henning JM, et al. Differences in urologist and patient assessments of health related quality of life in men with prostate cancer: results of the CaPSURE database. *J Urol* 1998;159:1988–1992.
30. Cronbach LJ. Coefficient alpha and the internal structure of tests. *Psychometrika* 1951;16:297–334.
31. Nunnally JC. *Psychometric theory,* 2nd ed. New York: McGraw-Hill, 1978.
32. Messick S. The once and future issues of validity: assessing the meaning and consequences of measurement. In: Wainer H, Braun HI, eds. *Test validity.* Hillside, NJ: Lawrence Erlbaum Associates, 1988.
33. Zwinderman AH. The measurement of change of quality of life in clinical trials. *Stat Med* 1990;9:931–942.
34. Olschewski M, Schumacher M. Statistical analysis of quality of life data in cancer clinical trials. *Stat Med* 1990;9:749–763.
35. Sprangers MA. Response-shift bias: a challenge to the assessment of patients' quality of life in cancer clinical trials. *Cancer Treat Rev* 1996;22[Suppl A]:55–62.
36. Aseltine RH Jr., Carlson KJ, Fowler FJ Jr., et al. Comparing prospective and retrospective measures of treatment outcomes. *Med Care* 1995;33:AS67–AS76.
37. Emberton M, Neal DE, Black N, et al. The effect of prostatectomy on symptom severity and quality of life. *Br J Urol* 1996;77:233–247.
38. Emberton M, Challands A, Styles RA, et al. Recollected versus contemporary patient reports of pre-operative symptoms in men undergoing transurethral prostatic resection for benign disease. *J Clin Epidemiol* 1995;48:749–756.
39. Chouinard E, Walter S. Recall bias in case-control studies: an empirical analysis and theoretical framework. *J Clin Epidemiol* 1995;48:245–254.
40. Berney LR, Blane DB. Collecting retrospective data: accuracy of recall after 50 years judged against historical records. *Soc Sci Med* 1997;45:1519–1525.
41. Herrmann D. Reporting current, past, and changed health status. What we know about distortion. *Med Care* 1995;33: AS89–AS94.
42. Litwin MS. Health related quality of life in older men without prostate cancer. *J Urol* 1999;161:1180–1184.
43. Boyle P. Cultural and linguistic validation of questionnaires for use in international studies: the nine-item BPH-specific quality-of-life scale. *Eur Urol* 1997;32:50–52.
44. Sagnier PP, Richard F, Botto H, et al. [Adaptation and validation in the French language of the International Score of Symptoms of Benign Prostatic Hypertrophy.] *Prog Urol* 1994;4:532–538.
45. Vela Navarrete R, Martin Moreno JM, Calahorra FJ, et al. [Cultural and linguistic validation, in Spanish, of the International Prostatic Symptoms Scale (I-PSS).] *Actas Urol Esp* 1994;18:841–847.
46. Patrick DL, Deyo RA. Generic and disease-specific measures in assessing health status and quality of life. *Med Care* 1989;27:S217–S232.
47. Ware JE Jr., Sherbourne CD. The MOS 36-item short-form health survey (SF-36). I. Conceptual framework and item selection. *Med Care* 1992;30:473–483.
48. Ware JE, Kosinski M, Keller SK. *SF-36 physical and mental health summary scales: a user's manual.* Boston: The Health Institute, New England Medical Center, 1994.
49. Kaplan RM, Ganiats TG, Sieber WJ, et al. The Quality of Well-Being Scale: critical similarities and differences with SF-36 [see comments]. *Int J Qual Health Care* 1998;10: 509–520.
50. Anderson JP, Kaplan RM, Berry CC, et al. Interday reliability of function assessment for a health status measure. The Quality of Well-Being scale. *Med Care* 1989;27:1076–1083.
51. Bergner M, Bobbitt RA, Carter WB, et al. The Sickness Impact Profile: development and final revision of a health status measure. *Med Care* 1981;19:787–805.
52. Bergner M, Bobbitt RA, Pollard WE, et al. The sickness impact profile: validation of a health status measure. *Med Care* 1976;14:57–67.
53. McDowell IW, Martini CJ, Waugh W. A method for self-assessment of disability before and after hip replacement operations. *BMJ* 1978;2:857–859.
54. Martini CJ, McDowell I. Health status: patient and physician judgments. *Health Serv Res* 1976;11:508–515.
55. Ware JE, Kosinski M, Keller SD. *SF-12: how to score the SF-12 physical and mental health summary scales.* Boston, MA: The Health Institute, New England Medical Center, 1995.
56. Ware J Jr., Kosinski M, Keller SD. A 12-Item Short-Form Health Survey: construction of scales and preliminary tests of reliability and validity. *Med Care* 1996;34:220–233.
57. Kaplan RM, Sieber WJ, Ganiats TG. The quality of well-being scale: comparison of the interviewer-administered version with a self-administered questionnaire. *Psychology and Health* 1997;12:783–791.
58. Aaronson NK, Ahmedzai S, Bergman B, et al. The European Organization for Research and Treatment of Cancer QLQ-C30: a quality-of-life instrument for use in international clinical trials in oncology. *J Natl Cancer Inst* 1993;85: 365–376.
59. Groenvold M, Klee MC, Sprangers MA, et al. Validation of the EORTC QLQ-C30 quality of life questionnaire through combined qualitative and quantitative assessment of patient-observer agreement. *J Clin Epidemiol* 1997;50: 441–450.
60. Cella DF, Tulsky DS, Gray G, et al. The Functional Assessment of Cancer Therapy scale: development and validation of the general measure. *J Clin Oncol* 1993;11:570–579.
61. Schag CA, Heinrich RL. Development of a comprehensive quality of life measurement tool: CARES. *Oncology (Huntingt)* 1990;4:135–138.
62. Schag CA, Ganz PA, Heinrich RL. Cancer Rehabilitation Evaluation System—short form (CARES-SF). A cancer specific rehabilitation and quality of life instrument. *Cancer* 1991;68:1406–1413.
63. Curran D, Fossa S, Aaronson N, et al. Baseline quality of life of patients with advanced prostate cancer. European Organization for Research and Treatment of Cancer (EORTC), Genito-Urinary Tract Cancer Cooperative Group (GUT-CCG). *Eur J Cancer* 1997;33:1809–1814.

64. Schag CAC, Heinrich RL. *Cancer Rehabilitation Evaluation System (CARES) manual.* Los Angeles: CARES Consultants, 1988.
65. de Haes JC, van Knippenberg FC, Neijt JP. Measuring psychological and physical distress in cancer patients: structure and application of the Rotterdam Symptom Checklist. *Br J Cancer* 1990;62:1034–1038.
66. Litwin MS, Hays RD, Fink A, et al. The UCLA Prostate Cancer Index: development, reliability, and validity of a health-related quality of life measure. *Med Care* 1998;36:1002–1012.
67. Krongrad A, Perczek RE, Burke MA, et al. Reliability of Spanish translations of select urological quality of life instruments. *J Urol* 1997;158:493–496.
68. Esper P, Mo F, Chodak G, et al. Measuring quality of life in men with prostate cancer using the functional assessment of cancer therapy-prostate instrument. *Urology* 1997;50:920–928.
69. Shrader-Bogen CL, Kjellberg JL, McPherson CP, et al. Quality of life and treatment outcomes: prostate carcinoma patients' perspectives after prostatectomy or radiation therapy. *Cancer* 1997;79:1977–1986.
70. Helgason AR, Fredrikson M, Adolfsson J, et al. Decreased sexual capacity after external radiation therapy for prostate cancer impairs quality of life. *Int J Radiat Oncol Biol Phys* 1995;32:33–39.
71. Helgason AR, Adolfsson J, Dickman P, et al. Sexual desire, erection, orgasm and ejaculatory functions and their importance to elderly Swedish men: a population-based study. *Age Ageing* 1996;25:285–291.
72. Helgason AR, Adolfsson J, Dickman P, et al. Factors associated with waning sexual function among elderly men and prostate cancer patients. *J Urol* 1997;158:155–159.
73. Walsh PC, Donker PJ. Impotence following radical prostatectomy: insight into etiology and prevention. *J Urol* 1982;128:492–497.
74. Walsh PC. Radical prostatectomy, preservation of sexual function, cancer control. The controversy. *Urol Clin North Am* 1987;14:663–673.
75. Geary ES, Dendinger TE, Freiha FS, et al. Nerve sparing radical prostatectomy: a different view. *J Urol* 1995;154:145–149.
76. Goldstein I, Feldman MI, Deckers PJ, et al. Radiation-associated impotence. A clinical study of its mechanism. *JAMA* 1984;251:903–910.
77. Zelefsky MJ, Eid JF. Elucidating the etiology of erectile dysfunction after definitive therapy for prostatic cancer. *Int J Radiat Oncol Biol Phys* 1998;40:129–133.
78. Fowler FJ Jr., Barry MJ, Lu-Yao G, et al. Effect of radical prostatectomy for prostate cancer on patient quality of life: results from a Medicare survey. *Urology* 1995;45:1007–1013.
79. Talcott JA, Rieker P, Propert K, et al. Long-term complications of treatment for early prostate cancer: 2-year followup in a prospective, multi-institutional outcomes study (meeting abstract). *Proc Annu Meet Am Soc Clin Oncol* 1996;5:252.
80. Bolla M, Gonzalez D, Warde P, et al. Improved survival in patients with locally advanced prostate cancer treated with radiotherapy and goserelin. *N Engl J Med* 1997;337:295–300.
81. Clark JA, Rieker P, Propert KJ, et al. Changes in quality of life following treatment for early prostate cancer. *Urology* 1999;53:161–168.
82. Litwin MS, McGuigan KA, Shpall AI, et al. Recovery of health related quality of life in the year after radical prostatectomy: early experience. *J Urol* 1999;161:515–519.
83. Penson DF, Litwin MS, Lubeck DP, et al. Transitions in health-related quality of life during the first nine months after diagnosis with prostate cancer. *Prostate Cancer and Prostatic Diseases* 1998;1:134–143.
84. Perez MA, Meyerowitz BE, Lieskovsky G, et al. Quality of life and sexuality following radical prostatectomy in patients with prostate cancer who use or do not use erectile aids. *Urology* 1997;50:740–746.
85. Pedersen KV, Carlsson P, Rahmquist M, et al. Quality of life after radical retropubic prostatectomy for carcinoma of the prostate. *Eur Urol* 1993;24:7–11.
86. Lim AJ, Brandon AH, Fiedler J, et al. Quality of life: radical prostatectomy versus radiation therapy for prostate cancer [see comments]. *J Urol* 1995;154:1420–1425.
87. Braslis KG, Santa-Cruz C, Brickman AL, et al. Quality of life 12 months after radical prostatectomy. *Br J Urol* 1995;75:48–53.
88. Rossetti SR, Terrone C. Quality of life in prostate cancer patients. *Eur Urol* 1996;30[Suppl 1]:44–48.
89. Fowler FJ, Barry MJ, Lu-Yao GL, et al. Patient-reported complications and follow-up treatment after radical prostatectomy. *Urology* 1993;42:622–629.
90. Fowler FJ Jr., Barry MJ, Lu-Yao G, et al. Effect of radical prostatectomy for prostate cancer on patient quality of life: results from a Medicare survey. *Urology* 1995;45:1007–1013.
91. Herr HW. Quality of life of incontinent men after radical prostatectomy. *J Urol* 1994;151:652–654.
92. Fossa SD, Woehre H, Kurth KH, et al. Influence of urological morbidity on quality of life in patients with prostate cancer. *Eur Urol* 1997;31:3–8.
93. Jonler M, Madsen FA, Rhodes PR, et al. A prospective study of quantification of urinary incontinence and quality of life in patients undergoing radical retropubic prostatectomy. *Urology* 1996;48:433–440.
94. Borghede G, Sullivan M. Measurement of quality of life in localized prostatic cancer patients treated with radiotherapy. Development of a prostate cancer-specific module supplementing the EORTC QLQ-C30. *Qual Life Res* 1996;5:212–222.
95. Beard CJ, Propert KJ, Rieker PP, et al. Complications after treatment with external-beam irradiation in early-stage prostate cancer patients: a prospective multiinstitutional outcomes study. *J Clin Oncol* 1997;15:223–229.
96. Caffo O, Fellin G, Graffer U, et al. Assessment of quality of life after radical radiotherapy for prostate cancer. *Br J Urol* 1996;78:557–563.
97. Fransson P, Widmark A. Self-assessed sexual function after pelvic irradiation for prostate carcinoma. Comparison with an age-matched control group. *Cancer* 1996;78:1066–1078.
98. Roach M 3rd, Chinn DM, Holland J, et al. A pilot survey of sexual function and quality of life following 3D conformal radiotherapy for clinically localized prostate cancer. *Int J Radiat Oncol Biol Phys* 1996;35:869–874.
99. Widmark A, Fransson P, Tavelin B. Self-assessment questionnaire for evaluating urinary and intestinal late side

effects after pelvic radiotherapy in patients with prostate cancer compared with an age-matched control population. *Cancer* 1994;74:2520–2532.

100. Pilepich MV, Caplan R, Byhardt RW, et al. Phase III trial of androgen suppression using goserelin in unfavorable-prognosis carcinoma of the prostate treated with definitive radiotherapy: report of Radiation Therapy Oncology Group Protocol 85-31. *J Clin Oncol* 1997;15:1013–1021.
101. Pilepich MV, Krall JM, al-Sarraf M, et al. Androgen deprivation with radiation therapy compared with radiation therapy alone for locally advanced prostatic carcinoma: a randomized comparative trial of the Radiation Therapy Oncology Group. *Urology* 1995;45:616–623.
102. Dearnaley DP, Norman AR, Shahidi M. Re: Time to normalization of serum testosterone after 3-month luteinizing hormone-releasing hormone agonist administered in the neoadjuvant setting: implications for dosing schedule and neoadjuvant study consideration [letter]. *J Urol* 1999;162:170.
103. Immediate versus deferred treatment for advanced prostatic cancer: initial results of the Medical Research Council Trial. The Medical Research Council Prostate Cancer Working Party Investigators Group. *Br J Urol* 1997;79:235–246.

26A

MANAGEMENT CONSIDERATIONS OF URINARY INCONTINENCE AND ERECTILE DYSFUNCTION AFTER LOCAL THERAPY FOR PROSTATE CANCER

GRAEME SCOTT STEELE
MICHAEL O'LEARY

POSTPROSTATECTOMY INCONTINENCE

Urinary incontinence after radical prostatectomy (RP) can be a distressing complaint that can profoundly affect quality of life. Reported rates of postprostatectomy incontinence (PPI) vary greatly between centers, and, frequently, incontinence rates of less than 10% are quoted (1–5). However, several reports indicate significantly higher rates of PPI, ranging between 20% and 87% (6–9). In a recent survey of more than 1,000 patients who had undergone RP for clinically localized prostate cancer, the incidence of incontinence requiring protection was 33%, whereas the incidence of any PPI was 66% (10). Furthermore, a prospective study using strict urodynamic criteria to assess PPI reported continence rates of only 13% (11).

Although reasons for the wide variation in PPI rates have not been fully elucidated, a number of factors have been shown to play a role in this regard (12–16). PPI, as perceived by the patient, has been shown to correlate poorly with objective measurements of the degree of incontinence. In addition, physician-reported incontinence can be inconsistent with the degree of incontinence observed by the patient, although this is disputed by some (5,9,17). Furthermore, the inconsistent definition of PPI used by various investigators; differences in methodology used to evaluate patients, as well as differences in length of follow-up; and the subjective nature of postoperative evaluation also contribute to variation in the incidence of incontinence (18).

Despite this, PPI remains a perplexing clinical problem and a major contributor to deterioration in quality of life after therapy for localized prostate cancer. Moreover, PPI does not necessarily imply the presence of intrinsic urethral sphincter deficiency but is frequently due to other causes. Therefore, careful patient workup is a *sine qua non* if patient expectations are to be met and good clinical outcomes achieved.

Mechanisms of Continence

Under normal conditions, urinary continence in men is maintained by the proximal urethral sphincter, which includes the bladder neck and prostatic urethra up to the verumontanum (19). When the proximal sphincter mechanism is compromised—for example, after transurethral resection of the prostate—continence is maintained by the distal urethral sphincter (DUS), which extends from the verumontanum to the membranous bulbar urethral junction (20). At the time of RP, the proximal urethral sphincter, as well as the proximal third (verumontanum to membranous urethra) of the DUS, is excised.

Although PPI is usually present in the immediate postoperative period, the majority of patients reports significant improvement in urinary continence within 3 months to 1 year after RP. However, factors responsible for restoration of continence are unclear. Indeed, it is surprising that the majority of patients does achieve a degree of continence, considering the extensive extirpation of the urinary sphincter at the time of surgery.

Evidence suggests that urethral smooth muscle and elastic tissue in the distal third of the DUS are primarily responsible for passive continence post RP (21). It is important to note that significant PPI can occur in the presence of an intact striated sphincter, as evidenced by the ability of severely incontinent patients post RP to interrupt their urinary flow voluntarily. Functional integrity of the fibroelastic smooth muscle component of the membranous urethra (intrinsic component of distal sphincter), therefore, appears to play a crucial role in the continence mechanism post RP. Cadaveric dissections, radiologic assessment, and urodynamic measurements have revealed considerable individual variation in membranous urethral length that is unrelated to age, height, or body weight (22,23). These findings possibly account for the fact that there is marked individual variability in time to continence after RP.

Mechanisms of Postprostatectomy Incontinence

Urodynamic evaluation of post RP patients has demonstrated several parameters that play a role in continence (24–27). These include a longer mean functional profile length and a higher maximal resting urethral closure pressure (12). In addition, tubularization above the level of the external sphincter was noted on voiding cystourethrography in continent patients and was found to be absent in incontinent patients. The length of this tubularization was noted to range from 0.75 to 1.50 cm (12). Several other studies have alluded to a critical functional urethral length that is ultimately responsible for mucosal coaptation, resulting in a mucosal seal that leads to post-RP continence (16,28). Factors such as urethral scarring and shortening of this critical urethral segment are synonymous with PPI by preventing adequate mucosal coaptation over the required length of urethra.

PPI has two important mechanisms. First, intrinsic sphincter deficiency (ISD), due to reduction in length of the distal sphincter mechanism; fibrosis and scarring of the intrinsic sphincter, alterations in nerve or blood supply, or both, to the intrinsic sphincter; and, finally, mucosal changes within the intrinsic sphincter may all lead to loss of mucosal coaptation and, hence, absence of a mucosal water seal. ISD alone classically manifests as stress urinary incontinence (SUI) and, in its severest form, gravitational incontinence. ISD can be simply diagnosed by measuring intraabdominal pressure using a rectal catheter during a Valsalva maneuver. This pressure, at which the patient leaks, is known as the *abdominal leak point pressure* (ALPP), and, in general, low ALPPs are synonymous with poor intrinsic function.

Second, changes in detrusor muscle function can be the sole cause of PPI or contribute to PPI caused by ISD. Detrusor instability (DI) and reduced compliance have been shown to occur *de novo* after RP. In fact, DI reportedly is the sole cause of PPI in 25% to 50% of patients. Significant reduction in bladder compliance has also been reported after RP (15). The pathogenesis of this finding is presumed to be due to partial bladder denervation that may occur as a result of dissection around the seminal vesicles and bladder base at the time of RP. We found significant reduction in mean compliance (pre-RP compliance, 36 cm H_2O; post-RP compliance, 26 cm H_2O) after RP. In addition, we showed that maximal voiding pressure was significantly higher in continent patients post RP, suggesting outlet (anastomotic) obstruction in continent patients. It is therefore possible that a degree of bladder outlet obstruction (BOO) may augment the function of the DUS by preventing radial forces at the bladder neck from taking effect during filling and Valsalva maneuvers and, therefore, from compromising the coaptation mechanism that normally creates a water seal and thus ensures continence (29).

Therefore, the pathophysiology of PPI is multifactorial and includes bladder dysfunction and sphincter dysfunction, either alone or in combination. In addition, overflow incontinence has been reported to account for a small percentage of PPI (30). Controversy, however, abounds as to the precise mechanism of urinary continence post RP. A recent report described distal sphincter sensory fibers originating from the dorsal nerve of the penis that may constitute the afferent pathway for normal DUS function. The close proximity of these nerves to the prostatic apex, therefore, may result in injury during RP (31). However, several reports have indicated poor correlation between the number of neurovascular bundles spared during RP and postprostatectomy continence rates (2,31).

Continence-Preserving Techniques

Despite reports indicating that fewer than 10% of patients who undergo RP experience PPI, investigators have described modifications to the anatomic RP in the hope of achieving better urinary continence post RP (32–36). In this regard, preservation of one or both neurovascular bundles has not been shown to have a significant influence on PPI (3). In addition, bladder neck sparing, as well as bladder neck tubularization techniques, has been reported to produce shorter times to continence after RP; however, the long-term outcome in PPI was no different when compared to patients in whom bladder neck tubularization or preservation was not performed (32–35). Puboprostatic ligament preservation has also been shown to improve the rapidity with which continence returns post RP, but the overall continence rates when compared to patients in whom the puboprostatic ligaments were not preserved was no different (36). Furthermore, rates of PPI have been reported to be similar in patients undergoing retropubic versus perineal prostatectomy (37–39). PPI, however, has been reported to be higher in patients who have undergone RP after radiation therapy for prostate cancer, which is thought to induce sphincteric or neurologic injury in addition to adversely affecting bladder compliance (40).

Continence Recovery Period Postradical Prostatectomy

In general, by the first postoperative month, 20% of patients will have achieved urinary continence; thereafter, 50% of patients are continent by 3 months; 66% by 6 months; and, by 12 months, between 70% and 90% of patients are continent. In the second postoperative year, a further 5% of patients reportedly regain continence. Therefore, in general, surgical intervention is delayed for at least 6 to 9 months, depending on severity of symptoms during the first postoperative year. The reason for this prolonged recovery period in some patients is not fully apparent; suffice it to say that once the mechanism of urinary continence after RP is understood, then reasons for longer recovery periods in some patients might be explained.

Evaluation of Postprostatectomy Incontinence

The multifactorial nature of PPI makes it essential to perform urodynamic studies in patients with bothersome incontinence after RP, especially in those patients in whom symptoms persist beyond 6 to 12 months. In view of the fact that lower urinary tract symptoms are nonspecific, urodynamic studies are the only means to differentiate various causes of PPI. It is important to rule out BOO as well as reduced compliance, especially in those patients who are being considered for surgical intervention.

The treatment of PPI is dependent on the clinical and urodynamic findings, as well as on patient wishes and expectations. Therapy may be pharmacologic, behavioral, or surgical, depending on the cause of PPI, as well as on the patient's perception of his symptoms. Although some patients may hardly be bothered by mild SUI and the need to wear incontinence pads, other patients may be extremely bothered by even the slightest degree of urinary incontinence.

Clinical History and Physical Examination

The evaluation of PPI should include a full history and physical examination, paying particular attention to degree of bother, presence of irritative voiding symptoms, medication history, past medical and surgical history, as well as a full neurologic history. Nighttime and daytime incontinence suggest the possibility of an overactive bladder but may also be due to BOO or detrusor underactivity's resulting in overflow incontinence.

Preexisting risk factors for PPI should be ascertained, such as pelvic external beam radiotherapy, transurethral prostatectomy, DI, previous pelvic surgery, lumbar spondylosis, urethral stricture disease, diabetes mellitus, and preexisting neurologic diseases (30). A prospective study reported that 27% of patients who complained of PPI were incontinent before RP (41). Furthermore, the natural history and duration of PPI need to be carefully documented, keeping in mind that although PPI resolves in the majority of patients by one year, incontinence may take up to 2 years to improve in some patients.

Cystoscopy

A diagnosis based on history and examination needs objective confirmation, usually with a urethroscopy and urodynamic study. Anastomotic strictures, foreign bodies, and retained sutures can all be confirmed at the time of urethroscopy. In addition, urethroscopy is useful with respect to determining whether a patient is an appropriate candidate for collagen therapy (42).

Urodynamic Testing

The role of urodynamic evaluation is to distinguish between detrusor and sphincteric causes of incontinence (43). During the cystometry phase of the urodynamic study, compliance and cystometric capacity are measured, and DI may be noted. During the voiding phase of the study, detrusor pressures are measured, which might point to the presence of BOO or detrusor muscle failure. When detrusor and urethral pressures are simultaneously measured, the exact site of the obstruction can be recorded (44). Urethral pressure profilometry records resting urethral pressure, as well as maximum voluntary contraction pressure at the external sphincter during pelvic floor contraction and functional urethral length. Furthermore, the clinical sign of urinary incontinence with Valsalva maneuver (SUI) can be elicited in the urodynamics laboratory, and, at the same time, ALPP can be measured to gauge the severity of ISD in patients with SUI (45).

Treatment of Postprostatectomy Incontinence

Once the etiology of PPI has been defined, appropriate therapy can be entertained. Two general principles should be borne in mind. First, noninvasive therapy should generally be attempted initially, during which time the physician will have an opportunity to establish a relationship with the patient and to gauge severity and natural history of the patient's incontinence. Second, although in most patients continence post RP is achieved within 1 year, approximately 5% of patients fail to achieve continence by 1 year but do improve in the second year. Therefore, if a patient has the impression that his continence is improving, it is prudent to hold off with invasive procedures until such time as the condition stabilizes. However, very severe stress and gravitational incontinence that have been present for 12 months post RP are hardly likely to show significant improvement during the second postoperative year.

Behavioral Therapy

Behavioral biofeedback therapy is appropriate in patients with sphincteric incontinence and in patients with overactive bladders (46). In this regard, timed voiding, fluid restriction, and pelvic floor exercises may improve symptoms and at the same time give the patient the moral support he needs during this difficult aspect of the recovery period.

Pharmacologic Therapy

Pharmacologic agents can be used in combination with behavioral therapy and are appropriate in patients with symptoms of overactive bladders. Anticholinergic agents are the mainstays of drug therapy for overactive bladders but require at least 6 to 8 weeks of therapy to take effect. Some patients with overactive bladders benefit from selective α-receptor blocker therapy, especially in those patients with a degree of BOO that has been shown to increase the density of α-adrenoreceptors (47).

Electrostimulation

Electrostimulation, which theoretically improves tonic activity and strength of pelvic floor muscles, has been extensively investigated in incontinent patients. Unfortunately, the results have been disappointing and the technique is rarely used today (48).

Urethral Bulking Agents

After conservative measures fail to produce significant improvement in PPI, more invasive measures should be recommended. The role of bulking agents (collagen, fat, and polytetrafluoroethylene paste) is to increase resistance to urine outflow by enhancing the urethral mucosal seal in the region of the intrinsic sphincter.

Bovine glutaraldehyde cross-linked collagen, a biocompatible substance that does not cause a foreign body reaction, has recently been introduced as an injectable bulking agent (42,49,50). Collagen can be injected in retrograde or antegrade fashion, and reports indicate that between 20% and 70% of patients are either dry or significantly improved (42,49,51). However, patients require a mean of 4.4 injections to achieve acceptable continence at considerable cost. Moreover, those patients with anastomotic strictures requiring incision and those patients who have undergone external beam radiotherapy respond poorly to collagen therapy.

There appear to be few side effects with collagen therapy, and at present there are no reports of glutaraldehyde cross-linked collagen particles migrating. Collagen injection into the external sphincter, however, can cause extreme discomfort. The incidence of hypersensitivity is 2% to 5%; therefore, all patients must undergo hypersensitivity testing with a prepackaged syringe containing 0.1 mL of collagen. There are, however, isolated case reports of patients experiencing delayed hypersensitivity to collagen (52,53). Although comparable continence rates with polytetrafluoroethylene (Teflon) paste have been reported, migration of polytetrafluoroethylene particles has been described, and for this reason polytetrafluoroethylene is no longer widely used (54). An important consideration with respect to collagen use is cost, especially in view of the fact that most patients require three to four injections. The estimated Medicare cost of each outpatient (general or spinal anesthesia) injection of collagen is $4,300. Therefore, collagen potentially has a similar cost to artificial genitourinary sphincter placement (55).

Artificial Genitourinary Sphincter

Prosthetic devices for the treatment of PPI have been in existence for more than three decades. The earliest devices attempted to restore continence by passive bulbourethral compression, but this pressure was difficult to control, and these devices encountered problems with persistent incontinence due to inadequate pressure and urethral erosion to excessive pressure (56). Scott implanted the first reliable artificial urinary sphincter in the early 1970s (57). This device (AS 700 series), was able to deliver a constant physiologic pressure to compress the urethra and was also designed to open, allowing for bladder emptying. However, constant cuff pressure during the postoperative healing period has led to an unacceptably high rate of cuff erosion. Therefore, the device was improved by incorporating a deactivation mechanism whereby the cuff was activated 6 to 8 weeks after implantation. This device, the American Medical Systems-800 Artificial Genitourinary Sphincter (AGUS), was associated with a significantly lower complication rate and has been in use since 1982 (58).

Candidates for AGUS placement require careful urodynamic evaluation to determine their suitability for this procedure. Cystometry to measure cystometric capacity and compliance and to exclude DI and voiding studies to exclude significant BOO should be performed (59). The ideal candidate for an AGUS is a patient with bladder compliance higher than 25 mL per cm H_2O, cystometric capacity greater than 200 mL, and the absence of DI. Patients with DI, however, can be treated with an anticholinergic agent and then reevaluated to gauge their response. On rare occasions, bladder augmentation may be contemplated to improve cystometric capacity and compliance before sphincter placement; however, these patients usually have experienced significant lower urinary tract symptoms before RP and may represent a subset of patients who are poor candidates for RP in the first place.

Anastomotic strictures that require incision should remain open for at least 3 months before implantation and should easily accept passage of at least a 14-French catheter.

Patients with skin excoriation or severe dermatitis should have an indwelling Foley catheter for several weeks to reduce the bacterial count on the skin and to allow the skin to heal. Furthermore, patients who lack basic cognitive skills or manual dexterity are also poor candidates for artificial sphincter placement.

Published reports indicate that 90% of patients are significantly improved, whereas 83% of patients are reported to be clinically dry (59). However, fully one-third of patients requires surgical revisions for problems related to cuff compression, tubing kinks, cuff links, and other malfunctions. We believe that in view of the effectiveness of the AGUS, the device is relatively underused for PPI and that far more patients could and should benefit from this treatment.

Anastomotic Strictures Postradical Prostatectomy

The combination of an anastomotic stricture and SUI post RP requires careful and judicious management. Our study highlighted a relatively high incidence of outlet obstruction due to anastomotic strictures that may play a significant role in augmenting continence. Therefore, the need to manage anastomotic strictures in patients with PPI judiciously cannot be overemphasized because of the possibility of exacerbating the patient's symptoms. In this regard, the recommended treatment is gentle urethral dilatation in a controlled environment and then possibly proceeding to clean intermittent catheterization if the anastomotic stricture recurs within a relatively short time period.

Patients with very severe anastomotic strictures, usually a complication of anastomotic distraction by pelvic hematoma formation, may be candidates for wide stricture incision and artificial sphincter placement (60). In this subset of patients, the intrinsic sphincter tends to be replaced by fibrous tissue, resulting in significant and irreversible ISD.

Male Slings

Based on the success of vesicovaginal sling procedures in women for SUI, sling procedures have been carried out in male patients with PPI (61). Schaeffer and associates reported their results recently with a male bulbourethral sling that uses bolsters placed beneath the bulbar urethra to form a sling (62). In a series of 64 patients, they reported that 36 patients (56%) were dry, whereas five patients (8%) were significantly improved. Urodynamic studies were performed postoperatively to determine whether these patients had urodynamic features of bladder outflow obstruction. Although Valsalva LPP was significantly increased, there was no evidence of obstruction when preoperative pressure flow studies were compared to postoperative studies (63). Clearly, more investigation of male slings is required before these procedures become widely practiced.

Other Treatment Options

Finally, other treatment options, such as the condom catheter, penile compression devices (Cunningham clamp), and incontinence briefs, may prove to be appropriate in those patients in whom all else fails, as well as in patients in whom more invasive options are precluded by co-morbidities. Suffice it to say that in this latter category of patients, the penile clamp may have devastating sequelae if not managed appropriately.

POSTRADIOTHERAPY URINARY INCONTINENCE

Apart from disease progression with time, the most feared long-term complication of RP is urinary incontinence. Therefore, an appealing aspect of brachytherapy, apart from the minimally invasive nature of this technique, is the low rate of significant side effects. McCammon and associates compared the quality of life among patients with prostate cancer treated with external beam radiotherapy or RP. Although only 32% of the RP patients claimed no incontinence at all and 24% of patients used pads after surgery, 71% of patients who underwent radiotherapy reported no incontinence, and only 9% of this group required pads (64). Published studies report an incidence of postbrachytherapy incontinence of 0.0% to 12.9% (65,66). Ragde and associates reported a 5% risk of urinary incontinence in a study with a 7-year follow-up (67). More recently, Benoit and associates reported a 6.6% incidence of incontinence in a study involving all men in the Medicare population who underwent brachytherapy in 1991. In this study, only four patients (0.2%) underwent placement of an AGUS for urinary incontinence, and a further five patients underwent construction of a colostomy for prostatic rectal fistula (68).

Despite potentially serious side effects of radiotherapy, several reports indicate that salvage and adjuvant external beam radiotherapy are fairly well tolerated. In general, 10% to 15% of patients experience short-term complications of increased bowel and bladder irritability, but fewer than 5% of patients experience long-term morbidity related to lower urinary tract function (69,70). Furthermore, prospective long-term studies have found that salvage and adjuvant external beam radiotherapy do not significantly influence urinary incontinence (70). Diabetes mellitus, however, has been shown to be an independent predictor for late genitourinary and gastrointestinal complications after external beam radiotherapy. Given the high frequency of diabetes in the elderly prostate cancer population, physicians may consider treatment modifications for this group of patients (71).

Persistent urinary symptoms after radiotherapy (external beam and brachytherapy) for prostate cancer, although uncommon, present a therapeutic challenge. Reduced cystometric capacity and compliance, as well as outlet changes such as bladder neck stenosis and urethral stricture, should be borne in mind when managing this subset of patients. Urge urinary incontinence is generally managed by a combination of behavioral and anticholinergic therapy but unfortunately may prove to be resistant to this combination. Furthermore, persistent obstructive symptoms postbrachytherapy may require outlet surgery in the form of a bladder neck incision or transurethral resection of the prostate, which is associated with a significant reported incidence of stress and gravitational incontinence (72).

In addition, irradiated surgical fields present unique challenges with respect to tissue healing and infection after prosthetic surgery. Radiotherapy is known to increase the likelihood of nonmechanical complications, especially infection and cuff erosion. Extreme care must therefore be taken so that avoidable iatrogenic factors, such as improper urethral catheterization and endoscopic manipulation with an activated American Medical Systems-800 device *in situ*, are not the cause of failure (73).

CONCLUSION

The recent dramatic increase in the incidence of patients undergoing RP and radiation therapy for prostate cancer has resulted in increasing numbers of patients with morbidity related to voiding dysfunction. Although many patients regain their continence with time, a subset of patients will have persistent problems and will continue to challenge the therapeutic armamentarium of the urologic surgeon. Appropriate therapy can only be offered once the nature of the urinary symptom has been fully elucidated, which means that urodynamic studies are necessary in a significant subset of patients. Unfortunately, at present there is no therapy that is universally effective. In the future, the causes of urinary incontinence after RP and radiation therapy need to be better defined, and then it is hoped that we will be able to avoid this devastating complication.

ERECTILE DYSFUNCTION

RP rates have increased dramatically since 1989, particularly in younger men. This trend is due largely to increased detection. Perhaps because men seeking treatment are younger, there has been an increased interest in therapies that preserve sexual function. Nerve-sparing RP, first described in 1983, has become the standard surgical therapeutic modality for clinically localized prostate cancer (74).

Neurovascular bundle preservation has been associated with early return of sexual function in some men. Initial reports indicated that nerve-sparing surgery resulted in preservation of erectile function in more than 80% of patients (75). More recently, however, preservation of erectile function has been reported to be less than 20% after RP (10). A multicenter patient self-reporting questionnaire on impotence, incontinence, and stricture formation involving 1,069 patients found that the overall incidence of erectile dysfunction post RP was 88% (10). Similarly, Zimmern and associates reported that although 42% of patients were potent post RP, approximately half of these patients categorized their erections as weak or unpredictable (76). Stamey and associates reported that when patients were questioned about erectile function by individuals other than their physicians, potency was preserved in 32% of patients when both nerves were spared, whereas unilateral preservation of nerves resulted in 13% of patients reporting post-RP erections. If neither right nor left neurovascular bundle was spared, only 1% of patients reported being potent postoperatively (77). Furthermore, only one-half of men engaged in sexual activity more frequently than once a month after RP. Smaller series from community centers have also reported less favorable outcomes with regard to preservation of sexual function (78).

Patient self report in retrospective analyses has generally demonstrated lower rates of preservation of sexual function than in physician-generated analyses of erectile dysfunction post RP. Fowler and associates reported on more than 1,000 Medicare patients in a national sample who responded to queries about erections (79). Approximately 40% reported partial or full erections postoperatively. Because these were Medicare patients, this was an older population who might be expected to be less active sexually. Nevertheless, loss of sexual function has been found to be not particularly bothersome to the majority of patients post RP, the majority of whom indicates feeling positive about the results of surgery (81%) and 89% of whom indicate that they would choose surgical treatment again (10,80).

In addition to preservation of neurovascular bundles, other factors probably play important roles with respect to potency after RP. Quinlan and associates reported postoperative potency in 68% of men undergoing nerve-sparing RP and found that factors that correlated with early return of sexual function were age, and clinical and pathologic stage (81). Of men age 50 years and younger, 90% had return of erections whether nerves were spared unilaterally or bilaterally (81). Catalona and associates supported this concept in their report of a large cohort of patients who underwent RP for clinically localized prostate cancer (82). In this series of 1,870 men, they reported recovery of erections in 68% of men undergoing bilateral nerve-sparing procedures and 47% of men with unilateral nerve-sparing procedures. In addition, they reported that better post-RP potency results were achieved in younger men with organ-confined disease. Potency was preserved in 90% of men who underwent bilateral or unilateral nerve-sparing surgery treated in the 40s, 80% in their 50s, 60% in their 60s, and 47% in their 70s (82). Another reason younger men may do better in preserving sexual function postoperatively is that they may often have better prognostic features and less advanced cancers, allowing better preservation of the neurovascular bundles.

Talcott and associates, however, reported no apparent benefit of unilateral preservation of cavernosal nerves over non-nerve-sparing surgery (83). They evaluated a cohort of 279 men to assess complications of therapy for early prostate cancer. In this prospective study, patients completed self-reporting questionnaires regarding quality of life before therapy and at 3 and 12 months afterward. Erectile dysfunction that was present in one-third of men pretreatment was nearly universal at 3 months after surgery, and, at 12 months after surgery in this study, most men reported inadequate erections.

The mechanism of erectile dysfunction after RP is generally believed to be neurologic injury. However, Aboseif and associates have shown that 40% of men have arteriogenic impotence after RP, thus indicating that injury to cavernosal nerves is not the only cause of erectile dysfunction post RP (84). It has been postulated that injury to the accessory pudendal artery at the time of RP may be a cause of erectile dysfunction. This artery was carefully identified and preserved in 79% of 33 patients who underwent RP for clinically localized prostate cancer. Potency rates were found to be similar in men with or without preservation of accessory arteries; routine preservation was therefore deemed not to be productive because of associated bleeding encountered at the time of attempted preservation of this artery (85).

In general, the literature indicates that less than half of men undergoing nerve-sparing RP will be satisfied with their erections postoperatively, which translates into significant numbers of patients who are potentially candidates for therapy of erectile dysfunction after RP.

Treatment Options

Even with nerve-sparing techniques, recovery of erections may take weeks to months and, in certain cases, several years. Therefore, erectile dysfunction therapy should be offered to patients so that they may resume sexual activity in the interim. In general, these patients can be successfully treated with either sildenafil, penile injection therapy with vasoactive medication, or the vacuum erection device (VED). The penile prosthesis, on the other hand, is generally reserved for those patients who fail more conservative measures, are impotent before RP and have already failed conservative measures, as well as for those patients who prefer a prosthesis over sildenafil, injection therapy, and the VED.

One hypothesis holds that prolonged intervals of diminished penile cavernosal blood flow can result in irreversible hypoxic damage. Montorsi and associates treated post-radical nerve-sparing prostatectomy patients with three weekly intracavernosal injections of prostaglandin under the assumption that pharmacotherapy would increase cavernous oxygenation, avoiding the hypoxia-induced damage related to the early postoperative absence of spontaneous erections (86). Normal erection recovery rate was 67% in the treated group versus 20% in controls. Regardless of whether intracavernous prostaglandin is given early or late to men after RP, it is highly efficacious, even when the non-nerve-sparing approach is used.

Prostaglandin has also been delivered transurethrally. Costabile and associates studied post-RP patients with erectile dysfunction and determined that 40% achieved erections sufficient for intercourse with intraurethral prostaglandin E_1 (PGE_1) (87). Many of these patients also reported urethral pain or burning that may be due to postoperative sensitization of corporal nerves or increased retention of PGE_1 as a result of dorsal venous ligation during surgery.

Oral therapy (sildenafil) for erectile dysfunction has become first-line therapy for most patients. Although overall efficacy has been reported in the range of 70% in patients with ED of all causes, Zippe and associates reported that in 80% of men, postbilateral nerve-sparing RP had a positive response (88). However, this study only included 15 patients. No patients who had undergone non-nerve-sparing surgery responded to sildenafil. A recent study by Zippe and associates showed that the presence or absence of the neurovascular bundles influenced the ability to achieve vaginal intercourse. In the patients who had undergone bilateral nerve-sparing RP, 71.7% (38 of 53) responded to sildenafil, and, among those with unilateral nerve-sparing RP, 50% (6 of 12) responded to sildenafil, whereas only 15.4% (4 of 26) who underwent non-nerve-sparing RP responded. This study also showed that the response to sildenafil was not related to the interval between surgery and initiation of drug therapy but was rather related to dose (89). Furthermore, 71% of patients required titration of the dose of sildenafil from 50 to 100 mg for a positive response (89). In general, the majority of patients with good erectile function before RP who became dysfunctional after RP experienced a good response to sildenafil, especially those patients who underwent bilateral nerve-sparing surgery.

Penile injection therapy is the most effective therapy for neurogenic impotence and least effective for vasculogenic impotence, and, therefore, the majority of patients with adequate erectile function before RP responds well to injection therapy. This mode of therapy is preferred by younger patients over the VED and in general by patients who experience erectile dysfunction after RP.

Khoudary and associates recently reported total sexual rehabilitation in men undergoing RP for prostate cancer (90). Simultaneous placement of a penile prosthesis during RP was reported in 50 patients and found to result in early return to sexual function without apparent increase in morbidity. However, with the introduction of sildenafil, simultaneous placement of penile prosthesis at the time of RP is likely to be received with less enthusiasm by patients and physicians alike.

Erectile Dysfunction after Radiation Therapy

Radiation therapy, even with new conformal techniques, has been associated with impairment of erectile function. In general, external beam radiotherapy to the pelvis is associated with erectile dysfunction in 30% to 60% of patients.

Classically, erectile dysfunction begins months after completion of therapy. Radiation injury to the corporal epithelium and trabecular smooth muscle results in venous leak, and arterial inflow appears to be unchanged (91,92).

Turner and associates prospectively evaluated 290 men who were treated with radiation for localized prostate cancer. At 12 months after treatment, 62% were still able to obtain satisfactory erections. This percentage deteriorated to 41% at 24 months (93). Fowler and associates reported that 23% of radiated men younger than age 70 years complained of erectile dysfunction versus 56% who underwent surgery (94). Litwin evaluated 438 men who underwent radiation or surgery and found that sexual function improved over time in both groups during the first year but deteriorated in the radiation group during the second year, while continuing to improve in the surgery group (95).

Because of the association of erectile dysfunction with external beam radiotherapy, this modality should be discouraged for use in benign conditions of the pelvis.

Therapy in patients with erectile dysfunction after radiation therapy is challenging because of the fact that tissue healing may be impaired and patients may be prone to infection. Furthermore, corporal fibrosis may result in inadequate responses to injection therapy.

CONCLUSION

Sildenafil has dramatically changed the way erectile dysfunction post RP is managed. For those patients who fail with sildenafil, other options are available. Further progress in pharmacotherapy is anticipated, which may result in these other options' being used less frequently in the future.

REFERENCES

1. Goluboff ET, Saidi JA, Mazer S, et al. Urinary continence after radical prostatectomy: the Columbia experience. *J Urol* 1998;159:1276–1280.
2. Catalona WJ, Basler JW. Return of erections and urinary continence following nerve sparing radical retropubic prostatectomy. *J Urol* 1993;150:905–907.
3. Steiner MS, Morton RA, Walsh PC. Impact of anatomical radical prostatectomy on urinary continence. *J Urol* 1991; 145:512–515.
4. Feneley MR, Walsh PC. Incontinence after radical prostatectomy. *Lancet* 1999;353:2091–2092.
5. Walsh PC, Marschke P, Ricker DD, et al. Potency and continence following anatomic radical prostatectomy: patient versus physician outcomes. *J Urol* 1999;16:387.
6. Gray M, Petroni GR, Theodorescu D. Urinary function after radical prostatectomy: a comparison of the retropubic and perineal approaches. *Urology* 1999;53:881–890.
7. Fowler FL, Barry MJ, Lu-Yao G, et al. Effect of radical prostatectomy for prostate cancer on quality of life: results from a Medicare survey. *Urology* 1995;45:1007–1013.
8. Hautman RE, Sauter TW, Wenderoth UK. Radical retropubic prostatectomy: morbidity and urinary continence in 418 consecutive cases. *Urology* 1994;43[Suppl]:47–51.
9. Jonler M, Madsen FA, Rhodes PR, et al. A prospective study of quantification of urinary incontinence and quality of life in patients undergoing radical retropubic prostatectomy. *Urology* 1996;48:433–440.
10. Kao TC, Cruess DF, Garner D, et al. Multicenter patient self-reporting questionnaire on impotence, incontinence and stricture after radical prostatectomy. *J Urol* 2000;163: 858–864.
11. Rudy DC, Woodside JR, Crawford ED. Urodynamic evaluation of incontinence in patients undergoing modified Campbell radical retropubic prostatectomy: a prospective study. *J Urol* 1984;132:708–712.
12. Presti JC Jr., Schmidt RA, Narayan PA, et al. Pathophysiology or urinary incontinence after radical prostatectomy. *J Urol* 1990;143:975–978.
13. Abdel-Azim MS, Sullivan MP, Yalla SV. Urodynamics of post-radical prostatectomy incontinence. *J Urol* 1990;143: 359A.
14. Hutch JA, Fishe R. Continence after radical prostatectomy. *Br J Urol* 1968;40:62–67.
15. Hellstrom P, Lukkarien O, Konturri I. Urodynamics in radical retropubic prostatectomy. *Scand J Urol Nephrol* 1989; 23:21–24.
16. Hauri D. Urinary continence after radical prostatectomy: the urodynamic proof of an anatomical hypothesis. *Urol Int* 1977;32:149–160.
17. Talcott JA, Rieker P, Clark JA, et al. Patient-reported symptoms after primary therapy for early prostate cancer: results of a prospective cohort study. *J Clin Oncol* 1998;16:275–283.
18. Sullivan MP, Hutcheson JC, Yalla SV. Management of incontinence following radical prostatectomy. *J Urol* 1995.
19. Burnett AL, Mostwin JL. In situ anatomical study of the male urethral sphincteric complex: relevance to continence preservation following major pelvic surgery. *J Urol* 1998; 160:1301–1306.
20. Turner Warwick R. The sphincter mechanisms: their relation to prostatic enlargement and its treatment. In: Hinman F, ed. *Benign prostatic hypertrophy*. New York: Springer-Verlag, 1983:809–828.
21. Yalla SV, Dibenedetto M, Fam BA, et al. Striated sphincter participation in distal passive urinary continence mechanisms: studies in male subjects deprived of proximal sphincter mechanism. *J Urol* 1979;122:655–660.
22. Myers RP. Male urethral sphincter anatomy and radical prostatectomy. *Urol Clin North Am* 1991;18:211–227.
23. Shaw PJ, Abrams PH, Feneley RCL, et al. The influence of prostatic anatomy and the differing effects of prostatectomy according to the surgical approach. *Br J Urol* 1979;51:549–555.
24. Kleinhans B, Gerharz E, Melekos M, et al. Changes of urodynamic findings after radical retropubic prostatectomy. *Eur Urol* 1999;35:217–221.
25. Ficazzola MA, Nitti VW. The etiology of post-radical prostatectomy incontinence and correlation of symptoms with urodynamic findings. *J Urol* 1998;160:1317–1320.
26. Winters JC, Appell RA, Rackley RR. Urodynamic findings in postprostatectomy incontinence. *Neurourol Urodyn* 1998; 17:493–498.

27. O'Donnell RD, Finn BF. Continence following nerve sparing radical prostatectomy. *J Urol* 1989;142:1227–1228.
28. Leach GE, Yun SK. Post prostatectomy incontinence: part I and II. *Neurourol Urodyn* 1992;11:91.
29. Steele GS, Sullivan MP, Yalla SV. Changes in detrusor contractility, detrusor compliance and outlet properties after radical prostatectomy. *J Urol* 1998;159:461A.
30. Geary SA, Dendinger TE, Freiha FS, et al. Incontinence and vesical neck strictures following radical retropubic prostatectomy. *Urology* 1995;45:1000–1006.
31. Narayan P, Konety B, Aslam K, et al. Neuroanatomy of the external urethral sphincter: implications for urinary continence preservation during radical prostate surgery. *J Urol* 1995;153:337–341.
32. Gomez CA, Soloway MS, Civantos F, et al. Bladder neck preservation and its impact on positive surgical margins during radical prostatectomy. *Urology* 1993;42:689–693.
33. Lowe BA. Comparison of bladder neck preservation to bladder neck resection in maintaining post-prostatectomy urinary continence. *Urology* 1996;48:889–893.
34. Klein EA, Light MR. The impact of bladder neck preservation during radical prostatectomy on continence and cancer control. *J Urol* 1995;153:383A.
35. Seaman EK, Benson MC. Improved continence with tubularized bladder neck reconstruction following radical retropubic prostatectomy. *Urology* 1996;47:532–535.
36. Poore RE, McCullough DL, Jarow JP. Puboprostatic ligament sparing improves urinary continence after radical retropubic prostatectomy. *Urology* 1998;51:67–72.
37. Bales GT, Chodak GW, Palmer JS, et al. Morbidity of radical perineal prostatectomy. *J Urol* 1995;153:253A.
38. Krauss DJ, Paletsky LH, Lilien OM. Urodynamics of post radical perineal prostatectomy. *J Urol* 1980;124:263–265.
39. Gray M, Petroni GR, Theodorescu D. Urinary function after radical prostatectomy: a comparison of the retropubic and perineal approaches. *Urology* 1999;53:881–890.
40. Rogers E, Ohori M, Kassabian VS, et al. Salvage radical prostatectomy: outcome measured by serum prostate specific antigen levels. *J Urol* 1995;153:104–110.
41. Foote J, Yun S, Leach GE. Postprostatectomy incontinence. Pathophysiology, evaluation, and management. *Urol Clin North Am* 1991;18:229–241.
42. Cespedes RD, Leng WW, McGuire EJ. Collagen injection therapy for postprostatectomy incontinence. *Urology* 1999; 54:597–602.
43. Gudziak MR, McGuire EJ, Gormley EA. Urodynamic assessment of urethral sphincter function in post-prostatectomy incontinence. *J Urol* 1996;156:1131–1134.
44. Yalla SV, Sharma GV, Barsamian EM. Micturitional static urethral pressure profile: a method of recording urethral pressure profile during voiding and the implications. *J Urol* 1980;124:649–656.
45. McGuire EJ, Cespedes RD, O'Connell HE. Leak-point pressures. *Urol Clin North Am* 1996;23:253–262.
46. O'Donnell PD, Doyle R. Biofeedback therapy technique for treatment of urinary incontinence. *Urology* 1991;37: 432–436.
47. Restorick JM, Mundy AR. The density of cholinergic and alpha and beta adrenergic receptors in the normal and hyper-reflexic human detrusor. *Br J Urol* 1989;63:32–35.
48. Tanagho EA, Schmidt RA. Electrical stimulation in the clinical management of the neurogenic bladder. *J Urol* 1988;140:1331–1339.
49. Wainstein MA, Klutke CG. Antegrade techniques of collagen injection for post-prostatectomy stress urinary incontinence: the Washington University experience. *World J Urol* 1997;15:310–315.
50. McGuire EJ, English SF. Periurethral collagen injection for male and female sphincteric incontinence: indications, techniques, and result. *World J Urol* 1997;15:306–309.
51. Appell RA, Vasavada SP, Rackley RR, et al. Percutaneous antegrade collagen injection therapy for urinary incontinence following radical prostatectomy. *Urology* 1996;48:769–772.
52. Elson ML. The role of skin testing in the use of collagen injectable materials. *J Dermatol Surg Oncol* 1989;15:301–303.
53. Elson ML. Re: Delayed hypersensitivity and systemic arthralgia following transurethral collagen injection for stress urinary incontinence. *J Urol* 1999;161:610.
54. Malizia AA Jr., Reiman HM, Myers RP, et al. Migration and granulomatous reaction after periurethral injection of polytef (Teflon). *JAMA* 1984;251:3277–3281.
55. Brown JA, Elliott DS, Barrett DM. Postprostatectomy urinary incontinence: a comparison of the cost of conservative versus surgical management. *Urology* 1998;51:715–720.
56. Giesy JD, Barry JM, Fuchs EF, et al. Initial experience with the Rosen incontinence device. *J Urol* 1981;125:794–795.
57. Scott FB, Bradley WE, Timm GW. Treatment of urinary incontinence by implantable prosthetic sphincter. *Urology* 1973;1:252–259.
58. Motley RC, Barrett DM. Artificial urinary sphincter cuff erosion. Experience with reimplantation in 38 patients. *Urology* 1990;35:215–218.
59. Barrett DM, Parulkar BG, Kramer SA. Experience with AS 800 artificial sphincter in pediatric and young adult patients. *Urology* 1993;42:431–436.
60. Mark S, Perez LM, Webster GD. Synchronous management of anastomotic contracture and stress urinary incontinence following radical prostatectomy. *J Urol* 1994;151:1202–1204.
61. Stamey T. Perineal compression of the corpus spongiosum of the bulbar urethra. An operation for post-radical prostatectomy urinary incontinence. *J Urol* 1994;151:490A.
62. Schaeffer AJ, Clemens JQ, Ferrari M, et al. The male bulbourethral sling procedure for post-radical prostatectomy incontinence. *J Urol* 1998;159:1510–1515.
63. Clemens JQ, Bushman W, Schaeffer AJ. Urodynamic analysis of the bulbourethral sling procedure. *J Urol* 1999;162: 1977–1981.
64. McCammon KA, Kolm P, Main B, et al. Comparative quality-of-life analysis after radical prostatectomy or external beam radiation for localized prostate cancer. *Urology* 1999; 54:509–516.
65. Stock RG, Stone NN, DeWyngaert JK, et al. Prostate specific antigen findings and biopsy results following interactive ultrasound guided transperineal brachytherapy for early stage prostate carcinoma. *Cancer* 1996;77:2386–2392.
66. Kaye KW, Olson DJ, Payne JT. Detailed preliminary analysis of 125iodine implantation for localized prostate cancer using percutaneous approach. *J Urol* 1995;153:1020–1025.

67. Ragde H, Blasko JC, Grimm PD, et al. Interstitial iodine-125 radiation without adjuvant therapy in the treatment of clinically localized prostate carcinoma. *Cancer* 1997;80:442–453.
68. Benoit RM, Naslund MJ, Cohen JK. Complications after prostate brachytherapy in the Medicare population. *Urology* 2000;55:91–96.
69. Formenti SC, Lieskovsky G, Simoneau AR, et al. Impact of moderate dose of postoperative radiation on urinary incontinence and potency in patients with prostate cancer treated with nerve sparing prostatectomy. *J Urol* 1996;155:616–619.
70. Van Cangh PJ, Richard F, Lorge F, et al. Adjuvant radiation therapy does not cause urinary incontinence after radical prostatectomy: results of a prospective randomized study. *J Urol* 1998;159:164–166.
71. Herold DM, Hanlon AL, Hanks GE. Diabetes mellitus: a predictor for late radiation morbidity. *Int J Radiat Oncol Biol Phys* 1999;43:475–479.
72. Gelblum DY, Potters L, Ashley R, et al. Urinary morbidity following ultrasound-guided transperineal prostate seed implantation. *Int J Radiat Oncol Biol Phys* 1999;45:59–67.
73. Martins FE, Boyd SD. Post-operative risk factors associated with artificial urinary sphincter infection-erosion. *Br J Urol* 1995;75:354–358.
74. Walsh PC, Lepor H, Eggleston JC. Radical prostatectomy with preservation of sexual function: anatomical and pathological considerations. *Prostate* 1983;4:473–485.
75. Walsh PC, Mostwin JL. Radical prostatectomy and cystoprostatectomy with preservation of potency. Results using a new nerve-sparing technique. *Br J Urol* 1984;56:694–697.
76. Zimmern PE, Kaswick J, Leach GE. How potent is potent before nerve sparing radical retropubic prostatectomy? *J Urol* 1995;154:1100–1101.
77. Geary ES, Dendinger TE, Freiha FS, et al. Nerve sparing radical prostatectomy: a different view. *J Urol* 1995;154:145–149.
78. Gaylis FD, Friedel WE, Armas OA. Radical retropubic prostatectomy outcomes at a community hospital. *J Urol* 1998;159:167–171.
79. Fowler FJ Jr., Barry MJ, Lu-Yao G, et al. Outcomes of external-beam radiation therapy for prostate cancer: a study of Medicare beneficiaries in three surveillance, epidemiology, and end results areas. *J Clin Oncol* 1996;14:2258–2265.
80. Fowler FJ. Patient reports of symptoms and quality of life following prostate surgery. *Eur Urol* 1991;20[Suppl 1]:44–49.
81. Quinlan DM, Epstein JI, Carter BS, et al. Sexual function following radical prostatectomy: influence of preservation of neurovascular bundles. *J Urol* 1991;145:998–1002.
82. Catalona WJ, Carvalhal GF, Mager DE, et al. Potency, continence and complication rates in 1,870 consecutive radical retropubic prostatectomies. *J Urol* 1999;162:433–438.
83. Talcott JA, Rieker P, Propert KJ, et al. Patient-reported impotence and incontinence after nerve-sparing radical prostatectomy. *J Natl Cancer Inst* 1997;89:1117–1123.
84. Aboseif S, Shinohara K, Breza J, et al. Role of penile vascular injury in erectile dysfunction after radical prostatectomy. *Br J Urol* 1994;73:75–82.
85. Polascik TJ, Walsh PC. Radical retropubic prostatectomy: the influence of accessory pudendal arteries on the recovery of sexual function. *J Urol* 1995;154:150–152.
86. Montorsi F, Guazzoni G, Strambi LF, et al. Recovery of spontaneous erectile function after nerve-sparing radical retropubic prostatectomy with and without early intracavernous injections of alprostadil: results of a prospective, randomized trial. *J Urol* 1997;158:1408–1410.
87. Costabile RA, Spevak M, Fishman IJ, et al. Efficacy and safety of transurethral alprostadil in patients with erectile dysfunction following radical prostatectomy. *J Urol* 1998; 160:1325–1328.
88. Zippe CD, Kedia AW, Kedia K, et al. Treatment of erectile dysfunction after radical prostatectomy with sildenafil citrate (Viagra). *Urology* 1998;52:963–966.
89. Zippe CD, Jhaveri FM, Klein EA, et al. Role of Viagra after radical prostatectomy. *Urology* 2000;55:241–245.
90. Khoudary KP, DeWolf WC, Bruning CO 3rd, et al. Immediate sexual rehabilitation by simultaneous placement of penile prosthesis in patients undergoing radical prostatectomy: initial results in 50 patients. *Urology* 1997;50:395–399.
91. Hall SJ, Basile G, Bertero EB, et al. Extensive corporeal fibrosis after penile irradiation. *J Urol* 1995;153:372–377.
92. Mittal B. A study of penile circulation before and after radiation in patients with prostate cancer and its effect on impotence. *Int J Radiat Oncol Biol Phys* 1985;11:1121–1125.
93. Turner SL, Adams K, Bull CA, et al. Sexual dysfunction after radical radiation therapy for prostate cancer: a prospective evaluation. *Urology* 1999;54:124–129.
94. Fowler FJ Jr., Barry MJ, Lu-Yao G, et al. Outcomes of external-beam radiation therapy for prostate cancer: a study of Medicare beneficiaries in three surveillance, epidemiology, and end results areas. *J Clin Oncol* 1996;14: 2258–2265.
95. Litwin MS. Examining health-related quality of life in men treated for prostate cancer. *World J Urol* 1999;17:205–210.

26B

MANAGEMENT OF RADIATION INJURY TO THE BOWEL

ELIZABETH BREEN
DAVID C. BROOKS

The delivery of radiation therapy to the pelvis during the course of treatment of prostate cancer can inadvertently injure neighboring nonneoplastic tissue. This chapter outlines the potential injuries to the gastrointestinal tract and treatments to alleviate the symptoms these injuries cause.

PATHOPHYSIOLOGY OF INJURY

The cells of the gastrointestinal tract are very sensitive to the effects of radiation. There are acute and chronic effects of radiation on the bowel. During the delivery of radiation therapy, the mucosal cells of the bowel are acutely injured directly and indirectly, resulting in a leakage of fluid and electrolytes into and out of the cells, crypt cell damage, and mucosal slough. Visibly, this results in edema and ulceration of the bowel mucosa. The further lack of regeneration of epithelial cells perpetuates this injury and exacerbates the symptoms. The symptoms of acute radiation injury to the bowel include abdominal cramping, diarrhea, mucous discharge, bleeding, tenesmus, urgency, and fecal incontinence (1,2). Although these symptoms occur in nearly all patients receiving radiation therapy to the pelvis, most experience resolution within 2 to 3 months of completion of the radiation therapy (3).

The chronic effects of radiation to the bowel, although less common than the acute effects, are more troubling because of the difficulty in treating the symptoms they cause. This late radiation injury to the bowel results from progressive occlusive endarteritis and diffuse collagen deposition within the bowel wall, causing bowel ischemia (4). The ischemia results in telangiectasias, necrotic ulcers, strictures, and fistulas (5).

The late sequelae of radiation injury to the bowel have been reported to occur in 5% to 12% of patients who receive radiation to the pelvis. This chronic injury and the symptoms it causes, however, often do not develop for months to years after completion of the radiation (3,6,7). The chances of developing chronic radiation injury to the bowel increases with several factors. Technically, the risk of injury increases with an increased total dose and dose per fraction of the radiation (8). One study reports no chronic effects of radiation in patients who underwent less than 40 Gy of radiation but injury in 20% of patients who received 60 Gy and injury in up to 60% of those patients who received 70 Gy (9).

The risk of late effects of radiation injury to the bowel varies not only with technical factors of the delivery of the radiation but also with patient variation. Situations that make patients more vulnerable to ischemia increase their risk of chronic radiation injury. This includes co-morbidities such as diabetes, hypertension, and increased patient age. Previous radiation to the pelvis or previous pelvic surgery that immobilizes loops of bowel in the pelvis also increases the risk of injury (7).

Symptoms

The symptoms of chronic radiation injury to the bowel vary according to the bowel affected and the degree of injury. Radiation injuries to the small bowel occur most often to the terminal ileum, especially in cases of previous pelvic surgery. The symptoms can range from diarrhea and bleeding to obstruction, leading to fistulization or perforation.

The rectum, owing to its proximity to the prostate and its fixed position within the pelvis, is the most common segment of bowel injured during pelvic irradiation (10). The symptoms range from bleeding proctitis to obstruction and fistulization from strictures. Some patients also suffer from fecal incontinence. The etiology of fecal incontinence is multifactorial, combining the poor compliance of the stiff rectum with an unmasking of poor sphincter tone or radiation injury directly to the pelvic nerves (11). Whether there is any direct effect of the radiation on the anal sphincter is controversial, with a recent study from Birnbaum et al. refuting such injury (12).

Diagnosis

The diagnosis of radiation injury to the bowel is determined via history and physical examination often in combination with endoscopy or radiographic studies, or both. During acute injury, the patients are often currently undergoing radiation therapy, although most patients do not suffer symptoms until they have received a minimum of 30 Gy (3). Endoscopy in this situation reveals hyperemia and mucosal edema.

When taking patient history, the majority of patients suffering from chronic effects of radiation injury to the bowel describe an onset of symptoms within 6 to 24 months of their radiation therapy; the remaining 15% describe the passage of many years since their treatment. In the case of proctitis, endoscopic findings have been graded into three stages. Stage one reveals vascular congestion and friable mucosa; stage two shows ulcerative, thickened mucosa with exudate; and stage three reveals ischemia, endarteritis, and necrosis (13). Other endoscopic findings include telangiectasias and ulcers. When diagnosing strictures, a digital rectal exam may reveal anal stenosis or a fixed pelvis, whereas endoscopy can reveal a noncompliant rectum with a fibrotic narrow lumen. Small bowel series can depict areas of stricture, dilatation, and fistulization. Barium enemas demonstrate shortened and narrowed bowel with or without strictures. Patients with fecal incontinence can also be evaluated with anorectal manometry and nerve studies.

TREATMENT OF RADIATION INJURY TO THE BOWEL

Treatment of Acute Injury

The treatment of the acute effects of radiation on the bowel are mainly supportive. Patients are rehydrated, fed a low-residue diet, and given antidiarrheals. Occasionally, patients are treated with oral or topical 5-ASA products, steroids, or sucralfate. For refractory symptoms, patients may need a temporary cessation of treatment.

Treatment of Chronic Injury

Although the symptoms caused by the chronic effects of radiation therapy occur in far fewer patients than the symptoms of acute injury, they are much more problematic to treat. In fact, because there is no perfect treatment for the symptoms of chronic radiation injury to the bowel, there are many treatments described. The success rate of most of these treatments alone can be lower than desired, requiring the trial of many forms of therapy for any one patient, beginning with the least invasive and moving to more invasive. Up to 20% of patients require operative intervention (3).

Treatment of Chronic Injury to the Rectum

Treatment of Bleeding Radiation Proctitis

The first effort to treat the injured mucosa in bleeding from radiation proctitis is to apply topical medication. Medications used include steroids, 5-ASA, and sucralfate. Steroid preparations consist of a 10% solution of hydrocortisone in an enema or foam solution that is delivered anally and retained overnight. The medication is usually tapered, because an abrupt withdrawal of the therapy can result in rebound bleeding. Topical 5-ASA, a treatment for ulcerative colitis, is usually delivered as a suppository or enema. Results unfortunately have not been very promising, with one series reporting only a transient benefit in one of five patients treated (14). Sucralfate, an aluminum hydroxide complex of sulfated sucrose often used to protect the gastric mucosa from acid damage, has been used in a ratio of 2 g in 20 mL of tap water delivered twice a day to treat the bleeding. In a series of three case reports, benefit was seen in each patient (15). Another topical therapy described is short-chain fatty acid enemas. Short-chain fatty acids, produced by bacteria in the lumen of the colon, are the primary fuel of colonocytes (16,17). Because of this, several groups have proposed treating the rectum directly by bathing it with short-chain fatty acids. Results have been mixed. One group reported a decrease in patients' bleeding but no endoscopic or pathologic improvement after the administration of a 60 mL enema containing 40-mM sodium butyrate twice a day, retained for 30 minutes for 4 weeks (18). Another series, however, reported no significant improvement in a small group of patients in a randomized double-blind trial of butyric acid enemas versus placebo (19).

A recent and promising topical therapy for bleeding radiation proctitis is the application of 4% formalin directly against the affected mucosa. Described techniques vary from diffuse irrigation of all rectal mucosa to specific swabbing of affected mucosa. Bleeding has been reported to cease in up to 75% of patients (20). Several applications may be required and there is a risk of development of painful fissures (21).

The next treatment offered after failure of relief by topical therapy is to use some of the same medications in an oral form. This includes oral steroids, sulfasalazine, or sucralfate. The theory here is that systemic medication might provide a more effective delivery of the medication to the damaged area in patients who may not be able to retain the topical medication. Results, again, however, have not been overly successful (22,23).

A less frequently used noninvasive form of treatment is hyperbaric oxygen. In one brief report, a 60% response rate was described (24).

If the desired response is not achieved with topical or oral medications, then more invasive options often are tried. This includes endoscopic laser ablation of the damaged mucosa. Because of the increased risk in this type of therapy, it is often reserved for patients whose blood loss is symptomatic enough to require blood transfusion. The lasers used, neodymium:yttrium-aluminum-garnet and argon, aim to superficially treat the mucosa, although there is risk of ulceration. Despite the initial decrease in bleeding seen in up to two of three of patients, the bleeding can recur and the treatment often has to be repeated (25–28).

Those patients with significant bleeding that does not respond to any of the previously mentioned treatments are faced with the option of surgical intervention. Surgical options range from simple diversion, which may not stop the bleeding 20% to 40% of the time (29,30), to resection with a stoma or resection with a primary anastomosis. Morbidity and mortality rates are high, reported from 12% to 65% and 0% to 13%, respectively. Risks involved include bleeding, and ureteral and other injury possible during complicated pelvic dissection and anastomotic leaks (27).

Treatment of a Rectal Stricture

Although some symptomatic rectal strictures can be treated by dilation, clinically significant strictures from radiation damage often respond only to surgical intervention. The simplest surgical option is to divert the fecal stream away from the stricture with a permanent stoma, being careful to use nonirradiated bowel to create the stoma (13). If the stricture is resected, then the decision about whether to reanastomose the bowel has to be addressed. In a technique popularized by Parks et al., the dissection to resect the stricture is carried down to the pelvic floor and the anastomosis is hand-sewn via the anus (31). The risk of complications is high, ranging from 25% to 50%. These include pelvic abscesses and anastomotic strictures. Even without such complications, the ultimate function from such a low anastomosis can be poor. Some patients experience overwhelming frequency, urgency, and even fecal incontinence. In one series, 25% to 37% of patients described disturbed continence after a coloanal anastomosis, and 15% required a permanent colostomy to obtain satisfaction (32,33). Even the surgical option of completely resecting the rectum and anus, creating a permanent colostomy, carries significant risk. In this situation, there is the risk of a nonhealing perineal wound. An option to avoid this is to dissect past the stricture, leaving a very short defunctionalized rectum and anus in place and avoiding the creation of a perineal wound.

Despite the risk of surgery in these patients, the severity of their symptoms and the scarcity of other options can leave patients with little choice. When surgery is necessary, adherence to certain principles can increase the success. One principle is to have an accurate preoperative assessment of the status of the original tumor and the extent of the radiation injury, including injury to other bowel or the urologic system. Assessment of the anal sphincter may help predict postoperative function. Attention should also be given to the patient's overall nutritional status (3). During the operation itself, principles such as using a midline incision to preserve all potential stoma sites and minimal mobilization to avoid potential injury to the bowel help avoid complications.

Treatment of Chronic Injury to the Small Bowel

The other area of bowel that can sustain chronic injury from pelvic irradiation is the small bowel. This occurs primarily in the area of the terminal ileum, particularly in patients who have adhesions from previous abdominal surgery.

Treatment of Diarrhea

Treatment of the diarrhea that results from chronic injury to the small bowel is aimed at supportive care as well as treating the etiology of the diarrhea. Patients are often placed on a low residue diet, antispasmodics, and antidiarrheals. If lack of bile salt reabsorption appears to be the problem, then patients often experience relief of their diarrhea by taking a binding resin, namely cholestyramine (34). For patients with bacterial overgrowth from stasis, a course of antibiotics often provides relief. For patients with significant malnutrition, enteral feeds or even parenteral nutrition can be used to improve their nutritional status.

Treatment of Strictures, Obstruction, and Fistulization

The degree of symptoms patients experience from a partial obstruction or fistula from a radiation stricture may respond to the medical treatment outlined earlier, but, after establishing adequate nutrition, some patients will require surgical intervention (35). Unfortunately, the surgical options for these patients carry morbidity and mortality rates of up to 65% and 45%, respectively (35). One difficult choice to be made when operating on a symptomatic stricture of the small bowel is whether to resect the stricture with a primary anastomosis or to simply bypass the strictured segment of bowel. There are no randomized studies attempting to answer this question. There is, however, much support for bypass operations, citing less morbidity, mainly from averting anastomotic leaks, and better symptomatic relief (36). Other studies, however, especially those published since improvements in parenteral nutrition and critical care have been made, support resection of strictures. Support is strongest for resection of strictures associated with bowel fistulas, as long as at least one limb of nonirradiated bowel is used in the anastomosis (37). In the unfortunate situation of a free perforation resulting from injury to small bowel, the creation of an ostomy is believed to be the safest course of action. Technically, when operating on radiation injury to the small bowel, gentle handling of the tissue and caution against overzealous enterolysis is indicated to avoid creation of more problems than are attempting to be fixed (38).

CONCLUSION

Although most patients suffer from acute injury to the bowel while undergoing radiation to the pelvis, these symptoms can often be successfully treated with careful medical management. Fortunately, symptoms from chronic injury to the rectum and small bowel are rare. For those patients who do suffer symptomatic injury, however, the treatment is often frustrating and vexing, as the effectiveness of many of the noninvasive forms of treatment are inconsistent, whereas surgical treatment carries a high risk of morbidity and mortality.

REFERENCES

1. Berthrong M. Pathologic changes secondary to radiation. *World J Surg* 1986;10:155.
2. Novak JM, Collins JJ, Donowitz M, et al. Effects of radiation on the human gastrointestinal tract. *J Clin Gastroenter* 1979;1:9–39.
3. Otchy DP, Nelson H. Radiation injuries of the colon and rectum. *Surg Clin N Am* 1994;73:1017–1035.
4. Galland RB, Spencer J. Natural history and surgical management of radiation enteritis. *Br J Surg* 1987;74:742.
5. Haselton PS, Carr N, Schefield PF. Vascular changes in radiation bowel disease. *Histopathology* 1985;9:517–534.
6. Perez CA, Lee HK, Georgiou A, et al. Technical factors affecting morbidity in definitive irradiation for localized carcinoma of the prostate. *Int J Radiat Oncol Biol Phys* 1990;18:841–848.
7. Mameghan H, Fisher R, Mameghan J, et al. Bowel complications after radiotherapy for carcinoma of the prostate: the volume effect. *Int J Radiat Oncol Biol Phys* 1990;18:315–320.
8. Roswit B, Malsky S, Reid C. Severe radiation injuries of the stomach, small intestine, colon and rectum. *Am J Roentgenol Radium Ther Nucl Med* 1972;114:460.
9. Strockbine MF, Hancock JE, Fletcher GH. Complications in 831 patients with squamous cell carcinoma of the intact uterine cervix treated with 3,000 rads or more whole pelvis irradiation. *Am J Roentgenol* 1970;108:293.
10. Schmidt EH, Symmonds RE. Surgical treatment of radiation-induced injuries of the intestine. *Surg Gynecol Obstet* 1981;153:896–900.
11. Varma JS, Smith AN, Busuttil A. Function of the anal sphincter after chronic radiation injury. *Gut* 1986;27:528.
12. Birnbaum EH, Dreznik Z, Myerson RJ, et al. Early effect of external beam radiation therapy on the anal sphincter: a study using anal manometry and transrectal ultrasound. *Dis Colon Rectum* 1992;35:757–761.
13. DeCosse JJ, Rhodes RS, Wente WB, et al. The natural history and management of radiation induced injury of the gastrointestinal tract. *Ann Surg* 1969;170:369.
14. Triantafillidis JK, Dadioti P, Nicolakis D, et al. High doses of 5-aminosalicylic acid enemas in chronic radiation proctitis: comparison with betamethasone enemas. *Am J Gastroenterol* 1990;85:1537–1538.
15. Kochar R, Sharma SC, Gupta BB. Rectal sucralfate in radiation proctitis. *Lancet* 1988;2;400.
16. McNeil NI, Cummings JH, James WPT. Short chain fatty acid absorption by the human large intestine. *Gut* 1978;19:819–822.
17. Cummings JH, Pomare EW, Branch WJ, et al. Short chain fatty acids in human large intestine, portal, hepatic and venous blood. *Gut* 1987;78:1221–1227.
18. Al-Sabbagh R, Sinicrope FA, Sellin JH, et al. Evaluation of short-chain fatty acid enemas: treatment of radiation proctitis. *Am J Gastroenterol* 1996;91:1814–1816.
19. Talley NA, Chen F, King D, et al. Short-chain fatty acids in the treatment of radiation proctitis. *Dis Colon Rectum* 1997;40:1046–1050.
20. Saclarides TJ, King DG, Franklin JL, et al. Formalin instillation for refractory radiation-induced hemorrhagic proctitis: report of 16 patients. *Dis Colon Rectum* 1996;39:196–199.
21. Roche B, Chautems R, Marti MC. Application of formaldehyde for treatment of hemorrhagic radiation-induced proctitis. *World J Surg* 1996;20:1092–1095.
22. Gilinsky NH, Khoury J, Thorton JJ. Treatment of chronic radiation enteritis and colitis with salicylazosulfapyridine and systemic corticosteroids. *Am J Gastroenterol* 1979;70: 62–65.
23. Sasai T, Hiraishi H, Suzuki Y, et al. Treatment of chronic post-radiation proctitis with oral administration of sucralfate. *Am J Gastroenterol* 1998;93:1593–1594.
24. Warren DC, Feehan P, Slade JB, et al. Chronic radiation proctitis treated with hyperbaric oxygen. *Undersea Hyperbar Med* 1997;24:187–189.
25. Alquist DA, Gostout CJ, Viggiano TR. Laser therapy for severe radiation-induced rectal bleeding. *Mayo Clin Proc* 1986;61:927–931.
26. Taylor JG, DiSario JA, Buchi KN. Argon laser therapy for hemorrhagic radiation proctitis: long-term results. *Gastro Endosc* 1993;39:641–644.
27. Lucarotti ME, Mountford RA, Bartolo DC. Surgical management of intestinal radiation injury. *Dis Colon Rectum* 1991;34:865.
28. Carbatzas C, Spencer GM, Thorpe SM, et al. Nd:YAG laser treatment for bleeding from radiation proctitis. *Endoscopy* 1996;28:497–500.
29. Gilinsky NH, Burns DG, Barbezat GO, et al. The natural history of radiation induced proctosigmoiditis: an analysis of 88 patients. *Q J Med* 1983;205:40.
30. Jao SW, Beart RW, Gunderson LL. Surgical treatment of radiation injuries of the colon and rectum. *Am J Surg* 1986;151:272.
31. Parks AG, Allen CL, Frank JD, et al. A method of treating post-irradiation rectovaginal fistulas. *Br J Surg* 1978;65:417.
32. Browning GG, Varma JS, Smith AN, et al. Late results of mucosal proctectomy and colo-anal sleeve anastomosis for chronic irradiation rectal injury. *Br J Surg* 1987;74:31–34.

33. Varma JS, Smith AN. Anorectal function following coloanal sleeve anastomosis for chronic radiation injury to the rectum. *Br J Surg* 1986;73:285–289.
34. Heusinkveld RS, Manning AR, Aristizabal SA. Control of radiation-induced diarrhea with cholestyramine. *Int J Radiol Oncol Biol Phys* 1978;4:687.
35. Russell JC, Welch JP. Operative management of radiation injuries of the intestinal tract. *Am J Surg* 1979;137:433.
36. Swan RW, Fowler WC Jr., Boronow RC. Surgical management of radiation injury to the small intestine. *Surg Gynecol Obstet* 1976;142:325–327.
37. Harling H, Balslev I. Radical surgical approach to radiation injury of the small bowel. *Dis Colon Rectum* 1986;29:371–373.
38. Galland RB, Spencer J. Surgical management of radiation enteritis. *Surgery* 1986;99:133–139.

27

MANAGEMENT CONSIDERATIONS FOR THE PATIENT WITH LOW-RISK DISEASE

GRAEME SCOTT STEELE
JEROME P. RICHIE

The increase in the number of patients diagnosed with prostate cancer from the late 1980s to the mid-1990s was larger than for any other solid malignancy. This increase is related to a variety of factors, including increased physician and patient awareness, development of the prostate-specific antigen (PSA) blood test, and the relative ease and accuracy with which the prostate gland can be biopsied. Recent data indicate that the number of patients who underwent radical prostatectomy (RP) from 1982 to 1992 increased by 100%, whereas the number of patients presenting with advanced disease during this time period declined by 60% (1).

This increase in number of patients diagnosed with clinically localized disease has resulted in prostate cancer management's assuming greater prominence among physicians and the lay public alike. Treatment options for patients with clinically localized prostate cancer, however, remain controversial. RP; radiotherapy, in the form of external beam radiotherapy or brachytherapy; androgen deprivation therapy (ADT); and watchful waiting (WW) are well recognized and generally accepted forms of therapy.

However, surgery and radiotherapy expose patients to a number of short- and long-term side effects that can be notoriously difficult to treat. Furthermore, local therapy for prostate cancer can be associated with significant failure rates, especially in those patients with poorly differentiated disease, high pretreatment PSA values, and clinically nonlocalized tumors (cT3) (2,3). Persistence of prostate carcinoma cells in the pelvis after primary treatment may ultimately lead to biochemical failure and subsequent clinical progression. Furthermore, adjuvant and second therapies are associated with significant morbidity and may prove to be ineffective in controlling progression of disease (4).

In most cases, the natural history of clinically localized prostate cancer involves a protracted clinical course, with clinical progression occurring several years after the initial diagnosis. This fact has contributed to the controversy regarding the management of low-stage prostate cancer. Aggressive local therapy in patients with a low risk of dying of disease has the potential to seriously adversely affect quality of life; nonetheless, potentially curative therapy should not be denied to patients with high risk of disease progression and subsequent death from prostate cancer. Therefore, the single most important aspect of avoiding inappropriate therapy and subsequent morbidity is patient selection. In this regard, only those men diagnosed with clinically localized prostate cancer who are in general good health, with a minimum life expectancy of 10 years, should be considered for definitive local therapy.

This overview discusses management of patients with low-risk prostate cancer and attempts to emphasize selection criteria for those patients who are most likely to benefit from a WW protocol.

NATURAL HISTORY OF PROSTATE CANCER

Opponents to prostate cancer screening point to the natural history of prostate cancer as a slow-growing disease with a prolonged subclinical course. Indeed, some reports indicate that most men demise with, but not of, prostate cancer. For example, George followed a cohort of 120 patients (mean age, 74.8 years; range, 62 to 90 years) with localized prostate cancer. The local tumor increased to palpable dimensions in 100 patients (84%), but metastatic disease developed in only 13 patients (10%). Although five patients died of prostatic cancer, the disease was not responsible for 48 additional deaths (5).

On the other hand, the literature is replete with studies that contradict the apparent benign nature of prostate cancer. Gronberg and associates examined records of almost 7,000 men with prostate cancer detected in northern Sweden and compared their survival to an age-matched group (6). Relative survival of men with prostate cancer was only 45% at 10 years. Furthermore, the decrease in survival was greater in younger men and in those with higher-grade cancers. Patients diagnosed before the age of 60 years had an

80% risk of dying of prostate cancer, whereas those older than 80 years of age at diagnosis had less than a 50% risk of prostate cancer–related death. Overall, men with prostate cancer lost an average of 40% of their expected longevity.

Therefore, despite evidence that, in some patients, the diagnosis of prostate cancer is most likely insignificant and represents a low risk to longevity, the majority of patients diagnosed with prostate cancer probably has clinically significant disease, which by definition requires definitive local therapy if disease progression is to be prevented.

Prostate cancer, therefore, cannot be considered a uniformly benign neoplasm with an indolent course. Only a subset of patients with localized prostate cancer has low-risk disease that, if observed, would run an indolent and benign course.

DEFINING LOW-RISK PROSTATE CANCER

Low-risk prostate cancer can be defined according to the following:

- Tumor grade and volume in stage T1 disease:
  - Stage T1a (A1) disease
  - Stage T1c disease
- Tumor grade and patient age

LOW-RISK PROSTATE CANCER—STAGE T1a DISEASE

In 1975, Jewett subdivided stage A prostate cancer based on observed differences in their clinical course into stage T1a (A1, focal) and stage T1b (A2, diffuse) disease (7). In this important article, he stated that stage T1a cancer, which by definition is both low grade and volume, should be left well alone, whereas stage T1b cancer should be treated. This surgical principle endures to this day.

Stage T1a prostate cancer denotes cancer not suspected clinically on digital rectal examination but detected on histologic examination of pathology specimens after transurethral resection of the prostate (TURP) or open prostatectomy and, therefore, usually occurring in the transition zone of the prostate. These tumors are low grade, not suspected clinically but rather found incidentally at TURP or open prostatectomy and comprising 5% or less of the total surgical specimen.

Incidence of Stage A1 Prostate Cancer

The number of patients undergoing surgery for symptomatic benign prostatic hyperplasia (BPH) has declined over the 1990s, owing to increased use of medical and minimally invasive therapy. Nevertheless, approximately 10% of patients who undergo prostatectomy for presumed BPH are found to have prostate cancer (8). The rate of cancer detection has been shown to be directly related to the volume of tissue examined. Moore and associates examined every chip of tissue submitted from TURP specimens and found prostate cancer in 25% of patients, whereas Murphy and associates found cancer in 17.2% of patients after analysis of all prostate tissue (9,10). It should be emphasized, however, that the vast majority of T1a and T2b cancers are diagnosed by analysis of the first 12 g of tissue, and, for that reason, most pathologists opt not to perform complete histologic analysis of the entire specimen.

Natural History of Stage A Prostate Cancer

Jewett's observations that the clinical courses of stage T1a and T1b disease differ have been corroborated by other authors. Cantrell and associates reported that only 2% of patients with stage T1a disease progressed when followed over a 4-year period (11). However, other investigators have reported higher rates of progression of stage T1a disease and in addition have pointed to the unreliability of TURP in defining stage T1a disease. Epstein and associates reported a 16% progression rate when patients with stage T1a disease were followed for 8 years (12).

Staging Error in Stage A Prostate Cancer

Variability in progression rates of stage T1a disease is related, at least in part, to the staging error. Zincke and associates pointed out that only 63% of patients with clinical stage T1a disease who underwent RP had pathologic stage T1a disease (13). Furthermore, 12% of patients with stage T1a disease were found to have pathologic stage T3 disease at time of RP (15). In addition, the Mayo Clinic experience showed that 26% of patients younger than 60 years of age with stage T1a disease progressed when followed for a prolonged period of time (mean follow-up, 10.2 years).

Larsen and associates studied 64 RP specimens of stage T1a prostate cancer. Although cancer was not detected in 6% of specimens, cancer was detected in minimal amount in 74% of specimens and in significant amount in 20% of specimens (14). Paulson and associates reported that 11 of 18 patients (61%) with stage T1a disease were upstaged to T1b and T3 disease after histologic analysis of the RP specimen (15). Voges and associates performed morphometric analysis on 44 RP specimens performed for clinical stage T1 disease. In 32 patients (73%), unsuspected cancers unrelated to the TURP tumor were found in the RP specimen, of which 87% were non–transition zone tumors (16).

Predicting Progression—Tumor Grade, Ploidy, and Volume

Tumor grade and volume are generally believed to be important prognostic variables when defining stage T1 disease. However, experience has shown that approximately

50% of stage T1a tumors that progressed are low grade, and approximately 75% are low volume (less than 1%). Greene and associates reported that most cancers of transition origin are diploid, whereas the majority of cancers that arise in the transition are nondiploid (17). Borre and associates studied ploidy in patients diagnosed with prostate cancer by TURP or open prostatectomy and reported that flow cytometric–determined diploidy was associated with disease-specific survival (18). The role of DNA ploidy in staging prostate cancer is controversial; generally, DNA ploidy provides little additional independent information to conventional staging criteria (19).

Larsen and associates showed that TURP tumor volume and grade were not statistically correlated with residual tumor volume found in RP specimens. They reported that Gleason scores 2 to 4 versus 5 to 7 tumors on TURP showed no difference in predicting residual tumor or minimal versus significant tumor volume at the time of RP. They also showed that substantial tumor volume exists in approximately 20% of patients with clinical stage T1a prostate cancer (16). This residual tumor is located in the peripheral zone of the prostate and therefore is inaccessible with the resectoscope at the time of TURP.

Greene and associates reported the presence of an associated peripheral zone cancer in 12 of 13 patients who underwent RP for stage T1a disease (20). The grade of the peripheral zone tumor was frequently higher than that of the transition tumor resected at time of TURP, and, in addition, the peripheral tumors tended to be larger. These observations imply that the greatest threat to patients with stage T1a disease is the presence of a second peripheral zone tumor, which is often of a higher grade than the incidental tumor removed at the time of TURP (36).

Staging T1a (A1) Prostate Cancer

Repeat Transurethral Resection of the Prostate

The use of repeat TURP for assessing probability of disease progression is a controversial topic. Repeat TURP could potentially be used to upgrade the stage of T1a disease to T1b disease and, in the process, identify those patients requiring early definitive treatment. Lowe and Barry reported that patients without residual tumor at repeat TURP did not develop disease progression and therefore suggested that staging TURP for incidental stage T1a disease provided important prognostic information (21).

However, Ingerman and associates reviewed the records of 24 patients with stage T1a disease on initial resection who underwent repeat TURP. Three (13%) of the patients progressed despite the fact that residual disease was not detected in a single patient (22). Zhang and associates supported this data by their findings that 3 of 38 patients without any evidence of residual cancer at repeat TURP developed disease progression, whereas only 3 of 12 patients with residual disease progressed (41).

Although available literature suggests that 10% of patients with stage T1a disease will be upstaged by repeat TURP, the significance of finding no residual disease is unclear, especially in view of the fact that disease progression is well described in this subset of patients. It is apparent that disease that is inaccessible at the time of the initial resection may be of a higher grade and volume than the tumor removed at initial TURP, and this unrecognized tumor determines the natural history of the disease. The majority of clinically significant prostate cancers arises in the peripheral zone, an area not amenable to tissue sampling with the resectoscope. Furthermore, Terris and associates have shown that a significant percentage of residual prostate cancers occur in the anterior fibromuscular stroma, as well as in the apical area. Once again, these areas are usually beyond the confines of the resectoscope in experienced hands (23). For this reason, it is generally believed that repeat resection does not effectively evaluate the risks of disease progression and has therefore largely fallen out of favor.

Transrectal Ultrasound of the Prostate

Transrectal imaging of the prostate has been proposed as a means of staging T1a and T1b disease. Grupps and associates prospectively reviewed the diagnostic accuracy of transrectal ultrasound (TRUS) in evaluation of incidental prostate cancers (24). They performed TRUS on 466 patients before prostatectomy and compared their results with the pathologic findings. Although TRUS correctly predicted tumors in 83% of patients, there was a significant discrepancy between stages. Only 3 of 21 patients with stages T1a and T1b were correctly identified by TRUS. Lee and associates correctly identified only 11 of 54 cases (20%) of residual transition zone cancer using TRUS alone (25).

Sheth and associates compared TRUS with pathologic examination of specimens obtained at TURP in 29 patients with clinical stage T1 disease (26). The overall sensitivity of TRUS was only 55%, and specificity was 37%. In seven patients, post-TURP scarring was reported as a hypoechoic lesion, and the authors therefore concluded that TRUS diagnosis of stage T1 disease was problematic. Egawa and associates reported that tumor size was an important factor with respect to determining the ability of TRUS to diagnose residual prostate cancer; none of the 54 lesions less than 0.1 mL in volume was identified by TRUS (27).

Magnetic Resonance Imaging

Carroll and associates evaluated the role of magnetic resonance imaging (MRI) for monitoring patients with low-volume cancer after TURP or open prostatectomy who subsequently underwent radical surgery (28). Seventeen patients underwent MRI scanning before undergoing RP, and the results of MRI scans were compared to pathology findings. For cancers originating in the peripheral zone, the overall sensitivity of detection was 80%. However, MRI proved to be unable to diagnose transition zone cancers. Prostate cancer in the transition zone was found to produce a heterogenous signal on T2-weighted images, which made visualization of low-intensity signals from prostate cancer difficult to discern. Endorectal coils have encountered similar problems in this regard, being unable to distinguish transition zone tumors from normal surrounding prostatic tissue (29). Furthermore, after TURP, the prostatic parenchyma has been found to give rise to a uniformly reduced signal that makes delineation of tumors from surrounding tissue problematic (30).

Although newer MRI techniques have yielded improved results and reduced interobserver variability, it must be borne in mind that MRI technology is expensive, accessibility is limited, and sensitivity still has not reached levels at which this technology can be comfortably used to accurately predict pathologic stage in patients with incidental prostate cancer (31).

Needle Biopsy of the Prostate

Transrectal needle biopsy of the prostate in patients with stage T1a disease has been well described by the Stanford group (25,32). Terris and associates reported the role of needle biopsy as an adjunct to TRUS and showed that needle biopsy improved ability to diagnose residual tumor (23). Diertick and associates found that needle biopsy core cancer lengths of 3 mm or more on one or two needle biopsies accurately predicted tumor volume of larger than 0.5 mL, thus implying that these tumors were by definition not clinically insignificant (34).

Serum Prostate-Specific Antigen Values in Stage A Disease

Most patients with stage T1a disease have normal serum PSA values at the time of TURP. Cohen and associates reported a mean serum PSA value of 2.3 ng per mL in patients with stage T1a disease, with more than 90% of such patients having a serum PSA value of less than 4 ng per mL (33). Belville and associates also analyzed serum PSA values in patients on WW protocols with a mean interval from diagnosis of 13 years. They found that 96% of patients recorded serum PSA values of less than 3 ng per mL, and nearly 60% had values less than 1 ng per mL (34). Voges and associates reported that post-TURP serum PSA values were elevated with increasing total residual cancer volume in the RP specimen (18).

Feneley and associates evaluated the role of serial serum PSA measurement after TURP in patients with stage T1a prostate cancer. They found that an incremental rise in serum PSA exceeding 20% per year yielded a sensitivity of 90% and specificity of 79% for biopsy-proven residual disease and concluded that serial PSA measurement (PSA velocity) could identify most patients with residual disease (35).

Although there are no currently available studies to examine the use of ratios between free and total serum PSA values in patients with incidental prostate cancer, free to total serum PSA ratios have been used in combination with needle biopsy findings in stage T1c prostate cancer to determine whether disease is potentially insignificant and therefore low risk (36). This subset of patients is discussed later in greater detail.

Tumor De-Differentiation in Stage A Prostate Cancer

Brawn reported that prostate cancer could de-differentiate with time, a finding that may have important implications with respect to WW protocols in patients with stage T1a disease, especially those patients in a younger age group (37). He analyzed 54 patients with stage T1a prostate cancer who underwent two TURP procedures, separated by a mean of 11 years, to establish whether histologic appearance of prostate cancer remained the same over a period of time. Brawn graded prostate cancer into four grades (grades 1 through 4) and reported that 73% of grade 1, 75% of grade 2, and 88% of grade 3 tumors dedifferentiated, which may partly explain the relatively high progression rates in some series of patients with stage T1a disease.

Progression of Stage A1 Disease

Zhang and associates followed 132 patients with stage T1a disease for 5 to 23 years; 13 patients (10%) had either progressed locally or systemically with long-term follow-up (38).

Similarly, Blute and associates reported disease progression in 4 of 15 patients (27%) younger than 60 years of age with stage T1a disease, followed for an average of 10.2 years, whereas Roy and associates noted disease progression in 3 of 14 patients (21%) with stage T1a disease when followed for more than 10 years (39,40).

Therefore, although at first glance stage T1a prostate cancer may appear to be a relatively innocuous disease, this is clearly not necessarily the case, and a blanket policy of WW for all patients with a diagnosis of stage T1a disease is obviously not an appropriate option. With this in mind, however, it is also important to note that, despite significant rates of disease progression in patients with stage T1a disease, mortality-related disease rates remain low.

Mortality in Stage A1 Disease

Brawn and associates reviewed 134 patients with stage A prostate cancer diagnosed between 1972 and 1986 at a single Veterans Administration Medical Center. The survival of patients with stages T1a and T1b disease was compared to a cohort of patients from the same institution with a diagnosis of BPH. Survival and tumor progression were similar for patients with stage T1a prostate cancer and for those patients with BPH in three age groups studied (younger than 65 years, 65 to 74 years, and older than 74 years of age). Stage T2b disease, however, was associated with significantly worse survival rates (41). Thompson and associates reported a 5% disease-specific mortality rate among 60 patients with stage T1a disease followed for a mean of 7.5 years (42).

Despite the fact that the Mayo Clinic experience showed that a relatively high percentage of patients with stage T1a disease have more advanced disease at time of RP, none of their stage T1a patients died of disease in the follow-up period (42).

Clearly, many (but not all) patients with a presumptive diagnosis of stage T1a prostate cancer do well with their disease. Despite the fact that there is biochemical evidence of disease progression, clinical progression may be absent and longevity unaltered by a slowly progressing tumor. Therefore, patient selection remains the key to avoiding unnecessary morbidity associated with curative therapy for early disease. This principle was enunciated succinctly by Whitmore, who stated, "In prostate cancer, is cure necessary in those in whom it is possible, and is cure possible in those in whom it is necessary?" (43).

LOW-RISK PROSTATE CANCER—STAGE T1c DISEASE

Although the incidence of stage T1a prostate cancer has declined, owing to current trends that prefer medical and minimally invasive therapy for patients with symptomatic BPH, during this same time period there has been a significant increase in the incidence of stage T1c prostate cancer.

The increase in the number of patients with clinically localized prostate cancer has been accompanied by an increased incidence in patient morbidity related to curative therapies. Physicians have therefore been prompted to investigate whether a subset of T1c prostate cancers poses little or no threat to the patient and might therefore be observed by a surveillance protocol (44–50).

In general, insignificant stage T1c prostate cancer is defined as low-volume disease (less than 0.5 mL) with a Gleason score of 6 or less. The frequency of insignificant stage T1c prostate cancer is reported to be between 6% and 30%. Despite the variation in reported incidence (likely due to variation in calculation of tumor volume), these percentages represent significant numbers of patients who are potential candidates for WW protocols.

D'Amico and associates have investigated the relationship between calculated prostate cancer volume and risk of progression. They reported that whereas only 15% of patients with a maximum tumor diameter of less than 1 mL progressed, patients with tumor volumes of 4 mL or greater had significantly higher rates of tumor progression, irrespective of the T stage of disease (51–53).

Epstein and associates studied 163 stage T1c RP specimens in which free to total serum PSA values were determined (39). In this study, insignificant prostate cancers were defined as organ confined, Gleason score less than 7 and tumor volume less than 0.5 mL. Of the tumors, 30% were found to be insignificant. The best model to predict preoperatively the presence of an insignificant tumor was a free to total serum PSA ratio of 0.15 or greater and favorable needle biopsy findings (less than 3 cores involved, in which no core had greater than 50% tumor involvement and a Gleason score of less than 7). Of 163 cases with stage T1c prostate cancers studied, almost one-third turned out to have insignificant disease, whereas 50% and 20% turned out to have moderate and advanced tumors, respectively.

Goto and associates evaluated the ability of commonly used diagnostic methods to predict the presence of insignificant T1c prostate cancer and found that a maximum cancer length of less that 2 mm in any core, combined with a PSA density of less than 0.1, predicted insignificant tumors in three-fourths of patients with these parameters.

Although Epstein and associates have reported an incidence of insignificant disease ranging from 17% to 30%, other authors have reported a much lower incidence of insignificant disease (39,52). Douglas and associates analyzed 67 stage T1c prostate cancers and reported insignificant disease in only 6% of patients. This low incidence may have been contributed to by a more stringent definition of insignificant disease (less than 0.2 mL) (48). Similarly, Lerner and associates reported that the majority of stage T1c prostate cancers was significant (more than 90%) (50).

In summary, the vast majority of patients with stage T1c prostate cancer has clinically significant disease that has the potential to impact on their longevity. A subset of stage T1c prostate cancers, however, is potentially not life threatening and therefore unlikely to affect longevity, especially in older patients. In the final analysis, patient age and comorbidity play an overriding role in selection of treatment options for clinically localized disease, especially in older patients whose longevity is estimated to be less than one decade.

LOW-RISK PROSTATE CANCER—PATIENT AGE

Serum PSA testing has led to a dramatic stage migration of prostate cancer and has resulted in an increase in incidence of patients diagnosed with early-stage disease. The earlier diagnosis of prostate cancer is especially relevant in younger patients who are most likely to benefit from curative therapies owing to their projected longevity. However, the diagnosis of low-stage prostate cancer in patients older than the age of 70 to 75 years has presented physicians with a therapeutic conundrum. Serum PSA testing in elderly patients has often been blamed as the culprit in this regard.

Before the advent of serum PSA screening, more than half of prostate cancers detected were clinically advanced at time of diagnosis, and distant metastases were noted in approximately 25% of patients. In elderly men, therefore, therapeutic choices were often between ADT introduced before clinical symptoms and ADT at the time of onset of bothersome clinical disease. Presently, however, an increased incidence of clinically diagnosed prostate cancer among elderly patients has prompted debate regarding the role of aggressive local therapy in patients with life expectancies less than 10 years.

Prostate cancer is therefore somewhat unique among human malignancies because of the marked discrepancy between the prevalence of histologic cancer and that of clinically evident disease. Although a 50-year-old man has an approximately 10% risk of developing clinically significant prostate cancer during his lifetime, the incidence of histologic presence of prostate cancer is much higher (54). Montie and associates showed that 40% of men in their 60s undergoing cystoprostatectomy for bladder cancer have histologic evidence of prostate cancer, whereas, in octogenarians, the incidence of histologic disease approaches 80% (55). Therefore, most elderly men die with, and not from, prostate cancer, so patient age and longevity at time of diagnosis need to be carefully factored into the therapeutic equation, especially in patients with clinically localized disease.

Because of these concerns, some physicians have been hesitant to carry out clinical testing for prostate cancer, especially in older men, hoping to avoid detection of unimportant disease that may then be subject to aggressive therapy. Ohori and associates, however, compared the pathologic features of incidental cystoprostatectomy prostate cancers to those of clinically detected (serum PSA, digital rectal examination, ultrasound) prostate cancers treated with RP. They found that all cystoprostatectomy prostate cancers were unimportant or curable, of lower grade, and less likely to extend beyond the confines of the prostate, whereas the RP specimens were of higher grade, more advanced, and less likely to be unimportant cancers. In fact, only 9% of the RP tumors were unimportant, as opposed to 78% of the cystoprostatectomy prostate cancers (56).

Albertsen and associates analyzed a series of men with prostate cancer who were managed conservatively (60). They found that men with low-grade disease (Gleason scores 2 to 4) faced minimal risk of dying from prostate cancer at 15 years. However, men with poorly differentiated disease (Gleason scores 7 to 10) faced a high risk of dying from disease, and this was even applicable to men diagnosed at age 74 years. Men with moderate-grade tumors (Gleason scores 5 to 6) faced only a modest risk of dying of their disease, which increased slowly over a 15-year period. Therefore, a 78-year-old man with a clinically localized Gleason score 5 tumor is unlikely to develop clinically significant advanced disease during his lifetime, in contrast to a 40-year-old man with the same tumor.

Fifteen-year outcome tables of patients with clinically localized prostate cancer indicate that only approximately 10% of patients 70 to 74 years of age with low-grade disease die from their tumors, and, therefore, this subset of patients can be reasonably presumed to have low-risk prostate cancer (60).

In summary, elderly men have a high incidence of histologic prostate cancer, and the majority of these tumors is clinically unimportant. For those elderly men with clinical evidence of disease, the majority of tumors is potentially significant, but tumor significance is dependent on factors such as co-morbidity and longevity. Although it is true to say that most men die with, rather than of, prostate cancer, knowledge of the presence of prostate cancer may allow the physician to institute timely palliative therapy that may significantly improve quality of life.

MANAGEMENT OF LOW-RISK PROSTATE CANCER

When interviewing a patient with a diagnosis of prostate cancer, it is important to bear in mind that there is no best single treatment, only options. Although each treatment choice has a number of unique advantages for the patient, each option has a unique set of complications and side effects. Until the inception of the Prostatectomy Intervention versus Observation Trial, comparing RP to observation, no well-designed, appropriately powered, prospective study had been completed to compare treatment options for localized prostate cancer.

In 1995, the Prostate Cancer Panel of the American Urological Association determined that, because of differences in patient selection and outcomes reporting among different series, it was impossible to make comparisons between treatment options with regard to efficacy and side effects (57). The panel concluded that all commonly available options, such as surveillance, RP, external beam radiotherapy, and brachytherapy, should be offered to all patients with newly diagnosed clinically localized prostate cancer.

In general, the determination of the best treatment option for a patient with newly diagnosed prostate cancer requires information about tumor stage, aggressiveness, patient life expectancy, co-morbidities, and, finally, patient preferences.

Although at first glance the presence of low-risk disease implies a conservative approach, for a variety of reasons this may not necessarily be the case. De-differentiation and progression of stage T1a prostate cancer are well described, and, therefore, patients entered into surveillance protocols require long-term follow-up, especially in younger patients (40). In addition, an appreciable subset of patients with stage T1a disease may be upstaged by restaging as described earlier and, therefore, may no longer be appropriate candidates for observation protocols. Retrospective studies, however, demonstrate that only 10% to 27% of patients with stage T1a disease will progress (41,42). Therefore, the majority of patients with stage T1a disease does well without treatment. A subset of patients may find the concept of surveillance undesirable and wish to proceed with curative therapy at a time that a cure can almost definitely be achieved. Surveillance can often effectively take advantage of the long symptom-free interval in low-risk disease in combination with shortened life expectancy in older patients (6,58).

Watchful Waiting for Low-Risk Prostate Cancer

Three recent reports have described the outcomes of WW protocols in approximately 2,000 men with prostate cancer. Their findings regarding older patients with low-grade disease are generally relevant to all patients with low-risk disease (59,60,62).

The report by Chodak and associates involved a metaanalysis of survival of 828 men with prostate cancer in several nonrandomized series of WW. In this report, the 10-year disease-specific actuarial survival rates were 87%, 87%, and 34% for grades 1, 2, and 3 disease, respectively. This study included patients with a median age of 69 years and a predominance of low-grade, low-stage tumors (for which it drew criticism); nevertheless, the study substantiated the concept that a significant subset of older men with low-risk disease do well on surveillance (61).

Albertsen and associates reported on 451 prostate cancer patients (mean age, 71 years) with a mean follow-up of 15.5 years (60). Patients received either no treatment or immediate or delayed hormonal therapy. The age-adjusted survival of men with Gleason scores 2 to 4 tumors was not significantly different from that of the general population. It should be borne in mind, however, that Gleason grade 2 tumors are rarely seen today in the United States. However, estimated loss-of-life expectancy among patients with Gleason scores 5 to 7 tumors was 4 to 5 years, and this subset of patients comprised 80% of the total group. Although this study showed that older men with well-differentiated disease do well with a WW approach, it can also be concluded that men with moderately and poorly differentiated disease had significantly decreased survival compared to a control population.

Similarly, a recent study by Johansson and associates involving 642 men with prostate cancer (there was a predominance of patients with favorable pathology) diagnosed between 1977 and 1984 reported that only 11% of 300 patients with clinically localized disease died of prostate cancer (62). The corrected 15-year survival rate was reported to be similar among patients treated by WW protocols and those treated at time of diagnosis.

Although it is generally well accepted that men with a life expectancy of fewer than 10 years are candidates for WW protocols, other reports have questioned a blanket policy of WW protocols for patients with low-risk disease. In this regard, Gronberg and associates reviewed 6,514 patients diagnosed with prostate cancer managed conservatively between 1971 and 1987, of whom approximately 85% died during the 7 to 23 years of follow-up (8). Prostate cancer–specific mortality was estimated to be 55%, and age at diagnosis was found to be a strong predictor of prostate cancer death. Patients diagnosed before the age of 60 years had an 80% risk of dying of prostate cancer, whereas those older than 80 years of age at diagnosis had less than a 50% risk of prostate cancer–related death.

McLaren and associates also reported high rates of clinical progression in patients with clinical T1 and T2 disease who were entered into WW protocols. Approximately 40% of T1 patients and 52% of T2 patients had clinical progression by 2 years (63).

Therefore, although advocates of WW protocols for clinically localized prostate cancer point out the advantages of avoiding potential morbidities from radical local therapies, it should also be borne in mind that WW protocols are not without significant potential problems. In a review of 514 patients with prostate cancer managed by WW protocols, Aus and associates reported that 319 patients (62%) died of prostate cancer. Of the patients who died of prostate cancer, 61% required one or more palliative therapies (TURP, external beam radiotherapy, or upper urinary tract diversion) before death. Furthermore, an average of 5 weeks was spent in the hospital because of prostate cancer (64).

It is generally well accepted that men with low-risk disease and a life expectancy of fewer than 10 years are candidates for WW protocols. However, younger patients with low-risk disease who enter WW protocols should only do so in the knowledge that there are risks of tumor de-differentiation and progression.

Recommendations for Treating Stage T1a Prostate Cancer

All patients with a presumptive diagnosis of stage T1a prostate cancer require restaging, as described earlier. For those patients in whom restaging confirms the presence of stage T1a disease, further management is generally made according to patient age and preference. Older men with a life expectancy of fewer than 10 to 12 years can be offered WW and restaged at a later date if there are clinical features of disease progression. Younger patients with life expectancies of 15 years or greater should be counseled regarding the possibility of disease progression, as described previously. In general, RP, external beam radiotherapy, and brachytherapy are all appropriate options in this subset of patients in view of their considerable life expectancy. The caveat is that these local therapies all carry with them the risk of significant side effects, whereas the risk of disease progression with time may remain low.

Recommendations for Treating Low-Risk Stage T1c Prostate Cancer

Low-volume disease on prostate needle biopsy, in combination with a Gleason score of less than 7 and a free to total serum PSA ratio that exceeds 15%, has a high positive predictive value with respect to predicting the presence of insignificant disease, as described earlier (39). Once again, therapy in this subset of patients is determined by patient age and preference. Therefore, just as with stage T1a disease, WW, RP, external beam radiotherapy, and brachytherapy are all options. In addition, ADT may be offered to some patients who desire treatment but remain skeptical regarding local therapies owing to possibilities of side effects. WW is appropriate for older patients, especially for those whose life expectancy is less than 10 to 12 years.

Recommendations for Treating Low-Risk Prostate Cancer in Older Men

Men older than the age of 70 years diagnosed with stage T1a, low-risk T1c disease or well-differentiated stage T2 disease are appropriate candidates for WW, especially if they have significant co-morbidities. Depending on patient preference and the treating physician's philosophy regarding early versus late ADT, some patients may elect to have no therapy until clinical evidence of disease progression occurs. By electing WW, the majority of such patients can optimize quality of life by avoiding side effects of local therapy or ADT, or both, which is especially advantageous in those patients whose prostate cancer never progresses clinically, which is probably the case in the majority of patients. Aggressive local therapy is probably inappropriate in this subset of patients.

CONCLUSION

Patients with newly diagnosed prostate cancer are often confronted with the difficult task of trying to understand their disease as well as the various treatment options. For patients with low-risk prostate cancer, the concept that their tumor may live in harmony with them is sometimes disturbing to patients and their families. The task of the physician, therefore, is to educate their patients in this regard, not only by spending time in the office, but also by recommending educational materials. Although this may be a time-consuming process, the patient with low-risk prostate cancer should be reminded that, by definition, time is on his side and that surveillance is in fact an active form of treatment.

REFERENCES

1. Newcomer LM, Stanford JL, Blumenstein BA. Temporal trends in rates of prostate cancer: declining incidence of advanced stage disease 1974 to 1994. *J Urol* 1997;158:1427–1430.
2. Catalona WJ, Smith DS. Cancer recurrence rates and survival rates after anatomic radical retropubic prostatectomy for prostate cancer: intermediate-term results. *J Urol* 1998;160: 2428–2434.
3. Walsh PC. Anatomic radical retropubic prostatectomy: evolution of the surgical technique. *J Urol* 1998;160:2418–2424.
4. Fowler FJ Jr., Barry MJ, Lu-Yao G, et al. Effect of radical prostatectomy for prostate cancer on patient quality of life: results from a Medicare survey. *Urology* 1995;45:1007–1013.
5. George NJ. Natural history of localised prostatic cancer managed by conservative therapy alone. *Lancet* 1988;1: 494–497.
6. Gronberg H, Damber L, Jonson H, et al. Prostate cancer mortality in northern Sweden, with special reference to tumor grade and patient age. *Urology* 1997;49:374–378.
7. Jewett HJ. The present status of radical prostatectomy for stages A and B prostatic cancer. *Urol Clin North Am* 1975;2: 105–124.
8. Sheldon CA, Williams RD, Fraley EE. Incidental carcinoma of the prostate: a review of the literature and critical reappraisal of classification. *J Urol* 1980;124:626–631.
9. Moore GH, Lawshe B, Murphy. Diagnosis of adenocarcinoma in transurethral resectates of the prostate gland. *Am J Surg Pathol* 1986;10:165–169.
10. Murphy WM, Dean PJ, Brasfield JA, et al. Incidental carcinoma of the prostate. How much sampling is adequate? *Am J Surg Pathol* 1986;10:170–174.
11. Cantrell BB, DeKlerk DP, Eggleston JC, et al. Pathological factors that influence prognosis in stage A prostatic cancer: the influence of extent versus grade. *J Urol* 1981;125:516–520.
12. Epstein JI, Paull G, Eggleston JC, et al. Prognosis of untreated stage A1 prostatic carcinoma: a study of 94 cases with extended followup. *J Urol* 1986;136:837–839.
13. Zincke H, Blute ML, Fallen MJ, et al. Radical prostatectomy for stage A adenocarcinoma of the prostate: staging errors and their implications for treatment recommendations and disease outcome. *J Urol* 1991;146:1053–1058.
14. Larsen MP, Carter HB, Epstein JI. Can stage A1 tumor extent be predicted by transurethral resection tumor volume, per cent or grade? A study of 6 stage A1 radical prostatectomies with comparison to prostate removed for stages A2 and B disease. *J Urol* 1991;146:1059–1063.
15. Paulson DF, Robertson JE, Daubert LM, et al. Radical prostatectomy in stage A prostatic adenocarcinoma. *J Urol* 1998;140:535–539.
16. Voges GE, McNeal JE, Redwine EA, et al. The predictive significance of substaging stage A prostate cancer (A1 versus A2) for volume and grade of total cancer in the prostate. *J Urol* 1992;147:858–863.
17. Greene DR, Rogers E, Wessels EC, et al. Some small prostate cancers are nondiploid by nuclear image analysis: correlation of deoxyribonucleic acid ploidy status and pathological features. *J Urol* 1994;151:1301–1307.
18. Borre M, Hoyer M, Nerstrom B, et al. DNA ploidy and survival of patients with clinically localized prostate cancer treated without intent to cure. *Prostate* 1998;36:244–249.
19. Brinker DA, Ross JS, Tran TA, et al. Can ploidy of prostate carcinoma diagnosed on needle biopsy predict radical prostatectomy stage and grade? *J Urol* 1999;162:2036–2039.
20. Greene DR, Egawa S, Neerhut G, et al. The distribution of residual cancer in radical prostatectomy specimens in stage A prostate cancer. *J Urol* 1991;145:324–328.

21. Lowe BA, Barry JM. The predictive accuracy of staging transurethral resection of the prostate in the management of stage A cancer of the prostate: a comparative evaluation. *J Urol* 1990;143:1142–1145.
22. Ingerman A, Broderick G, Williams RD, et al. Negative repeat transurethral resection of prostate fails to identify patients with stage A1 prostatic carcinoma at lower risk of progression: a long-term study. *Urology* 1993;42:528–532.
23. Terris MK, McNeal JE, Stamey TA. Transrectal ultrasound imaging and ultrasound guided prostate biopsies in the detection of residual carcinoma in clinical stage A carcinoma of the prostate. *J Urol* 1992;147:864–869.
24. Grups JW, Gruss A, Wirth M, et al. Diagnostic value of transrectal ultrasound in tumor staging and in the detection of incidental prostatic cancer. *Urol Int* 1990;45:38–40.
25. Lee F, Torp-Pedersen ST, Carroll JT, et al. Use of transrectal ultrasound and prostate-specific antigen in diagnosis of prostatic intraepithelial neoplasia. *Urology* 1989; 34(6 Suppl):4–8.
26. Seth S, Hamper UM, Walsh PC, et al. Stage A adenocarcinoma of the prostate: transrectal US and sonographic-pathologic correlation. *Radiology* 1991;179:35–39.
27. Egawa S, Greene DR, Flanagan WF, et al. Transrectal ultrasonography in stage A prostate cancer: detection of residual tumor after transurethral resection of prostate. *J Urol* 1991;146:366–371.
28. Carroll PR, Sugimura K, Cohen MB, et al. Detection and staging of prostatic carcinoma after transurethral resection or open enucleation of the prostate: accuracy of magnetic resonance imaging. *J Urol* 1992;147:402–406.
29. Milestone BN, Seidman EJ. Endorectal coil magnetic resonance imaging of prostate cancer. *Semin Urol* 1995;13:113–121.
30. Quinn SF, Franzini DA, Demlow TA, et al. MR imaging of prostate cancer with an endorectal surface coil technique: correlation with whole-mount specimens. *Radiology* 1994; 190:323–327.
31. Yu KK, Scheidler J, Hricak H, et al. Prostate cancer: prediction of extracapsular extension with endorectal MR imaging and three-dimensional proton MR spectroscopic imaging. *Radiology* 1999;213:481–488.
32. Dietrick DD, McNeal JE, Stamey TA. Core cancer length in ultrasound-guided systematic sextant biopsies: a preoperative evaluation of prostate cancer volume. *Urology* 1995; 45:987–992.
33. Cohen MK, Riggs MW, Brawn PN, et al. Serum prostate-specific antigen levels in stage A1 prostatic cancer. *Am J Clin Pathol* 1993;100:127–129.
34. Belville WD, Vaccaro JA, Kiesling VJ Jr. Prostate-specific antigen and digital rectal examination in long-term follow-up of stage A1 prostate carcinoma. *Urology* 1992;39:586–588.
35. Feneley MR, Webb JA, McLean A, et al. Post-operative serial prostate-specific antigen and transrectal ultrasound for staging incidental carcinoma of the prostate. *Br J Urol* 1997;75:14–20.
36. Epstein JI, Chan DW, Sokoll LJ, et al. Nonpalpable stage T1c prostate cancer: prediction of insignificant disease using free/total prostate specific antigen levels and needle biopsy findings. *J Urol* 1998;160:2407–2411.
37. Brawn PN. The dedifferentiation of prostate cancer. *Cancer* 1983;52:246–251.
38. Zhang G, Wasserman NF, Sidi AA, et al. Long-term followup results after expectant management of stage A1 prostatic cancer. *J Urol* 1991;146:99–102.
39. Blute ML, Zincke H, Farrow GM. Long-term followup of young patients with stage A adenocarcinoma of the prostate. *J Urol* 1986;136:840–843.
40. Roy CR 2nd, Horne D, Raife M, et al. Incidental carcinoma of prostate, long-term follow-up. *Urology* 1990;36: 210–213.
41. Brawn PN, Johnson EH, Speights VO, et al. Long-term survival of stage A prostate carcinoma, atypical hyperplasia/adenosis and BPH. *Br J Cancer* 1994;69:1098–1101.
42. Thompson IM, Zeidman EJ. Extended follow-up of stage A1 carcinoma of prostate. *Urology* 1989;33:455–458.
43. Whitmore WF Jr., Warner JA, Thompson IM Jr. Expectant management of localized prostatic cancer. *Cancer* 1991;67: 1091–1096.
44. Elgamal AA, Van Poppel HP, Van de Voorde WM, et al. Impalpable invisible stage T1c prostate cancer: characteristics and clinical relevance in 100 radical prostatectomy specimens—a different view. *J Urol* 1997;157:244–250.
45. Douglas TH, McLeod DG, Mostofi FK, et al. Prostate-specific antigen-detected prostate cancer (stage T1c): an analysis of whole-mount prostatectomy specimens. *Prostate* 1997;32:59–64.
46. Goto Y, Ohori M, Arakawa A, et al. Distinguishing clinically important from unimportant prostate cancers before treatment: value of systematic biopsies. *J Urol* 1996;156: 1059–1063.
47. Lerner SE, Seay TM, Blute ML, et al. Prostate specific antigen detected prostate cancer (clinical stage T1c): an interim analysis. *J Urol* 1996;155:821–826.
48. Humphrey PA, Keetch DW, Smith DS, et al. Prospective characterization of pathological features of prostatic carcinomas detected via serum prostate specific antigen based screening. *J Urol* 1996;155:816–820.
49. Epstein JI, Walsh PC, Carmichael M, et al. Pathologic and clinical findings to predict tumor extent of nonpalpable (stage T1c) prostate cancer. *JAMA* 1994;271:368–374.
50. Carter HB, Sauvageot J, Walsh PC, et al. Prospective evaluation of men with stage T1C adenocarcinoma of the prostate. *J Urol* 1997;157:2206–2209.
51. D'Amico AV, Renshaw AA, Schultz D, et al. The impact of the biopsy Gleason score on PSA outcome for prostate cancer patients with PSA < or = 10 ng/ml and T1c,2a: implications for patient selection for prostate-only therapy. *Int J Radiat Oncol Biol Phys* 1999;45:847–851.
52. Renshaw AA, Richie JP, Loughlin KR, et al. Maximum diameter of prostatic carcinoma is a simple, inexpensive, and independent predictor of prostate-specific antigen failure in radical prostatectomy specimens. Validation in a cohort of 434 patients. *Am J Clin Pathol* 1999;111:641–644.
53. D'Amico AV, Chang H, Holupka E, et al. Calculated prostate cancer volume: the optimal predictor of actual cancer volume and pathologic stage. *Urology* 1997;49:385–391.
54. Mikuz G. Pathology of prostate cancer. Old problems and new facts. *Adv Clin Path* 1997;1:21–34.

55. Montie JE, Wood D Jr., Pontes E, et al. Adenocarcinoma of the prostate in cystoprostatectomy specimens removed for bladder cancer. *Cancer* 1989;63:381–385.
56. Ohori M, Wheeler TM, Dunn JK, et al. The pathological features and prognosis of prostate cancer detectable with current diagnostic tests. *J Urol* 1994;152:1714–1720.
57. Middleton RG, Thompson IM, Austenfeld MS, et al. Prostate Cancer Clinical Guidelines Panel Summary report on the management of clinically localized prostate cancer. The American Urological Association. *J Urol* 1995;154:2144–2148.
58. Wasson JH, Cushman CC, Bruskewitz RC, et al. A structured literature review of treatment for localized prostate cancer. Prostate Disease Patient Outcome Research Team [Published erratum appears in *Arch Fam Med* 1993;2:1030]. *Arch Fam Med* 1993;2:487–493.
59. Chodak GW, Thisted RA, Gerber GS, et al. Results of conservative management of clinically localized prostate cancer. *N Engl J Med* 1994;330:242–248.
60. Albertsen PC, Fryback DG, Storer BE, et al. Long-term survival among men with conservatively treated localized prostate cancer. *JAMA* 1995;274:626–631.
61. Klopukh BV, Djavan B, Kadesky K, et al. High false positive rates of fine needle aspiration leads to overly optimistic assessment of outcomes of conservative treatment for localized prostate cancer. *J Urol* 1995;153:496A.
62. Johansson JE, Holmberg L, Johansson S, et al. Fifteen-year survival in prostate cancer. A prospective, population-based study in Sweden [Published erratum appears in *JAMA* 1997;278:206]. *JAMA* 1997;277:467–471.
63. McLaren DB, McKenzie M, Duncan G, et al. Watchful waiting or watchful progression? Prostate specific antigen doubling times and clinical behavior in patients with early untreated prostate carcinoma. *Cancer* 1998;82:342–348.
64. Aus G, Hugosson J, Norlen L. Need for hospital care and palliative treatment for prostate cancer treated with non-curative intent. *J Urol* 1995;154:466–469.

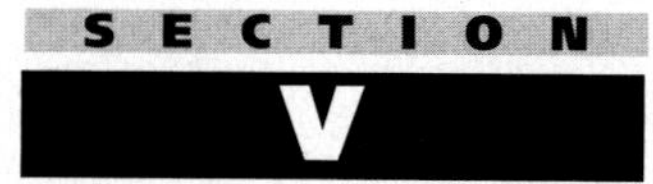

EARLY PROSTATE CANCER—MULTIMODALITY TREATMENT

28

COMBINED EXTERNAL BEAM RADIATION THERAPY OR BRACHYTHERAPY AND HORMONES

JOYCELYN L. SPEIGHT
MACK ROACH III

The nonsurgical management of prostate cancer has increased dramatically over the last decade. The vast majority of patients managed without surgery receive some form of radiotherapy with or without hormone replacement therapy (HRT). The expanding interest in radiotherapy may arise in part from the fact that long-term survival rates with radiotherapy appear to be equivalent to those achieved with radical prostatectomy (8,46,48,49,62,88,89). The optimal management of clinically localized prostate cancer is one of the most common, challenging, and controversial areas for patients and physicians. For no other site is there so much disagreement among "experts" as to who should have surgery, radiotherapy, or receive HRT alone or in combination with one of these other modalities. To make matters more confusing, there are numerous ways to deliver therapeutic radiation, including external photon radiotherapy, intensity-modulated radiotherapy, proton and neutron beam irradiation, and brachytherapy, with no clear consensus as to which radiotherapy option is best. What is clear is that certain patients may be better suited for one or another or, in fact, a combination of these modalities.

This chapter attempts to summarize the existing literature defining the role of HRT combined with two of the most commonly used types of radiotherapy: x-ray–based external beam radiation therapy (EBRT) and brachytherapy.

SELECTION PRINCIPLES FOR TREATMENT

The patient who would derive the greatest survival benefit from treatment of clinically localized prostate cancer is the patient who has the highest risk of dying from prostate cancer. It will be difficult to identify a therapeutic intervention that reduces the prostate-specific mortality by 50% in low-risk patients, because such large numbers of patients would be required just to detect a decrease in risk from 10% to 5%. Furthermore, the impact of therapy is diluted when patients cured of their prostate cancer die of other causes. This fact grows out of a reality that competing causes of death dictate the overall survival (OS) in the first 10 to 15 years for men who have low-risk disease.

Albertsen et al. (2) retrospectively evaluated the risk of death from expectantly managed prostate cancer in a cohort of men stratified by age and tumor histology [Gleason score (GS)]. Evaluated in the context of treatment outcome data, their data support the notion that the patients for whom a survival benefit from treatment can be demonstrated are those who have the greatest risk of dying from prostate cancer. Men ages 55 to 74 years with well-differentiated tumors (GS 2 to 5) have minimal risk of death from prostate cancer and are much more likely to die from competing causes, such as heart disease, during the first 15 years after diagnosis. Conversely, during this same period, men with poorly differentiated tumors (GS 7 to 10) have the highest risk for death, regardless of their age at the time of diagnosis. Men with GS 6 tumors have an intermediate risk, with approximately 50% of men younger than 55 to 64 years alive at 15 years after diagnosis, whereas most older men (65 to 74 years) have died of competing causes (2). Aus et al. (5) and Chodak et al. (16) also demonstrated the impact of histologic grade on survival with lower cause-specific and disease-specific survival (DSS) rates seen in men with high-grade tumors.

In light of the effect of histologic grade on DSS and cause-specific survival, it can be surmised that the radiotherapy dose needed to achieve maximal prostate-specific antigen (PSA) suppression may vary with risk as determined by pretreatment prognostic variables, such as PSA, GS, and stage.

DEFINING HIGH-RISK DISEASE

Having concluded that the benefit of treatment varies with the risk for recurrence or death due to prostate cancer, it is important to define how risk is determined and assigned to patients. This is particularly important, because risk estimates are often central to the treatment choices that are recommended.

Several studies have demonstrated that pretreatment PSA level and GS are predictive of biochemical failure or death. Pretreatment PSA, although a very important screening tool, has not been validated as a surrogate to predict death. Other studies have identified DNA ploidy, the number of positive biopsies, p53 status, and prostatic acid phosphatase levels as having prognostic significance; however, these have not been widely validated.

Multivariate analysis of patients with clinically localized prostate cancer treated with EBRT alone on phase III Radiation Therapy Oncology Group (RTOG) trials between 1975 and 1992 (90,91,106) showed that centrally reviewed GS, clinical stage, and pathologic lymph node status correlate with DSS and OS. In this analysis, four distinct prognostic subgroups were defined, each with a predictable risk of death from prostate cancer. Each prognostic group and the 5-, 10-, and 15-year rates after EBRT treatment for each group are summarized in Table 28-1. Definitions of risk have typically used one or several of these variables to identify low-, intermediate-, and high-risk subgroups; however, no uniform definition for the determination of risk exists. This lack of consensus often makes it difficult to make meaningful comparisons between treatments and studies. The choice of a uniform risk model is one central issue that must be resolved before we can objectively decide what subgroups of patients will benefit from which of the available treatments. The current American Joint Committee on Cancer staging system does not appear to be very reliable in terms of defining the risk of recurrence after radiotherapy.

One of the first and most widely used nomograms to predict risk was developed by Partin (71,72). Kattan et al. subsequently developed nomograms to predict outcome

TABLE 28-1. DISEASE-SPECIFIC SURVIVAL BY RISK GROUPS: RADIATION THERAPY ONCOLOGY GROUP RANDOMIZED TRIALS, RADIOTHERAPY ALONE (1975–1992)

Group	Death/no.	5 yr (%)[a]	10 yr (%)[a]	15 yr (%)[a]
1	53/363	96 (94–98)	86 (82–90)	72 (62–83)
2	84/232	94 (92–97)	75 (70–81)	61 (51–72)
3	92/338	83 (79–87)	62 (55–70)	39 (26–60)
4	154/324	64 (58–70)	34 (27–42)	27 (20–37)

Note: Group 1 includes patients with a Gleason score (GS) = 2–6 and T1-2Nx; group 2 includes GS 2–6, T3Nx or N+, or GS 7, T1-2Nx; group 3 includes GS 7, T3Nx or N+, or GS 8–10, T1-2Nx; and group 4 includes GS 8–10, T3Nx, or N.

[a]95% confidence intervals in parentheses.

Modified from Roach M 3rd, Lu J, Pilepich MV. Four prognostic subgroups predict long-term survival from prostate cancer following radiotherapy alone on Radiation Therapy Oncology Group trials. *Int J Radiat Oncol Biol Phys* 2000;47:609–615.

after prostatectomy and, more recently, to predict relapse-free survival after three-dimensional conformal radiation therapy (3D CRT) treatment, based on pretreatment PSA and using dose as a variable (50). This model, although intriguing, is limited by its heavier weighting of PSA over GS, stage, and even the use of HRT. Several analyses have demonstrated that histologic grade is the single most predictive variable for outcome in the management of prostate cancer (77,90,91). Stage has also been validated as a significant independent variable, and the use of HRT to date has demonstrated the greatest impact on DSS and OS. Also of concern is the assumption that radiotherapy dose has a uniform effect for all patient subgroups. Several reports have already indicated that this is not the case. No dose effect has been demonstrated for patients whose disease features would classify them into low- or high-risk subgroups (44,81,100). Ultimately, this nomogram may not reliably predict death due to prostate cancer.

The inclusion of PSA as a continuous variable in a predictive model is important; however, although PSA may predict failure, as previously mentioned, it has not been validated as a surrogate for DSS or OS (59,78,92). Based on the published literature to date, the single most consistent factors that define patients with a high risk of death due to prostate cancer include GS of 7 or greater, lymph node status, and bulky palpable disease. Pretreatment serum PSA greater than 20 ng per mL correlates with increased risk of distant metastases and the need for salvage hormone therapy. With longer follow-up times, PSA greater than 20 ng per mL may indeed be predictive for survival.

TREATMENT STRATEGIES

Historically, clinically assessed rates of local control and disease-free status underestimated local failure rates, owing to the presence of occult disease. The incidence of positive biopsies after radiotherapy treatment has been reported to range from 21% to 93% in various series (7,18,53,70,94–96). Prostate biopsy status at 24 to 36 months postradiotherapy is an independent predictor of outcome, although its accuracy is confounded by the high percentage of indeterminate biopsies (19).

Many attempts to decrease local failure rates have been focused on dose escalation to overcome the "intrinsic resistance" of prostate cancer cells (28). Several retrospective (Table 28-2) studies and prospective, nonrandomized dose escalation trials (Table 28-3) have suggested improvements in PSA response, freedom from PSA failure, and disease-free survival (DFS) with the use of higher radiation doses in some patient subgroups. The optimum dose has not yet been determined; however, it is apparent that treating to higher radiotherapy doses alone is not the complete solution for the question of how to improve local control with EBRT for some patient subgroups. Retrospective analyses

TABLE 28-2. PROSPECTIVE RADIOTHERAPY DOSE ESCALATION TRIALS

Author (ref)	Results	Comments
Zelefsky et al. (114)	Intermediate- and high-risk patients did better with doses ≥75.6 Gy	Sequential dose escalation, with shorter median follow-up for higher doses.
Pollack et al. (83)	Improved biochemical control for patients with PSA >10 ng/mL	Only published randomized trial; used conventional and conformal techniques.
Michalski et al. (68,69)	Better than expected tolerance to higher doses (79.2 Gy max)	Phase II randomized trial.
Bey et al. (9)	Higher probability of achieving PSA nadir ≤1 ng/mL with doses >74 Gy	All 3D CRT; sequential dose escalation. Significantly shorter follow-up in high-dose group (17.5 mo vs. 30 mo).

3D CRT, three-dimensional conformal radiation therapy; max, maximum; PSA, prostate-specific antigen.

have failed to identify a benefit to biochemical no evidence of disease (bNED) from higher radiotherapy doses for high-risk patients (100,101). Mounting evidence from randomized and nonrandomized trials suggests that the addition of neoadjuvant or adjuvant therapies may be part of the answer. HRT has been the most widely evaluated adjuvant therapy to date.

RATIONALE FOR COMBINED HORMONE THERAPY AND EXTERNAL BEAM RADIATION THERAPY

For more than 50 years, androgen ablation has been recognized as an important tool in the management of locally advanced prostate cancer. The hormone-responsive nature of prostate cancer was first recognized in 1941 by Huggins and Hodges (47), who demonstrated that advanced prostate cancer responded to surgical castration. Pharmacologic agents that modify androgen production or its ability to interact with prostate cancer cells, or both, have provided nonsurgical alternatives to orchiectomy. The historical evolution of the studies, which have led to the widespread interest in the use of HRT, has been elegantly described elsewhere.

Androgen deprivation significantly reduces the volume of the hormone-responsive tumor. *In vivo*, androgen-sensitive tumors show a significant regression in volume (greater than 90%) after orchiectomy. *In vitro*, a cessation of cell division was noted in Shinogyi cell lines when grown in an androgen-free medium (61,111). Tumor cytoreduction resulted in improved oxygenation and an associated increase in radiosensitivity (80). *In vivo* and *in vitro* experiments have documented a decrease in the radiotherapy dose needed to kill 50% of a tumor cell population (TCD50) when androgen suppression is administered before radiation. The greatest incremental decrease in TCD50 is seen when EBRT is applied at the point of maximal androgen suppression and tumor shrinkage (111).

TABLE 28-3. RETROSPECTIVE STUDIES DEMONSTRATING A DOSE RESPONSE WITH RADIOTHERAPY IN INTERMEDIATE- AND HIGH-RISK PATIENTS

Author (ref)	Risk groups	Results
Roach et al. (88)	Gleason score 8–10, PSA <20 ng/mL	Improve bNED rates with dose >71.5 Gy
Pollack et al. (82)	PSA ≥4–10 ng/mL, PSA >10 ng/mL	Improved bNED with dose >67–77 Gy for PSA >4–10 and >77 Gy for PSA >20ng/mL
Hanks et al. (43)	PSA >10 ng/mL	Improved 5-year bNED with dose >75.52 Gy
Fiveash et al. (29)	T1-T2, Gleason score 8–10	Improved bNED with dose > 70 Gy
Pinover et al. (79)	PSA <10 ng/mL, T2b-T3, GS ≥7, or PNI	Improved bNED with dose ≥76 Gy
Hanks et al. (42)	Unfavorable PSA <10 ng/mL, unfavorable PSA = 10–19.9 ng/mL, and favorable PSA >20 ng/mL	Improved 5-yr bNED rates with 75–80 Gy for unfavorable patients with PSA <20 ng/mL and favorable patients with PSA levels >20 ng/mL
Kupelian (54)	Essentially all subgroups, most noticeable for GS ≥7	Improved bNED and DFS with dose ≥72 Gy
Pollack et al. (81)	T1-T2, PSA >10 ng/mL	Improved bNED with dose >67–77, no benefit with dose >77 Gy
Speight et al. (100)	Essentially all groups except <0% or >35% risk of lymph node involvement	Improved freedom from PSA failure with dose >69 Gy, no benefit with dose >77 Gy
Valecenti et al. (106)	Gleason score 8–10	Improved DSS and OS with dose >66 Gy

bNED, biochemical no evidence of disease; DFS, disease-free survival; DSS, Disease-specific survival; GS, Gleason score; OS, overall survival; PNI, perineural invasion; PSA, prostate-specific antigen.

The distinct mechanisms of action of radiotherapy and hormone ablation suggest a rationale for their combined use. The pathophysiologic mechanism of EBRT is the formation of nonrepairable DNA double strand breaks (40) and the induction of programmed cell death or apoptosis (99). Cytoreduction induced by hormone blockade may improve radiocurability by decreasing the number of logs of cell kill required for tumor sterilization. Studies have confirmed an inverse ratio between tumor volume and control with EBRT (42). Clinical trials appear to support this finding and are discussed later. The combined use of androgen ablation and EBRT appears to cause additive or augmented cell killing, or both. Neoadjuvant androgen ablation in effect "primes" the machine to sterilize androgen-dependent cell clones. Androgen-independent cells remain susceptible to EBRT-mediated DNA damage, as well as EBRT-induced activation of the apoptotic pathway. Experimental and clinical data support the existence of a synergistic interaction between EBRT and total androgen suppresion (TAS), with combined modality treatment yielding better treatment responses than either modality alone.

The theoretical basis, then, for combined HRT and EBRT is derived from experimental and clinical data that suggest a synergistic interaction between hormonal deprivation therapy and radiation therapy that leads to increased local and regional cell killing (99,109,111). This hypothesis has been confirmed in animal models (99,111).

HORMONE THERAPY AND EXTERNAL BEAM RADIATION THERAPY

Retrospective evaluations comparing androgen deprivation given in conjunction with radiotherapy compared to radiotherapy alone for patients with clinically localized prostate cancer have noted significant improvements in local control and DFS. An OS benefit has not, however, been consistently demonstrated.

Since the first randomized, multiinstitutional trial from Del Regato (23), the preponderance of data from prospective randomized trials demonstrates improvements in OS and DSS with the use of androgen-suppressive therapy alone or in conjunction with radiotherapy. Table 28-4 summarizes the results of several prospective randomized trials.

The Medical Research Council of Great Britain (66) completed one of the first randomized trials to demonstrate a survival advantage for the use of early HRT in patients with locally advanced and metastatic disease. This study reinforced the concept of hormone ablation as a first-line therapy in the management of prostate cancer.

RTOG 85-31 evaluated the effect of long-term goserelin monotherapy after radiotherapy compared with radiotherapy alone. A significant improvement in local control, biochemical control, rate of distant metastases, and cause-specific survival was demonstrated for patients with nonbulky, stage T3 disease and node-positive disease at 5 and 8 years. A subset analysis demonstrated a significant survival advantage to long-term goserelin monotherapy for GS 8 to 10 patients treated with primary radiotherapy (74,76).

The results of RTOG 86-10, which evaluated the use of 4 months of combined hormone ablation with goserelin and flutamide in men with bulky T2 and T3 tumors, were initially reported in 1995. Improvements in local control, DFS, distant metastasis–free survival, and biochemical control were seen at 5 years of follow-up (75). An update of 86-10 showed a significant improvement in absolute survival at 8 years for patients with GS 2 to 6 tumors (72% vs. 52%, $p = .015$) who received 2 months of neoadjuvant hormone ablation followed by 2 months of therapy administered concurrently with EBRT (76). Hormone suppression–related improvements in local control, rate of distant metastases, and cause-specific mortality remained significant. No benefit from short-term androgen ablation was seen for patients with bulky GS 7 to 10 tumors.

Laverdiere et al. reported a 65% incidence of positive biopsies at 2 years for patients treated with radiotherapy alone, compared to a 28% positive biopsy rate when 3 months of HRT preceded radiotherapy. More impressive was the significant decrease in incidence of positive biopsies when hormonal ablation therapy was continued after the completion of radiotherapy, for a total of 10 months (28% vs. 5%, $p < .0001$) (57). This study not only demonstrated the benefit of the use of hormone therapy in patients with earlier stages of disease, but also was one of the first studies to demonstrate the inadequacy of conventional doses of radiation (64 Gy) for tumor eradication.

The EORTC incorporated 1 month of neoadjuvant androgen blockade before radiotherapy followed by 3 years of a gonadotropin-releasing hormone agonist after the completion of EBRT. Statistically significant improvements in local control, DFS, and OS were noted at 5 years (12) for patients receiving hormone ablation over those treated with radiotherapy alone ($p = .001$).

Preliminary results from RTOG 92-02, a prospective randomized trial evaluating the duration of androgen ablation in stage T2c-T4 patients, demonstrated a significant improvement in DFS, time to clinical local progression, freedom from distant metastases, biochemical control, and OS with long-term (26-month) hormone suppression therapy. This trial establishes long-term HRT as the standard of care for locally advanced (GS 8 to 10) patients (42).

These studies have predominantly evaluated patients with locally advanced disease. The data support the use of long-term adjuvant HRT in this group of patients. One significant question that remains unanswered is whether patients with earlier stages of disease will benefit from HRT. RTOG 94-08, a four-arm phase III trial evaluating the role of endocrine therapy in good-prognosis, locally confined prostate adenocarcinoma, addresses this question. Until the results of this study are available, some insight may be gleaned from retrospective analyses.

TABLE 28-4. RANDOMIZED TRIALS: ANDROGEN BLOCKADE + EXTERNAL BEAM RADIATION THERAPY VERSUS EXTERNAL BEAM RADIATION THERAPY ALONE

Study	Study design	Results
Medical Research Council [MRC (1997) (66)]	Immediate vs. delayed androgen suppression (orchiectomy + GRHa) for locally advanced M0 and M1 patients	Improved OS for M0 disease at 10 yr
RTOG 85-31 (58,74,76)	EBRT + adjuvant GRHa vs. EBRT alone	Improved LC, DFS, and decreased DM with adjuvant GRHa, improved OS for GS 8–10 patients
RTOG 86-10 (76)	nCAB × 2 mo then CAB + EBRT vs. EBRT alone	Improved LC, PFS, and time to DM with 4 mo, CAB at 5 yr, improved OS in T3, GS 2–6 patients at 8 yr, no benefit to short-term CAB in GS 7–10
Canadian trial [Laverdiere et al. (1997) (57)]	nCAB × 3 mo then EBRT vs. nCAB + EBRT then CAB × 6 mo vs. EBRT alone	Decreased positive biopsy rates at 6 and 12 mo with CAB, long-term better than short-term; decreased median PSA at 12 mo with CAB
EORTC trial [Bolla et al. (1997) (12)]	EBRT + CAB[a] × 1 mo then GRHa × 3 yr vs. EBRT alone	Improved LC, time to progression, DFS, and OS at 5 yr with GRHa
Swedish study [Granfors et al. (1998) (39)]	Orchiectomy + EBRT vs. EBRT alone for T1-4, pN0-3, M0 patients	Improved PFS, DFS, and OS for orchiectomy + EBRT; early androgen deprivation better than delayed
RTOG 92-02 [Hanks et al. (2000) (42)]	4 mo neoadjuvant/concurrent CAB + EBRT with vs. without 2-yr adjuvant CAB	Improved DFS and OS at 5 yr with long-term CAB for GS 8–10

CAB, combined androgen blockade (GRHa + flutamide); DFS, disease-free survival; DM, distant metastases; EBRT, external beam radiation therapy; EORTC, European Organization for Research and Treatment of Cancer; GRHa, gonadotropin-releasing hormone agonist; GS, Gleason score; LC, local control; OS, overall survival; PFS, progression-free survival; RTOG, Radiation Therapy Oncology Group.
[a]CAB = GRHa + Androcur.

Improved local-regional control and freedom from PSA relapse have been reported in intermediate- and high-risk patients treated with hormone suppression and EBRT (21,91,107). D'Amico et al. evaluated 5-year PSA outcome after EBRT with or without 6 months of HRT. A significant advantage was seen from the use of HRT in intermediate-risk (stage T2b, GS 7, or PSA 10.1 to 20.0 ng per mL) and high-risk (stage T2c, GS 8, or PSA greater than 20 ng per mL) patients. There was a trend for improved biochemical control for low-risk patients treated with combined modality therapy ($p = .09$) (21).

Vicini et al. reviewed the literature on androgen deprivation and EBRT in patients with localized prostate cancer. Conflicting results were obtained regarding a beneficial effect of hormone suppression on OS; however, a trend toward improved local-regional control and freedom from PSA relapse was identified (107).

A metaanalysis of men treated on RTOG trials from 1975 to 1992 supports the use of short-term (4-month) hormone suppression in risk group 2 (T3Nx, GS 2 to 6 or N+, GS 2 to 6 or T1-2Nx, or GS 7) patients. A DSS advantage is noted at 5 and 8 years; however, no overall specific survival was seen (Fig. 28-1) (91). The absence of a significant survival benefit may be owing to the wide variation in risk across the subgroup, which includes early (stage T1-T1) and locally advanced (T3, N+) patients. When the

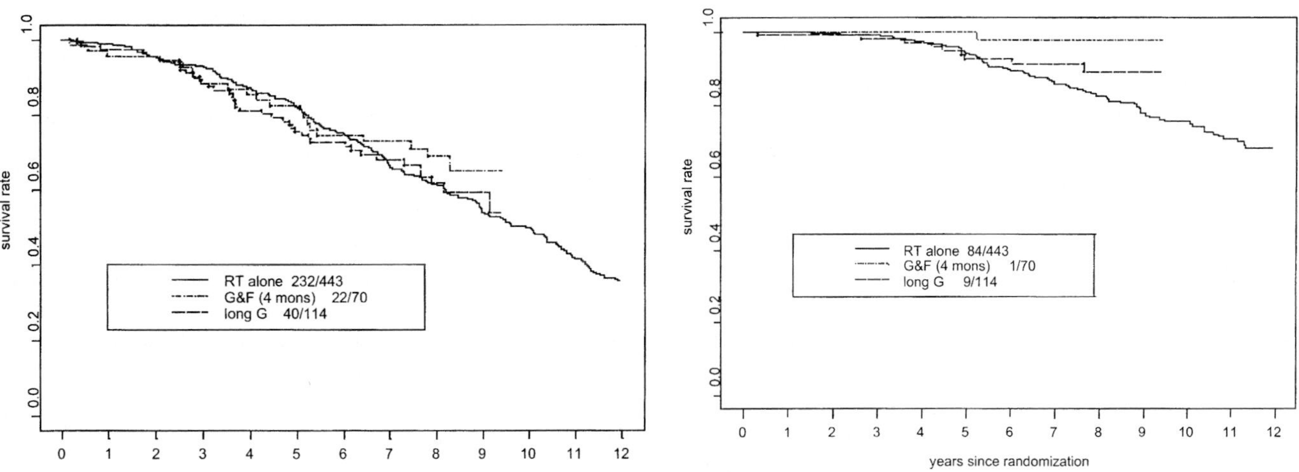

FIGURE 28-1. **A, B:** Overall and disease-specific survival for groups 1 and 2 by treatment type. F, flutamide; G, goserelin; RT, radiation therapy.

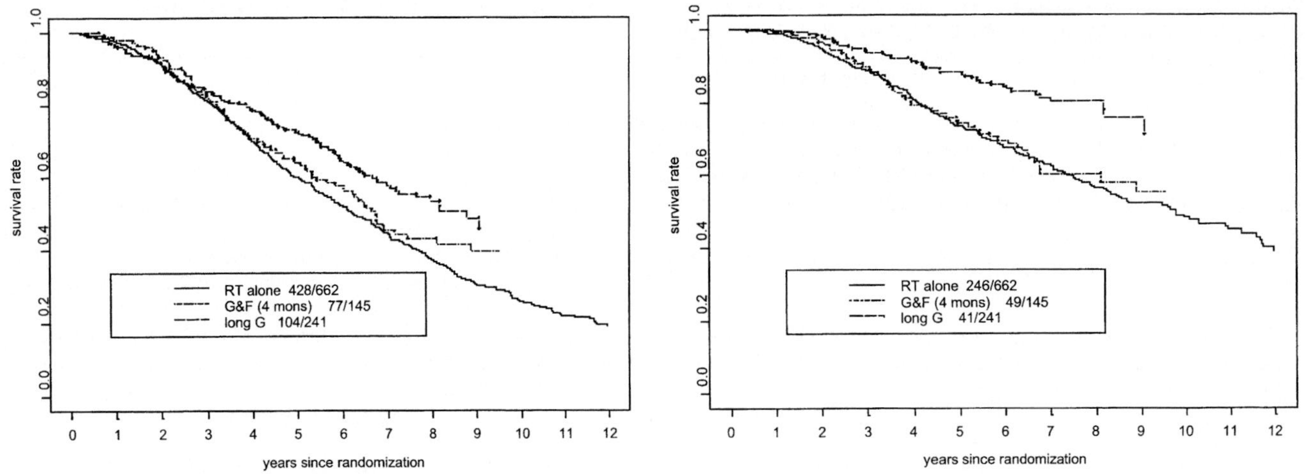

FIGURE 28-2. A, B: Overall and disease-specific survival for groups 3 and 4 by treatment type. F, flutamide; G, goserelin; RT, radiation therapy.

analysis is limited to patients with bulky tumors, the same group of patients evaluated in RTOG 86-10, a statistically significant survival advantage becomes apparent. This corroborates the findings of RTOG 86-10 (76). "High-intermediate"–risk group 3 patients (T3Nx, GS 7 or N+, GS 7 or T1-2, or GS 8 to 10) did not benefit from 4 months of hormone ablative therapy (Fig. 28-2).

HORMONE THERAPY AND EXTERNAL BEAM RADIATION THERAPY IN NODE-POSITIVE PATIENTS

The outcomes for patients with node-positive disease treated with regional therapy alone have been disappointing. The vast majority of patients treated with radiotherapy alone has evidence of local regional failure or biochemical failure at 5 years (45). Trials examining the use of HRT in conjunction with radiotherapy have been more promising (93,108,110).

A subset analysis of pathologic node-positive patients enrolled in RTOG 85-31 showed better rates of PSA control with the use of HRT plus radiotherapy compared to radiotherapy alone (55% vs. 11%) (58). Two randomized trials have confirmed a survival advantage for the early use of hormone ablation in locally advanced and lymph node–positive patients. Surgically staged node-positive patients (T1-4, N1-N3, and M0) who were treated with orchiectomy and radiotherapy had significantly reduced mortality (p = .02) and improved cause-specific survival (p = .06) and time to disease progression, compared to node-positive patients treated with radiotherapy alone (39). The work of Messing et al. (67) further supports early hormone-suppressive therapy over delayed therapy. Postprostatectomy, node-positive patients treated with immediate androgen ablation had better OS (p = .02), DFS (p <.01), and bNED survival (p <.001) compared to similar patients who did not receive ablative therapy until disease progression (67).

HORMONE THERAPY AND BRACHYTHERAPY

Several studies have suggested that low-risk patients (stage T2a or less, PSA less than 10, or GS of 6 or less) have equivalent PSA control rates when treated with seed implants or EBRT (13,113,115). Biochemical control rates for intermediate- and high-risk patients (stage T2b or greater, PSA 10 or greater, GS of 7 or greater) have been reported in some studies to be higher when treated with the addition of EBRT compared to implant alone (13,20,38,87). Other analyses have failed to find a benefit for brachytherapy plus EBRT in this same group of patients (10,84). High-risk patients (GS 8 to 10 or PSA less than or equal to 20 ng per mL) have better biochemical control with EBRT. Neither treatment alone is effective for patients with PSA greater than 20, regardless of stage or GS (13). One small series reported by King et al. found that patients treated with seed implants did better than patients treated with EBRT (52). However, the patients treated with EBRT in this series received suboptimal radiation doses, and a higher percentage of the patients had high-risk features.

No randomized trials have been completed that examine the role of hormone suppression for patients treated with brachytherapy. A retrospective matched pair analysis failed to identify an improvement in OS or relapse-free survival for relatively low-risk patients treated with hormone suppression and brachytherapy compared to those treated with brachytherapy alone. Stratification by GS, pretreatment PSA, and stage also failed to identify a subgroup that benefits from hormone suppression (85).

Prospective studies have examined the efficacy of androgen ablation given in conjunction with EBRT and brachytherapy.

In a series from the Seattle Prostate Institute, the addition of hormone suppression did not significantly increase freedom from PSA failure (103); however, patient numbers were small, and follow-up was short at the time of reporting. Stone and Stock reported significant improvement in freedom from biochemical failure at 4 years for intermediate-risk patients (stage T2b or greater, GS greater than 6, PSA greater than 10 ng per mL) treated with 5 months of hormone ablation in addition to brachytherapy over a similar group of patients treated with brachytherapy alone (102). An update reported significant improvements in biochemical control for high-risk patients (two or more high-risk features) treated with hormone ablation with brachytherapy versus brachytherapy alone (60).

At this time, the primary benefit from the short-term use of HRT before brachytherapy in low-risk patients appears to be limited to volume reduction of the prostate. This helps to eliminate pubic arch interference, decrease urinary morbidity, and improve dosimetric coverage. Intermediate- and high-risk patients may benefit from the addition of HRT when treated with brachytherapy. High-risk patients, however, probably require more aggressive management, and the addition of EBRT is warranted. Randomized trials have been planned that will address this question.

COMBINED ANDROGEN BLOCKADE VERSUS MONOTHERAPY

Several studies have documented the presence and intraprostatic effect of dihydrotestosterone (DHT), the 5-alpha reduction product of testosterone and active intraprostatic androgen (4,30–37,55,56,98). Based on animal data, it has been recognized that although only 5% of serum DHT comes from the adrenal glands, approximately 40% of intraprostatic DHT is derived from the conversion of the adrenal androgens within the prostate gland (30,55,56).

Medical and surgical castration reduce serum testosterone levels by 90% to 95%; however, moderate intraprostatic DHT levels exist, suggesting that plasma androgens, which remain detectable in this setting, may be a relatively significant source of DHT. High levels of DHT have been demonstrated in prostate tissue samples obtained from men at the time of relapse after monotherapy (36). Even low levels of DHT within the gland may prevent maximal tumor suppression within the prostate, and the previously mentioned studies provide a strong rationale for the use of combined hormone blockade in men with prostate cancer.

The results of randomized trials comparing combined androgen blockade (CAB) therapy to monotherapy for metastatic disease have been inconclusive (Table 28-5). Eighteen trials have reported no significant difference in OS with the use of CAB (1). Three of these 18 trials, however, did report a trend toward improved survival, favoring CAB (17,24,26). Three other trials have suggested a significant advantage for OS with maximal hormone suppression, with median increase in survival ranging from 3.7 to 7.0 months and an increase in 5-year survival ranging from 3% to 9% (17,24,26). Two metaanalyses of CAB studies were also contradictory. The first, published in *Lancet* (86), found only a 2- to 3-month survival advantage to the use of CAB. The analysis by Chaubet et al.

TABLE 28-5. SELECTED CLINICAL TRIALS COMPARING MONOTHERAPY VERSUS COMBINED ANDROGEN BLOCKADE

Author (yr) (ref)	Type of study	Subgroups	Comments
Tyrell (1991) (105)	Prospective randomized multicenter	T3-T4 or any T, M + goserelin + flutamide vs. goserelin alone	No difference in relapse rate, time to progression or overall survival at 2 yr; 57% patients had distant metastasis
Crawford (1990) (17)	Randomized	D2, leuprolide + flutamide vs. leuprolide + placebo	Longer progression-free survival and increased median duration of survival with CAB, greatest benefit in patients with minimal disease
Denis (1998) (24)	Phase III prospective randomized	Any T, M + goserelin + flutamide vs. orchiectomy	Improved PFS, duration of survival, time to first progression with CAB
Dijkman (1997) (26)	Randomized, double-blind multicenter	Any T, M + orchiectomy + nilutamide vs. orchiectomy + placebo	Longer median survival with CAB, better OS at 2 and 5 yr with CAB
Eisenberger (1998) (27)	Randomized	Any T, M + orchiectomy + flutamide vs. orchiectomy + placebo	No difference in overall survival, no benefit for patients with minimal disease
Boccardo (1999) (11)	Randomized multicenter	C or D Biclutamide vs. flutamide + goserelin	Overall no difference in PFS,OS; small patient number with short follow-up (median = 38 mo); stage C and D initially combined for evaluation, then study design altered during trial to exclude stage D patients; patients in treatment arms not comparable

Note: C, D, M, T, indicate clinical stages.
CAB, combined androgen blockade; OS, overall survival; PFS, progression-free survival.

(15) demonstrated a clear survival benefit to androgen ablation. In perhaps the most comprehensive review thus far, the Agency for Health Care Policy and Research conducted a metaanalysis of 21 randomized trials to address this question. This analysis showed a statistically significant survival advantage for CAB at 5 years (hazard ratio, 0.871; 95% confidence interval, 0.805 to 0.942) (1). No significant advantage was noted for good prognosis patients with CAB; however, only six trials stratified patients by prognostic group, and the definitions of risk were not uniform. Little data exist comparing the effect of CAB versus monotherapy on quality of life (QOL).

CAB decreases the risk of progression and overall death and increases cause-specific survival for patients with metastatic disease. It is reasonable to suspect that patients with localized prostate cancer will respond differently to hormone deprivation than patients with metastatic disease, and minimizing DHT activity in these patients may have a greater impact on disease control than that seen in patients with metastatic disease (37). The data, overall, support the use of CAB over monotherapy.

Many other questions remain regarding the use of hormone ablation, such as the optimal duration of hormone use before radiotherapy. The question of how high the radiation dose should be in the presence or absence of HRT has not been answered. Several randomized trials currently ongoing from the RTOG, when completed, will address these issues. Furthermore, the role of HRT with or without higher doses has been alluded to but never directly addressed.

EXTERNAL BEAM RADIATION THERAPY, HORMONE THERAPY, AND QUALITY OF LIFE

QOL is now seen as an independent variable to be assessed, distinct from the more customary end points when evaluating treatment paradigms. Previously published studies have documented that prostate cancer and its treatment significantly impact many different QOL issues, and several studies have attempted to quantify the nature and the magnitude of posttreatment sequelae. Scott et al. (97) analyzed quality adjusted time without symptoms and toxicity for patients treated on RTOG 86-10 (EBRT with or without TAS). No difference in a 5-year rate of toxicity was seen for the two groups. Furthermore, the average time to distant metastases and toxicity and the quality adjusted survival time were significantly longer for patients treated with TAS, except in the highest risk group (p <.05).

Several chronic sequelae deserve independent consideration.

Potency

The etiology of erectile dysfunction resulting from radiation therapy is most probably multifactorial. Susceptible tissues include small blood vessels, nerve bundles, the corporal and bulbar structures, and the corporal smooth muscle. Studies using venous duplex ultrasonography to evaluate patients with postradiotherapy erectile dysfunction suggest that the primary pathophysiology is arteriogenic, resulting in disrupted blood flow to the corpora cavernosa and corpus spongiosum (112). Other mechanisms may include radiation-related alterations in nitric oxide synthesis and release by endothelial cells or a decline in serum androgen levels secondary to internal radiation scatter. Several confounding variables influence the rate of potency preservation, including age older than 70 years; comorbid chronic conditions, such as vascular disease or diabetes; and pretreatment erectile dysfunction (16,112). Treatment technique and radiation dose have been shown to influence outcome (64,73,115).

Androgen suppressive therapy has also been identified as a cause of impotence when given as a sole therapy and in conjunction with radiation. Neoadjuvant androgen suppression in conjunction with radiotherapy is associated with higher incidence of secondary impotence compared to radiotherapy alone (43% vs. 27%, p <.001) (114). The mechanism, however, appears to be distinct from that of radiation. Animal studies demonstrate an association between androgen suppression and down-regulation in the number of nitrous oxide receptors and the production of nitrous oxide (6). There is also evidence of a correlation between the absence of testosterone and decreased intracavernosal pressures (6).

Postradiation erectile dysfunction can be satisfactorily managed in several ways (63). Sildenafil improves the ability to achieve and maintain an erection in most patients (51,115). Patients with partial or moderate erectile function are more likely to benefit. Intracavernosal pharmacotherapy has yielded 65% erectile response (112).

Bone Loss: Incidence, Risk, and Prevention

A reduction in bone mineralization and the development of osteoporosis has been demonstrated in men with hypogonadism, regardless of etiology. Low testosterone levels have been closely correlated with osteoporosis in older men. Although the link between these two variables is not fully understood, the presence of androgen receptors on osteoblast cells has been demonstrated (3,14). Diamond et al. quantitated the effect of CAB on bone density in men receiving HRT for metastatic prostate cancer after 6 and 12 months of treatment. Combined treatment with GRH agonists and antiandrogen therapy resulted in a 6.6% decrease and 6.5% decrease in lumbar spine and femoral neck bone mineral density, respectively, which was greater than expected when compared to age-matched controls (25).

Insufficiency fractures secondary to irradiation have been described primarily in the literature in postmenopausal women treated with pelvic radiation for gynecologic malignancy. Little is known about the incidence of insufficiency fractures in men treated with pelvic irradiation for prostate cancer. The mechanism for destruction is believed to be late-onset injury of the microcirculation and impairment in the function of osteoblasts, resulting in increased susceptibility to traumatic and stress fractures. Increased rates of bone turnover and trabecular plate perforation have also been documented.

It is highly likely that the synergism between radiotherapy and hormone ablation will extend to include increased treatment-related toxicity. Based on published data and case reports documenting greater risks of osteoporotic fracture in hypogonadal men (22,65,104), it appears that the most potentially debilitating side effect is osteoporosis and the increased risk for skeletal fracture.

Clinical studies suggest that bisphosphonates, a class of drugs that reduce bone reabsorption by reducing osteoclast activity or causing apoptosis of osteoclast cells (22), may be helpful for prevention or treatment, or both, of osteoporosis secondary to hormone ablation. Studies evaluating the use of adjuvant cyclical intermittent etidronate administered during hormone ablation in patients treated for metastatic prostate cancer and osteoporosis have shown decreased rates of bone turnover, reversal of spinal bone loss, and slowed loss from femoral bones (22). The significance of the effects of TAS, both positive (improved OS) and negative (increased risk of fracture), has led to proposals for upcoming prospective QOL trials.

SUMMARY

Neoadjuvant and adjuvant hormone suppression combined with radiotherapy improve local control, prolong DFS, delay the time to the development of metastatic disease, and prolong OS in some subsets of patients. HRT does not appear to significantly increase survival for very low-risk patients; however, a trend for improved survival with 6 months of androgen ablation has been suggested (21). Another role for HRT in this subgroup is cytoreduction to overcome problems with pubic arch interference for patients seeking permanent seed implant. Frequently, this category of patient is seeking brachytherapy in the hopes of maintaining potency. Because potency may be impaired by the use of even short-term HRT, and there does not appear to be a survival benefit, cautious use of hormone-suppressive therapy is advisable.

The most comprehensive randomized data accumulated and analyzed to date demonstrate a benefit for the use of HRT in conjunction with EBRT in intermediate- and high-risk patients. Intermediate-risk patients benefit from 4 months of neoadjuvant CAB. Patients receiving EBRT will have additional benefit for improved local and biochemical control from the use of higher doses of radiation [D_{max} (maximum dose recieved) greater than 69 to 77 Gy] and 3D CRT techniques (81,100,101). High-risk patients benefit from long-term androgen ablation (44,74,76). The optimal duration of hormone use remains to be determined, but based on the information we have to date, 24 to 36 months seems reasonable. Early HRT appears to offer significant survival advantages over delayed HRT (39,67).

In evaluating patients for the use of neoadjuvant HRT, there are patients for whom the presence or absence of a survival benefit has not been completely defined. The absence of a demonstrable survival benefit in various analyses, including the RTOG metaanalysis, may be a result of the manner in which the analyses were performed. Specifically, many of the patients were treated before the availability of PSA. For example, low-risk patients who have a poor prognostic feature, such as PSA greater than 20 ng per mL, and who may have a greater than 50% incidence of positive biopsies after radiotherapy, may in fact benefit from the use of HRT. Additional studies are needed to answer these questions.

REFERENCES

1. Agency for Health Care Policy and Research. Evidence report/technology assessment, publication no. 4. Relative effectiveness and cost-effectiveness of methods of androgen suppression in the treatment of advanced prostate cancer, 1999.
2. Albertsen PC, Hanley JA, Gleason DF, et al. Competing risk analysis of men aged 55–74 years at diagnosis managed conservatively for clinically localized prostate cancer. *JAMA* 1998;280:975–980.
3. Anderson DC. Osteoporosis in men. *BMJ* 1992;305:489–490.
4. Anderson KM, Liao S. Selective retention of dihydrotestosterone by prostatic nuclei. *Nature* 1968;219:277–279.
5. Aus G, Hugosson J, Norlen L. Long term survival and mortality in prostate cancer treated with non-curative intent. *J Urol* 1995;154:460–465.
6. Baba K, Yajima M, Carrier S, et al. Delayed testosterone replacement restores nitric oxide synthase-containing nerve fibres and the erectile response in rat penis. *BJU Int* 2000; 85:953–958.
7. Babain RJ, Kojima M, Saitoh M, et al. Detection of residual prostate cancer after external radiotherapy. *Cancer* 1995;75: 2153–2158.
8. Bagshaw MA, Cox RS, Ray GR. Status of prostate cancer at Stanford University. *NCI Monogr* 1988;7:47–60.
9. Bey P, Carrie C, Beckendorf V, et al. Dose escalation with 3D CRT in prostate cancer: French study of dose escalation with conformal 3D radiotherapy I prostate cancer—preliminary analysis. *Int J Radiat Oncol Biol Phys* 2000;48:513–517.
10. Blasko JC, Grimm PD, Sylvester JE, et al. Palladium-103 brachytherapy for prostate carcinoma. *Int J Radiat Oncol Biol Phys* 2000;46:839–850.
11. Boccardo F, Rubagotti A, Barrichello M, et al. Biclutamide monotherapy versus prostate cancer plus Goserelin in prostate cancer patient: results of an Italian prostate cancer project study. *J Clin Oncol* 1999;17:2027–2038.
12. Bolla M, Gonzalez D, Warde P, et al. Improved survival in patients with locally advanced prostate cancer treated with radiotherapy and Goserelin. *N Engl J Med* 1997;337:295–300.
13. Brachman DG, Thomas T, Hilbe J, et al. Failure free survival following brachytherapy alone or external beam irradiation alone for T1-2 prostate tumors in 222 patients: results from a single practice. *Int J Radiat Oncol Biol Phys* 2000;48:111–117.

14. Broulik PD, Starka L. Effect of antiandrogens Casodex and epitestosterone on bone composition in mice. *Bone Vol* 1997; 20:473–475.
15. Chaubet JF, Tosteson TD, Dong EW, et al. Maximum androgen blockade in advanced prostate cancer: a meta-analysis of published randomized controlled trials using non-steroidal antiandrogens. *Urology* 1997;49:71–78.
16. Chodak GW, Thisted RA, Gerber GS, et al. Results of conservation management of clinically localized prostate cancer. *N Engl J Med* 1994;330:242–248.
17. Crawford ED, Blumenstein BA, Goodman PJ, et al. Leuprolide with and without Flutamide in advanced prostate cancer. *Cancer* 1990;66(1 Suppl):1039–1044.
18. Crooks J, Robertson S, Collin G, et al. Clinical relevance of trans-rectal ultrasound, biopsy and serum prostate specific antigen following external beam radiotherapy for carcinoma of the prostate. *Int J Radiat Oncol Biol Phys* 1993;27:31–37.
19. Crooks J, Malone S, Perry G, et al. Postradiotherapy biopsies: what do they really mean? Results for 498 patients. *Int J Radiat Oncol Biol Phys* 2000;48:355–367.
20. D'Amico AV, Whittington R, Malkowicz SB, et al. Biochemical outcome after radical prostatectomy, external; beam radiation therapy or interstitial radiation therapy for clinically localized prostate cancer. *JAMA* 1998;280:969–974.
21. D'Amico AV, Schultz D, Loffredo M. Biochemical outcome following external beam radiation therapy with or without androgen suppression therapy for clinically localized prostate cancer. *JAMA* 2000;284:1280–1283.
22. Daniell HW. Osteoporosis after orchiectomy for prostate cancer. *J Urol* 1997;157:439–444.
23. Del Regato. Long term curative results of radiotherapy for patients with inoperable prostatic adenocarcinoma. *Radiology* 1979;131:271–291.
24. Denis LJ, Keuppens F, Smith PH, et al. Maximal androgen blockade: final analysis of EORTC phase III trial 30853. EORTC genito-urinary tract cancer cooperative and the EORTC data cancer. *Eur Urol* 1998;33:144–151.
25. Diamond T, Campbell J, Bryant C, et al. The effect of combined androgen blockade on bone turnover and bone mineral densities in men treated for prostate cancer. *Cancer* 1998;83:1561–1566.
26. Dijkman GA, Jankegt RA, Reijike TM, et al. Long-term efficacy and safety of nilutamide plus castration in advanced prostate cancer and the significance of early PSA normalization. International Anandron Study Group. *J Urol* 1997;158:160–163.
27. Eisenberger MA, Blumenstein BA, Crawford ED, et al. Bilateral orchiectomy with or without Flutamide for metastatic prostate cancer. *N Engl J Med* 1998;339:1036–1042.
28. Suit HD, Baumann M, Skates S, et al. Clinical interest in determinations of cellular radiation sensitivity. *Int J Radiat Biol* 1989;56:725–737.
29. Fiveash JB, Hanks GE, Roach MR, et al. 3D conformal radiation therapy (3D CRT) for high-grade prostate cancer: a multi-institutional review. *Int J Radiat Biol* 2000;47:335–342.
30. Geller J, Albert J. DHT in prostate cancer tissue—a guide to management and therapy. *Prostate* 1985;6:19–25.
31. Geller J, Albert J. Effects of castration compared with total androgen blockade on tissue dihydrotestosterone (DHT) concentration in benign prostatic hyperplasia. *Urol Res* 1987;15:151–153.
32. Geller J, Candari C. Comparison of dihydrotestosterone levels in prostatic cancer metastases and primary prostate cancer. *Prostate* 1989;15:171–175.
33. Geller J, Albert J, Vik A. Advantages of total androgen blockade in the treatment of advanced prostate cancer. *Semin Oncol* 1988;15(2 Suppl):53–61.
34. Geller J, Partido L, Sionit L, et al. Comparison of androgen-independent growth and androgen-dependent growth in BPH and cancer tissue from the same radical prostatectomies in sponge-gel matrix histoculture. *Prostate* 1997;312: 250–254.
35. Geller J. Basis for hormonal management of advanced prostate cancer. *Cancer* 1993;71:1039–1045.
36. Geller J. Rationale for blockade of adrenal as well as testicular androgens in the treatment of advanced prostate cancer. *Semin Oncol* 1985;12(1 Suppl):28–35.
37. Geller J, Liu J, Albert J, et al. Relationship between human prostatic epithelial cell protein synthesis and tissue dihydrotestosterone (DHT) level. *Clin Endocrinol* 1987;26:155–161.
38. Grado GL, Larson TR, Balch CS, et al. Actuarial disease-free survival after prostate cancer brachytherapy using interactive techniques with biplane ultrasound and fluoroscopic guidance. *Int J Radiat Oncol Biol Phys* 1998;42:289–298.
39. Granfors T, Modig H, Damber JE, et al. Combined orchiectomy and external beam radiotherapy versus radiotherapy alone for non-metastatic prostate cancer with or without pelvic lymph node involvement: a prospective randomized study. *J Urol* 1998;159:2030–2034.
40. Hall EJ. *Radiobiology for the radiobiologist*, 4th ed. Philadelphia: JB Lippincott Co, 1994.
41. Reference deleted by author.
42. Hanks GE, Lu JD, Machtay M, et al. RTOG PROTOCOL 9202: a phase III trial of the use of long-term total androgen suppression following neoadjuvant hormonal cytoreduction and radiotherapy in locally advanced carcinoma of the prostate. *Int J Radiat Oncol Biol Phys* 2000;48:112.
43. Hanks GE, Hanlon AL, Schultheiss TE, et al. Dose escalation with 3D conformal treatment: five year outcomes, treatment optimization, and future directions *Int J Radiat Oncol Biol Phys* 1998;41:501–510.
44. Hanks GE, Hanlon AL, Pinover WH, et al. Dose selection for prostate cancer patients based on dose comparison and dose response studies. *Int J Radiat Oncol Biol Phys* 2000;46: 823–832.
45. Hanks GE, Buzydlowski JW, Perez CA, et al. The 10-year outcome of pathologic and imaging node positive patients treated with irradiation in Radiation Therapy Oncology Group (RTOG)-7506. *J Urol* 1996;155(Suppl):611A.
46. Hanks GE, Martz KL, Diamond J. The effect of dose on local control of prostate cancer. *Int J Radiat Oncol Biol Phys* 1988;5:1299.
47. Huggins C, Hodges CV. Studies on prostate cancer: I. The effects of castration, of estrogen and of androgen injection on serum phosphatases in metastatic carcinoma of the prostate. *Cancer Res* 1941;1:293–297.
48. Iselin CE, Robertson JE, Paulson DF. Radical prostatectomy: oncological outcome during a 20 year period. *J Urol* 1999;161:163–168.
49. Jacobson SJ, Bergstrahl EJ, Zincke H, et al. Population based study of comorbidity and survival following a diagnosis of prostate cancer. *J Urol* 1996;155(Suppl):324A.

50. Kattan MW, Zelefsky MJ, Kupelian PA, et al. Pre-treatment nomogram for predicting the outcome of three-dimensional conformal radiotherapy in prostate cancer. *J Clin Oncol* 2000;18:3352–3359.
51. Kedia S, Zippe CD, Agarwal A, et al. Treatment of erectile dysfunction with sildenafil citrate (Viagra) after radiation therapy for prostate cancer. *Urology* 1999;54:308–312.
52. King CR, Sanzone J, Anderson KR, et al. Definitive therapy for stage T1/T2 prostate carcinoma: PSA-based comparison between surgery, external beam and implant radiotherapy. *J Brachyther Int* 1998; 14:169.
53. Kuban DA, El-Mahdi AM, Schelhammer PF. The significance of post-irradiation prostate biopsies with long term follow up. *Int J Radiat Oncol Biol Phys* 1992;24:409–414.
54. Kupelian PA, Mohan DS, Lyons J, et al. Higher than standard radiation doses (≥72 Gy) with or without androgen deprivation in the treatment of localized prostate cancer. *Int J Radiat Oncol Biol Phys* 2000;46:567–574.
55. Labrie F, Dupont A, Belanger A. Complete androgen blockade for the treatment of prostate cancer. In Devita VT, Hellman S, Rosenberg, eds. *Important advances in oncology.* Philadelphia: Lippincott, 1985:193–217.
56. Labrie F. Combined androgen blockade: its unique efficacy for the treatment of localized prostate cancer. *PPO Updates* 1999;13:1–9.
57. Laverdiere J, Gomez JL, Cusan L, et al. Beneficial effect of combination hormonal therapy administered prior and following external beam irradiation therapy in localized prostate cancer. *Int J Radiat Oncol Biol Phys* 1997;37:247–252.
58. Lawton CA, Winter K, Byhardt R, et al. Androgen Suppression plus radiation vs. radiation alone for patients with D1(pN+) adenocarcinoma of the prostate (results based on a national prospective randomized trial RTOG 85-31). *Int J Radiat Oncol Biol Phys* 1997;38:931–939.
59. Lee WR, Hanks GE, Hanlon A. Increasing prostate-specific antigen profile following definitive radiotherapy for localized prostate cancer: clinical observations. *J Clin Oncol* 1996;15:230–238.
60. Lee LN, Stock RG, Stone NN. The impact of hormonal therapy on outcome in moderate to high risk prostate cancer treated with permanent radioactive seed implantation. *Int J Radiat Oncol Biol Phys* 2000:116.
61. Lim JD, Hasegawa M, Sikes C, et al. Supra-additive apoptotic response of R3327-G rat prostate tumors to androgen ablation and radiation *Int J Radiat Oncol Biol Phys* 1997;38:1071–1078.
62. Lu-Yao GL, Yao SL. Population-based study of long-term survival in patients with clinically localized prostate cancer. *Lancet* 1997;349:906-918.
63. Lue TF. Erectile dysfunction. *N Engl J Med* 2000;342: 1802–1813.
64. Mantz CA, Song P, Farhangi E, et al. Potency probability following conformal megavoltage radiotherapy using conventional doses for localized prostate cancer. *Int J Radiat Oncol Biol Phys* 1997;37:551–557.
65. McGrath SA, Diamond T. Osteoporosis as a complication of orchiectomy in two elderly men with prostatic cancer. *J Urol* 1995;154:535–536.
66. Medical Research Council Prostate Cancer Working Party Investigators Group. Immediate versus deferred treatment for advanced prostate cancer: initial results of the Medical Research Council Trial. *Br J Urol* 1997;79: 235–246.
67. Messing EM, Manola J, Sarosody M, et al. Immediate hormonal therapy compared with observation after radical prostatectomy and pelvic lymphadenectomy in men with node-positive prostate cancer. *N Engl J Med* 1999;341:1781–1788.
68. Michalski JM, Purdy JA, Winter K, et al. Preliminary report of toxicity following 3D radiation for prostate cancer on 3DOG/RTOG 9406. *Int J Radiat Oncol Biol Phys* 2000;46:391–402.
69. Michalski JM, Winter K, Purdy JA, et al. Update of toxicity following 3D radiation for prostate cancer on RTOG 9406. *Int J Radiat Oncol Biol Phys* 2000;48(3 Suppl):228.
70. Miller EB, Ladaga LE, El-Mahdi AM, et al. Reevaluation of prostate biopsy after definitive radiation therapy: frequency and prognostic significance of positive results of post-irradiation biopsy after definitive radiation therapy. *Urology* 1993;41:311–316.
71. Partin AW, Kattan MW, Subong EN, et al. Combination of PSA, clinical stage and Gleason score to predict pathological stage in men with localized prostate cancer: a multi-institutional update. *JAMA* 1997;277:1445–1451.
72. Partin AW, Yoo J, Carter HB, et al. The use of prostate specific antigen, clinical stage and Gleason score to predict pathological stage in men with localized prostate cancer. *J Urol* 1994;151:172–173.
73. Pickett B, Fisch BM, Weinberg VK, et al. Dose to the bulb of the penis is associated with the risk of impotence following radiotherapy for prostate cancer. *Int J Radiat Oncol Biol Phys* 1997;35(3 Suppl):1011.
74. Pilepich MV, Caplan R, Byhardt RW, et al. Phase III trial of androgen suppression using Goserelin in unfavorable prognosis carcinoma of the prostate treated with definitive radiotherapy: report of Radiation Therapy Oncology Group Protocol 85-31. *J Clin Oncol* 1997;15:1013–1021.
75. Pilepich MV, Sause WT, Shipley WU, et al. Androgen deprivation with radiation therapy compared with radiation therapy alone for locally advanced prostatic carcinoma: a randomized comparative trial of the Radiation Therapy Oncology Group. *Urology* 1995;45:616–623.
76. Pilepich MV, Winter K, Byhardt RW, et al. Androgen ablation adjuvant to definitive radiotherapy in carcinoma of the prostate: year 2000 update of RTOG phase III studies 8610 and 8531. *Int J Radiat Oncol Biol Phys* 2000:114.
77. Pilepich MV, Krall JM, Sause WT, et al. Prognostic factors in carcinoma of the prostate—Analysis of RTOG study 75-06. *Int J Radiat Oncol Biol Phys* 1987;13:339–349.
78. Pinover WH, Hanlon AL, Hanks GE. bNED control: praying to a false God? *Int J Radiat Oncol Biol Phys* 1997;39:218–219.
79. Pinover WH, Hanlon AL, Horwitz EM, et al. Defining the appropriate radiation dose for pretreatment PSA ≤10ng/ml prostate cancer. *Int J Radiat Oncol Biol Phys* 2000;47:649–654.
80. Pollack A, Zagars GK, Kopplin S. Radiotherapy and androgen ablation for clinically localized, high risk prostate cancer. *Int J Radiat Oncol Biol Phys* 1995;32:13–20.
81. Pollack A, Smith LG, Von Eschenbach AC. External beam radiotherapy dose response characteristics of 1127 men with prostate cancer treated in the PSA era. *Int J Radiat Oncol Biol Phys* 2000;48:507–512.
82. Pollack A, Zagars GK. External beam radiotherapy dose response of prostate cancer. *Int J Radiat Oncol Biol Phys* 1997; 39:1011–1018.

83. Pollack A, Zagars GK, Smith LG, et al. Preliminary results of a randomized dose-escalation study comparing 70 Gy to 78 Gy for the treatment of prostate cancer. *Int J Radiat Oncol Biol Phys* 1999;45(3 Suppl):146.
84. Potters L, Cha C, Ashley R, et al. The role of external beam irradiation in patients undergoing prostate brachytherapy. *Urol Oncol* 2000;5:112–117.
85. Potters L, Torre T, Ashley R, et al. Examining the role of neoadjuvant deprivation I patients undergoing prostate brachytherapy. *J Clin Oncol* 2000;18:1187–1192.
86. Prostate Cancer Trialists' Collaborative Group. Maximum androgen blockade in advanced prostate cancer: an overview of 22 randomised trials with 3,283 deaths in 5,710 patients. *Lancet* 1995;346:265–269.
87. Ragde H, Elgamal AA, Snow PE, et al. Ten-year disease-free survival after transperineal sonography guided iodine-125 brachytherapy with or without 54 gray external beam irradiation in the treatment of patients with clinically localized, low to high Gleason grade prostate carcinoma. *Cancer* 1998;83:989–1001.
88. Roach M 3rd, Meehan S, Kroll S, et al. Radiotherapy for high grade clinically localized adenocarcinoma of the prostate. *J Urol* 1996;156:1719–1723.
89. Roach M 3rd, Lu J, Pilepich MV, et al. Long-term survival years after radiotherapy alone: RTOG prostate cancer trials. *J Urol* 1999;161:864–868.
90. Roach M 3rd, Lu J, Pilepich MV. Four prognostic subgroups predict long-term survival from prostate cancer following radiotherapy alone on Radiation Therapy Oncology Group trials. *Int J Radiat Oncol Biol Phys* 2000;47:609–615.
91. Roach M 3rd, Lu J, Pilepich MV. Predicting long-term survival and the need for hormonal therapy: a meta-analysis of RTOG Prostate cancer trials. *Int J Radiat Oncol Biol Phys* 2000;47:617–627.
92. Sandler HM, Dunn RL, McLaughlin PW, et al. Overall survival after prostate-specific antigen detected recurrence following conformal radiation therapy. *Int J Radiat Oncol Biol Phys* 2000;48:629–633.
93. Sands ME, Pollack A, Zagars GK. Influence of radiotherapy on node-positive prostate cancer treated with androgen ablation. *Int J Radiat Oncol Biol Phys* 1995;31:13–19.
94. Scardino PT. The prognostic significance of biopsies after radiotherapy for prostatic cancer. *Semin Urol* 1983;1:243–252.
95. Scardino PT, Wheeler TM. Local control of prostate cancer with radiotherapy: frequency and prognostic significance positive results of post-irradiation biopsy. *NCI Monogr* 1988;7:95–103.
96. Schelhammer PF, El-Mahdi AM, Higgins EM, et al. Prostate biopsy after definitive treatment by interstitial 125-Iodine implant or external beam radiation therapy. *J Urol* 1987;137:897–901.
97. Scott C, Roach M, Lawton C, et al. Q-twist analysis for prostate cancer treatment with or without hormonal therapy: RTOG 86-10. 1998 *Int J Radiat Oncol Biol Phys* (abst).
98. Siiteri PK, Wilson JD. Dihydrotestosterone metabolism in prostate hypertrophy. I. The formation of content of dihydrotestosterone in the hypertrophic prostate of man. *J Clin Invest* 1970;49:1737–1745.
99. Sklar GN, Eddy HA, Jacobs SC, et al. Combined anti-tumor effect of suramin plus irradiation in human prostate cancer cells: the role of apoptosis. *J Urol* 1993;150:1526–1532.
100. Speight JL, Weinberg VK, McLaughlin PW, et al. Three dimensional conformal radiotherapy and dose >69 Gy improve PSA failure-free survival in intermediate risk prostate cancer. *J Clin Oncol* (*in press*).
101. Speight JL, Weinberg VK, McLaughlin PW, et al. 3D conformal radiotherapy improves PSA failure rates for intermediate risk patients at conventional doses. In: Cox J, ed. *Proceedings of the American Society for Therapeutic Radiology and Oncology*. San Antonio, TX, 1999:346.
102. Stone N, Stock RG. Prostate brachytherapy: treatment strategies. *J Urol* 1999;162:421–426.
103. Sylvester JE, Blasko JC, Grimm PD, et al. 125-iodine/103-palladium brachytherapy with or without neoadjuvant androgen ablation for early stage prostate cancer. *Int J Radiat Oncol Biol Phys* 2000;48(3 Suppl):310.
104. Townsend MF, Sanders WH, Northway RO, et al. Bone fractures associated with luteinizing hormone-releasing hormone-agonists used in the treatment of prostate carcinoma. *Cancer* 1997;79:545–550.
105. Tyrell CJ, Altwein JE, Klippel F, et al. A multicenter randomized trial comparing the luteinizing hormone-releasing hormone analogue Goserelin acetate alone with flutamide in the treatment of advanced prostate cancer. *J Urol* 1991;146:1321–1326.
106. Valecenti R, Lu J, Pilepich MV, et al. Survival advantage from higher-dose radiation therapy for clinically localized prostate cancer treated on the Radiation Therapy Oncology Group. *J Clin Oncol* 2000;18:2740–2746.
107. Vicini FA, Kini VR, Spenser W, et al. The role of androgen deprivation in the definitive management of clinically localized prostate cancer treated with radiation therapy. *Int J Radiat Oncol Biol Phys* 1999;43:707–713.
108. Whittington R, Malkowicz SB, Machtay M, et al. Combined hormonal and radiation therapy for lymph node positive prostate cancer. *Urology* 1995;46:213–219.
109. Widmark A, Damber JE, Bergh A, et al. Estramustine potentiates the effects of irradiation on the Dunning (R3327) rat prostatic adenocarcinoma. *Prostate* 1994;24:79–83.
110. Zagars GK, Pollack A, Von Eschenbach AC. Unfavorable local-regional prostate cancer management with radiation and androgen ablation. *Cancer* 1997;80:764–775.
111. Zeitman AL, Nakfoor BM, Prince EA, et al. The effect of androgen deprivation and radiation therapy on an androgen-sensitive murine tumor: an *in vitro* and *in vivo* study. *Cancer J Sci Am* 1997;3:31–36.
112. Zelefsky MJ, Eid JF. Elucidating the etiology of erectile dysfunction after definitive therapy for prostate cancer. *Int J Radiat Oncol Biol Phys* 1998;40:129–133.
113. Zelefsky MJ, Hollister T, Raben A. Five-year biochemical outcome and toxicity with transperineal CT-planned permanent I-125 implantation for patients with localized prostate cancer *Int J Radiat Oncol Biol Phys* 2000;47:1261–1266.
114. Zelefsky MJ, Leibel SA, Gaudin PB, et al. Dose escalation with three-dimensional conformal radiation therapy affects the outcome in prostate cancer. *Int J Radiat Oncol Biol Phys* 1998;41:491–500.
115. Zelefsky MJ, Wallner KE, Ling CC, et al. Comparison of the 5-year outcome and morbidity of three-dimensional conformal radiotherapy versus transperineal permanent iodine-125 implantation for early stage prostate cancer. *J Clin Oncol* 1999;17:517–522.

29

COMBINATION EXTERNAL BEAM RADIATION THERAPY AND BRACHYTHERAPY FOR CLINICALLY LOCALIZED PROSTATE CANCER

MICHAEL J. ZELEFSKY

One of the many treatment options used for patients with localized prostate cancer is the combination of external beam radiation therapy (EBRT) and interstitial implantation. Series reporting outcomes of this combination treatment approach have included patients with various prognostic features. Although there is no consensus at this time as to which patients are best suited for combination therapy, many investigators have favored such an approach for patients with more aggressive disease, reserving monotherapy (implantation or EBRT alone) for those with favorable risk disease. Combination therapy can be accomplished when EBRT is integrated with either permanent interstitial implantation or temporary brachytherapy using afterloading catheters. This chapter discusses the rationale for using combination therapy, summarizes the outcome of EBRT combined with either low-dose rate (LDR) or high-dose rate (HDR) brachytherapy and, finally, makes recommendations as to which patients are best suited for these treatment approaches.

RATIONALE FOR COMBINATION THERAPY

Especially among patients with intermediate- and unfavorable-risk prostate cancer, several reports have documented improved outcomes with higher radiation doses when using external beam three-dimensional conformal radiation therapy (3D CRT) (1–3). Although excellent prostate-specific antigen (PSA) relapse-free survival (RFS) rates have been achieved for patients with favorable risk disease using transperineal implantation (TPI) alone (4–7), results have been generally suboptimal for patients with adverse prognostic features treated with this approach. Table 29-1 demonstrates the PSA RFS outcomes for several series that have reported outcome with TPI alone among patients with adverse prognostic features. Although the characteristics of treated patients vary from series to series and confound attempts to make direct comparisons, these reports nevertheless highlight the fact that implantation alone is not sufficient therapy for locally advanced prostate cancer. The likely explanation for the inferior outcome with TPI alone in these patients may be related to an insufficient radiation dose or dose rate to overcome radioresistant tumor clonogens. In addition, TPI alone may not deliver adequate dose to the periprostatic tissues in such patients with higher risks of extraprostatic disease involvement. It would therefore appear that the rationale for incorporating EBRT with interstitial implantation for patients with adverse prognostic risk factors is related to the need to deliver escalated radiation doses to this cohort of patients. Combining EBRT with a brachytherapy boost (in the form of interstitial permanent implantation or temporary implantation with afterloading catheters) may represent equally effective approaches for delivering higher radiation doses that are now recognized as critical for achieving optimal tumor control.

OUTCOME OF COMBINED EXTERNAL BEAM RADIATION THERAPY AND LOW-DOSE-RATE BRACHYTHERAPY

Ragde et al. (8) reported on 54 patients treated with conventional EBRT to 45 Gy followed by a permanent iodine 125 (^{125}I) implant delivering 120 Gy. With a median follow-up time of 119 months, the 10-year likelihood of maintaining a PSA level less than 0.4 ng per mL was 75%. However, among these 54 patients, only 24% and 41% had Gleason scores higher than 7 and PSA levels greater than 10 ng per mL, respectively. Dattoli et al. (9) reported on 73 patients

TABLE 29-1. FIVE-YEAR PROSTATE-SPECIFIC ANTIGEN (PSA) RELAPSE-FREE SURVIVAL FOR INTERMEDIATE- AND UNFAVORABLE-RISK PROSTATE CANCER TREATED WITH INTERSTITIAL IMPLANTATION ALONE

Authors	Patient cohort	Treatment	Follow-up (mo)	Outcome (%)
Blasko	PSA >10–20	^{103}Pd	42	80
	PSA >20	^{103}Pd		67
Grado	PSA >10–20	^{125}I/^{103}Pd	46	72
	PSA >20			57
Brachman	PSA >10–20	^{125}I/^{103}Pd	51	55
	PSA >20			48
Stock	Intermediate	^{125}I	19	60
Potters	Intermediate	^{125}I/^{103}Pd	41	74
	Unfavorable			55
D'Amico	Intermediate	^{125}I	41	33
	Unfavorable			5
Zelefsky	Intermediate	^{125}I	48	77
	Unfavorable	^{125}I		38

treated with EBRT to 41 Gy followed by a permanent palladium 103 (^{103}Pd) implant delivering an additional 80 Gy. In this group, 49% had clinical T3 disease, 55% had Gleason scores higher than 7, and 44% had PSA levels greater than 15 ng per mL. Although excellent biochemical outcome was reported, the median follow-up was too short to draw meaningful conclusions. Singh et al. from Memorial Sloan-Kettering Cancer Center (10) reported on 65 patients with intermediate- or unfavorable-risk prostate cancers treated with 3D CRT and ^{103}Pd and were followed for a median of 2 years. The 3-year PSA RFS was 87% with a median PSA value at last follow-up of 0.25 ng per mL. The PSA RFS was 90% for patients who had an initial PSA less than 10 ng per mL and 80% for those who had an initial PSA greater than 10 ng per mL. Critz et al. (11) reported on 689 patients with early-stage prostate cancer treated with transperineal ultrasound-guided implantation using ^{125}I followed 3 weeks later by the delivery of 45 Gy of conventional EBRT. The pretreatment PSA levels were 10 ng per mL or less and Gleason scores less than 7 in 73% and 76% of patients, respectively. No patients received neoadjuvant or adjuvant hormonal therapy. PSA relapse was defined as a PSA nadir level greater than 0.2 ng per mL or a subsequent rising PSA above this level. The median follow-up in that report was 4 years. The actuarial 5-year PSA RFS rates for patients with pretreatment PSA levels 0 to 4 ng per mL (n = 50), 4 to 10 ng per mL (n = 451), greater than 10 to 20 ng per mL (n = 144), and greater than 20 ng per mL (n = 44) were 94%, 93%, 75%, and 69%, respectively. These results appear to be at least comparable to what can be achieved with high-dose 3D CRT alone for this prognostic risk group. Nevertheless, longer follow-up will be necessary in all these studies to fully assess the durability of biochemical control among patients with adverse prognostic features treated by combination therapy.

TOLERANCE OF COMBINED EXTERNAL BEAM RADIATION THERAPY AND LOW-DOSE-RATE BRACHYTHERAPY

There is a paucity of information regarding the long-term tolerance of combined EBRT and brachytherapy for patients with localized prostate cancer. Critz et al. (12) reported grade 2 or greater rectal toxicities in 23% and grade 2 or greater urinary toxicities in 20% of treated patients using this approach. The higher toxicity rates in this report may have been attributed to their use of a retropubic rather than the TPI technique. With a median follow-up of 2 years, Dattoli et al. (9) observed a 3% incidence of post-treatment urethral strictures requiring transurethral resection, and one patient developed moderate urinary incontinence. No rectal toxicities were reported.

The tolerance profile for patients treated with combined EBRT and TPI at Memorial Sloan-Kettering Cancer Center was recently summarized (Fig. 29-1) (10). Four patients (6%) with acute urinary retention required Foley catheterization within 48 hours of the implant procedure. Twenty-three patients (42%) developed grade 2 urinary symptoms after completion of therapy requiring alpha-blocker medications. Three patients (4%) noted rare stress incontinence, and no patient described urge incontinence. Of the 65 patients treated, 45 (68%) reported at their last follow-up that their urinary symp-

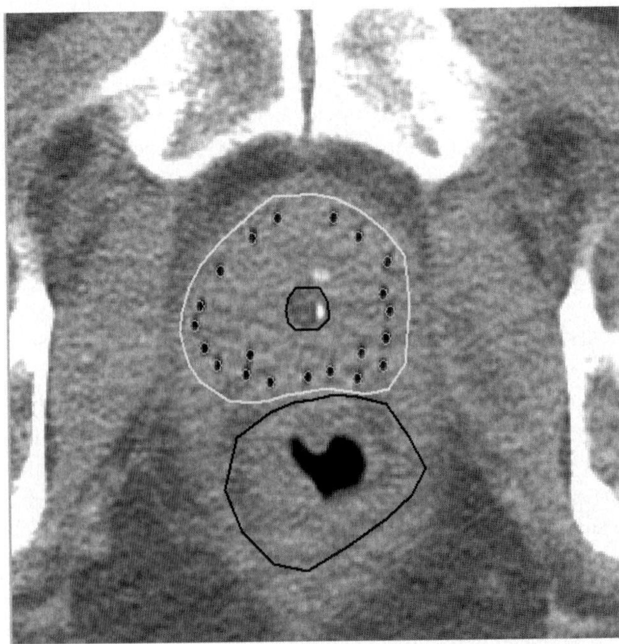

FIGURE 29-1. Peripheral catheter distribution for high-dose-rate brachytherapy at Memorial Sloan-Kettering Cancer Center.

toms had resolved. Eight patients (13%) developed grade 2 rectal bleeding within 6 months from the completion of therapy. No grade 3 or 4 rectal toxicities have been observed. Five patients (8%) reported increased frequency of bowel movements, which were managed with conservative measures. Forty-four of the patients (66%) were potent before the initiation of treatment. Of these, 17 (26%) developed erectile dysfunction.

COMBINED EXTERNAL BEAM RADIATION THERAPY AND HIGH-DOSE-RATE BRACHYTHERAPY: RATIONALE AND OUTCOME

HDR brachytherapy has been used in combination with EBRT for the treatment of locally advanced prostate cancer (13–16). In general, for this approach, patients undergo transperineal placement of afterloading catheters within the prostate under ultrasound guidance (Fig. 29-1). After computed tomography–based treatment planning, several high-dose fractions, ranging from 4 to 6 Gy each, are administered over an interval of 24 to 36 hours using iridium 192 (^{192}Ir). This treatment is followed by supplemental EBRT directed to the prostate and periprostatic tissues to a dose of 45.0 to 50.4 Gy using conventional fractionation.

HDR brachytherapy offers several potential advantages over other techniques. Taking advantage of an afterloading approach, the radiation oncologist and physicist can more easily optimize the delivery of radiotherapy to the prostate and compensate for potential regions of underdosage (*cold spots*) that may be present with permanent interstitial implantation (Fig. 29-2). Doses can also be constrained to effectively limit the volume of rectum and urethra exposed to the high radiation doses (Fig. 29-3). Furthermore, this technique reduces radiation exposure to the radiation oncologist and others involved in the procedure, compared with permanent interstitial implantation. Finally, HDR brachytherapy boosts may be radiobiologically more efficacious in terms of tumor cell kill for patients with increased tumor bulk or adverse prognostic features, compared to LDR boosts such as ^{125}I or ^{103}Pd.

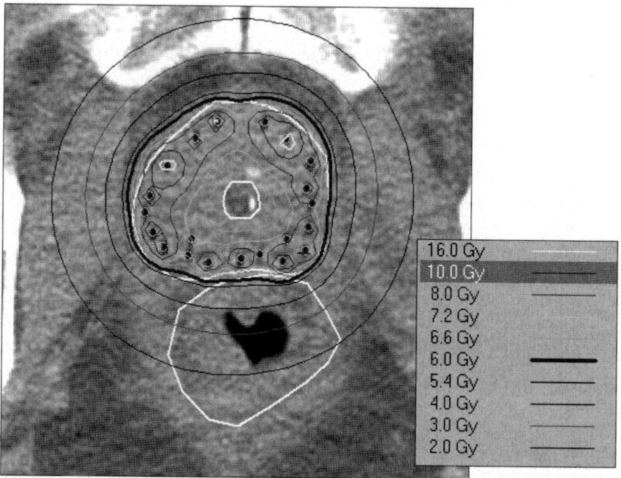

FIGURE 29-2. Dose distribution demonstrating excellent coverage of the prostate with the 6-Gy prescription isodose line. High-dose regions are restricted from the urethra.

Kovacs et al. (13) recently presented their HDR brachytherapy experience in 171 patients with varying clinical stages and tumor differentiation. Approximately one-third of the treated patients had T3 or high-grade disease. A total of 50 Gy of external radiation therapy was delivered, followed by two HDR ^{192}Ir boosts consisting of 15 Gy each. With a median follow-up of 52 months, the 5-year PSA RFS was 79%. Sixteen percent of patients experienced chronic proctitis, and 11% reported chronic cystitis. Mate et al. (14) reported 104 patients who were treated with 4 fractions of HDR ^{192}Ir followed by 50.4 Gy of EBRT. The majority of their patients had stage T1-2 disease with a median pretreatment PSA level of 8.1 ng per mL. With a median follow-up of 45 months, the 5-year actuarial PSA RFS for patients with pretreatment PSA levels less than 20 ng per mL was 84%. The 5-year actuarial incidence of urethral stricture development was 8%. No other grade 3 or 4 toxicities were observed.

Martinez et al. have used fractionated outpatient HDR brachytherapy boosts interdigitated throughout the course of EBRT (15,16). Real-time intraoperative planning from the intraoperative ultrasound image was performed, and each of three HDR boost treatments was delivered in the operating room under anesthesia. A dose escalation study was implemented to gradually increase the dose per fraction delivered with the HDR boost from 5.5 Gy × 3 fractions to 10.5 Gy × 3 fractions. Four percent of patients experienced grade 3 acute toxicities that included dysuria, urinary frequency, perineal pain, diarrhea, and urinary retention. The incidence of late grade 2 urinary and rectal toxicities was 9% and 5%, respectively (Fig. 29-3). The 5-year actuarial incidence of late grade 3 urinary toxicity was 8%. In a recent matched-pair analysis comparing patients treated with this program and conventional EBRT, the 5-year PSA RFS rate for patients treated with HDR boost combined with EBRT was 67%, compared to 44% for those treated with EBRT alone (p <.001) (16). A multivariate analysis also demonstrated that the addition of an HDR boost was an independent predictor for an improved biochemical outcome.

TREATMENT RECOMMENDATIONS

In the absence of randomized prospective trials, it is difficult to clearly define the clinical indications and benefits of combined EBRT and TPI. Specifically, further studies are needed to determine whether the combined approach achieves sig-

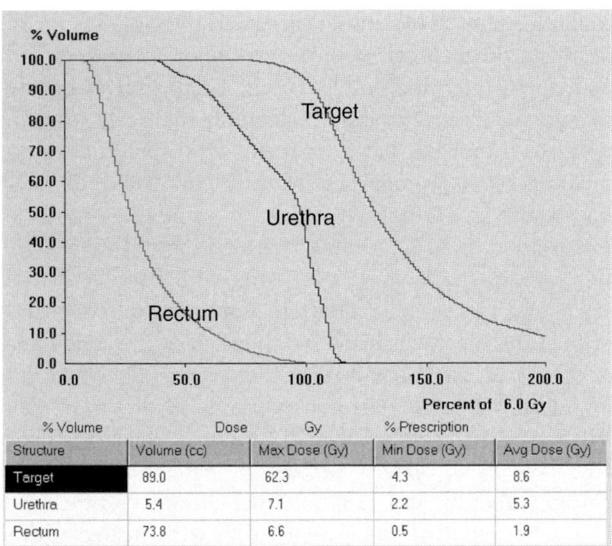

Structure	Volume (cc)	Max Dose (Gy)	Min Dose (Gy)	Avg Dose (Gy)
Target	89.0	62.3	4.3	8.6
Urethra	5.4	7.1	2.2	5.3
Rectum	73.8	6.6	0.5	1.9

FIGURE 29-3. Dose volume histogram display for the target, urethra, and rectum demonstrating high dose for the target with restricted doses to the urethra and rectum.

nificantly superior biochemical outcomes for patients with adverse prognostic features compared to TPI alone or high-dose 3D CRT. It also remains unclear whether the combined approach is necessary for patients with favorable risk disease in whom the results of monotherapy alone have been excellent. In recent retrospective comparisons (4,17,18), no differences in biochemical outcome have been observed in patients with favorable-risk prognostic features treated with TPI alone, compared to combined EBRT and TPI. At the present time, combined EBRT and TPI should be reserved for selected patients with intermediate- or high-risk prognostic features, whereas monotherapy appears to be sufficient for those with favorable risk features. In addition, such combined approaches would be appropriate for patients who have bowel-overlying portions of the target volume, in whom escalated doses cannot be safely given with EBRT alone, and a brachytherapy procedure would need to be incorporated to safely deliver higher doses of therapy.

REFERENCES

1. Zelefsky MJ, Leibel SA, Gaudin PB, et al. Dose escalation with three-dimensional conformal radiation therapy affects the outcome in prostate cancer. *Int J Rad Oncol Biol Phys* 1998;41:491–500.
2. Hanks GE, Lee WR, Hanlon AL, et al. Conformal technique dose escalation for prostate cancer: biochemical evidence of improved cancer control with higher doses in patients with pretreatment prostate-specific antigen >10 ng/ml. *Int J Rad Oncol Biol Phys* 1996;35:862–868.
3. Pollack A, Zagars GK. External beam radiotherapy dose response of prostate cancer. *Int J Rad Oncol Biol Phys* 1997; 39:1011–1018.
4. D'Amico AV, Whittington R, Malkowicz SB, et al. Biochemical outcome after radical prostatectomy, external beam radiation therapy, or interstitial radiation therapy for clinically localized prostate cancer. *JAMA* 1998;280:969–974.
5. Grimm PD, Blasko JC, Ragde H, et al. Does brachytherapy have a role in the treatment of prostate cancer? *Hematol Oncol Clin North Am* 1996;10:653–673.
6. Zelefsky MJ, Hollister T, Raben A, et al. Five year biochemical outcome and toxicity with transperineal CT-planned permanent I-125 prostate implantation for patients with localized prostate cancer. *Int J Radiat Oncol Biol Phys* 2000;47:1261–1266.
7. Potters L, Cha C, Oshinsky G, et al. Risk profiles to predict PSA relapse-free survival for patients undergoing permanent prostate brachytherapy. *Cancer J Sci Am* 1999;5:301–306.
8. Ragde H, Elgamal AA, Snow PB, et al. Ten year disease free survival after transperineal sonography-guided I-125 brachytherapy with or without 45 gray external beam irradiation in the treatment of patients with clinically localized, low to high Gleason grade prostate carcinoma. *Cancer* 1998;83:989–1001.
9. Dattoli M, Wallner K, Sorace R, et al. Palladium 103 brachytherapy in the treatment of cancer of the prostate. *Int J Radiat Biol Phys* 1996;33:875–879.
10. Singh A, Zelefsky MJ, Raben A, et al. Combined 3-dimensional conformal radiotherapy and transperineal Pd-103 permanent implantation for patients with intermediate and unfavorable risk prostate cancer. *Int J Cancer* 2000;90:275–280.
11. Critz FA, Williams WH, Levinson AK, et al. Simultaneous irradiation for prostate cancer: intermediate results with modern techniques. *J Urol* 2000;164:738–741.
12. Critz FA, Levinson K, Williams WH, et al. Prostate-specific antigen nadir of 0.5 ng/ml or less defines disease freedom for surgically staged men irradiated for prostate cancer. *Urology* 1997;49:668–672.
13. Kovacs G, Galalae R, Loch T, et al. Prostate preservation by combined external beam and HDR brachytherapy in nodal negative prostate cancer. *Strahlenther Onkol* 1999;175:87–88.
14. Mate TP, Gottesman JE, Hatton J, et al. High dose-rate afterloading 192Iridium prostate brachytherapy: feasibility report. *Int J Radiat Oncol Biol Phys* 1998;41:525–533.
15. Martinez A. High dose rate brachytherapy for prostate cancer. In: Greco C, Zelefsky MJ, eds. *Radiotherapy for prostate cancer*. Amsterdam, Netherlands: Harwood Academic Publishers, 2000.
16. Kestin LL, Martinez AA, Stromberg JS, et al Matched-pair analysis of conformal high-dose rate brachytherapy boost versus external-beam radiation therapy alone for locally advanced prostate cancer. *J Clin Oncol* 2000;18:2869–2880.
17. Zelefsky MJ, Wallner KE, Ling CC, et al. Comparison of the 5-year outcome and morbidity of three dimensional conformal radiotherapy versus transperineal permanent iodine-125 implantation for early-stage prostatic cancer. *J Clin Oncol* 1999;17:517–522.
18. Stokes SH. Comparison of biochemical disease-free survival of patients with localized carcinoma of the prostate undergoing radical prostatectomy, transperineal ultrasound-guided radioactive seed implantation or definitive external beam irradiation. *Int J Radiat Oncol Biol Phys* 2000;47:129–136.

30

PROTON BEAM THERAPY IN PROSTATE CANCER

ANTHONY L. ZIETMAN
WILLIAM U. SHIPLEY

Since the late 1980s, early detection strategies have meant that prostate cancer is routinely detected at a stage that, in all likelihood, it is still locally confined. The efficacy of the local measure is therefore of paramount importance, as therapy is potentially curative (1). Dose escalation is the most intuitive tool available to the radiation oncologist to maximize the chance for cure, but its execution requires the development of highly accurate dose delivery systems. The 1990s have seen a remarkable evolution in photon planning and treatment, with documented evidence of reduced morbidity and the early suggestion of greater antitumor efficacy (2–5). Despite this, it remains true that photons are fundamentally constrained by an inherent property, their depth-dose profile. Regardless of beam energy or intensity, the intrinsic shape of this profile is the same with a maximal dose relatively close to the skin and an exponential decrease in dose beyond this point. This latter property ensures that radiation will always stream beyond the target like a tail. By contrast, heavy, charged, subatomic particles, such as protons, demonstrate a quite different depth-dose profile (Fig. 30-1). Early experiments in water showed that the dose deposited by a beam of monoenergetic protons *increases* slowly with depth but reaches a sharp maximum near the end of the particles' range (the Bragg peak). The dose falls to zero after the Bragg peak at the end of the particles' range (6). If one could determine with accuracy the location of a tumor within the body and also the densities of the tissues surrounding it, then it should be possible to design exquisitely conformed treatments for tumors that deliver lower integral radiation doses than can ever be achieved with photons (7). The great attraction of the photon beam comes from these physical properties. Commercially developed cyclotrons now produce 150- to 250-megavolt (MeV) beams, which are of considerable interest to the clinician. These energies correspond to a range in tissue of 15 to 30 cm, sufficient to reach most human tumors.

The physical properties of protons are distinctive, and the biologic properties are not. The radiobiologic equivalent of protons is indistinguishable from 250-kV x-rays and, thus, only approximately 10% more effective than a megavoltage linear accelerator beam. Dose is expressed as cobalt gray equivalent, or CGE.

In the early days of proton therapy, treatment facilities were few, beam energies were low, and planning was laborious. This modality was therefore reserved for tumors in a limited number of relatively accessible sites in which the benefits of a rapid dose fall-off were self evident (e.g., choroidal melanomas, pituitary neoplasms, and tumors of the skull base and spine). Despite these limitations, much evidence has been accumulated to demonstrate the efficacy of proton therapy for localized solid tumors and to demonstrate that dose escalation could routinely be attained with a proportionate increase in normal tissue morbidity (8). Two dedicated hospital-based cyclotron facilities now exist in the United States, with several more in the planning or construction stages. Randomized trials are under way for tumors in several sites, and the hypothesis that dose escalation can be achieved with reduced normal tissue injury, on which all conformal radiation strategies are predicated, is now being put to the test.

COMPARING PROTONS WITH CONTEMPORARY CONFORMAL PHOTONS

Beam-for-beam and plan-for-plan protons always generate a more attractive dose distribution than photons (unless skin sparing is a crucial issue). For the same target dose, protons put fewer doses outside the target than x-rays, such that the integral dose will always be less than with photons (Fig. 30-2). On the average, this "dose bath" is approximately half that of x-rays. Likewise, for the same extra-tumoral dose, protons can deliver a higher target radiation dose. The crucial test for proton planning comes when it is compared with intensity-modulated x-ray beams. Uniform x-ray beams deliver approximately

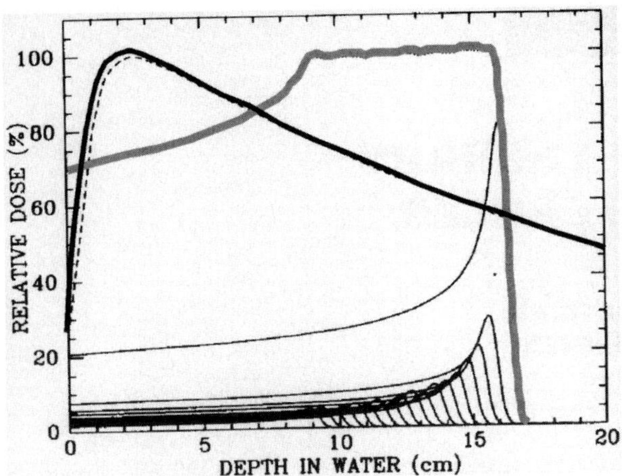

FIGURE 30-1. Depth-dose profiles for a proton beam (with a spread Bragg peak) and a 10-megavolt photon beam.

uniform doses to the boundary of the target and tend to fill any concavities, such as those that may exist when a tumor encircles a critical nontarget structure. If multiple nonuniform beams are delivered, however, then a concavity in the dose distribution becomes possible. This has been a considerable recent advance in photon therapy. However, what is applicable to a photon beam is also applicable to a proton beam. If proton beams are substituted for x-ray beams and matched for dose in the target region and with the same intensity profiles, then we get a plan that is identical in the target volume but that features even less dose elsewhere. What is more, this may not even be the best proton plan possible! Actually, proton therapy has featured intensity modulation almost from its inception, in the sense of range modulation with spreading of the Bragg peak. Just as intensity-modulated x-ray plans outperform uniform-field x-ray plans, so will intensity-modulated proton plans outperform uniform-field proton plans.

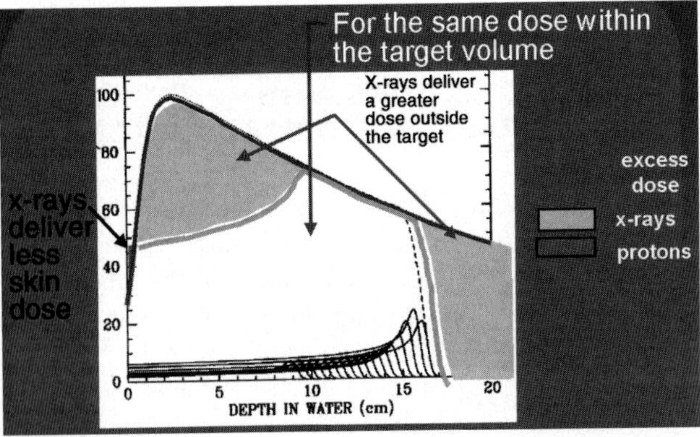

FIGURE 30-2. Single beam plans for protons and 10-megavolt photons matched in a target region between 10- and 16-cm deep. Note that for the same target volume photons deliver a greater dose outside the target volume than protons, except in the skin.

A second major issue concerning proton radiation is its potential cost. The most appropriate yardstick against which this must be measured is that of contemporary three-dimensional conformal radiation. In most aspects, the costs will be the same. The patient work-up and preparation (the imaging studies and interdisciplinary consultations) do not differ. The treatment planning will likewise not differ (the delineation of target and normal volumes), nor will the development of the plan or the archiving of the data. Quality assurance will be identical. The only difference comes in the capital cost and maintenance of the facility, which will be more. With the passage of time, however, and with a large throughput of patients, this cost will be progressively amortized. Ultimately, proton therapy need only be fractionally more expensive than conformal x-ray therapy.

PROTON BEAM AND PROSTATE CANCER

First Clinical Trial

The earliest clinical trial of the proton beam in prostate cancer was the phase III study reported by Shipley et al. in 1979 (9). Seventeen patients with locally advanced tumors were treated at the Harvard Cyclotron and Massachusetts General Hospital with pelvic photons to a dose of 50.4 Gy and a perineal proton boost to a total of 75.6 CGE. The perineal approach was necessitated by the range limitation imposed by the Harvard Cyclotron's 16-MeV proton beam. The morbidity profile was favorable with only two urethral strictures in patients who had had prior transurethral resections of the prostate and no severe late rectal complications.

First Randomized Trial

In the pre-prostate-specific antigen (PSA) era, the majority of cases of apparently localized prostate cancer presenting to physicians were what we would now regard as locally advanced disease. This was therefore the focus of much research effort at that time. From 1982 to 1992, 202 men with T3-T4 tumors were randomized in a phase III trial at the Massachusetts General Hospital (10). All patients received 50.4 Gy using conventional photons and a four-field box beam arrangement. Half were randomized to receive a boost to 67.2 Gy using conventional photons through lateral portals, and the other half were boosted to a total dose of 77.2 CGE with perineal protons (Fig. 30-3). Ninety-three of 103 patients randomized to the high-dose arm, and 96 of 99 in the conventional-dose arm received their assigned dose. The end points were clinical local failure based on a digital rectal exam, a positive posttreatment transurethral resection of the prostate specimen, or a positive rebiopsy (performed on a minority of patients with negative digital rectal examination). After 1989, PSA was used in follow-up, allowing for a biochemical evaluation of outcome. There was a trend to an improvement in local

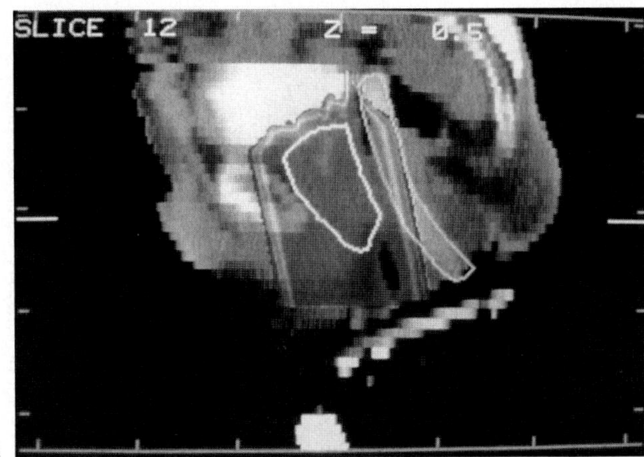

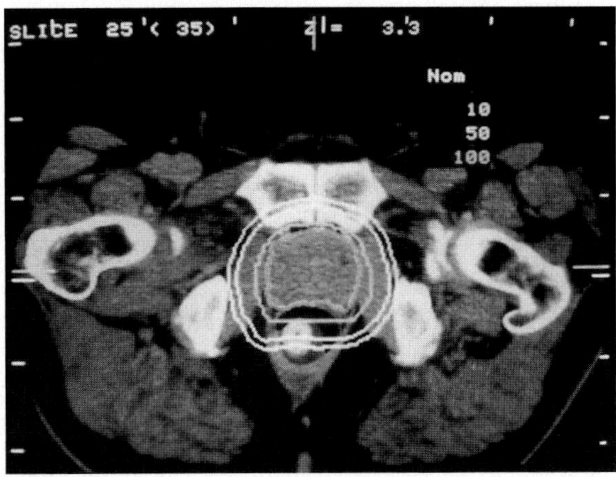

FIGURE 30-3. **A:** Sagittal computed tomography reconstruction with isodoses of a perineal proton field used at the Massachusetts General Hospital (MGH) to boost prostatic tumors. Note the lucite tube and water balloon within the rectum. These serve to displace the posterior rectal wall from the path of the beam and immobilize the prostate. **B:** Transverse computed tomography view through the prostate with isodoses demonstrating the MGH perineal boost.

control at 8 years, but this did not reach statistical significance (73% high dose vs. 59% low dose, p = .09). There was, however, a statistically significant improvement in local disease control at 5 and 8 years for the subset with Gleason 7 to 10 tumors treated in the high-dose arm (94% and 84% vs. 64% and 19%). The percentage of positive rebiopsies was also lower for this subset in the high-dose arm, although biases will have been introduced here by the fact that not all men with negative digital rectal examinations consented to rebiopsy. This gain in local control was not seen for men with lower Gleason grade tumors.

The improved local outcome for men did not translate into a gain in terms of disease-free survival (biochemical or clinical) or overall survival. In retrospect, this is not surprising. All men had large tumors, and most were randomized before the use of PSA screening. Many would have PSA levels surely indicative of metastatic disease and, in a comparable contemporary trial, would not have been included, as they could not stand to gain from an improved local measure. Other explanations are that the trial was underpowered with, or that the dose escalation was simply insufficient for, that stage of disease.

Perhaps the most useful information to emerge from this trial came from the subsequent analysis of treatment-related morbidity (10,11). It must be remembered that all patients received full pelvic photon treatment, so no difference would be expected, nor was it seen in terms of small bowel toxicity. The sites of greatest interest were the bladder, urethra, and rectum. The actuarial incidence of urethral stricture was seen in 19% of those in the high-dose arm and only 8% in the low-dose arm (p = .07). This was usually relieved by urologic intervention, such that it was only a persistent problem in 2% of patients in each arm. Corresponding figures for late hematuria were 14% and 8%, respectively. Among the 78 patients fully potent before irradiation who had not had endocrine therapy for a relapse, the risk of subsequent impotence was equal at 60% and 62%.

The actuarial rates of rectal bleeding were higher in the high-dose arm (32% vs. 12%), but in only one patient did this represent a grade 4 problem (Fig. 30-4). To gain greater insight into the relationship between dose and rectal bleeding, a dose-volume histogram analysis was performed on the patients receiving a proton boost, 41 of whom had bled (12). Patients receiving at least 76.5 CGE to at least 40% of their anterior rectal wall had an 81% actuarial risk of rectal bleeding as compared with 25% who received this dose to less than 40% (Fig. 30-5). It was also of note that the bleed-

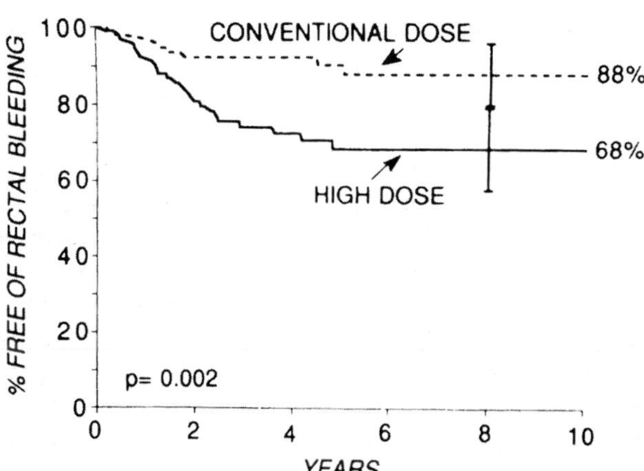

FIGURE 30-4. Actuarial incidence of rectal bleeding for patients treated with 67.2-Gy photons or 77.2-colbalt gray equivalent protons or photons in the Massachusetts General Hospital randomized trial. (From Shipley WU, Verhey LJ, Munzenrider JE, et al. Advanced prostate cancer: the results of a randomized comparative trial of high dose irradiation boosting with conformal protons compared with conventional dose irradiation using photons alone. *Int J Radiat Oncol Biol Phys* 1995;32:3–12, with permission.)

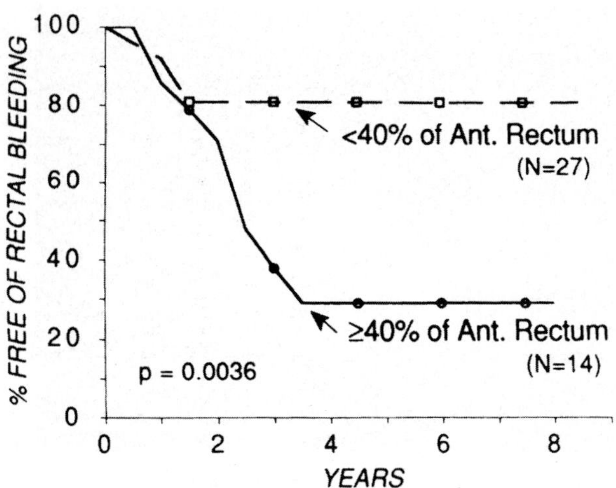

FIGURE 30-5. Actuarial risk of rectal bleeding for the high-dose patients in the Massachusetts General Hospital randomized trial. This graph shows the significance of the volume of anterior (Ant.) rectal wall receiving full dose.

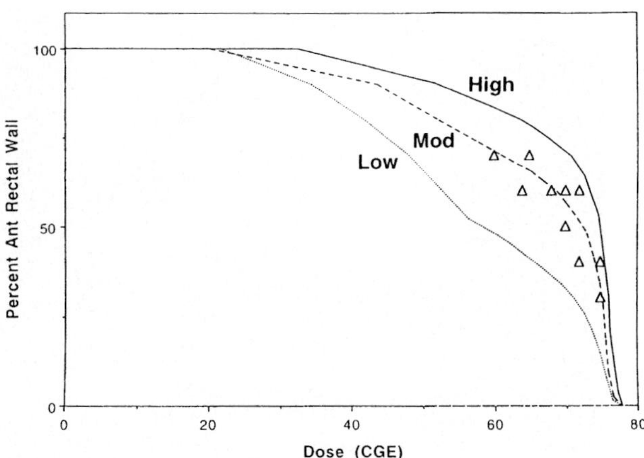

FIGURE 30-6. The risk of rectal bleeding in the high-dose arm of the Massachusetts General Hospital trial depending on lower-dose areas within the rectal dose volume histogram and not just the volume receiving full dose. Hartford et al. (12) have derived three risk groups according to dose-volume histogram shape. Ant, anterior; CGE, cobalt gray equivalent; Mod, moderate.

ing risk is not uniquely correlated with the volume receiving the highest dose of radiation, because there is also synergy with other parts of the dose-volume histogram. Thus, for a given, fixed high dose and volume, the risk increases according to the larger volume receiving a lower dose. A particularly potent synergy comes when greater than 60 Gy is given to more than 70% of the anterior rectal wall (Fig. 30-6). No subportion of the dose-volume histogram dominates, and Hartford et al. have made tables of statistically significant and equivalent risk combinations (12).

PROTON BEAM AND PROSTATE CANCER IN THE PROSTATE-SPECIFIC ANTIGEN ERA

In 1991, patients with more "contemporary" prostate cancer began to be treated in large numbers at the dedicated hospital-based facility at Loma Linda University Medical Center in California. Patients were treated with a combination of pelvic photons and a proton boost or with protons alone to their prostate, depending on their estimated risk of nodal disease. All proton treatments were given using opposed lateral 225- to 250-MeV beams that, together with the regular use of a water-filled rectal balloon, allowed for good rectal sparing. The total prostate dose was usually 74 to 75 CGE in 37 to 40 daily fractions. Between 1991 and 1995, 643 men were treated. The median follow-up at the time of their first retrospective analysis was 43 months (13). Using three successive rises in PSA as a surrogate end point, they reported 4.5-year biochemical no evidence of disease (bNED) rates of 100%, 89%, 72%, and 53% for men with pretreatment PSA values of less than 4, 4 to 10, 10.1 to 20.0, and greater than 20 ng per mL, respectively. These figures are certainly competitive with those seen after radical prostatectomy, high-dose conformal photon therapy, or brachytherapy but can only be regarded as preliminary. The definition of failure used in most studies of high-dose therapy is three successive rises in PSA. Longer follow-up will be required to avoid artefactual elevations in bNED rates. They are nevertheless very promising.

The study also examined toxicity using the Radiation Therapy Oncology Group criteria. Grade 2 rectal bleeding was seen in 21% of patients at 3 years. No grade 3 toxicity was seen. Grade 2 genitourinary (GU) toxicity was seen in 5.4% at 3 years and was usually macroscopic hematuria. No urethral strictures were seen. The very nature of GU morbidity is that its incidence increases with the passage of years, and the figure quoted will surely rise with time. Nevertheless, these data support the hypothesis that modest dose escalation may be safely achieved using conformal proton beams.

SECOND RANDOMIZED TRIAL

In 1995, the Massachusetts General Hospital and Loma Linda University Medical Center decided to launch a common venture to answer the critical question in prostate cancer: Does dose matter? Although the answer has certainly been assumed by some authors, new data have emerged, indicating that conventional doses of external radiation may be very effective in eradicating the very early–stage prostate cancer so commonly seen in the PSA era (14). This begs the question, Can we justify the time, expense, and risk of dose escalation in terms of improved cancer control? Under the auspices of the National Cancer Institute and the Proton Radiation Oncology Group (PROG), we initiated PROG 95-09. This trial randomized 390 men with T1-2N0-XM0 adenocarcinoma of the prostate and a pretreatment PSA of less than 15 ng per mL to receive a 19.8- or 28.8-CGE proton boost to the prostate to be followed without interruption by 50.4 Gy using three-dimensional conformal photons to the prostate and seminal vesicles. Although accrual is now complete, the results in terms of freedom from local failure (by planned rebiopsy) or biochemical failure are still many years off. It is of note that 97% of men in both arms completed protocol treatment, suggesting that even high doses of radiation are very acutely tolerable. In the first analysis of objective toxicity, 3 years after the first patient was accrued, 242 patients could be evaluated. Combined grade 3 GU and rectal toxicity was seen in 6.6% of those randomized to 70.2 CGE and 2.5% of those randomized to 79.2 CGE. Only one grade 4 toxicity was seen: temporary urinary retention in a man in the high-dose arm.

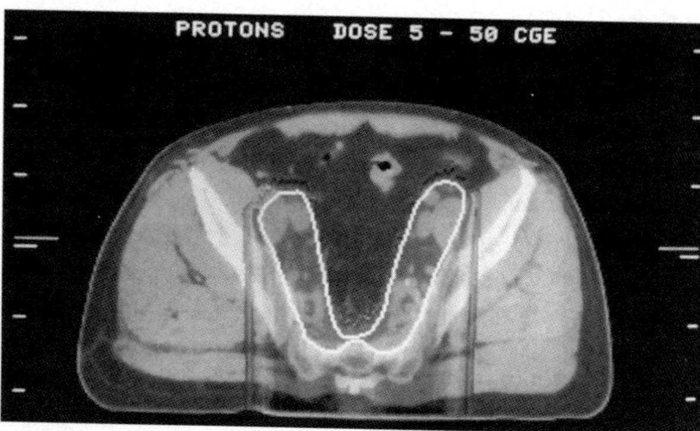

FIGURE 30-7. Dose distribution for treatment to the pelvic lymph nodes using a posterior intensity modulated proton beam. Note the limited bowel irradiation compared with treatments using photons. CGE, cobalt gray equivalent.

NEW PROTOCOLS

The collaborative randomized trial completed in 1999 certainly gives no reason to suspect that the minimum tolerated dose has yet been achieved for prostate radiation using the proton beam. A new phase I/II study is being activated in which men with early-stage prostate cancer will be treated using protons alone to a total dose of 84.6 CGE. If this dose level is tolerable, then it will be tested in a randomized fashion against a dose midway between the two arms of the first trial, 75.6 CGE. Eighty patients will be accrued to the phase II study over the next 12 months, but safety, for the purpose of initiating the phase III study, will not be declared until there has been 18 months' median follow-up.

It is also time to reexamine the issue of dose escalation in locally advanced prostate cancer. The work of Fuks et al. has shown quite clearly that a second "wave" of metastasis follows local failure and is likely the cause of it (15). Thus, not all the metastases so commonly seen after the treatment of T3 disease are the consequence of occult micrometastases present at diagnosis, and some may be preventable by better local control. Local failure is seen in up to 50% of patients treated conventionally for T3 disease, and a persistent tumor may be found on rebiopsy of a significant proportion of the remainder (16). Neoadjuvant androgen deprivation seems to offer some help in this regard and is now a standard part of treatment for this stage of disease (17). Neoadjuvant therapy may be combined with dose escalation and is a potentially beneficial approach. A phase I/II PROG trial will also soon begin looking at the safety of pelvic nodal treatment plus a proton boost to the prostate and, if indicated, the seminal vesicles to a total dose of 84.6 CGE. These doses will be given against a background of androgen deprivation. Treating more advanced disease to high doses presents a greater planning challenge than the treatment of early-stage disease, for the reasons indicated by Hartford et al. (12). Although the volumes of the anterior rectal wall receiving full dose can be kept small, the need for wider field treatment to obturator nodes and seminal vesicles does increase the rectal volume receiving lower doses and consequently increases the risk of bleeding. This problem challenges all who use three-dimensional conformal therapy for locally advanced tumors but wider field treatment is the one to which protons are perhaps best suited.

The ability of the proton beam to treat a concave volume may also be exploited in the treatment of pelvic lymph nodes (Fig. 30-7). A modulated posterior beam can be used to almost entirely avoid the small bowel. This approach may also have application in cancer of the uterine cervix or rectum.

CONCLUSION

Proton beam radiation is currently the most conformal of all available conformal therapies and outperforms photons plan for plan. Conformal proton beam therapy has demonstrated safety and efficacy in the treatment of tumors in difficult radiation dose–limited situations, such as the central nervous system and eye, and in situations in which integral dose is critical, such as pediatrics. The prostate is likewise a target needy of higher dose but surrounded by sensitive structures, and National Cancer Institute–sponsored studies are now under way to evaluate the role of proton beam. Several new centers are being established in the United States, and advances in accelerator technology are starting to reduce the cost of these units. It is therefore likely that proton beam therapy will be brought within the reach of an increasing number of prostate cancer patients over the coming years.

REFERENCES

1. Zietman AL. Radiation therapy or prostatectomy: an old conflict revisited in the PSA era. *Semin Radiat Oncol* 1998;8:81–86.
2. Ten Haken RK, Perez-Tamayo C, Tesser RJ, et al. Best treatment of the prostate using shaped fixed fields. *Int J Radiat Oncol Biol Phys* 1989;6:193–200.
3. Dearnaley DP, Khoo VS, Norman AR, et al. Comparison of radiation side-effects of conformal and conventional radio-

therapy in prostate cancer: a randomized trial. *Lancet* 1999; 353:267–273.

4. Zelefsky MJ, Leibel SA, Gaudin PB, et al. Dose escalation with 3-D conformal radiation therapy affects the outcome in prostate cancer *Int J Radiat Oncol Biol Phys* 1998;41: 491–500.
5. Hanks GE, Hanlon AL, Schultheiss TE, et al. Dose escalation with 3-D conformal treatment: 5 year outcomes, treatment optimization, and future directions. *Int J Radiat Oncol Biol Phys* 1998;41:501–510.
6. Archambeau J, Bennett G, Levine G. Proton radiation therapy. *Radiology* 1974;110:445–447.
7. Suit HD, Urie M. Proton beams in radiation therapy. *J Natl Cancer Inst* 1992;84:155–164.
8. Munzenrider JE, Gragoudas E, Seddon J, et al. Conservative treatment of uveal melanoma: probability of eye retention after proton treatment. *Int J Radiat Oncol Biol Phys* 1988; 15:553–558.
9. Shipley WU, Tepper JE, Pront GR, et al. Proton radiation as boost therapy for localized prostatic carcinoma. *JAMA* 1979;241:1912–1915.
10. Shipley WU, Verhey LJ, Munzenrider JE, et al. Advanced prostate cancer: the results of a randomized comparative trial of high dose irradiation boosting with conformal protons compared with conventional dose irradiation using photons alone. *Int J Radiat Oncol Biol Phys* 1995; 32:3–12.
11. Benk V, Adams J, Shipley WU, et al. Late rectal bleeding following combined x-ray and proton high dose irradiation for patients with stages T3-4 prostate carcinoma. *Int J Radiat Oncol Biol Phys* 1996;26:551–557.
12. Hartford AC, Niemierko A, Adams JA, et al. Conformal irradiation of the prostate: estimating long-term rectal bleeding risk using dose-volume histograms. *Int J Radiat Oncol Biol Phys* 1996;36:721–730.
13. Slater JD, Yonemoto LT, Rossi CJ, et al. Conformal proton therapy for prostate carcinoma. *Int J Radiat Oncol Biol Phys* 1998;42:299–304.
14. Shipley WU, Thames HD, Sandler HM, et al. Radical radiation therapy: long-term results. *JAMA* 1999;281:1598–1601.
15. Fuks Z, Leibel SA, Walker KE, et al. The effect of local control on metastatic dissemination in carcinoma of the prostate. *Int J Radiat Oncol Biol Phys* 1991;21:537–547.
16. Zietman AL, Westgeest JC, Shipley WU. Radiation based approaches in the management of T3 adenocarcinoma of the prostate. *Semin Urol Oncol* 1997;15:230–238.
17. Pilepich MV, Krall JM, Al-Sarraf M, et al. Androgen deprivation with radiation therapy alone for locally advanced adenocarcinomas of the prostate: a randomized comparative trial of the RTOG. *Urology* 1995;45:616–623.

31

NEOADJUVANT ANDROGEN DEPRIVATION BEFORE RADICAL PROSTATECTOMY FOR PROSTATE ADENOCARCINOMA

JEFF A. WIEDER
MARK S. SOLOWAY

Androgen deprivation is a systemic hormone therapy that induces programmed cell death (apoptosis) and inhibition of cell proliferation in malignant prostate tissue (1). When this therapy is applied before definitive treatment for prostate cancer, it is called *neoadjuvant androgen deprivation* (NAD). The use of NAD before radical prostatectomy is controversial. However, review of the literature may provide insight into its application before surgery.

BACKGROUND

In 1941, Huggins and Hodges (2) described the first evidence of androgen sensitivity in prostate cancer. NAD was initially reported by Vallett (3) in 1944 and was accomplished by bilateral orchiectomy before perineal prostatectomy. Subsequently, several clinicians used bilateral orchiectomy or estrogen, or both, before radical prostatectomy for locally advanced prostate carcinoma (4–11). One investigator reported a similar 15-year disease-free survival between radical prostatectomy for clinically organ-confined prostate cancer and NAD followed by radical prostatectomy for locally advanced prostate cancer (11). Despite these promising results, NAD did not gain widespread acceptance because of the irreversibility of orchiectomy and the cardiovascular risks associated with estrogens. With the advent of luteinizing hormone releasing hormone (LHRH) agonists, reversible androgen suppression could be achieved with minimal toxicity. Renewed interest in NAD prompted modern investigations, including prospective randomized trials.

RATIONALE FOR NEOADJUVANT ANDROGEN DEPRIVATION

The rationale for using NAD before radical prostatectomy is to eradicate malignant androgen-dependent cells in the hope that sufficient tumor regression will permit complete resection of residual cancer. NAD may benefit men with (a) presumed organ-confined prostate cancer, (b) locally advanced cancer, and (c) occult metastatic cancer.

Radical prostatectomy is most likely to cure patients with organ-confined prostate adenocarcinoma. However, predicting which patients have organ-confined disease is difficult, because clinical stage does not accurately reflect the extent of tumor. Approximately 50% of men with clinical stage T1 or T2 prostate cancer have extension of tumor outside the prostate capsule (12–14). Furthermore, 20% to 30% of patients with clinical stage T1 or T2 cancer have positive surgical margins at prostatectomy (15). Therefore, many men undergoing radical prostatectomy for clinically localized disease have an unfavorable pathologic outcome. Perhaps NAD can improve the prognosis of these patients by increasing the chances of complete resection.

Patients with locally advanced prostate cancer are usually not considered candidates for radical surgery, because complete resection is rarely achieved (15). Preoperative hormone therapy to reduce tumor bulk may permit total resection in these patients. Occult metastatic prostate cancer may occur in some patients who are thought to have localized tumors. If NAD can eradicate micrometastatic disease, then radical prostatectomy can cure these patients.

SIDE EFFECTS OF NEOADJUVANT ANDROGEN DEPRIVATION

The specific side effects of NAD depend on the form of therapy administered. Adverse reactions of the more common agents are summarized here. Estrogens may cause gynecomastia, impotence, peripheral edema, and altered fat distribution (14,16). The most serious complications of estrogen therapy are deep venous thrombosis, pulmonary embolism, cerebrovascular accident, and myocardial infarction, which have been reported in up to 5% of patients (14,16). LHRH agonists can cause testicular atrophy, loss of libido, impotence, hot flashes, body fat redistribution, and weight gain (16–19). A potentially serious side effect of an LHRH agonist is the flare phenomenon. LHRH agonists may cause an initial transient increase in testosterone that may induce cancer growth and exacerbate tumor-related symptoms (i.e., the cancer "flares" up) (17–19). Occasionally, the flare generates serious sequela, such as ureteral obstruction (17,18), spinal cord compression (18,19), or possibly death. The clinical impact of the flare phenomenon is obviously stage dependent. The increase in testosterone (above the pre-NAD level) peaks in 3 to 4 days and lasts for approximately 7 days (17–19). Thereafter, testosterone continuously declines until castrate levels are reached, in approximately 30 days (17–19). Administering an antiandrogen before the LHRH agonist may eliminate the "flare" (20). Some clinicians start the antiandrogen and LHRH agonist at the same time; however, it may be beneficial to have a steady state level of antiandrogen before starting the LHRH agonist. To reach steady state, the antiandrogen should be started four half-lives before giving the LHRH agonist. The antiandrogen should be continued for at least 1 week after the LHRH agonist, because the increase in testosterone above pretreatment levels lasts approximately 1 week. However, some clinicians continue the antiandrogen for at least 1 month after the LHRH agonist, because it takes approximately 30 days (17–19) for testosterone to reach castrate levels.

Side effects may vary among the nonsteroidal antiandrogens. Most of these agents can cause hot flashes, breast pain, and gynecomastia (16,21). Diarrhea is more frequent with flutamide (16,21). Rare, serious side effects include hepatitis and cholestatic jaundice (16,21). Because a nonsteroidal antiandrogen is often administered with an LHRH agonist (combined androgen blockade), side effects of NAD may represent a mixture of those from the antiandrogen and the LHRH agonist.

CLINICAL EFFECTS OF NEOADJUVANT ANDROGEN DEPRIVATION

Serum Prostate-Specific Antigen

In nearly all patients (22,23), serum prostate-specific antigen (PSA) declines by approximately 90% with up to 3 months of NAD (12,14,23–32). When longer intervals of NAD are administered, serum PSA decreases even further (32–35). PSA declines rapidly over the first 1 to 2 months, followed by a slower decline from 3 to 8 months (33–35). PSA nadir is reached in 22% to 34% of patients after 3 months of NAD and 84% to 86% after 8 months (33–35). Time to PSA nadir is not related to the pretreatment PSA (33,35). Undetectable PSA is achieved in 27% to 55% of patients after 3 months of NAD (22,28,32,33,35). Continuing NAD achieves undetectable PSA in 60% to 88% of patients at 6 months (33,35) and 66% to 73% at 8 months (32,33). Rarely, the PSA may not change, despite castrate levels of testosterone (33,35).

Downsizing of the Prostate

Several studies demonstrate that the transrectal ultrasound (TRUS)–determined prostate volume decreases by approximately 30% (range, 12% to 52%) after NAD (12,14,23–26,28,31,32,36–41). This reduction in volume probably occurs by atrophy of benign and malignant elements (42). Extending the duration of NAD from 3 to 8 months results in significantly greater reduction in TRUS prostate volume (32).

Decreased Size of the Radiographic Lesion

In patients with radiographic evidence of cancer, the size of the radiographic lesion decreases by approximately 30% (38) in at least half of the subjects receiving NAD (25,36,40,43). D'Amico et al. (36) found that a reduction in endorectal magnetic resonance imaging tumor volume was significantly associated with organ-confined disease at prostatectomy.

Clinical Downstaging of Prostate Cancer

Clinical downstaging is defined as a decrease in the patient's clinical tumor stage after NAD. Clinical downstaging is noted in 40% of men with cT1-T2 tumors (25) and 32% to 90% of men with cT2-T3 tumors (26,31,44) after 3 months of NAD. In patients with cT2b tumors, none had clinical downstaging after 1.5 months of NAD (14). Downstaging from cT3 to cT2 cancer occurs in 48% to 60% of subjects receiving NAD (14,39). In the authors' experience, the prostate feels more normal (smaller and smoother) in the vast majority of patients undergoing NAD. A small portion of subjects (5.1% to 8.3%) are clinically upstaged after NAD (14,25).

PATHOLOGIC EFFECTS OF NEOADJUVANT ANDROGEN DEPRIVATION

Problems with Pathologic Interpretation

Accurate histologic assessment is only possible when the pathologist is aware of the factors that may have altered the prostate. Therefore, the clinician must notify the pathologist when a patient has received NAD. The histologic changes induced by androgen deprivation can make pathologic interpretation difficult and may lead to misinterpretation by the pathologist. Misinterpretation is generally manifested by inappropriate tumor grading or missed tumor foci.

Multiple studies report that tumor grade is higher in prostates exposed to NAD compared to those without preoperative treatment (27,33,41,45–48). This "upgrading" is paradoxic, because it implies that a more aggressive tumor develops during hormone therapy, when the tumor actually shows marked atrophy (49) and minimal proliferative activity (41). This paradox exists because androgen deprivation significantly affects two of Gleason's (50) criteria: tumor gland size and the amount of stroma between the tumor glands (49). Androgen deprivation decreases tumor gland size and increases stroma, giving the tumor a high-grade appearance (41,49). Thus, a favorable finding (marked response to hormonal therapy) may be misinterpreted as an unfavorable finding (high-grade tumor). With more experience, most pathologists can differentiate between androgen withdrawal effect and high-grade tumor (51). Nonetheless, standard Gleason scoring in androgen-deprived prostate cancer may result in artificially high scores. Therefore, Civantos et al. (49) proposed (a) not assigning a Gleason score to prostates that have undergone androgen deprivation or (b) using a modified Gleason score that excludes criteria based on gland size and stroma. Using this modified scoring system, they found that the variation between biopsy grade and prostatectomy grade was the same in treated and untreated subjects (49).

The pathologist may overlook foci of residual cancer for several reasons. First, cytoarchitectural changes may be so extreme that neoplastic elements may not be recognized (41,42,52,53). For example, NAD clears the cytoplasm (42,49,52) and reduces the size of the nuclei (41,42,49,52,54) and nucleoli (41,42,47,49,52,55). Thus, valuable criteria for determining malignancy (nuclear size and prominent nucleoli) may be lost after NAD. Second, tumors may shrink so much that they become difficult to identify by conventional hematoxylin and eosin (H & E) staining (33,34,41,42,52–54). In fact, Gleave et al. (33,34), Witjes et al. (26), and Bazinet et al. (54) reported that patients initially classified as pT0 based on H & E staining were found to have microscopic foci of tumor after staining for prostatic acid phosphatase (PAP). Third, incomplete or inadequate sectioning of the prostate may contribute to missing positive surgical margins (15) or small foci of cancer (49,56). Fourth, the pathologist may not have experience in examining prostates exposed to NAD and, thus, may miss the diagnosis (51).

Several studies of NAD have attempted to identify unrecognized prostate cancer cells by using additional sectioning (49,56) or special stains (26,33,34,41–43,54,57). In specimens originally classified as pT0 based on H & E staining, PAP staining revealed microscopic foci of the tumor (26,33,34,54). Bazinet et al. (54) used immunohistochemical cytokeratin staining with AE AE1/AE3, which stains benign and malignant prostatic epithelial cells, to demonstrate that conventional H & E staining resulted in missing 40% of positive margins and 33% of capsular penetration.

Problems in identifying residual cancer after NAD engender questions regarding the validity of all studies that show no residual tumor, decreased positive margins, and decreased capsular penetration. Perhaps these pathologic changes are not true effects of NAD but rather misinterpretation of the pathologic specimen. The problems in identifying residual cancer after NAD should be kept in mind when reviewing the literature. Thorough examination of the prostate and recognition of histologic changes caused by NAD are crucial to determining the existence of a residual tumor. Special stains and additional sectioning may be necessary to accurately determine pathologic stage.

Positive Surgical Margins

NAD effects on the prostate may make it difficult to identify the tumor at the resection margin. Karakiewicz et al. (57) and Bazinet et al. (54) demonstrated that monoclonal cytokeratin antibody staining showed a higher rate of positive margins compared to conventional H & E staining. However, Gleave et al. (34) showed no difference in positive margins when comparing conventional H & E staining with cytokeratin and PAP staining. Thus, the need for special stains to determine margin status remains controversial. Nonetheless, thorough pathologic sectioning should be performed (15).

Many randomized and nonrandomized studies demonstrate that NAD significantly decreases the rate of positive margins (Tables 31-1 and 31-2). The reason for this may include (a) a reduction in prostate volume (12,14,23–26,28,31,32,36–41) that permits resection of wider surgical margins (62); (b) pathologic downstaging of the tumor (13,26,44,61,63), resulting in regression of cancer that would have been at the resection margin; (c) local tissue reaction that results in better definition of surgical planes, thus permitting a more effective resection; and (d) misinterpretation by the pathologist (26,54).

The effectiveness of NAD in reducing positive margins depends on clinical tumor stage and biopsy Gleason score. NAD significantly decreases positive margins in clinical stage T1 and T2 prostate cancers (Tables 31-1 and 31-2) (12,14,21,24–26,37,49). Prospective randomized studies (14,26,64), nonrandomized case-controlled studies (30,60), and uncontrolled studies (43) have shown that NAD does not reduce the high incidence of positive margins in clinical stage T3 cancer (Tables 31-1 and 31-2). In most studies, NAD has been administered for the same duration regardless of tumor stage. Because high-stage tumors correlate with large tumor volume (65), T3 cancers may require a longer duration of NAD to achieve the same effects seen in smaller, lower-stage tumors. Men with biopsy Gleason score greater than 7 have a less dramatic reduction in positive margins with NAD (34). Thus, high-grade tumors may be less responsive to androgen withdrawal (48,52). The relationship between pretreatment PSA and positive margins is

TABLE 31-1. PROSPECTIVE RANDOMIZED TRIALS COMPARING PATHOLOGIC FINDINGS BETWEEN RADICAL PROSTATECTOMY ALONE AND NEOADJUVANT ANDROGEN DEPRIVATION (NAD) FOLLOWED BY RADICAL PROSTATECTOMY

Prospective randomized trials	No. of patients		Clinical stage	NAD duration (mo)	Type of NAD	% Positive margins		*p* Value for margins	% Positive SV		*p* Value for SV	% Positive nodes		*p* Value for nodes
	RP only	NAD + RP				RP only	NAD + RP		RP only	NAD + RP		RP only	NAD + RP	
Clinical stage T1-T2														
Kava et al. (24)	74	63	T1-T2	3	CAB	32	16	.04	—	—	—	—	—	—
Fair et al. (12)	66	65	T1-T2	3	CAB	36	17	—	—	—	—	—	—	—
Dalkin et al. (58)	28	28	T1c-T2b	3	LHRH	—	—	NS	—	—	—	3.6	3.6	NS
Goldenberg et al. (25)	101	91	T1b-T2c	3	CPA	64.8	27.7	.001	14.3	27.7	.035	3.3	6.9	NS
van Poppel et al. (14)	36	37	T2b	1.5	Estramustine	—[a]	—[a]	<.01	—	—	—	—	—	—
Soloway et al. (21)	138	144	T2b	3	CAB	48	18	<.001	22	15	NS	6	6	NS
Witjes et al. (26)	92	107	T2	3	CAB	36	14	<.01	—	—	—	16	4	—
Clinical stage T2-T3														
Labrie et al. (13)	90	71	B,C	3	CAB	33.8	7.8	<.001	—	—	—	—	—	—
Witjes et al. (26)	164	190	T2,T3	3	CAB	46	27	<.01	—	—	—	23	12	.01
Clinical stage T3														
van Poppel et al. (14)	29	25	T3	1.5	Estramustine	—[b]	—[b]	—	—	—	—	—	—	—
Witjes et al. (26)	72	83	T3	3	CAB	59	43	NS	—	—	—	32	16	—
Clinical stage T1-T3														
Aus et al. (59)	59	63	T1b-T3a	3	LHRH	45.5	23.6	.013	—	—	—	14	15	—

CAB, combined androgen blockade with luteinizing hormone releasing hormone agonist and flutamide; CPA, cyproterone acetate; LHRH, luteinizing hormone releasing hormone agonist; NS, not statistically significant; RP, radical prostatectomy; SV, seminal vesicle.

[a]Percent of subjects having positive margins was not reported (subjects may have had more than one positive margin). However, percent of the total number of positive margins was significantly less in the NAD + RP group.

[b]The incidence of positive margins increased with NAD (no *p* value reported).

TABLE 31-2. NONRANDOMIZED CONTROLLED TRIALS COMPARING PATHOLOGIC FINDINGS BETWEEN RADICAL PROSTATECTOMY ALONE AND NEOADJUVANT ANDROGEN DEPRIVATION (NAD) FOLLOWED BY RADICAL PROSTATECTOMY

Nonrandomized controlled trials	No. of patients		Clinical Stage	NAD duration (mo)	Type of NAD	% Positive margins		*p* Value for margins	% Positive SV		*p* Value for SV	% Positive nodes		*p* Value for nodes
	RP only	NAD + RP				RP only	NAD + RP		RP only	NAD + RP		RP only	NAD + RP	
Clinical stage T2														
Civantos et al. (49)	60	113	T2	3	CAB	43	19	.00076	23	22	NS	5	6	NS
Fair et al. (12)	53	49	T2	3	CAB	34	8	—	—	—	—	10	8	—
Lee et al. (37)	12	119	B	3	CAB	33.3	9.2	.025	—	—	—	—	—	—
Clinical stage T2-T3														
Schulman and Sassine (39)	60	40	T2-T3	2–12	CAB	57	32	—	—	—	—	—	—	—
Oesterling et al. (30)	21	21	B2-C	1–4	LHRH ± flutamide	38	86	<.01	43	60	NS	29	29	NS
Vaillancourt et al. (47)	49	47	B-C	3	CAB	27	2	.002	6	0	NS	—	—	—
Clinical Stage T3														
Bergstralh et al. (60)	144	72	T3	—	CAB, DES, or orch	63	57	NS	—	—	—	36	39	—
Clinical stage T1-T3														
Cookson et al. (28)	72	69	T1b-T3	3	CAB	33	10	<.01	—	—	—	10	7	—
Abbas et al. (27)	120	40	T1c-T3a	3–20	LHRH ± flutamide	40.8	22.5	<.05	15	22.5	NS	1.6	2.5	NS
Solomon et al. (38)	119	156	T1-T3	3	CAB	35.3	11.5	—	—	—	—	—	—	—
Fair et al. (12,29)	72	69	T1-T3	3	CAB	33	10	—	—	—	—	10	8	—
Wood et al. (61)	918	99	—	—	—	22	13	.06	—	—	—	—	—	—

CAB, combined androgen blockade with luteinizing hormone releasing hormone agonist and flutamide; DES, diethylstilbestrol; LHRH, luteinizing hormone releasing hormone agonist; NS, not statistically significant; orch, bilateral orchiectomy; RP, radical prostatectomy; SV, seminal vesicle.

inconsistent. In men with pretreatment PSA greater than 10 ng per mL, Gleave et al. (34) found that NAD was not effective in reducing positive margins, whereas Kava et al. (24) found a significant reduction in positive margins. Dalkin et al. (58) reported no relation between pretreatment PSA and pathologic outcome.

After NAD, the most common sites of positive margins after radical prostatectomy are the apex (25) and posterolateral (14). In cT1 or cT2 tumors treated with NAD, apical (14,25,38), posterolateral (14), lateral (25), and urethral positive margins (21) occur significantly less often than without neoadjuvant therapy, whereas the rate of positive margins at the bladder neck (prostate base) (14,21,25), anterior (25), and posterior (25) are not affected by NAD. In cT3 tumors, NAD did not decrease positive margins at the apex, posterolateral, or base (14).

In summary, NAD decreases the incidence of positive margins in clinical stage T1 and T2 tumors. Men with clinical stage T3 cancer and Gleason score greater than 7 are at high risk for positive margins despite NAD.

Capsule Penetration

NAD decreases the rate of capsular penetration and therefore increases the incidence of organ-confined cancer (12,13,21,25–29,47,61,66,67).

Pelvic Lymph Node Metastasis

Witjes et al. (26) reported a significantly lower rate of pelvic lymph node metastasis in patients receiving NAD compared to those receiving only radical prostatectomy (12.8% vs. 23.2%, respectively; p <.01). However, the majority of studies reveals no significant difference in the incidence of pelvic lymph node metastasis (Tables 31-1 and 31-2) (12,21,25,27–29,60). Thus, it is unlikely that NAD affects lymph node status.

Seminal Vesical Invasion

Goldenberg et al. (25) reported a significantly higher rate of seminal vesicle invasion in subjects receiving NAD compared to those receiving no pretreatment (27.7% vs. 14.3%, respectively; p = .035). However, most studies report no difference in seminal vesical invasion between subjects receiving and not receiving NAD (Tables 31-1 and 31-2) (21,27,47,68). Thus, NAD does not reduce the incidence of seminal vesical invasion.

Pathologic Downstaging

Pathologic downstaging occurs when the pathologic stage is lower than the pretreatment clinical stage. Although one study reported that NAD results in no significant pathologic downstaging compared to surgery alone (58), most others show significant pathologic downstaging with NAD (13,14,26,61,63). In a metaanalysis of seven randomized trials, Bonney et al. (63) reported that pathologic downstaging occurred significantly more often after NAD. Approximately 13% to 55% of patients are pathologically downstaged after NAD (13,14,26,31,37,39,45). Approximately 6% (range, 0% to 18%) of subjects receiving NAD are downstaged to pT0 (12,13,21,25,26,35,37,39,43,44,47,54,66,69,70). As stated previously, these patients may be classified erroneously as pT0 because of misinterpretation by the pathologist. Nevertheless, it is possible that some subjects have complete tumor regression after NAD (43), although this is probably rare.

Pathologic Upstaging

Pathologic upstaging occurs in approximately 9% to 54% of subjects undergoing NAD before radical prostatectomy (13,14,39). Upstaging may be caused by poor response to NAD, development of androgen insensitive tumor, or inaccurate pretreatment clinical staging.

Gleason Score and Tumor Grade

Multiple studies report that tumor grade is higher in prostates exposed to NAD than in those without preoperative treatment (27,33,45–48). As stated previously, this "upgrading" is artificial and may be confusing to the clinician. Civantos et al. (49) proposed (a) not assigning a Gleason score on prostates that have undergone androgen deprivation or (b) using a modified Gleason score that excluded criteria based on gland size and stroma.

Additional Histologic Findings

NAD does not affect all areas of the prostate equally. In fact, up to 43% of prostates treated with NAD had areas of tumor that were not affected (52). The histologic changes induced by NAD are less prominent in high-grade tumors (48,52). The most common histologic effects of NAD are summarized in Table 31-3. In benign prostate tissue, NAD increases gland atrophy, basal cell prominence or hyperplasia, vacuolization of the inner cell layer, squamous metaplasia, and transitional metaplasia but reduces the occurrence of high-grade prostatic intraepithelial neoplasia. In malignant prostate tissue, NAD increases gland atrophy, cytoplasmic vacuolization, cytoplasmic clearing, nuclear condensation, stroma between glands, squamous metaplasia, and lymphocytic infiltration but reduces the prominence of the nucleoli. NAD significantly decreases the incidence of neural invasion (37,47) but does not influence vascular invasion (47). NAD rarely induces necrosis (37,48,49,52).

NAD causes many different architectural patterns in malignant prostate tissue. The most common pattern is characterized by decreased size and density of neoplastic

TABLE 31-3. HISTOLOGIC EFFECTS OF NEOADJUVANT ANDROGEN DEPRIVATION (NAD) ON BENIGN AND MALIGNANT PROSTATE TISSUE

Changes in benign tissue associated with NAD
- Increased non–tumor gland atrophy (37,42,47,49,52,70)
- Increased basal cell hyperplasia/prominence (37,41,42,47,49,52,55,70)
- Vacuolated inner cell layer (41,47,49,52,70)
- Increased squamous metaplasia (37,42,47,49,52,55,70)
- Increased transitional metaplasia (49,52,70)
- Decreased high-grade prostatic intraepithelial neoplasm (42,46,47,49,52,55,71)

Changes in malignant tissue associated with NAD
- Increased cytoplasmic vacuolization (23,37,41,42,47,49,52,54,55,70)
- Increased cytoplasmic clearing (42,49,52)
- Increased nuclear pyknosis/condensation (41,42,49,52,54,55)
- Increased squamous metaplasia (42,49,52)
- Increased tumor gland atrophy (42,48,49,52,70)
- Increased stroma between glands (decreased gland density) (42,48,49,52)
- Increased lymphocytic infiltrate of tumor (42,49,52)
- Loss of nucleolar prominence (41,42,47,55)
- Decreased neural invasion (37,47)

glands and is usually associated with increased stroma between glands (49,52,70). This pattern has been referred to as the *LHRH effect* (49,52). The second most common pattern, initially described as hemangiopericytoma-like (70), consists of branching clefts lined with tumor cells (52,70). A third pattern exhibits lymphocytic infiltration and large tumor cells with clear or vacuolated cytoplasm (42,49,52). Occasionally, NAD results in markedly dilated tumor glands that may mimic benign atrophic glands (41,70).

Circulating Prostate Cancer Cells

Investigations using reverse transcriptase-polymerase chain reaction demonstrate that NAD decreases circulating prostate cancer cells in the blood (72) and bone marrow (43,68). Thus, NAD may eliminate micrometastatic disease. Su et al. (72) reported that circulating prostate cancer cells increased immediately after radical prostatectomy, then gradually declined. This trend existed regardless of whether the patient received NAD, suggesting that prostate manipulation during surgery causes hematogenous dissemination of tumor. Nonetheless, circulating prostate cancer cells occurred less frequently with NAD at each time point compared to surgery alone, implying that NAD may reduce dissemination from surgical manipulation. These studies suggest that NAD may be capable of eliminating hematogenous micrometastasis that occurs before surgery and those that occur from surgical manipulation. However, follow-up data are needed to determine whether these findings will improve survival.

In patients with prostate cancer cells in their bone marrow, Wood et al. (68) found organ-confined cancer in 45% of subjects receiving NAD, compared to 6% in men undergoing surgery alone (p = .018). This indicates that some men undergoing NAD have local tumor regression, resulting in what appears to be organ-confined cancer, but still have circulating micrometastatic disease. In other words, NAD may influence the local tumor more than the metastasis. This may explain why NAD before radical prostatectomy has not improved disease-free survival.

EFFECT OF NEOADJUVANT ANDROGEN DEPRIVATION ON SURGERY, HOSPITAL STAY, AND COMPLICATIONS

With a large prostate, NAD may facilitate resection by reducing prostate volume and creating more space for a surgeon to operate. However, a moderate or small-size prostate may recede further under the pubic bone during NAD, making access to the prostate more difficult and the dissection, especially at the apex, more arduous (Solway, *unpublished observations*, 2000). The authors have observed extensive periprostatic fibrosis in some patients who have received NAD. When this fibrosis is present, the apical dissection is often more difficult. Seminal vesical adherence to the periprostatic tissue may occasionally make radical prostatectomy more difficult after NAD (21). However, most authors report no difference in the difficulty between radical prostatectomy alone and surgery after NAD (14,25). In addition, the ability to perform nerve sparing does not appear to be altered by NAD (21,25). However, when NAD induces periprostatic fibrosis, nerve sparing may be more difficult (Solway, unpublished observations, 2000). NAD before radical prostatectomy does not significantly alter mean hospital stay (21,26), operative time (14,21,26,31,44), surgical blood loss (14,21,25,26,31), volume of blood transfused (21), or the number of patients requiring transfusion (25).

Rectal and ureteral injuries, which rarely occur during radical prostatectomy, occurred even less often after NAD in a multiinstitutional study (21). Gleave et al. (25) reported no difference in intraoperative complications between men receiving and not receiving NAD. The incidence and type of postoperative complications are not significantly different (25,26).

SURVIVAL AFTER NEOADJUVANT ANDROGEN DEPRIVATION AND RADICAL PROSTATECTOMY

Positive surgical margins and capsular penetration are associated with an increased risk of progression (15). Because NAD decreases the incidence of positive margins and capsular penetration, clinicians hoped these pathologic findings would translate into improved survival. However, prospective randomized (59,64,71,73–75) and nonran-

TABLE 31-4. TRIALS COMPARING BIOCHEMICAL PROGRESSION BETWEEN RADICAL PROSTATECTOMY ALONE AND NEOADJUVANT ANDROGEN DEPRIVATION (NAD) FOLLOWED BY RADICAL PROSTATECTOMY

Initial studies	Most recent follow-up study	Clinical stage	NAD duration (mo)	Type of NAD	Minimum follow-up (yr)	% Biochemical progression: RP only	% Biochemical progression: NAD + RP	p Value
Prospective randomized trials								
Fair et al. (12)[a]	Balaji et al. (71)[a]	T1-T2	3	CAB	2.7[b]	14.8	18.7	NS
Goldenberg et al. (25,69)	Klotz et al. (73)	T1b-T2c	3	CPA	3	30.1	40.2	NS
Witjes et al. (26)	Witjes et al. (74)	T2	3	CAB	3–4	18	14	NS
Soloway et al. (21)	Soloway et al. (75)	T2b	3	CAB	2	21.6	21	NS
van Poppel et al. (14)	Baert et al. (64)	T2,T3	3	CAB	3.3[c]	Comparable		NS
Schulman et al. (44) and Witjes et al. (26)	Witjes et al. (74)	T2,T3	3	CAB	3–4	23	19	NS
Witjes et al. (26)	Witjes et al. (74)	T3	3	CAB	3–4	Comparable		NS
Hugosson et al. (76) and Pedersen et al. (77)	Aus et al. (59)	T1b-T3a	3	LHRH + CPA	2.5	Comparable in subjects with negative nodes		NS
Nonrandomized case-controlled trials								
Hellstrom et al. (78)[d]	—	T1b-T3	3	LHRH	3	16	43	<.05
Cookson et al. (28)	—	T1b-T3	3	CAB	2.9[b]	Comparable		NS

CAB, combined androgen blockade with luteinizing hormone releasing hormone agonist and flutamide; CPA, cyproterone acetate; LHRH, luteinizing hormone releasing hormone agonist; NS, not statistically significant; RP, radical prostatectomy.
[a]Approximately 25% of the patients were from a prospective nonrandomized case-controlled phase II study.
[b]Median years of follow-up.
[c]Mean years of follow-up.
[d]Control group did not have stage T3 subjects, but NAD group had T3 subjects and a higher proportion of high-grade tumors.

domized case-controlled (28) studies have shown no difference in disease-free survival between NAD and no neoadjuvant treatment with up to 4 years of follow-up (Table 31-4). Furthermore, no study has demonstrated a difference in overall survival. The reasons why NAD has not improved survival may include (a) follow-up has not been long enough to detect a difference in survival; (b) the decrease in positive margins or capsular penetration, or both, is spurious; (c) the pathologic findings are accurate, but androgen deprivation leaves behind islands of tumor outside the limits of resection; or (d) NAD may produce androgen-insensitive clones that metastasize before radical prostatectomy.

In subjects receiving NAD, biochemical failure rate is higher in those with positive margins (34,73) and higher pathologic stage (12,34,73). With NAD before radical prostatectomy, the effect of pretreatment PSA on recurrence is unclear. Some studies could not predict recurrence based on pretreatment PSA (45,69). Gleave et al. (34) reported a higher biochemical failure rate in men with pretreatment PSA greater than 10 ng per mL, whereas Klotz et al. (73) found that men with PSA of 25 to 50 ng per mL failed less often. In subjects receiving NAD, the effect of pretreatment Gleason score on progression is also unclear. Seventeen percent of subjects with a Gleason score of 7 or greater recurred biochemically, compared to 6% with a Gleason score less than 7 (34). However, other studies have demonstrated no difference in progression based on Gleason score (73). Note that pathologic Gleason score after NAD may be artificially high and may confound comparisons of Gleason score and progression.

Although NAD decreases capsular penetration and positive margins, improved pathologic outcome has not translated into longer survival with approximately 4 years follow-up. Men with positive margins and high pathologic stage are more likely to recur despite NAD.

WHO SHOULD BE TREATED WITH NEOADJUVANT ANDROGEN DEPRIVATION?

Based on the literature, it is impossible to determine which patients, if any, should receive NAD. However, the following observations may help identify the men who are likely to benefit from NAD.

NAD significantly reduces positive margins in clinical stage T1 and T2 cancer (Tables 31-1 and 31-2) (12,14,24,25,37,49). Although these findings have not translated into improved disease-free survival, the improved pathologic outcome may eventually provide a long-term benefit. Although NAD has not decreased positive margins in clinical stage T3 cancer (14,26,30,60,64), these patients may still derive an unrecognized benefit through reduction in total tumor burden.

Among men with clinical stage T1-T2, well- or moderately differentiated prostate cancer and PSA less than or equal to 4 ng per mL, Rabbani et al. (79) found that 89% of patients had organ-confined, margin-negative specimens. In a study with more than 90% of subjects having well- or moderately differentiated clinical stage T1c or T2a tumors and PSA less than 20 ng per mL, Dalkin et al. (58) reported no statistically significant difference in the pathologic outcome between men treated and not treated with 3 months of NAD. Thus, subjects with well- or moderately differentiated clinical stage T1 or T2a tumors and low PSA rarely achieve improved pathologic outcome after 3 months of NAD and, therefore, are unlikely to benefit from NAD. We await the results of the Canadian Uro-Oncology Group trial (32) to determine whether these patients benefit from a longer duration of NAD. Avoiding NAD in men who have a high likelihood of organ-confined disease can prevent the side effects associated with hormone therapy (80).

Because NAD has not improved disease-free or overall survival, we do not recommend it. If the clinician is considering NAD, then we recommend enrolling the patient in a clinical trial, if possible. Men with low-stage, low- or moderate-grade tumors, and low PSA are unlikely to benefit from NAD. We consider NAD before radical prostatectomy for men with clinical stage T2c or T3a prostate cancer, because they are at high risk for a positive surgical margin (15). We do not perform nerve sparing in these patients because of the high risk of capsular penetration into the neurovascular bundle in these stages (15).

WHAT IS THE OPTIMUM AGENT(S) FOR NEOADJUVANT ANDROGEN DEPRIVATION?

The type of NAD varies considerably. Some of the most recent agents include LHRH agonist alone (27,78), LHRH agonist with antiandrogen (13,21,24,26,27,33,44,59, 75–77), cyproterone acetate (25,69,73), cyproterone acetate and diethylstilbestrol (33,35), and estramustine (14). Gomella et al. (45) found no difference in the biochemical recurrence rate between men receiving neoadjuvant LHRH agonist alone and men receiving LHRH agonist with flutamide. However, this study was nonrandomized and examined only 21 patients. There have been no prospective randomized studies comparing regimens. Therefore, the optimum NAD agent is unknown.

WHAT IS THE OPTIMUM DURATION OF NEOADJUVANT ANDROGEN DEPRIVATION?

The optimum duration of NAD is not clear. In fact, the end point that indicates adequate preoperative response to NAD has not been elucidated. Currently, two end points are applied: (a) PSA nadir (43) and (b) completion of a specific duration of NAD.

Prostate-Specific Antigen Nadir

Theoretically, ablation of androgen-sensitive tumor cells is completed when PSA nadir is achieved. However, it is unclear whether the serum PSA reflects the degree of apoptosis (81). Soloway et al. (21) demonstrated that preoperative PSA nadir after NAD did not correlate with the incidence of positive surgical margins, suggesting that PSA nadir may not be an appropriate end point. In addition, the PSA nadir is not related to the presence of circulating prostate cancer cells (68).

Perhaps patients do not benefit from NAD unless they achieve an undetectable serum PSA. However, McLeod et al. (22) showed that there was no difference in positive margins between subjects achieving an undetectable preoperative PSA and those with a detectable PSA after NAD. They concluded, "Our series supports the contention that it is not necessary to achieve an undetectable level of PSA prior to surgery."

Specific Duration of Neoadjuvant Androgen Deprivation

Most studies have investigated 3 months of NAD. However, this duration of treatment is somewhat arbitrary. The clinician must balance the time to achieve maximum tumor reduction and apoptosis with the time to emergence of androgen-insensitive tumors.

During androgen deprivation in humans, apoptosis in the prostate begins in 2 weeks and reaches completion by approximately 8 weeks (81). This observation suggests that administering NAD for more than 3 months will not achieve additional tumor cell death. In addition, Van der Kwast et al. (82) demonstrated that extending NAD therapy to 6 months did not result in further reduction of prostate weight.

Some clinicians suggest that continuing NAD for more than 3 months is preferable. PSA nadir is reached in only 22% to 34% of patients after 3 months of NAD, compared to 84% to 86% after 8 months (33). When NAD therapy is extended from 3 to 8 months, TRUS-determined prostate volume continues to decline (32). In addition, median pathologic tumor volume was 60% less in men treated with 6 months compared to 3 months of NAD (82). A smaller prostate and lower tumor volume may imply a greater chance of complete excision. In fact, Gleave et al. (32) showed a significantly lower positive margin and capsular penetration rate after 8 months of NAD compared to 3 months. Similar findings were reported after 6 months of NAD (9.1% positive margins after 6 months of NAD vs. 27.8% after 3 months), although this difference was not statistically significant (82). Gleave et al. (32) reported no difference in the occurrence and seriousness of adverse events when NAD was continued for 8 months.

In the Shionogi mouse mammary carcinoma, an androgen-sensitive cell line, androgen independence develops after approximately 30 days of androgen withdrawal (56). Recent studies on the LNCap cell line indicate that androgen resistance may develop in a little as 2 weeks (83). These findings fuel concern that androgen-insensitive tumor cells may rapidly proliferate during NAD in humans, resulting in preoperative metastases or poor pathologic outcome at prostatectomy. With 3 months of NAD, Civantos et al. (49) found that 43% of prostatectomy specimens contained tumors that appeared unresponsive to hormone therapy. Using MIB-1 immunostaining for proliferative activity, Van der Kwast et al. (82) reported no evidence of androgen insensitivity after 3 months of NAD, but 2 of 17 tumors appeared hormone resistant after 6 months of NAD. In subjects undergoing 8 months of NAD, Gleave et al. (33) found no increase in proliferative activity between the prostatectomy specimen and the pretreatment prostate biopsy (based on staining with prolifera-tion cell nuclear antigen and Ki-67). In fact, Ki-67 was markedly suppressed after 8 months of NAD, suggesting that androgen-insensitive cells did not develop with up to 8 months of NAD.

Based on limited and somewhat conflicting data, androgen-independent tumors may or may not develop with up to 8 months of NAD. Although androgen-insensitive clones may develop during short periods of NAD, it is unclear whether these clones are clinically significant.

WHAT ARE THE POTENTIAL ADVANTAGES OF NEOADJUVANT ANDROGEN DEPRIVATION?

NAD may have several potential advantages, including decreased serum PSA, reduction in prostate size, clinical downstaging, pathologic downstaging, decreased positive surgical margins, decreased capsular penetration, and decreased circulating prostate cancer cells. None of these findings has translated into improved disease-free or overall survival. Perhaps long-term benefit is not apparent, because duration of follow-up is inadequate.

WHAT ARE THE POTENTIAL DISADVANTAGES OF NEOADJUVANT ANDROGEN DEPRIVATION?

Problems in identifying residual cancer after NAD engender questions regarding the validity of all studies that show improved pathologic outcome. Although clinicians consistently report improved pathologic parameters after NAD, it rarely eliminates the neoplasm completely and has not altered survival. Without demonstrable long-term benefit, patients receiving NAD may assume unnecessary risks and experience needless side effects. NAD adds substantial cost and may make surgical dissection more difficult. Furthermore, some patients may experience psychological distress from delayed definitive treatment.

CONCLUSION

NAD has consistently improved clinical and pathologic parameters in prostate cancer treated with radical prostatectomy. NAD induces a 90% decline in serum PSA, shrinks the prostate by approximately 30%, and causes clinical downstaging. NAD does not appear to affect intraoperative blood loss, hospital stay, surgical complications, or difficulty of surgery; however, it does add substantial cost to treatment and causes side effects (albeit rarely serious). NAD consistently improves pathologic outcome after radical prostatectomy in patients with clinical stage T1 or T2 prostate cancer by pathologic downstaging, reducing positive margins, and increasing organ confinement. NAD may be capable of eliminating hematogenous micrometastasis that occur before surgery and those that occur from surgical manipulation. Despite these observations, NAD has not altered survival with up to 4 years of follow-up.

Currently, there is insufficient information regarding the following key aspects of NAD: (a) the end point that determines adequate preoperative response to NAD; (b) the optimum NAD regimen; (c) the population, if any, in which NAD before radical prostatectomy should be used; (d) the development of androgen-insensitive clones during NAD and their clinical significance; and (e) the question, Will survival improve with longer follow-up? To help elucidate these issues, men receiving NAD should be considered for clinical trials when possible.

REFERENCES

1. Kyprianou N, English HF, Isaacs JT. Programmed cell death during regression of PC-82 human prostate cancer following androgen deprivation. *Cancer Res* 1990;50:3753.
2. Huggins C, Hodges CV. Studies on prostate cancer I: the effect of castration, of estrogen, and of androgen injection on serum phosphatase in metastatic carcinoma of the prostate. *Cancer Res* 1941;1:293.
3. Vallett BS. Radical perineal prostatectomy subsequent to bilateral orchiectomy. *Del Med J* 1944;16:9.
4. Scott WW, Benjamin JA. The role of bilateral orchiectomy in the treatment of carcinoma of the prostate gland: a report of 82 cases. *Bull N Y Acad Med* 1945;21:307.
5. Colston JA, Brendler H. Endocrine therapy in carcinoma of the prostate; preparation of patients for radical perineal prostatectomy. *JAMA* 1947;134:848.
6. Parlow AL, Scott WW. Hormone control therapy as a preparation for radical perineal prostatectomy in advanced carcinoma of the prostate. *N Y J Med* 1949;49:629.
7. Guitierrez R. New horizons in the surgical management of carcinoma of the prostate gland. *Am J Surg* 1949;78:147.
8. Scott WW. An evaluation of endocrine control therapy followed by radical perineal prostatectomy in selected cases of advanced prostatic carcinoma. *Cancer* 1953;6:248.
9. Scott WW. An evaluation of endocrine therapy plus radical perineal prostatectomy in the treatment of advanced carcinoma of the prostate. *J Urol* 1964;91:97.

10. Chute R, Fox BM. Non-resectable carcinoma of the prostate rendered resectable by endocrine therapy. *J Urol* 1966;95:577.
11. Scott WW, Boyd HL. Combined hormonal control therapy and radical prostatectomy in the treatment of selected cases of advanced carcinoma of the prostate: a retrospective study based upon 25 years of experience. *J Urol* 1969;101:86.
12. Fair WR, Cookson MS, Stroumbakis N, et al. The indications, rationale, and results of neoadjuvant androgen deprivation in the treatment of prostatic cancer: Memorial Sloan-Kettering Cancer Center results. *Urology* 1997;49(Suppl 3A):46.
13. Labrie F, Cusan L, Gomez JL, et al. Neoadjuvant hormonal therapy: the Canadian experience. *Urology* 1997;49(Suppl 3A):56.
14. Van Poppel H, de Ridder D, Elgamal AA, et al. Neoadjuvant hormonal therapy before radical prostatectomy decreases the number of positive surgical margins in stage T2 prostate cancer: interim results of a prospective randomized trial. *J Urol* 1995;154:429.
15. Wieder JA, Soloway MS. Incidence, etiology, location, prevention, and treatment of positive margins after radical prostatectomy for prostate cancer. *J Urol* 1998;160:299.
16. Daneshgari F, Crawford ED. Endocrine therapy of advanced carcinoma of the prostate. In: Das S, Crawford ED, eds. *Cancer of the prostate.* New York: Marcel Dekker Inc, 1993:333.
17. Smith JA Jr., Glode LM, Wettlaufer JN, et al. Clinical effects of gonadotropin-releasing hormone analogue in metastatic carcinoma of the prostate. *Urology* 1985;25:106.
18. Debruyne FM, Denis L, Lunglmayer G, et al. Long-term therapy with a depot luteinizing hormone-releasing hormone analogue (Zoladex) on patients with advanced prostatic carcinoma. *J Urol* 1988;140:775.
19. Soloway MS. Efficacy of buserelin in advanced prostate cancer and comparison with historical controls. *Am J Clin Oncol* 1988;11(Suppl 1):S29.
20. Labrie F, Dupont A, Belanger A, et al. Flutamide eliminates the risk of disease flare in prostatic cancer patients treated with a luteinizing hormone-releasing hormone agonist. *J Urol* 1987;138:804.
21. Soloway MS, Sharifi R, Wajsman Z, et al. Randomized prospective study comparing radical prostatectomy alone versus radical prostatectomy preceded by androgen blockade in clinical stage B2 (T2bNxMx) prostate cancer. *J Urol* 1995; 154:424.
22. McLeod DG, Johnson CF, Klein E, et al. PSA levels and the rate of positive surgical margins in radical prostatectomy specimens preceded by androgen blockade in clinical B2 (T2bNxM0) prostate cancer. *Urology* 1997;49:70.
23. Andros EA, Danesghari F, Crawford ED. Neoadjuvant hormonal therapy in stage C adenocarcinoma of the prostate. *Clin Invest Med* 1993;16:510.
24. Kava BR, Stroumbakis N, Dalbagni G, et al. Prospective randomized clinical trial comparing primary therapy with Zoladex + flutamide and radical prostatectomy versus radical prostatectomy alone in patients with clinically localized prostate cancer. *J Urol* 1997;157(Suppl)253:(abst).
25. Goldenberg SL, Klotz LH, Srigley J, et al. Randomized, prospective, controlled study comparing radical prostatectomy alone and neoadjuvant androgen withdrawal in the treatment of localized prostate cancer. *J Urol* 1996;156:873.
26. Witjes WP, Schulman CC, Debruyne FM. Preliminary results of a prospective randomized study comparing radical prostatectomy versus radical prostatectomy associated with neoadjuvant hormonal combination therapy in T2-3N0M0 prostatic carcinoma. *Urology* 1997;49(Suppl 3A):65.
27. Abbas F, Kaplan M, Soloway MS. Induction androgen deprivation therapy before radical prostatectomy for prostate cancer—initial results. *Br J Urol* 1996;77:423.
28. Cookson MS, Sogani PC, Sheinfeld RJ, et al. Pathologic staging and biochemical recurrence after neoadjuvant androgen deprivation therapy in combination with radical prostatectomy in clinically localized prostate cancer: results of a phase II study. *Br J Urol* 1997;79:432.
29. Fair WR, Aprikian AG, Cohen D, et al. Use of neoadjuvant androgen deprivation therapy in clinically localized prostate cancer. *Clin Invest Med* 1993;16:516.
30. Oesterling JE, Andrews PE, Suman VJ, et al. Preoperative androgen deprivation therapy: artificial lowering of serum prostate specific antigen without downstaging of the tumor. *J Urol* 1993;149:779.
31. Macfarlane MT, Abi-Aad A, Stein A, et al. Neoadjuvant hormonal deprivation in patients with locally advanced prostate cancer. *J Urol* 1993;150:132.
32. Gleave M, Goldenberg SL, Warner J, et al. Randomized comparative study of 3 vs. 8 months of neoadjuvant hormonal therapy prior to radical prostatectomy: biochemical and pathologic effects. *J Urol* 1999;161(Suppl):154(abst).
33. Gleave ME, Goldenberg SL, Jones EC, et al. Biochemical and pathological effects of 8 months of neoadjuvant androgen withdrawal therapy before radical retropubic prostatectomy in patients with clinically confined prostate cancer. *J Urol* 1996;155:213.
34. Gleave M, Goldenberg SL, Jones E, et al. Biochemical and pathological effects of eight months of neoadjuvant androgen withdrawal therapy—an update on 125 consecutive patients. *J Urol* 1997;157:390.
35. Sullivan L, Gleave M, Goldenberg L, et al. Long-term neoadjuvant hormonal therapy prior to radical prostatectomy in localized prostate cancer. *J Urol* 1994;151(Suppl):435A.
36. D'Amico AV, Chang E, Garnick M, et al. Assessment of prostate cancer volume using endorectal coil magnetic resonance imaging: a new predictor of tumor response to neoadjuvant androgen suppression therapy. *Urology* 1998;51:287.
37. Lee F, Siders DB, Newby JE, et al. The role of transrectal ultrasound-guided staging biopsy and androgen ablation therapy prior to radical prostatectomy. *Clin Invest Med* 1993; 16:458.
38. Solomon MH, McHugh TA, Dorr RP, et al. Hormone ablation therapy as neoadjuvant treatment to radical prostatectomy. *Clin Invest Med* 1993;16:532.
39. Schulman CC, Sassine AM. Neoadjuvant hormonal deprivation before radical prostatectomy. *Clin Invest Med* 1993;16:523.
40. Pinault S, Têtu B, Gagnon J, et al Transrectal ultrasound evaluation of local prostate cancer in patients treated with LHRH agonist and in combination with flutamide. *Urology* 1992;39:254.
41. Armas OA, Aprikian AG, Melamed J, et al. Clinical and pathobiological effects of neoadjuvant total androgen ablation therapy on clinically localized prostatic adenocarcinoma. *Am J Surg Pathol* 1994;18:979.

42. Reuter VE. Pathological changes in benign and malignant prostatic tissue following androgen deprivation therapy. *Urology* 1997;49(Suppl 3A):16.
43. Kollerman MW, Pantel K, Enzmann T, et al. Supersensitive PSA-monitored neoadjuvant hormone treatment of clinically localized prostate cancer: effects on positive margins, tumor detection and epithelial cells in the bone marrow. *Eur Urol* 1998;34:318.
44. Schulman CC, Oosterhof GO, van Cangh PJ, et al. Multicenter study of neoadjuvant combined androgen deprivation therapy in T2-3, N0, M0 prostatic carcinoma. *J Urol* 1994;151(Suppl):435A.
45. Gomella LG, Liberman SN, Mulholland SG, et al. Induction androgen deprivation plus prostatectomy for stage T3 disease: failure to achieve prostate-specific antigen-based freedom from disease status in a phase II trial. *Urology* 1996;47:870.
46. Ferguson J, Zincke H, Ellison E, et al. Decrease of prostatic intraepithelial neoplasia following androgen deprivation therapy in patients with stage T3 carcinoma treated by radical prostatectomy. *Urology* 1994;44:91.
47. Vaillancourt L, Têtu B, Fradet Y, et al. Effect of neoadjuvant endocrine therapy (combined androgen blockade) on normal prostate and prostatic carcinoma. *Am J Surg Pathol* 1996; 20:86.
48. Murphy WM, Soloway MS, Barrows GH. Pathologic changes associated with androgen deprivation therapy for prostate cancer. *Cancer* 1991;68:821.
49. Civantos F, Marcial MA, Banks ER, et al. Pathology of androgen deprivation therapy in prostate carcinoma. *Cancer* 1995;75:1634.
50. Gleason DF. Histologic grading of prostate cancer: a perspective. *Hum Pathol* 1992;23:273.
51. Smith DM, Murphy WM. Histologic changes in prostate carcinomas treated with leuprolide (luteinizing hormone-releasing hormone effect). *Cancer* 1994;73:1472.
52. Civantos F, Soloway MS, Pinto JE. Histopathological effects of androgen deprivation in prostate cancer. *Semin Urol Oncol* 1996;14(Suppl 2):22.
53. McNeal JE. Effect of LHRH agonist therapy on the histologic identification and grading of prostatic carcinoma. *Monogr Urol* 1997;18:83.
54. Bazinet M, Zheng W, Begin LR, et al. Morphological changes induced by neoadjuvant androgen ablation may result in underdetection of positive surgical margins and capsular involvement by prostatic carcinoma. *Urology* 1997;49:721.
55. Montironi R, Schulman CC. Pathologic changes in prostate lesions after androgen manipulation. *J Clin Pathol* 1998; 51:5.
56. Bruchovsky N, Rennie PS, Coldman AJ, et al. Effects of androgen withdrawal on the stem cell composition of the Shionogi carcinoma. *Cancer Res* 1990;50:2275.
57. Karakiewicz PI, Begin LR, Bazinet M. Use of monoclonal cytokeratin antibodies after neoadjuvant androgen ablation leads to pathologic upstaging of radical prostatectomy specimens compared with conventional histopathologic assessment. *Monogr Urol* 1997;18:84.
58. Dalkin BL, Ahmann FR, Nagle R, et al. Randomized study of neoadjuvant testicular androgen ablation therapy before radical prostatectomy in men with clinically localized prostate cancer. *J Urol* 1996;155:1357.
59. Aus G, Hugosson J, Abrahamsson PA, et al. Pretreatment with triptorelin before radical prostatectomy: a 3-year follow-up. *J Urol* 1997;157(Suppl):393(abst).
60. Bergstralh EJ, Amling CL, Martin SK, et al. Long-term outcome following preoperative androgen deprivation therapy for clinical stage T3 prostate cancer. *J Urol* 1997;157(Suppl): 332(abst).
61. Wood D, Sakr WA, Grignon DJ, et al. "Down staging" with neoadjuvant hormone treatment: the more organ confined prostate does not translate into lower PSA failure. *J Urol* 1997;157:388.
62. Hachiya T, Nogaki J, Ishida H, et al. A study on androgen deprivation therapy prior to radical prostatectomy with special reference to the tumor volume. *Nippon Rinsho* 1998;56: 2157.
63. Bonney WW, Schned AR, Timberlake DS. Neoadjuvant androgen ablation for localized prostatic cancer: pathology methods, surgical end points and meta-analysis of randomized trials. *J Urol* 1998;160:1754.
64. Baert LV, Goethuys HJ, De Ridder DJ, et al. Neoadjuvant treatment before radical prostatectomy decreases the number of positive margins in cT2-T3 but has no impact on PSA progression or survival in cT2-T3. *J Urol* 1998;159(Suppl): 61(abst).
65. Scardino PT, Shinohara K, Wheeler TM, et al. Staging of prostate cancer. Value of ultrasonography. *Urol Clin North Am* 1989;16:713.
66. Cohen DW, Aprikian A, Russo P, et al. Neoadjuvant androgen ablation combined with radical prostatectomy for clinically localized carcinoma of the prostate. *J Urol* 1994; 151(Suppl):435A.
67. Cookson MS, Fair WR. Neoadjuvant androgen deprivation therapy and radical prostatectomy for clinically localized prostate cancer. *AUA Update Series* 1997;16:98.
68. Wood DP Jr., Beaman A, Banerjee M, et al. Effect of neoadjuvant androgen deprivation on circulating prostate cells in the bone marrow of men undergoing radical prostatectomy. *Clin Cancer Res* 1998;4:2119.
69. Goldenberg SL, Klotz L, Jewett M, et al. A randomized trial of neoadjuvant androgen withdrawal therapy prior to radical prostatectomy: 24 month post-treatment PSA results. *J Urol* 1997;157:92.
70. Tetu B, Srigley JR, Boivin JC, et al. Effect of combination endocrine therapy (LHRH agonist and flutamide) on normal prostate and prostatic adenocarcinoma. *Am J Surg Pathol* 1991;15:111.
71. Balaji KC, Rabbani F, Tsai H, et al. Effect of neoadjuvant hormonal therapy on prostatic intraepithelial neoplasia and its prognostic significance. *J Urol* 1999;161(Suppl): 154(abst).
72. Su SL, Heston WD, Perroti M, et al. Evaluating neoadjuvant therapy effectiveness on systemic disease: use of a prostatic-specific membrane reverse transcription polymerase chain reaction. *Urology* 1997;49(Suppl 3A):95.
73. Klotz LH, Goldenberg SL, Jewett M, et al. CUOG randomized trial of neoadjuvant androgen ablation before radical prostatectomy: 36 month posttreatment PSA results. *Urology* 1999;53:757.

74. Witjes WP, Schulman CC, Debruyne FM, et al. Neoadjuvant combined androgen deprivation therapy in locally confined prostatic carcinoma: 3 to 4 years of follow up of a European randomized trial. *J Urol* 1998;159(Suppl):254(abst).
75. Soloway M, Sharifi R, Wajsman Z, et al. Radical prostatectomy alone versus prostatectomy preceded by androgen blockade in cT2b prostate cancer—24 month results. *J Urol* 1997;157:160.
76. Hugosson J, Abrahamsson PA, Ahlgren G, et al. The risk of malignancy in the surgical margin at radical prostatectomy reduced almost three-fold in patients given neo-adjuvant hormone treatment. *Eur Urol* 1996;29:413.
77. Pedersen KV, Lundberg S, Hugosson J, et al. Neoadjuvant hormonal treatment with triptorelin versus no treatment prior to radical prostatectomy: a prospective randomized multicenter study. *J Urol* 1995;153(Suppl):391A(abst).
78. Hellstrom M, Haggman M, Pedersen K, et al. A 3-year follow-up of patients with localized prostate cancer operated on with or without pre-treatment with the GnRH-agonist triptorelin. *Br J Urol* 1996;78:432.
79. Rabbani F, Sullivan LD, Goldenberg SL, et al. Neoadjuvant androgen deprivation therapy before radical prostatectomy: Who is unlikely to benefit? *Br J Urol* 1997;79:221.
80. Wieder JA, Soloway MS. Interstitial pneumonitis associated with neoadjuvant leuprolide and nilutamide for prostate cancer. *J Urol* 1998;159:2099.
81. Berges RR, Kassen A, Sommerfeld HJ, et al. Kinetics of androgen ablation induced programmed cell death in human prostatic epithelial cells. *J Urol* 1998;159(Suppl):6(abst).
82. Van der Kwast TH, Têtu B, Candas B, et al. Prolonged neoadjuvant combined androgen blockade leads to a further reduction of prostatic tumor volume: three versus six months of endocrine therapy. *Urology* 1999;53:523.
83. Belldegrun A, McBride W, Tso CL. Hormone deprivation treatment induces selective growth of super aggressive prostate cancer clones. *J Urol* 1999;161(Suppl):127(abst).

32

MANAGEMENT OF HIGH-RISK PROSTATE CANCER

BRENT K. HOLLENBECK
JAMES E. MONTIE
MARTIN G. SANDA

A significant proportion of prostate cancers is progressive and lethal if untreated. One of the greatest challenges facing the practicing physician in managing prostate cancer is to identify which prostate cancer patients require therapy and to determine the best treatment for each individual case. With a paucity of data from prospective trials randomizing patients to local regional therapy versus observation, physicians are often left basing decisions regarding whether or not to treat on large, nonrandomized series confounded by selection bias and varying definitions of treatment failure. Moreover, much of the published data has reported biochemical recurrence as the principal end point, yet, the relationship between biochemical failure and overall or cancer-specific survival remains poorly defined (1,2).

In 1998, approximately 200,000 men were diagnosed with prostate cancer (3), and nearly 40,000 men died from the disease. The majority of newly diagnosed prostate cancer is clinically localized, and such cancers can be categorized as being curable by local therapy (low risk) or likely to recur after local regional treatment (high risk). The purposes of this chapter are to identify clinical parameters indicative of prostate cancer that are at high risk for progressing after radiation or surgery, to characterize the natural history of this relatively aggressive form of prostate cancer, and to examine adjuvant and neoadjuvant treatment options for such high-risk cancers.

PARAMETERS FOR IDENTIFYING HIGH-RISK CANCERS

There have been numerous attempts to define the clinical course of prostate cancer. Because of the aforementioned unknowns in treating these patients, it is important to identify a subset of individuals who are likely to progress regardless of the local regional therapeutic modality and to concentrate efforts toward improving survival in this patient population. Patients with a low biopsy Gleason sum, low prostate-specific antigen (PSA), and clinically localized prostate cancer have superior results with only subtle differences among various therapies (1,2,4–6). As summarized later, those individuals with a high PSA, high Gleason sum, and advanced-stage prostate cancer tend to have a poor prognosis after local regional therapy. Strategies to improve survival in this subset of patients are needed.

Clinical Stage as a High-Risk Parameter

Given the widespread use of PSA as a screening tool, the proportion of prostate cancer with advanced clinical stage has decreased; however, its overall incidence remains unchanged (3). Locally advanced adenocarcinoma of the prostate (clinical stage T3-4) is defined as a tumor that extends through the prostate capsule or invades adjacent organs (including the seminal vesicles). Historically, at the time of pelvic lymphadenectomy, approximately 35% to 46% of patients with clinical T3 cancers harbored positive lymph nodes (7,8), and, in men with high-grade T3 prostate cancer, the likelihood of nodal involvement approached 93% (7).

At least three observational cohorts demonstrate that the natural history of clinical stage T3 cancers portends a worse prognosis than stage T1-T2 cancers. In 1993, Adolfsson (9) reported on 50 men with clinical stage T3 prostate cancer who were managed conservatively, with 58% receiving androgen deprivation for progression. Cancer-specific survival for this cohort was favorably skewed by predominance of lower-grade cancers, advanced age of the patients at diagnosis, and competing early non–cancer-related mortality. Nevertheless, 9-year cancer-specific survival was 70% in those patients with T3 cancers, which is significantly lower than the 90% 10-year cancer-specific survival (10) reported by the author in a T1-2 cohort managed in a similar fashion. Johansson (11) retrospectively reviewed 642 patients with prostate cancer managed conservatively with observation followed by androgen deprivation for progression. Cancer-specific survivals were 85% for stage T1-2 disease compared to 66% for stage T3-4 disease at 10 years of follow-up. Interestingly, patients younger than 61 years accounted for 44% of the prostate cancer deaths, demonstrating that competing (non-cancer) mortality for older men (e.g., older than 65 to 70 years of age) can favorably skew cancer-specific survival data and consequently underestimate the cancer risk in selected observation cohorts. Finally, Rana reviewed 199 patients with T2-4NxM0 prostate cancer and found a 50% to 70% 10-year cancer-specific survival for stages T3-4 (12) compared to 85% to 90% (9,11) for stages T1-2, despite 86% of these patients having received early hormonal therapy.

These findings indicate that clinical stage T3-4 prostate cancer has a more aggressive natural course than clinical stage T1-2 cancer. The aggressive nature of locally advanced disease is associated with a decrease in cancer-specific survival and should be regarded as a risk factor for disease progression.

Biopsy Gleason Score as a High-Risk Parameter

The Gleason score is consistently associated with survival independent of clinical stage or other factors. In 1994, Chodak (13) reviewed 828 patients with clinically localized prostate cancer treated with delayed hormonal therapy or observation in a metaanalysis of six previously published series. The 10-year cancer-specific survival for Gleason sum 2 to 7 tumors was 87%, compared to only 34% for Gleason sum 8 to 10 cancers. Despite possible selection bias affecting the series as a whole, the survival data indicate the disparity in the disease-free survival between poorly differentiated and well-differentiated tumors.

The largest single cohort study to assess the natural history of prostate cancer not having undergone definitive local regional therapy is comprised of the analyses of the Connecticut Tumor Registry reported by Albertsen (4,14). Gleason sum 8 to 10 cancers comprised only 10% of the cohort but accounted for 25% of the cancer deaths. Fifteen-year cancer-specific survivals for Gleason sums of 7 or less were found to be as high as 70% to 96% and 30% to 58%, respectively, compared to only 23% to 40% survival for Gleason sums 8 to 10 cancers (Fig. 32-1). The pivotal role of high tumor grade in identifying patients with poor prognosis was confirmed by Johansson (11), who reported that 68% of patients with high-grade prostate cancer died of this disease compared to fewer than 38% of those with lower-grade cancers.

In summary, biopsy Gleason sum 8 to 10 prostate cancer is a harbinger of adverse outcome among men receiving definitive surgery or radiation, and many such men die of their cancer before 10 to 15 years of follow-up. Conservative management (i.e., observation without any intervention) for Gleason sum 8 to 10 tumors should not be

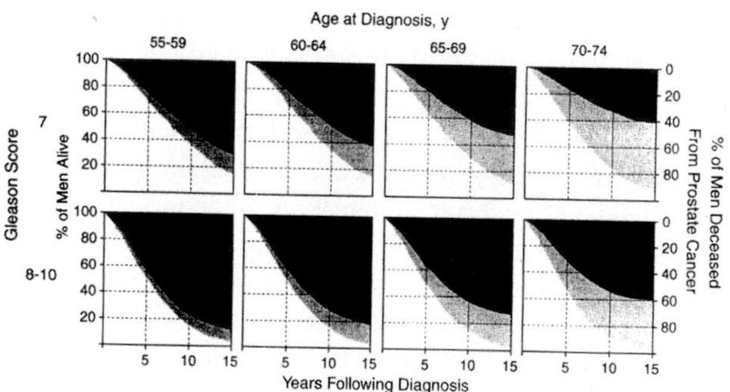

FIGURE 32-1. Prostate cancer mortality is significant among Gleason sum 7 or Gleason sum 8 to 10 tumors at all ages when managed conservatively (without surgery or radiation). The black-shaded area represents a proportion of conservatively treated patients dying of prostate cancer based on age at diagnosis. The gray-shaded areas represent death from competing causes in this cohort. Notice that overall 15-year mortality is consistently 85% for patients with conservatively managed Gleason sum 8 to 10 cancer cases who did not undergo surgery or radiation. Observed reduction in prostate cancer–specific mortality at later ages appears, simply owing to increasing risk of competing mortality; thus, these data do *not* support the notion that prostate cancer risk is reduced with advancing age at diagnosis. (From Albertsen PC, Hanley JA, Gleason DF, et al. Competing risk analysis of men aged 55 to 74 years at diagnosis managed conservatively for clinically localized prostate cancer. *JAMA* 1998; 280:975–980, with permission.)

considered the standard of care regardless of age for patients with life expectancies greater than 10 years. Figure 32-1 illustrates the high cancer mortality in the Connecticut Tumor Registry cohort all of whom were managed expectantly (4), and demonstrates the detrimental impact of high-grade prostate cancer at all ages.

Prostate-Specific Antigen as a High-Risk Parameter

Serum PSA level is commonly used as a screening tool to detect prostate cancer in its early stages. PSA was used to detect 68% of prostate cancers in 1990 compared to only 5.8% in 1984 (15). To our knowledge, however, there is no published long-term survival data for patient cohorts managed by observation and evaluated in the context of serum PSA at diagnosis. Owing to the paucity of data examining the overall survival among men with elevated PSA managed expectantly, the use of PSA as a marker for adverse prognosis can instead be evaluated in context of the association of PSA greater than 20 ng per mL with adverse pathology (i.e., seminal vesicle invasion or the presence of lymph node metastases) as a surrogate measure of local regional therapy failure.

Partin et al. found that preoperative serum PSA levels were significantly elevated in patients with nodal spread or seminal vesicle invasion (6). However, the predictive value of elevated PSA is low: Although serum PSA levels higher than 20 ng per mL are associated with a four times higher risk of seminal vesicle or lymph node involvement, only 20% and 17% of patients, respectively, with PSA greater than 20 ng per mL had such adverse pathology. Thus, although nodal involvement and seminal vesicle invasion are much more likely to occur in men with a PSA greater than 20 ng per mL, selected men with such elevated PSA in surgical cohorts may, nevertheless, be effectively treated by surgery. Therefore, pretreatment PSA in the moderately elevated range (20 to 50 ng per mL) has limited use for identifying cancers at a high risk of progression, unless such PSA values are evaluated in the context of other variables, such as Gleason score. The use of PSA in identifying high-risk cancers has been enhanced by models combining Gleason sum, clinical stage, and pretreatment (6,16–19). These models are, at present, limited by the use of biochemical progression rather than survival as an end point (20).

Summary of Parameters to Identify High-Risk Prostate Cancers

In summary, review of natural history data and information regarding predictive factors suggests that a Gleason sum greater than 7, a clinical stage greater than T2, and a serum PSA at diagnosis greater than 20 are factors that contribute significantly to the risk of prostate cancer progression. Patients harboring either Gleason sum higher than 7 or clinical stage greater than T2 cancers are at high risk of progression and cancer death, and this risk is magnified by serum PSA greater than 20 ng per mL at diagnosis. These patients are more likely to have progressive disease, may die of their cancer if managed expectantly, and can require additional therapies beyond the usual standard of surgery or radiation monotherapies, as discussed later.

STANDARD PRIMARY THERAPIES FOR HIGH-RISK PROSTATE CANCER

Hormonal Therapy

Each of the prostate cancer series that has been studied to define the natural history of high-risk disease includes patients who, at some point during their clinical course, received some form of androgen deprivation therapy. This concept stemmed from the investigations by Huggins and Hodges (21) in 1941 that describe significant clinical responses in men with metastatic prostate cancer treated with androgen ablation.

In the late 1960s and early 1970s, the Veterans Administration Cooperative Urological Research Group (VACURG) revisited the effects of hormonal therapy on locally advanced and metastatic prostate cancer. In study 1, patients with locally advanced prostate cancer (stage III) and patients with metastatic disease or elevated acid phosphatases (stage IV) were randomized to receive a placebo, diethylstilbestrol (DES), orchiectomy, or DES and orchiectomy (22). The study's findings challenged the long-held belief that androgen deprivation conferred a survival benefit to patients with advanced prostate cancer. A trend toward a cancer-specific survival benefit (although not significant in overall survival) was seen for castration in stage IV cancers, whereas administration of a placebo resulted in higher survival than DES in stage III patients, likely related to the cardiotoxicity of DES.

The results from study 2 showed a survival advantage for hormonal therapy in stage IV but not in stage III cancers, despite DES cardiotoxicity (23). The VACURG findings implied that, although patients with advanced prostate cancer may not incur a survival advantage when treated with chronic hormonal therapy using DES instituted early during their cancer management (stage III), they may sustain an overall survival benefit when treated with androgen deprivation at some later point during their clinical course (stage IV). However, the VACURG studies lacked statistical power to assess negative effects, and the cardiovascular toxicity of high-dose DES contaminated the overall survival results.

The Medical Research Council (MRC) enrolled patients with locally advanced or asymptomatic metastatic prostate cancer in a randomized study to compare immediate and delayed hormonal therapy (24). The MRC study noted that 67% of all deaths were attributed to prostate cancer, reiterating that patients with advanced prostate cancer do not have an indolent disease. Interestingly, the study noted a statistically significant difference in prostate cancer mortality between deferred and immediate treatment groups, 55% versus 43%. The overall mortality was also statistically significant, 78% versus 70%. Patients who received deferred therapy were also three times as likely to require a transurethral resection of the prostate and twice as likely to have spinal cord compression or pathologic fractures. These findings suggest a possible benefit to initiating hormonal therapy in high-risk prostate cancer patients before clinical or symptomatic progression.

However, a definitive recommendation regarding when to begin hormonal therapy in patients with asymptomatic, high-risk prostate cancer is elusive. Certainly, men with local or distant symptoms from their prostate cancer should receive hormonal therapy, and it may be beneficial to begin hormonal therapy before the onset of symptomatic progression. Although the MRC study suggested a benefit in survival to patients receiving early hormonal therapy, no studies have yet incorporated asymptomatic PSA progression as criteria for instituting hormonal therapy. The ability to assess asymptomatic progression of high-risk cancers by evaluating serum PSA changes therefore represents an opportunity for further refining hormone therapy initiative and is in need of prospective evaluation in clinical trials.

Radical Prostatectomy

Radical prostatectomy can cure some, but not all, high-risk prostate cancers (as defined by the criteria of Gleason sum higher than 7, clinical stage greater than T2, or PSA greater

TABLE 32-1. PROGRESSION-FREE SURVIVAL AFTER RADICAL PROSTATECTOMY IN HIGH-RISK PATIENTS

Risk factor	Study (ref)	5-yr PSA-free survival (%)
High grade	D'Amico et al. (5)	31
(Gleason 8–10)	Pound et al. (1)	41
Clinical stage T3	Gerber et al. (30)	11–29
	Lerner et al. (26)	58
	Pound et al. (1)	61
PSA >20 ng/mL	Pound et al. (1)	54

PSA, prostate-specific antigen.

than 20 ng per mL). It has been suggested that even when not curative, radical prostatectomy may prolong survival in such cases (25–29). This section focuses on the results of radical prostatectomy in individuals with such high-risk cancers (Table 32-1) (Fig. 32-2).

Radical Prostatectomy for High Gleason Sum Cancers

Tumor grade clearly affects the likelihood of recurrent-free survival and overall survival after radical prostatectomy. In a retrospective review pooling data from eight universities, Gerber (30) found that the 10-year cancer-specific survivals were significantly different for Gleason sum 2 to 4 (low-grade), Gleason sum 5 to 7 (intermediate-grade), and Gleason sum 8 to 10 (high-grade) tumors for men undergoing radical prostatectomy for clinically localized prostate cancer. The 10-year cancer-specific survival for men with high-grade tumors was only 77%, compared to 94% in men with low-grade prostate cancer. This effect was reflected in similar trends in 5-year PSA-free survival in other studies (Table 32-1). The important role of the biopsy Gleason sum as an adverse factor for cancer-free survival at 10 years after radical prostatectomy was affirmed by recent data from The Johns Hopkins Hospital (1). Among patients who underwent radical prostatectomy by Walsh, the 5-year PSA-free survivals were 92% for cancers with Gleason scores less than 7 and 66% for Gleason scores equal to 7, compared to 41% for Gleason score 8 to 10 cancers (1). D'Amico found similar trends for patients treated at Harvard or the University of Pennsylvania, as shown in Figure 32-2 (5). It is notable that only half of such men with PSA recurrence develop clinical metastases by 5 years after their first postsurgical rise in PSA (20). Despite lower rates of durable cancer-free survival after radical prostatectomy for high-grade cancers (compared to lower-grade cancers), a significant proportion of men do experience significant cancer control after surgery as monotherapy for these cancers (Table 32-1). Indeed, cancer control by surgery for high-grade prostate cancer is no worse than (and may be better than) that of alternative primary therapies, such as radiation (Fig. 32-2) (Table 32-2). The significant likelihood of postsurgical progression in high Gleason sum cancers does warrant the development of successful systemic adjuvants. Nevertheless, surgery is a reasonable initial treatment option for Gleason score 8 to 10 cancers in patients without competing co-morbidities.

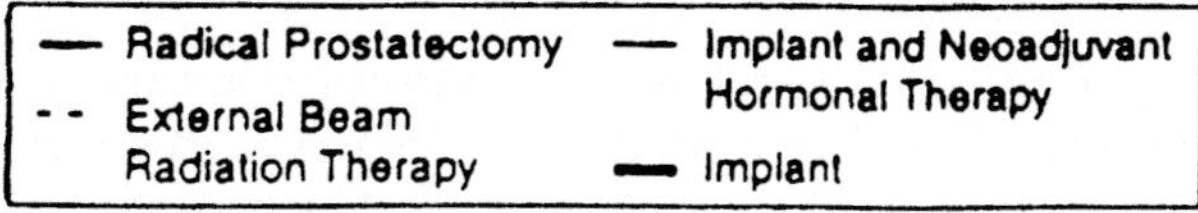

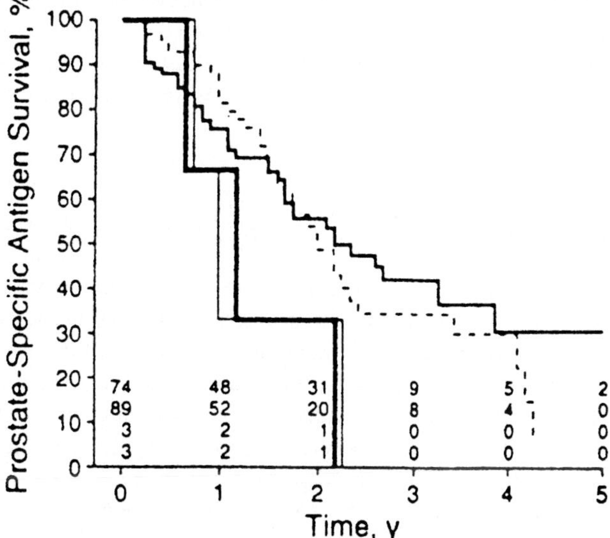

FIGURE 32-2. Progression-free survival after radical prostatectomy or external beam radiation suggests more favorable outcome than that after brachytherapy for Gleason score higher than 7 cancers (surgery vs. brachytherapy, $p = .06$; radiation vs. brachytherapy, $p = .05$). (From D'Amico AV, Whittington R, Malkowicz B, et al. Biochemical outcome after radical prostatectomy, external beam radiation therapy, or interstitial radiation therapy for clinically localized prostate cancer. *JAMA* 1998;280:969–974, with permission.)

Radical Prostatectomy for Locally Advanced Prostate Cancer (Clinical Stage T3)

Radical prostatectomy is not commonly used as a means to eradicate disease in patients with clinical T3 to T4 disease.

TABLE 32-2. PROGRESSION-FREE SURVIVAL AFTER RADIATION THERAPY IN HIGH-RISK PATIENTS

Risk factor	Study (ref)	5-yr PSA-free survival (%)
High grade	D'Amico et al. (5)	<10
(Gleason 8–10)	Zagars et al. (55)	<44[a]
	Pilepich et al. (61)	46
	Fiveash et al. (59)	63
Clinical stage T3	Zietman et al. (54)	42
	Zagars et al. (55)	43
PSA >20 ng/mL	Shipley et al. (2)	47

PSA, prostate-specific antigen.
[a]Four-year PSA-free survival.

Nevertheless, some T3 cancers can be cured by radical prostatectomy, as evidenced by outcomes in at least three recent large cohort studies at leading centers. At The Johns Hopkins Hospital, Pound (1) found that patients with clinical T3a prostate cancers treated by radical prostatectomy had an 8-year recurrence-free rate of 52%. Although a less favorable outcome than for earlier stage (T1-2) cancers, such survival without the elimination of cancer in half of the cases suggested some efficacy of radical prostatectomy as therapy for select T3a cancers (Table 32-1). At the Mayo Clinic, Lerner (26) reviewed 812 patients with clinical T3 prostate cancer who underwent radical prostatectomy. The 10-year cancer-specific survival in this large cohort was 80%, and, at 15 years, only 31% of these patients had died of their prostate cancer. The results are somewhat confounded by the fact that 60% of the population received some form of adjuvant therapy. A notable finding in the Mayo series was that 17% of patients thought to have extraprostatic extension on rectal exam (clinical T3) were found to have organ-confined cancers on surgical pathology (pathologic stage T2). The effectiveness of surgery or radiation in selected clinical stage T3 cases, therefore, can partially be explained by the inaccuracy of digital rectal examinations and consequent overestimation of clinical stage in some cases. In a retrospective multiinstitutional pooled analysis, Gerber (25) reviewed results in 298 men with clinical T3 prostate cancer who intended to undergo radical prostatectomy. Eighty-one percent of these men had a radical prostatectomy with bilateral lymph node dissection, whereas the remainder had a pelvic lymph node dissection alone. Ten-year cancer-specific survival in all patients managed surgically was only 57%. However, patients with clinical T3 disease who underwent bilateral pelvic lymph node dissection in addition to radical prostatectomy had a 10-year cancer-specific survival of 70%, suggesting a possible survival benefit with radical prostatectomy in select cases. Absence of even a biochemical recurrence in a significant proportion of such T3 cases 5 years after radical prostatectomy further attests to a potential role for surgery in select cases (Table 32-1).

Radical Prostatectomy for Patients with High Prostate-Specific Antigen

Widespread use of screening PSA and, consequently, preoperative PSA information have been widely available only in the past 10 years, and, hence, preoperative PSA has been used principally to predict pathologic outcome and postoperative recurrence, with little data available regarding overall survival. Favorable pathology (i.e., organ-confined prostate cancer) in the radical prostatectomy specimen is much less frequent in patients with a preoperative PSA greater than 20 ng per mL. The presence of such adverse pathology after radical prostatectomy has been correlated with decreased survival (25,28,29). For example, patients with PSA values greater than 20 ng per mL have been noted to have a 5-year PSA-free survival of only 54% (Table 32-1), compared to 72% to 94% in men with preoperative PSA values less than or equal to 20 ng per mL (1). The median time from biochemical failure to the onset of metastatic disease in this cohort was 8 years, and the subsequent time to death was 5 years (20). Despite the higher risk of postsurgical recurrence for patients with preoperative PSA greater than 20 ng per mL, a subset of such individuals nevertheless remains free of clinical cancer at 10 years, providing the rationale for using radical prostatectomy as an option for definitive therapy in these patients.

Summary: Radical Prostatectomy as Monotherapy for High-Risk Cancers

In summary, selected high-risk prostate cancer patients with clinical stage T3, biopsy Gleason sum 8 to 10, or markedly elevated PSA (who have a life expectancy greater than 10 years) may benefit from radical prostatectomy and should be offered surgery with a curative intent (Table 32-1). However, due to the significant possibility of progression by such cancers after radical prostatectomy, the possible role of systemic adjuvant therapy merits comment (31).

Hormone Therapy as an Adjuvant for Radical Prostatectomy

Radical prostatectomy provides excellent pelvic control of pathologic stage T3 or greater prostate cancer, and recurrences are usually distant (32,33). Hence, high-risk prostate cancers could potentially benefit from an effective systemic adjuvant. One such approach entails hormonal therapy administered as a neoadjuvant; an alternative approach entails use of hormonal therapy as a postsurgical adjuvant in select high-risk cases.

Neoadjuvant Hormonal Therapy before Radical Prostatectomy for High-Risk Cancers

Hypothetical rationale supporting the use of hormonal therapy as a neoadjuvant before radical retropubic prostatectomy includes prompt apoptosis and growth inhibition of the hormonally responsive subset of prostate cancer cells. It has been speculated that this effect may render locally advanced cancers amenable to complete resection (34). However, the flaw of this hypothesis is suggested by the presence of hormonally independent components in such locally aggressive cancers. Figure 32-3 demonstrates that neoadjuvant hormonal therapy (before radical prostatectomy) would be expected to cause an artifact of apparently reduced pathology stage due to elimination of hormonally sensitive cells. However, the distribution of androgen-independent cancer cells (within and beyond the surgical margin) is not changed by the hormonal neoadjuvant, and, therefore, systemic recurrence (due to persistence of fatal, androgen-resistant

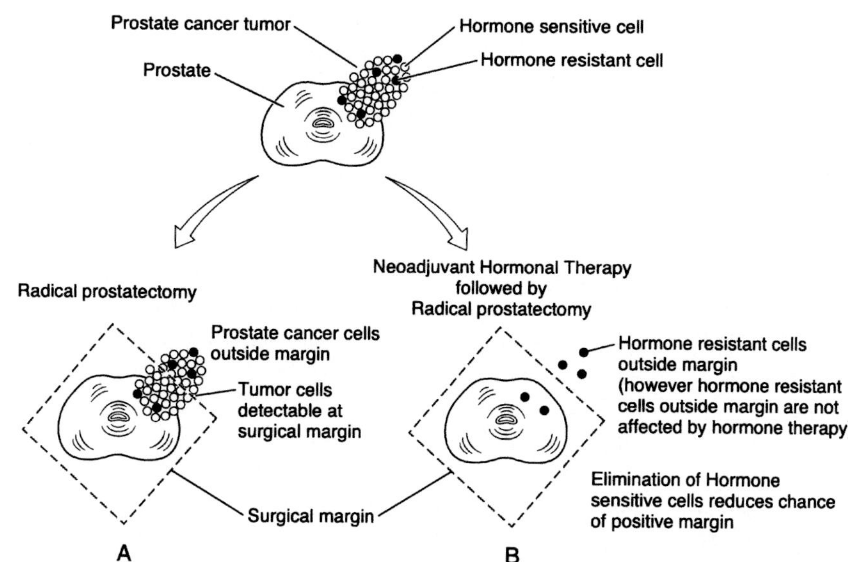

FIGURE 32-3. Flaws in the hypothesis of neoadjuvant hormonal therapy before radical prostatectomy. Hormonal treatment decreases tumor size and eradicates hormone-sensitive cells before surgery **(A)**. Androgen-insensitive prostate cancer cells are not affected by androgen deprivation and can remain around the margins of resection to facilitate a local recurrence **(B)**.

cells) is not affected by the hormonal neoadjuvant despite a predictable, misleading pathologic "downstaging" that is due to artifact (Fig. 32-3). This flaw in the hypothetical benefit of hormonal neoadjuvant before radical prostatectomy has been confirmed in clinical studies: Despite the artifactual misleading effects of hormonal neoadjuvant on reducing apparent pathology stage and margin status, clinical recurrence and progression are not changed by the hormonal neoadjuvant in retrospective and prospective, as well as randomized, clinical trials (35–45). Moreover, neoadjuvant hormonal therapy can delay the time to definitive (surgical) treatment and needlessly expose patients to significant hormonal side effects in the absence of demonstrated benefit. We therefore recommend against the routine use of neoadjuvant hormonal therapy before radical prostatectomy, even in the setting of high-risk cancers.

Hormone Therapy as a Postsurgical Adjuvant

Postsurgical adjuvant hormonal therapy, in contrast, enables the practitioner to offer systemic therapy continuously and specifically to those who are at risk for progression after radical prostatectomy based on pathologic stage. The potential benefit of postsurgical hormonal adjuvant therapy was recently shown in a randomized prospective trial of continuous postsurgical androgen deprivation for prostate cancer with lymph node involvement (46). Men who had undergone radical prostatectomy and had prostate cancer extension to the pelvic lymph nodes were randomized to receive immediate hormonal therapy (orchiectomy or goserelin) or hormonal therapy at the time of disease progression (radiographically evident metastases or symptomatic local recurrence). At a mean follow-up of 7.2 years, only 4.3% of patients who received immediate androgen deprivation died of prostate cancer compared to 31% of men who were managed with deferred treatment. Clinical progression and biochemical recurrence rates for immediate and delayed hormonal therapy were 9% and 56% and 11% and 19%, respectively. Thus, only 20% of patients who were treated with postsurgical adjuvant hormonal therapy recurred, compared to 75% of those in whom hormonal therapy was delayed. Although the cohort was relatively small (n = 98), the results suggested a significant survival benefit related to immediate and continuous adjuvant hormonal therapy in men with regional lymph node metastases.

In summary, neoadjuvant hormonal therapy before radical prostatectomy lacks evidence of survival benefits despite its artifactual effect on pathologic stage and margin status (Fig. 32-3). Conversely, patients who are noted to have lymph node involvement at the time of the radical prostatectomy appear to gain a survival advantage from continuous postsurgical hormonal adjuvant therapy. The latter (postsurgical) hormonal adjuvant strategy differs from the neoadjuvant approach in the disease severity of the treated cases as well as in the duration of hormonal therapy. Regardless of whether analogous postsurgical adjuvant hormonal therapy will yield similar benefits in patients with high-risk cancers (e.g., defined by high Gleason score, clinical stage, or markedly elevated PSA) awaits appropriate studies.

Radiation Therapy for High-Risk Prostate Cancer

Radiation therapy has been an acceptable treatment for localized prostate cancer and is currently used in approximately 25% of these patients (47). It is also the most used local regional treatment modality in men with locally advanced disease. Since the advent of PSA, however, the use of conventional external beam radiation has been criticized. Local failure rates of 38% have been reported in patients fol-

TABLE 32-3. CANCER CONTROL WITH SALVAGE PROSTATECTOMY FOR LOCALIZED PROSTATE CANCER RECURRENCE AFTER RADIATION THERAPY

Study (ref)	% PSA-free survival (actuarial follow-up)	% Cancer-specific survival (actuarial follow-up)
Lerner et al. (47)	43% (10 yr)	70% (10 yr)
Tefilli et al. (68)	44% (3 yr)	—
Rogers et al. (63)	55% (5 yr)	95% (5 yr)
	33% (8 yr)	87% (8 yr)

PSA, prostate-specific antigen.
Note: Complications: incontinence, 50% (Lerner), 63% (Tefilli), 58% (Rogers); urethrovesical stricture, 11% (Tefilli), 28% (Rogers).

lowed prospectively with transrectal ultrasound-guided biopsies after standard external beam radiotherapy (48). To achieve an acceptable PSA-free survival, Schellhammer (49) proposed that conventional radiation therapy be reserved for patients with a clinical stage T1-2a, Gleason sum of 6 or less prostate cancers with pretreatment PSA less than or equal to 10 to 15 ng per mL. Patients with clinical characteristics other than these would benefit from the addition of hormonal therapy or dose escalation, or both. This section reviews the results of conventional and conformal radiotherapy in men with high-risk prostate cancers (Table 32-3).

Ten-year clinical disease-free survivals for patients undergoing conventional radiation therapy for clinical stage T1-2 range from 60% to 81%, whereas clinical stage T3-4 patients have been reported to be as low as 17% to 55% (50–52). When PSA values are used as an end point, these failure rates increase by 10% to 35% (53). The Massachusetts General Hospital experience included 1,044 patients with T1-4NxM0 treated between 1977 and 1991 (54). These men received a total tumor dose of 68.4 Gy. The 10-year biochemical disease-free survival for T1-2 patients was 40%, whereas only 18% of men with clinical stage T3-4 prostate cancer remained free from PSA recurrence. When analyzing these subsets and including only high-grade patients, the same survivals fall to 20% and 10%, respectively. The results of 707 patients with clinical stage T1-4NxM0 prostate cancer treated with conventional radiation therapy with total doses ranging from 60 to 70 Gy were reported (55). Approximately half of men with clinical stage T3-4 or high-grade prostate cancer (including Gleason sum 7) remained free from any recurrence at 5 years, compared to almost 75% of patients with clinically localized tumor or Gleason sums 2 to 6 prostate cancer. Of note, only 23% of individuals with a pretreatment PSA greater than 20 ng per mL were without recurrence at 5 years, whereas 84% of patients with a PSA less than 4 ng per mL were free of disease. Given that conventional radiation has failed to demonstrate durable results in the treatment of high-risk prostate cancer, newer techniques, including whole-pelvic and dose-escalating three-dimensional conformal radiotherapy, have been used in attempts to overcome some of the shortcomings of the traditional delivery methods.

Whole-pelvic radiotherapy, in addition to prostatic radiotherapy, has been studied to determine whether there is any added benefit to its use. It is commonly used and, in theory, is thought to add a tumor-killing benefit to patients with microscopically disseminated disease in the regional lymph nodes (56). The majority of series that have examined whole-pelvic versus prostate radiation alone have concluded that there is no added benefit to treating the entire pelvis (53). A recent series noted that men who received whole-pelvic radiotherapy had a higher biochemical recurrence rate at 5 years (53%) than those who received prostate radiotherapy alone (38%) (57). Hence, whole-pelvic radiotherapy, although commonly used, has an unknown role in treating men suspected of having node-positive prostate cancer. Until data from randomized prospective trials are available, patients suspected of having nodal involvement would best be served by treatment with radiotherapy and adjuvant hormones for which there is a proven survival benefit (58).

Conformal techniques were developed to improve on some of the shortcomings of conventional methods. Conformal radiation therapy allows for a higher dose delivery to the prostate and seminal vesicles while minimizing the deleterious effects on the bladder and rectum. Fiveash (59) reported the results of a multiinstitutional series of high-risk patients who received conformal radiation therapy. The patient population consisted of men with high-grade prostate cancer, 42% of whom had locally advanced disease. The 5-year PSA-free survival for patients with T1-2 prostate cancer was 79% compared to only 45% in men with T3-4 disease. Results from other cohorts are less promising. A report on 707 men with prostate cancer treated with conformal techniques (57) noted that only 23% of clinical stage T3-4 patients were free from any recurrence at 5 years. Eighty-eight percent of patients with preradiation therapy PSA values of less than or equal to 4 ng per mL were free of disease, compared to only 30% of patients with a PSA greater than 20 ng per mL. Patients with Gleason sums 2 to 6 and Gleason sums 8 to 10 had 5-year biochemical disease-free survivals of 61% and 34%, respectively. These data reiterate the suboptimal results of contemporary radiation approaches to high-risk patients. Nonetheless, conformal radiation therapy appears to result in improved biochemical survival when compared to conventional radiotherapy techniques.

Radiation Therapy Combined with Hormonal Therapy

Results using radiation therapy for clinical stage T3-4 prostate cancers are poor, with durable cure rates as low as 17%. Unacceptable failure rates have driven investigators to search for a means to augment the efficacy of radiation therapy. Hormonal therapy induces apoptosis in prostate cancer cells, potentially increasing radiation sensitivity and cancer control at a given radiation dosage. Proponents of adjuvant and neoadjuvant hormonal therapy in addition to radiation therapy cite three randomized prospective trials that point to statistically significant biochemical and metastases-free survivals and, in one, overall survival.

In 1995, preliminary results from the Radiation Therapy Oncology Group (RTOG) 86-10 trial were reported (60). Four hundred seventy-one patients with clinical stage T2b-T4Nx-2M0 and a tumor volume greater than 25 cm^2 by digital rectal examination were randomized to receive either whole-pelvic radiotherapy with a prostate boost to a total of 65 to 70 Gy or the aforementioned plus neoadjuvant hormonal therapy with goserelin and flutamide beginning two months before and continuing throughout radiation therapy. Biochemical disease-free and metastases-free survival were significantly improved in the neoadjuvant hormone arm. The 5-year local control rate in the neoadjuvant hormone arm was significantly higher at 54% compared to only 29% in the radiation only arm. However, 5-year overall survivals for the neoadjuvant hormonal therapy and radiation alone groups were both approximately 60%.

In 1997, Pilepich (61) reported results of RTOG 85-31, which was designed to determine the effects of adjuvant hormonal therapy on patients treated with definitive radiation therapy. In this study, 977 patients with T3Nx-0M0, T1-4N1-3M0, or pT3N0-3M0 were randomized to receive whole-pelvic radiation with a prostate boost (prostatic fossa irradiation only in postprostatectomy patients) or radiation with adjuvant goserelin beginning the last week of therapy and lasting indefinitely or until progression. Like RTOG 86-10, significant improvements in the 5-year local control rates, biochemical disease-free, and metastases-free survivals were noted in the adjuvant treatment group. Once again, however, overall survivals in the adjuvant hormonal therapy group and radiation alone group were no different—75% and 71%, respectively. However, a significant overall survival benefit was noted in men who received adjuvant hormonal therapy with Gleason score 8 to 10 prostate cancer.

The most convincing data supporting the use of androgen deprivation in conjunction with radiation were reported in the European Organization for the Research and Treatment of Cancer (EORTC) 22863 (58). The population consisted of high-risk patients with T1-2N0-xM0 and World Health Organization grade 3 or T3-4N0-xM0 prostate cancer. A total of 415 patients were randomized to undergo whole-pelvic radiation with a prostate boost or radiation plus adjuvant goserelin beginning the first day of radiation and lasting for 3 years. Cyproterone acetate was given during the first month to prevent androgen flare effects. A significant difference in overall survival was noted for patients who received adjuvant therapy when compared to those who underwent radiation therapy alone. Five-year overall survival for the two groups was 79% and 62%, respectively (p = .001).

Each of these three randomized prospective trials cites significant benefits associated with hormonal neoadjuvant for radiation therapy as measured by 5-year recurrence or progression-free survival, whereas only one study showed an overall survival benefit. This discrepancy in overall survival effects of hormonal neoadjuvant can be reconciled based on the RTOG 85-31 observation of a survival benefit limited to high-risk patients. The 5-year survival of 62% noted in EORTC 22863 (58) for patients treated with radiation alone is much lower than similar survivals (71% to 78%) reported by the RTOG (60,61), suggesting that the EORTC 22863 cohort may have included more high-risk cancers than the RTOG studies. If the hormonal neoadjuvant benefit is limited to high-risk cases (as seen in RTOG 85-31), then a predominance of high-risk cases in EORTC 22863 can explain the overall survival differences. Irrespective of how these different studies are reconciled, evidence from at least two randomized studies points to a survival benefit from hormonal therapy as a neoadjuvant to radiation. Despite the possible benefits of such neoadjuvants, the ability of radiation therapy to control high-risk prostate cancers does not appear to be very different than that of radical prostatectomy (Tables 32-1 and 32-2) (Fig. 32-2).

Brachytherapy is mentioned only for completeness in this setting, because patients with high-risk disease generally do not fair well with modality of treatment. D'Amico (5) reported on 1,872 patients with clinically localized prostate cancer who were treated with radical prostatectomy, external beam radiation therapy, or interstitial radiation implants with or without neoadjuvant hormone therapy. The patients were divided into low- (T1c-2a, PSA less than or equal to 10 ng per mL, and Gleason sum of 6 or less); intermediate- (T2b, PSA 10 to 20 ng per mL, or Gleason sum 7); and high- (T2c, PSA greater than 20 ng per mL, or Gleason sum of 8 or higher) risk groups. PSA failure was defined as three consecutive rises in PSA measured at least 3 months apart. Patients undergoing brachytherapy in the intermediate- and high-risk groups had a three times higher risk of cancer progression at 5 years when compared to radical prostatectomy, and this was not improved by adding neoadjuvant hormonal therapy (Fig. 32-2). Therefore, brachytherapy may not be as effective as radical prostatectomy or conformal radiation therapy in treating high-risk prostate cancer. Use of brachytherapy for such cancers should at present be limited to an investigational setting. Progression free survival rates observed in the retrospective cohort analysis by D'Amico et al. also failed to show any advantage over radiation therapy compared to radical prostatectomy in controlling high-risk cancers, regardless of whether neoadjuvant hormonal therapy was used (Fig. 32-2). These data again demonstrate no distinct advantage of either surgery or external beam radiation therapy in treating high-risk prostate cancers, although each appears to be more effective than brachytherapy.

SALVAGE THERAPY FOR LOCALLY RECURRENT PROSTATE CANCER

Patients who fail definitive local therapy for their prostate cancer are, by definition, high-risk patients. Salvage radical prostatectomy or radiation therapy should be offered to select individuals who have recurrent local disease but have no indications of metastatic cancer. In general, all men who are considered for salvage therapy should be fully evaluated for the presence of metastatic disease with a bone scan; CT scan of the abdomen and pelvis; PSA; and, possibly, prostatic acid phosphatase. Patients should also be counseled on higher complication rates associated with salvage therapy.

Salvage Radical Prostatectomy

Patients treated with radiation therapy have evidence of locally persistent prostate cancer in as much as 38% of patients biopsied, with a potentially significant rate of local recurrence and related progression at 10 years of follow-up (47,48). Thus, select patients who are found to have persistent localized prostate cancer without evidence of a distant recurrence may be considered for salvage therapy.

Salvage radical prostatectomy for locally recurrent or persistent cancers after radiation therapy may be associated with significant subsequent cancer control but is also associated with significant morbidity (Table 32-3). The evidence supporting an effect of salvage radical prostatectomy in controlling or eliminating such cancers is based on retrospective analyses of small surgical cohorts in which significant associations with improved recurrence-free survival based on risk stratification were observed. Tefilli (64) reported results on 27 patients who received either radical prostatectomy (n = 24) or radical cystectomy (n = 3) for radioresistant prostate cancer. All patients had histologic confirmation of persistent prostate cancer more than 18 months after radiation therapy and had a preradiation PSA of less than 20 ng per mL. After salvage surgery, 44% of patients were biochemically free of disease (PSA less than 0.4 ng per mL) at a median follow-up of 34 months. Pathologic organ confinement among these cases was associated with improved progression-free survival: All ten cases with organ-confined cancers showed no biochemical evidence of disease, whereas only 2 of 17 individuals with extraprostatic disease did not progress. Despite a rather lengthy (18 months) pause after primary radiation, these results suggest that salvage radical prostatectomy can be associated with subsequent cancer control in select cases.

Other studies have corroborated the association of salvage radical prostatectomy with subsequent cancer progression–free survival. The 10-year cancer-specific survival among 108 patients with recurrent prostate cancer treated with salvage prostatectomy at the Mayo Clinic was 70% (47). Similarly, Rogers et al. found a nonprogression rate of 55% at 5 years reported among 40 men who underwent salvage prostatectomy after definitive radiotherapy (63). In this study, a subset of patients who had a preoperative PSA of less than 10 ng per mL had a more favorable outcome (87% 5-year PSA-free survival). These findings suggest that early intervention in patients with a rising PSA after radiation therapy may afford better cancer control than surgery delayed until PSA is greater than 10 ng per mL. Of interest, however, pathologically organ-confined cancer was found even in some (albeit only 15%) patients with PSA greater than 10 ng per mL before salvage radical prostatectomy. Therefore, elevated PSA greater than 10 ng per mL does not preclude possibly effective cancer therapy via salvage radical prostatectomy in a small subset of cases.

Morbidity associated with salvage prostatectomy, however, is higher than that seen with primary radical prostatectomy. Complications including incontinence, vesicle neck contracture, and rectal injury were reported to be 50% to 63% (47,62–64), 11% to 28%, and 15%, respectively. Nonetheless, high local recurrence rates for radiation-resistant prostate cancers mandate that select men with isolated localized tumors be considered for surgical treatment at a time when cure remains possible.

Salvage Radiation Therapy

Men with locally recurrent prostate cancer after radical prostatectomy may be candidates for salvage radiation therapy. However, only a small proportion of men who undergo radical prostatectomy subsequently develop regionally confined recurrence amenable to radiation. For example, Pound et al. found that fewer than 5% of patients selected for radical prostatectomy at The Johns Hopkins Hospital were found to have such local regional recurrence at 10 years' follow-up (1). In this series, 129 men developed rising PSA after prostatectomy, and the vast majority (84%) of such recurrences were systemic. Nevertheless, the remaining subset of men with local regional recurrence may benefit from radiation salvage. Risk factors for local recurrence amenable to radiation salvage have included PSA recurrence more than 2 years after surgery, Gleason sum less than 8, and absence of seminal vesicle or lymph node extension at the time of radical prostatectomy (65,66). A review of salvage radiation therapy cohorts followed for 13 to 50 months found a PSA response as high as 64% (67). However, the effectiveness of radiation alone in these postsurgical patients is confounded by the fact that many received hormonal therapy at some point. Tefilli (64) reported on a cohort of 43 patients treated with salvage radiotherapy, none of whom received neoadjuvant or adjuvant hormonal therapy. The mean time to PSA recurrence in these patients after surgery was 24 months. At a mean follow-up of 31 months after salvage radiotherapy, 74% were found to have an undetectable PSA. The authors concluded that salvage radiotherapy is best suited for patients with node-negative prostate cancer whose postprostatectomy PSA has not risen above 2 ng per mL.

In contrast to salvage radical prostatectomy (for which prior radiation compounds the subsequent morbidity of surgery), the morbidity of salvage radiation therapy does not appear to be compounded by the prior surgery (64–68) and is associated with quality of life effects similar to those of standard radiation. Moreover, a retrospective analysis of a single cohort, in which outcomes of salvage surgery after radiation were compared to outcomes of salvage radiation after surgery, found significantly better quality of life when radical prostatectomy preceded radiation (68).

In summary, salvage therapy may be offered to select individuals with a PSA recurrence at least 2 years after definitive local therapy. Patients should be thoroughly evaluated for metastatic disease with a bone scan and abdominal pelvic CT scan, and, if these studies are negative, patients having previously received radiation should undergo prostate biopsy not earlier than 18 months after radiation therapy is completed. PSA rise immediately after radiation or surgery is a harbinger of high likelihood of metastatic cancer not as likely to respond to local salvage. Once the 2-year initial follow-up of the primary therapy has been completed, salvage therapy is most effective if implemented early after biochemical recurrence (as delay is likely to result in further progression). Finally, consideration must be given to the patient's overall health and co-morbidities, and quality of life benefits may be optimized if surgery precedes radiation rather than if radiation precedes surgery. Salvage therapy should not be offered to patients who are not expected to outlive their prostate cancer if left untreated.

CONCLUSION

Natural history data suggest that criteria for defining high-risk prostate cancer include high biopsy grade (Gleason scores 8 to 10), clinical stage T3, and markedly elevated serum PSA (greater than 20 ng per mL). Review of published series and comparative studies indicates that either radical prostatectomy or external beam radiation therapy can provide adequate cancer control for patients with such high-risk prostate cancers. Neither of these therapies (surgery or external beam radiation) shows a clear advantage over the other with regard to cancer control. Conversely, surgery, as well as external beam radiation, may be more effective at controlling high-risk cancers than less aggressive approaches, such as brachytherapy. Hormonal therapy has modest efficacy as a neoadjuvant with radiation for high-risk cancers in general or as a postsurgical adjuvant after radical prostatectomy for cancers with lymph node involvement. However, progression-free survival data (as well as tenets of androgen-independent mechanisms of prostate cancer progression) do not support the use of hormone therapy as a surgical neoadjuvant. Finally, retrospective quality of life outcome data suggest that salvage therapy strategies for combining surgical therapy and external beam radiation may be best accomplished when surgical removal is performed before later radiation salvage, as needed. New therapies for use as systemic adjuvants for high-risk prostate cancer are clearly needed, but radical prostatectomy or external beam radiation can nevertheless achieve cancer control in a significant proportion of these cancers.

REFERENCES

1. Pound CR, Partin AW, Epstein AI, et al. Prostate-specific antigen after radical retropubic prostatectomy. *Urol Clin North Am* 1997;24:395–406.
2. Shipley WU, Thames HD, Sandler HM, et al. Radiation therapy for clinically localized prostate cancer—a multi-institutional pooled analysis. *JAMA* 1999;281:1598–1604.
3. Landis SH, Murray T, Bolden S, et al. Cancer statistics, 1998. *Cancer J Clin* 1998;48:6–29.
4. Albertsen PC, Hanley JA, Gleason DF, et al. Competing risk analysis of men aged 55 to 74 years at diagnosis managed conservatively for clinically localized prostate cancer. *JAMA* 1998;280:975–980.
5. D'Amico AV, Whittington R, Malkowicz B, et al. Biochemical outcome after radical prostatectomy, external beam radiation therapy, or interstitial radiation therapy for clinically localized prostate cancer. *JAMA* 1998;280:969–974.
6. Partin AW, Kattan MW, Subong ENP, et al. Combination of prostate-specific antigen, clinical stage, and Gleason score to predict pathological stage of localized prostate cancer. *JAMA* 1997;277:1445–1451.
7. Fallon B, Williams RD. Current options in the management of clinical stage C prostate carcinoma. *Urol Clin North Am* 1990;17:853–866.
8. Lynch JH, Graham CW. Management of stage C adenocarcinoma of the prostate. *Br J Urol* 1992;79(Suppl 1):50–56.
9. Adolfsson J. Deferred treatment of low grade stage t3 prostate cancer without distant metastases. *J Urol* 1993;149: 326–329.
10. Adolfsson J, Steineck G, Hedlund P. Deferred treatment of clinically localized low-grade prostate cancer: actual 10-year and projected 15-year follow-up of the Karolinska series. *Urology* 1997;50:722–726.
11. Johansson JE, Holmberg L, Johansson S, et al. Fifteen-year survival in prostate cancer. *JAMA* 1997;277:467–471.
12. Rana A, Chisholm GD, Khan M, et al. Conservative management with symptomatic treatment and delayed hormonal manipulation is justified in men with locally advanced carcinoma of the prostate. *Br J Urol* 1994;74:637–641.
13. Chodak GW, Thisted RA, Gerber GS, et al. Results of conservative management of clinically localized prostate cancer. *N Engl J Med* 1994;330:242–248.
14. Albertsen PC, Fryback DG, Storer BG, et al. Long-term survival among men with conservatively treated prostate cancer. *JAMA* 1995;274:626–631.
15. Perrotti M, Rabbani F, Russo P, et al. Early prostate caner detection and potential for surgical cure in men with poorly differentiated tumors. *Urology* 1998;52:106–110.
16. D'Amico AV, Whittington R, Malkowicz B, et al. Pretreatment nomogram for prostate-specific antigen recurrence

after radical prostatectomy or external-beam radiation therapy for clinically localized prostate cancer. *J Clin Oncol* 1999;17:168–172.

17. Pisansky TM, Kahn MJ, Rasp GM, et al. A multiple prognostic index predictive of disease outcome after irradiation for clinically localized prostate carcinoma. *Cancer* 1997;79: 337–344.
18. Kattan MW, Eastham JA, Stapleton MF, et al. A preoperative nomogram for disease recurrence following radical prostatectomy for prostate cancer. *J Natl Cancer Inst* 1998;90: 766–771.
19. D'Amico AV, Desjardin A, Chung A, et al. Assessment of outcome prediction models for patients with localized prostate carcinoma managed with radical prostatectomy or external beam radiation therapy. *Cancer* 1998;82:1887–1896.
20. Pound CR, Partin AW, Eisenberger MA, et al. Natural history of progression after PSA elevation following radical prostatectomy. *JAMA* 1999;281:1591–1597.
21. Huggins C, Hodges CV. The effect of castration of estrogen and of androgen injection on serum phosphatases in metastatic carcinoma of the prostate. *Cancer Res* 1941;1:293–297.
22. VACURG. Treatment and survival of patients with cancer of the prostate. The Veterans Administration Cooperative Urological Research Group. *Surg Gynecol Obstet* 1967;124: 1011–1017.
23. Byar DP. Proceedings: the Veterans Administration Cooperative Urological Research Group's studies of cancer of the prostate. *Cancer* 1973;32:1126–1130.
24. The MRC Prostate Cancer Working Party Investigators Group. Immediate versus deferred treatment for advanced prostatic cancer: initial results of the Medical Research Council. *Brit J Urol* 1997;79:235–246.
25. Gerber GS, Thisted RA, Chodak GW, et al. Results of radical retropubic prostatectomy in men with locally advanced prostate cancer: multi-institutional pooled analysis. *Eur Urol* 1997;32:385–390.
26. Lerner SE, Blute ML, Zincke H. Extended experience with radical prostatectomy for clinical stage T3 prostate cancer: outcome and contemporary morbidity. *J Urol* 1995;154: 1447–1452.
27. Steinberg GD, Epstein JI, Piantadosi S, et al. Management of stage D1 adenocarcinoma of the prostate: the Johns Hopkins experience 1974 to 1987. *J Urol* 1990;144:1425–1432.
28. Oefelein MG, Smith ND, Grayhack JT, et al. Long-term results of radical retropubic prostatectomy in men with high grade carcinoma of the prostate. *J Urol* 1997;158:1460–1465.
29. Golimbu M, Provet J, Al-Askari S, et al. Radical prostatectomy for stage D1 prostate cancer. *Urology* 1987;30:427–435.
30. Gerber GS, Thisted RA, Scardino PT, et al. Results of radical prostatectomy in men with clinically localized prostate cancer. *JAMA* 1996;276:615–619.
31. Gomez JL, Cusan L, Diamond P, et al. Long-term treatment of clinical stage C/T3 prostate cancer with flutamide and castration: 6-year median follow-up. *Br J Urol* 1997;80(Suppl 2):1080.
32. Scott WW, Boyd HL. Combined hormone control therapy and radical prostatectomy in the treatment of selected cases of advanced carcinoma of the prostate: a retrospective study based upon 25 years of experience. *J Urol* 1961;101:86–92.
33. Lowe BA, Lieberman SF. Disease recurrence and progression in untreated pathologic stage T3 cancer: selecting the patient for adjuvant therapy. *J Urol* 1997;158:1452–1456.
34. Wieder JA, Soloway MS. Incidence, etiology, location, prevention and treatment of positive surgical margins after radical prostatectomy for prostate cancer. *J Urol* 1998;160: 299–315.
35. Fair WR, Cookson MS, Stroumbakis N, et al. The indications, rationale, and results of neoadjuvant androgen deprivation in the treatment of prostate cancer: Memorial Sloan-Kettering Cancer Center results. *Urology* 1997;49(Suppl 3A):46–55.
36. Narayan P, Lowe BA, Carroll PR, et al. Neoadjuvant hormonal therapy and radical prostatectomy for clinical stage C carcinoma of the prostate. *Br J Urol* 1994;73:544–548.
37. Gomella LG, Liberman SN, Mulholland G, et al. Induction androgen deprivation plus prostatectomy for stage T3 disease: failure to achieve prostate-specific antigen-based freedom from disease status in a phase II trial. *Urology* 1996;47: 870–877.
38. Cher ML, Shinohara K, Vapnek BJ, et al. High failure rate associated with long-term follow-up of neoadjuvant androgen deprivation followed by radical prostatectomy for stage C prostate cancer. *Br J Urol* 1995;75:771–777.
39. Aprikan AG, Fair WR, Reuter VE, et al. Experience with neoadjuvant diethylstilboestrol and radical prostatectomy in patients with locally advanced prostate cancer. *Br J Urol* 1994;74:630–636.
40. Kennedy TJ, Sonneland AM, Marlett MM, et al. Luteinizing hormone-releasing hormone downstaging of clinical stage C prostate cancer. *J Urol* 1992;147:891–893.
41. Witjes WP, Schulman CC, Debruyne FM. Preliminary results of a prospective randomized study comparing radical prostatectomy versus radical prostatectomy associated with neoadjuvant hormonal combination therapy in T2-3N0M0 prostate cancer. *Urology* 1997;49(Suppl 3A):65–69.
42. Aus G, Abrahamsson PA, Ahlgren G, et al. Hormonal treatment before radical prostatectomy: a 3-year followup. *J Urol* 1998;159:2013–2017.
43. Soloway MS, Sharifi R, Wajsman Z, et al. Randomized prospective study comparing radical prostatectomy alone versus radical prostatectomy preceded by androgen blockade in clinical stage B2 (T2bNxM0) prostate cancer. *J Urol* 1995; 154:424–428.
44. Van Poppel H, De Ridder D, Elgamal AA, et al. Neoadjuvant hormonal therapy before radical prostatectomy decreases the number of positive surgical margins in stage T2 prostate cancer: interim results of a prospective randomized trial. *J Urol* 1995;154:429–434.
45. Fair WR, Scher HI. Neoadjuvant hormonal therapy plus surgery for prostate cancer. *Surg Oncol Clin North Am* 1997;6:831–845.
46. Messing E, Manola J, Wilding G, et al. Immediate hormonal therapy vs. observation for node positive prostate cancer following radical prostatectomy and pelvic lymphadenectomy: a randomized phase III ECOG/INTER group trial. *J Urol* 1998;161:175.
47. Lerner SE, Amling CL, Kaynan AM, et al. The role for salvage surgery in radio-recurrent/resistant carcinoma of the prostate. *AUA Update Series* 1999;18:58–63.

48. Crook JM, Choan E, Perry GA, et al. Serum prostate-specific antigen profile following radiotherapy for prostate cancer: implications for patterns of failure and definition of cure. *Urology* 1998;51:566–572.
49. Schellhammer PF, El-Mahdi AM, Kuban DA, et al. Prostate-specific antigen after radiation therapy. *Urol Clin North Am* 1997;24:407–414.
50. Perez CA, Lee HK, Georgiou A, et al. Technical and tumor-related factors affecting outcome of definitive irradiation of localized carcinoma of the prostate. *Int J Radiat Oncol Biol Phys* 1993;26:581–591.
51. Perez CA, Pilepich MV, Zivnuska F. Tumor control in definitive irradiation of localized carcinoma of the prostate. *Int J Radiat Oncol Biol Phys* 1986;12:523–531.
52. Arcangeli G, Micheli A, Arcangeli G, et al. Definitive radiation therapy for localized prostate adenocarcinoma. *Int J Radiat Oncol Biol Phys* 1991;20:439–446.
53. Stock RG, Ferrari AC, Stone NN. Does pelvic irradiation play a role in the management of prostate cancer? *Oncology* 1998;12:1467–1472.
54. Zietman AL, Coen JJ, Dallow KC, et al. The treatment of prostate cancer by conventional radiation therapy: an analysis of long-term outcome. *Int J Radiat Oncol Biol Phys* 1995;32:287–292.
55. Zagars GK, Pollack A, Kavadi VS, et al. Prostate-specific antigen and radiation therapy for clinically localized prostate cancer. *Int J Radiat Oncol Biol Phys* 1995;32:293–306.
56. Gervasi LA, Mata J, Easley JD, et al. Prognostic significance of lymph node metastases in prostate cancer. *J Urol* 1989;142:332–335.
57. Fukunaga-Johnson N, Sandler HM, McLaughlin PW, et al. Results of 3D conformal radiotherapy in the treatment of localized prostate cancer. *Int J Radiat Oncol Biol Phys* 1997;38:311–317.
58. Bolla M, Gonzalez D, Warde P, et al. Improved survival in patients with locally advanced prostate cancer treated with radiotherapy and goserelin. *N Engl J Med* 1997;337:295–300.
59. Fiveash JB, Hanks G, Roach M 3rd, et al. 3D conformal radiation therapy for high grade prostate cancer: a multi-institutional review. *Int J Rad Oncol Biol Phys* 2000;47:335–342.
60. Pilepich MV, Sause WT, Shipley WU, et al. Androgen deprivation with radiation therapy compared with radiation therapy alone for locally advanced prostatic carcinoma: a randomized comparative trial of the RTOG. *Urology* 1995; 45:616–623.
61. Pilepich MV, Caplan R, Byhardt RW, et al. Phase III trial of androgen suppression using goserelin in unfavorable-prognosis carcinoma of the prostate treated with definitive radiotherapy: report of RTOG protocol 85-31. *J Clin Oncol* 1997;15:1013–1021.
62. Pontes JE, Montie J, Klein E, et al. Salvage surgery for radiation failure in prostate cancer. *Cancer* 1993;71:976–980.
63. Rogers E, Ohori M, Kassabian VS, et al. Salvage radical prostatectomy: outcome measured by serum prostate specific antigen levels. *J Urol* 1995;153:104–110.
64. Tefilli MV, Gheiler EL, Tiguert R, et al. Salvage surgery or salvage radiotherapy for locally recurrent prostate cancer. *Urology* 1998;52:224–229.
65. Cadeddu JA, Partin AW, DeWeese TL, et al. Long-term results of radiation therapy for prostate cancer recurrence following radical prostatectomy. *J Urol* 1998;159:173–177.
66. Rodgers R, Grossfeld GD, Roach M 3rd, et al. Radiation therapy for the management of biopsy proved local recurrence after radical prostatectomy. *J Urol* 1998;160:1748–1753.
67. Forman JD, Velasco J. Therapeutic radiation in patients with a rising post-prostatectomy PSA level. *Oncology* 1998; 12:33–39.
68. Tefilli MV, Gheiler EL, Tiguert R, et al. Quality of life in patients undergoing salvage procedures for locally recurrent prostate cancer. *J Surg Oncol* 1998;69:156–161.

33

ADJUVANT EXTERNAL BEAM RADIATION THERAPY POSTPROSTATECTOMY

ALAN POLLACK
LEWIS G. SMITH

DEFINING ADJUVANT TREATMENT

Adjuvant postprostatectomy treatment is defined here as the administration of radiotherapy for high-risk pathologic features in the setting of an undetectable prostate-specific antigen (PSA). Some have categorized the treatment of patients with a detectable PSA postprostatectomy that have undergone radiotherapy within 6 months of surgery as adjuvant (1). However, this is more appropriately classified as an attempt at salvage (2–4). Those with a detectable PSA postprostatectomy are at a much higher risk of harboring regional or distant metastasis, a considerable local tumor burden, or both. Although the use of radiotherapy in the treatment of patients with a persistently elevated postprostatectomy PSA is consistent with the concept of adjuvant therapy, it is difficult to determine the extent of regional or distant spread, using available imaging methods. The main focus of this chapter is on the outcome of patients who are candidates for, or have received, adjuvant radiotherapy.

The premise for the use of adjuvant external beam radiation therapy (EBRT) postprostatectomy is that, in the setting of adverse pathologic findings, surgery usually does not result in the complete extirpation of the tumor, and residual prostate cancer cells remain in the surgical bed. As has been pointed out by Anscher (5), leaving behind 10^6 to 10^7 tumor cells without any normal prostate tissue would result in a serum PSA of approximately 0.035 ng per mL [calculated from estimates that 1 cc of prostate cancer results in a serum PSA of 3.5 ng per mL (6)]. This PSA level is below the threshold of detection for most assays. The rationale for the administration of adjuvant radiotherapy within 6 months of radical prostatectomy for high-risk pathologic features is that a significant percentage of these patients will eventually develop local recurrence, and local recurrence will predispose to metastatic disease and reduce survival. The correlation of local prostate cancer recurrence to distant metastasis is well established (7–9). The discussion below is divided into two sections. A summary of the surgical data relating to the incidence of and outcome associated with adverse pathologic features is described first, followed by a discussion of the results of adjuvant radiotherapy.

SELECTION OF PATIENTS FOR ADJUVANT RADIOTHERAPY

Biochemical Failure as a Surrogate for Clinical Relapse

The use of the detectable or rising PSA profile as an early indicator of relapse has greatly augmented the characterization of high-risk pathologic features at prostatectomy. Although PSA is secreted in small amounts by some nonprostatic tissues (10), for all practical purposes, a detectable serum PSA after radical prostatectomy is consistent with eventual clinical failure (9). The same conclusions hold using ultrasensitive PSA assays that measure levels below 0.1 ng per mL (11,12). Most genitourinary specialists consider a PSA of greater than 0.2 to 0.4 ng per mL as evidence of failure to control the disease surgically. A rise in PSA above this threshold postoperatively is an excellent predictor of future clinically detectable disease. PSA has been shown to rise 3 to 5 years before clinical relapse occurs (13,14).

There are several lines of evidence that document a strong correlation between biochemical failure and clinical outcome. After prostatectomy for clinical T1-T2 (cT1-T2) disease, the PSA drops to undetectable in more than 95%. When biochemical failure is manifest, vesicourethral anastomosis and prostatic fossa biopsies are positive in the majority (15,16). In the series by Pound et al. (9), no man developed local or distant failure without an elevation in PSA. They reported that the median time to distant metastasis after biochemical failure was 8 years. The main correlates of the development of distant metastasis were postprostatectomy PSA doubling time and time from surgery to a rise in PSA. A rise in PSA postprostatectomy is the earliest and most consistent evidence of tumor progression.

Determinants of Recurrence after Prostatectomy

The main local pathologic risk factors associated with increased clinical or biochemical failure, or both, are extracapsular extension (ECE), seminal vesicle invasion (SVI), high Gleason score (higher than 6), and a positive margin (margin+) (13,17–20). There are clearly interactions between these factors. For example, the combination of ECE and Gleason score higher than 6 is associated with higher failure rates than ECE with Gleason scores of 6 or less (13,17–19). Also, the prognostic value of the extent of margin positivity (focal vs. extensive or single vs. multiple) is affected by Gleason score (17).

The detection of regional metastasis in the lymph nodes [lymph node invasion (LNI)] constitutes another distinct high-risk group. In the majority of cases, planned prostatectomy has been aborted with the finding of LNI on frozen section, although enthusiasm for completing surgery combined with long-term androgen ablation is gaining strength (21,22). Radiotherapy combined with androgen ablation as primary treatment for LNI has also been used with success (23). Because there is limited information available on the role of adjuvant radiotherapy postprostatectomy in this cohort (24), this topic is not discussed further.

The incidence of ECE ranges from 32% to 61% in clinically organ-confined (cT1-T2) prostate cancer (Table 33-1) (25–34). SVI is approximately 10%, and lymph node positivity is approximately 5%. Margin positivity, which is the strongest determinant of relapse after radical prostatectomy in seminal vesicle–negative and lymph node–negative cases, is seen in 15% to 43%. It should be noted that SVI [pT3c, 1992 American Joint Committee on Cancer (AJCC) staging system (35)] is a subset of ECE. Because the prognosis associated with ECE without SVI (pT3a,b; 1992 AJCC staging system) is much better than that with ECE with SVI (pT3c), these entities should be segregated. Considerable stage migration has been observed since PSA was introduced as a screening tool. The incidence of ECE (27,36,37), margin positivity (17), and lymph node involvement (36,37) has declined.

The risk of adverse pathologic features is a function of clinical stage. The AJCC 1992 staging system discriminates the risk of such adverse features to a greater degree than the 1997 system. Han et al. (38) reported rates of ECE, SVI, and LNI of 47.1%, 5.5%, and 3.5% for category cT2a, whereas for category cT2b the rates were 54.1%, 7.8%, and 11.4%. Likewise, Ramos et al. (29), Kupelian et al. (33), and Stamey et al. (39) have found a higher incidence of pT3 disease for category cT2b over cT2a. The rates of pT3 for cT2b and cT2c were similar in all of these series. The differences described for cT2a and cT2b also extend to rates of positive margins and biochemical outcome.

Table 33-2 (40–42) displays the relationships of the adverse pathologic features and the risk of biochemical failure. The 5- and 10-year freedom from biochemical failure rates related to ECE are variable and affected by margin positivity, SVI, Gleason score, and nodal involvement. When the seminal vesicles and lymph nodes are not involved, margin positivity is the most important pathologic determinant of outcome. The risk of biochemical failure is approximately 40% to 60% at 5 years, with additional failures seen between 5 and 10 years. That many of these patients have an isolated local recurrence is clear. In summary, the rationale for adjuvant radiotherapy is based on sound observations that patients with adverse pathologic features are at high risk

TABLE 33-1. INCIDENCE OF ADVERSE PATHOLOGIC FEATURES IN PROSTATECTOMY SPECIMENS FROM CT1-T2 PATIENTS

Author (ref)	n	% ECE	% SV+	% LN+	% Margin+
Blute et al. (25)	2,475	32	15	7	—
Cheng et al. (26)	339	35	14	6	24
Jhaveri et al. (27)	731	54	—	—	—
Gilliland et al. (28)	1,395	47	7	3	33
Ramos et al. (29)[a]	1,620	32	7	1	24
Bauer et al. (30)	378	57	—	—	—
Pound et al. (19)	1,623	52	6	7	—
Dillioglugil et al. (31)	611	39	11	6	—
Lowe et al. (32)	583	35	4	3	15
Epstein et al. (18)	721	58	7	8	23
Kupelian et al. (33)	337	61	18	8	43
Ohori et al. (34)	478	43	12	5	16
Weighted average:		41	9	5	24

ECE, extracapsular extension; LN, lymph node; SV, seminal vesicle.
[a]T1-T2b (T2c excluded).

TABLE 33-2. RELATIONSHIP OF EXTRACAPSULAR EXTENSION (ECE) AND MARGIN POSITIVITY TO FREEDOM FROM BIOCHEMICAL FAILURE

	Freedom from biochemical failure rates			
	% 5 yr		% 10 yr	
Author (ref)	ECE	Margin+	ECE	Margin+
Grossfeld et al. (40)	—	52	—	—
Kupelian et al. (20)	~43	~35	—	—
Dillioglugil et al. (31)	79	—	79	—
Epstein et al. (17,18)	78[a]	64	68	55
Anscher et al. (40)	—	66	—	—
Zietman et al. (41)	27	26	—	—
Paulson (42)	—	42	—	38

[a]Established ECE and 4-year rate.

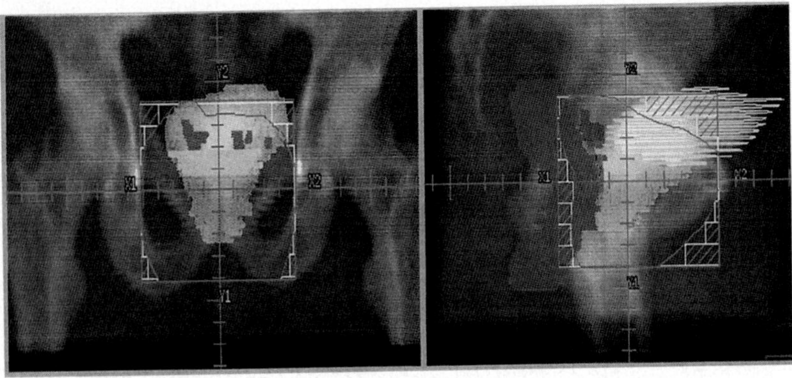

A,B

FIGURE 33-1. Example of adjuvant conformal radiation therapy fields. **A:** Anterior-posterior view. **B:** Right lateral view. (See also color Figure 33-1.)

of eventual disease relapse and that local recurrence, although not readily apparent, is a prominent component of failure, as defined by a rising PSA.

ADJUVANT RADIOTHERAPY

Radiotherapy Technique and Dose

Typically, a four-field arrangement is used for the adjuvant treatment of prostate cancer postprostatectomy. There is a trend to move away from specifying dose to the isocenter and specify dose to a planning target volume, which is consistent with the International Commission on Radiation Units and Measurements criteria (43). In addition, three-dimensional (3D) treatment planning and conformal radiation therapy (CRT) is being applied more frequently in the postoperative setting (44–45). Figure 33-1 shows examples of anterior and lateral fields planned using 3D CRT. In the example shown, the bladder neck, which has been pulled down into the prostatic fossa, has been outlined as an estimate of the planning target volume. The periprostatic surgical clips have also been outlined as a guide to defining the surgical bed. Radiation doses have traditionally been lower in adjuvant, as compared to salvage, treatment. Doses have ranged from 45 Gy to more than 60 Gy (Table 33-3) (46–52). Recently, Valicenti and colleagues (53) described a dose response for patients treated adjuvantly for pT3N0 prostate cancer. They divided patients into those treated to less than or equal to 61.2 Gy (n = 14) versus those treated to greater than 61.2 Gy (n = 38). The 3-year biochemical no evidence of disease (bNED) rate for the low-dose group was 64%, compared to 90% for those who received the higher dose (p = .015). Because small numbers of patients were used in this study, the investigators were unable to perform a multivariate analysis controlling for the possible unequal distribution of prognostic factors. Petrovich et al. (47) have advocated doses of 45 to 54 Gy depending on pathologic criteria with reasonable results. However, in their latest publication, no difference in outcome was found between patients treated adjuvantly to these doses and a group of high-risk prostatectomy patients not treated with radiation from their institution. The need for doses above 61.2 Gy is uncertain but is recommended until other dose-response evidence is forthcoming.

The timing of radiotherapy after radical prostatectomy in the adjuvant setting has not been studied in any detail. Most investigators classify treatment as adjuvant when radiotherapy is administered within 3 to 6 months of radi-

TABLE 33-3. FREEDOM FROM BIOCHEMICAL FAILURE AFTER ADJUVANT EXTERNAL BEAM RADIATION THERAPY

Author (ref)	n	pStage	% Margin+	Follow-up (mo)	Dose (Gy)	% bNED (yr)
Leibovich et al. (46)	76	T2N0	100[a]	29	63	88 (5)
Nudell et al. (3)	36	T2-T3	97	~23	68	~58 (5)
Petrovich et al. (47)	201	T3N0	41	68	48	67 (5)
Vicini et al. (4)	38	T2c-T4	—	49	59.4	67 (5)
Valicenti et al. (45)	52	T3N0	83	39	64.8	82 (5)
Valicenti et al. (48)	15	T3cN0	20	~38	64.8	86 (3)
Morris et al. (49)	40	T3N0	85	31	60–62	88 (3)
Coetzee et al. (50)	30	T2-T3c	100	33	66–70	50 (4)
Schild et al. (51)	60	T3N0	82	32	62	57 (5)
Zietman et al. (52)	68[b]	T3N0	94	NS	60–64	64 (5)

bNED, biochemical no evidence of disease; NS, not significant.
[a]Single positive margin.
[b]Only 27 confirmed to have undetectable prostate-specific antigen.

cal prostatectomy. In our experience, 3 months may not be enough in many cases to allow for return of urinary continence. Our policy is to wait for the return of urinary continence but to administer radiation within 6 months of radical prostatectomy, even if urinary incontinence persists.

Clinical Failure after Adjuvant Radiotherapy

A number of series, mainly from the pre-PSA era, have found that local failure is reduced after adjuvant radiotherapy for high-risk features postprostatectomy (46,54–58). Anscher et al. (5,57) reported that local control at 10 years was 92% for those receiving adjuvant radiotherapy versus 60% for those who did not receive any adjuvant treatment. The difference in local control was much greater at 10 years than at 5 years, illustrating the need for long-term follow-up using this end point. The effect on local control usually has translated into a benefit in overall disease freedom, but there is no evidence that adjuvant radiotherapy impacts distant metastasis or survival. The problem with relating improved local control to a reduction in distant metastasis and death due to progression is that large numbers of patients are required. This is particularly true for prostate cancer studies, because androgen ablation effectively prolongs the time to the development of distant metastasis and patients are elderly, often dying of intercurrent disease before there is evidence of progression. The small retrospective studies performed to date have been inadequate to address the effect of adjuvant radiotherapy on distant metastasis and survival.

Biochemical Failure after Adjuvant Radiotherapy

Biochemical failure occurs years before the manifestation of clinical relapse (13,14) and is a strong correlate of local relapse and metastasis (9). Very few patients demonstrate distant metastasis in the absence of a rising PSA (9,31,33). Biochemical failure after radiotherapy is clearly a harbinger of disease relapse and has proven invaluable in assessing the success of adjuvant radiotherapy. In the setting of postoperative radiotherapy, the same criteria that are used to define biochemical failure—namely, a rise in PSA to above 0.2 to 0.4 ng per mL—should be used. It is inappropriate to use less stringent definitions. Table 33-3 shows a summary of several representative PSA era series. In distinction to the results achieved with a radical prostatectomy alone for high-risk patients based on pathologic features (Table 33-2), there appears to be a reduction in biochemical failure at 5 years an average of 50% to 30%. Table 33-4 summarizes contemporary series in which direct comparisons of freedom from biochemical failure were made between high-risk patients treated with radical prostatectomy alone and those treated with radical prostatectomy plus adjuvant radiotherapy. In some analyses, matched pair comparisons have been made. In all but one study, in which statistical comparisons were done, adjuvant radiotherapy reduced biochemical failure significantly. As mentioned earlier, the University of Southern California group (47) uses a lower dose of radiation that may have influenced the lack of effect they observed. They note, however, that the radiotherapy group in their analysis had more adverse pathologic features than the surgical control group.

TABLE 33-4. ADJUVANT EXTERNAL BEAM RADIATION THERAPY POSTPROSTATECTOMY: RECENT COMPARATIVE STUDIES

Author (ref)	n	Dose (Gy)	% bNED (yr)	*p* value
Leibovich et al. (46)[a]	76	—	59 (5)	.005
	76	63	88 (5)	
Petrovich et al. (47)	40	—	69 (5)	NS
	201	48	68 (5)	
Valicenti et al. (45)[a]	36	—	66 (3)	NA
	36	64.8	93 (3)	
Schild (61)	~228	—	40 (5)	.0003
	~60	60–67	90 (5)	
Valicenti (48)[b]	20	—	48 (3)	.01
	15	64.8	86 (3)	

bNED, biochemical no evidence of disease; NA, not available; NS, not significant.
[a]Matched pair analysis.
[b]pT3cN0 patients.

Efficacy of Adjuvant Radiotherapy for Seminal Vesicle Invasion

The limitations of available data related to the efficacy of adjuvant radiotherapy for prostatectomy patients at high risk of relapse based on pathologic criteria are considerable. The stage designation of pT3N0 includes two distinct risk groups, those with ECE without SVI and those with SVI. These risk groups have rarely been analyzed separately and, when they have, the number of SVI patients has been small. Valicenti and colleagues (48) directly addressed the question of the efficacy of adjuvant postoperative radiotherapy for pT3cN0 disease. There were 53 men identified from a cohort of 375 men who underwent radical prostatectomy at their institution between 1989 and 1995. Of these, 35 had an undetectable PSA postoperatively, and 15 were treated adjuvantly with radiotherapy only. The bNED rate at 3 years for the group receiving adjuvant radiotherapy was 86% versus 48% for the 20 patients who were observed.

There is no question that pT3c disease is associated with a high risk of biochemical and clinical recurrence, with a significant distant failure rate; however, not all patients with SVI have a dismal prognosis. There are other modifying factors besides lymph node involvement (59). Although patients with seminal vesicle invasion are at high risk of harboring lymph node or distant metastasis, local recurrence has been identified as a major site of failure

(54,60). Patients with pT3cN0 disease who have an undetectable PSA after radical prostatectomy appear to constitute a favorable subset that may be effectively consolidated through irradiation of the prostatic fossa. In contrast, the salvage of pT3c patients with a persistently elevated PSA after a radical prostatectomy has been poor (48,51,61). The benefit of radiotherapy for pT3cN0 disease appears to be restricted to those in whom PSA has been reduced to undetectable levels post prostatectomy.

Complications of Adjuvant Radiotherapy

Severe complications from adjuvant radiotherapy using modern techniques and beam energies of 10 MV or greater are rare but have been reported (2). The complication rate from the combination of radical prostatectomy plus radiation therapy is approximately the same as for radical prostatectomy alone (51,58). However, there is a higher rate of urethral and bladder neck stricture and proctitis from adjuvant radiotherapy. The frequency of these effects does not appear to be different than that observed from definitive prostate treatment. Despite the fact that a significant proportion of the bladder is irradiated because it is pulled down into the prostatic fossa, the bladder complication rates have been acceptable. Grade 3 or above acute urinary or bowel complications are unusual and may be reduced with the use of 3D CRT (45). In fact, urinary irritative or obstructive symptoms or incontinence, or both, seem to be lower for patients receiving adjuvant radiotherapy after radical prostatectomy as compared to definitive radiotherapy. Residual incontinence from radical prostatectomy may actually improve during radiotherapy, owing to radiation-induced edema, but typically returns to baseline levels approximately a month after radiotherapy is completed. The incidence of grade 2 or higher late bladder complications is on the order of 5% (44). Late rectal complications are lower and are in line with those observed from definitive prostate radiation treatment.

Adjuvant versus Salvage Radiotherapy

A number of groups have compared the results of adjuvant and salvage radiotherapy postprostatectomy (2,4,49,50). In nearly every series, the results of salvage radiotherapy have been worse. However, there are clearly two groups of patients who receive salvage treatment. The prognosis of those who have a persistently elevated PSA after radical prostatectomy has generally been found to be worse than those with a low, slowly rising PSA occurring years after radical prostatectomy (44,61,62–64). In contrast, Garg and associates (65) have argued that equivalent results may be obtained if salvage radiotherapy is begun when PSA is less than 2 ng per mL. However, the number of patients with a persistently elevated PSA was small, and the results, although not significant, suggested that these patients have a worse prognosis than those with delayed biochemical failure.

For the cohort of patients who initially achieved an undetectable PSA postprostatectomy, the efficacy of salvage radiotherapy has been shown to be dependent on the preradiotherapy PSA level. Forman et al. (66,67) have consistently shown improved results when treatment is initiated before the PSA rises above 2 ng per mL. Other investigators have also documented that the PSA level before the administration of salvage radiotherapy is an important determinant of outcome. Wu et al. (63) used a PSA to a cut point of 2.5, Schild et al. (61,62) a cut point of 1.1, Morris et al. (49) a cut point of 1.7, and Zelefsky et al. (44) a PSA cut point of 1 ng per mL. Freedom from failure for patients in whom salvage radiotherapy was administered when the PSA was below these cut points has been much higher than for those with PSAs above these levels. There is no clear-cut answer to the question of whether patients should be treated adjuvantly or at salvage. Because at least 50% of pathologic high-risk patients will require salvage later and adjuvant treatment may necessitate a lower dose, adjuvant treatment may be preferable, particularly in younger men. Hypothetically, leaving cancer cells behind with the chance to mutate and spread distantly is disconcerting when there is an effective treatment available with low morbidity.

CLINICAL TRIALS

There are two randomized prospective trials designed to evaluate the use of adjuvant EBRT after prostatectomy. The first is Southwest Oncology Group 8794 (Radiation Therapy Oncology Group 90-19, IG–0086), which was begun by the Southwest Oncology Group in 1987 and is now closed. This trial was designed to compare disease-free survival and to assess the toxicities of therapy among resected pT3N0M0 patients treated with or without adjuvant EBRT. The other trial is from the European Organization for Research and Treatment of Cancer 22911 and was opened in 1992. This trial was designed to compare the local recurrence rates, acute and late morbidity, overall survival, disease-free survival, and cancer-related survival of patients with pT3N0 adenocarcinoma of the prostate randomized to postoperative radiation therapy or observation.

RECOMMENDATIONS

The weight of the data supports the use of adjuvant radiotherapy in the setting of high-risk pathologic attributes postprostatectomy. There have been improvements in treatment planning and delivery that have reduced side effects. The lack of an obvious effect on survival should not be considered in the decision to use adjuvant radiotherapy, because the small retrospective series that has examined this issue has not had the power to detect a survival benefit. The fact that biochemical failure rates are significantly reduced with adjuvant radiotherapy, while morbidity is low, supports this approach. Doses above 60 Gy are recommended. There also may be additional benefit from the use of androgen ablation in combination with adjuvant radiotherapy (68).

REFERENCES

1. Zietman AL, Coen JJ, Shipley WU, et al. Adjuvant irradiation after radical prostatectomy for adenocarcinoma of prostate: analysis of freedom from PSA failure. *Urology* 1993;42: 292–299.
2. Valicenti RK, Gomella LG, Ismail M, et al. Durable efficacy of early postoperative radiation therapy for high-risk pT3N0 prostate cancer: the importance of radiation dose. *Urology* 1998;52:1034–1040.
3. Nudell DM, Grossfeld GD, Weinberg VK, et al. Radiotherapy after radical prostatectomy: treatment outcomes and failure patterns. *Urololgy* 1999;54:1049–1057.
4. Vicini FA, Ziaja EL, Kestin LL, et al. Treatment outcome with adjuvant and salvage irradiation after radical prostatectomy for prostate cancer. *Urology* 1999;54:111–117.
5. Anscher MS. Adjuvant therapy for pathologic stage C prostate cancer: A casualty of the PSA revolution? *Int J Radiat Oncol Biol Phys* 1996;34:745–747.
6. Stamey TA, Kabalin JN, Mcneal JE, et al. Prostate specific antigen in the diagnosis and treatment of adenocarcinoma of the prostate. II. Radical prostatectomy treated patients. *J Urol* 1989;141:1076–1083.
7. Zagars GK, von Eschenbach AC, Ayala AG, et al. The influence of local control on metastatic dissemination of prostate cancer treated by external beam megavoltage radiation therapy. *Cancer* 1991;68:2370–2377.
8. Fuks Z, Leibel SA, Wallner KE, et al. The effect of local control on metastatic dissemination in carcinoma of the prostate: long-term results in patients with ^{125}I implantation. *Int J Radiat Oncol Biol Phys* 1991;21:537–547.
9. Pound CR, Partin AW, Eisenberger MA, et al. Natural history of progression after PSA elevation following radical prostatectomy. *JAMA* 1999;281:1591–1597.
10. Iwakiri J, Grandbois K, Wehner N, et al. An analysis of urinary prostate specific antigen before and after radical prostatectomy: evidence for secretion of prostate specific antigen by the periurethral glands. *J Urol* 1993;149:783–786.
11. Haese A, Huland E, Graefen M, et al. Ultrasensitive detection of prostate specific antigen in the followup of 422 patients after radical prostatectomy. *J Urol* 1999;161:1206–1211.
12. Witherspoon LR, Lapeyrolerie T. Sensitive prostate specific antigen measurements identify men with long disease-free intervals and differentiate aggressive from indolent cancer recurrences within 2 years after radical prostatectomy. *J Urol* 1997;157:1322–1328.
13. Paulson DF. Impact of radical prostatectomy in the management of clinically localized disease. *J Urol* 1994;152:1826–1830.
14. Pollack A, Zagars GK, Kavadi VS. Prostate specific antigen doubling time and disease relapse after radiotherapy for prostate cancer. *Cancer* 1994;74:670–678.
15. Connolly JA, Shinohara K, Presti JC Jr., et al. Local recurrence after radical prostatectomy: characteristics in size, location, and relationship to prostate-specific antigen and surgical margins. *Urology* 1996;47:225–231.
16. Shekarriz B, Upadhyay J, Wood DP Jr., et al. Vesicourethral anastomosis biopsy after radical prostatectomy: predictive value of prostate-specific antigen and pathologic stage. *Urology* 1999;54:1044–1048.
17. Epstein JI. Incidence and significance of positive margins in radical prostatectomy specimens. *Urol Clin North Am* 1996;23:651–663.
18. Epstein JI, Partin AW, Sauvageot J, et al. Prediction of progression following radical prostatectomy. A multivariate analysis of 721 men with long-term follow-up. *Am J Surg Pathol* 1996;20:286–292.
19. Pound CR, Partin AW, Epstein JI, et al. Prostate-specific antigen after anatomic radical retropubic prostatectomy. *Urol Clin North Am* 1997;24:395–406.
20. Kupelian PA, Katcher J, Levin HS, et al. Stage T1-2 prostate cancer: a multivariate analysis of factors affecting biochemical and clinical failures after radical prostatectomy. *Int J Radiat Oncol Biol Phys* 1997;37:1043–1052.
21. Messing EM, Manola J, Sarosdy M, et al. Immediate hormonal therapy compared with observation after radical prostatectomy and pelvic lymphadenectomy in men with node-positive prostate cancer. *N Engl J Med* 1999;341:1781–1788.
22. Ghavamian R, Bergstralh EJ, Blute ML, et al. Radical retropubic prostatectomy plus orchiectomy versus orchiectomy alone for pTxN+ prostate cancer: a matched comparison. *J Urol* 1999;161:1223–1227.
23. Zagars GK, Pollack A, von Eschenbach AC. Unfavorable local-regional prostate cancer management with radiation and androgen ablation. *Cancer* 1997;80:764–775.
24. Wiegel T, Bressel M, Carl UM. Adjuvant radiotherapy following radical prostatectomy—results of 56 patients. *Eur J Cancer* 1995;31A:5–11.
25. Blute ML, Bergstralh EJ, Partin AW, et al. Validation of Partin tables for predicting pathological stage of clinically localized prostate cancer. *J Urol* 2000;164:1591–1595.
26. Cheng L, Slezak J, Bergstralh EJ, et al. Preoperative prediction of surgical margin status in patients with prostate cancer treated by radical prostatectomy. *J Clin Oncol* 2000;18: 2862–2868.
27. Jhaveri FM, Klein EA, Kupelian PA, et al. Declining rates of extracapsular extension after radical prostatectomy: evidence for continued stage migration. *J Clin Oncol* 1999;17: 3167–3172.
28. Gilliland FD, Hoffman RM, Hamilton A, et al. Predicting extracapsular extension of prostate cancer in men treated with radical prostatectomy: results from the population based prostate cancer outcomes study. *J Urol* 1999;162:1341–1345.
29. Ramos CG, Carvalhal GF, Smith DS, et al. Clinical and pathological characteristics and recurrence rates of stage T1C versus T2A or T2B prostate cancer. *J Urol* 1999;161: 1525–1529.
30. Bauer JJ, Connelly RR, Seterheinn IA, et al. Biostatistical modeling using traditional preoperative and pathological prognostic variables in the selection of men at high risk for disease recurrence after radical prostatectomy for prostate cancer. *J Urol* 1998;159:929–933.

31. Dillioglugil O, Leibman BD, Kattan MW, et al. Hazard rates for progression after radical prostatectomy for clinically localized prostate cancer. *Urology* 1997;50:93–99.
32. Lowe BA, Lieberman SF. Disease recurrence and progression in untreated pathologic stage T3 prostate cancer: selecting the patient for adjuvant therapy. *J Urol* 1997;158:1452–1456.
33. Kupelian P, Katcher J, Levin H, et al. Correlation of clinical and pathologic factors with rising prostate-specific antigen profiles after radical prostatectomy alone for clinically localized prostate cancer. *Urology* 1996;48:249–260.
34. Ohori M, Wheeler TM, Kattan MW, et al. Prognostic significance of positive surgical margins in radical prostatectomy specimens. *J Urol* 1995;154:1818–1824.
35. American Joint Committee on Cancer. *Manual for staging of cancer*, 4th ed. Philadelphia: JB Lippincott Co, 1992:181–186.
36. Amling CL, Blute ML, Lerner SE, et al. Influence of prostate-specific antigen testing on the spectrum of patients with prostate cancer undergoing radical prostatectomy at a large referral practice. *Mayo Clin Proc* 1998;73:401–406.
37. Stamey TA, Donaldson AN, Yemoto CE, et al. Histological and clinical findings in 896 consecutive prostates treated only with radical retropubic prostatectomy: epidemiologic significance of annual changes. *J Urol* 1998;160:2412–2417.
38. Han M, Walsh PC, Partin AW, et al. Ability of the 1992 and 1997 American Joint Committee on Cancer staging systems for prostate cancer to predict progression-free survival after radical prostatectomy for stage T2 disease. *J Urol* 2000;164:89–92.
39. Stamey TA, Sozen TS, Yemoto CM, et al. Classification of localized untreated prostate cancer based on 791 men treated only with radical prostatectomy: common ground for therapeutic trials and TNM subgroups. *J Urol* 1998;159:2009–2012.
40. Grossfeld GD, Tigrani VS, Nudell D, et al. Management of a positive surgical margin after radical prostatectomy: decision analysis. *J Urol* 2000;164:93–100.
41. Zietman AL, Edelstein RA, Coen JJ, et al. Radical prostatectomy for adenocarcinoma of the prostate: the influence of preoperative and pathologic findings on biochemical disease-free outcome. *Urology* 1994;43:828–833.
42. Paulson DF. Impact of radical prostatectomy in the management of clinically localized disease. *J Urol* 1994;152:1826–1830.
43. ICRU Report 50. Prescribing, recording, and reporting photon beam therapy. Bethesda, MD: International Commission on Radiation Units and Measures. *ICRU Reports* 1993;9:1–72.
44. Zelefsky MJ, Aschkenasy E, Kelsen S, et al. Tolerance and early outcome results of postprostatectomy three-dimensional conformal radiotherapy. *Int J Radiat Oncol Biol Phys* 1997;39:327–333.
45. Valicenti RK, Gomella LG, Ismail M, et al. The efficacy of early adjuvant radiation therapy for pT3N0 prostate cancer: a matched-pair analysis. *Int J Radiat Oncol Biol Phys* 1999;45:53–58.
46. Leibovich BC, Engen DE, Patterson DE, et al. Benefit of adjuvant radiation therapy for localized prostate cancer with a positive surgical margin. *J Urol* 2000;163:1178–1182.
47. Petrovich Z, Lieskovsky G, Langholz B, et al. Comparison of outcomes of radical prostatectomy with and without adjuvant pelvic irradiation in patients with pathologic stage C (T3N0) adenocarcinoma of the prostate. *Am J Clin Oncol* 1999;22:323–331.
48. Valicenti RK, Gomella LG, Ismail M, et al. Pathologic seminal vesicle invasion after radical prostatectomy for patients with prostate carcinoma. *Cancer* 1998;82:1909–1914.
49. Morris MM, Dallow KC, Zietman AL, et al. Adjuvant and salvage irradiation following radical prostatectomy for prostate cancer. *Int J Radiat Oncol Biol Phys* 1997;38:731–736.
50. Coetzee LJ, Hars V, Paulson DF. Postoperative prostate-specific antigen as a prognostic indicator in patients with margin-positive prostate cancer, undergoing adjuvant radiotherapy after radical prostatectomy. *Urology* 1996;47:232–235.
51. Schild SE, Wong WW, Grado GL, et al. The results of radical retropubic prostatectomy and adjuvant therapy for pathologic stage C prostate cancer. *Int J Radiat Oncol Biol Phys* 1996;34:535–541.
52. Zietman AL, Coen JJ, Shipley WU, et al. Adjuvant irradiation after radical prostatectomy for adenocarcinoma of prostate: analysis of freedom from PSA failure. *Urology* 1993;42:292–298.
53. Valicenti RK, Gomella LG, Ismail M, et al. Effect of higher radiation dose on biochemical control after radical prostatectomy for PT3N0 prostate cancer. *Int J Radiat Oncol Biol Phys* 1998;42:501–506.
54. Gibbons RP, Cole BS, Richardson RG, et al. Adjuvant radiotherapy following radical prostatectomy: results and complications. *J Urol* 1986;135:65–68.
55. Meier R, Mark R, St Royal L, et al. Postoperative radiation therapy after radical prostatectomy for prostate carcinoma. *Cancer* 1992;70:1960–1966.
56. Cheng WS, Frydenberg M, Bergstralh EJ, et al. Radical prostatectomy for pathologic stage C prostate cancer: influence of pathologic variables and adjuvant treatment on disease outcome. *Urology* 1993;42:283–291.
57. Anscher MS, Robertson CN, Prosnita LR. Adjuvant radiotherapy for pathologic stage T3/4 adenocarcinoma of the prostate: ten-year update. *Int J Radiat Oncol Biol Phys* 1995;33:37–43.
58. Syndikus I, Pickles T, Kostashuk E, et al. Postoperative radiotherapy for stage pT3 carcinoma of the prostate: improved local control. *J Urol* 1996;155:1983–1986.
59. Tefilli MV, Gheiler EL, Tiguert R, et al. Prognostic indicators in patients with seminal vesicle involvement following radical prostatectomy for clinically localized prostate cancer. *J Urol* 1998;160:802–806.
60. Anscher MS, Prosnitz LR. Multivariate analysis of factors predicting local relapse after radical prostatectomy—possible indications for postoperative radiotherapy. *Int J Radiat Oncol Biol Phys* 1991;21:941–947.
61. Schild SE. Radiation therapy after prostatectomy: Now or later? *Semin Radiat Oncol* 1998;8:132–139.
62. Schild SE, Buskirk SJ, Wong WW, et al. The use of radiotherapy for patients with isolated elevation of serum prostate specific antigen following radical prostatectomy. *J Urol* 1996;156:1725–1729.
63. Wu JJ, King SC, Montana GS, et al. The efficacy of post-prostatectomy radiotherapy in patients with an isolated elevation of serum prostate-specific antigen. *Int J Radiat Oncol Biol Phys* 1995;32:317–323.
64. McCarthy JF, Catalona WJ, Hudson MA. Effect of radiation therapy on detectable serum prostate specific antigen levels following radical prostatectomy: early versus delayed treatment. *J Urol* 1994;151:1575–1578.

65. Garg MK, Tekyi-Mensah S, Bolton S, et al. Impact of postprostatectomy prostate-specific antigen nadir on outcomes following salvage radiotherapy. *Urology* 1998;51: 998–1002.
66. Forman JD, Meetze K, Pontes E, et al. Therapeutic irradiation for patients with an elevated post-prostatectomy prostate specific antigen level. *J Urol* 1997;158:1436–1439.
67. Forman JD, Velasco J. Therapeutic radiation in patients with a rising post-prostatectomy PSA level. *Oncology (Huntingt)* 1998;12:33–39.
68. Eulau SM, Tate DJ, Stamey TA, et al. Effect of combined transient androgen deprivation and irradiation following radical prostatectomy for prostatic cancer. *Int J Radiat Oncol Biol Phys* 1998;41:735–740.

34

ADJUVANT HORMONAL THERAPY FOR PROSTATE CANCER

BRIAN I. RINI
NICHOLAS J. VOGELZANG

Since the landmark observations of Huggins and Hodges in 1941 regarding the efficacy of androgen suppression in prostate carcinoma, hormone therapy has been a mainstay of treatment (1). There has been, however, considerable debate and investigation concerning the optimal timing of such therapy. One particular area of interest is the use of hormonal ablation as adjuvant treatment after radiation or prostatectomy. With continued stage migration seen as a result of the introduction of routine screening prostate-specific antigen (PSA) measurements, there will be a greater number of patients with organ-confined and otherwise nonmetastatic disease. As such, thorough knowledge of the risks and benefits of immediate hormonal ablation versus such therapy at progression is of critical importance and will affect the care of great numbers of men with prostate cancer. This chapter defines *adjuvant treatment* as that given after primary treatment for a neoplasm to treat any possible residual tumor. As will be seen later, in the description of the studies, many studies use hormonal ablation outside that strict definition. First, we examine androgen ablation therapy as studied in a prostate cancer cell line. Second, we have investigated all major relevant studies, including those studying concomitant or neoadjuvant hormone treatment, or both, because of the lack of data from trials that used hormonal ablation in a truly adjuvant setting. Third, we provide a historical perspective on adjuvant hormone therapy in various stages and high-risk subgroups via careful examination of the major trials of hormonal ablation that have thus far shaped our thinking about adjuvant therapy. Last, we mention future trials that will hopefully answer the many questions that still remain. The data thus far provide some general guidelines for current treatment and, more important, guide future randomized trial designs to better define the role of adjuvant therapy in prostate carcinoma.

PRECLINICAL STUDIES

Clinically meaningful therapy is often first studied in a preclinical model to allow for examination of effectiveness and issues such as timing, dose, duration, and other variables. The most applicable model of androgen ablation therapy in the adjuvant setting was reported in the Dunning R-3327 rat prostatic adenocarcinoma model by Isaacs in the early 1980s (1a). The effect of timing of androgen ablation was studied with respect to the response of the tumor and subsequent survival of the host. Fifty intact and ten castrated male rats were inoculated subcutaneously with 1.5×10^6 viable tumor cells on day 0. At 100, 150, 200, and 250 days, respectively, ten of the intact tumor-bearing rats were castrated. All rats were allowed to live out their lives, and tumor growth and survival data were collected. It required between 140 and 160 days before tumors became palpable in rats castrated at day 0 versus 40 and 50 days observed in intact hosts. This delay in tumor growth translated into a substantial increase in overall host survival, as day 0 castrated rats lived an average of 470 ± 25 days versus 350 ± 15 days for intact hosts. As the time to castration was increased, tumor regrowth rate was greater and survival shorter for each subgroup. These results support the contention that the timing of androgen ablation has a direct effect on the therapeutic benefit of such therapy as measured by tumor growth and host survival. It must be noted, however, that all animals eventually relapsed into an androgen-unresponsive state, indicating, according to the authors, the need for upfront therapy directed at androgen-independent cells.

EARLY ADJUVANT TRIALS

As described later, many trials allowed for hormonal treatment at progression in patients not originally given hormones. Thus, many randomized trials of adjuvant hormones actually compared early versus delayed hormonal treatment. It is thus important to understand the most important trial of immediate versus delayed treatment for advanced prostate cancer. The Medical Research Council trial accrued 938 patients from 1985 to 1993 before the widespread use of PSA to diagnose and follow prostate cancer patients forced the study's premature closure (2). This study randomized hormone-naïve patients with locally advanced (defined as T2-4) or metastatic prostate cancer to immediate hormone treatment [orchiectomy or luteinizing hormone releasing hormone (LHRH) analog] or to the same treatment at progression. This trial was not a purely adjuvant trial, as 30% to 40% of patients had metastatic disease at the onset. Nonetheless, the results have applications for the use of adjuvant hormones. Significant differences in favor of immediate hormonal treatment were seen with respect to disease-free survival, overall survival, and development of major complications, including pathologic fractures, spinal cord compression, ureteric outlet obstruction, and development of metastases (Tables 34-1 and 34-2). Thus, the principle of early hormonal ablation for advanced prostate cancer was supported by these data. Interestingly, the benefit in terms of prostate cancer death was largely seen in M0 patients. Such a retrospective subgroup analysis does not prove the principle of early adjuvant hormone therapy, as most patients did not undergo therapeutic radiation or surgery for localized disease before hormonal treatment. It does, however, provide a hypothesis that those patients with locally advanced, nonmetastatic prostate cancer (and thus a smaller burden of disease) may achieve the most benefit with early therapy. Extending this hypothesis, such therapy given with minimal residual disease in the truly adjuvant setting may exploit the benefits of hormonal ablation.

TABLE 34-1. MAJOR COMPLICATION RATE OF IMMEDIATE AND DELAYED HORMONAL TREATMENT IN THE MEDICAL RESEARCH COUNCIL TRIAL

	Immediate (n = 469)	Delayed (n = 465)
Pathologic fracture		
M0	3	6
Mx	1	4
M1	7	11
Total	11	21
Cord compression		
M0	3	3
Mx	1	6
M1[a]	5	14
Total[b]	9	23
Ureteric obstruction[c]		
M0	22	28
Mx[d]	1	12
M1	10	15
Total[b]	33	55
Extraskeletal metastases		
M0	17	26
Mx	7	9
M1	13	20
Total[a]	37	55

[a]2*p* <.05: otherwise not statistically significant.
[b]2*p* <.025: otherwise not statistically significant.
[c]Excludes seven patients receiving local radiotherapy to the prostate.
[d]2*p* <.005: otherwise not statistically significant.
Adapted from Adib RS, Anderson JB, Ashken MH, et al. Immediate versus deferred treatment for advanced prostatic cancer: initial results of the Medical Research Council trial. *Br J Urol* 1997;79:235–246.

TABLE 34-2. CAUSES OF DEATH FOR IMMEDIATE AND DELAYED HORMONAL TREATMENT IN THE MEDICAL RESEARCH COUNCIL TRIAL

	Overall (n = 934)	Immediate (n = 469)	Delayed (n = 465)
All deaths			
M0[a]	321	150	171
Mx	144	67	77
M1	224	111	113
Total[a]	689	328	361
Deaths from prostate cancer (% of all deaths)[b]			
M0[c]	200 (62)	81 (54)	119 (70)
Mx	86 (60)	38 (57)	48 (62)
M1	174 (78)	84 (76)	90 (80)
Total[c]	460 (67)	203 (62)	237 (71)

[a]2*p* <.01 for immediate versus deferred treatment otherwise statistically not significant.
[b]Includes 17 deaths from unknown causes.
[c]2*p* <.001 for immediate versus deferred treatment otherwise statistically not significant.
Adapted from Adib RS, Anderson JB, Ashken MH, et al. Immediate versus deferred treatment for advanced prostatic cancer: initial results of the Medical Research Council trial. *Br J Urol* 1997;79:235–246.

The earliest studies looking at the use of adjuvant hormonal therapy in prostate cancer were conducted by the Veterans Administration Cooperative Urological Research Group (VACURG) between 1960 and 1975 (3,4). It is of importance to understand the details of these three important trials because they provided the foundation for future study of adjuvant hormone therapy. Patients were staged in the pre-PSA era as follows: stage 1 included patients with incidentally found microscopic cancer; stage II, palpable cancer by rectal examination not beyond the prostatic capsule; stage III, local extension beyond the capsule; and stage IV, elevated prostatic acid phosphatase (PAP) or demonstrable metastases. No patients had staging laparotomies or bone scans. As well, staging was purely clinical, and no information obtained at open operation was used to restage patients. Thus, it is likely that many patients were understaged. The authors do provide data that indicate that overall and disease-specific death were equal in patients with only elevated PAP compared to those patients with proven metastases, indicating that elevated PAP represents nondetectable metastases. Also, in all the VACURG studies, the treating physician could change treatment because of symptoms or disease progression. Nearly half of all patients who originally received placebo were subsequently "crossed over" to hormonal treatment. Thus, comparisons with the placebo group may more accurately be comparisons of early versus delayed endocrine treatment. Nonetheless, the three VACURG studies described in the following paragraphs gave the first insight into the role of adjuvant hormone therapy for prostate cancer.

TABLE 34-3. DEATHS BY STAGE, TREATMENT, AND CAUSE IN THE FIRST VETERANS ADMINISTRATION COOPERATIVE UROLOGICAL RESEARCH GROUP STUDY

Stage	I		II		III				IV			
Treatment	Px + P	Px + E	Px + P	Px + E	P	E	O + P	O + E	P	E	O + P	O + E
n	60	60	85	94	262	265	266	257	223	211	203	216
Prostate cancer	3	2	8	2	46	18	35	25	105	82	97	82
Cardiovascular	20	25	255	32	88	112	95	108	55	76	56	59
Other causes	7	10	9	12	43	50	54	48	29	23	29	40
Total deaths	30	37	42	46	177	180	184	181	189	181	182	181

E, 5.0 mg diethylstilbestrol daily; O, orchiectomy; P, placebo; Px, radical prostatectomy.
Adapted from Byar DP. The Veterans Administration Cooperative Urological Research Group's studies of cancer of the prostate. *Cancer* 1973;32:1126–1130.

The first VACURG study began in 1960 and randomized 120 stage I patients and 179 stage II patients to receive radical prostatectomy (RP) followed by placebo or 5 mg daily of diethylstilbestrol (DES). Stage I patients who received DES had a significantly worse overall survival compared to placebo-treated patients secondary to increased cardiovascular events. There were no significant differences in disease-specific or overall survival for stage II patients (Table 34-3). Thus, this portion of the study, in which hormones were used in a truly adjuvant setting, failed to demonstrate benefit for this particular hormonal treatment, albeit with a relatively underpowered study.

The first VACURG study also randomized 1,050 stage III and 853 stage IV patients to placebo, 5 mg DES, orchiectomy plus placebo, or orchiectomy plus 5 mg DES. The three endocrine treatment arms had significantly less progression (defined as first increase in PAP, first metastasis, or death from prostate carcinoma) than the placebo group. This delayed progression did not translate into an overall survival benefit, partially because of the increased cardiovascular deaths in the DES groups. Important, however, is that the phenomenon of delayed progression (including decreased prostate cancer death) not translating into a survival benefit would be redemonstrated in later studies. Even comparing placebo alone versus orchiectomy plus placebo (and thus eliminating the DES-induced cardiovascular mortality) fails to translate decreased progression into overall survival benefit, largely because of competing, noncancer deaths in the orchiectomy group. In summary, the first VACURG study demonstrated that early hormonal therapy was effective in slowing the progression of prostate cancer, but its benefits were offset by unacceptable side effects and competing causes of death.

The second VACURG study began in 1967 and randomized 1,506 stage III and IV patients to placebo, 0.2 mg, l mg, or 5 mg of DES daily. The study was stopped in 1969 because of, and excess of, cardiovascular deaths in the 5-mg DES arm. This study demonstrated that l mg and 5 mg of DES significantly delayed progression of stage III patients to stage IV, and patients who took l mg of DES had a significantly greater overall survival than the other groups. The delayed progression seen in the 5-mg DES group did not translate into a survival benefit because of the excess cardiovascular deaths (Table 34-4). Subsequent covariate analysis revealed that immediate estrogen therapy would be most beneficial for younger patients (younger than 75 years) with high-grade tumors (Gleason 7 to 10). This study was important in that it showed that l mg of DES was as effective and less toxic than 5 mg and that early hormonal therapy could delay progression and increase overall survival in a subset of prostate cancer patients. The authors recommend delay in initiation of hormonal therapy with DES because of toxicity.

TABLE 34-4. DEATHS BY STAGE, TREATMENT, AND CAUSE IN THE SECOND VETERANS ADMINISTRATION COOPERATIVE UROLOGICAL RESEARCH GROUP STUDY

Stage	III				IV			
Treatment (mg/d)	Placebo	0.2 DES	1.0 DES	5.0 DES	Placebo	0.2 DES	1.0 DES	5.0 DES
n	75	73	73	73	53	52	55	54
Prostate cancer	11	9	3	3	21	28	17	14
Cardiovascular	15	14	18	31	10	7	10	10
Other causes	11	19	14	7	9	1	4	7
Total deaths	37	42	35	41	40	36	31	31

DES, diethylstilbestrol.
Adapted from Byar DP. The Veterans Administration Cooperative Urological Research Group's studies of cancer of the prostate. *Cancer* 1973;32:1126–1130.

TABLE 34-5. SUMMARY RESULTS FROM THE THIRD VETERANS ADMINISTRATION COOPERATIVE UROLOGICAL RESEARCH GROUP STUDY

	n	No. of deaths: Prostate cancer	Cardiovascular	Other	% 5-yr survival
Stage I					
Placebo	98	1	10	17	61
1-mg DES	107	4	29	12	45
Stage II					
Placebo	45	3	16	3	48
1-mg DES	48	4	7	3	75

DES, diethylstilbestrol.
Adapted from Byar DP, Corle DK. Hormone therapy for prostate cancer: results of the Veterans Administration Cooperative Urological Research Group studies. *NCI Monogr* 1988;7:165–170.

The third VACURG study was from 1969 to 1975 and randomized 205 stage I and 93 stage II patients to l mg of DES or placebo without prior surgery or radiation. Peculiar results were obtained in that DES produced an excess of cardiovascular deaths in stage I but not stage II patients. The authors are unable to account for such results. As well, DES decreased progression and increased 5-year overall survival (Table 34-5). In summary, the VACURG studies provide more information about early versus delayed hormonal therapy than about true adjuvant treatment, but the disease progression benefit seen in some patient subgroups provides an impetus for including early hormonal treatment in subsequent trials, although then and even now many look to this trial as favoring delayed therapy.

LOCALLY ADVANCED DISEASE

Adjuvant Treatment after Surgery

Beyer et al. provided one of the first examinations of the efficacy of adjuvant treatment after RP (5). Two hundred ninety-three pathologically staged T1-4 patients treated from 1977 to 1990 underwent RP. Sixty-four patients had positive lymph nodes. Adjuvant therapy was given at the discretion of the operating surgeon to 29% of patients (89% unspecified endocrine treatment and 11% radiation therapy). The nontreated group had a greater projected 5-year survival and a longer time to progression, but this likely reflected a greater proportion of nonadjuvant patients with lower-stage disease. Subgroup analysis of T3N0 and all N+ patients failed to demonstrate any significant differences in progression or survival. Strong selection bias forcing a retrospective subgroup analysis, variable adjuvant treatment, and short follow-up preclude meaningful conclusions from being drawn.

The Mayo Clinic reported on their experience before 1989 in pathologic stage C (defined as capsular perforation or seminal vesicle invasion) patients who had undergone bilateral pelvic lymphadenectomy and radical retropubic prostatectomy (6). Eight hundred ninety-four such patients were subjected to either no further treatment (660 patients), adjuvant external radiation therapy (XRT) (131 patients), or adjuvant orchiectomy (103 patients) at the discretion of the treating surgeon. Many observation patients were treated with some form of hormonal therapy at progression. The adjuvant group included more patients with increased tumor bulk, higher grade, and seminal vesicle involvement. Multivariate analysis that adjusted for these factors demonstrated a significantly lower local and systemic progression rate for patients who received either form of adjuvant treatment. There was no difference between the XRT and orchiectomy groups, and there was no advantage to adjuvant treatment for disease-specific or overall survival.

Adjuvant Treatment after Radiotherapy

An early study similar to the VACURG studies was conducted by Zagars et al. from 1967 to 1973 (7). Seventy-eight previously untreated patients with clinical stage C prostate carcinoma were randomized to XRT alone (40 patients) or XRT plus estrogen (38 patients). Patients received variable doses of estrogen as the study progressed because of emerging data from other studies. Twenty patients received 5 mg of DES, 12 received 2 mg of DES, 2 received 12 mg of chlorotrianisene, and 4 never received any estrogen for a variety of reasons. Also of note, of the 27 XRT-only patients who relapsed, 26 received some form of hormone treatment. Significant advantages in disease-free survival and freedom from metastasis were seen in favor of the combined treatment group when analyzed by intent to treat and by treatment actually received. This benefit held up with 15 years of follow-up, suggesting that early hormonal treatment, when combined with radiotherapy, may provide durable long-term benefits. No overall survival advantage was demonstrated. Cardiovascular deaths numbered ten in the estrogen group and six in the XRT group and therefore were unlikely to account for the lack of survival benefit with disease control. The authors postulate that a low cancer-related death rate, regardless of disease status, and a greater prolongation of life with hormone treatment in previously untreated patients, could explain the lack of overall survival difference. This early study is important in that it was one of the first to demonstrate the benefits of early hormonal treatment combined with radiotherapy in locally advanced disease.

Another study with significance to this field was conducted in the early 1970s by a Dutch radiotherapy group (8). Patients with clinical stage T3-4NxM0 prostate cancer were analyzed retrospectively by treatment received. Twenty-six patients were treated with orchiectomy followed by 1 mg DES daily, 30 patients were treated with radiotherapy alone, and 30 were treated with a combination of these therapies. Patients in the radiotherapy-only group had a significantly greater overall survival at 4 years than the other groups. Again, there were ten cardiovascular deaths in the groups treated with hormones, likely accounting for the decreased survival. As well, the combined therapy group had a significantly greater percentage of patients with poorly differentiated tumors. It is difficult to draw meaningful conclusions from this small, nonrandomized study, but it was an early attempt to investigate the effect of adjuvant hormonal treatment.

A randomized study examining the addition of orchiectomy to radiation was reported by Fellows et al. (9). Two hundred seventy-seven patients with clinical stage T2-4NxM0 prostate cancer were randomized to receive radiotherapy alone, orchiectomy alone, or a combination of the two. The groups were comparable with respect to age, performance status, Gleason score, and T stage. The incidence of distant metastases was significantly higher in the radiotherapy alone group compared to the groups that included orchiectomy, but no difference in overall survival was seen. As these patients were clinically staged only, it is likely that many had nodal involvement. The benefit to orchiectomy may thus be from undetected nodal or metastatic disease, or both, at the beginning of therapy. The small sample sizes make it difficult to evaluate the true value of adjuvant hormonal therapy from these data.

The M. D. Anderson Cancer Center retrospectively examined pathologic T1-4N0M0 prostate cancer patients treated with XRT alone from 1987 to 1991 (81 patients) or XRT plus hormonal treatment between 1990 to 1992 (38 patients) (10). Patients were considered high risk on the basis of pretreatment PSA greater than 30 ng per mL or tumor grade 3 or 4. The hormone group was very heterogeneous in regards to treatment, as 14 underwent orchiectomy and 24 received monthly leuprolide. As well, 15 received androgen ablation before XRT (mean time of 2.7 months) and 11 were given flutamide initially. Mean duration of hormone treatment after completion of XRT was 1.7 months. Thirty-six of the 51 patients in the XRT group were treated with androgen ablation at relapse. Although the hormone group had more patients with adverse prognostic features including age, grade, and Gleason score, there was a significant advantage in terms of freedom from PSA relapse, local control, and freedom from any relapse for the hormone group. Again, no differences with regard to distant metastasis or overall survival were seen.

These early studies investigating hormone therapy after radiotherapy prompted larger randomized trials that attempted to more precisely define the best use of adjuvant hormonal treatment. Many of the studies described later use hormones neoadjuvantly or concomitantly, or both, as well as adjuvantly, and, therefore, distinguishing the beneficial effects of true adjuvant therapy is impossible. Nonetheless, these are the most recent, largest trials, and they provide insight into the use of adjuvant therapy. Laverdiere et al. randomized clinical stage B and C patients to XRT alone, XRT plus 3 months of neoadjuvant combination therapy (LHRH agonist plus flutamide), or combination therapy 3 months before, during, and 6 months after XRT (11). The three well-matched groups of approximately 40 patients each were analyzed by prostate biopsies and corresponding serum PSA measurement at 12 and 24 months after XRT. Interim analysis revealed that patients treated with one of the hormonal therapy schemes had a significantly lower percentage of positive biopsies and lower median PSA values at both time points. As well, only one patient in the last group had residual neoplasm at 24 months, suggesting that prolonged therapy before, during, and after XRT may have a benefit over neoadjuvant therapy alone. The authors suggest that decreased tumor volume with androgen blockade allowed for greater local control with the same radiation dose. Long-term follow-up is needed to determine whether this hormone therapy had a suppressive or a curative effect. This trial suffers from a high relapse rate in the XRT only group as well as small numbers of patients but, like most of the trials described, adds information in judging the value of adjuvant therapy.

Another recent retrospective review was reported by Anderson et al. in 1997 (12). Fifty-six patients were treated between 1988 and 1993 with XRT plus hormones and compared to 56 patients matched for stage, grade, and pretreatment PSA levels who were treated with radiotherapy alone. All patients were clinical stage T1-3NxM0 with a median follow-up of 41 months. Hormonal treatment included an LHRH analog with or without flutamide for a median of 3 months given before or during XRT, or both, as well as after therapy. A patient was considered to be biochemically without evidence of disease [biochemical no evidence of disease (bNED)] if there was no clinical or radiographic evidence of disease, and serum PSA was less than 1.5 ng per mL and not rising on two consecutive occasions. Five-year bNED control was significantly greater in the hormone group (55%) versus the radiotherapy alone group (31%), with a 20-month delay in disease progression favoring the hormone group as well. This significant advantage in terms of bNED control was most notable in the T2C/T3, Gleason score 7 to 10, and pretreatment PSA greater than 15 ng per mL patient subgroups who received hormonal therapy. Despite these benefits, no overall survival advantage could be demonstrated. This trial adds strength to the notion that hormonal ablation around the time of radiotherapy is beneficial for disease control. It also introduces the variables of type and duration of hormonal ablation.

The most notable trial that examined adjuvant therapy after radiation for localized prostate cancer was reported by Bolla et al. for the European Organization for the Research and Treatment of Cancer (EORTC) (13). Between 1987 and 1995, 401 patients with clinically localized disease (T1-2, grade 3 or T3-4, any grade, N0M0) were randomized to radiotherapy alone or radiotherapy plus 3.6 mg of goserelin every 4 weeks beginning on the first day of radiation. Hormone therapy was continued in the vast majority of patients for 3 years or until progression or death. A steroid antiandrogen cyproterone acetate was given for 1 month starting 1 week before the first dose of goserelin. The groups were well matched with regard to age, performance status, clinical stage, grade, and pretreatment PSA levels (median on study PSA of 30 ng per mL). Five-year overall survival in the combined treatment group was 79% versus 62% in the radiotherapy group (p = .001) (Fig. 34-1). Significant advantages to adjuvant hormone therapy were also seen with respect to disease-free survival and local control (Fig. 34-2). It is worth noting, however, that the confidence intervals for the survival data did barely overlap, and survival in the radiotherapy group is low when compared to similar patients from other series. The poor outcome of the radiotherapy group was possibly because of the high median on study PSA. Hormone treatment was not without side effects, as 34% of hormone patients had more than three hot flashes per day, and the group had an unexplained significant increase in late grade 1 to 3 incontinence. This trial supports better disease control with adjuvant hormone therapy, and it is the first to show an overall survival advantage. It is unclear whether the extended duration of hormonal ablation or other factors account for this trial translating disease-free survival into an overall survival benefit or whether this trial will stand out as an aberrance as more data accumulate.

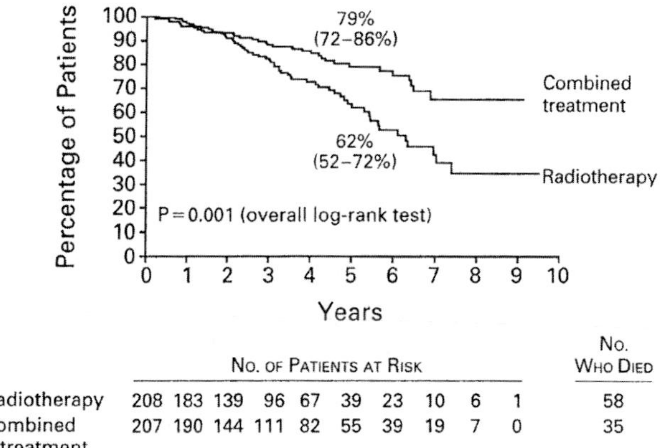

	No. of Patients at Risk										No. Who Died
Radiotherapy	208	183	139	96	67	39	23	10	6	1	58
Combined treatment	207	190	144	111	82	55	39	19	7	0	35

FIGURE 34-1. Kaplan-Meier estimate of overall survival. The overall survival rate at 5 years was 79% (95% confidence interval, 72% to 86%) for the combined treatment group and 62% (95% confidence interval, 52% to 72%) for the group treated only with radiotherapy. (From Bolla M, Gonzalez D, Warde P, et al. Improved survival in patients with locally advanced prostate cancer treated with radiotherapy and goserelin. *N Engl J Med* 1997;337:295–300, with permission.)

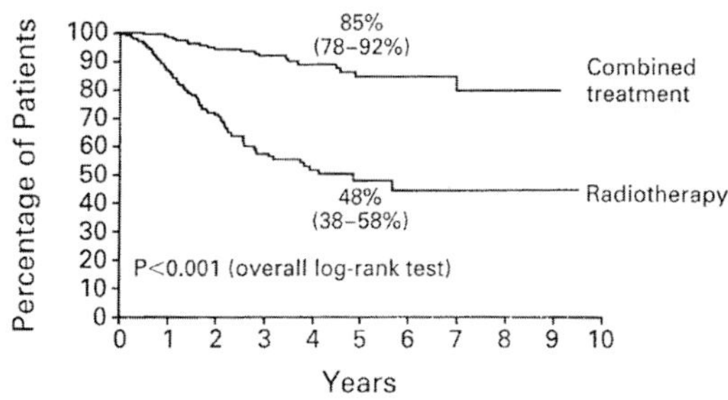

	No. of Patients at Risk										No. with Disease Progression
Radiotherapy	208	163	107	59	38	19	11	5	3	1	78
Combined treatment	207	189	138	108	78	51	36	16	5	0	20

FIGURE 34-2. Kaplan-Meier estimate of disease-free interval. This curve shows the proportion of surviving patients who were free of disease at each time point. The method takes the censoring process into account. The number of patients who are at risk for the event at each time point is the total number of patients minus the number in whom disease progressed or who were lost to follow-up. (From Bolla M, Gonzalez D, Warde P, et al. Improved survival in patients with locally advanced prostate cancer treated with radiotherapy and goserelin. *N Engl J Med* 1997;337:295–300, with permission.)

The largest trial that examined the role of adjuvant hormone therapy in locally advanced prostate cancer was conducted by the Radiation Therapy Oncology Group (85-31), reported by Pilepich et al. in 1997 (14) and updated by Lawton et al. at the 1999 American Society of Clinical Oncology meeting (15). Nine hundred seventy-seven patients with T3NxM0 or T1-2N+M0 prostate cancer were randomized to receive radiotherapy and either goserelin, 3.6 mg monthly to be started during the last week of XRT and continued indefinitely or until progression, or the same hormone therapy at relapse. Patients were well matched with respect to Gleason score, and just fewer than 30% of patients had involved lymph nodes. Significant advantages in favor of immediate adjuvant hormone therapy were seen for local and distant failure as well as clinical and bNED survival at 8 years of follow-up. This advantage was most prominent in Gleason scores 8 to 10 tumors. Overall survival had not significantly diverged at 5 years (75% vs. 72%) or 8 years (49% vs. 42%), although the numbers slightly favor the adjuvant group. This group of patients is similar to the group of patients reported by Bolla et al. with a greater percentage of node-positive patients, and adjuvant treatment was similar. The overall survival at 5 years for both treatment groups is similar to Bolla's adjuvant group, and thus the poor survival in the nonadjuvant group in the Bolla et al. study may account for the survival significance seen.

The previous studies looked mainly at locally advanced prostate cancer to determine the benefit of adjuvant hormone ablation after radiotherapy or RP. The early studies were promising in that estrogen was effective in treating prostate cancer, but unacceptable side effects made this treatment untenable. As newer forms of hormonal ablation developed, several, but not all, trials showed that adjuvant hormonal therapy was effective for disease control, especially in conjunction with radiotherapy. The timing and optimal type of treatment were developed through these most recent studies, with disease-specific and possibly overall survival benefits demonstrated.

NODE-POSITIVE PROSTATE CANCER

As patients are staged and treated with more aggressive surgical approaches, lymph node–positive patients can be rendered free of gross evidence of disease. Kramer et al. reported in 1981 on 44 patients with pathologically staged D1 prostate cancer treated with surgery, radiation, or delayed hormonal therapy (16). No advantage to an aggressive local therapy was seen, and medial survival was only 39.5 months. Although this study did not examine adjuvant therapy specifically, it underscores the systemic nature of node-positive prostate cancer and the inadequacy of local treatment alone for long-term disease control. Thus, stage D1 patients may be ideal candidates for adjuvant hormone therapy to eliminate micrometastatic disease. Below is a chronologic account of the major trials that have examined this issue.

Ninety-four patients with clinically localized prostate cancer underwent pelvic lymphadenectomy from 1977 to 1983, as described by van Aubel et al. (17). Gross or microscopic lymph node involvement, or both, was found in 30 patients who then underwent orchiectomy. Node-negative patients underwent RP alone. The authors reported a greater than 45-month median time to progression and a greater than 60-month median survival, both of which compare favorably to the historical delayed therapy controls presented in the study. The authors also maintain that the orchiectomy group had greater local control, leading to an improvement in symptoms and a better quality of life. Although these retrospective data are appealing, no prospective data were presented to support this contention. This small, nonrandomized study was a first look into adjuvant therapy for Dl prostate cancer.

A retrospective analysis of 68 pathologically staged N+M0 patients treated from 1966 to 1981 was reported by Kramolowsky (18). Thirty patients who received immediate therapy (either orchiectomy or exogenous hormone therapy) after treatment of the primary lesion were compared to the patients who received hormonal ablation at progression or not at all. This patient group is unusual in that some patients received cryosurgical ablation (14 in the immediate group and 12 in the delayed group), and two patients in the immediate group received no treatment for the primary lesion. Groups were well matched with respect to age, grade of lesion, and number of nodes involved. The subgroup of clinical stage B patients in the immediate treatment group had a significantly longer interval from diagnosis to progression, defined as change in bone scan or two consecutive elevated acid phosphatase levels, versus the delayed group (100 months vs. 43 months). No significant difference with respect to time from diagnosis to death was demonstrated. Subgroup analysis of patients younger than 65 years (20 patients in each group) demonstrated significant advantage in time to progression and median survival for the immediate treatment group. Again, a significant non–prostate cancer death rate may have contributed to the lack of benefit in overall survival.

DeKernion et al. also retrospectively analyzed 56 patients who underwent RP with pelvic lymph node dissection and pathologic lymph node involvement (19). Patients were given either immediate hormonal ablation (21 patients) or such therapy at progression (35 patients) at the discretion of the treating physician. Patients in the early therapy group had more advanced disease, as measured by the number and percentage of positive nodes and incidence of seminal vesicle invasion. Groups were otherwise matched for age, Gleason score, and volume of primary tumor. Biochemical disease-free survival was significantly better in the early therapy group without an overall survival advantage. Comparing both groups while correcting for Gleason score and percentage of positive nodes showed a 3.1-fold greater risk of progression or death for the non-early treatment group. All patients generally had low-volume nodal disease, as reflected in the excellent overall survival of the entire group (78% at 98 months). Therefore, aggressive surgical and hormonal management may be expected to benefit such patients most. The authors contend that such an approach may even have palliative value, although no hard data were presented to support this contention.

A large retrospective study that provided interesting data was reported by Zinke et al. from the Mayo Clinic in 1992 (20). Data were presented on 370 patients who underwent RP and bilateral pelvic lymphadenectomy from 1966 to 1988. Adjuvant hormonal therapy was given to 293 patients and was a significant favorable risk factor in multivariate analysis for local, systemic, and overall progression, including PSA as an end point. It was also significant for reducing the risk of prostate cancer death, but only in patients with DNA diploid tumors. The adjuvant treatment was variable and included mainly orchiectomy, although 53 patients received radiotherapy as well, and 58 received neoadjuvant hormonal ablation with an LHRH agonist. There was also a crude survival benefit seen with adjuvant hormone therapy for patients with diploid DNA as contrasted to aneuploid DNA in the tumor tissue. An accelerated death rate is noted after progression for patients with nondiploid tumors given early hormonal treatment, likely accounting for the survival differences seen. The authors postulate that increased tumor growth with time leads to more nondiploid cells, thus accounting for decreased responsiveness to delayed systemic hormonal therapy. The authors also speculate that improved local control with early hormone therapy translates into improved quality of life. This study is important in that it identifies a subclass of prostate tumors that may potentially achieve an overall survival benefit with adjuvant hormonal ablation. As well, it raises the important issue of quality of life, although more firm data must be collected to prove this benefit. In fact, a retrospective review of 139 patients reported in 1995 compared pelvic lymphadenectomy and androgen ablation with or without RP. Much greater local control was reported for the group that also received RP (21). Of patients who also received RP, 8% had local progression versus 69% in those patients without RP, although RP patients had a lower volume of nodal disease. This study, as in others that mention quality of life, uses local progression and the need for subsequent procedures as the main determinant of quality of life. Indeed, there are likely other factors that can be measured to give a more complete picture. These results also suggest that aggressive local therapy, surgery, or radiotherapy may be the major factor in local control, especially in patients with a lower volume of nodal disease, which in turn permits hormonal therapy to act on a lower tumor volume.

More recently, Messing et al. reported on immediate hormonal therapy versus observation for node-positive prostate cancer after RP and pelvic lymphadenectomy (22). This phase III Eastern Cooperative Oncology Group study randomized 98 men between 1988 and 1992 with clinical TI or T2 lesions and negative bone scans to bilateral orchiectomy or goserelin (patient's choice) or observation after surgery. Hormonal therapy was administered to observation patients on progression. Eighty percent of men had a PSA less than 0.4 ng per mL at randomization. At a mean follow-up of 7.2 years, biochemical or clinical progression (19.2% vs. 55.8%) and overall survival (85.0% vs. 64.7%) significantly favored the early hormonal therapy group. The results from this small trial are interesting in that they provide some evidence that early hormonal therapy after aggressive surgery for early-stage prostate cancer may confer an overall survival advantage.

It is readily apparent that no absolute conclusions can be drawn about the benefit of adjuvant therapy for locally advanced or node-positive prostate cancer. The studies described earlier were conducted over many years, during which advances in radiotherapy, surgical technique, and screening made prostate cancer a moving target. The larger studies, especially those conducted by Bolla and the Mayo Clinic, however, provide a foundation on which to base future randomized trials. The final section of this chapter looks at the rationale and design of the larger current and upcoming trials that will attempt to more clearly define the true role of adjuvant hormonal therapy in prostate cancer.

FUTURE TRIALS

The EORTC randomized phase III trial No. 30943 is investigating immediate versus deferred hormonal therapy in patients with persistently elevated or rising PSA after definitive therapy. Approximately 1,666 patients with T1-3 N0-xM0 asymptomatic prostate carcinoma will be enrolled over 4 years. Patients will be randomized to one of two arms. Arm 1 will be immediate treatment with one of four treatment regimes: orchiectomy alone, orchiectomy plus continuous antiandrogen, depot LHRH analog plus short-term antiandrogen, or depot LHRH analog plus continuous antiandrogen. Arm 2 is watchful waiting with hormonal treatment as in arm 1 initiated with documented symptomatic disease progression. End points include disease-free and overall survival, quality of life, and cost effectiveness. Such a study will tell us whether hormonal ablation initiated at first sign of biochemical relapse or begun with persistent biochemical disease after radical therapy is beneficial. It may also allow determination of the risk and benefit profiles of the various hormonal treatment regimens used.

The EORTC is trying to further confirm and extend the Bolla et al. data via a randomized, phase III trial of long-term hormonal treatment with LHRH analog versus no further treatment in locally advanced prostatic carcinoma treated by irradiation and 6 months of combined androgen blockade. Whether the 3 years of hormonal treatment given in the Bolla et al. study is required for full benefit or whether shorter adjuvant therapy is sufficient will be studied.

The Radiation Therapy Oncology Group trial 94-13 is a phase III trial that will investigate the timing of total androgen ablation in relation to radiotherapy. Patients with clinical stage T2C through T4 with a Gleason score greater than 6 and a PSA of 4 to 100 ng per mL will be randomized to total androgen suppression of goserelin or leuprolide and flutamide given 2 months before XRT until XRT completion or for 4 months beginning at the completion of XRT. Patients will also be randomized to whole-pelvic radiation followed by a prostate boost or XRT to the prostate only. Patients will be monitored for biochemical failure as well as disease-free and overall survival. The study is designed to enroll approximately 1,200 patients and to detect with 80% power an 8% difference in 5-year survival. This study will further define the importance of timing of androgen suppression in relation to radiotherapy, as well as necessary duration of therapy.

Probably the largest ongoing adjuvant trial is the bicalutamide (Casodex) Early Prostate Cancer program.

This international, multiinstitutional study is investigating the role of the oral antiandrogen bicalutamide given to patients with T1b-4, any N, nonmetastatic prostate carcinoma. The North America arm of the study requires patients to have had previous treatment of curative intent. In North America, more than 80% of patients had undergone radical surgery. Patients were randomized 1:1 to either 150 mg per day of bicalutamide or placebo after definitive therapy. Recruitment has been recently completed with 8,115 patients randomized between 1995 and 1998. Patients were allowed neoadjuvant hormonal therapy with a 6-week washout period after 5α-reductase inhibitors and 15-week washout after LHRH analog treatment. Principle end points are overall survival, time to clinical progression (both PSA based and non-PSA based), and safety and tolerability. No preliminary results are yet available. This trial will provide insight into the role of oral antiandrogens for early prostate cancer.

CONCLUSION

Treatment of prostate cancer with surgery or radiation followed by adjuvant hormonal treatment is a conceptually appealing concept. Success with this approach in breast cancer, as well as effective hormonal treatment in prostate cancer, have led to investigation in this area. This chapter has reviewed the major contributions to this field by examining adjuvant hormonal trials. It is clear that adjuvant hormonal treatment can feasibly be given to patients, and some such patients will respond to this treatment. Like many other cancer therapies, however, the risk to benefit ratio of therapy for a given patient is not entirely clear. The Medical Research Council, EORTC, Bolla et al., and Messing et al. data provide evidence that early therapy confers an advantage to disease-free and possibly overall survival. Nonetheless, the lack of high-quality, large-scale randomized studies and the published negative studies give caution to recommending early therapy for all patients. Clearly, ongoing and future studies must define the role of adjuvant therapy in terms of type of therapy, timing and duration of therapy, interaction with concomitant surgery and radiation, and need for other nonhormonal therapy. It is likely that there are subgroups with more aggressive disease (defined by certain patient and/or tumor characteristics) that would benefit most. Importantly, the other half of the equation must be emphasized (namely, the side effects borne by all patients). Quality of life for patients given early therapy must be evaluated in upcoming trials to provide patients and physicians with all the necessary data to make an informed decision about adjuvant hormonal therapy for prostate cancer. Active participation in these ongoing trials by patients and physicians caring for such patients is strongly encouraged.

REFERENCES

1. Huggins C. Endocrine-induced regression of cancers. *Science* 1967;156:1050–1054.

1a. Isaacs JT. The timing of androgen ablation therapy and/or chemotherapy in the treatment of prostatic cancer. *Prostate* 1984;5:1–17.

2. Adib RS, Anderson JB, Ashken MH, et al. Immediate versus deferred treatment for advanced prostatic cancer: initial results of the Medical Research Council trial. *Br J Urol* 1997;79:235–246.
3. Byar DP. The Veterans' Administration Cooperative Urological Research Group's studies of cancer of the prostate. *Cancer* 1973;32:1126–1130.
4. Byar DP, Corle DK. Hormone therapy for prostate cancer: results of the Veterans' Administration Cooperative Urological Research Group studies. *NCI Monogr* 1988;7:165–170.
5. Beyer A, Leitenberger A, Altwein JE. Adjuvant hormone therapy following radical prostatectomy. *Eur Urol* 1993;4: 51–56.
6. Chang WS, Frydenberg M, Bergstralh EJ, et al. Radical prostatectomy for pathologic stage C prostate cancer: influence of pathologic variables and adjuvant treatment on disease outcome. *Urology* 1993;42:283–291.
7. Zagars GK, Johnson DE, von Eschenbach AC, et al. Adjuvant estrogen following radiation therapy for stage C adenocarcinoma of the prostate: long-term results of a prospective randomized study. *Int J Radiat Oncol Biol Phys* 1988;14: 1085–1091.
8. van der Werf-Messing B, Sourek-Zikova V, Blonk DI. Localized advanced carcinoma of the prostate: radiation therapy versus hormonal therapy. *Int J Radiat Oncol Biol Phys* 1976;1:1043–1048.
9. Fellows GJ, Clark PB, Beynon LL, et al. Treatment of advanced localized prostatic cancer by orchiectomy, radiotherapy or combined treatment. *Br J Urol* 1992;70:304–309.
10. Pollack A, Zagars GK, Kopplin S. Radiotherapy and androgen ablation for clinically localized high-risk prostate cancer. *Int J Radiat Oncol Biol Phys* 1995;32:13–20.
11. Laverdiere J, Gomez JL, Cusan L, et al. Beneficial effect of combination hormonal therapy administered prior and following external beam radiation therapy in localized prostate cancer. *Int J Radiat Oncol Biol Phys* 1997;37:247–252.
12. Anderson PR, Hanlon AL, Movsas B, et al. Prostate cancer patient subsets showing improved 'bned' control with adjuvant androgen deprivation. *Int J Radiat Oncol Biol Phys* 1997;39:1025–1030.
13. Bolla M, Gonzalez D, Warde P, et al. Improved survival in patients with locally advanced prostate cancer treated with radiotherapy and goserelin. *N Eng J Med* 1997;337:295–300.
14. Pilepich MV, Byhardt RW, Lawton CA, et al. Phase III trial of androgen suppression using goserelin in unfavorable prognosis carcinoma of the prostate treated with definitive radiotherapy: report of the Radiation Therapy Oncology Group protocol 8531. *J Clin Oncol* 1997;15:1013–1021.
15. Lawton C, Winter K, Murray K, et al. Updated results of the phase III Radiation Therapy Oncology Group (RTOG) trial 85-31 evaluating the potential benefit of androgen deprivation following standard radiation therapy for unfavorable prognosis carcinoma of the prostate. American Society

of Clinical Oncology 35th Annual Meeting, Atlanta, 1999(abst).

16. Kramer SA, Cline WA, Farnham R, et al. Prognosis of patients with stage D1 prostatic adenocarcinoma. *J Urol* 1981; 125:817–819.
17. van Aubel OG, Hoekstra WJ, Schroder FH. Early orchiectomy for patients with stage D1 prostatic carcinoma. *J Urol* 1985;134:292–294.
18. Kramolowsky EV. The value of testosterone deprivation in stage D1 carcinoma of the prostate. *J Urol* 1988;139:1242–1244.
19. DeKernion JB, Neuwirth H, Stein A, et al. Prognosis of patients with stage D1 prostate carcinoma following radical prostatectomy with and without early endocrine therapy. *J Urol* 1990;144:700–703.
20. Zinke H, Bergstralh EJ, Larson-Keller JJ, et al. Stage D1 prostate cancer treated by radical prostatectomy and adjuvant hormonal treatment. *Cancer* 1992;70:311–323.
21. Frohmuller HG, Theiss M, Manseck A, et al. Survival and quality of life of patients with stage D1 (t1-3pN1-2M0) prostate cancer. *Eur Urol* 1995;27:202–206.
22. Messing EM, Manola J, Sarosdy M, et al. Immediate hormonal therapy compared with observation after radical prostatectomy and pelvic lymphadenectomy in men with node-positive prostate cancer. *N Engl J Med* 1999;341:1781–1788.

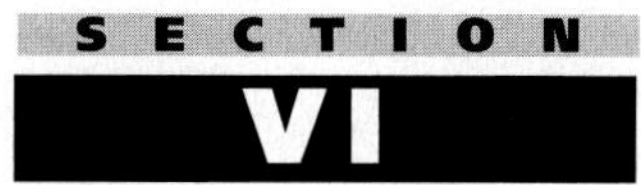

ADVANCED HORMONE-SENSITIVE DISEASE

35

DEFINING TREATMENT FAILURE AFTER LOCAL TREATMENT AND RESTAGING

HAKAN KUYU
M. CRAIG HALL
FRANK M. TORTI

Despite current treatment of radical prostatectomy or radiation therapy for clinically localized prostate cancer, a substantial portion of patients will experience relapse heralded by a detectable or rising serum prostate-specific antigen (PSA), or both (1–4). PSA has proven to be a sensitive means of monitoring the disease status of patients after treatment (5–8). A rise in serum PSA after definitive treatment of prostate cancer provides the earliest evidence of residual or recurrent disease in nearly all patients (9,10). PSA failure often precedes clinical recurrence by several months to years (11,12).

DEFINITION OF PROSTATE-SPECIFIC ANTIGEN PROGRESSION IN RADICAL PROSTATECTOMY PATIENTS

The serum PSA level of patients with organ-confined prostate cancer should fall to undetectable levels after radical prostatectomy. With the half-life of PSA estimated to be 3.2 days, undetectable levels are usually reached by 3 to 4 weeks after surgery (13). The limit of detection of PSA depends on currently available PSA assays. Some investigators define 0.1 ng per mL as the threshold PSA value after radical prostatectomy, above which there is a high risk of persistent disease. Vessella and Lange demonstrated that all patients with postprostatectomy PSA levels exceeding 0.1 ng per mL had subsequent higher elevations of PSA and biochemical failure (14). In another study among men whose PSA level was less than 0.4 ng per mL 3 to 6 months after radical prostatectomy, only 9% developed recurrent disease within 6 to 50 months. However, 100% of men with PSA levels of 0.4 ng per mL or greater after radical prostatectomy had evidence of recurrence within 6 to 49 months (10).

Although investigators have used various PSA cutoffs to determine biochemical recurrence after radical prostatectomy, a rising serum PSA is the ultimate confirmation of relapse (11,15–21).

The use of an ultrasensitive assay may detect recurrent cancer 9 to 12 months earlier than the conventional assays (22,23). Klee et al. showed that with the ultrasensitive IMx PSA assay, only 38% of postradical prostatectomy patients had nondetectable values compared to 60% with the tandem-R PSA assay (24). Although newer second-generation assays can measure PSA levels as low as 0.008 ng per mL (25), the clinical usefulness of these assays remains to be defined. For example, using an ultrasensitive immunoassay, Yu and Diamandis evaluated 1,064 female sera for PSA and determined that 17% of women had detectable levels of PSA, including 1.5% (16 women) with levels of 0.1 ng per mL or greater (26). At Wake Forest University, we generally accept PSA levels exceeding 0.1 ng per mL with subsequent rise as evidence of biochemical relapse.

DEFINITION OF PROSTATE-SPECIFIC ANTIGEN PROGRESSION IN RADIATION-TREATED PATIENTS

PSA levels after radiation therapy decline more slowly when compared to treatment with surgery and many times may not reach undetectable levels, due to PSA secretion from the prostate left *in situ* (27–29). The American Society for Therapeutic Radiology and Oncology Consensus Panel recently published guidelines concerning PSA recurrence after radiation therapy (30):

- Biochemical failure is not justification *per se* to initiate additional treatment. It is not equivalent to clinical failure. It is, however, an appropriate early end point for clinical trials.
- Three consecutive increases in PSA are a reasonable definition of biochemical failure after radiation therapy. For

clinical trials, the date of failure should be the midpoint between the postirradiation nadir PSA and the first of three consecutive rises.

- The use of three rather than two consecutive values reduces the risk of falsely declaring biochemical failure due to "bouncing" PSAs. This phenomenon results when sequential PSA determinations show one or two rises followed by a fall and a subsequent failure to rise again.
- No definition of PSA failure has, as yet, been shown to be a surrogate for clinical progression or survival.
- Nadir PSA is a strong prognostic, but no absolute level is a valid cut point for separating such successful and unsuccessful treatments. Nadir PSA is similar in prognostic value to pretreatment prognostic variables.

The Consensus Panel also provided guidelines for studies presented for publication in prostate cancer. They recommended a minimum observation period of 24 months, PSA determinations to be obtained every 3 or 4 months during the first 2 years after completion of radiation therapy, and every 6 months thereafter. It was suggested that patients with only one or two consecutive rises in PSA be reported separately.

CLINICAL AND RADIOGRAPHIC EVALUATION OF EARLY PROSTATE-SPECIFIC ANTIGEN PROGRESSION AFTER DEFINITIVE TREATMENT

Once biochemical relapse after definitive local therapy is documented, it is useful to attempt to differentiate between local or pelvic recurrences versus distant metastases. In general, PSA relapse occurs earlier, and PSA doubling time is more rapid with distant metastases. In contrast, biochemical failure tends to be delayed, and the doubling time is more prolonged in the setting of local recurrence (31,32). PSA relapse in the first year postoperatively, as well as the presence of seminal vesicle invasion after prostatectomy, is also predictive for distance relapse. Tools available for the evaluation of patients with biochemical relapse are summarized in Table 35-1.

Digital rectal exams (DREs) may reveal evidence of local recurrence or progression in the setting of biochemical failure but are often unreliable because of difficulty in distinguishing recurrent tumors from postoperative changes (33–35). Palpatory abnormalities after radiation therapy may also persist and make interpretation difficult (36–38). In one study, the location of recurrent disease was evaluated in 63 patients who had abnormal levels of PSA (0.4 ng per mL or greater) 6 to 240 months after radical prostatectomy (39). Among 57 patients without evidence of disease by methods including DRE by three urologists, needle biopsies of the anastomosis revealed local disease in 42%. No local disease was discovered in 30 postradical prostatectomy patients with normal PSA levels. There was a wide range of transrectally palpable contours after radical prostatectomy in patients with and without elevated PSA levels.

TABLE 35-1. EVALUATION OF PATIENTS WITH BIOCHEMICAL RELAPSE

Digital rectal examination
Transrectal ultrasound
Technetium-99m bone scintigraphy
Scintigraphic radiolabeled monoclonal antibody imaging (indium-111 capromab pendetide)
Computed tomography scan
Magnetic resonance imaging
Positron emission tomography scan

Transrectal ultrasound is useful in guiding biopsies of the vesicouretral anastomosis after prostatectomy or of the prostate after radiation therapy (7,9). Most investigators, however, do not recommend biopsy unless it would impact treatment options. It is not our practice to biopsy the vesicourethral anastomosis. We biopsy the prostate after radiation therapy only when consideration is being given to either salvage surgery or radiation.

Technetium-99m bone scintigraphy is the method of choice for diagnosis of skeletal metastases (9,40,41). It is indicated in the setting of a rapidly increasing PSA (short doubling time) and bone pain. Although the bone scan is very sensitive for detecting skeletal metastases, it is not specific. Especially in patients with undetectable or low (20 ng per mL or less) PSA levels, a bone scan usually does not provide any additional information (42). In a recent study, 93 patients were evaluated for PSA recurrence with bone scans (43). The lowest PSA value associated with a positive bone scan was 46 ng per mL. The authors did not recommend bone scans to be used unless PSA value was greater than 40 ng per mL. We usually obtain a baseline bone scan for further follow-up if PSA is 20 ng per mL or greater.

Indium-111 capromab pendetide (ProstaScint) is a new U.S. Food and Drug Administration–approved scintigraphic radiolabeled monoclonal antibody imaging study that detects prostate-specific membrane antigen. A recent multicenter study enrolled 183 men who had PSA relapse after radical prostatectomy in whom PSA later increased (44). Immunoscintigraphy revealed disease in 108 of 181 patients (60%). The antibody was localized most frequently to the prostatic fossa (34%), abdominal lymph nodes (23%), and pelvic lymph nodes (22%). The authors concluded that this new scan could assist in determining the location and extent of disease in patients who have increasing PSA after prostatectomy. Babaian et al. studied 19 patients with prostate cancer using ProstaScint and reported a 76% accuracy with sensitivity and specificity of 44% and 86%, respectively (45). The negative predictive value was 83%, and the positive predictive value was 50%. They suggested that the detection threshold of this antibody scan was disease foci 5 mm or greater. In a study of 14 patients, monoclonal antibody imaging was found to have a positive predictive value of 60%, negative predictive value of 75%, and sensitivity of 86% (46). The interpretation of these scans is at times difficult. Where and when this imaging modality should be applied in the work-up and follow-up of prostate cancer remains an area of active investigation.

Computed tomography (CT) is commonly used to evaluate patients with biochemical relapse but has a very low yield in this setting. In a recent German study, the sensitivity of CT to detect recurrence after radical prostatectomy was evaluated (47). In more than 500 patients who had undergone radical prostatectomy for carcinoma of the prostate, CT examinations of the pelvis were retrospectively evaluated. In 22 cases of local recurrence confirmed by biopsy, positive results on CT were found in eight patients (36%) and negative results in nine patients (41%). In the remaining five cases (23%), no distinction could be made between scar and local recurrence. This study suggests that sensitivity of CT scans for evaluation of local recurrence of prostate cancer after surgery is low. Although the literature regarding the role of CT scan for the evaluation of patients with PSA relapse after definite treatment is limited, there are several studies evaluating its usefulness for staging before radical prostatectomy. Levran et al. studied 861 patients with newly diagnosed prostate cancer (48). Only 13 (1.5%) of these men had positive pelvic CT scans. The authors did not recommend the use of pelvic CT for clinical staging in patients with a PSA level of 20 ng per mL or less because of the low yield and the absence of cost effectiveness.

Magnetic resonance imaging (MRI) has been shown to be helpful in the diagnosis of bone metastases, especially when other radiographic examinations are inconclusive or spinal cord compression is suspected (49–53). Fujii et al. evaluated 36 prostate cancer patients with MRI and bone scan (52). Twenty-seven patients were untreated, and nine patients were thought to have hormone-refractory cancer. The MRI was able to detect bone metastases that were not found by bone scan in seven patients. The MRI successfully identified areas of spinal cord compression in five patients with spinal metastases and associated neuropathy.

Positron emission tomography (PET) is currently being studied as a diagnostic method for prostate cancer (54,55). Shreve et al. evaluated the accuracy of the PET scan in 34 patients with biopsy-proven prostate cancer with known or suspected metastatic disease (56). In 202 untreated osseous metastases in 22 patients, the sensitivity of PET was 65% with a positive predictive value of 98%. The conclusion of the authors was that PET scans can help to identify osseous and soft tissue metastases of prostate cancer with a high positive predictive value but are less sensitive than bone scans in the identification of osseous metastases.

RECOMMENDATIONS FOR RESTAGING AT THE TIME OF PROGRESSION DOCUMENTED BY PROSTATE-SPECIFIC ANTIGEN

Based on our assessment of the literature and current practice, we recommend the following restaging work-up:

1. Complete history and physical examination. DRE is often unreliable.
2. Routine laboratory studies, especially assessment of PSA velocity.
3. Judicious use of radiologic methods. A bone scan is often helpful as a baseline for further follow-up if PSA is 20 ng per mL or greater. It is the method of choice for diagnosis of skeletal metastases. MRI may be able to detect bone metastases that are not found by bone scan. MRI is also very useful to evaluate for spinal cord compression. We do not recommend routine use of CT scan for evaluation of biochemical relapse, especially if PSA is less than 20 ng per mL. More studies are needed to determine the role of indium-111 capromab pendetide and PET scan.
4. We do not recommend biopsy of vesicourethral anastomosis, as this does not impact on treatment options after radical prostatectomy. We biopsy the prostate if salvage surgery or radiation is considered.

REFERENCES

1. Stephenson RA. Population based prostate cancer trends in the PSA era: data from the Surveillance, Epidemiology, and End Results (SEER) program. *Monogr Urol* 1998;19:1–19.
2. Moul JW. Rising PSA after local therapy failure: immediate vs deferred treatment. *Oncology (Huntingt)* 1999;13:985–993.
3. Catalone WJ, Smith DS. 5-year tumor recurrence rates after anatomical radical retropubic prostatectomy for prostate cancer. *J Urol* 1994;152:1837–1842.
4. Trapasso JG, DeKernion JB, Smith RB, et al. The incidence and significance of detectable levels of serum prostate specific antigen after radical prostatectomy. *J Urol* 1994;152: 1821–1825.
5. Goad JR, Chang SJ, Ohori M, et al. PSA after definitive radiotherapy for clinically localized prostate cancer. *Urol Clin North Am* 1993;20:727–736.
6. Stamey TA, Yang N, Hay AR, et al. Prostate-specific antigen as a serum marker for adenocarcinoma of the prostate. *N Engl J Med* 1987;317:909–916.
7. Babaian RJ, Kojima M, Saitah M, et al. Detection of residual prostate cancer after external radiotherapy. Role of prostate specific antigen and transrectal ultrasonography. *Cancer* 1995;75:2153–2158.
8. Partin AW, Oesterling JE. The clinical usefulness of prostate specific antigen: update 1994. *J Urol* 1994;152:1358–1368.
9. Ferguson JK, Oesterling JE. Patient evaluation if prostate-specific antigen becomes elevated following radical prostatectomy or radiation therapy. *Urol Clin North Am* 1994:21:677–685.
10. Leibman BD, Dillioglugil O, Wheeler TM, et al. Distant metastasis after radical prostatectomy in patients without an elevated scum prostate specific antigen level. *Cancer* 1995;76: 2530–2534.
11. Frazier HA, Robertson JE, Humphrey PA, et al. Is prostate specific antigen of clinical importance in evaluating outcome after radical prostatectomy? *J Urol* 1993;149:516–518.

12. Lange PK, Ercole CJ, Lightner DJ, et al. The value of serum prostate specific antigen before and after radical prostatectomy. *J Urol* 1989;141:873–879.
13. Oesterling JE, Chan DW, Epstein JL, et al. Prostate specific antigen in the preoperative and postoperative evaluation of localized prostatic cancer treated with radical prostatectomy. *J Urol* 1988;139:766–772.
14. Vessella RL, Lange PH. Issues in the assessment of PSA immunoassays. *Urol Clin North Am* 1993;20:607–619.
15. Stock RG. Locoregional therapies for early stage prostate cancer. *Oncology* 1995;9:803–811.
16. Tapasso JG, DeKernion JB, Smith RB, et a1. The incidence and significance of detectable levels of serum prostate specific antigen after radical prostatectomy. *J Urol* 1994;152: 1821–1825.
17. Paulson DF. Impact of radical prostatectomy in the management of clinically localized disease. *J Urol* 1994;152:1826–1830.
18. Zincke H, Oesterling JE, Blute ML, et al. Long-term (15 years) results after radical prostatectomy for clinically localized (stage T2c or lower) prostate cancer. *J Urol* 1994;15: 1850–1857.
19. Dillioglugil O, Leibman BD, Kattan M, et al. Hazard rates for progression, determined by PSA, after radical prostatectomy for T1-2 prostate cancer. *J Urol* 1995;153:391A.
20. Partin AW, Pound CR, Clemens IQ, et al. Serum PSA after anatomic radical prostatectomy. *Urol Clin North Am* 1993; 20:713–725.
21. Catalona WJ, Smith DS. 5-year tumor recurrence rates after anatomical radical retropubic prostatectomy for prostate cancer. *J Urol* 1994;152:1837–1842.
22. Takayama TK, Kreiger JN, True LD, et al. The enhanced detection of persistent disease after prostatectomy with a new prostate c antigen immunoassay. *J Urol* 1993;150:374–378.
23. Haese A, Huland E, Graefen M, et al. Ultrasensitive detection of prostate specific antigen in the follow-up of 422 patients after radical prostatectomy. *J Urol* 1999;161:1206–1211.
24. Klee GG, Dodge LA, Zincke H, et al. Measurement of serum prostate specific antigen using IMx prostate specific antigen assay. *J Urol* 1994;151:94–98.
25. Klee GG, Preissner CM, Oesterling JE. Development of a highly sensitive immunochemiluminometric assay for prostate specific antigen (PSA). *Urology* 1994;44:76–82.
26. Yu H, Diamandis EP. Measurement of serum prostate specific antigen levels in women and in prostatectomized men with an ultrasensitive immunoassay technique. *J Urol* 1995;153:1004–1008.
27. Zagars GK, Pollack A. The fall and rise of prostate-specific antigen. Kinetics of serum prostate-specific antigen levels after radiation therapy for prostate cancer. *Cancer* 1993;72:832–842.
28. Zagars GK, Sherman NE, Babaian RJ. Prostate-specific antigen and external beam radiation therapy in prostate cancer. *Cancer* 1991;67:412–420.
29. Critz FA, Levinson AK, Williams WH, et al. Prostate specific antigen nadir achieved by men apparently cured of prostate cancer by radiotherapy. *J Urol* 1999;161:1199–1205.
30. American Society for Therapeutic Radiology and Oncology Consensus Panel. Consensus statement: guidelines for PSA following radiation therapy. *Int J Radiat Oncol Biol Phys* 1997;37:1035–1041.
31. Danella J, Steckel J, Dorey F, et al. Detectable prostate-specific antigen levels following radical prostatectomy: relationship of doubling time to clinical outcome. *J Urol* 1993; 149:447(abst).
32. Partin AW, Pearson JD, Landis PK, et al. Evaluation of serum prostate specific antigen velocity after radical prostatectomy to distinguish local recurrence from distant metastases. *Urology* 1994;43:649–659.
33. Connolly JA, Shinohara K, Presti JC. Local recurrence after radical prostatectomy: characteristics in size, location, and relationship to prostate-specific antigen and surgical margins. *Urology* 1996;47:225–231.
34. Takayama TK, Lange PH. Radiation therapy for local recurrence of prostate cancer after radical prostatectomy. *Urol Clin North Am* 1994;21:687–700.
35. Foster LS, Jajodia P, Fournier G, et al. The value of prostate specific antigen and transrectal ultrasound guided biopsy in detecting prostatic fossa recurrences following radical prostatectomy. *J Urol* 1993;149:1024–1028.
36. Kabalin JN, Hodge KY, McNeal JE, et al. Identification of residual cancer in the prostate following radiation therapy: Role of transrectal ultrasound guided biopsy and prostate specific antigen. *J Urol* 1989;142:326–331.
37. Egawa S, Carter SC, Wheeler TM, et al. Ultrasonographic changes in the normal and malignant prostate after definitive radiotherapy. *Urol Clin North Am* 1989;16:741–749.
38. Crook J, Perry G, Robertson S, et al. Routine prostate biopsies following radiotherapy for prostate cancer: results for 226 patients. *J Urol* 1995;153:502A.
39. Lightner DJ, Lange PH, Reddy PK, et al. Prostate specific antigen and local recurrence after radical prostatectomy. *J Urol* 1990;144:921–926.
40. Crook J, Robertson S, Collin G, et al. Clinical relevance of transrectal ultrasound, biopsy, and serum prostate-specific antigen following external beam radiotherapy for carcinoma of the prostate. *Int J Radiat Oncol Biol Phys* 1993;27:31–37.
41. Barichello M, Gion M, Bonazza A, et al. Prostate specific antigen as a unique routine test in monitoring therapy for inoperable prostate cancer. Comparison with radionuclide bone scan and prostatic acid phosphatase. *Eur Urol* 1995; 27:295–300.
42. Miller PD, Eardley I, Kirby RS. Prostate specific antigen and bone scan correlation in the staging and monitoring of patients with prostatic cancer. *Br J Urol* 1992;70:295–298.
43. Bianco FJ, Lam JS, Davis LP, et al. Limited role of radionuclide bone scan inpatients with prostate cancer recurrent after radical prostatectomy. *J Urol* 1998;159:288(abst).
44. Kahn D, Williams RD, Manyak M, et al. ^{111}Indium capromab pendetide in the evaluation of patients with residual or recurrent prostate cancer after radical prostatectomy. *J Urol* 1998;159:2041–2047.
45. Babaian RJ, Sayer J, Podoloff DA, et al. Radioimmunoscintigraphy of pelvic nodes with ^{111}Indium-labeled monoclonal antibody cyt-356. *J Urol* 1994;152:1952–1955.
46. Haseman MK, Reed NL, Rosenthal SA. Monoclonal antibody imaging of occult prostate cancer in patients with elevated prostate-specific antigen. Positron emission tomography and biopsy correlation. *Clin Nucl Med* 1996;21:704–713.
47. Kramer S, Gorich J, Gottfried HW, et al. Sensitivity of computed tomography in detecting local recurrence of pros-

tatic carcinoma following radical prostatectomy. *Br J Radiol* 1997;70:995–999.
48. Levran Z, Gonzales JA, Diakno AC, et al. Are pelvic computed tomography, bone scan and pelvic lymphadenectomy necessary in the staging of prostatic cancer. *Br J Urol* 1995;75:778–781.
49. Algra PR, Bloem JL, Tissing H, et al. Detection of vertebral metastases: comparison between MR imaging and bone scintigraphy. *Radiographics* 1991;11:219–232.
50. Avrahumi E, Tadmor R, Dally O, et al. Early MR demonstration of spinal metastases in patients with normal radiographs and CT and radionuclide bone scans. *J Comput Assist Tomogr* 1989;13:598–602.
51. Smoker WR, Bodershy JC, Knutzon RK, et al. The role of MR imaging in evaluating metastatic spinal disease. *AJR Am J Roentgenol* 1987;149:1241–1248.
52. Fujii Y, Higashi Y, Owada F, et al. Magnetic resonance imaging for the diagnosis of prostate cancer metastatic to bone. *Br J Urol* 1995;75:54–58.
53. Turner JW, Hawes DR, Williams RD. Magnetic resonance imaging for detection of prostate cancer metastatic to bone. *J Urol* 1993;149:1482–1484.
54. Hoh CK, Seltzer MA, Franklin J, et al. Positron emission tomography in urological oncology. *J Urol* 1998;159:347–356.
55. Effert PJ, Bares R, Handt S, et al. Metabolic imaging of untreated prostate cancer by positron emission tomography with 18F-fluorine-labeled deoxyglucose. *J Urol* 1996;155:994–998.
56. Shreve PD, Grossman HB, Gross MD, et al. Metastatic prostate cancer: initial findings of PET with 2-deoxy-2-(F-18) fluoro-D-glucose. *Radiology* 1996;199:751–752.

36

LOCAL THERAPY FOR RECURRENT PROSTATE CANCER

MAXWELL V. MENG
KATSUTO SHINOHARA
GARY D. GROSSFELD
PETER R. CARROLL

Although prostate cancer remains the most common malignancy and is the second leading cause of cancer-specific deaths in American men, advances in the diagnosis and treatment have increased opportunities for cure. Use of prostate-specific antigen (PSA) screening in combination with digital rectal examination and transrectal ultrasound (TRUS) has allowed earlier detection of prostate cancer, resulting in considerable stage migration and an increased incidence of organ-confined disease (1,2). Nonpalpable prostate cancer (T1c) associated with an increased level of serum PSA is the most common clinical stage of disease currently detected (3).

Despite earlier diagnosis of prostate cancer and improved treatment modalities, there still exists a significant risk of disease recurrence after therapy. The pathologic extent of disease is clinically understaged in as many as 50% of patients undergoing radical prostatectomy, with 30% to 40% of such patients showing evidence of extraprostatic spread (4). A recent analysis of patients enrolled in a disease registry of prostate cancer patients demonstrated that 22% of patients who received initial treatment with radical prostatectomy, radiation therapy, or cryotherapy required a second form of prostate cancer treatment within 3 years of initial therapy (5). The majority of these treatments was administered in a therapeutic (nonadjuvant) fashion for apparent evidence of disease recurrence. Four percent of patients received adjuvant therapy within 3 months, presumably in those men at high risk for primary local treatment failure. Differences existed between the frequency, as well as form, of secondary treatments among the initial treatment types, even when controlling for cancer stage, Gleason grade, and serum PSA. Patients managed with radical prostatectomy had the lowest rate of second cancer treatment. Similar results have been reported by others, with at least 16% to 35% of radical prostatectomy patients and 24% of radiotherapy patients receiving second cancer treatments within 5 years of primary treatment (6–8). However, there are no adequate studies comparing outcomes of these secondary treatments, and the specific indications and optimal timing for additional therapy are equally undefined. Herein, we discuss the identification of local recurrence after initial treatment for prostate cancer, as well as the various treatment options with definitive, curative intent in patients whose cancers recur locally after radical prostatectomy, radiation therapy, or cryosurgery.

RISK FACTORS FOR RECURRENCE

Multiple studies have examined predictors of recurrence after definitive treatment for prostate cancer. The majority of this data is derived from an analysis of the outcomes of patients treated by radical prostatectomy (Table 36-1). Pretreatment clinical features that correlate with prognosis include T stage, biopsy Gleason score, and serum PSA level (9). As one would expect, higher stage, the presence of Gleason pattern 4 or greater or a Gleason sum greater than 7, and PSA levels exceeding 10 ng per mL are associated with an increased risk of progression after surgery. These elements have been combined to more accurately predict tumor extent or pathologic stage and, therefore, prognosis; such probability tables and multivariate models have been based on a large number of men who have undergone radical prostatectomy (10–12). In addition to clinical parameters, more precise prognosis can be made from analysis of the radical prostatectomy specimen. Pathologic criteria, which are independent factors, include tumor grade, surgical margin status, and the presence of extracapsular disease, seminal vesicle invasion, or involvement of pelvic lymph nodes (i.e., pathologic stage greater than T2N0M0) (13). Patients with Gleason sum 8 to 10 fare poorly when compared to patients with Gleason sum 2 to 4 and 5 to 6; those with a Gleason score of 7 have an intermediate prognosis

TABLE 36-1. RISK FACTORS FOR RECURRENCE AFTER RADICAL PROSTATECTOMY

Pretreatment features
Higher stage (14,105–110)
Biopsy Gleason grade (any pattern 4, sum >7) (14,105–110)
Preoperative prostate-specific antigen (>10 ng/mL) (14,105–110)
Greater number of positive biopsies (111)
Pathologic features
Higher stage (seminal vesicle, lymph node involvement) (14,107,109,112,113)
Higher tumor Gleason grade (14,105,112,114)
Positive surgical margin (14,112,115,116)
DNA ploidy (117)

(14). However, cure is possible even in patients with high-grade cancer (Gleason sum greater than 7), if confined to the prostate pathologically. Approximately 50% of men with positive surgical margins progress after radical prostatectomy; yet, if disease is localized, then recurrence-free rates of more than 80% have been reported (15). Patients with organ-confined, low- to intermediate-grade prostate cancer have 5-year disease-free recurrence rates greater than 80%, whereas this falls to less than 40% in patients with seminal vesicle involvement (pT3) or positive lymph nodes (13,14). Prostate cancer volume correlates with risk of extraprostatic disease and treatment outcomes. Although pretreatment tumor volume is difficult to assess, recent studies demonstrate that the number of positive biopsies, as well as percent of biopsy cores, involved with cancer can predict risk of extracapsular cancer and disease recurrence after radical prostatectomy (16–18). Similarly, in patients receiving radiation therapy and cryotherapy, risks of recurrence are associated with pretreatment serum PSA, tumor grade, and clinical stage. In addition, PSA nadir after treatment predicts risk for treatment failure (19). Thus, multiple predictors are available to help identify patients receiving definitive therapy for localized prostate cancer who are at increased risk for disease recurrence.

IDENTIFYING RECURRENCE AND ITS SITE

Prostate-Specific Antigen

PSA is a powerful tool, not only in the diagnosis of prostate cancer, but also in the monitoring of patients after definitive treatment of clinically localized prostate cancer. Typically, biochemical failure precedes clinical disease by 6 to 48 months (20). Pound et al. characterized disease progression after PSA elevation in patients undergoing radical prostatectomy. Actuarial time to metastases was 8 years from the time of PSA failure and was predicted by time to biochemical failure, Gleason score, and PSA doubling time (21). The serum PSA of patients after radical prostatectomy should fall to undetectable levels, and initial testing should begin at 2 to 3 months. Serial PSA measurements provide the most reliable method in detecting recurrence, as tumor progression rarely occurs in the absence of PSA elevation. Likewise, PSA is used as an end point in monitoring outcomes after radiotherapy and cryotherapy. In these cases, however, PSA declines to low but often detectable levels, and the PSA response to treatment is unpredictable (22). As a result, definitions of treatment success and failure are variable, and no consensus exists. Recent recommendations from the American Society of Therapeutic Radiology and Oncology define recurrence after radiotherapy as three consecutive rises in serum PSA independent of PSA nadir (23). Only a single study has validated this definition by correlation with clinical outcomes (24). Critz et al. propose a PSA nadir of 0.5 ng per mL or more as the end point for brachytherapy treatment failure, demonstrating significant 5- and 10-year disease-free survival rates in those with nadir PSA values less than 0.5 ng per mL (25,26). However, the prognostic value of this nadir depends on most men's achieving a nadir of 0.2 ng per mL or less (27). Time to reach PSA nadir varies with treatment modality. PSA nadir is typically achieved within 6 weeks after radical prostatectomy or cryosurgery. After radiation therapy, time to PSA nadir ranges from 8 to 18 months and even longer with brachytherapy. Ragde et al. reported an average of 42 months to PSA nadir in a series of 152 patients receiving brachytherapy. In our evaluation of cryosurgical ablation, we have defined biochemical failure as PSA nadir 0.5 ng per mL or greater, or PSA nadir less than 0.5 ng per mL with a subsequent increase in PSA of at least 0.2 ng per mL on two consecutive measurements (28). Patterns of PSA failure, such as time to failure, nadir PSA reached, time to nadir PSA level, and PSA velocity, are current methods to further evaluate for treatment failure (25,26,29,30). Thus, despite the widespread use of PSA to monitor disease activity after radiotherapy and cryotherapy, controversy exists regarding exact definitions of treatment failure.

Distinguishing between local recurrence and distant failure is crucial in subsequent treatment decisions (Fig. 36-1). Physical examination of the prostate or surgical bed by digital rectal examination is neither sensitive nor specific in detection or localization of low-volume disease recurrence because of irradiated and postsurgical changes in the prostatic fossa. Changes in serial examinations over time, however, may help to detect local disease (31). More recently, the need for anastomotic biopsy has been questioned. Preliminary data from our patients receiving radiotherapy after prostatectomy show no differences in outcomes between those treated for biochemical failure alone and those treated for biopsy-proven recurrence, suggesting that biopsy may not be necessary to define patients most appropriate for salvage therapy (32).

PSA kinetics, in conjunction with pathologic stage and Gleason grade, may provide the best means of identifying the location of tumor failure. Patients with low-grade disease generally have local recurrence, whereas those with seminal vesicle invasion or positive lymph nodes are more likely to fail distantly. PSA velocity less than 0.75 ng per

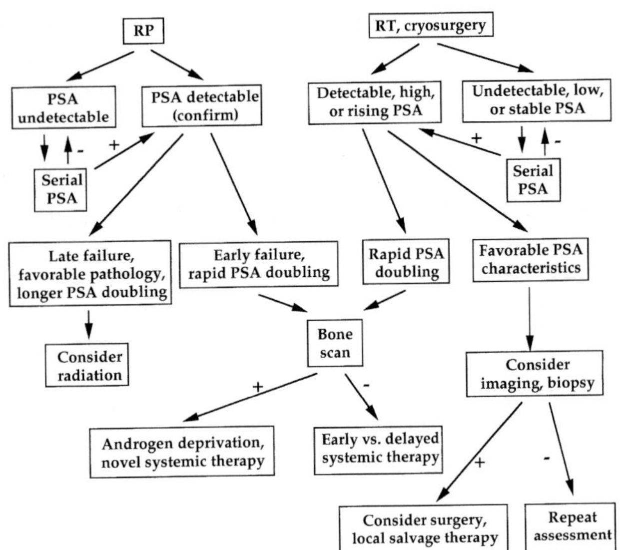

FIGURE 36-1. Algorithm for evaluation, diagnosis, and treatment of recurrent prostate cancer. PSA, prostate-specific antigen; RP, radical prostatectomy; RT, radiation therapy.

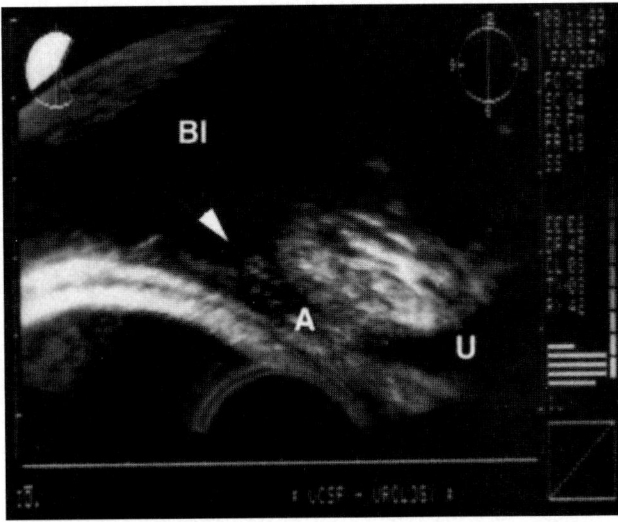

FIGURE 36-2. Normal transrectal ultrasound after radical prostatectomy. Longitudinal image of the prostatic fossa. A, vesicourethral anastomosis; arrowhead, bladder neck; Bl, bladder; U, bulbar urethra.

mL per year was observed in 94% of patients with local recurrence (33). Conversely, more than 50% of men with metastatic disease had a PSA velocity greater than 0.75 ng per mL per year. In the same study, earlier postoperative elevations in PSA within two years were associated with distant disease. Clearly, PSA doubling time less than 6 months suggests distant disease. Trapasso et al. described a median PSA doubling time of 4.3 months in patients ultimately progressing with distant failure, whereas those patients with clinically detected local failure or biochemical failure only had a PSA doubling time of 11.7 months (34). Shorter PSA doubling times also predict increased risk for and shorter time to the appearance of clinical disease (35).

Imaging

Imaging studies complement clinical and pathologic information in localizing primary treatment failure. These modalities include TRUS, pelvic computed tomography (CT), magnetic resonance imaging (MRI) and spectroscopy (MRS), positron emission tomography (PET), and single photon emission CT (SPECT).

The overall probability of a positive anastomotic biopsy performed for an elevated PSA is between 40% and 50% and is not dependent on rectal findings (36–38). TRUS alone does not increase detection of local recurrence, but merely guides needle placement to the vesicourethral anastomosis. Pelvic anatomy as seen by TRUS after radical prostatectomy has been well described (Fig. 36-2) (38–40). Bladder neck tissue can be seen as a homogeneous, hyperechoic ring at the level of the anastomosis. Recurrent disease is usually seen as a hypoechoic mass posterior or posterolateral to the anastomosis; recurrences elsewhere are less common (38). Nonmalignant postoperative tissue may also appear hypoechoic, decreasing the sensitivity and specificity for identifying local recurrence. In addition, up to one-third of recurrences may have an isoechoic appearance. Posttreatment changes of the *in situ* organ after radiation or cryotherapy make the use of TRUS even more difficult in these patients with recurrence. Radiation creates a small hyperechoic gland with distortion of normal tissue planes, whereas the prostate after cryoablation appears "fuzzy" (36). Nonetheless, local recurrences can be visualized as peripheral hypoechoic lesions. As mentioned earlier, TRUS-guided biopsies may not be necessary to confirm local recurrence after radical prostatectomy. Indications for TRUS-guided biopsy after radiation or other forms of focal therapy, such as cryotherapy, are not clear. Most would agree that such biopsies should be considered in those patients treated with radiation or cryotherapy who show serial elevations in serum PSA after reaching a PSA nadir. Nadir levels of PSA are usually reached within 8 to 18 months after radiation and within 3 months after cryotherapy, as stated previously.

Technology in cross-sectional imaging (CT and MRI) continues to evolve, and so does its role in visualizing locally recurrent cancer. CT has virtually replaced lymphography in detecting enlarged lymph nodes with sensitivities ranging from 30% to 80% but does not play a significant role in examining local disease (41). MRI is useful in imaging local and metastatic disease (42,43). Endorectal coil MRI increases resolution to 3 mm, appreciably greater than TRUS. Most recurrences after radical prostatectomy appear at the vesicourethral anastomosis as isointense lesions on T1-weighted images relative to the surrounding levator ani muscles and as areas of reduced signal intensity on T2-weighted images in the normally high-

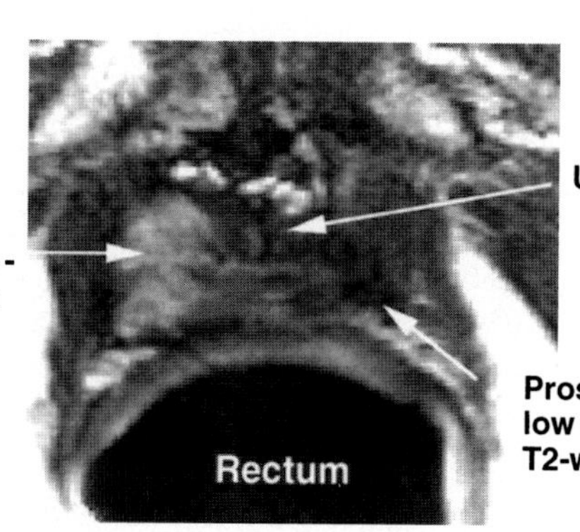

FIGURE 36-3. Magnetic resonance imaging (MRI) demonstrating recurrent prostate cancer after radiation therapy. T2-weighted image showing an irregular soft tissue mass on the left side, representing likely tumor recurrence.

signal-intensity peripheral zone. After radiotherapy, tumor recurrences have similar characteristics—hyperintense on T2-weighted images when compared to the levator ani muscles but hypointense relative to the peripheral zone (Fig. 36-3) (44). Another promising avenue is the use of three-dimensional hydrogen-1 MRS in detecting differences in citrate and choline levels in malignant and benign prostate cells (Fig. 36-4) (45). However, further studies are required to document the use of routine MRI and MRS in evaluating treatment failure.

PET, although used routinely in brain and cardiac imaging, is not well described in prostate cancer. Imaging takes advantage of differential cellular uptake and metabolism of a radiolabeled compound, such as the glucose analog 18-fluoro-2-deoxyglucose (46). Theoretically, the increased positron emission by tumor cells is detected and allows localization; however, high 18-fluoro-2-deoxyglucose activity is seen in the urinary bladder as well as in benign prostatic hyperplastic tissue. Thus, the use of PET in recurrent prostate cancer, especially after radiotherapy and cryotherapy, is unclear (47–49).

Clinical use of antibody imaging and SPECT in prostate cancer is a recent development, with U.S. Food and Drug Administration approval in 1996 for use in postprostatectomy patients with biochemical recurrence but no detectable site of recurrence by conventional imaging (50). The indium-111 (^{111}In) capromab pendetide (ProstaScint) scan is based on a murine monoclonal antibody, recognizing prostate-specific membrane antigen conjugated to a linker-chelator and the radioisotope ^{111}In. Results do not indicate a clear role for ProstaScint imaging, with overall sensitivity and specificity ranging from 44% to 92% and 36% to 86%, respectively (51). However, although inferior to bone scintigraphy for detecting bone metastases, ProstaScint is able to detect prostatic fossa recurrence with reasonable accuracy. Kahn et al. reported on SPECT findings and ability to predict response to salvage radiotherapy in 32 patients (52). Seventy percent of those patients with a normal scan or evidence of only local disease had a durable, complete response to radiotherapy, whereas only 22% with ProstaScint findings outside the prostatic fossa responded.

RECURRENCE AFTER RADICAL PROSTATECTOMY

Despite earlier diagnosis, improved patient selection, and evolution in surgical technique, as many as 35% to 50% of patients undergoing radical prostatectomy develop biochemical recurrence after treatment. Up to half of these

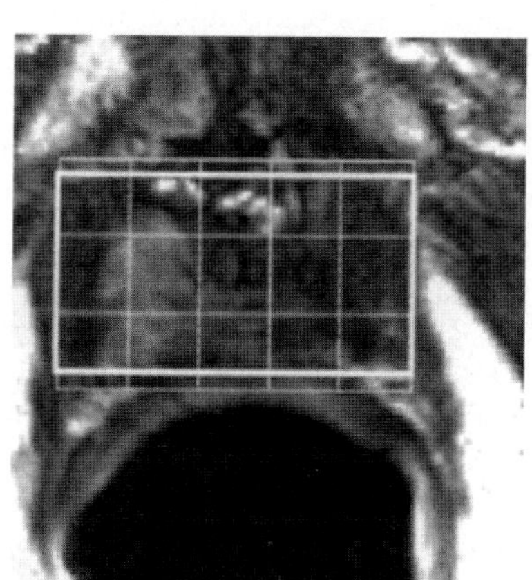

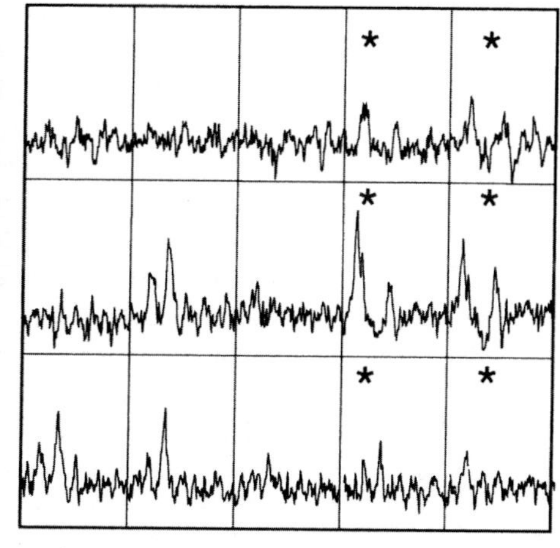

FIGURE 36-4. Magnetic resonance spectroscopy of the prostate shown in Figure 36-3 **(A)**. Areas in which (choline+creatine)/citrate >0.74 suggest prostate cancer **(B)**.

men have local recurrence, with the remainder having distant disease alone or combined local and distant failure (53). Therefore, it is important to define the role of regional therapy in patients after radical prostatectomy who may potentially benefit from further treatment.

External beam radiation therapy has been used in an adjuvant fashion in men with adverse pathologic characteristics at increased risk for recurrence and a therapeutic fashion in men with biochemical PSA failure or biopsy proven recurrence. Older data with significant follow-up were obtained before the widespread use of PSA. Gibbons et al. compared outcomes between patients receiving adjuvant radiation therapy and those merely followed for disease progression (54). Although local recurrence in the untreated group was higher, no statistically significant survival advantage was noted in the treated group. There was a suggestion that immediate adjuvant therapy was superior to delayed therapy for clinically detectable local recurrence in preventing metastases and cancer-specific deaths.

More recent studies suggest that 51% to 94% of patients receiving adjuvant radiotherapy will maintain a persistently undetectable PSA (Table 36-2) (54–58). In addition, local recurrence rates appear to be decreased in such patients compared to similar patients who did not receive adjuvant radiation. Nevertheless, a clear survival benefit still has not been demonstrated, and the role of adjuvant radiotherapy in those patients at risk for failure remains controversial. The rationale for early adjuvant radiation includes more effective treatment of a smaller tumor volume. The potential for unnecessary therapy, however, exists in these patients. One particular area of controversy involves those men with positive surgical margins. Although at risk for local recurrence, up to half of these men remain disease free at 10 years and would not benefit from additional radiation. Recently, we analyzed this question by creating a decision analytic model, comparing early adjuvant radiotherapy with surveillance in patients with positive surgical margins at the time of radical prostatectomy (59). The decision analysis demonstrated an outcome benefit for adjuvant radiation in patients with low to intermediate Gleason grade and no seminal vesicle invasion. Furthermore, surveillance was favored in patients with a single positive margin, but improved outcome values were associated with adjuvant radiation for multiple positive margins. Other data support the decision analysis and suggest a benefit to adjuvant therapy in some patients. Bullock et al. analyzed 544 men with undetectable postoperative PSA levels but adverse pathologic features (60). Adjuvant radiotherapy demonstrated a statistically significant improvement in 7-year recurrence-free survival only in the group with positive surgical margins. Valicenti et al. compared prostatectomy patients with stage pT3N0 in a matched-pair analysis (61). Those men receiving adjuvant radiation therapy had a 5-year disease-free rate of 89%—an 83% reduction in the risk of biochemical failure. Until data from prospective randomized trials are available regarding survival, this information merely aids the physicians and patients in determining management strategy after surgery. Currently, the European Organization for Research and Treatment of Cancer, the National Cancer Institute, and the Southwest Oncology Group have trials under way comparing radical prostatectomy and observation with radical prostatectomy and adjuvant radiotherapy in men with pathologic stage T3 prostate cancer (62).

TABLE 36-2. RESULTS OF RADIOTHERAPY AFTER PROSTATECTOMY

Study	n	% with undetectable PSA	Length of follow-up
Adjuvant radiotherapy (delivered immediately for adverse pathologic features)			
McCarthy et al. (55)	27	83	40 mo
Morris et al. (66)	40	81	3 yr
Petrovich et al. (57)	63	85	5 yr
Zietman et al. (58)	68	77	5 yr
Grossfeld et al. (59)	36	80	3 yr
Therapeutic radiotherapy (delivered in a delayed fashion for biochemical relapse)			
Hudson et al. (64)	21	29	12.6 mo
Schild et al. (63)	46	50	5 yr
Wu et al. (67)	53	23	2 yr
McCarthy et al. (55)	37	54	27.5–36 mo
Morris et al. (66)	48	47	3 yr
Forman et al. (68)	47	73	36 mo
Cadeddu et al. (70)	30	37	At least 2 yr
vander Kooy et al. (65)	30	56	8 yr
Coetzee et al. (56)	45	51	33 mo
Nudell et al. (32)	47	41	3 yr

PSA, prostate-specific antigen.

Treatment of biochemical disease recurrence with radiation can often result in an undetectable PSA. In general, freedom from biochemical recurrence has been reported in 30% to 65% of men after therapeutic or salvage radiotherapy (Table 36-2) (63–68). Schild et al. reported an overall 50% disease-free survival at 3 years; however, 78% of those patients with a preradiation PSA less than 1 ng per mL were disease free, whereas only 18% of men with PSA greater than 1 ng per mL remained disease free (63). Forman et al. also reported improved disease-free survival in patients with lower preradiation PSA (less than 2 ng per mL) (68). Other investigators have reported no differences between adjuvant and therapeutic radiotherapy in patients with initially undetectable PSA after surgery. Similarly, Coetzee et al. noted a more durable response to radiation in men who failed after an initial undetectable PSA when compared to men with a persistently detectable PSA (66% at 40 months vs. 20% at 12 months, respectively) (56). We recently evaluated our experience with radiation after radical prostatectomy in 105 patients at the University of California, San Francisco (UCSF) (32). The overall 5-year disease-free survival rate was 43%, with failure after radiation defined as PSA greater

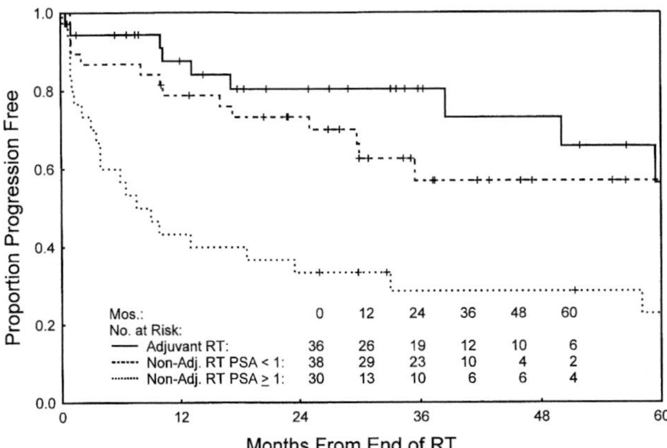

FIGURE 36-5. Prostate-specific antigen (PSA) progression-free survival by preradiotherapy PSA. Comparison of the interval to biochemical disease recurrence in patients treated with adjuvant radiation therapy (RT), therapeutic RT with pre-RT PSA <1 ng per mL, and therapeutic RT with pre-RT PSA ≥1 ng per mL. The number of patients at risk according to the indication for RT is given below the curves. (From Nudell DM, Grossfeld GD, Weinberg VK, et al. Radiotherapy following radical prostatectomy: treatment outcomes and patterns of failure. *Urology* 1999;54:1049, with permission.)

than 0.2 ng per mL. Outcomes were equivalent in those men receiving adjuvant and salvage radiotherapy when therapeutic radiation was initiated with a low serum PSA (less than 1 ng per mL) (Fig. 36-5). There were no differences between the two groups with respect to preprostatectomy PSA, tumor grade, or pathologic stage. Our data, as well as that from Vicini et al., also demonstrate the indication for radiotherapy (adjuvant vs. therapeutic) as an independent prognostic factor associated with biochemical control (69). However, no other clinical-, pathologic-, or treatment-related factors were associated with 5-year outcome in their patients. Cadeddu et al. present more pessimistic data (70). Only 21% of men had an undetectable PSA for more than 2 years after therapeutic radiation after prostatectomy. No patients with Gleason score of 9 or greater, positive seminal vesicles, or positive lymph nodes had undetectable PSA levels more than 2 years. Finally, early treatment (i.e., at lower PSA or isolated PSA elevation without documented local recurrence) did not predict a favorable response to therapy. Thus, although it appears that adjuvant radiotherapy is a viable option in patients at higher risk for local recurrence, radiation may be used with efficacy in a therapeutic fashion when tumor volume, as reflected by serum PSA, is low. Patients most likely to benefit from salvage radiation after prostatectomy include those with low- to moderate-grade tumors with an undetectable postoperative PSA that rises after more than 1 year later. The exact timing of radiation has yet to be determined, although a PSA cut point of 2 ng per mL currently appears reasonable.

Morbidity of adjuvant or therapeutic external beam radiation has not been carefully reported. Typically, 45 to 65 Gy is delivered to the prostatic bed and is generally well tolerated. Short-term complications, including bowel and bladder irritability, are seen in approximately 10% of patients, whereas long-term and significant complications are less well defined (71). A retrospective study of 294 men analyzed the effects of adjuvant external beam radiation on urinary continence and potency after nerve-sparing prostatectomy (72). With a median follow-up of 2.6 years, no significant impact of postoperative radiation was seen on urinary continence or erectile dysfunction. A more recent study evaluated quality of life in patients undergoing salvage procedures (73). When compared to patients undergoing salvage prostatectomy after initial radiotherapy, patients treated with radiation after prostatectomy fared better in measures of physical well-being and urinary continence. Both groups, however, reported a high incidence of impotence and similar satisfaction with their quality of life.

Other forms of treatment for locally recurrent disease after radical prostatectomy have been reported but are not well characterized. These include brachytherapy and cryosurgical ablation. Kotrouvelis et al. treated five patients with salvage brachytherapy after prostatectomy with acceptable morbidity and results (74). At UCSF, we have treated three cases of local recurrence after prostatectomy with cryoablation; one patient has had an undetectable PSA for 3 years. Another patient had salvage brachytherapy after prostatectomy, and, 18 months after the procedure, his PSA was 0.03 ng per mL. Improvements in technology may lead to improved outcomes with these modalities. However, further studies are required before their routine use after radical prostatectomy can be recommended.

RECURRENCE AFTER RADIATION THERAPY

Radiation therapy (external beam or brachytherapy) has been used with increasing frequency for organ-confined prostate cancer (75). As with surgery, a certain percentage of patients receiving radiation may fail locally due to inadequate localization of the target, inadequate dose, or radiation resistance. Therefore, issues of detection and localization of recurrence after radiation and subsequent treatment options are important to elucidate.

As mentioned earlier, PSA definitions of radiation failure have varied among the studies. Nevertheless, any rising PSA level after radiation therapy may signal active residual disease. An exception may be those who have been treated with neoadjuvant hormonal therapy in whom androgen levels may rise after stopping androgen deprivation. In addition, an interesting phenomenon has been noted in approximately one-third of patients who receive brachytherapy but not other forms of radiation. A self-limited, temporary rise in serum PSA often occurs 12 to 18 months after the procedure; this benign PSA flare is unrelated to tumor progression (76). As many as one-third of patients may demonstrate rising PSA levels at 3 years, and as many as half may fail clinically within 5 to 7 years after external beam radiation (77–79). Recurrence rates appear to have decreased through the use of radiation techniques that target the prostate better and allow for delivery of higher doses. In those patients with recurrent or persistent localized disease, the curative therapeutic options traditionally included salvage prostatectomy or cryoablation. Most commonly, however, androgen ablation was instituted with postradiation recurrence. We have found that androgen deprivation is the most common form (88%) of secondary treatment after radiotherapy, suggesting limited curative options for those patients currently failing initial radiation. Innovative forms of treatment have emerged in recent years that may increase potentials for cure with secondary treatments.

Salvage prostatectomy after radiotherapy has been approached cautiously in the past. It may be technically difficult but has been demonstrated to be feasible with acceptable morbidity and cure rates. Several reports document the efficacy of salvage surgery (80–82). Overall, cancer-specific survival and disease-free rates have ranged from 70% to 90% and 30% to 50% at 8 to 10 years, respectively. Pathologically organ-confined disease is found in 20% to 50% of cases and is an important prognostic factor. In a series from Tefilli et al., all patients with organ-confined disease were disease free at 34 months (83). Amling et al. (84) reported a 10-year disease-free survival of 43% in 108 patients, similar to results from Rogers et al. and Moul et al. (82,85). DNA ploidy and preoperative serum PSA were significant predictors of outcome after surgery. Another study also reported radical prostatectomy Gleason score as an independent predictor of cancer-specific survival (86). Other factors influencing outcomes of salvage prostatectomy include preradiation clinical stage and preoperative PSA (87). Data suggest that PSA levels less than 10 ng per mL before surgery may predict pathologically localized disease and reduced recurrence. Currently, the Cancer and Leukemia Group B is evaluating salvage radical prostatectomy in a prospective fashion. Criteria for inclusion are men with biopsy-proven local disease at least 18 months after initial radiotherapy for PSA less than 20 ng per mL and Gleason sum less than 8 (71). In general, salvage prostatectomy after radiation should be reserved for men with low co-morbidity and a 10-year life expectancy in who recurrence is not locally advanced. Parameters guiding the decision include Gleason sum of 7 or less, PSA less than 10 ng per mL, and clinical stage T2 or less at the time of radiation and surgery. However, accurate presurgical staging is often difficult after radiation and may make appropriate patient selection difficult.

Complications of salvage prostatectomy are more common when compared to primary prostatectomy. Urinary incontinence is seen in 20% to 60% of patients, bladder neck contracture in approximately 20%, and impotence is virtually universal. Rectal injury occurs in fewer than 10% of patients and rarely necessitates fecal diversion (80,82,88,89). Contemporary series report better outcomes owing to improved patient selection, earlier identification of failure, and improved surgical technique. Nevertheless, patients must be informed of all potential outcomes, including cystoprostatectomy and urinary diversion, temporary diverting colostomy, and inoperability secondary to pelvic desmoplasia. Some have proposed planned salvage cystoprostatectomy or urinary diversion, or both, at the time of salvage surgery to maximize subsequent lower urinary tract function (90–92). Careful preoperative evaluation is necessary to identify manifestations of radiation injury, such as intractable hematuria, low-capacity bladder, and irritative lower urinary tract symptoms, which may alter treatment decisions.

Interest in primary and salvage cryosurgical ablation of the prostate has reemerged with technical innovations and the desire for minimally invasive procedures. High-resolution TRUS allows precise placement of the probes and real-time visualization of the freezing process. In addition, freezing may cause greater tumor destruction of a heterogeneous, radioresistant cell population even outside the prostate in adjacent tissues, when compared to other modalities. Reported results, however, have been modest with the largest series of patients treated at the M. D. Anderson Cancer Center (93). Seventy-seven percent of patients had negative sextant biopsies 6 months after cryoablation, but only 45 of 150 patients (31%) had persistently undetectable PSA with a mean follow-up of 13.5 months. A double freeze-thaw cycle appeared more effective than a single cycle in reducing positive posttreatment biopsy and biochemical failure rates. Bales et al. noted only a 9% disease-free rate after salvage cryotherapy (94). PSA characteristics in monitoring outcome after cryotherapy, either primary or salvage, are not well defined. Early evidence suggests that PSA nadir (less than 0.5 ng per mL) is currently the best prognostic indicator of biochemical- and biopsy-proved failure. Furthermore, it was noted that even small fluctuations in PSA might signify subsequent biochemical failure (95). Other variables, such as initial clinical stage, number of probes, and operator experience, may play a role in salvage outcomes.

Morbidity of salvage cryotherapy, similar to salvage prostatectomy, may be significant. A majority of men will experience problems with incontinence, and up to 50% may require transurethral resection for urinary retention and obstructive voiding symptoms. Impotence occurs in approximately 70% of men. Cespedes et al. stress the importance of effective urethral warming and the potential of improvements in incontinence up to 1 year after therapy in these patients (96). Complications such as urethrorectal fistula, abscess formation, and urethral stricture are fortunately rare.

Salvage brachytherapy after primary radiotherapy has been proposed as a promising treatment modality (97). In the past, concerns centered on the risk of injury to the urethra, bladder, and rectum with additional radiation as well as the questionable biologic response in a tumor with possible radioresistant elements, given failure of standard external beam radiotherapy. However, further investigation is warranted in light of improvements in imaging, treatment planning, and delivery methods as well as the documented morbidity of alternatives (i.e., prostatectomy and cryoablation). Grado et al. followed 49 patients treated with brachytherapy after biopsy-proven primary radiotherapy failure (97). Actuarial biochemical-free survival was 34% at 5 years and was associated with a postsalvage PSA nadir below 0.5 ng per mL. Local disease control was 98%—only a single patient demonstrated local clinical failure. These results are encouraging, especially given the treatment population. The median age was 73.3 years, and 71% had locally advanced disease at initial presentation; 90% of the cancers were moderately to poorly differentiated on prebrachytherapy biopsies. Complications were similar to those patients undergoing primary brachytherapy.

Innovative forms of therapy are being developed that may play a role in salvage therapy. High-intensity focused ultrasound and radiofrequency interstitial ablation are being studied and appear to have promise in local control of prostate cancer (98–100). These methods induce coagulative necrosis of the tissue within the confines of the prostatic capsule. In preliminary studies, primary high-intensity focused ultrasound achieved local control in 60% to 80% of patients (101). Radiofrequency ablation was able to produce predictable lesions of *in vivo* prostates before radical prostatectomy. Although these modalities hold promise as relatively noninvasive methods to treat recurrent cancer, their long-term efficacy and morbidity require further definition.

RECURRENCE AFTER CRYOTHERAPY

Cryosurgical ablation of the prostate has evolved greatly over the past 30 years. Early experience revealed limited local and overall control with significant treatment morbidity. More contemporary data provide a better understanding of the technique. We have performed cryoablation in 176 patients over a 5-year period with a mean follow-up of 31 months (28). Nadir PSA was undetectable in almost half of the patients, and biopsies were positive in 38%. *Treatment success*, defined as a PSA nadir less than 0.5 ng per mL that did not rise by more than 0.2 ng per mL on two consecutive measurements, was seen in 43% of men. Pretreatment PSA less than 10 ng per mL and undetectable PSA nadir after cryotherapy predicted for biochemical recurrence-free survival. Similar results have been reported by Long et al. (102). Although it appears that a substantial number of patients fail cryotherapy, the majority was at high risk for disease recurrence based on pretreatment stage, serum PSA, and Gleason grade. Results of cryotherapy may be comparable to other forms of primary therapy when accounting for the unfavorable patient population.

For those patients whose cancers recur after cryotherapy, the choice of secondary treatment is not well defined. Repeat freezing has been reported, as well as salvage prostatectomy. In the subset of patients at UCSF who underwent multiple cryotherapy procedures, 67% had no cancer on subsequent biopsies, but only 33% achieved long-term, favorable PSA values (28). Grampas et al. successfully performed radical perineal prostatectomy in six patients after initial cryotherapy (103). Pisters et al. used cryotherapy in a neoadjuvant fashion with radical prostatectomy in patients with locally advanced cancer (104). Of seven patients treated, only one failed by PSA criteria, one had positive surgical margins, and four had stage pT0. Substantial morbidity with respect to incontinence and impotence was reported. Radiation treatment can be given after cryoablation. Unlike cryotherapy after radiation, salvage radiation after cryotherapy appears to be associated with minimal morbidity.

FUTURE DIRECTIONS

Recurrence after definitive treatment for prostate cancer is a significant problem. Inadequate trials exist to determine the optimal diagnostic and treatment strategies after radical prostatectomy, radiation therapy, or cryosurgical ablation in which there is potential for or documented evidence of local disease. Limited curative options are available in many situations. We await the development of more efficacious and perhaps less morbid treatment options.

Other promising areas of research concern detection of disease relapse and molecular characterization of disease. Use of the ultrasensitive PSA assay may allow earlier determination of biochemical failure and prompt institution of salvage therapy. This lead time may increase efficacy of second treatments, such as radiotherapy after prostatectomy, by minimizing tumor burden. Pathologic and immunohistochemical markers can add additional information to prognosis. It remains to be determined whether certain genetic markers can predict for disease recurrence or metastatic potential; if found, this information could direct the type and timing of additional interventions. In addition, it must be recognized that not all patients who fail initial treatment as evidenced by biochemical relapse will experience disease-specific morbidity or mortality. Better discrimination of such patients may spare them the inconvenience, cost, and morbidity of complex testing or treatment, or both.

Finally, many patients fail primary and salvage therapy because of undetected metastatic or micrometastatic disease. Development of novel systemic treatment may address this issue by affecting local and distant prostate cancer cells. New approaches currently undergoing evaluation, such as antiangiogenesis agents or immunotherapy, may revolutionize therapy of prostate cancer.

REFERENCES

1. Newcomer LM, Stanford JL, Blumstein BA, et al. Temporal trends in rates of prostate cancer: declining incidence of advanced stage disease, 1974–1994. *J Urol* 1997;158:1427.
2. Carter HB, Partin AW. Diagnosis and staging of prostate cancer. In: Walsh PC, Retik AB, Vaughan ED Jr., et al., eds. *Campbell's urology*, 7th ed. Philadelphia: WB Saunders, 1998:2519.
3. Humphrey PA, Keetch DW, Smith DS, et al. Prospective characterization of pathological features of prostatic carcinomas detected via serum prostate specific antigen based screening. *J Urol* 1996;155:816.
4. Johansson JE, Holmberg L, Johansson S, et al. Fifteen-year survival in prostate cancer. A prospective, population-based study in Sweden. *JAMA* 1997;277:467.
5. Grossfeld GD, Stier DM, Flanders SC, et al. Use of second treatment following definitive local therapy for prostate cancer: data from the CaPSURE database. *J Urol* 1998;160:1398–1404.
6. Lu-Yao GL, Potosky AL, Albertsen PC, et al. Follow-up prostate cancer treatments after radical prostatectomy: a population-based study. *J Natl Cancer Inst* 1996;88:166.
7. Fowler FL Jr., Barry MJ, Lu-Yao G, et al. Patient-reported complications and follow-up treatment after radical prostatectomy. The National Medicare Experience: 1988–1990 (updated June 1993). *Urology* 1993;42:622.
8. Fowler FJ Jr., Barry MJ, Lu-Yao G, et al. Outcomes of external-beam radiation therapy for prostate cancer: a study of Medicare beneficiaries in three surveillance, epidemiology, and end results areas. *J Clin Oncol* 1996;14:2258.
9. Nasseri KK, Austenfeld MS. PSA recurrence after definitive treatment of clinically localized prostate cancer. *AUA Update Series* 1997;16:82.
10. Partin AW, Subong ENP, Walsh PC, et al. Combination of prostate-specific antigen, clinical stage, and Gleason score to predict pathological stage of localized prostate cancer: a multi-institutional update. *JAMA* 1997;277:1445.
11. Kattan MW, Wheeler TM, Scardino PT. Postoperative nomogram for disease recurrence after radical prostatectomy for prostate cancer. *J Clin Oncol* 1999;17:1499.
12. D'Amico AV, Chang H, Holoupka E. Calculated prostate cancer volume: the optimal predictor of the actual prostate cancer volume. *Urology* 1997;49:385.
13. Epstein JI. Pathology of adenocarcinoma of the prostate. In: Walsh PC, Retik AB, Vaughan ED Jr., et al., eds. *Campbell's urology*, 7th ed. Philadelphia: WB Saunders, 1998:2497.
14. Eastham JA, Scardino PT. Radical prostatectomy. In: Walsh PC, Retik AB, Vaughan ED Jr., et al., eds. *Campbell's urology*, 7th ed. Philadelphia: WB Saunders, 1998:2547.
15. Epstein JI. Incidence and significance of positive margins in radical prostatectomy specimens. *Urol Clin North Am* 1996;23:651.
16. Borirakchanyavat S, Bhargava V, Shinohara K, et al. Systematic sextant biopsies in the prediction of extracapsular extension at radical prostatectomy. *Urology* 1997;50:373.
17. Presti JC Jr., Shinohara K, Bacchetti P, et al. Positive fraction of systematic biopsies predicts risk of relapse after radical prostatectomy. *Urology* 1998;52:1079.
18. Wills ML, Sauvageot J, Partin AW, et al. Ability of sextant biopsies to predict radical prostatectomy stage. *Urology* 1998;51:759.
19. Goad JR, Chang SJ, Ohori M, et al. PSA after definitive radiotherapy for clinically localized prostate cancer. *Urol Clin North Am* 1993;20:727.
20. Lange PH, Ercole CJ, Lightner DJ, et al. The value of serum prostate specific antigen determinations before and after radical prostatectomy. *J Urol* 1989;141:873.
21. Pound CR, Partin AW, Eisenberger MA, et al. Natural history of progression after PSA elevation following radical prostatectomy. *JAMA* 1999;281:1591.
22. Polascik TJ, Oesterling JE, Partin AW. Prostate-specific antigen 1998: what we have learned and where we are going. Part II: detection, staging, and monitoring of prostate cancer. *AUA Update Series* 1998;17:218.
23. American Society for Therapeutic Radiology and Oncology Consensus Panel. Consensus statement: guidelines for PSA following radiation therapy. *Int J Radiat Oncol Biol Phys* 1997;37:1035.
24. Horwitz EM, Vicini FA, Ziaja EL, et al. The correlation between the ASTRO consensus panel definition of biochemical failure and clinical outcome for patients with prostate cancer treated with external beam irradiation. American Society of Therapeutic Radiology and Oncology. *Int J Radiat Oncol Biol Phys* 1998;41:267.
25. Critz FA, Levinson AK, Holladay D, et al. Prostate-specific antigen nadir of 0.5 ng/mL or less defines disease freedom for surgically staged men irradiated for prostate cancer. *Urology* 1997;49:668.
26. Critz FA, Levinson AK, Williams WH, et al. The PSA nadir that indicates potential cure after radiotherapy for prostate cancer. *Urology* 1997;49:322.
27. Critz FA, Levinson AK, Williams WH, et al. Prostate specific antigen nadir achieved by men apparently cured of prostate cancer by radiotherapy. *J Urol* 1999;161:1199.
28. Koppie TM, Shinohara K, Grossfeld GD, et al. The efficacy of cryosurgical ablation of prostate cancer: the University of California, San Francisco experience. *J Urol* 1999;162:427.
29. Zagars GK. Serum PSA as a tumor marker for patients undergoing definitive radiation therapy. *Urol Clin North Am* 1993;20:737.
30. Goad JR, Chang S, Ohori M, et al. PSA after definitive radiotherapy for clinically localized prostate cancer. *Urol Clin North Am* 1993;20:727.
31. Schellhammer PF, Kuban DA, el-Mahdi AM. Local failure after definitive radiation or surgical therapy for carcinoma of the prostate and options for prevention and therapy. *Urol Clin North Am* 1991;18:485.
32. Nudell DM, Grossfeld GD, Weinberg VK, et al. Radiotherapy following radical prostatectomy: treatment outcomes and patterns of failure. *Urology* 1999;54:1049.
33. Partin AW, Pearson JD, Landis PK, et al. Evaluation of serum prostate-specific antigen velocity after radical prostatectomy to distinguish local recurrence from distant metastases. *Urology* 1994;43:649.
34. Trapasso JG, deKernion JB, Smith RB, et al. The incidence and significance of detectable levels of serum prostate serum antigen after radical prostatectomy. *J Urol* 1994;152:1821.
35. Patel A, Dorey F, Franklin J, et al. Recurrence patterns after radical retropubic prostatectomy: clinical usefulness of prostate specific antigen doubling times and log slope prostate specific antigen. *J Urol* 1997;158:1441.

36. Lightner DJ, Lange PH, Reddy PK, et al. Prostate specific antigen and local recurrence after radical prostatectomy. *J Urol* 1990;144:921.
37. Foster LS, Jajodia P, Fournier G, et al. The value of prostate specific antigen and transrectal ultrasound guided biopsy in detecting prostatic fossa recurrence following radical prostatectomy. *J Urol* 1993;149:1024.
38. Connolly JA, Shinohara K, Presti JC Jr., et al. Local recurrence after radical prostatectomy: characteristics in size, location, and relationship to prostate-specific antigen and surgical margins. *Urology* 1996;47:225.
39. Goldenberg SL, Carter M, Dashefsky S, et al. Sonographic characteristics of the urethrovesical anastomosis in the early post-radical prostatectomy patient. *J Urol* 1992;147:1307.
40. Parra RO, Wolf RM, Huben RP. The use of transrectal ultrasound in the detection and evaluation of local pelvic recurrences after a radical urological pelvic operation. *J Urol* 1990;144:707.
41. Oyen RH, Van Poppel HP, Ameye FE, et al. Lymph node staging of localized prostatic carcinoma with CT and CT-guided fine-needle aspiration biopsy: prospective study of 285 patients. *Radiology* 1994;190:315.
42. Huch Boni RA, Meyenberger C, Lundquist JP, et al. Value of endorectal coil versus body coil MRI for diagnosis of recurrent pelvic malignancies. *Abdom Imaging* 1996;21:345.
43. Algra PR, Bloem JL, Tissing H, et al. Detection of vertebral metastases: comparison between MR imaging and bone scintigraphy. *Radiographics* 1991;11:219.
44. Silverman JM, Krebs TL. MR imaging evaluation with transrectal surface coil of local recurrence of prostatic cancer in men who have undergone radical prostatectomy. *Am J Radiol* 1997;168:379.
45. Kurhanewicz J, Vigneron DB, Hricak H, et al. Three-dimensional H-1 MR spectroscopic imaging of the in situ human prostate with high (0.24-0.7-cm^3) spatial resolution. *Radiology* 1996;198:795.
46. Hoh CK, Seltzer MR, Franklin J, et al. Positron emission tomography in urological oncology. *J Urol* 1998;159:347.
47. Effert PJ, Bares R, Handt S, et al. Metabolic imaging of untreated prostate cancer by positron emission tomography with 18 fluorine-labeled deoxyglucose. *J Urol* 1996;155:994.
48. Laubenbacher C, Hofer C, Avril N, et al. F-18 FDG PET for differentiation of local recurrent prostate cancer and scar. *J Nucl Med* 1995;36:198P.
49. Shreve PD, Grossman HB, Gross MD, et al. Metastatic prostate cancer: initial findings of PET with 2-deoxy-2-[F-19]fluoro-D-glucose. *Radiology* 1996;199:751.
50. Texter JH Jr., Neal CE. The role of monoclonal antibody in the management of prostate adenocarcinoma. *J Urol* 1998;160:2393.
51. Elgamal AA, Troychak MJ, Murphy GP. ProstaScint scan may enhance identification of prostate cancer recurrences after prostatectomy, radiation, or hormone therapy: analysis of 136 scans of 100 patients. *Prostate* 1998;37:261.
52. Kahn D, Williams RD, Haseman MK, et al. Radioimmunoscintigraphy with In-111-labeled capromab pendetide predicts prostate cancer response to salvage radiotherapy after failed radical prostatectomy. *J Clin Oncol* 1998;16:284.
53. Partin AW, Oesterling JE. The clinical usefulness of prostate specific antigen: update 1994. *J Urol* 1994;152:1358.
54. Gibbons RP, Cole BS, Richardson RG, et al. Adjuvant radiotherapy following radical prostatectomy: results and complications. *J Urol* 1985;135:65.
55. McCarthy JF, Catalona WJ, Hudson MA. Effect of radiation therapy on detectable serum prostate specific antigen levels following radical prostatectomy: early versus delayed treatment. *J Urol* 1994;151:1575.
56. Coetzee LJ, Hars V, Paulson DF. Postoperative prostate-specific antigen as a prognostic indication in patients with margin-positive prostate cancer, undergoing adjuvant radiotherapy after radical prostatectomy. *Urology* 1996;47:232.
57. Petrovich Z, Lieskovsky G, Freeman J, et al. Surgery with adjuvant irradiation in patients with pathologic stage C adenocarcinoma of the prostate. *Cancer* 1995;76:1621.
58. Zietman AL, Coen JJ, Shipley WU, et al. Adjuvant irradiation after radical prostatectomy for adenocarcinoma of prostate: analysis of freedom from PSA failure. *Urology* 1993;42:292.
59. Grossfeld GD, Tigrani VS, Nudell D, et al. Management of a positive surgical margin after radical prostatectomy: decision analysis. *J Urol* 2000;164:93–99.
60. Bullock AD, Carvalhal GF, Ramos CG, et al. Post-prostatectomy adjuvant radiotherapy for pathologically advanced prostate cancer: impact on recurrence rates. *J Urol* 1999;161:386A.
61. Valicenti RK, Gomella LG, Ismail M, et al. The efficacy of early adjuvant radiation therapy for pT3N0 prostate cancer: a matched-pair analysis. *J Urol* 1999;161:337A.
62. Thompson IM, Seay TM. Will current clinical trials answer questions about prostate adenocarcinoma? *Oncology* 1997;11:1109.
63. Schild SE, Buskirk SJ, Won WW, et al. The use of radiotherapy for patients with isolated elevation of serum prostate specific antigen following radical prostatectomy. *J Urol* 1996;156:1725.
64. Hudson MA, Catalona WJ. Effect of adjuvant radiation therapy on prostate specific antigen following radical prostatectomy. *J Urol* 1990;143:1174.
65. vander Kooy MJ, Pisanski TM, Cha SS, et al. Irradiation for locally recurrent carcinoma of the prostate following radical prostatectomy. *Urology* 1997;49:65.
66. Morris MM, Dallow KC, Zietman AL, et al. Adjuvant and salvage irradiation following radical prostatectomy for prostate cancer. *Int J Radiat Oncol Biol Phys* 1997;38:731.
67. Wu JJ, King SC, Montana GS, et al. The efficacy of post-prostatectomy radiotherapy in patients with an isolated elevation of serum prostate-specific antigen. *Int J Radiat Oncol Biol Phys* 1995;32:317.
68. Forman JD, Wharam MD, Lee DJ, et al. Definitive radiotherapy following prostatectomy: results and complications. *Int J Radiat Oncol Biol Phys* 1986;12:185.
69. Vicini FA, Ziaja EL, Kestin LL, et al. Treatment outcome with adjuvant and salvage irradiation after radical prostatectomy for prostate cancer. *Urology* 1999;54:111.
70. Cadeddu JA, Partin AW, DeWeese TL, et al. Long-term results of radiation therapy for prostate cancer recurrence following radical prostatectomy. *J Urol* 1998;159:173.
71. Ornstein DK, Oh J, Herschman JD, et al. Evaluation and management of the man who has failed primary curative therapy for prostate cancer. *Urol Clin North Am* 1998;25:591.

72. Formenti SC, Lieskovsky G, Simoneau AT, et al. Impact of moderate dose of postoperative radiation on urinary continence and potency in patients with prostate cancer treated with nerve sparing prostatectomy. *J Urol* 1996;155:616.
73. Tefilli MV, Gheiler EL, Tiguert R, et al. Quality of life in patients undergoing salvage procedures for locally recurrent prostate cancer. *J Surg Oncol* 1998;69:156.
74. Kotrouvelis PG, Katz SE, Lailas N, et al. Salvage CT guided brachytherapy for recurrent prostate cancer. *J Urol* 1999; 161:297A.
75. Mettlin C. The American Cancer Society National Prostate Cancer Detection Project and national patterns of prostate cancer detection and treatment. *CA Cancer J Clin* 1997;47:265.
76. Ragde H, Elgamal AA, Snow PB, et al. Ten-year free survival after transperineal sonography-guided iodine-125 brachytherapy with or without 45-gray external beam irradiation in the treatment of patients with clinically localized, low to high Gleason grade prostate carcinoma. *Cancer* 1998;83:989.
77. Lee WR, Hanlon AL, Hanks GE. Prostate specific antigen nadir following external beam radiation therapy for clinically localized prostate cancer: the relationship between nadir level and disease free survival. *J Urol* 1996;156:450.
78. Stamey TA, Ferrari MK, Schmid HP. The value of serial prostate specific antigen determinations 5 years after radiotherapy: steeply increasing values characterize 80 percent of patients. *J Urol* 1993;150:1856.
79. Zietman AL, Coen JJ, Dallow KC, et al. The treatment of prostate cancer by conventional radiation therapy: an analysis of long-term outcome. *Int J Radiat Oncol Biol Phys* 1995;32:287.
80. Lerner SE, Blute ML, Zincke H. Critical evaluation of salvage surgery for radiorecurrent/resistant prostate cancer. *J Urol* 1995;154:1103.
81. Pontes JE. Role of surgery in managing local recurrence following external-beam radiation therapy. *Urol Clin North Am* 1994;21:701.
82. Rogers E, Ohori M, Kassabian VS, et al. Salvage radical prostatectomy: outcome measure by serum prostate specific antigen levels. *J Urol* 1995;153:104.
83. Tefilli MV, Gheiler EL, Tiguert R, et al. Salvage surgery or salvage radiotherapy for locally recurrent prostate cancer. *Urology* 1998;52:224.
84. Amling CL, Lerner SE, Martin SK, et al. Deoxyribonucleic acid ploidy and serum prostate specific antigen predict outcome following salvage prostatectomy for radiation refractory prostate cancer. *J Urol* 1999;161:857.
85. Moul JW, Paulson DF. The role of radical surgery in the management of radiation recurrent and large volume prostate cancer. *Cancer* 1991;68:1265.
86. Cheng L, Sebo TJ, Slezak J, et al. Predictors of survival for prostate carcinoma patients treated with salvage radical prostatectomy after radiation therapy. *Cancer* 1998;83:2164.
87. Gheiler EL, Tefilli MV, Tiguert R, et al. Predictors for maximal outcome in patients undergoing salvage surgery for radio-recurrent prostate cancer. *Urology* 1998;51:789.
88. Pontes LE, Montie J, Klein E, et al. Salvage surgery for radiation failure in prostate cancer. *Cancer* 1993;71:976.
89. Zincke H. Radical prostatectomy and exenterative procedures for local failure after radiotherapy with curative intent: comparison of outcomes. *J Urol* 1992;147:894.
90. Bochner BH, Figueroa AJ, Skinner EC, et al. Salvage radical cystoprostatectomy and orthotopic urinary diversion following radiation failure. *J Urol* 1998;160:29.
91. Gheiler EL, Wood DP Jr., Montie JE, et al. Orthotopic urinary diversion is a viable option in patient undergoing salvage cystoprostatectomy for recurrent prostate cancer after definitive radiation therapy. *Urology* 1997;50:580.
92. Pisters LL, English SF, Dinney CPN, et al. Salvage prostatectomy with continent catheterizable urinary reconstruction: a novel approach to recurrent prostate cancer following radiation therapy. *J Urol* 1999;161:335A.
93. Pister LL, von Eschenbach AC, Scott SM, et al. The efficacy and complications of salvage cryotherapy of the prostate. *J Urol* 1997;157:921.
94. Bales GT, Williams MJ, Sinner M, et al. Short-term outcomes after cryosurgical ablation of the prostate in men with recurrent prostate carcinoma following radiation therapy. *Urology* 1995;46:676.
95. Greene GF, Pisters LL, Scott SM, et al. Predictive value of prostate specific antigen nadir after salvage cryotherapy. *J Urol* 1998;160:86.
96. Cespedes RD, Pisters LL, von Eschenbach AC, et al. Long-term follow up of incontinence and obstruction after salvage cryosurgical ablation of the prostate: results in 143 patients. *J Urol* 1997;157:237.
97. Grado GL, Collins JM, Kriegshauser JS, et al. Salvage brachytherapy for localized prostate cancer after radiotherapy failure. *Urology* 1999;53:2.
98. Madersbacher S, Pedevilla M, Vingers L, et al. Effect of high-intensity focused ultrasound on human prostate cancer in vivo. *Cancer Res* 1995;55:3346.
99. Beerlage HP, van Leenders GJ, Oosterhof GO, et al. High-intensity focused ultrasound (HIFU) followed after one to two weeks by radical retropubic prostatectomy: results of a prospective study. *Prostate* 1999;39:41.
100. Zlotta AR, Djavan B, Matos C, et al. Percutaneous transperineal radiofrequency ablation of prostate tumour: safety, feasibility and pathological effects of human prostate cancer. *Br J Urol* 1998;81:265.
101. Gelet A, Chapelon JY, Bouvier R, et al. Local control of prostate cancer by transrectal high intensity focused ultrasound therapy: preliminary results. *J Urol* 1999;161:156.
102. Long JP, Fallick ML, LaRock DR, et al. Preliminary outcomes following cryosurgical ablation of the prostate in patients with clinically localized prostate carcinoma. *J Urol* 1998;159:477.
103. Grampas SA, Miller GJ, Crawford ED. Salvage radical prostatectomy after failed transperineal cryotherapy: histologic findings from prostate whole-mount specimens correlated with intraoperative transrectal ultrasound images. *Urology* 1995;45:936.
104. Pisters LL, Dinney CP, Pettaway CA, et al. A feasibility study of cryotherapy followed by radical prostatectomy for locally advanced prostate cancer. *J Urol* 1999;161:509.
105. Partin AW, Pound CR, Clemens JQ, et al. Prostate-specific antigen after anatomic radical prostatectomy: the Johns Hopkins experience after ten years. *Urol Clin North Am* 1993;20:713.
106. Zincke H, Oesterline JE, Blute ML, et al. Long-term (15 years) results after radical prostatectomy for clinically local-

ized (stage T2c or lower) prostate cancer. *J Urol* 1994;152: 1850.

107. D'Amico AV, Whittington R, Malkowicz SB, et al. A multivariate analysis of clinical and pathological factors that predict for prostate specific antigen failure after radical prostatectomy for prostate cancer. *J Urol* 1995;154: 131.
108. Zietman AL, Edelstein RA, Coen JJ, et al. Radical prostatectomy for adenocarcinoma of the prostate: the influence of preoperative and pathologic findings on biochemical disease-free outcome. *Urology* 1994;43:828.
109. Catalona WJ, Smith DJ. Five-year tumor recurrence rates after anatomic radical retropubic prostatectomy for prostate cancer. *J Urol* 1994;152:1837.
110. Ohori M, Goad JR, Wheeler TM, et al. Can radical prostatectomy alter the progression of poorly differentiated prostate cancer? *J Urol* 1994;152:1843.
111. Presti JC Jr., Shinohara K, Bacchetti P, et al. Positive fraction of systematic biopsies predicts risk of relapse after radical prostatectomy. *Urology* 1998;52:1079.
112. Epstein JI, Pizov G, Walsh PC. Correlation of pathologic findings with progression after radical retropubic prostatectomy. *Cancer* 1993;71:3582.
113. Epstein JI, Partin AW, Sauvageot J, et al. Prediction of progression following radical prostatectomy: a multivariate analysis of 721 men with long-term follow-up. *Am J Surg Pathol* 1996;20:286.
114. Epstein JI, Carmichael MJ, Pizov G, et al. Influence of capsular penetration on progression following radical prostatectomy: a study of 196 cases with long-term follow-up. *J Urol* 1993;150:135.
115. Ohori M, Wheeler TM, Kattan MW, et al. Prognostic significance of positive surgical margins in radical prostatectomy specimens. *J Urol* 1995;154:1818.
116. Montie JE. Significance and treatment of positive margins or seminal vesicle invasion after radical prostatectomy. *Urol Clin North Am* 1990;17:803.
117. Carmichael MJ, Veltri RW, Partin AW, et al. Deoxyribonucleic acid ploidy analysis as a predictor of recurrence following radical prostatectomy for stage T2 disease. *J Urol* 1995;153:1015.

37

SALVAGE RADIATION AFTER RADICAL PROSTATECTOMY

WILLIAM U. SHIPLEY
ANTHONY L. ZIETMAN

For men with pathologic stage T1 and T2 prostate cancer, the incidence of residual disease within the tumor bed is low, and the probability of a surgical cure is high. Unfortunately, extracapsular disease (pathologic stage T3 [pT3]) is commonly found in the final pathologic specimen of these men (1), because the uncertainty inherent in clinical and radiologic evaluations makes it difficult to determine with precision those individuals with organ-confined disease. Surgical series suggest that only half of all men with clinical stage T1-2 prostate cancer have organ-confined disease at surgery (2–7). The higher the tumor stage, the greater the likelihood that clinical staging will prove to be an underestimate. Up to 26% of patients with clinical T1c disease will ultimately prove to have extracapsular disease, compared with 33% of patients with clinical T2a disease and 68% of those with clinical T2b-c disease (3,6).

Men with pT3 disease are at higher risk for local and distant relapse than are those with organ-confined disease, but the degree of risk varies with histologic feature and the presence or absence of detectable postoperative serum prostate-specific antigen (PSA) level. Not all patients with pT3 disease need or are good candidates for postprostatectomy radiation therapy. Defining the optimal therapy for these patients requires clear answers to the following important questions:

1. Is it possible to predict which men are at particular risk for local rather than distant failure?
2. If so, can immediate adjuvant local irradiation prevent a predictable postoperative rise in PSA level?
3. Can salvage irradiation effectively suppress a PSA level that has already begun to rise?
4. Is immediate adjuvant irradiation any more effective than deferring radiation until a relapse is detected?

Although the rates of radical prostatectomy have declined somewhat from a high of 206 per 100,000 men in 1992, the overall fall in rates obscures important age-related trends. The largest decrease has occurred among older men, dropping 51% in men 70 to 74 years of age and 71% in men 75 years of age or older. In contrast, prostatectomy rates in younger men increased between 1992 and 1995, rising 42% in men 45 to 49 years of age and 18% in men 50 to 54 years of age (8). The answers to the questions presented earlier are of utmost importance to all men who undergo prostatectomy as well as for the clinicians who will treat them. But they are especially important for the increasing number of younger men who face many years of life after prostatectomy, many of whom will be confronted with the troubling problem of what course to take when cancer recurs after prostatectomy.

FAILURE PATTERNS OF PATHOLOGIC T3 PATIENTS

Historic Clinical Outcome Studies

Extracapsular disease clearly increases the risk of local failure, with long-term studies reporting rates ranging 25% (9) and higher (Table 37-1). Myers and Fleming reported 10-year local recurrence figures of 46% when the capsule was "perforated" (6), whereas an actuarial analysis by Anscher and Prosnitz gave a risk of 51% at 10 years and 68% at 15 years (10,11). In the multivariate analysis performed by these investigators, the strongest independent predictors of local failure were positive surgical margins, high tumor grade, and an elevated serum acid phosphatase level. Capsular penetration alone did not have predictive value.

Seminal vesicle involvement also predicts recurrence. For local failure, Gibbons et al. (9) and Schellhammer (1) reported rates of 44% when seminal vesicles were involved. In an effort to disentangle seminal vesicle involvement from positive surgical margins, Anscher and Prosnitz used a multivariate analysis (11). They determined that seminal vesicle invasion was not an independent predictor for local

TABLE 37-1. CLINICAL LOCAL FAILURE RATES AFTER RADICAL PROSTATECTOMY WITH POSTOPERATIVE RADIATION IN THOSE JUDGED TO BE AT HIGH RISK: PT3, NO

	Surgery alone				Surgery + radiation therapy			
Primary author (ref)	n	5 yr (%)	10 yr (%)	15 yr (%)	n	5 yr (%)	10 yr (%)	15 yr (%)
Single-institution comparative studies								
Gibbons (9)	23	30	—	—	22	5	—	—
Anscher[a] (10)	113	25	51	68	46	4	4	4
Jacobson (33)	24	17	—	—	26	0	—	—
Shevlin[a] (41)	57	20	28	—	16	0	0	—
Ray (27)	—	—	—	—	13	23	—	—
Pilepich (36)	—	—	—	—	18	0	—	—
Forman[a] (25)	—	—	—	—	16	0	—	—
Hanks (26)	—	—	—	—	11	0	—	—
Lange (42)	—	—	—	—	24	0	—	—
Petrovich (34)	—	—	—	—	78	3	—	—

Note: Results of mature series.
[a]Actuarial data (all others crude rates).

failure but was the strongest predictor for distant metastasis. This fits with the grave prognosis that seminal vesicle invasion has long been recognized to carry—of 17 patients reported by Jewett et al. to have unsuspected seminal vesicle involvement, none was alive at 15 years (5). Thus, although the actuarial percentages for local failure may be high when the seminal vesicles are involved, the actual numbers are relatively low because of the substantial mortality due to distant metastasis or the introduction of androgen suppression when metastases arise.

Contemporary Prostate-Specific Antigen Outcome Studies

In recent years, PSA failure has come to be regarded as an early signal of failure and a trigger for subsequent therapy. Among patients with organ-confined disease, a steadily rising PSA is seen in less than 20% of cases. Among those with extensive extracapsular disease, positive margins, or seminal vesicle invasion, up to 75% may ultimately relapse (Table 37-2). A rising PSA level may signal one of three possibilities: the first sign of a local failure, metastatic disease, or local failure plus metastatic disease. Local therapy such as tumor bed irradiation can benefit only those patients with truly local disease, whereas a more global approach, such as androgen suppression, is called for when metastatic disease is present.

Although extraprostatic disease is classified as stage pT3, patients with extracapsular disease confined to the specimen may well differ from those with positive surgical margins. In one series from Duke University Medical Center, 68% of men with specimen-confined disease were biochemically free of disease at 4 years, compared with only 34% of those with positive margins, a group that comprised 23% of all prostatectomies (12). At Boston University Medical Center, only 25% of patients with positive margins were biochemically disease free at 5 years (13) (Fig. 37-1). Using a scrupulous step-sectioning process, the

TABLE 37-2. DISEASE-FREE SURVIVAL OF PT3, NO PATIENTS OVERALL

Institution (ref)	n	% of all RP pT3, N0	% pT3 + margins	% pT3 + SV	% Freedom from prostate-specific antigen failure
Receiving no adjuvant treatment					
Duke University (12)	124	55	43	46	51
UCLA (43)	230	50	NS	15	41
Boston University (13)	32	52	81	19	27
The Johns Hopkins University (17)	956	59	6 extensive	6	73 (+ margins, Gleason score <7)
			62 focal		30 (+ margins, ≥7)
Receiving adjuvant radiation therapy					
MGH (29)	40	—	85	30	81 (4 yr)
USC (31)	95	—	39	34	66 (5 yr)
Washington University (39)	40	—	NS	NS	75 (7 yr)

+ margin, positive surgical margin; MGH, Massachusetts General Hospital; NS, not stated; RP, radical prostatectomy; SV, seminal vesicle; UCLA, University of California, Los Angeles; USC, University of Southern California.

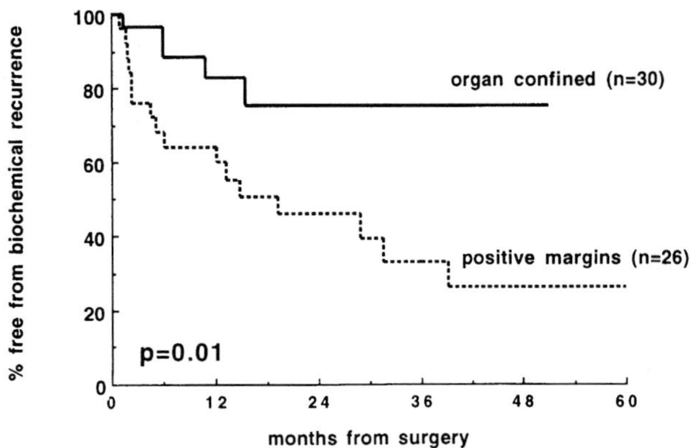

FIGURE 37-1. Freedom from subsequent failure by final pathologic stage for node-negative patients treated by radical prostatectomy at the Boston University Medical Center. (From Zietman AL, Edelstein RA, Coen JJ, et al. Radical prostatectomy for adenocarcinoma of the prostate: the influence of preoperative and pathologic findings on biochemical disease-free outcome. *Urology* 1994;43:828, with permission.)

Johns Hopkins and Stanford groups have drawn a prognostic distinction between focal and extensive positive margins that may prove useful in further refining the subgroup at particular risk of relapse (14–17). This work suggests that the high proportion of patients with focally positive margins has a 40% risk of progression at 5 years, compared to the smaller proportion of patients with extensively positive margins who face a 65% risk of progression. These numbers are reflected in the failure rate of men with positive margins in the Duke and Boston University series, in which such distinctions were not made. The very low incidence of extensively positive margins at Johns Hopkins is the consequence of good case selection—relatively few patients with bulky disease, high-grade disease, or high preoperative PSA values undergo radical prostatectomy.

There is considerable overlap in risk among men with positive margins and men with extensive extracapsular disease. For patients with "established" extracapsular disease regardless of margin status, Partin et al. showed only 20% freedom from relapse, although those with positive margins failed significantly faster (16,18). In addition to extraprostatic involvement, high Gleason sum (7 or greater) is a powerful predictor of PSA failure.

The timing and rate of rise of the PSA level after surgery may be used to distinguish occult local failure from occult distant failure. Of 51 postprostatectomy patients who were followed from an increase in PSA level to the development of clinical failure, 16 (31%) developed local disease and 35 (69%) distant disease (19). If the 21 patients with positive lymph nodes (all of whom developed distant failure) were excluded, then 53% developed local disease and 47% developed distant disease. At the time of local failure, the average PSA level was only 7 ng per mL, compared to 123 ng per mL at the time of distant failure.

Contemporary Rebiopsy Series

Certain pathologic features are clearly associated with PSA failure. The source of this PSA may well be residual disease in the prostatic fossa. Evidence supporting this comes from studies in which systematic attempts have been made to rebiopsy the fossa. In a study of 63 men with postoperative PSA elevations, Lange determined that only six had distant metastases determined by bone or computed tomography (CT), and 40% of the remaining 57 had positive biopsies at the urethrovesical junction (20). Of 30 men with a normal PSA level, none had positive biopsies. Lange's group also reported that pelvic radiotherapy reduced PSA levels in 80% of those who received it; PSA levels fell to undetectable levels in 53% (21). This study offers solid evidence that a substantial proportion of men with elevated postoperative PSA levels have residual disease within the pelvis. Whether this is the *only* site of disease recurrence may be determined largely by the presence or absence of seminal vesicle invasion and the histologic grade.

In a later study of 114 men with rising PSA levels and no evidence of metastatic disease by bone and CT scan, Connolly et al. report that 54% had locally persistent/recurrent disease on careful rebiopsy. Of these, 20% had been reported as having organ-confined disease at the time of prostatectomy, and 66% had positive margins (22).

Pelvic irradiation is more likely to durably suppress PSA levels in the presence of positive margins than it is in the presence of seminal vesicle involvement, which seems to confirm the clinical suspicion that relapse is more often distant rather than local for patients with seminal vesicle involvement. Patients with nodal disease are at particularly high risk of dissemination and are not considered in this discussion.

RESULTS WITH POSTOPERATIVE SALVAGE RADIATION THERAPY FOR ISOLATED RISES IN PROSTATE-SPECIFIC ANTIGEN LEVELS

At many institutions, adjuvant irradiation is not routinely given to those at substantial risk of local failure on the grounds that routine adjuvant therapy would irradiate some men unlikely to benefit from it—namely, those with no disease and those with occult metastatic disease. It is reserved instead as salvage therapy if the PSA level should subsequently rise. Such a "wait and watch" policy has been made possible by the use of PSA criteria in defining relapse, which allows for faster detection and earlier treatment of failure. The timing and the rate of rise of postoperative PSA level may be used to discriminate between occult local failure and occult distant failure. In a study by Partin et al., only 1 of 17 men with a rising PSA level in the first year after surgery went on to develop local failure (19). This increased to 9 of 23 in the second and third years and to 6 of 11 after the

TABLE 37-3. RESULTS OF SALVAGE IRRADIATION FOR PATIENTS WITH DETECTABLE PROSTATE-SPECIFIC ANTIGEN (PSA) LEVELS AFTER RADICAL PROSTATECTOMY AND NO RADIOLOGIC EVIDENCE OF METASTASES

Institution (ref)	n	Follow-up (median, yr)	% Freedom from PSA failure (yr)
Delayed rise in PSA level (initially undetectable)			
The Johns Hopkins University (44)	66	9	10 (5)
Washington University (44)	44	6.5	36 (6)
Mayo (AZ/FL) (45)	33	3.5	56 (5)
MGH (24)	25	3.5	35 (4)
Stanford (32)	13	2.5	54 (3)
Persistently detectable postoperative PSA level			
University of Minnesota (20)	15	>1.5	26 (2)
Stanford (32)	12[a]	2.5	8 (3)
Washington University (39)	22	6.5	18 (6)
MGH (24)	30	3.5	35 (4)
Mayo (AZ/FL) (45)	13	3.5	18 (5)
All detectable postoperative PSA levels (series not separating A from B)			
Washington University (39)	68	6.5	30 (6)
The Johns Hopkins University (17)	82[b]	9	10 (5)
Mayo (AZ/FL) (39)	121	3.5	45 (5)
MGH (24)	55	4	27 (5)
Wayne State (39)	82	2	60 (4)
UCSF (40)	34[b]	3	48 (3)
Duke (46)	53	1.3	26 (2)

MGH, Massachusetts General Hospital; UCSF, University of California, San Francisco.
[a]Seven of 12 were node positive.
[b]All biopsy-proven local recurrence.

third year. The majority (15 of 16) with local failure had a PSA velocity of less than 0.75 ng per mL per year.

A component of local failure is evident in a substantial proportion of men with isolated PSA rises after radical prostatectomy, with minimum estimates from rebiopsy studies of 40% to 54%. It is therefore no surprise that a majority of patients with a rising PSA level and a negative metastatic workup (usually isotope bone scan and pelvic CT scan) respond to local measures, such as salvage radiation (21). Whether the response is durable is the subject of much debate (Table 37-3). An early study by McCarthy et al. reported a high (68%) 3-year freedom from biochemical failure in men given salvage irradiation for isolated PSA failure (23). Although longer follow-up reveals a continued increase in failure, 36% of patients in this series remained biochemically disease free at 6 years. We have observed a similar phenomenon among patients at Massachusetts General Hospital (MGH)—1% of selected patients initially responded to radiation with PSA levels falling to less than 0.5 ng per mL, but this was maintained in only 27% at 5 years (24). It thus appears that salvage radiation therapy is effective in the long term only for a minority of treated patients.

McCarthy et al. noted that a lower proportion of durable responses was seen when the original pathology had shown organ-confined disease, as compared to those who had been pT3 (23). This suggests that the small number of patients with organ-confined disease who do relapse do so more commonly with metastatic disease.

Immediate Adjuvant or Salvage Irradiation?

The lively debate on the relative merits of immediate adjuvant radiation therapy versus delayed salvage irradiation is fueled by conflicting evidence on this topic. Historical studies suggest that beginning therapy after the appearance of gross local recurrence may be too late. In these studies, crude local control rates for locally recurrent tumors range from 58% to 100% at 5 years, with a mean of 70% (9,25–28). These data suggest, not surprisingly, that it is more difficult to control a gross recurrence than a microscopic residuum. At the MGH, fewer than 40% of men irradiated for palpable local recurrence of prostate cancer were biochemically disease free 2 years after irradiation (29). Equally dismal is clinical disease-free survival, with less than 20% survival 10 years after irradiation. Cure after gross local failure is thus most unlikely.

Three older long-term studies suggest a benefit of adjuvant irradiation in terms of clinical disease-free survival compared to historical controls with deferred salvage (10,30,31). However, these studies were generally performed before the use of PSA testing was common, and, thus, salvage therapy would not have been given until relatively late. Today, the widespread use of PSA levels in follow-up allows for earlier detection of failure and thus may reduce the impact of deferred irradiation.

Data from a number of studies suggests that durable suppression of PSA level is inversely related to the PSA level at the time of irradiation (Table 37-4). This can be explained two ways: First, the PSA level correlates with local tumor volume and the probability of metastases. Allowing a tumor to regrow locally to a significant size also allows a second chance for metastasis to occur. Second, the PSA level at the time of radiation may reflect the rate of rise, with early rapid rises correlated far more strongly with ultimate metastasis than with clinical local failure (19).

Persistently Detectable Prostate-Specific Antigen Levels after Prostatectomy

Patients whose PSA levels do not decline to undetectable levels after prostatectomy comprise a subgroup with a particularly poor prognosis (Table 37-3). Although this may reflect a large bulk left within the tumor bed, it more likely represents the presence of metastatic disease. In the series of

TABLE 37-4. RELATIONSHIP BETWEEN PROSTATE-SPECIFIC ANTIGEN (PSA) VALUE AT THE TIME OF SALVAGE IRRADIATION AND THE LIKELIHOOD OF DISEASE CONTROL

Institution (ref)	n	Follow-up (yr)	PSA at time of irradiation	% Freedom from PSA failure
Stanford (32)	21	2.5	<3[a]	89
			>3	8
Mayo (AZ/FL) (45)	46	3.5	<1.1	76
			>1.1	26
MGH (24)	55	3.5	<1.7	66
			>1.7	29
UCSF (40)	34	3	<4	58
			>4	15
Wayne State (39)	82	2	<2	72
			>2	22
Duke (46)	53	1.3	<2.5	52
			>2.5	8

MGH, Massachusetts General Hospital; UCSF, University of California, San Francisco.
[a]Yang assay.

Partin et al., none of the patients with a PSA level detectable in the first 6 months after surgery developed local failure, whereas all of those observed without treatment went on to develop metastases (19). Lange et al. reported that only 26% of patients with detectable PSA levels after prostatectomy had durably depressed PSA levels after radiation (21), McCarthy et al. reported only 18% (23), and Link et al. saw a durable response in only 1 patient of 12 (32).

Although radiation may be offered to men whose PSA levels fail to drop into the undetectable level after prostatectomy on the small chance of cure, the major clinical issue for them is whether to begin androgen deprivation early or on clinical relapse.

RADIATION TECHNIQUE

Target Volume

The careful ultrasound-guided rebiopsy studies reported by Connolly et al. clearly document the likely sites of local failure in the perianastomotic region 66% of the time, usually posterior or lateral; at the bladder neck in 16% of cases; and within the retrovesical space in 13% (22). This relatively small area makes up the target volume for salvage or adjuvant radiation (Fig. 37-2). There is no need for elective pelvic radiation, because lymph nodes in this region were sampled during prostatectomy and found negative. Larger nodal fields would greatly increase the morbidity of postoperative treatment.

Radiation Dose and Morbidity

An appropriate concern of urologic surgeons is that postoperative radiotherapy will interfere with healing and thus exacerbate complications such as incontinence, stricture formation, impotence, and edema. Several reports now testify that doses of 60 to 65 Gy, which give excellent local control, have an acceptably low risk of complications (9,10,24–26,33–37).

In most comparative studies, adjuvant radiotherapy does not increase the incidence of incontinence or stricture, both of which run between 5% and 15%. Meticulous morbidity data, compiled and reported by the University of Southern California (USC) group, compare 95 irradiated patients with 293 who were not irradiated over the same time period (31). Perfect continence or only mild stress incontinence was achieved in 87% of those irradiated and 88% of those not irradiated, and no urethral strictures were seen in either group. In a European randomized trial of 52 men undergoing radical prostatectomy alone and 48 receiving adjuvant radiation, no difference in continence rates were observed, with 83% and 77% totally dry, respectively (38).

In the USC series, adjuvant radiation therapy did reduce potency rates, with only 18% of men who underwent nerve-sparing prostatectomy and adjuvant irradiation retaining potency sufficient for intercourse compared to 46% of the unirradiated patients. At Washington University, adjuvant irradiation was associated with a 50% or higher reduction in potency (39). In an effort to moderate the impact of adjuvant irradiation on potency, the USC group has been using radiation doses lower than those used at the MGH (45 to 55 Gy vs. 60 to 64 Gy). Elsewhere, men who wish to remain sexually active are being offered the option of having the pump and reservoir components of an inflatable penile prosthesis implanted during prostatectomy.

Edema of the genitals and lower limbs was once believed to be more common with adjuvant or salvage irradiation, with reports of incidence between 0% and 21% (median, 9%). Edema was most common when pelvic irradiation was given to patients who had had pelvic lymphadenectomies or treatment with high radiation doses via cobalt machines (27,33). With awareness of these risk factors, the incidence of radiation-associated edema has been reduced to near zero in a number of reports (9,24,34,36). Bowel complications, usually grade 1 to 2 rectal bleeding, are also uncommon, with a reported incidence of 0% to 12% (median, 4%).

Schild et al. and Forman et al. have reported (39) that radiation doses greater than 65 Gy may be more effective than lower doses for tumor eradication (40). Although both of these small series reported little morbidity, the median follow-up was relatively short. Doses above 65 Gy raise increasing concerns about complications that may take years to develop, particularly involving the bladder.

The optimal dose for salvage irradiation of the prostatic bed is the one that maximizes tumor control with the minimum of morbidity. Outside of a protocol setting, the recommended dose is 64 to 66 Gy with conventional fractionation.

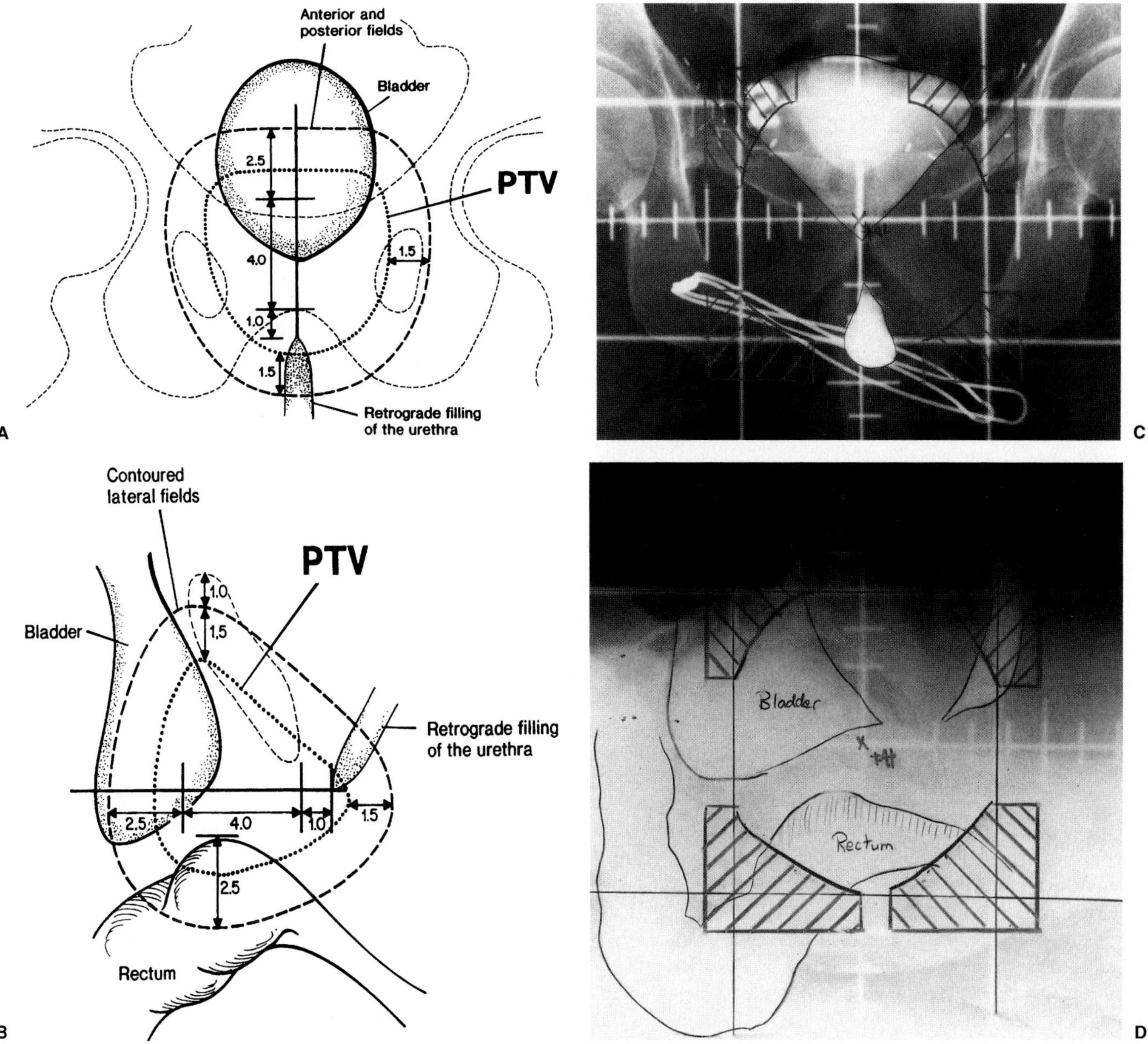

FIGURE 37-2. **A** and **B:** Schematic diagrams showing anteroposterior and lateral fields used to deliver radiation therapy after radical prostatectomy. **C** and **D:** Anteroposterior and lateral simulation films corresponding to **(A)** and **(B)**. Rectal barium, a cystogram, and a urethrogram are routinely used to define target and nontarget structures. PTV, planning target volume.

CANDIDATES FOR SALVAGE IRRADIATION

Among patients with a detectable PSA level after radical prostatectomy and no radiologic evidence of metastases, our experience has shown that salvage radiation therapy has a higher chance of success when (Fig. 37-3)

- Initial pathology shows positive surgical margins.
- Initial pathology shows no seminal vesicle invasion.
- PSA level is low (less than 2 to 3 ng per mL).
- PSA level begins rising more than 1 year after surgery.
- Rate of rise in PSA level is slow.

Salvage radiation therapy has a lower chance of success when

- Initial pathology shows seminal vesicle invasion.
- Initial pathology shows organ-confined tumor.
- Initial pathology shows Gleason score 8 to 10 tumor.
- PSA level is high (greater than 2 to 3 ng per mL).
- PSA level is persistently detectable after surgery.
- Rate of rise in PSA level is rapid.

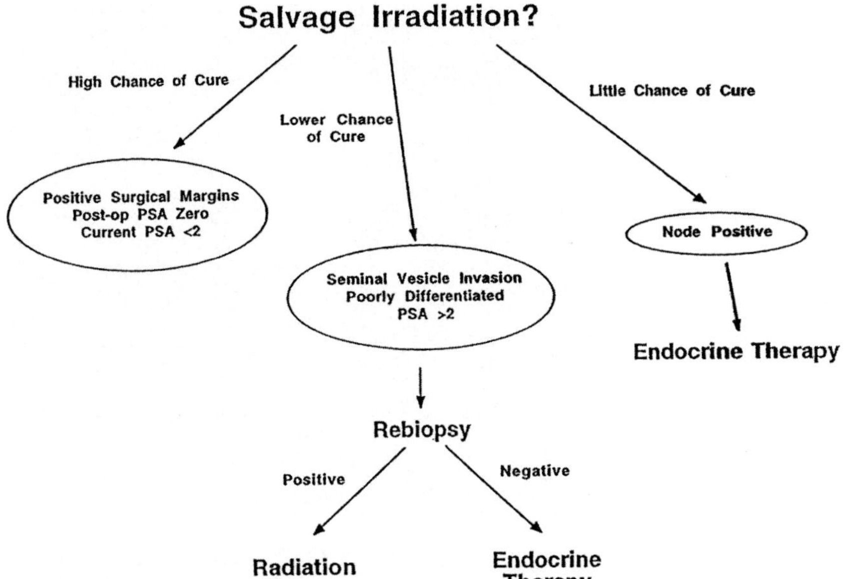

FIGURE 37-3. Schema to determine which patients with isolated late rises in serum prostate-specific antigen (PSA) after radical prostatectomy may benefit from salvage irradiation. Post-op, postoperative.

To help identify suitable candidates for salvage irradiation, ultrasound-guided biopsy of the prostatic bed or indium-111–labeled cyt-356 scintigraphy may be used. Negative results from this test, however, should not preclude irradiation if other criteria strongly suggest locally recurrent disease. Biopsy results may be of more benefit in deciding between radiation and endocrine therapy for those individuals in whom the success of salvage radiation is likely to be low.

An open study randomizing men with postoperative PSA values between 0.2 and 4.0 ng per mL to salvage radiation with or without long-term androgen deprivation using high-dose bicalutamide is currently being conducted by the Radiation Therapy Oncology Group (96-01). The dual aims of this trial are to obtain a valid and prospectively gathered measure of the efficacy of salvage radiation and to answer an important question about the value of early androgen deprivation.

AMERICAN SOCIETY FOR THERAPEUTIC RADIOLOGY AND ONCOLOGY RECOMMENDATIONS

A consensus panel convened by the American Society for Therapeutic Radiology and Oncology in 1997 examined the use of radiation therapy among men with a rising PSA level after radical prostatectomy. The panelists considered relevant data from four institutions that had experience (published and unpublished) in treating men with this presentation and also cross examined the presenters. The four institutions and presenters included MGH, Anthony L. Zietman, M.D.; Washington University School of Medicine, M'Liss A. Hudson, M.D.; Mayo Clinic of Scottsdale, Arizona, Steven A. Schild, M.D.; and Wayne State University, Jeffrey D. Forman, M.D. Follow-up in these four series ranged from a median of 2.0 years to 5.5 years. The consensus statement from the panel, published in full in the *Journal of Clinical Oncology* (39), is reproduced below:

- The rate of complete biochemical remission depends on patient selection. In the data presented to the consensus panel, approximately 70% of patients had complete PSA remission after salvage radiation. The data were insufficient, however, to judge the durability of this remission, with actuarial biochemical failure-free survival rates at 5 years ranging from 27% to 45%.
- Among prostatectomy patients for who pathology findings indicate a high probability of local cure, waiting for secure evidence of biochemical failure (PSA level rising to 0.5 mg per mL) likely does not reduce the chances of successful salvage irradiation. In fact, waiting until the PSA level begins rising affords solid evidence of a true relapse that requires further therapy. The panel noted that the PSA level at the time of salvage irradiation may make a difference in outcome, with better results occurring before a PSA threshold of 1.5 ng per mL.
- The panel concluded that there are, at present, no subgroups of patients (based on preprostatectomy PSA level or pathologic findings from the prostatectomy specimen) for who salvage radiation therapy is clearly more or less effective.
- It is justifiable to give the highest radiation dose possible that does not cause morbidity. Based on data presented at the conference, an effective dose is 64 Gy or slightly higher with standard fractionation (1.8 to 2.0 Gy per fraction).
- To date, the impact of androgen suppression among patients with or without radiation therapy after prostatectomy is unclear, and, in this setting, it should be considered investigational.

CONCLUSION

When radical prostatectomy fails to cure prostate cancer, salvage radiation therapy is an option for some men. The type of patient for whom salvage radiation appears most promising is a man whose pathologic specimen shows positive surgical margins but no seminal vesicle invasion, PSA level begins rising more than 1 year after surgery and rate of rise is slow, and PSA level is below 3 ng per mL.

Logically, it seems that postprostatectomy irradiation should offer the greatest benefit if performed when the residual tumor volume is at its smallest. This means treating men at greatest risk for subsequent local failure as soon as possible after surgery, possibly even before the PSA level becomes detectable. The difference between a good prognosis and a bad one often depends on a remarkably small difference in PSA level, somewhere between 1.0 and 4.0 ng per mL. If the follow-up policy is casual or the patient poorly compliant, then this window of opportunity—and thus the last chance for cure—may easily be missed. Until the ultrasensitive PSA assay becomes widely available, a policy of early treatment may, on balance, be safest.

REFERENCES

1. Schellhammer PF. Radical prostatectomy. Patterns of local failure and survival in 67 patients. *Urology* 1988;31:191–197.
2. Catalona WJ, Stein AJ. Staging errors in clinically localized prostatic cancer. *J Urol* 1982;127:452–456.
3. Catalona WJ, Smith DS. Cancer recurrence and survival rates after anatomic radical retropubic prostatectomy for prostate cancer: intermediate-term results. *J Urol* 1998;160: 2428–2434.
4. Eggleston JC, Walsh PC. Radical prostatectomy with preservation of sexual function: pathological findings in the first 100 cases. *J Urol* 1985;134:1146–1148.
5. Jewett HJ, Eggleston JC, Yawn DH. Radical prostatectomy in the management of carcinoma of the prostate: probable causes of some therapeutic failures. *J Urol* 1972;107:1034–1040.
6. Myers RP, Fleming TR. Course of localized adenocarcinoma of the prostate treated by radical prostatectomy. *Prostate* 1983;4:461–472.
7. Zincke H, Blute ML, Fallen MJ, et al. Radical prostatectomy for stage A adenocarcinoma of the prostate: staging errors and their implications for treatment recommendations and disease outcome. *J Urol* 1991;146:1053–1058.
8. Ellison LM, Heaney JA, Birkmeyer JD. Trends in the use of radical prostatectomy for treatment of prostate cancer. *Eff Clin Pract* 1999;2:228–233.
9. Gibbons RP, Cole BS, Richardson RG, et al. Adjuvant radiotherapy following radical prostatectomy: results and complications. *J Urol* 1986;135:65–68.
10. Anscher MS, Prosnitz LR. Postoperative radiotherapy for patients with carcinoma of the prostate undergoing radical prostatectomy with positive surgical margins, seminal vesicle involvement and/or penetration through the capsule. *J Urol* 1987;138:1407–1412.
11. Anscher MS, Prosnitz LR. Multivariate analysis of factors predicting local relapse after radical prostatectomy—possible indications for postoperative radiotherapy. *Int J Radiat Oncol Biol Phys* 1991;21:941–947.
12. Frazier HA, Robertson JE, Humphrey PA, et al. Is prostate specific antigen of clinical importance in evaluating outcome after radical prostatectomy? *J Urol* 1993;149:516–518.
13. Zietman AL, Edelstein RA, Coen JJ, et al. Radical prostatectomy for adenocarcinoma of the prostate: the influence of preoperative and pathologic findings on biochemical disease-free outcome. *Urology* 1994;43:828–833.
14. Epstein JI, Pizov G, Walsh PC. Correlation of pathologic findings with progression after radical retropubic prostatectomy. *Cancer* 1993;71:3582–3593.
15. McNeal JE, Villers AA, Redwine EA, et al. Capsular penetration in prostate cancer. Significance for natural history and treatment. *Am J Surg Pathol* 1990;14:240–247.
16. Partin AW, Borland RN, Epstein JI, et al. Influence of wide excision of the neurovascular bundle(s) on prognosis in men with clinically localized prostate cancer with established capsular penetration. *J Urol* 1993;150:142–146.
17. Pound CR, Partin AW, Epstein JI, et al. Prostate-specific antigen after anatomic radical retropubic prostatectomy. Patterns of recurrence and cancer control. *Urol Clin North Am* 1997;24:395–406.
18. Partin AW, Piantadosi S, Sanda MG, et al. Selection of men at high risk for disease recurrence for experimental adjuvant therapy following radical prostatectomy. *Urology* 1995;45: 831–838.
19. Partin AW, Pearson JD, Landis PK, et al. Evaluation of serum prostate-specific antigen velocity after radical prostatectomy to distinguish local recurrence from distant metastases. *Urology* 1994;43:649–659.
20. Lange PH. Prostate-specific antigen for staging prior to surgery and for early detection of recurrence after surgery. *Urol Clin North Am* 1990;17:813–817.
21. Lange PH, Lightner DJ, Medini E, et al. The effect of radiation therapy after radical prostatectomy in patients with elevated prostate specific antigen levels. *J Urol* 1990;144:927–932.
22. Connolly JA, Shinohara K, Presti JC Jr., et al. Local recurrence after radical prostatectomy: characteristics in size, location, and relationship to prostate-specific antigen and surgical margins. *Urology* 1996;47:225–231.
23. McCarthy JF, Catalona WJ, Hudson MA. Effect of radiation therapy on detectable serum prostate specific antigen levels following radical prostatectomy: early versus delayed treatment. *J Urol* 1994;151:1575–1578.
24. Morris MM, Dallow KC, Zietman AL, et al. Adjuvant and salvage irradiation following radical prostatectomy for prostate cancer. *Int J Radiat Oncol Biol Phys* 1997;38:731–736.
25. Forman JD, Wharam MD, Lee DJ, et al. Definitive radiotherapy following prostatectomy: results and complications. *Int J Radiat Oncol Biol Phys* 1986;12:185–189.
26. Hanks GE, Dawson AK. The role of external beam radiation therapy after prostatectomy for prostate cancer. *Cancer* 1986;58:2406–2410.
27. Ray GR, Bagshaw MA, Freiha F. External beam radiation salvage for residual or recurrent local tumor following radical prostatectomy. *J Urol* 1984;132:926–930.

28. Zietman AL, Shipley WU, Willett CG. Residual disease after radical surgery or radiation therapy for prostate cancer. Clinical significance and therapeutic implications. *Cancer* 1993;71:959–969.
29. Zietman AL, Coen JJ, Shipley WU, et al. Adjuvant irradiation after radical prostatectomy for adenocarcinoma of prostate: analysis of freedom from PSA failure. *Urology* 1993;42: 292–298.
30. Meier R, Mark R, St. Royal L, et al. Postoperative radiation therapy after radical prostatectomy for prostate carcinoma. *Cancer* 1992;70:1960–1966.
31. Freeman JA, Lieskovsky G, Cook DW, et al. Radical retropubic prostatectomy and postoperative adjuvant radiation for pathological stage C (PcN0) prostate cancer from 1976 to 1989: intermediate findings. *J Urol* 1993;149:1029–1034.
32. Link P, Freiha FS, Stamey TA. Adjuvant radiation therapy in patients with detectable prostate specific antigen following radical prostatectomy. *J Urol* 1991;145:532–534.
33. Jacobson GM, Smith JA Jr., Stewart JR. Postoperative radiation therapy for pathologic stage C prostate cancer. *Int J Radiat Oncol Biol Phys* 1987;13:1021–1024.
34. Petrovich Z, Lieskovsky G, Langholz B, et al. Radiotherapy following radical prostatectomy in patients with adenocarcinoma of the prostate. *Int J Radiat Oncol Biol Phys* 1991;21: 949–954.
35. Petrovich Z, Lieskovsky G, Langholz B, et al. Radical prostatectomy and postoperative irradiation in patients with pathological stage C (T3) carcinoma of the prostate. *Int J Radiat Oncol Biol Phys* 1998;40:139–147.
36. Pilepich MV, Walz BJ, Baglan RJ. Postoperative irradiation in carcinoma of the prostate. *Int J Radiat Oncol Biol Phys* 1984;10:1869–1873.
37. Valicenti RK, Gomella LG, Ismail M, et al. Durable efficacy of early postoperative radiation therapy for high-risk pT3N0 prostate cancer: the importance of radiation dose. *Urology* 1998;52:1034–1040.
38. Van Cangh PJ, Richard F, Lorge F, et al. Adjuvant radiation therapy does not cause urinary incontinence after radical prostatectomy: results of a prospective randomized study. *J Urol* 1998;159:164–166.
39. American Society for Therapeutic Radiology and Oncology (ASTRO) Consensus Panel. Consensus statements on radiation therapy of prostate cancer: guidelines for prostate rebiopsy after radiation and for radiation therapy with rising prostate-specific antigen levels after radical prostatectomy. *J Clin Oncol* 1999;17:1155–1163.
40. Rogers R, Grossfeld GD, Roach M 3rd, et al. Radiation therapy for the management of biopsy proved local recurrence after radical prostatectomy. *J Urol* 1998;160:1748–1753.
41. Shevlin BE, Mittal BB, Brand WN, et al. The role of adjuvant irradiation following primary prostatectomy, based on histopathologic extent of tumor. *Int J Radiat Oncol Biol Phys* 1989;16:1425–1430.
42. Lange PH, Moon TD, Narayan P, et al. Radiation therapy as adjuvant treatment after radical prostatectomy: patient tolerance and preliminary results. *J Urol* 1986;136:45–49.
43. Stein A, deKernion JB, Smith RB, et al. Prostate specific antigen levels after radical prostatectomy in patients with organ confined and locally extensive prostate cancer. *J Urol* 1992;147:942–946.
44. Cadeddu JA, Partin AW, DeWeese TL, et al. Long-term results of radiation therapy for prostate cancer recurrence following radical prostatectomy. *J Urol* 1998;159:173–177.
45. Schild SE, Buskirk SJ, Wong WW, et al. The use of radiotherapy for patients with isolated elevation of serum prostate specific antigen following radical prostatectomy. *J Urol* 1996;156:1725–1729.
46. Wu JJ, King SC, Montana GS, et al. The efficacy of postprostatectomy radiotherapy in patients with an isolated elevation of serum prostate-specific antigen. *Int J Radiat Oncol Biol Phys* 1995;32:317–323.

38

SYSTEMIC MANAGEMENT OF THE PATIENT WITH PROSTATE CANCER AND A RISING PROSTATE-SPECIFIC ANTIGEN AFTER DEFINITIVE TREATMENT

DEREK RAGHAVAN

Although prostate cancer is one of the most common malignancies in Western society, it has been shown that patients with this disease are underrepresented in participation in clinical trials (1). As a result, it is difficult to make definitive evidence-based statements about several issues in clinical management, including the timing of treatment. It is even difficult to establish what constitutes optimal therapy for several common clinical scenarios (2).

The debate regarding optimal primary treatment of localized prostate cancer has been addressed in sections IV and V. It is clear that several options of appropriate care are available, including radical surgery, external beam irradiation (with a range of technical variations), and brachytherapy. The possibility of watchful waiting is also widely practiced but remains controversial. The heterogeneity of prostate cancer with respect to presentation and natural history has fueled this controversy. Nevertheless, the fact that it appears safe to follow *some* patients with prostate cancer expectantly opens for discussion the issue of timing of treatment at relapse.

DEFINITION OF PROGRESSIVE DISEASE AFTER DEFINITIVE PRIMARY TREATMENT

Although there is no complete consensus regarding the definition of progressive cancer after primary therapy, this issue has been addressed to some extent. The American Society for Therapeutic Radiology and Oncology has published guidelines for the identification of failure of primary radiotherapy (3). The American Society for Therapeutic Radiology and Oncology panel concluded that

- Biochemical failure is not equivalent to clinical failure but does constitute an appropriate early end point for clinical trials.
- Three serial increases in prostate-specific antigen (PSA) constitute an appropriate definition of biochemical failure after radiotherapy.
- No specific definition of PSA failure has been proven to be a surrogate for clinical progression or survival.
- The nadir of PSA is a useful prognostic determinant, although no specific nadir level has been identified that defines likely success of treatment.

Clinical practice has defined that a nadir PSA level of less than 0.1 ng per mL is an appropriate end point after radical prostatectomy (4), and it generally appears that failure to achieve that nadir level correlates with subsequent relapses (5). There is no standard approach to follow-up after radical surgery. However, a recent survey of members of the American Urological Association revealed a wide spectrum of clinical practice but a general consensus that follow-up should consist of digital rectal examination, urinalysis, and PSA measurement three to four times in the first year, with reducing frequency in subsequent years (6). This is an interesting pattern in view of the previously documented lack of accuracy and reproducibility of digital rectal examination for prostate cancer in untreated patients (7). However, the true use of digital rectal examination after prostatectomy has not been studied in a structured fashion. In this survey, most urologists did not report the frequent use of more complex blood tests or imaging studies in the routine follow-up of their patients. Prior studies had confirmed a very limited role for routine radionuclide bone scintigraphy for surveillance after prostatectomy unless the PSA level is more than 30 to 40 ng per mL (8).

Although there are no specific guidelines that define failure of surgery, our usual practice is to define three serially rising, detectable levels of PSA as indicative of residual or reactivated prostate cancer. There has been

TABLE 38-1. FACTORS IN DECISION ON EARLY TREATMENT OF ASYMPTOMATIC RISING PROSTATE-SPECIFIC ANTIGEN (PSA)

Factor	Disease-free survival benefit	Overall survival benefit
Rate of rise of PSA	Yes	No?
Absolute level of PSA	Yes?	No?
Young age of patient (≤65 yr)	No	Yes?
Documented site(s) of disease	Yes	No?
Tumor grade	Yes	Yes?
Length of disease-free interval	Yes?	?
Serious intercurrent illnesses	?	No
Patient preference/anxiety	Yes	No

some controversy as to whether the rate of rise of PSA at the time of relapse after radical prostatectomy actually predicts the time of onset of clinical relapse (9,10). To date, studies that have assessed the use of perioperative sampling of circulating tumor cells via reverse transcriptase-polymerase chain reaction have not shown useful correlations with outcome, although the follow-up has been relatively short (11).

Analogous to the situation after radical radiotherapy, there is no consensus regarding the optimal timing of "salvage" treatment in this context (Table 38-1). However, many patients who have been attuned to meticulous PSA surveillance before and after prostatectomy find it unacceptable merely to watch and wait, believing that they are losing a chance for potential cure. If one believes that cure is still possible after failure of primary treatment, then this is a reasonable approach. However, given the relatively disappointing long-term results of salvage radiotherapy after failure of surgery or of the approaches to failed primary radiotherapy (12), this may not be a very realistic view.

ASSESSMENT OF THE PATIENT WITH RISING PROSTATE-SPECIFIC ANTIGEN AFTER DEFINITIVE LOCAL THERAPY

There are three dominant clinical patterns of relapse after local therapy: (a) locoregional relapse in the prostatic bed and adjacent tissues, (b) systemic failure, and (c) synchronous failure at both local and distant sites. In general, a relatively standard approach can be used for the assessment of patients with a rising PSA after local therapy irrespective of the modality that has been used initially. Although case selection bias often leads to patients with less extensive prostate cancer being selected for radical prostatectomy, the patterns of local relapse after surgery or radiotherapy can be approached in similar fashion. Clinical examination for evidence of local recurrence and distant spread is usually accompanied by biochemical assessment of circulating levels of PSA, serum alkaline phosphatase (13) and renal function, and measurement of hematologic indices for evidence of bone marrow involvement or anemia. Transrectal ultrasonography and biopsy may define the presence of local relapse (14) and may indicate the grade of the tumor, although sampling error can yield artifacts of interpretation. Of importance, a negative biopsy does not rule out the possibility of local recurrence, and we usually regard persistently rising serum PSA as an indicator of relapse, notwithstanding an inability to identify the actual site of recurrence. We do not usually perform a biopsy of the prostatic bed unless further local therapy is planned. D'Amico and Hanks have illustrated that the PSA doubling time is a relatively reliable predictor for the onset of clinical symptoms after failure of local therapy (15). We generally apply this concept regarding a sudden and dramatic change in the rate of rise of PSA as a relative indication to commence therapy.

Radionuclide bone scanning is often used to screen for bone metastases (16), although the yield for this test is relatively low in the asymptomatic patient, especially if the serum alkaline phosphatase is normal and the PSA is less than 5 ng per mL (17). In one series, bone scans were uniformly negative in patients who relapsed after radical prostatectomy in whom PSA levels were less than 40 ng per mL (18). In some programs, chest radiography and computed tomography scanning of the abdomen and pelvis are routinely used but are usually normal, unless the PSA is significantly elevated (i.e., unless neuroendocrine elements dominate the pattern of relapse). More recently, investigative protocols have suggested that the site of relapse may be identified by radionuclide scanning with radiolabeled antibodies against prostate-specific membrane antigen, the so-called ProstaScint scan (19) or by positron emission tomography scanning.

Similar considerations obtain in the patient with a rising PSA after radiotherapy, and, in general, the approach to restaging is similar. After radical radiotherapy, clinical assessment of the prostatic bed may be more difficult because of the posttreatment induration. Although transrectal ultrasound can identify a local mass, it is somewhat unreliable in distinguishing between postradiation scarring and local recurrence. In this situation biopsy may be helpful, although the biopsy after radiotherapy is often characterized by extensive fibrosis making interpretation more difficult.

If local relapse is identified after radiotherapy, then salvage prostatectomy may have a role in achieving cure, although the procedure has significant morbidity (12), as discussed elsewhere in this volume (Chapter 36). Conversely, salvage radiotherapy may achieve cure in up to 50% of cases after failure of radical prostatectomy (20,21). As a rising PSA after definitive local therapy is frequently a harbinger of systemic relapse, the current discussion is focused predominantly on options of systemic treatment for this problem.

TIMING AND IMPACT OF SYSTEMIC TREATMENT FOR LOCALIZED AND METASTATIC DISEASE: IS THIS A SURROGATE FOR TREATING EARLY RELAPSING DISEASE?

Studies of the Veterans Administration Cooperative Urological Research Group

The value of early systemic intervention for prostate cancer remains highly controversial. The early studies of the Veterans Administration Cooperative Urological Research Group (VACURG) were carried out before the availability of PSA as a surrogate of response and before the use of bone and computed tomography scans and other sophisticated staging techniques (22). Nevertheless, for patients with raised circulating levels of prostatic acid phosphatase or with radiologic or biopsy evidence of metastases, the VACURG conducted a trial (study 1) in which patients were randomly allocated to treatment by placebo, estrogens, orchiectomy plus placebo, or orchiectomy plus estrogens. In their initial report in 1967 with follow-up until 5 years, these investigators noted a slightly lower survival in the group treated with placebo, although this result did not achieve statistical significance. It is possible that the lack of a statistically significant difference was due to the relatively small number of cases treated, as each of the arms had only approximately 200 cases entered. With further follow-up to a maximum of 9 years, it became clear that the cancer-related outcomes were somewhat obscured by the proportion of cardiovascular deaths among patients treated with estrogens (23). If one considers only deaths from cancer, then a higher proportion of cancer-related deaths was found in the placebo-treated group, although the absolute differences were still relatively small. Of course, this can only be a hypothesis-generating approach, as retrospective subset analysis is flawed by a substantial potential to introduce bias.

The significance of the VACURG studies was furthermore obscured by the fact that investigators were allowed to change treatment—thus, if a patient progressed on placebo therapy, he could be treated with estrogens. It is therefore possible that some of the outcomes actually reflected the comparison of *early* versus *late* hormonal therapy rather than representing a true comparison of placebo versus hormone treatment. When reviewing the late results of their studies with follow-up until 12 years, Byar and Corle noted that the impact of cardiovascular deaths was less in patients with stage III–IV disease. However, this analysis did not make available the crude data or survival curves for patients with stage III–IV disease in each of the treatment subgroups (24).

In VACURG study 2, which compared placebo against three doses of estrogen, the lowest death rate from cancer among patients with stage N disease was found in the group treated with 5 mg diethylstilbestrol daily, although this group also had the highest cardiovascular mortality rate (23). With the increased availability of predicting morbidity from estrogen therapy as well as the potential to overcome such problems via prophylactic anticoagulation, the use of systemic estrogen therapy is being reevaluated and may even find a role in adjuvant treatment protocols.

Trials of the British Medical Research Council

More recently, the British Medical Research Council has reported the results of an important clinical trial assessing the timing of hormone therapy for advanced prostate cancer. In this study, patients with locally advanced and metastatic prostate cancer were randomly allocated to systemic hormonal therapy at the time of presentation or to a policy of observation with hormonal therapy at the time of onset of symptoms (25). A total of 938 patients was recruited, with follow-up information available on 934. Fifty-one patients on the delayed therapy arm died of causes other than cancer before the need to start treatment for cancer and thus were not subjected unnecessarily to the side effects of castration. Most of these patients were older than 70 years of age. A greater number of deaths and complications from cancer occurred in the deferred therapy group. Thus, at first reading, this study supports the early introduction of hormonal therapy—the actuarial cancer-specific survival for the group classified as nonmetastatic, treated early, was approximately 35% at 10 years, compared to approximately 20% for those in the delayed therapy group (survival estimates from published curves). However, overall survival curves for the two groups showed only a small difference owing to the proportion of cases who died of intercurrent disease before relapse (and thus before the initiation of hormonal therapy).

However, closer review raises important issues that could have an impact on the use of these data as a model for early intervention after relapse of primary therapy (3). The study was conducted in the United Kingdom, in which there is considerable rationing of health care resources. Even in the published paper, it was noted that some patients did not have access to radionuclide bone scans for the staging procedure. In the United Kingdom, access to health care is frequently delayed in the National Health System. This is particularly important, as the follow-up protocol for this trial was not symmetric for both treatment groups but rather was at the discretion of the investigators. Thus, there was a selection bias against the delayed group wherein these patients could have experienced delayed therapy for metastatic disease as a consequence of the random follow-up schedule and potential associated delays from the health system.

Also germane are data from a British Medical Research Council study that compared radiotherapy and orchiectomy alone and combined therapy for previously untreated patients with T2-T4 NxMo prostate cancer (26). In this study, 277 patients were randomly allocated to receive treatment between 1980 and 1985. Patients underwent staging tests that included a chest radiography and radionuclide bone scan, but lymph node staging was not required. Patients were excluded if prostatic acid phosphatase level was elevated but PSA was not measured. Once again, the incidence of metastases was higher in the group of patients treated with radiotherapy alone, but there was no statistically significant difference in survival between the groups. At first reading, this would imply no benefit for early hormonal therapy. However, it is emphasized that there were only approximately 90 cases in each group, severely limiting the power of the study to detect small but important differences. Of interest, although not statistically significant, the observed/expected death rate in the radiotherapy treated group was 1.19, compared to 0.94 for orchiectomy alone and 0.90 for combined therapy, although the median survival figures were all clustered at approximately 4 years. By contrast, there appeared to be an absolute deficit of survival of approximately 10% at 7 years for patients treated with radiotherapy alone, although this was not statistically significant. One potentially crucial flaw in the design of this important trial was the lack of standardization of radiotherapy dose and fractionation—this was left to the discretion of individual clinicians, and the publication did not even specify the range of dose and fractionation from the clinicians at 23 treatment centers. Given the clear evidence that radiation doses of less than 70 Gy yield substantially inferior local control and survival for stages T1 through T2 disease, it is possible that this could have influenced the worse results in this trial of therapy for stage T3 disease.

Scandinavian Urological Collaborative Group

Similar data were reported by a Scandinavian collaborative group that assessed the role of early hormonal therapy versus observation and salvage hormones for patients with previously untreated, localized prostate cancer (27). In this study, 285 men were randomized to receive estrogens, estramustine phosphate, or surveillance followed by endocrine therapy at progression. Because of a high cardiovascular complication rate, the trial was altered after 5 years to reduce the dose of estrogens. Similarly to many trials of that time, insufficient patients were entered to allow definitive statements to be made for each trial subgroup. Nevertheless, a trend in favor of early hormonal therapy was noted with respect to the probability of developing metastases and death from prostate cancer. Analogous to the VACURG study, the impact of protection on death from prostate cancer was substantially reduced by the prevalence of deaths from cardiovascular disease in the early treatment groups, and the overall conclusion was that there was no significant saving of life from the early introduction of hormone therapy.

National Prostatic Cancer Project

The National Prostatic Cancer Project has also addressed the role of systemic treatment for localized prostate cancer but with an emphasis on early use of cytotoxics rather than hormonal therapy (28). In these trials, patients underwent open bilateral pelvic lymph node dissection followed by radical prostatectomy or cryosurgery (protocol 900) or radiotherapy (protocol 1000). Patients were then randomized to receive adjuvant cyclophosphamide, estramustine, or observation. With an average follow-up of 11 years (range, 7 to 14 years), these studies showed prolonged disease-free survival from adjuvant estramustine therapy for patients treated by radiotherapy but with a less clear impact in the surgically treated groups. It appears that there was no significant impact on overall survival. A subsequent report in a non–peer-reviewed publication provided follow-up at a mean of 14.3 years (range, 11 to 18 years), confirmed the previous findings, and emphasized that the greatest impact on progression-free survival was found in lymph-node–positive cases (29).

Systemic Hormones for Locally Extensive Disease: Is There a Survival Benefit?

The primary management of locally extensive prostate cancer (stage C or T3) is predicated on biologic considerations that are similar to those that obtain for the first locoregional relapse after primary therapy. The tumors share characteristics of increased robustness, decreased differentiation, aneuploidy, and an increased propensity for occult metastasis.

For patients with more extensive nonmetastatic prostate cancer, there appears to be a general consensus that systemic hormonal therapy adds to the impact of radiotherapy (30–32), although the issue of survival benefit is not yet resolved. Bolla et al. (30) have reported that prolonged adjunctive therapy with hormones confers a survival benefit, whereas the study reported in manuscript form by the Radiation Therapy and Oncology Group (RTOG) has shown only a disease-free survival benefit thus far (31). However, at the Annual Scientific Meeting of the American Society of Clinical Oncology in May 2000, the RTOG updated their data to show an overall survival benefit from combined therapy for some categories of prostate cancer, although this analysis is flawed owing to its emphasis on retrospective subsets (33). A similar survival benefit from the combination of systemic hormonal therapy and prostatectomy has not yet been demonstrated in any study (34,35), despite evidence of downstaging after neoadjuvant hormonal therapy (36–38). This difference may be explained by the differences in the duration of hormonal therapy, as the majority of studies involving combined radiotherapy and hormones has used longer schedules of hormone suppression. Nevertheless, it also suggests that early systemic treatment is not a panacea for early prostate cancer.

These issues are of importance, as they provide some of the surrogate information regarding timing of treatment. In the absence of specific data from relevant clinical trials of salvage treatment after failure of local treatment (radiotherapy and prostatectomy), some information can also be gained from studies assessing the use of early systemic therapy in other contexts.

WHAT ARE THE IMPLICATIONS FOR MANAGEMENT OF RELAPSING PROSTATE CANCER AFTER LOCAL THERAPY?

The critical issue in deciding on when to start treatment for the patient with asymptomatic rising PSA is to define whether the proposed intervention will improve overall survival or quality of life. It makes intuitive sense that early therapy is likely to impact on disease-free survival. This can certainly contribute to improved quality of life, provided that the side effects of therapy do not counterbalance this benefit. For example, it is difficult to balance the respective weighting of reduced anxiety due to a falling PSA level versus increased anxiety regarding impaired sexuality due to hormonal therapy.

The synthesis of the data presented previously is highly complex and reflects the heterogeneity of patient populations, trial design, and relatively short follow-up of these trials in many instances. No randomized trial data are available to allow dissection of the impact of case selection bias and lead-time bias in evaluating the nonrandomized trials in the literature. Case selection bias may occur owing to the nature of the patient and tumor involved in trials of early intervention—for example, the better-educated, more health conscious patient responding quickly to a rising PSA. Lead-time bias can occur in the following way: The identification of rising PSA allows the documentation of relapsing occult disease followed by early treatment but without actually lengthening absolute life expectancy (compared to the course of events if treatment had been withheld until symptoms had identified the recurrence).

On balance, genuine equipoise still exists, and there is no simple answer to resolve questions regarding the timing and necessity of treatment for asymptomatic rising PSA. The trials reported earlier clearly do not provide a consistent set of data regarding the use of early hormonal intervention or other systemic therapy. It is clear that early hormonal therapy is associated with earlier onset of symptoms and toxicity; the potential for development of late complications, such as osteoporosis; and prolongation of disease-free interval. What is not clear is whether early systemic therapy (with hormones or cytotoxics) actually confers an overall survival benefit. At present, it seems most likely that early intervention does not improve overall survival provided that a patient is under scrutiny, with assessment of evolving tumor progression and the potential complications of that process.

FUTURE TRIALS

The pattern of relapse after local therapy is predictable, based on a series of prognostic factors, such as advanced T stage, high grade, and PSA (see chapters 16 through 20). Using these prognostic factors to identify high-risk cases, many of the cooperative cancer trial groups have designed trials that will help to resolve some of the uncertainties about optimal management of this problem. For example, the RTOG is currently assessing the use of bicalutamide (Casodex) when added to salvage radiotherapy for patients with rising PSA after failure of surgery for stage T3 prostate cancer (RTOG protocol 96-01). This group is also preparing studies focused on adjuvant treatment for patients at high risk of relapse. The National Cancer Institute of Canada and the Southwest Oncology Group are studying the use of intermittent androgen blockade in patients with rising PSA after definitive local radiotherapy (protocol JPR-7). Similarly, these groups are designing trials that will incorporate chemotherapy or bisphosphonates, or both, for the adjuvant treatment of patients after definitive therapy of high-risk disease.

REFERENCES

1. Chlebowski RT, Curti M, Lillington L. Trends in prostate and breast cancer clinical research as reported in the ASCO proceedings. *Proc Am Soc Clin Soc* 1999;18:315a.
2. Raghavan D. Prostate cancer management under scrutiny: one man's meta-analysis is another man's Poisson. *J Clin Oncol* 1999;17:3371–3373.
3. American Society for Therapeutic Radiology and Oncology Consensus Panel. Guidelines for PSA following radiation therapy. *Int J Radiat Oncol Biol Phys* 1997;37:1035–1041.
4. Takayama TK, Vessella RL, Brawer MK, et al. The enhanced detection of persistent disease after prostatectomy with a new prostate specific antigen immunoassay. *J Urol* 1993;150:374–378.
5. Cheng WS, Bergstralh EJ, Frydenberg M, et al. Prostate-specific antigen levels after radical prostatectomy and immediate adjuvant hormonal treatment for stage D1 prostate cancer are predictive of early disease outcome. *Eur Urol* 1994;25:189–193.
6. Oh J, Colberg JW, Ornstein DK, et al. Current followup strategies after radical prostatectomy: a survey of American Urological Association urologists. *J Urol* 1999;161:520–523.
7. Angulo JC, Montie JE, Bukowsky T, et al. Interobserver consistency of digital rectal examination in clinical staging of localized prostatic carcinoma. *Urol Oncol* 1995;1:199–205.
8. Cher ML, Bianco FJ, Lam JS, et al. Limited role of radionuclide bone scintigraphy in patients with prostate specific antigen elevations after radical prostatectomy. *J Urol* 1998;160:1387–1391.
9. Patel A, Dorey F, Franklin J, et al. Recurrence patterns after radical retropubic prostatectomy: clinical usefulness of prostate specific antigen doubling times and log slope prostate specific antigen. *J Urol* 1997;158:1441–1445.

10. Pruthi RS, Johnstone I, Tu I-P, et al. Prostate-specific antigen doubling times in patients who have failed radical prostatectomy: correlation with histologic characteristics of the primary cancer. *Urology* 1997;49:737–742.
11. Oefelein MG, Ignatoff JM, Clemens JQ, et al. Clinical and molecular followup after radical retropubic prostatectomy. *J Urol* 1999;162:307–311.
12. Zerati M, Pontes JE. Treatment of local failure of prostate cancer after radiotherapy and surgery. In: Raghavan D, Scher HI, Leibel SA, et al., eds. *Principles and practice of genitourinary oncology*. Philadelphia: Lippincott–Raven Publishers, 1997:567–571.
13. Urwin GH, Percival RC, Yates AJ, et al. Biochemical markers and skeletal metabolism in carcinoma of the prostate. *Br J Urol* 1985;57:711–714.
14. Fowler JE, Brooks J, Prabhakar P, et al. Variable histology of anastomotic biopsies with detectable prostate specific antigen after radical prostatectomy. *J Urol* 1995;153:1011–1014.
15. D'Amico AV, Hanks GE. Linear regressive analysis using prostate-specific antigen doubling time for predicting tumor biology and clinical outcome in prostate cancer. *Cancer* 1993;72:2638–2643.
16. Merrick MV, Ding CL, Chisholm GD, et al. Prognostic significance of alkaline and acid phosphatase and skeletal scintigraphy in carcinoma of the prostate. *Br J Urol* 1985;57: 715–721.
17. Miller PD, Eardley M, Kirby R. Prostate specific antigen and bone scan correlation in the staging and monitoring of patients with prostatic cancer. *Br J Urol* 1992;70:295–298.
18. Bianco FJ, Lam JS, Davis LP, et al. Limited role of radionuclide bone scan in patients with prostate cancer recurrence after radical prostatectomy. *J Urol* 1998;159:288.
19. Kahn D, Williams RD, Manyak MJ, et al. 111Indium-capromab pendetide in the evaluation of patients with residual or recurrent prostate cancer after radical prostatectomy. *J Urol* 1998;159:2041–2047.
20. Wu JJ, King SC, Montana GS, et al. The efficacy of post-prostatectomy radiotherapy in patients with an isolated elevation of serum prostate specific antigen. *Int J Radiat Oncol Biol Phys* 1995;32:317–323.
21. Forman JE, Meetze K, Pontes JE, et al. Therapeutic irradiation for patients with an elevated post-prostatectomy PSA level. *J Urol* 1997;158:1436–1440.
22. Veterans Administration Co-operative Urological Research Group. Treatment and survival of patients with cancer of the prostate. *Surg Gynecol Obstet* 1967;124:1011–1017.
23. Byar DP. The Veterans Administration Cooperative Urological Research Group's studies of cancer of the prostate. *Cancer* 1973;32:1126–1130.
24. Byar DP, Corle DK. Hormone therapy for prostate cancer: results of the Veterans Administration Cooperative Urological Research Group studies. *NCI Monogr* 1988;7:165–170.
25. Medical Research Council Prostate Cancer Working Party Investigators Group. Immediate versus deferred treatment for advanced prostatic cancer: initial results of the Medical Research Council trial. *Br J Urol* 1997;79:235–246.
26. Fellows GJ, Clark PB, Beynon LL, et al. Treatment of advanced localised prostatic cancer by orchiectomy, radiotherapy, or combined treatment. *Br J Urol* 1992;70:304–309.
27. Lundgren R, Nordle O, Josefsson K, et al. Immediate estrogen or estramustine phosphate therapy versus deferred endocrine treatment in nonmetastatic prostate cancer: a randomized multicenter study with 15 years of followup. *J Urol* 1995;153:1580–1586.
28. Schmidt JD, Gibbons RP, Murphy GP, et al. Adjuvant therapy for clinical localized prostate cancer treated with surgery or irradiation. *Eur Urol* 1996;29:425–433.
29. Schmidt JD, Gibbons RP, Murphy GP, et al. Adjuvant estramustine phosphate treatment for localized prostate cancer. *PPO Updates: Principles and Practice of Oncology*. Philadelphia: Lippincott 1997;11: 1–9.
30. Bolla M, Gonzalez D, Warde P, et al. Improved survival in patients with locally advanced prostate cancer treated with radiotherapy and goserelin. *N Engl J Med* 1997;337:295–300.
31. Pilepich MV, Sause WT, Shipley WU, et al. Androgen deprivation with radiation therapy compared with radiation therapy alone for locally advanced prostatic carcinoma. A randomized comparative trial of the Radiation Therapy Oncology Group. *Urology* 1995;45:616–623.
32. Granfors T, Modig H, Damber J-E, et al. Combined orchiectomy and external radiotherapy versus radiotherapy alone for nonmetastatic prostate cancer with or without pelvic lymph node involvement: a prospective randomized study. *J Urol* 1998;159:2030–2034.
33. Pilepich MV, Winter KA, Roach M, et al. Phase III Radiation Therapy Oncology Group (RTOG) trial 86-10 of androgen deprivation before and during radiotherapy in locally advanced carcinoma of the prostate. An updated report. *Proc Am Soc Clin Oncol* 2000 (*in press*).
34. Aprikian AG, Fair WR, Reuter VE, et al. Experience with neoadjuvant diethylstilboestrol and radical prostatectomy in patients with locally advanced prostate cancer. *Br J Urol* 1994;74:630–636.
35. Dalkin BL, Ahmann FR, Nagle R, et al. Randomized study of neoadjuvant testicular androgen ablation therapy before radical prostatectomy in men with clinically localized prostate cancer. *J Urol* 1996;155:1357–1360.
36. Goldenberg SL, Klotz LH, Srigley J, et al. Randomized, prospective, controlled study comparing radical prostatectomy alone and neoadjuvant androgen withdrawal in the treatment of localized prostate cancer. *J Urol* 1996;156: 873–877.
37. Van Poppel H, De Ridder D, Elgamal AA, et al. Neoadjuvant hormonal therapy before radical prostatectomy decreases the number of positive surgical margins in stage T2 prostate cancer: Interim results of a prospective randomized trial. *J Urol* 1995;154:429–434.
38. Soloway MS, Roohollah S, Wajsman Z, et al. Randomized prospective study comparing radical prostatectomy alone versus radical prostatectomy preceded by androgen blockage in clinical stage B2 (T2bNxMo) prostate cancer. *J Urol* 1995;154:424–428.

39

PROGNOSTIC FACTORS FOR RESPONSE AND SURVIVAL WITH HORMONE THERAPY

MENACHEM LAUFER
MARIO A. EISENBERGER

Metastatic prostate cancer is incurable by any therapeutic modality available at the present time; the clinical course is characteristically progressive and eventually fatal. Androgen deprivation treatment (ADT) remains the mainstay for the treatment of patients with metastatic disease. Extensive data derived from prospective trials have shown that the median survival of cohorts of patients with hormone-naïve metastatic disease has remained relatively stable from 1950 to 2000 (1–4). Although ADT results in major therapeutic benefits in approximately 80% of patients with metastasis, virtually all patients develop hormone refractory disease for which no treatment has shown to improve survival (5,6).

The purpose of this chapter is to describe and critically discuss the currently known prognostic factors for response and survival in hormone-naïve metastatic prostate cancer (TxNxM1). Data derived from prospectively randomized clinical trials have shown a marked heterogeneity in the outcome of these patients. A number of important disease and host-related factors have been shown to profoundly influence the outcome of patients with metastatic disease (7–9). Adequate characterization of such factors is critical for the design and interpretation of results of clinical trials and allows clinicians to plan their therapeutic approach based on a careful estimate of outcome in individual patients.

During the past several years, widespread clinical use of the prostate-specific antigen (PSA) test has provided the opportunity to identify evidence of disease activity before the development of overt clinical and radiologic signs and symptoms of metastasis. This resulted in a significant increase in the proportion of patients presenting with early stages of disease and at the same time a progressive reduction in the incidence of cases with newly diagnosed stage D2 disease (stage migration) (10). Similarly, treatment patterns have changed during the last decade as a result of PSA-based decisions for implementation of therapeutic interventions. Patients who demonstrate a rising serum PSA level as the only manifestation of disease activity are often initiated on ADT. This increasingly common treatment practice, although of unproven long-term benefit, has further contributed to a sharp decrease in the proportion of patients presenting with newly diagnosed stage D2 disease.

Several traditional clinical and laboratory parameters have been evaluated with regard to their prognostic role in patients with metastatic disease (11–24). In view of the changes in treatment practices, some of the traditional prognostic factors, such as performance status (PS), weight loss, and bone pain, are less commonly seen in current populations of hormone-naïve patients in whom ADT is instituted. A new set of prognostic clinical and especially laboratory factors, such as various measurements of serum PSA (e.g., different definitions of PSA velocity), other potential markers in the blood, as well as several tumor- and host-related molecular and biologic determinants, are likely to substitute for the more traditional clinical factors in the future.

The reports included in this review are based on the experience reported in patients enrolled in studies conducted over the past few decades (11–24). It is important to note that the studies illustrated herein used a whole spectrum of hormonal interventions that could explain some of the different findings in outcome reported with the same parameters. Methods of analysis also varied. A substantial amount of data is derived from prospectively analyzed data of large-scale randomized studies, but many reports represent a retrospective evaluation of uncontrolled data using multivariate analyses. With the previously mentioned caveats, the reader will be able to assess the wealth of information accumulated on prognostic factors in patients with metastatic disease over the years that undoubtedly remains clinically useful (Table 39-1).

TABLE 39-1. PROGNOSTIC FACTORS

Prognostic factor	Author (ref)	No. of M1/total	Outcome measure	*p* value	Source or type of therapy
T-stage of primary tumor	de Voogt et al. (13)	232/232	Survival	<.001	Two EORTC trials on 1976–1981
	Johansson et al. (14)	62/150	PFS	.04	Estrogen vs. orchiectomy (ORCH)
			Survival	.02	
	Sylvester et al. (12)	313/313	Survival	.006	EORTC 30853
Grade of primary tumor (WHO or Gleason)	Wilson et al. (20)	88/88	Survival	.002	ORCH or other Hx
	Veronesi et al. (16)	NR	Survival	NR	Buserelin
	Berner et al. (21)	116/116	Survival	NR	NR
	Miller et al. (29,39)	97/97	Survival	<.005	ORCH
	Oosterlinck et al. (24)	NA	PFS	NA	Combined androgen blockade (CAB)
	Sylvester et al. (12)	354/354	Survival	.003	EORTC 30843
	Furuya et al. (27)	139	NR	NR	NR
	Palmberg et al. (28)	236	Survival	NR	NR
Other cellular and molecular factors					
DNA ploidy	Miller et al. (29,39)	97/97	Survival	<.001	ORCH
c-erbB-2 expression	Morote et al. (31)	70/70	Survival	<.03	NR
Tissue PSA content	Stege et al. (32)	14/67	PFS	.001	ORCH/LHRH-A/estrogen
Acid phosphatase expression	Berner et al. (21)	116/116	Survival	NR	NR
Nuclear texture analysis	Jorgensen et al. (18)	262/262	Survival	<.001	Scandinavian ORCH vs. CAB
Lewis (x) adhesion molecule	Jorgensen et al. (18)	262/262	Survival	<.01	Scandinavian ORCH vs. CAB
Neuroendocrine differentiation	Di Sant'Agnese (35)	NA	PFS and survival	NA	Multiple series
Androgen receptor content	Takeda et al. (33)	62/62	PFS and survival	NR	NR
Extent of bone disease (semiquantitative grading)	Ishikawa et al. (37)	110/110	PFS	.05	Multiple hormonal interventions
	Ernst et al. (22)	162/162	Survival	.003	Multiple hormonal combinations
	Lukkarinen et al. (17)	NA/82	PFS	<.00001	LHRH-A
	Waaler et al. (19)	73/73	Survival	NR	NR
	Takeda et al. (33)	62/62	Survival PFS	NR	NR
Combined bone and soft tissue	Eisenberger et al. (11)	603/603	Survival	.03	INT 036, leuprolide vs. CAB
Performance status	Chodak et al. (8)	NR/240	Survival	NR	Goserelin vs. castration
	Sylvester et al. (12)	354/354	Survival	.0001	EORTC 30843
	Mulders et al. (15)	NR/175	NR	NR	NR
	Oosterlinck et al. (24)	N/A	PFS	n.s.	CAB
	Cipolla et al. (38)	43/43	PFS	NR	NR
Pain	Chodak et al. (8)	?/240	Survival	NR	Goserelin vs. castration
	Eisenberger et al. (11)	603/603	Survival	<.001	INT 0036
	Sylvester et al. (12)	313/313	Survival	.002	EORTC 30853
	Veronesi et al. (16)	NR	Survival	NR	Buserelin
Anemia	Eisenberger et al. (11)	603/603	Survival	.008	INT 0036
	Sylvester et al. (12)	313/313	Survival	.0001	EORTC 30853
	Mulders et al. (15)	NR/175	NR	NR	NR
	Jorgensen et al. (18)	262/262	Survival	<.05	Scandinavian ORCH vs. CAB
	Cipolla et al. (38)	43/43	PFS	.006	NR
			Survival	.02	NR
PSA	Cooper et al. (39a)	60/60	Survival	NR	Preliminary of EORTC 30853
	Matzkin et al. (30)	57/57	PFS	<.001	Several Hx combinations
Acid phosphatase	Lukkarinen et al. (17)	NA/82	PFS	<.005	LHRH-A
	Waaler et al. (19)	73/73	Survival	NR	NR

EORTC, European Organization for Research and Treatment of Cancer; Hx, history; INT, intermediate; LHRH-A, luteinizing hormone releasing hormone antigen; NA, not applicable; NR, not reported; n.s., not significant; PFS, progression-free survival; PSA, prostate-specific antigen; WHO, World Health Organization.

CLINICAL END POINTS: CONTEMPORARY ISSUES

Target End Points Response, Progression, and Survival

The most commonly targeted end point in prognostic factor analyses is overall survival or cancer-specific survival. Indeed, the majority of the reports in this review evaluated various clinical and laboratory factors as predictors of survival. Other less frequently used end points include response to treatment, duration of response or progression-free survival, or both. In prostate cancer, it is recognized that the assessment of response and progression in patients with metastatic disease is usually confounded by the well-known inherent difficulties to reliably quantify the status of disease in bone (25). Various reports correlated a variety of candidate prognostic factors with response-dependent end points, such as progression-free survival and duration of response, which are particularly troublesome in this disease for the reasons indicated earlier. Furthermore, even in other tumor types, in which assessments of response in measurable metastatic sites can be more reliably performed, the correlation between response and survival has not been conclusively established. With this in mind, the reader should recognize that no single definition of response has been adequately validated as a surrogate for survival, and, although the benefits derived from response to treatment are of clinical significance, it should be considered as a separate entity.

During the past several years, PSA changes have been commonly used as the main indicator of response to hormonal therapy in prostate cancer (26–30). The majority of the patients with hormone-naïve metastatic disease frequently demonstrate a dramatic decline in serum PSA after adequate gonadal ablation. As has been shown in recent studies, approximately 75% of patients with distant metastasis will demonstrate declines below 4 ng per mL (4). Exploratory retrospective analyses conducted by various investigators independently suggested that a variety of measurements of PSA declines of different durations and at various time points after ADT could predict for the magnitude of progression-free and overall survival. However, the correlation between PSA response and survival has not been conclusively validated in prospective randomized clinical trials (see later). The use of serum PSA in contemporary clinical trials has also affected the definition and timing of disease progression. Several studies in this review used non–PSA-driven criteria to define disease progression, and this should be differentiated from measurements relying on PSA-driven criteria. Data derived from current prospective trials involving ADT indicate that PSA relapses are observed almost invariably several months before other evidence of disease progression, such as new bone, soft tissue and/or visceral disease, or new symptoms (50).

TUMOR-RELATED PROGNOSTIC FACTORS

Tumor Stage

Tumor stage (clinical T category) at the start of the hormonal treatment was reported as an independent predictor of survival by three authors (12–14), whereas several others failed to demonstrate this relationship (17–21). All three studies indicating a positive relationship between T stage and survival were conducted before the availability of PSA, when a much larger proportion of patients had evidence of metastatic disease at the time of initial diagnosis. Proportions ranging from 60% to 75% of these patients were reported to present with T3-size lesions or higher, and most had no prior treatment given to their primary tumors. This is contrary to what is observed in contemporary series, in which most patients with prostate cancer present with evidence of localized or regional disease (10) and receive some type of local treatment that prevents adequate assessment of the prognostic role of local T stage when metastatic disease becomes evident.

Tumor Grade and Related Markers

The histologic grade tumors were investigated by numerous groups (9,12–28). The method of grading varied among the various reports; some used the original World Health Organization (WHO) system with three levels of differentiation, and more recent reports used primarily the Gleason grading system. Eight different reports, including a recent analysis of a large prospectively randomized study (European Organization for Research and Treatment of Cancer 30843), indicated that tumor grade is an independent prognostic factor (12,14,18–21,24,28,29). Interestingly, all these studies used the WHO grading system. One group actually compared the two grading systems and concluded that the WHO criteria were superior to the Gleason scoring system in predicting survival outcome in patients with metastatic disease (19). The data on histologic grading have not been reported in several of the largest contemporary studies, including the two large National Cancer Institute (NCI)–sponsored studies investigating the effects of complete androgen blockade (intergroup trials 0036 and 0105) (4,11).

Contrary to the compelling findings in early stages of prostate cancer, several studies reported no significant correlation between histologic grading and survival outcome in patients with metastatic disease (13–17,20). The explanation for this relatively unexpected finding and the difference in the results between studies in metastatic disease is unclear. It should be noted, however, that the only source of tissue available on these patients was the biopsy of the primary tumor or prostatectomy specimens many times obtained several years before the actual studies, which may not correspond to the grading of the metastatic disease. This is furthermore supported by the findings by Pound et al. (9) in their study on the natural history of patients with evidence of biochemical relapses after radical prostatectomy, indicating that the Gleason score of the primary tumors did not accurately predict the outcome of patients who subsequently demonstrated evidence of bone metastasis. It is well known that tumors often demonstrate changes in differentiation from their original pattern to higher grades at the time of progression. This may also explain the lack of relationship between the original grading pattern with the survival outcome of patients with metastatic disease measured from the time of development of metastasis.

Several investigators reported that various cellular and molecular markers, commonly used as outcome predictors in localized prostate cancer, might be useful in metastatic disease. Various prognostic factors in this group include DNA ploidy (29), chromatin texture by image analysis (18), expression of the adhesion molecules sialyl Lewis (x) (18), c-erbB-2 expression (31), tissue expression of PSA (32) or tissue prostatic acid phosphatase (PAP) (21), and androgen receptor content (33).

Uncommon histologic variants of prostate cancer, such as the presence of small cell carcinoma, and poorly differentiated tumors expressing neuroendocrine markers are believed to respond poorly to ADT, behave more aggressively, and are usually associated with poor prognosis (34,35).

EXTENT OF METASTATIC DISEASE

Minimal versus Extensive Disease

The prognostic significance of extent of disease (EOD) is well documented in prostate cancer (11). Two different methods of evaluating the EOD have been described in the literature. The NCI 0036 (11) and 0105 (4) trials (monotherapy vs. combined androgen blockade) stratified patients using a qualitative method based on bone and soft tissue involvement. *Minimal disease* is defined as axial skeleton involvement (pelvis and spine) or soft tissue nodal involvement, or both, whereas the extensive disease subset includes patients with appendicular skeleton (extremities, skull, ribs) or visceral involvement, or both. The distribution of disease sites has shown a relatively good correlation with the definition of EOD used. The vast majority of patients with extensive disease (more than 80%) demonstrated evidence of pelvic and axial skeleton involvement. The prognostic significance of EOD by this method was demonstrated in a retrospective analysis of the results of trial 0036 (11). Indeed, EOD was seen to be a significant predictor for survival in univariate analysis, was strongly associated with other important prognostic parameters, and, along with other prognostic factors, such as anemia, anorexia, weight loss, and bone pain, was among the significant factors on multivariate analyses (Cox hazard model) (11).

Other trials in stage D2 patients used a definition of EOD based on the number of positive areas on bone scan (12,36). Subgroups were empirically developed based on the number of metastatic lesions reported on bone scans. This semiquantitative method was retrospectively validated in the context of several trials with ADT, in which the necessary baseline bone scan information was available for adequate analysis (17,19,22,23,31).

HOST DISEASE INTERACTION

PS is one of the strongest predictors of outcome in metastatic prostate cancer (8,12,15,22,38). Some reports indicated that PS is significant in univariate but not in multivariate analysis, probably because this parameter is closely related to other established prognostic factors (18,25,37).

A variety of host factors have been shown to predict for survival outcome in studies conducted several years ago (11). It is important to recognize that currently, the impact of some of these factors is relatively minor primarily owing to patient selection. Among other significant parameters are anemia (12,17,20,38), pain (8,12,16), and the presence of co-morbidity (11,13). Age at diagnosis was widely investigated and was found by three authors to be an independent prognostic factor, using multivariate analysis (14,20,21). In these studies, younger patients usually present with a variety of other unfavorable findings, and it is generally agreed that the death hazard ratio in patients with ages far below the median of the population evaluated is indeed significantly increased. Age at diagnosis was widely investigated and was found by three authors to be an independent prognostic factor, using multivariate analysis (16,22,23). In these studies, younger age was associated with worse prognosis findings, and it is generally agreed that the death hazard ratio in patients with ages far below the median of the population evaluated is indeed significantly increased.

PRETREATMENT SERUM MARKERS

Serum Prostate-Specific Antigen

The significance of the pretreatment PSA value has been extensively evaluated as a prognostic factor in all stages of prostate cancer. Although in clinically localized prostate cancer there is clear correlation between PSA levels, volume and probability of organ-confined disease, and, consequently, outcome, this relationship in patients with metastatic disease is much less well defined. Cooper et al. (39a) found that pretreatment PSA was related to survival in a preliminary report on 60 patients enrolled in a large clinical trial. A "cutoff" level of 300 ng per mL discriminated between poor- and better-risk groups. Matzkin et al. (30), using a variety of hormonal interventions including single agent antiandrogen, reported that the baseline PSA level was predictive of time to disease progression in 57 patients with stage D2 disease. A similar correlation with overall survival was demonstrated in 789 patients of the Southwest

Oncology Group (SWOG) 0105 trial (50). However, we identified several published reports in which pretreatment PSA was not an independent prognostic factor (9,13,20, 22,32,45). Also, it should be noted that the proportion of patients currently presenting with very high PSA levels (i.e., greater than 300 ng per mL) is relatively small; therefore, the importance of pretreatment total PSA needs to be further evaluated.

Different measurements of PSA and other prostatic antigens are currently under intensive investigation (41,42). These include free PSA, complexed PSA, free/total PSA ratio, prostate-specific membrane antigen, and kallikrein 2. Little is known about the prognostic role of these markers in metastatic disease. Bjork et al. (46) recently reported their experience with the free/total PSA ratio in 66 patients with various stages of the disease, of whom 48 received hormonal therapy. Using multivariate analysis, the authors found that the free/total PSA ratio was a significant prognostic factor for survival.

Various methods of posttreatment changes of PSA, such as the time to PSA recurrence after local therapy, PSA velocity, or doubling time, have been reported to predict for the probability of development of metastatic disease after local treatment (47,48). However, Pound et al. (9) recently reported that neither the PSA doubling time nor time of biochemical recurrence has significant correlation with survival in patients with established metastatic disease.

Prostatic Acid Phosphatase

PAP is currently considered less sensitive than serum PSA as a marker for the detection and follow-up of prostate cancer. Two separate groups reported a statistically significant correlation between pretreatment PAP and prognosis (17,19). The majority of reports, however, failed to confirm these findings (13–15,18,22,30), nor did they appear to enhance the prognostic role of PSA.

Alkaline Phosphatase

Based on its association with bone metastasis, numerous groups investigated the role of pretreatment alkaline phosphatase (ALP) and survival. Most investigators reported that pretreatment ALP was at least as significant as extent of bone disease, pain or PS, and other serum markers in predicting the prognosis of stage D2 patients (8,11–13,15,17,18,31,43).

OTHER LABORATORY PARAMETERS

Serum Testosterone

Wilson et al. (20) showed that low testosterone levels before the initiation of medical or surgical castration were associated with a worse prognosis. This observation was confirmed by other investigators (8,22,23,43). A plausible explanation for this observation is that tumors that already survived and progressed in relatively androgen-deficient environments respond less favorably to androgen withdrawal therapy. Interestingly, one group reported that patients with normal pretreatment testosterone had better prognosis (p >.01) than patients with high testosterone levels (17).

Miscellaneous Laboratory Parameters

A multitude of laboratory parameters were evaluated as possible prognostic factors before hormonal therapy in patients with metastatic disease. These include serum creatinine, lactic dehydrogenase, liver function tests, fibrinogen, and erythrocyte sedimentation rate. Only the latter has been consistently reported as a strong predictive factor. Increased risk was observed with erythrocyte sedimentation rates greater than 20 mm (14,18).

Posttreatment Prostate-Specific Antigen Response

Sequential serum PSA determinations constitute routine clinical practice in patients undergoing systemic treatments for prostate cancer. It is routinely used to assess the effects of treatment in this disease. In patients with symptomatic metastatic disease, ADT results in major benefits in up to 80% of patients (5). In the more common asymptomatic patient, serum PSA determinations usually represent the only measure for evaluation of response to ADT during the initial phase of treatment. Evidence of improvement in bone scans is usually a slow process, and measurable disease is uncommon. The majority of the patients with hormone-naïve metastatic prostate cancer demonstrates a PSA decline with appropriate gonadal ablation (4,39).

Cooper et al. (39a) reported that PSA declines to less than or equal to 10 ng per mL at 3 to 6 months of treatment combined with EOD were highly predictive for time to progression. Various authors evaluated PSA declines to ≤4 ng per mL at various time points after the institution of ADT, such as 2 (45), 3 (26,27), 3 to 6 (24), or 6 months (31,42,44), all of which showed a strong predictive role for time to progression and survival using multivariate analysis. Various investigators reported that a PSA nadir below 4 ng per mL at any time after treatment was a significant, favorable prognostic indicator (30,50), using multivariate analyses. Indeed, Eisenberger et al. (50) reported that the posttreatment PSA nadir below 4 ng per mL represented the most powerful predictor for time to disease progression and survival in a preliminary analysis of the initial 232 patients enrolled in a prospective trial comparing surgical castration with or without flutamide, conducted by the SWOG and Eastern Cooperative Oncology Group. In fact, using multivariate analysis, the posttreatment PSA decline was the most significant among various other prognostic factors, including pretreatment EOD (minimal vs. extensive) and PS (11,50). However, the final results of the study demonstrated that despite a significant difference observed in the proportion of patients with PSA normalization on the flutamide arm, the figures of progression-free and overall survival were not significantly different between arms. This critical observation underscores the preliminary nature of retrospective multivariate analyses and stresses the importance of proper validation in prospective trials. At this time, although the hypothesis of PSA surrogacy for survival remains a reasonable one, the precise changes, including the optimal nadir and possibly duration of PSA decline, that reflect the required target for clinical trials remain undefined. The relationship between the various changes in PSA and other, more traditional end points (progression-free and overall survival) needs to be carefully defined in prospective randomized trials (surrogacy test).

Arai et al. (42) made the initial observation that a PSA decline of at least 80% after 1 month of treatment predicts longer time to progression (more than 2 years). Similarly, two other groups reported that a 90% decrease in 2, 3, and 6 months was predictive of progression-free survival (30) or survival (43). Recently, Palmberg et al. (28) performed a multivariate analysis on PSA at 12 months from the commencement of hormonal therapy. The authors combined the rate and absolute level of PSA decline and defined various groups of patients with regard to their outcome. On one side of the spectrum was a good-risk group, in which patients had an undetectable PSA, and on the other side there was a poor-risk group, in which patients had a PSA decline of less than 50%. This report also emphasizes the importance of duration of PSA response.

Other markers have been assessed as prognostic factors after ADT. Matzkin et al. (30) found that posttreatment PAP has a similar predictive value as PSA. Pelger et al. (49) reported that a "flare" (increase) in ALP activity at 1 month was an independent predictor for progression-free survival.

MATHEMATIC MODELS

This approach for evaluating the risk of individual patients gained more popularity in early-stage prostate cancer before or after local treatment. In metastatic disease, only one group of investigators recently reported on the developing of a mathematic model for risk evaluation. Based on two European Organization for Research and Treatment of Cancer trials, 30843 and 30853 (monotherapy vs. combined androgen blockade), Sylvester et al. (12) performed a multivariate analysis and identified three independent factors in 30843 (grade, PS, and ALP) and four independent factors in 30853 (hemoglobin, ALP, pain, and T stage). In their formula, every factor received a numeric value, and a total score was calculated for each patient. Using this model, patients with higher or lower scores demonstrated a median survival of 1.75 and 3.50 years, respectively. Furthermore, evaluation of this model requires adequate validation in prospective randomized trials.

AFRICAN-AMERICAN MEN

African-American men have the highest incidence of prostate cancer and a higher than average mortality (128% higher than white men) (59). The influence of race in the outcome of prostate cancer is a subject of major controversy. Some studies have suggested a similar survival outcome in patients with advanced disease when issues such as patient numbers and type of treatment practices are controlled for (60,61). The analysis of the NCI intergroup 0105 suggests that ethnicity was an independent prognostic factor for survival (62). Interestingly, ethnicity also increased the hazard ratio in baseline QOL parameters in that same study. The influence of ethnicity in the outcome of prostate cancer remains controversial; however, evolving experience indicates that intrinsic, unique biologic characteristics of the disease can be race related (63–66), and these may support the hypothesis of ethnical differences in the outcome of prostate cancer. However, the influence of diagnosis and treatment remains an open question.

FUTURE DIRECTIONS

There are several factors that require careful prospective assessments; among these are various histopathologic and molecular markers in the primary biopsy or prostatectomy specimens or preferably obtained from secondary biopsy at the time of disease progression. Few studies have reported their findings, and some are illustrated in Table 39-1. Such markers were evaluated for prediction of PSA recurrence and survival after local therapy for early-stage prostate cancer. Tissue markers include p53 mutation, *bcl-2* expression, and expression of Ki-67, p27, apoptotic index, microvessel density, and various growth factors, including the vascular endothelial growth factor and insulin growth factor super family, among others.

Another area that deserves further investigation is the large variety of alterations in the androgen receptor gene and expression. Low androgen receptor content was shown to correlate with poor prognosis by one group (31). However, the status and function of the androgen receptor are complex and dynamic processes that deserve further study.

Various growth factors and related proteins are believed to play a role in the progression of prostate cancer (51–54). Serum and plasma levels of vascular endothelial growth factors, insulin growth factors, and cytokines (interleukin-6) were recently shown to be elevated in prostate cancer, especially in metastatic stage (55–58). Furthermore, investigation on possible prognostic value of these proteins is warranted.

SUMMARY

Our review of the literature revealed several widely accepted, independent, and established prognostic factors. These include extent of metastatic disease, PS, anemia, pain, pretreatment ALP, and testosterone and posttreatment PSA decline. The issue of primary histologic grade and ethnicity remains highly controversial. Clearly, there is need for new validated prognostic factors in this patient population. Future directions may incorporate novel molecular markers, serum and/or plasma growth, and angiogenic factors and new serum prostate cancer markers.

REFERENCES

1. Huggins C, Stevens RE, Hodges CV. Studies on prostatic cancer: II. The effects of castration on advanced carcinoma of the prostate gland. *Arch Surg* 1941;43:209–222.
2. Veterans Administration Cooperative Urological Research Group. Factors in the prognosis of carcinoma of the prostate: a cooperative study. *J Urol* 1968;100:59–62.
3. The Leuprolide Study Group. Leuprolide versus diethylstilbestrol for metastatic prostatic cancer. *N Engl J Med* 1984;311:1281–1286.
4. Eisenberger MA, Blumenstein BA, Crawford ED, et al. A randomized and double blind comparison of bilateral orchiectomy with or without flutamide for the treatment of patients with stage D2 prostate cancer: results of NCI Intergroup Study 0105. *N Engl J Med* 1998;339:1036–1042.
5. Waselenko JK, Dawson NA. Management of progressive metastatic prostate cancer. *Oncology* 1997;11:1551–1559.
6. Eisenberger MA. Chemotherapy for prostate carcinoma. *NCI Monogr* 1988;7:151–163.
7. Emrich LJ, Priore RL, Murphy GP, et al. Prognostic factors in patients with advanced stage prostate cancer. *Cancer Res* 1985;45:5173–5179.
8. Chodak GW, Vogelzang NJ, Caplan RJ, et al. Independent prognostic factors in patients with metastatic (stage D2) prostate cancer. The Zoladex Study Group. *JAMA* 1991; 265:618–621.
9. Pound CR, Partin AW, Eisenberger MA, et al. Natural history of progression after PSA elevation following radical prostatectomy. *JAMA* 1999;281:1591–1597.
10. Landis SH, Murray T, Bolden S, et al. Cancer statistics, 1999. *CA Cancer J Clin* 1999;49:8–31.
11. Eisenberger MA, Crawford ED, Blumenstein BA, et al. Prognostic factors in stage D2 prostate cancer; important implication for future trials: results of a cooperative intergroup study (INT 0036). *Semin Oncol* 1994;21:613–619.
12. Sylvester R, Denis LJ, de Voogt HJ. The importance of prognostic factors in the interpretation of two EORTC metastatic prostate cancer trials. *Eur Urol* 1998;33:134–143.
13. de Voogt HJ, Suciu S, Sylvester R, et al. Multivariate analysis of prognostic factors in patients with advanced prostatic cancer: results from 2 European Organization for Research on Treatment of Cancer trials. *J Urol* 1989;141:883–888.
14. Johansson JE, Andersson SO, Holmberg L, et al. Prognostic factors in progression-free survival and corrected survival in patients with advanced prostatic cancer: results from a randomized study comprising 150 patients treated with orchiectomy or estrogens. *J Urol* 1991;146:1327–1332.
15. Mulders PF, Dijkman GA, Fernandez del Moral P, et al. Analysis of prognostic factors in disseminated prostatic cancer: an update Dutch Southeastern Urological Cooperative Group. *Cancer* 1990;65:2758–2761.
16. Veronesi A, Lo Re G, Dal Bo V, et al. Buserelin treatment of advanced prostatic carcinoma: prognostic factor analysis. *Eur Urol* 1992;21:274–279.
17. Lukkarinen O, Lehikoinen K. Prognostic factors of advanced prostatic carcinoma. *Ann Chir Gynecol Suppl* 1993;206:9–13.
18. Jorgensen T, Kanagasingam Y, Kaalhus O, et al. Prognostic factors in patients with metastatic (stage D2) prostate cancer: experience from the Scandinavian Prostatic Cancer Group Study-2. *J Urol* 1997;158:164–170.
19. Waaler G, Nilssen MO. Prognostic factors in disseminated prostatic cancer, with special emphasis on extent of disease. *Urol Int* 1994;53:130–134.
20. Wilson DW, Harper ME, Jensen HM, et al. Prognostic index for the clinical management of patients with advanced prostatic cancer: a British Prostate Study Group investigation. *Prostate* 1985;7:131–141.
21. Berner A, Harvei S, Tretil S, et al. Prostatic carcinoma: a multivariate analysis of prognostic factors. *Br J Cancer* 1994; 69:924–930.
22. Ernst DS, Hanson J, Venner PM. Analysis of prognostic factors in men with metastatic prostate cancer. Uro-Oncology Group of Northern Alberta. *J Urol* 1991;146:372–376.
23. Crawford ED, Blumenstein B. Proposed substages for metastatic prostate cancer. *Urology* 1997;50:1027–1028.
24. Oosterlinck W, Mattelaer J, Casselman J, et al. PSA evolution: a prognostic factor during treatment of advanced prostatic carcinoma with total androgen blockade. Data from a Belgian multicentric study of 546 patients. *Acta Urol Belg* 1997;65:63–71.
25. Dreicer R. Metastatic prostate cancer: assessment of response to systemic treatment. *Semin Urol Oncol* 1997;15:28–32.
26. Dijkman GA, Janknegt RA, De Reijke TM, et al. Long-term efficacy and safety of nilutamide plus castration in advanced prostate cancer, and the significance of early prostate specific antigen normalization. International Anandron Study Group. *J Urol* 1997;158:160–163.
27. Furuya Y, Akimoto S, Akakura K, et al. Response of prostate-specific antigen after androgen withdrawal and prognosis in men with metastatic prostate cancer. *Urol Int* 1998;60: 28–32.
28. Palmberg C, Koivisto P, Visakorpi T, et al. PSA decline is an independent prognostic marker in hormonally treated prostate cancer. *Eur Urol* 1999;36:191–196.
29. Miller JI, Ahmann FR, Drach GW, et al. The clinical usefulness of serum prostate specific antigen after hormonal therapy of metastatic prostate cancer. *J Urol* 1992;147:956–961.

30. Matzkin H, Eber P, Todd B, et al. Prognostic significance of changes in prostate-specific markers after endocrine treatment of stage D2 prostatic cancer. *Cancer* 1992;70:2302–2309.
31. Morote J, de Torres I, Caceres C, et al. Prognostic value of immunohistochemical expression of the c-erbB-2 oncoprotein in metastatic prostate cancer. *Int J Cancer* 1999;84:421–425.
32. Stege R, Tribukait B, Lundh B, et al. Quantitative estimation of tissue prostate specific antigen, deoxyribonucleic acid ploidy and cytological grade in fine needle aspiration biopsies for prognosis of hormonally treated prostatic carcinoma. *J Urol* 1992;148:833–837.
33. Takeda H, Akakura K, Masai M, et al. Androgen receptor content of prostate carcinoma cells estimated by immunohistochemistry is related to prognosis of patients with stage D2 prostate carcinoma. *Cancer* 1996;77:934–940.
34. Randolph TL, Amin MB, Ro JY, et al. Histologic variants of adenocarcinoma and other carcinomas of prostate: pathologic criteria and clinical significance. *Mod Pathol* 1997;10:612–629.
35. di Sant'Agnese PA. Neuroendocrine differentiation in carcinoma of the prostate. Diagnostic, prognostic, and therapeutic implications. *Cancer* 1992;70:254–268.
36. Soloway MS, Hardeman SW, Hickey D, et al. Stratification of patients with metastatic prostate cancer based on extent of disease on initial bone scan. *Cancer* 1988;61:195–202.
37. Ishikawa S, Soloway MS, Van der Zwaag R, et al. Prognostic factors in survival free of progression after androgen deprivation therapy for treatment of prostate cancer. *J Urol* 1989;14:1139–1142.
38. Cipolla B, Guille F, Moulinoux JP, et al. Erythrocyte polyamines and prognosis in stage D2 prostatic carcinoma patients. *J Urol* 1994;151:629–633.
39. Miller J, Horsfall DJ, Marshall VR, et al. The prognostic value of deoxyribonucleic acid flow cytometric analysis in stage D2 prostatic carcinoma. *J Urol* 1991;145:1192–1196.
39a. Cooper EH, Armitage TG, Robinson MR, et al. Prostatic specific antigen and the prediction of prognosis in metastatic prostatic cancer. Cancer 1991;66:1025–1028.
40. Smith JA Jr., Lange PH, Janknegt RA, et al. Serum markers as a predictor of response duration and patient survival after hormonal therapy for metastatic carcinoma of the prostate. *J Urol* 1997;157:1329–1334.
41. Brawer MK, Benson MC, Djavan H, et al. Prostate serum markers. In: Murphy G, Khouri S, Partin A, et al., eds. *Report from the 2nd International Consultation in prostate cancer.* Monte Carlo, Monaco: Health Publication, 1999:139–160.
42. Arai Y, Yoshiki T, Yoshida O. Prognostic significance of prostate specific antigen in endocrine treatment for prostatic cancer. *J Urol* 1990;144:1415–1419.
43. Reynard JM, Peters TJ, Gillatt D. Prostate-specific antigen and prognosis in patients with metastatic prostate cancer—a multivariable analysis of prostate cancer mortality. *Br J Urol* 1995;675:507–515.
44. Evans CP, Gajendran V, Tewari A, et al. The proportional decrease in prostate specific antigen level best predicts the duration of survival after hormonal therapy in patients with metastatic carcinoma of the prostate. *Br J Urol* 1996;78:426–431.
45. Kawakami S, Takagi K, Yonese J, et al. Prognostic significance of prostate-specific antigen levels two months after hormonal manipulation of metastatic prostate cancer. *Eur Urol* 1997;32:58–63.
46. Bjork T, Lilja H, Christensson A. The prognostic value of different forms of prostate specific antigen and their ratios in patients with prostate cancer. *BJU Int* 1999;84:1021–1027.
47. Pound CR, Partin AW, Epstein JI, et al. Prostate-specific antigen after anatomic radical retropubic prostatectomy. Patterns of recurrence and cancer control. *Urol Clin North Am* 1997;24:395–406.
48. Patel A, Dorey F, Franklin J, et al. Recurrence patterns after radical retropubic prostatectomy: clinical usefulness of prostate specific antigen doubling times and log slope prostate specific antigen. *J Urol* 1997;158:1441–1445.
49. Pelger RC, Lycklama A, Nijeholt GA, et al. The flare in serum alkaline phosphatase activity after orchiectomy: a valuable negative prognostic index for progression-free survival in prostatic carcinoma. *J Urol* 1996;156:122–126.
50. Eisenberger M, Crawford ED, Blumenstein B, et al. The prognostic significance of PSA in stage D2 prostate cancer. *Proc Am Society Clin Oncol* 1995;14:235(abst).
51. Kaicer EK, Blat C, Harel L. IGF-I and IGF-binding proteins: stimulatory and inhibitory factors secreted by human prostatic adenocarcinoma cells. *Growth Factors* 1991;4:231–237.
52. Culig Z, Hobisch A, Cronauer MV, et al. Androgen receptor activation in prostatic tumor cell lines by insulin-like growth factor-I, keratinocyte growth factor, and epidermal growth factor. *Cancer Res* 1994;54:5474–5478.
53. Ferrer FA, Miller LJ, Lindquist R, et al. Expression of vascular endothelial growth factor receptors in human prostate cancer. *Urology* 1999;54:567–572.
54. Joseph IB, Isaacs JT. Potentiation of the antiangiogenic ability of linomide by androgen ablation involves down-regulation of vascular endothelial growth factor in human androgen-responsive prostatic cancers. *Cancer Res* 1997;57:1054–1057.
55. Kanety H, Madjar Y, Dagan Y, et al. Serum insulin-like growth factor-binding protein-2 (IGFBP-2) is increased and IGFBP-3 is decreased in patients with prostate cancer: correlation with serum prostate-specific antigen. *J Clin Endocrinol Metab* 1993;77:229–233.
56. Chan JM, Stampfer MJ, Giovannucci E, et al. Plasma insulin-like growth factor-I and prostate cancer risk: a prospective study. *Science* 1998;279:563–566.
57. Drachenberg DE, Elgamal AA, Rowbotham R, et al. Circulating levels of interleukin-6 in patients with hormone refractory prostate cancer. *Prostate* 1999;41:127–133.
58. Duque JL, Loughlin KR, Adam RM, et al. Plasma levels of vascular endothelial growth factor are increased in patients with metastatic prostate cancer. *Urology* 1999;54:523–527.
59. Marwick C. ACS sets blueprint for action against prostate cancer in African Americans. *JAMA* 1998;279:418–419.
60. Bergan RC, Walls RG, Figg WD, et al. Similar clinical outcomes in African-American males and non–African-American males treated with suramin for metastatic prostate cancer. *J Natl Med Assoc* 1997;89:622–628.

61. Optenberg SA, Thompson IM, Friedichs P, et al. Race, treatment and long term survival from prostate cancer in an equal access medical care delivery system. *JAMA* 1995;274: 1599–1605.
62. Thompson IN, Eisenberger MA, Crawford ED et al.
63. Devgan SA, Henderson BE, Yu MC, et al. Genetic variation of 3 beta-hydroxysteroid dehydrogenase type II in three racial/ethnic groups: implications in prostate cancer risks. *Prostate* 1997;33:9–12.
64. Reichardt JK, Madrikakis N, Henderson BE, et al. Genetic variability of the human SRD5A2 gene: implications in prostate cancer risk. *Cancer Res* 1995;55:1937–1940.
65. Irvine SA, Yu MC, Ross RK. The CAG and GGC microsatellites of the androgen receptor gene are in linkage disequilibrium in men with prostate cancer. *Cancer Res* 1995;55:1937–1940.
66. Ingles SA, Coetzee GA, Ross RK, et al. Associations of prostate cancer with vitamin D receptor haplotypes in African Americans. *Cancer Res* 1998:58:1620–1623.

40

ANDROGEN ABLATION FOR PROSTATE CANCER: MECHANISMS AND MODALITIES

DANIEL P. PETRYLAK
JUDD W. MOUL

Sixty years have passed since the initial report by Huggins and Hodges that prostate cancer is an androgen-sensitive tumor (1,2). Significant palliation of bone pain due to metastatic disease, relief of urinary tract obstruction, as well as resolution of spinal cord compression can be noted after castration in men with metastatic prostate cancer. However, despite this revolutionary concept (at that time) for which the lead authors received the Nobel Prize in 1966, controversy regarding the timing of the initiation of the androgen blockade [asymptomatic prostate-specific antigen (PSA) rises vs. symptomatic metastatic disease], the best regimen (monotherapy vs. combined blockade) once the decision is made to treat the patient, and the duration of androgen blockade (continuous vs. intermittent therapy) remains. Despite these controversies, the median time to progression for men treated with hormone therapy for metastatic disease remains between 18 and 24 months. This chapter reviews the major effects of androgen blockade at the cellular level and clinical level and summarizes the methods available to the urologist or oncologist to achieve androgen blockade.

COMPOSITION OF ANDROGENS IN HUMANS

Testosterone and its metabolites play the primary role of growth regulation of normal and cancerous prostate. These steroid molecules stimulate prostate cancer cell growth and inhibit cell death by binding to the androgen receptor, which is located in the nucleus of the prostate cancer cell (3). Circulating testosterone is in effect a prohormone. Once testosterone enters the stroma of the prostate, it is irreversibly metabolized by 5α-reductase to dihydrotestosterone, which is approximately ten times more active than its parent molecule (4). This androgen metabolite is then transported into the prostate epithelial cells. Dihydrotestosterone then binds to the androgen-binding region of the androgen receptor, inducing phosphorylation of the receptor. The DNA-binding region of the androgen receptor then binds to androgen-responsive genes, thus promoting transcription (5). Other androgens, such as androstenedione, dehydroepiandrosterone, and dehydroepiandrosterone sulfate, are peripherally converted to dihydrotestosterone. Adrenal androgens account for approximately 10% of androgens found in men; however, they are insufficient to prevent prostate cell death (6), and their contribution to prostate cancer cell growth is controversial.

Testicular androgen secretion is regulated by the hypothalamus through the pituitary gonadotropin luteinizing hormone (LH), a protein comprised of two subunits with a molecular weight of 28,000 kd. The secretion of LH is regulated by LH releasing hormone (LHRH), a decapeptide that in turn stimulates the anterior pituitary gland to release LH. LHRH release is pulsatile, with bursts occurring approximately every hour. LH stimulates the Leydig cells of the testes to secrete testosterone. LH secretion is controlled by a feedback loop; exogenous administration of androgens will down-regulate LH secretion.

CELLULAR MECHANISM OF ANDROGEN BLOCKADE

Prostate cancer cells deprived of androgen undergo *apoptosis*, otherwise termed *programmed cell death*, as well as a decrease in cellular proliferation. Morphologically, changes can be detected in normal and cancerous prostate tissue after the androgen blockade. In the rat ventral prostate, glandular involution is observed rapidly after castration. Cytoplasmic apoptotic bodies and autolytic vacuoles can be detected with the ventral lobe of the prostate responding more rapidly than the lateral or dorsal lobes. Normal, human prostate cancer tissue deprived of androgen will demonstrate atrophy, basal cell prominence, vacuolated luminal cell layer, and squamous and transitional cell metaplasia. The most common effect of androgen ablation that is observed is the presence of small tumor glands separated by stroma, thus resulting in an overall decrease in volume of the prostate gland. Pyknosis and branching empty spaces are less frequent. These volume changes are particularly important in considering the response to androgen blockade, as volume changes can be mistaken for actual tumor shrinkage. Large, clear tumor cells within an inflammatory response were a third histologic pattern. Apparently unaltered tumor areas were observed in 43% of prostates tissue exposed to androgen deprivation therapy, suggesting that this treatment is not curative (7).

The altered relationship between cellular proliferation and death can also be detected at the molecular level. A variety of different cellular proteins are expressed in a temporal fashion after androgen withdrawal. The selection factors necessary for cellular survival are achieved through clonal selection of cells preadapted to survive without androgen, as well as induction of genes stimulated by androgen withdrawal that results in proteins that confer a survival advantage. These molecular changes may contribute to the eventual hormone-resistant state as well as progression of disease after androgen ablation and may be in part responsible for the relative drug resistance that has been observed in prostate cancer. There is the suggestion that this pathway is different in normal, when compared to malignant, prostate tissue. One molecular marker that remains relatively constant in expression after androgen blockade is the androgen receptor. This implies that the apoptotic pathway that the androgen receptor controls is intact, and over time this axis is lost. In the Dunning R3327 prostate adenocarcinoma model, testosterone-repressed prostate messenger 2 was induced by androgen withdrawal in the rat ventral prostate 2 to 5 days post–androgen ablation but not in the androgen-sensitive implanted tumors (8). This protein is associated with resistance to apoptosis. In animal models, castration results in the induction of protein synthesis, particularly in the antiapoptotic protein called Bcl-2. Bcl-2 can delay the time to androgen independence, and increased expression has been noted in androgen-ablated prostate tissue. Patterns of growth factor receptor expression are changed—for example, the expression of transforming growth factor alpha shifts from the stroma in untreated tissue to the tumor cell in treated tissue, suggesting an autocrine growth factor loop. There is an increase in epidermal growth factor receptors noted in benign tissue. In the CWRU-22 prostate cancer xenograft model after castration, an increase in expression of p53, p21/WAF1, and a decrease in the Ki-67 proliferative index without activation of apoptosis implies that the primary mechanism may be cell cycle arrest (9). Furthermore, evidence suggests that the tumor vasculature may differ significantly before and after androgen blockade by an indirect response of the prostatic parenchyma to an ischemic/hypoxic environment caused by a drastic reduction of blood flow to the tissue that occurs when androgens are withdrawn (10,11).

METHODS OF ANDROGEN ABLATION

Orchiectomy

Bilateral orchiectomy has been the gold standard for the treatment of metastatic prostate cancer. Two techniques exist: total orchiectomy and subcapsular orchiectomy. *Subcapsular orchiectomy* spares the tunica albuginea and epididymis and will preserve some tissue in the scrotum and thus may lessen the psychological effect of orchiectomy. Although the possibility exists of persistent testosterone-producing cells remaining in the patient after subcapsular orchiectomy, comparative studies to total orchiectomy have found no difference in testosterone levels and pituitary hormones (12,13).

Because no compensatory adrenal androgen synthesis occurs, castration is permanent (14,15). Serum testosterone levels are reduced by 95% within 3 hours of castration (16). As the hypothalamus senses a rapid decline in testosterone levels, there is a permanent rise in LH and follicle-stimulating hormone (FSH) after orchiectomy. Although the outcome of orchiectomy is equivalent to that of LHRH agents, most patients now prefer monthly or longer duration LHRH injections to castration (17). This is primarily owing to psychological reasons; a past study has demonstrated that patients prefer LHRH to orchiectomy because of the psychological implications of the loss of testicles. In this era of managed care, one important difference between orchiectomy and medical castration is that orchiectomy also offers the advantage of lower cost (18).

Estrogens

Estrogens affect castration primary by down-regulating the secretion of LH and FSH by the pituitary and thus decreasing testosterone secretion by Leydig cells. Castrate levels of testosterone are achieved generally between 3 and 9 weeks (19). Duration of exposure to estrogens is important to the durability of response, with rapid escape from suppression occurring with patients on short-term therapy (20). The effect is dependent on dose: One mg of diethylstilbestrol (DES) will not consistently induce castration, whereas 5 mg will almost universally result in testosterone levels less than 50 ng per dL. Adrenal androgens remain unaffected by estrogen treatment (21). Other direct cytotoxic effects on prostate cancer cells may involve nonhormonal mechanisms, such as the disruption of cytoplasmic microtubules (22). Side effects of estrogens include nausea, vomiting, gynecomastia, fluid retention, and cardiovascular events. Investigators have attempted to reduce the rate of thrombosis in patients treated with 2 or 3 mg of DES by administering 1 mg of coumadin prophylactically; no reduction in thromboembolic events was observed (23).

DES is the most extensively evaluated estrogen for the treatment of metastatic prostate cancer. Two randomized studies performed by the Veterans Administration Cooperative Research Group demonstrated the effectiveness of DES but at cost of toxicity. The first randomized 2,052 patients received either 5 mg DES or placebo (24). Overall, 45% of patients who were randomized to placebo eventually received DES, and no difference in survival was noted between the two arms. The second study randomized patients to receive 0.2, 1.0, or 5.0 mg of DES and was terminated early owing to an excess of cardiovascular side effects noted in the 5-mg arm (25). This trial concluded equivalent rates of disease control for 1 and 5 mg of DES.

Parentally administered estrogens, such as polyestrol phosphate, have a lower rate of cardiovascular events than orally administered estrogens (26).

Antiandrogens

Two classes of antiandrogens are used in the treatment of prostate cancer: steroidal and nonsteroidal. Steroidal antiandrogens include cyproterone acetate and megestrol acetate. Both drugs act by two mechanisms of action: (a) inhibition of C21-9 decarboxylase, an enzyme responsible for adrenal androgen synthesis, and (b) inhibition of gonadotropin release (27). Cyproterone acetate is not approved for the treatment of advanced prostate cancer in the United States.

Nonsteroidal antiandrogens competitively block the binding of dihydrotestosterone to its receptor. Three are commonly available in the United States: flutamide (Eulexin), bicalutamide (Casodex), and nilutamide (Nilandron) (Anandron). Single-agent administration of these agents will decrease the intracellular levels of testosterone and dihydrotestosterone; however, in contrast to steroidal antiandrogens, serum levels of testosterone will increase owing to a compensatory increase in LHRH (28). Flutamide is converted to a hydroxy metabolite that is approximately five times more effective in binding to the androgen receptor than its parent compound (29). Diarrhea is the most common toxicity observed with flutamide and may be related to the lactose with which flutamide is diluted. The most severe toxicity observed with flutamide is hepatotoxicity (30). This can be reversible if detected early; however, it can be fatal. Bicalutamide has a longer half-life than flutamide and a lower rate of diarrhea. Three unique side effects of nilutamide are a flushing reaction, difficulty in visual adaptation to dark with prolonged treatment, and pulmonary fibrosis (31). All of these agents when administered as single agents can cause significant gynecomastia, primarily due to peripheral conversion of androgen to estrogen.

The role of antiandrogen monotherapy is controversial. Metaanalysis of trials comparing antiandrogen monotherapy to orchiectomy or LHRH agonists for patients with metastatic disease found no difference or a modest benefit for LHRH or orchiectomy. A recent randomized study comparing 150 mg of bicalutamide to orchiectomy or goserelin in patients with T3 or T4 prostate cancer demonstrated equivalent survival with an improvement of sexual function and physical capacity for those patients treated with bicalutamide (32). For those patients who initially opt for monotherapy, it is clear that secondary responses can be obtained using castration after bicalutamide monotherapy. In a retrospective study of 54 patients, Kasimis et al. demonstrated that after failing bicalutamide therapy at a dosage of 50 mg, 34% of men responded to surgical or medical castration (33). This apparently does not affect survival; an overall median survival of 119 months was observed, which is comparable to the median survivals reported in combined androgen blockade studies. Because potency is preserved in patients treated with bicalutamide, this sequential approach may preserve potency for a time during androgen blockade and may be a possible alternative to maximal androgen blockade in younger patients who wish to preserve their potency (33).

Gonadotropin-Releasing Hormone Analogs

Chemical castration can be affected by inhibition of LH secretion. This has become the preferred method of androgen ablation. As noted earlier, LHRH secretion is pulsatile. Administration of LHRH agonists interferes with this pulsatile secretion through a negative feedback. LHRH agonists differ from LHRH in the substitution of D leucine for glycine at position 6. Two LHRH formulations are approved for use in the United States. Leuprolide acetate (Lupron) is available in daily subcutaneous and monthly, every-3-months, or every-4-months intramuscular injections, whereas goserelin acetate (Zoladex) is available as a monthly or every-3-months subcutaneous implant that is usually given into the abdominal wall. Recently, a one-year leuprolide implant has become available (Viadur). When these agonists are administered, an initial rise in LH and FSH is observed. The surge of LH results in a down-regulation of LHRH receptors in the pituitary gland, resulting in a decline in testosterone secretion in 2 to 3 weeks. This decline in serum testosterone is preceded by a testosterone surge. Unless antiandrogens are administered, symptoms such as bone pain, urinary obstruction, and, in the most extreme case, spinal cord compression, can result in patients with metastatic disease.

A recent metaanalysis of monotherapies concluded that the survival of patients treated with LHRH agonists was equivalent to those patient treated with orchiectomy. There was no difference in the effectiveness of different LHRH agonists (34).

Timing of the Institution of Hormonal Therapy

The original Veterans Administration Cooperative Research Group studies did not demonstrate a survival advantage to hormonal therapy focused on treatment when a patient developed metastatic disease (24). However, these results cannot be generalized to patients with early-stage prostate cancer and those who have only marker elevations. There are no prospective data to guide the clinician in starting androgen blockade. In fact, some of the most controversial areas are when to treat a patient with locally advanced prostate cancer, whether patients with lymph-node-positive disease should be treated, and what to do about a rising PSA after definitive local therapy. This is particularly important in light of the fact that patients who fail local therapy often have a long course until they develop symptomatic disease (35). In fact, 68% of nearly 400 urologists surveyed stated that they recommend androgen blockade for nonmetastatic rising PSAs postprostatectomy. Of note, a similar pattern of response was found from urologists who responded to the same questionnaire in men with metastatic disease, and 81% believe that such treatment prolongs survival in men with stage C disease (36). Of note, half of urologists surveyed who believe that androgen blockage given in this setting does not prolong survival were found to administer androgen ablation to these patients. There is no clear answer, and any treatment decision that the clinician has to offer must be made with the natural history of the disease in mind. Recent data from Johns Hopkins indicate that it takes a median of 8 years for a patient to develop metastatic disease after his PSA begins to rise (35). The most controversial question is when to initiate hormonal therapy in a patient with a rising PSA level after prior local therapy (36a). Because a survival benefit was not observed in the original Veterans Administration studies, the prevailing wisdom was that hormonal therapy should start when patients became symptomatic (24). However, more recent randomized studies of combined androgen blockade demonstrate a tail in the survival curves, implying that a small fraction of patients enjoy a durable long-term survival past the median of 18 to 24 months observed in other studies. The patients who appeared to survive the longest in the Southwest Oncology Group 89-10 were those with few lesions on bone scan, good performance status, and who underwent combined androgen blockade. Whether this represents patients who have a less biologically aggressive form of prostate cancer or earlier treatment remains problematic. In conclusion, there are no guidelines for the institution of androgen blockade.

Messing et al. randomized men with node-positive disease to undergo observation or to undergo androgen blockade (37). This trial was terminated early owing to the fact that patients could not be accrued after the implementation of routine PSA screening. However, in the 98 patients enrolled, those who received immediate hormonal therapy had a significantly better cancer-specific survival at 7 year follow-up than those men who were observed until clinical progression.

Alternative Hormonal Therapies: PC-SPES

PC-SPES (38) is a compound that is comprised of eight herbs: chrysanthemum, isatis, licorice, ganoderam lucidum, *Panax* pseudo-ginseng, *Rabdosia rubescens*, saw palmetto, and Scutellaria (skullcap). *In vitro* antitumor activity has been demonstrated against hormone-sensitive as well as -insensitive human prostate cancer cell lines. PC-SPES has a toxicity profile similar to that of estrogen (39). The estrogenic activity of PC-SPES is significant, with a 1 to 200 dilution of an extract of one 320-mg capsule resulting in estrogenic activity equivalent to 1 nm of estradiol. However, this may not be the only mechanism of PC-SPES antitumor activity. Four different peaks on high-pressure liquid chromatography have been identified (40). The relative contribution of each of these components to its antitumor activity is not known. Although the mixture had definite clinical activity, no studies have been performed comparing this compound to maximal androgen blockade, antiandrogen monotherapy, or DES.

SIDE EFFECTS OF ANDROGEN BLOCKADE

Osteoporosis

Withdrawal of hormones can result in osteoporosis. Chemical or surgical castration in men with prostate cancer is usually followed by accelerated bone loss that may be superimposed on an already depleted bone mass (41). This effect is becoming particularly more relevant to quality of life issues as patients are being treated earlier in the natural history of prostate cancer with androgen ablation, thus increasing the risk of osteoporosis and skeletal-related events.

Androgen ablation increases the risk of pathologic fracture. Daniel et al. examined the records of a total of 235 men with non–stage A prostate cancer diagnosed between 1983 and 1990 for risk factors for osteoporosis, including orchiectomy (41,42). Of these patients, 13.6% treated with orchiectomy had a pathologic fracture, compared to 1.1% who did not undergo this procedure. The 17 castrated men alive in 1995 were interviewed, and femoral neck bone mineral density was compared to that of 23 controls of similar age before hormonal therapy, demonstrating a decrease in bone mineral density (42). A study by Townsend et al. found the rate of osteoporotic fractures post–LHRH treatment to be 5% (43). Whether bisphosphates or other agents that can inhibit bone resorption will prevent bone loss is currently under investigation. Prospective evaluation of bone mineral density is warranted.

Anemia

Anemia appears to be a significant problem and develops regardless of the stage of a patient's prostate cancer at the initiation of hormone therapy. This is due to the fact that androgens directly stimulate hematopoietic stem cells, resulting in a normochromic, normocytic anemia (44). In a study by Strum et al. of 142 patients who received combined hormonal blockade (CHB), hemoglobin levels declined significantly in all patients from a mean baseline of 149 g per L to a mean of 139 g per L, 132 g per L, and 131 g per L at 1, 2, and 3 months postandrogen blockade, respectively (45). Hemoglobin levels continued to decline during CHB to a mean nadir of 123 g per L at a mean of 5.6 months postinitiation of CHB, representing a mean absolute hemoglobin decline at a nadir of 25.4 g per L. A hemoglobin decline of more than 10% was noted in 120 of the 133 (90%) patients, whereas 13% of patients demonstrated a more severe decline of more than 25%. Significant symptoms related to anemia occurred in 17 patients (13%). Symptoms in these patients were easily corrected with the subcutaneous administration of recombinant human erythropoietin (45).

Sexual Function

Androgen blockade leads to the loss of potency and libido. For those patients stopping androgen blockade, recovery is variable and can take up to 1 year, with approximately 25% of patients still castrate at 1 year. Sexual function may be maintained using antiandrogen monotherapy, as noted in the earlier section Antiandrogens.

Hot Flushes

All forms of testicular androgen ablation will result in hot flushes. Some studies have found that approximately two-thirds of men experience symptoms including a feeling of heat, usually localizing in the upper body and face; peripheral vasodilation; and profuse sweating (46). These symptoms parallel those of women with menopause; however, although in men testosterone levels decrease with age, hot flushes are almost never observed in healthy men. The mechanism of hot flushes is unclear; however, it may be related to the spontaneous release of catecholamines from the hypothalamus (47). It is postulated that chronically low testosterone levels decrease the release of opioid peptides from the hypothalamus, leading to an increase in intrahypothalamic levels of catecholamines. Release of these catecholamines can be precipitated by changes in the environmental temperature, ingestion of hot liquids, or changes in body position. Treatments for hot flushes include inhibition of central adrenergic activity with clonidine, megestrol (20 mg twice a day), as well as DES and can result in complete resolution of hot flushes in 70% of patients (48). However, fewer side effects, particularly in thromboembolic events, are observed with megestrol. Future studies will focus on the use of antidepressants, which have been demonstrated to reduce the rate of hot flashes in women with breast cancer.

REFERENCES

1. Huggins C, Hodges CV. Studies in prostate cancer. I. The effect of estrogen and androgen injections on serum phosphastats in metastatic carcinoma of the prostate. *Cancer Res* 1941;1:243.
2. Huggins C, Stevens RE, Hodges CV. Studies in prostatic cancer. II. The effect of castration on advanced carcinoma of the prostate gland. *Arch Surg* 1941;43:209.
3. Brolin J, Lowhagen T, Skoog L. Immunocytochemical detection of the androgen receptor in fine-needle aspirates from benign and malignant prostate tissue. *Cytopathology* 1992;3:351–357.
4. Silver RI, Wiley EL, Davis DL, et al. Expression and regulation of steroid 5 a reductase activity in prostate disease. *J Urol* 1994;152:433–437.
5. Kuiper GC, Faber PW, van Rooij HC, et al. Structural organization of the human androgen receptor gene. *J Mol Endocrinol* 1989;2:1–4.
6. Osterling JE, Epstein JI, Walsh PC. The inability of adrenal androgens to stimulate the adult prostate: an autopsy evaluation of men with hypogonadism and panhypopituitarism. *J Urol* 1986;136:103–104.
7. Civantos F, Marcial MA, Banks ER, et al. Pathology of androgen deprivation therapy in prostate carcinoma. A comparative study of 173 patients. *Cancer* 1995;75:1634–1641.
8. Miyake H, Nelson C, Rennie PS, et al. Overexpression of insulin-like growth factor binding protein-5 helps accelerate progression to androgen-independence in the human prostate LNCaP tumor model through activation of phosphatidylinositol 3'-kinase pathway. *Endocrinology* 2000;141:2257–2265.
9. Agus DB, Cordon-Cardo C, Fox W, et al. Prostate cancer cell cycle regulators: response to androgen withdrawal and development of androgen independence. *J Natl Cancer Inst* 1999;91:1869–1876.
10. Buttyan R, Ghafar MA, Shabsigh A. The effects of androgen deprivation on the prostate gland: cell death mediated by vascular regression. *Curr Opin Urol* 2000;10:415–420.
11. Geck P, Maffini MV, Szelei J, et al. Androgen-induced proliferative quiescence in prostate cancer cells: the role of AS3 as its mediator. *Proc Natl Acad Sci U S A* 2000;97:10185–10190.
12. Zhang XY, Donavan MP, Williams BT, et al. Comparison of subcapsular orchiectomy and total orchiectomy for the treatment of metastatic prostate cancer. *Urology* 1996;47:402–404.
13. Bergman B, Damber JE, Tomic R. Effects of total and subcapsular orchidectomy on serum concentrations of testosterone and pituitary hormones in patients with carcinoma of the prostate. *Urol Int* 1996;37:139–144.

14. Robinson MR, Thomas BS. Effects of hormonal therapy on plasma testosterone levels in prostatic carcinoma. *BMJ* 1971;4:391–394.
15. Young HH, Kent JR. Plasma testosterone levels in patients with prostatic cancer before and after treatment. *J Urol* 1968;99:788–792.
16. Grayhack JT, Keeler TC, Kozlowsku JM. Carcinoma of the prostate: hormonal therapy. *Cancer* 1987;60:589–591.
17. Cassielth BR, Soloway M, Vogelzang NJ. Patients' choice of treatment in stage D prostate cancer. *Urology* 1989; 33:57–62.
18. Chon JK, Jascobs SC, Nasulnd MJ, et al. The cost value of medical vs. surgical hormonal therapy for metastatic prostate cancer. *J Urol* 2000;164:737–737.
19. Cox LE, Crawford ED. Estrogens in the treatment of prostate cancer. *J Urol* 1995;154:1991–1998.
20. Beck PH, McAnnich JW, Goebel JL, et al. Plasma testosterone levels in patients receiving diethylstilbestrol. *Urology* 1993;11:577.
21. Geller J, Albert JD. Comparison of various hormonal therapies for prostatic carcinoma. *Semin Oncol* 1983;10: 34–41.
22. Robertson CN, Roberson KM, Padilla GM, et al. Induction of apoptosis by diethylstilbestrol in hormone-insensitive prostate cancer cells. *J Natl Cancer Inst* 1996;88:908–917.
23. Klotz L, McNeill I, Fleisher N. A phase 1-2 trial of diethylstilbestrol plus low dose warfarin in advanced prostate carcinoma. *J Urol* 1999;16:169–172.
24. The Veterans Administration Cooperative Urological Research Group. Carcinoma of the prostate: treatment comparisons. *J Urol* 1967;96:516.
25. Cox RL, Crawford ED. Estrogens in the treatment of prostate cancer. *J Urol* 1995;154;1991–1998.
26. Iverson P. Orchidectomy and oestrogen therapy revisted. *Eur Urol* 1998;34(Suppl):7–11.
27. Neuman F, Graf K. Discovery, development, mode of action and clinical use of cyproterone acetate. *J Int Med Res* 1982; 3:1–9.
28. Migliari R, Balzano S, Scarpa RM. Short-term effects of flutamide administration on hypothalamic-pituitary–testiclar axis in men. *J Urol* 1988;139:637–639.
29. Belanger A, Giasson M, Couture J, et al. Plasma levels of hydroxy-flutamide in patients with prostatic cancer receiving the combined hormonal therapy: an LHRH agonist and flutamide. *Prostate* 1988;12:79–84.
30. Wysowski DK, Freiman JP, Tourtelot JB, et al. Fatal and nonfatal hepatotoxicity associated with flutamide. *Ann Intern Med* 1993;118:860–864.
31. Sarosdy MF. Which is the optimal antiandrogen for use in combined androgen blockade of advanced prostate cancer? The transition from first to second generation antiandrogen. *Anticancer Drugs* 1999;10:791–796.
32. Iversen P, Tyrrell CJ, Kaisary AV, et al. Bicalutamide monotherapy compared with castration in patients with nonmetastatic locally advanced prostate cancer: 6.3 years of followup. *J Urol* 2000;164:1579–1582.
33. Kasimis B, Wilding G, Kries W, et al. Survival of patients who had salvage castration after failure on bicalutamide monotherapy for stage D2 prostate cancer. *Cancer Invest* 2000;18:602–608.
34. Seidenfeld J, Samson DJ, Hassselblad V, et al. Single-therapy androgen suppression in men with advanced prostate cancer: a systematic review and meta-analysis. *Ann Int Med* 2000;132:566–567.
35. Pound CR, Partin AW, Eisenberger MA, et al. Natural history of progression after PSA elevation following radical prostatectomy. *JAMA* 1999;281:1591–1597.
36. Wasson J, Fowler FJ, Barry MJ. Androgen deprivation therapy for asymptomatic advanced prostate cancer in the prostate specific antigen era: a national survey of urologist beliefs and practices. *J Urol* 1998;159:1993–1997.

36a. Moul JW. Prostate specific antigen only progression of prostate cancer. *J Urol* 2000;163:1632–1642.

37. Messing EM, Manola J, Sarosdy M, et al. Immediate hormonal therapy compared with observation after radical prostatectomy and pelvic lymphadenectomy in men with node-positive prostate cancer. *N Engl J Med* 1999;341:1781–1788.
38. Kubota T, Hisatake J, Hisatake Y, et al. HPPC-SPES: a unique inhibitor of proliferation of prostate cancer cells in vitro and in vivo. *Prostate* 2000;42:163–171.
39. DiPaola RS, Zhang H, Lambert GH, et al. Clinical and biologic activity of an estrogenic herbal combination (PC-SPES) in prostate cancer. *N Engl J Med* 1998;339:785–791.
40. Hsieh T, Chen SS, Wang X, et al. Regulation of androgen receptor (AR) and prostate specific antigen (PSA) expression in the androgen-responsive human prostate LNCaP cells by ethanolic extracts of the Chinese herbal preparation, PC-SPES. *Biochem Mol Biol Int* 1997;42:535–544.
41. Daniell HW, Dunn SR, Ferguson DW, et al. Progressive osteoporosis during androgen deprivation therapy for prostate cancer. *J Urol* 2000;163:181–186.
42. Daniell HW. Osteoporosis after orchiectomy for prostate cancer. *J Urol* 1997;157:439–444.
43. Townsend MF, Sanders WH, Northway RO, et al. Bone fractures associated with luteinizing hormone-releasing hormone agonists used in the treatment of prostate carcinoma. *Cancer* 1997;79:545–550.
44. Fonseca R, Rajkumar SV, White WL, et al. Anemia after orchiectomy. *Am J Hematol* 1998;59:230–233.
45. Strum SB, McDermed JE, Scholz MC, et al. Anemia associated with androgen deprivation in patients with prostate cancer receiving combined hormone blockade. *Br J Urol* 1997;79:933–941.
46. The Leuprolide Study Group. Leuprolide versus diethylstilbestrol for metastatic prostate cancer. *N Engl J Med* 1989; 311:181.
47. Casper RF, Yen SS. Neuroendocrinology of menopausal hot flushes: an hypothesis of the flush mechanism. *Clin Endocrinol* 1985;22:293–312.
48. Smith JA. A prospective comparison of treatments for symptomatic hot flushes following endocrine therapy for prostate cancer. *J Urol* 1994;152:132–134.

41

COMBINED ANDROGEN BLOCKADE FOR THE TREATMENT OF METASTATIC CANCER OF THE PROSTATE

PAUL F. SCHELLHAMMER

Although Surveillance, Epidemiology, and End Results data from the Utah registry show that the incidence of prostate cancer has continued to decline from a peak age-adjusted incidence of 250 cases to 100,000 in 1992, and the American Cancer Society has decreased its incidence projections from 334,500 in 1997 to 179,300 in 1999, prostate cancer continues to account for 29% of all cancers diagnosed in the U.S. male population (1,2). Disease prevalence, the pool from which incident cancers arise, is indeed astounding. Autopsy findings in older men indicate that the incidence of prostate cancer nearly doubles with each decade of life after age 50 years—from 10% of men in their fifties to 70% of men in their eighties (3,4). In addition, recent studies have identified microscopic cancer in a large percentage of very young men. An autopsy series of men aged 10 to 49 years identified prostatic intraepithelial neoplasia in 9%, 20%, and 44% and a small foci of histologic cancer in 0%, 27%, and 34% of men in their third, fourth, and fifth decades, respectively (5).

However, in the face of this prevalent disease burden, the dynamics of prostate-specific antigen (PSA) early detection have changed incidence demographics. As a consequence of early PSA detection, prevalent cases have been culled from the population so that currently the number of new diagnoses is not the sum of prevalent and incident cases but essentially a reflection of the latter. Therefore, the incidence of prostate cancer has diminished to less than 200,000 cases per year. As a result of PSA detection, the proportion of patients with metastatic disease at diagnosis has also further diminished. Data from the National Cancer Database of the American College of Surgeons Commission on Cancer and from the National Cancer Institute's (NCI) Surveillance, Epidemiology, and End Results Program for the years 1984 through 1991 indicate that 30% of men have advanced (regional or metastatic) disease at the time of diagnosis (6,7). Recent data have shown a dramatic decrease in M1 disease to 8% of newly diagnosed cancers (2). This decreasing absolute and proportion of incidence in advanced disease is an experience common to all urologists.

As an example, the percent of patients with M1 disease presenting to a community medical school practice (Eastern Virginia Medical School) in 1985 was 32%, 11% in 1994, and 10% in 1998 (8). The experience extends to Europe. The large European screening trial found a 2% incidence of metastatic disease at diagnosis, compared to the metastatic disease incidence of 22% in the 1989 to 1995 time period (9).

Although this migration to early-stage disease at detection will reduce the number of patients receiving androgen deprivation therapy as initial treatment, the pool of patients with a rising PSA after definitive therapy is expanding and will represent a large population for whom androgen deprivation therapy will be considered and most often applied. In support of this, a recent poll of urologists indicated that 69% were likely to use androgen deprivation when PSA rises were detected after local therapy (10). In the final analysis, a large proportion of men with prostate cancer will eventually experience androgen deprivation—those who do present with advanced disease initially; those with local disease treated with neoadjuvant or adjuvant androgen deprivation, or both, in addition to definitive local therapy; and, finally, the largest population, namely those with local therapy who evidence biochemical disease progression.

The hormonal dependency of cancer of the prostate was established in 1941 by Huggins and colleagues (11,12). They demonstrated the dramatic response to surgical castration in men with metastatic disease. However, after this dramatic clinical response, prostate cancer became refractory to hormonal treatment with a median progression-free survival of 18 to 24 months and a median survival of 24 to 30 months (13,14). Further application of hormonal manipulation was investigated. It was recognized that, although surgical castration removed the source of 95% of total testosterone production, androgenic substances are

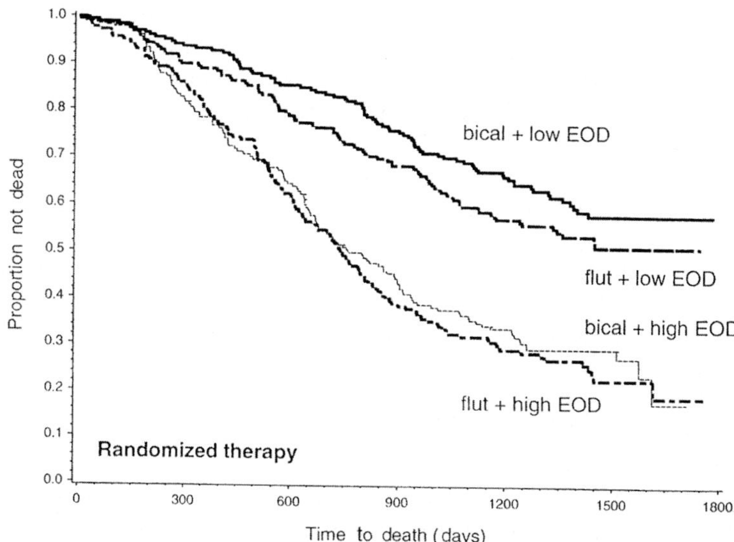

FIGURE 41-1. Comparison of extent of disease (EOD) for patients with combined androgen blockade with bicalutamide (bical) or flutamide (flut) as an antiandrogen. (From AstraZeneca, with permission.)

also produced by the adrenal gland. Huggins questioned whether these adrenal androgens were responsible for the observed relapses after orchiectomy. He tested the hypothesis by performing surgical adrenalectomy in patients with progressive prostate cancer after surgical castration (15). A rapid subjective and objective response was observed in some patients but was short lived. This initial foray into combined androgen blockade (CAB) was thwarted by the substantive surgical procedure of adrenalectomy in ill patients and was further complicated by the problems of postoperative hypoadrenalism. The concept of adrenal blockade, however, remained intriguing and was pursued by others who used adrenal biosynthesis inhibitors, such as aminoglutethimide (16). However, toxicity remained significant. The full exploration of the concept awaited the development of new pharmaceutical agents. It is important to recognize that coincidental with extensive exploration of these new agents was the previously mentioned stage migration to lesser disease volume even among patients with nominally M1 metastatic disease. Therefore, apparent advances in therapeutic results must always be tempered by the more favorable disease status of the populations treated. For example, the earlier detection of metastatic disease as a result of radiologic imaging prompted by PSA elevations has extended the survival interval after the initiation of androgen deprivation for M1 disease through the mechanism of lead-time bias. The median survival of patients with radiologically documented metastatic disease entering a large randomized trial using CAB exceeded 3 years (17). This prolonged response is explained by the minimal extent of disease present in 43% of patients. In fact, when analyzed by disease extent, the median survival for minimal disease had not been reached at 5 years (18) (Fig. 41-1). This extension of survival after initiation of androgen deprivation will be further amplified as therapy is initiated on the prompt of PSA rise alone, absent any physical, radiologic, or other laboratory evidence of disease.

NEW PHARMACOLOGIC AGENTS

The development of two classes of pharmacologic agents in the early 1970s set the stage for a reawakening in the interest and application of CAB. Readily applied and reversible and well-tolerated medical treatment regimens became available that circumvented the drawbacks of the surgical approach. Luteinizing hormone releasing hormone agonists (LHRHa) that could produce medical castration and nonsteroidal antiandrogens that could block adrenal androgen effect ushered in an era of CAB therapy. Parenthetically, it is of interest that the two Nobel prizes to grace urologic disease were received by Huggins and Schalley in recognition of their investigations on the hormonal therapy of prostate cancer.

Luteinizing Hormone Releasing Hormone Analogs

The biologic action of LHRH, which is released in a pulsatile fashion by the hypothalamus, is to induce the synthesis and release of LH by the pituitary, which in turn stimulates the testis to produce testosterone. However, chronic administration of potent synthetic analogs of LHRH causes a depletion of receptors and paradoxic decline in testosterone to castrate levels (19). LHRHa do not affect extratesticular androgen production. There is evidence suggesting a direct inhibitory effect of LHRHa on prostate cancer cells *in vitro* (20,21). LHRHa are peptides; thus, they cannot be administered orally. They are administered by daily or depot (long acting) injection. (Leuprolide acetate [Lupron] and goserelin acetate [Zoladex] are the most commonly injectable forms; buserelin is an LHRHa administered intranasally.) Clinical trials have demonstrated that daily treatment with LHRHa causes a decrease in serum testosterone by the third week of treatment in patients with advanced prostate cancer (22). Depot formulations of LHRHa are shown to be as effective (23,24). These long-acting preparations have obvious advantages related to patient comfort and treatment compliance.

LHRHa therapy has been compared to orchiectomy (25,26) and diethylstilbestrol (DES) (27,28). Patients with advanced prostatic carcinoma were treated with monthly injections of goserelin or orchiectomy in a prospective randomized trial. Castrate levels of testosterone were achieved by 4 weeks of goserelin therapy and were maintained during follow-up. Objective response was achieved in 82% of patients with goserelin versus 77% with orchiectomy. The two treatment groups did not differ significantly in time to treatment failure and survival (25,26). Studies comparing goserelin with 3-mg per day DES (27,28) found no significant difference in objective response rate, time to treatment failure, or survival but showed better patient tolerance of the goserelin treatment. Leuprolide has been compared with 3-mg per day DES. There was no statistically significant difference in objective response and 1-year survival rates (28).

The common side effect associated with LHRHa therapy is androgen deprivation. Rare complications include pituitary apoplexy (29) and renal failure (30). A flare phenomenon can be associated with the initiation of LHRHa. A transient overstimulation of receptors and a surge of testosterone secretion occur within the first few days of therapy. This may be associated with exacerbation of bone pain, upper and lower urinary obstruction (31), and neurologic symptoms in patients with spinal cord metastases. Sudden death due to disease flare has been reported (32). The flare phenomenon may be detrimental to the survival of patients with prostate cancer. Disease flare may be avoided by pretreating patients with antiandrogens (androgen receptor blockers). They may be initiated before or concurrent with the initiation of LHRHa treatment (17,33). One of the objections to the NCI 0036 study, as will be detailed later, was that flare was blocked in the LHRHa plus flutamide arm but not in the LHRHa only arm, thereby providing an advantage to the combination and a possible explanation for the improved survival in the combination arm. A large randomized trial of 813 patients began antiandrogen treatment simultaneously with LHRHa and recorded flare responses in less than 1% of patients (17,34). A chronic flare effect has also been postulated to occur with depot administration—namely, an intermittent asymptomatic testosterone flare with each injection. This disadvantage may be countered with the development of LHRH antagonists. Abarelix is an antagonist in clinical trial. Baseline and change from baseline testosterone, LH, and PSA were measured after LHRHa depot (4- and 12-week formulations) and compared to the same data after abarelix. Testosterone surge of 39% to 73% was measured with the LHRHa depot before returning to baseline at 9 to 11 days, whereas testosterone was 87% of baseline on the second day after abarelix (35,36); PSA levels fell by 43% at 2 weeks after abarelix, compared to only 5% after LHRHa depot. Therefore, more rapid androgen ablation without surge and more precipitous fall in PSA followed abarelix depot.

Although an overwhelming majority of patients treated with LHRHa does achieve castrate levels of testosterone, some do not (37,38), and, even in cases in which castration levels have been achieved, testosterone levels may subsequently increase (24,38). Therefore, when prostate cancer progresses during LHRHa therapy, a castrate testosterone serum level should be documented before the tumor is labeled androgen independent. Testosterone levels above castrate warrant surgical castration.

Antiandrogens

Antiandrogens are substances that block the androgen receptor sites at the target organs and exert their therapeutic action by blocking testosterone and dihydrotestosterone (DHT) from interacting with prostatic androgen receptors. The androgen receptor is a complex intracytoplasmic protein with three functional domains: the ligand-binding domain at the c-terminal, which binds androgens with high affinity; the DNA-binding domain; and the N-terminal domain. Androgen binding to the receptor causes a conformal change and translocation of the bound receptor to the nucleus that then binds to the DNA and initiates DNA transcription (39).

Antiandrogens may be steroidal or nonsteroidal in action. Cyproterone acetate (CPA), megestrol acetate, and medroxyprogesterone acetate are examples of steroidal antiandrogens. Of these, CPA, a potent antiandrogen and progestin, is commonly used to treat prostatic cancer (40). Steroidal antiandrogens, in addition to their ability to block the androgen receptor site in the prostate, also act like estrogen by inhibiting LH secretion in the pituitary and lowering serum testosterone to castrate levels. Experimental evidence also suggests that CPA may suppress adrenal secretion of androgens. The progestational property of CPA, while avoiding hot flashes, does lead to suppression of libido and erectile potency (41). Its steroidal properties also account for its propensity to cause cardiovascular side effects (42) and adversely affect serum lipoproteins (43). Hepatotoxicity has also been reported with CPA (44). Although used extensively in Canada and Europe, CPA is not U.S. Food and Drug Administration approved in the United States. In contrast, the family of nonsteroidal antiandrogens is devoid of progestational properties. Flutamide was the first nonsteroidal antiandrogen to be approved by the U.S. Food and Drug Administration. The active component is hydroxyflutamide, a metabolite of flutamide, which has a short half-life of 5.2 hours (45). Gastrointestinal intolerance, particularly diarrhea, is the most troublesome side effect associated with flutamide (46). Liver function abnormalities, including fatal hepatotoxicity, have been reported (47). The antiandrogen nilutamide (Nilandron) has a half-life of approximately 2 days (48). Side effects associated with nilutamide are abnormal light-dark adaptation and interstitial pneumonitis (49).

Bicalutamide (Casodex) is a nonsteroidal antiandrogen that has a 5- to 7-day half-life (50,51). Unlike flutamide, it does not require metabolic activation. Bicalutamide has relatively few side effects. Nonsteroidal antiandrogens have a high affinity and specificity for the androgen receptor without androgenic, estrogenic, progestational, or glucocorticoid properties. Theoretically, therefore, the androgen receptor blockade should fulfill the objective of complete androgen blockade, as the receptor is occupied and prevents ligand interaction from any source, whether from testes or adrenals. However, compared to testosterone and DHT, antiandrogens have a much lower affinity for the androgen receptor (50,51). Furthermore, antiandrogens act peripherally to inhibit androgen-stimulated prostate growth and centrally to inhibit the action of androgen on the hypothalamus and pituitary gland. The latter effect activates a positive feedback mechanism, leading to an increased secretion of LH and, consequently, an increased production of testosterone. On the one hand, this preservation of serum testosterone levels has the advantage of preserving libido and potency in two-thirds of patients with normal pretreatment sexual function. On the other hand, this rise in testosterone levels after antiandrogen administration may displace antiandrogens from the androgen receptors and negate their therapeutic effect. All of the antiandrogens have been tested in clinical trials in combination with medical or surgical castration to achieve CAB.

COMBINED ANDROGEN BLOCKADE

Geller initially described the phenomenon of elevated DHT in the prostatic cells of patients after surgical castration and postulated that adrenal androgens could provide a source of DHT and continued androgenic stimulus (52). The large body of basic science endocrinology that provided experimental evidence for this concept came from the laboratory of Dr. Ferdinand Labrie (52a). Labrie demonstrated that humans are unique among animal species in having adrenals that secrete large amounts of the inactive precursor steroids dehydroepiandrosterone (DHEA); its sulfate, DHEAS; and androstenedione. In accordance with Geller's concepts and findings, these adrenal androgens can be converted into more potent androgens in peripheral tissues, including the prostate. The plasma levels of DHEAS are 100- to 500-fold higher than testosterone and therefore, although qualitatively of relatively low potency, quantitatively they provide a substantial substrate for conversion into the more potent androgens by the prostate (53). Approximately 60% of total intraprostatic DHT originates from the testis, whereas 40% is of adrenal origin (53) (Fig. 41-2). Based on this clarification of physiology and endocrinology and the availability of LHRHa and antiandrogens, the stage was set for clinical testing of CAB in men with prostate cancer. Initial studies were conducted with the steroidal antiandrogen CPA. Bracci and Di Silverio described the use of a steroidal antiandrogen, CPA, in conjunction with bilateral orchiectomy in 1977 (54). In 1983, Labrie published a small phase-2 trial that included 37 previously untreated patients with stage C or D prostate cancer. He combined leuprolide with the nonsteroidal antiandrogen flutamide and reported an objective response in 29 of 30 evaluable patients (55). Labrie subsequently published a further successful application of combined therapy (56,57). As a result, CAB was widely publicized as an unqualified success as a primary treatment for patients with prostate cancer. However, there was cause for concern in that a natural experiment of nature seemed at odds with this success. Specifically, prostate cancer does not occur in men with intact adrenal function who had suffered traumatic or purposeful prepubertal castration. This objection was countered by the statement that adrenal androgens, although not capable of initiating prostate cancer, could conceivably sustain or support prostate cancer already initiated in the adult man; that prostate cancer cells are more "sensitive" to adrenal androgens; and that these sensitive clones, which survived castration effect, might be suppressed by the addition of antiandrogen to surgical or medical castration. Although androgen-independent cells also likely present *ab initio* and will eventually repopulate the tumor volume and result in hormone refractory disease and prostate cancer mortality, duration of response might be significantly prolonged with CAB, and this might be reflected in lengthened survival. A detailed discussion of the pros and cons surrounding these arguments has been thoroughly reviewed by Schröder et al. (58). Only randomized clinical trials could clarify the issue. Appropriately, these were constructed to test the hypothesis of clinical benefits for CAB.

For clarification, the terms *complete* or *total* androgen blockade, often used to describe the combination of castration plus an antiandrogen, are inaccurate. Although these latter two terms describe the intent of a combination of pharmacologic agents to negate androgenic effect, they do not assure that this end point completely or totally is indeed realized. The term *combination androgen blockade* is therefore a more accurate and appropriate descriptor of the regimen without overstating the end point.

RANDOMIZED CLINICAL TRIALS

The advantage of a new treatment strategy rests in the demonstration in a prospective, randomized trial of its superiority of efficacy or the demonstration of equal efficacy at reduced toxicity when compared to standard therapy.

The CAB concept has received as much attention as any with regard to testing in randomized controlled trials. It certainly has been the most intensively studied treatment protocol for prostate cancer. These investigations have not led to a unanimous opinion as to the advantage of combined therapy or its defined role in treatment, because some published studies have reported a significant treatment

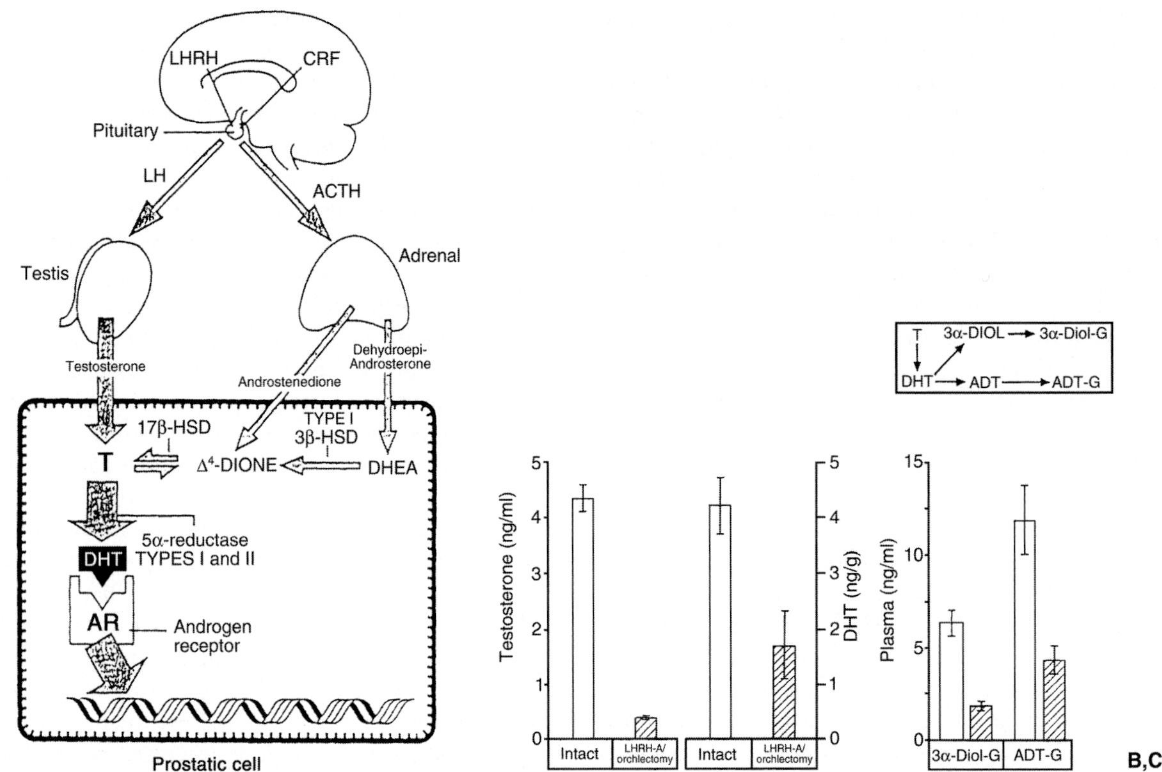

FIGURE 41-2. **A:** Intracrine activity in the human prostate or biosynthetic steps involved in the formation of the active androgen dihydrotestosterone (DHT) from testicular testosterone (T) as well as from the adrenal precursors dehydroepiandrosterone (DHEA), DHEA sulfate, and androstenedione (Δ^4-dione) in human prostatic tissue. The widths of the arrows indicate the relative importance of the sources of DHT in the human prostate; approximately 60% of total intraprostatic DHT originates from the testes, whereas 40% is of adrenal origin in a 65-year-old man. The testes secrete testosterone, which is transformed into the more potent androgen DHT by 5α-reductase in the prostate. Instead of screening T or DHT directly, the adrenal secretes very large amounts of precursors of DHT, namely DHEA and DHEA sulfate, as well as some Δ^4-dione, which are transported in the blood to the prostate and other peripheral tissues. These inactive precursors are then transformed locally into the active androgens T and DHT by intracrine activity. In fact, the enzymatic complexes DHEA sulfatase, 3β hydroxysteroid dehydrogenase/isomerase (3β-HSD), 17β hydroxysteroid dehydrogenase (17β-HSD), and 5α-reductase, and all are present in the prostatic cells, thus providing 40% of total DHT in this tissue. **B:** Effect of castration on the serum levels of T, on one hand, and on the concentration of the active androgen 5α-DHT remaining in prostatic cancer tissue after castration, on the other hand. Note the relatively small effect (approximately 60%) of castration on intraprostatic DHT concentration as compared to the 90% fall in serum T. **C:** Plasma concentrations of androstane-3α, 17β-diol glucuronide (3α-Diol-G), and androsterone glucuronide (ADT-G) on 20 intact and 18 castrated (*shaded area*) men with prostate cancer. Patients were of similar ages. ACTH, adrenocorticotropic hormone; CRF, corticotropin-releasing factor; LHRH-A, luteinizing hormone releasing hormone agonist. (From Labrie F, Belanger A, Dupont A, et al. Science behind total androgen blockade: from gene to combination therapy. *Clin Invest Med* 1993;16:475–492, with permission.)

effect in favor of CAB for advanced prostate cancer, whereas others have not. Many of the studies failing to show a superiority of CAB to castration monotherapy had inadequate statistical power to do so, based on insufficient patient populations or duration of follow-up, or both, or other methodologic weaknesses (59). It has been stated that to detect a clinically and statistically significant difference in survival end points between alternative treatments in patients with prostate cancer, it is necessary to accrue at least 300 patients to each treatment (60). The enrollment in many studies that failed to detect any advantage with CAB enrolled fewer patients. On the other hand, those trials that have shown significance to the combined therapy have been questioned as to the clinical importance and clinical impact of the statistical analysis (i.e., statistical significance without clinical relevance).

Trials Pre–National Cancer Institute 0105: Confirmatory of Combined Androgen Blockade

Spurred by the potential benefits of CAB, the NCI sponsored an intergroup cooperative study that was initiated in 1985. When published in 1989, this double-blind, ran-

TABLE 41-1. SUMMARY OF STUDIES THAT CONFIRM SURVIVAL BENEFIT WITH COMBINED ANDROGEN BLOCKADE THERAPY

Study (reference)	Study design	Population	Study drugs	n	Maximum/mean follow-up	Progression-free survival	Median length of survival (mo)
NCI INT-0036 (45,61)	DB, R, PC	Stage D2	LPL + FLT LPL + PLC	303 300	48 mo (max)	16.5 vs. 13.9 mo, $p = .039$	35.6 vs. 28.3, $p = .035$[a]
EORTC 00853 (62–67)	R	Stage M1	GSA + FLT SC alone	164 163	7.2 yr (med)	$p = .009$	34 vs. 27, $p = .008$[b] $p = .04$[a]
Anandron International Study Group (101,102)	DB, R, PC	Stage M1	Nil + SC SC alone	225 232	82–102 mo (range)	21.2 vs. 14.7 mo, $p = .002$	37 vs. 29.8, $p = .013$[b] $p = .033$[a]

DB, double-blind; EORTC, European Organization on Research and Treatment of Cancer; FLT, flutamide 250 mg 3 times a day orally; GSA, goserelin acetate 3.6 mg every 28 days subcutaneously; LPL, leuprolide 1 mg/day subcutaneously; max, maximum; NCI INT, National Cancer Institute Intergroup; Nil, nilutamide 300 mg/day for 1 mo followed by 150 mg/day subcutaneously; PC, placebo-controlled; PLC, placebo; R, randomized; SC, surgical castration.
[a]Overall survival.
[b]Cancer-specific survival.

domized, placebo-controlled NCI Intergroup study (NCI INT-0036), coordinated by the Southwest Oncology Group (SWOG) (45,61), was the largest trial on the subject. The maximum follow-up was 48 months. The final analysis of this study of 603 previously untreated patients with metastatic (stage D2) disease found that progression-free survival (16.5 months: 95% confidence interval (CI), 14.6 to 19.5) and median length of survival (35.6 months: 95% CI, 31.2 to 38.9) were significantly longer in patients treated with CAB (1 mg per day leuprolide subcutaneously plus 250 mg of flutamide three times a day orally) than in those treated with leuprolide plus placebo (13.9 months: 95% CI, 10.8 to 15.3; and 28.3 months: 95% CI, 25.7 to 30.6, respectively). The proportional hazards regression test for the difference in survival distribution was significant for progression-free survival ($p = .039$) and median length of survival ($p = .035$) (Table 41-2). Of interest is the fact that, although this trial was not initially powered by patient sample size to detect the 26% survival difference that was found (the original calculations included a 90% power to detect a 40% difference), the very rapid accrual of patients over 15 months provided enough events (deaths) at analysis to establish this lesser difference as statistically significant. In addition, the overall response rate (complete plus partial responses) as assessed by the National Prostatic Cancer Project criteria was higher, although not significantly, in the CAB group (43.6% vs. 35.3%). Post-study subgroup analysis found the greatest benefit from CAB for a small number of patients with a good performance status and minimal disease. The only adverse event, reported significantly more often in the CAB group, was diarrhea (13.6% vs. 4.9%, $p < .001$).

The urologic group of the European Organization on Research and Treatment of Cancer (EORTC) conducted a phase 3 randomized study comparing CAB (goserelin acetate, 3.6 mg every 4 weeks subcutaneously plus flutamide, 250 mg three times a day orally) with bilateral orchiectomy in 327 previously untreated patients with metastatic (stage M1) prostate cancer (EORTC 30853) (Table 41-1) (62–67). When initially reported with a median follow up of 2.5 years, there was no statistical advantage to CAB. However, final analysis, conducted at a median follow-up of 7.2 years, proved different (67). With 80% of patients expired, time to death due to malignant disease ($p = .008$) and time to first progression ($p = .009$) and progression-free survival ($p = .02$) were significantly longer in patients treated with CAB. As with the NCI trial, there was a statistically significant survival advantage in favor of CAB ($p = .04$); the medians for duration of survival with CAB and orchiectomy were 34 months and 27 months, respectively (Table 41-2). There were significantly fewer deaths due to malignant disease in patients treated with CAB (94

TABLE 41-2. NATIONAL CANCER INSTITUTE INT-0105 OUTCOMES

Overall survival and median time to progression: study INT-0105				
	All patients		Minimal disease subset	
Survival (mo)	CAB (n = 697)	Orchiectomy (n = 685)	CAB (n = 141)	Orchiectomy (n = 146)
Progression-free	20.4	18.6	48.1	46.2
Overall	33.5	29.9	52.1	51.0

CAB, combined androgen blockade.
Note: $p > .05$.

vs. 110), and the median time to death from malignant disease was 42 months with CAB and 29 months with orchiectomy (p = .008). Similar to the subgroup analysis in the NCI INT-0036 trial, CAB was particularly beneficial in patients with minimal disease. A rise in the PSA level predicted treatment failure and progression to lung or liver metastases was associated with extremely poor prognosis. The most frequently reported adverse events in both arms were hot flushes (70% CAB vs. 59% orchiectomy) and gynecomastia (22% vs. 8%), both anticipated pharmacologic effects of treatment. These gains in survival in the NIC and EORTC trials were achieved, therefore, with acceptable toxicity.

The first randomized controlled study that tested CAB was the EORTC Genitourinary (GU) Group protocol 30805 (68). This protocol was developed in 1979 before Labrie's initial study and report. It compared orchiectomy castration plus CPA, 150 mg per day, to orchiectomy alone. Treatment with DES, 1 mg daily, comprised a third arm; 335 patients with metastatic disease were accrued. The final analysis published in 1995 showed no difference in time to progression and overall survival among the three treatment arms. EORTC 30843 randomized 368 patients with M1 or M0N4 disease to orchiectomy or buserelin plus a short term (2 weeks) of CPA or continuous CPA. There was no difference in time to progression or survival between the treatment arms (69). The results of the trial 30853 differed from the prior CAB trials of the EORTC 30805 and 30843. Analysis of these trials revealed a difference in prognostic factors, which likely explained the outcome disparity between trials as discussed by Sylvester (70).

The multicenter, double-blind, randomized Anadron International Study Group trial compared nilutamide, 300 mg daily for 1 month, then 150 mg daily plus orchiectomy to orchiectomy plus placebo (Table 41-1) (71,72) in 457 patients with metastatic prostate cancer. At first analysis published in 1993, the follow-up for survival was approximately 4.5 years, and the median follow-up was 35 months. Statistically significant advantages favoring CAB were reported. The median interval to objective progression with CAB (20.8 months) was longer than that with orchiectomy alone (14.9 months); the difference in the survival distribution was significant (p = .0041). The overall response rate of 41%, similar to that in the NCI INT-0036 trial, was significantly (p <.001) higher than the 24% response rate with orchiectomy alone. The median intervals to death from all causes and from cancer were longer in the CAB group (27.3 months and 37.0 months, respectively), compared to the orchiectomy group (24.2 months and 30.0 months) but were not statistically different. An update of this trial was reported in 1997 (73). Patients continued taking study drug or placebo until progression or intolerance or withdrawal by personal consent. However, when progression occurred, only patients who had been on nilutamide continued the drug to permit a comparison according to maintained initial therapy. At second analysis, follow-up ranged from 82 to 102 months, which was 55 months longer than the first analysis for progression and 47 months longer than the first analysis for survival. The median intervals to progression were at 21.2 and 14.7 months for the combination versus the monotherapy arm, respectively. This 6.5-month difference was statistically significant (p = .002). The median intervals to death from prostate cancer were 37.0 and 29.8 months for the combination arm versus the monotherapy arm, respectively. This difference of 7 months was also statistically significant (p = .013). When all cause survival was analyzed, the advantage to the combination arm maintained statistical significance (p = .033). More patients in the CAB group than in the orchiectomy group had a decrease in pain (74% vs. 68%, p = .046) and normalization of prostatic acid phosphatase levels (51% vs. 32%, p = .027) at 1 month. Of interest in this study was the finding that normalization of PSA at 3- and 6-month intervals related to progression-free status and both cause-specific and all-cause mortality to a statistically significant degree. The finding is in contradistinction to the NCI orchiectomy with or without flutamide trial, NCI 0105, in which the normalization of PSA carried no statistically significant relationship to survival (74). In the nilutamide study, PSA levels were measured on only 272 of 457 patients. This might reduce the predicted accuracy as compared to the NCI study, which evaluated PSA levels in all 1,348 patients included on the study. A retrospective quality of life (QOL) evaluation was also performed for this trial (75). No instrument for QOL assessment had been available during the conduct of the trial. It was concluded that subjective improvement in pain and urinary symptoms and delayed subjective progression translated into an improvement in QOL. The nilutamide metaanalysis also supported a QOL advantage to CAB based on a statistically significant reduction in pain in the CAB arm. However, as described later, a prospective QOL assessment with validated instruments conducted as part of the INT-0105 trial clearly demonstrated a detriment to QOL in the combined arm that was highly significant (76). Once again, a caution is raised against translating retrospective analyses and hypotheses generating proposals into standard care without individual testing and confirmation in a randomized trial.

Inconclusive Studies

Several trials of CAB for the treatment of metastatic prostate cancer have been interpreted as not confirming the results of the NCI INT-0036, EORTC 30853, or the Anandron International Study Group trials (Table 41-3). However, the results of some of these trials are actually inconclusive, as they did not have sufficient statistical power to confirm the degree of survival benefit established in the NCI INT-0036 and other trials. These latter trials included smaller numbers of patients accrued over longer

TABLE 41-3. SUMMARY OF SELECTED STUDIES THAT DO NOT CONFIRM A SURVIVAL BENEFIT WITH COMBINED ANDROGEN BLOCKADE THERAPY

Study (reference)	Study design	Population	Study drugs	n	Maximum/mean follow-up	Progression-free survival	Median length of survival (mo)
IPSCG (77,78)	DB, R, PC	M0: 43%; M1: 57%	GSA + FLT GSA	287 284	56.2 mo (med)	NS between groups	42.2 vs. 37.7
DAPROCA (79–81)	R	M0: 7%; N,M0: 2%; M1: 91%	GSA + FLT SC alone	129 133	57 mo (med)	16.5 vs. 16.8 mo NS	22.7 vs. 27.6 NS
PONCAP (83)	R	C: 48%; D1: 7%; D2: 45%	GSA + FLT GSA	152 152	18 mo (med)	24 vs. 17 mo NS	NS between groups
Fourcade et al. (84)	DB, R, PC	M0: 17%; M+: 82%; Mx: 0.4%	GSA + FLT GSA + PLC	120 125	15 mo (med)	NS between groups	Not reached
Di Silverio et al. (85)	R	Stage M+, N+, T3/T4	GSA + CYA GSA	156 159	180 wk (mean) (interim analysis)	54 vs. 55 wk NS	NS between groups
Crawford et al. (87)	DB, R, PC	D2	LPL + Nil LPL + PLC	—	—	24.3 vs. 22.2 mo NS	—
Beland et al. (88)	DB, R, PC	—	ORCH + Nil ORCH + PLC	—	—	—	24.3 vs.18.9, $p = .137$

CYA, cyproterone acetate; DAPROCA, Danish Prostatic Cancer Study Group; DB, double-blind; FLT, flutamide; GSA, goserelin acetate 3.6 mg every 28 days subcutaneously; IPSCG, International Prostate Cancer Study Group; LPL, leuprolide 1 mg/day subcutaneously; Nil, nilutamide; NS, not significant; ORCH, orchiectomy; PC, placebo-controlled; PLC, placebo; PONCAP, Italian Prostatic Cancer Project; R, randomized; SC, surgical castration.

time intervals with fewer survival events available for analysis. They were not sufficiently powered to detect the 25% difference that was possible with the NCI trial. Low statistical power may be due to several factors, including an insufficient number of patients; an insufficient number of events; an accrual rate lower than anticipated in sample size calculations, which translates into fever events at analysis; and interval follow-up that is abbreviated. A review of the data from some of these trials is illustrative.

The International Prostate Cancer Study Group trial of 571 evaluable patients, which compared goserelin acetate and flutamide to castration monotherapy, did not confirm a beneficial effect of CAB by the parameters of objective response or survival (Table 41-3) (77,78). Objective response rates were 65% and 67%, respectively. The median duration of follow-up for survival at the final analysis of this trial was 56.2 months. The median length of survival was 42.2 months in the CAB group, compared to 37.7 months in patients treated with goserelin acetate alone. Analyses of survival were performed for all evaluable patients and separately for those with M0 and M1 disease. Forty-three percent of patients had M0 disease. The 300 patients with M1 disease whose median follow-up was 2 years were not numerically adequate to demonstrate the difference in survival found in the NCI INT-0036 trial. Of note was the finding that prostatic acid phosphatase and PSA exhibited a statistically greater decrease in the combination therapy arm.

The Danish Prostate Cancer Group (DAPROCA) compared goserelin acetate plus flutamide with orchiectomy in 262 previously untreated patients with advanced prostate cancer (DAPROCA 86) (79–81). Neither the interim analysis with median follow-up for survival of 30 months and 39 months nor the final analysis with a median follow-up for survival of 57 months found significant differences between treatment groups for time to progression of disease (16.5 months for CAB vs. 16.8 months for orchiectomy) or median length of survival (22.8 months vs. 27.6 months). The sample size determination for the DAPROCA 86 trial was based on detecting a 20% difference in response with 90% probability. The trial was not originally constructed to detect a difference in survival and could not, therefore, provide information regarding the 26% difference in survival found in the NCI INT-0036 trial. Although of identical construction as EORTC 3085, it also could not, for the same reasons, confirm EORTC 3085. In fact, the risk of overlooking a potential benefit from this trial has been calculated at 50% (82).

Analyses of studies by the Italian Prostatic Cancer Project investigators and a French group found no significant differences between CAB (goserelin acetate plus flutamide, doses as for EORTC 30853 trial) with respect to time to disease progression or survival based on a median follow-up of 18 months in 304 patients (83) and a follow-up period of 15 months in 245 patients (84). Based on sample size determinations, they will not have adequate statistical power to detect the treatment effect difference in survival of the NCI INT-0036 and EORTC 3085 trials.

An interim analysis (24 months) of an Italian cooperative multicenter trial found no significant differences in time to disease progression, overall survival, or response rates (objective and best response) between treatment with goserelin acetate, 3.6 mg every 28 days subcutaneously plus

TABLE 41-4. NATIONAL CANCER INSTITUTE INT-0036 OUTCOMES

Overall survival and median time to progression: study INT-0036				
	All patients		Minimal disease subset	
Survival (mo)	CAB (n = 303)	Leuprolide (n = 300)	CAB (n = 41)	Orchiectomy (n = 41)
Progression-free	16.5[a]	13.9	48.0	19.0
Overall	35.6[b]	28.3	61.0	42.0

CAB, combined androgen blockade.
[a] $p = .039$.
[b] $p = .035$.

200-mg CPA daily orally and goserelin acetate alone in 315 eligible patients (85,86).

Two U.S.- and Canadian-controlled, cooperative, randomized studies of CAB were published in 1990 and 1991. In a double-blind study involving 411 patients with newly diagnosed metastatic D2 prostate cancer, nilutamide (300 mg per day for 1 month, then 150 mg per day) was used as the antiandrogen in combination with leuprolide (1 mg per day subcutaneously), compared to leuprolide alone. A significantly better response rate (53% vs. 41%) and higher normalization of PSA (76% vs. 52% at 3 months) were associated with CAB (87). Additionally, at 6 months, CAB was significantly more effective for metastatic bone pain than was LHRHa alone. Although the median time to progression and survival was lengthened by the addition of nilutamide (24.3 vs. 22.2 months), the difference was not significant. These results were published before median progression-free or overall survival was reached. In a smaller, double-blind, randomized, multicenter, Canadian study, bilateral orchiectomy plus nilutamide was compared to orchidectomy alone in 208 patients with metastatic (stage D2) prostate cancer (88). Higher response rates (45% vs. 20%) were noted, and a greater proportion of patients had at least a 25% decrease in serum alkaline phosphatase (70% vs. 40% at 6 months) with CAB. However, there were no significant differences in time to progression or death, although the trend for overall survival favored CAB (24.3 vs. 18.9 months, $p = .137$). No subanalyses on patients with minimal disease were conducted in either of these studies.

Another factor that confounded the comparison of the various trials was the different modalities of castration (surgical vs. medical) and the different antiandrogen used (e.g., nilutamide, flutamide, or CPA). The question was raised: Is there enough difference between these agents within the same general family (specifically antiandrogens) to make a difference in treatment outcome?

The variable outcomes reported from these trials resulted in uncertainty and some confusion within the urologic community. Nevertheless, these variables served to awaken the interest in the statistical parameters and concepts that drive clinical trials—namely, clinical trial outcome needs to be understood in the context of sample size; events; size effect; confidence intervals, all calculated as part of initial trial design; and the omnipresent p value.

Retrospective subgroup analyses in the NCI INT-0036 and EORTC 30853 trials generated the hypothesis that particular benefit from CAB was seen in patients with minimal disease. To test this hypothesis would require a randomized trial to address this issue prospectively. To this end, and to confirm the NCI 0036 trial as well as answer some concerns about trial validity, two lines of further investigation followed: construction of a large confirmatory trial and combined evaluation of all individually reported trials by metaanalysis.

National Cancer Institute 0105

The NCI INT-0105 trial was initiated in December 1989 (Table 41-2). Accrual was completed in September 1994. It was a prospective study of the relative benefits of CAB and monotherapy based on the extent of disease for patients randomized to orchiectomy plus placebo or orchiectomy plus flutamide. With 1,378 patients accrued, this trial represents the largest to date to study the benefits of CAB (74). This trial was constructed to answer objections raised by the NCI INT-0036 trial. They were that daily subcutaneous injections of leuprolide may have driven a subclinical period of disease progression "flare" and that flutamide in the combination arm only served to block flare. The inference is that leuprolide alone may be inferior to surgical castration monotherapy. In addition was the concern that compliance with the required daily injection of leuprolide was not complete and the greater disadvantage that this imparts to the monotherapy arm compared to the combination arm, in which antiandrogen would buffer the detrimental effects of irregular compliance.

Based on the results of the NCI INT-0036 trial, the NCI INT-0105 trial was constructed to have a 90% power at a 0.05 level of significance (one sided) to detect a 25% improvement in survival from a median of 28.3 months (death hazard ratio of 1.25) (74). Information regarding treatment benefits for the subgroup of patients with minimal disease was considered of vital importance, as this subgroup of patients currently represents the majority of men with M1 disease as a result of the early complete radiologic evaluation triggered by a rising PSA profile.

For most physicians caring for patients with metastatic prostate cancer who based their treatment recommendations to use complete androgen blockade on the results of NCI trial 0036 published in the *New England Journal of Medicine* in 1989 (46), which showed a survival advantage to CAB, the final publication of NCI 0105 trial 10 years later in the same journal was quite startling, disturbing, and confusing. By the parameters used to construct the trial, there was no statistical advantage to orchiectomy plus flutamide versus orchiectomy alone (74). Although the trial did show an approximately 10% survival difference in favor of the combination (Fig. 41-3), this did not reach statistical significance, because the trial had been powered to demonstrate a 25% difference in survival between the two arms, a difference comparable to the NCI 0036 trial published 10 years before. However, it is important to recognize that a difference as large as 20% between the two groups could be missed. Furthermore, NCI 0105 had been constructed to randomize patients by performance status and extent of disease to monotherapy or combined therapy to test the validity of the hypothesis that patients with minimal disease would derive the greatest advantage from CAB, as had been noted in trial 0036. However, in NCI 0105, there was no statistically significant advantage to the combination for the good performance and minimal disease subgroups. Again, this outcome illustrated the danger of extrapolating post-trial subanalysis, no matter how logical or attractive, to standard practice without confirmation as a primary question in a subsequent randomized trial.

An interesting caveat to consider is the possible consequence of crossover to flutamide at the time of failure among patients taking placebo, which was permitted by trial design. Could this favorably modify the survival of the control arm so as to reduce the difference between the two arms? The nilutamide (Anandron) trial, which demonstrated survival superiority to CAB, did not permit addition of Anandron to the placebo arm at time of failure (72,73).

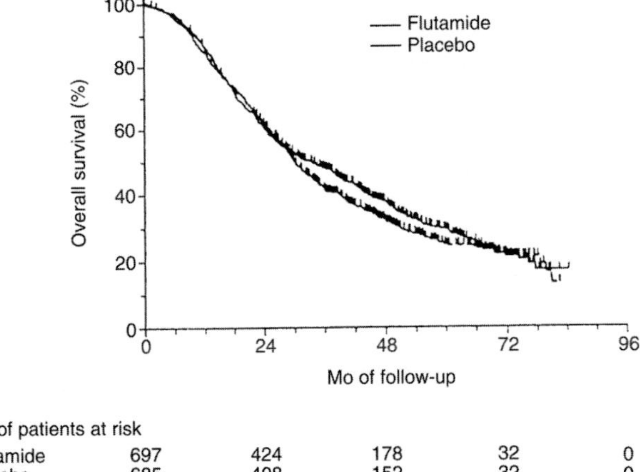

FIGURE 41-3. Overall survival among eligible patients with follow-up according to treatment assignment. (From Eisenberger MA, Blumenstein BA, Crawford ED, et al. Bilateral orchiectomy with or without flutamide for metastatic prostate cancer. *N Engl J Med* 1998;339:1040–1041, with permission.)

The NCI 0105 trial analysis also provided critically important information about the biomarker PSA. This was the first large trial to systematically include PSA as a marker of tumor status and response and to correlate its profile with survival end points. There was a statistically higher incidence of normalization to a PSA less than 4 (p = .018) in the combination arm. This intuitively might lead to the prediction that a better clinical and survival outcome was assured. If PSA response were truly a surrogate for survival, then this statistically significant reduction in PSA in the combination arm would predict a survival benefit for this arm. This was not the case, and, therefore, in the context of a large perspective randomized trial, which is the only mechanism for assigning surrogate end points, this discordance between PSA response and survival rendered PSA invalid as a surrogate end point. This fact calls into question the common reliance on serum PSA values as a meaningful predictor of long-term outcome. In fact, the discussion of results contained the statement "PSA has no role as surrogate marker for survival in patients with metastatic prostate cancer" (46). Questions and comments are pertinent with regard to the surrogate end point issue. Might there have been a correlation with survival if the stricter PSA end point of undetectable PSA had been used? Although PSA may not be a surrogate for survival in patients with hormone-naïve disease, in which PSA level decreases in response to cell death and gene down-regulation after androgen deprivation, it may be more "accurate" in the context of hormone refractory disease, in which PSA decrease is more related to a reduction in tumor cell population. However, the definition of surrogate end point is very precise, very restrictive, and most difficult to fulfill, as stated by Prentice and Flemming: "A valid surrogate end point must do two things: it must correlate with the end point of interest and it must, on interventions that change the end point, change accordingly. Thus, validation of surrogate end points can only occur in the context of trials that have studied interventions that are shown to effect change in end point" (89–91). As yet, no biomarker has achieved this level of surrogacy.

The NCI 0105 trial was also unique in that it measured QOL parameters and therefore was able to assess the incremental morbidity, if any, of combination therapy as compared to monotherapy. A separate publication analyzing QOL issues has been reported (74). A sobering conclusion was reached. Patients on the combination arms experienced a statistically higher incidence of gastrointestinal effects, anemia, and abnormality of liver function tests. In this setting, the patients receiving combination of orchiectomy and flutamide not only failed to achieve a response benefit but also paid a price both economically, the additional cost of the antiandrogen, and qualitatively, with depreciation in QOL. The attention to QOL in this clinical trial is especially important, because hormonal treatment of metastatic disease can be considered largely palliative rather than curative. Because relief of symptoms may be brought about at the expense of some treatment-related toxicity, it is important that overall QOL is maintained—namely, that the treatment will not worsen the patient's current status. As was done in this trial, QOL measurement should be gathered through patient-reported instruments. These instruments should also be collected at the same time for both treatment arms and should be administered so that patients feel no pressure to provide responses that might parallel their understanding of their disease response or the physician's attitude toward the same. Detailed knowledge of clinical response before a QOL evaluation might bias patients' reporting of their symptoms and QOL (i.e., favorable for an objective response and unfavorable if clinical response is lacking). Patients receiving flutamide reported more and worse emotional functioning at 3 and 6 months (p <.003) (Table 41-5). There were other QOL parameters that favored the group receiving placebo, although statistical significance was not reached. These data strongly suggest that QOL benefits within the first 6 months after treatment were reduced when flutamide was added to orchiectomy. The reason for the decrease in emotional functioning was unclear. It was postulated that emotional functioning might not only be mediated by symptoms' status but also by a direct effect. As already noted, receptors for antiandrogens are found in the central nervous system as has been documented from animal studies (50,51). The increases that occur in serum testosterone after the administration of flutamide support interaction with central nervous systems receptors that, by negative feedback, act to increase LH and testosterone. It is possible that the negative effects on emotional functioning that were observed are explained by the action of antiandrogens on androgen receptors in the brain, pituitary, and hypothalamus.

A specific side effect of CAB with flutamide, largely underappreciated, is the anemia that occurs in some patients. Strum et al. analyzed 133 patients at baseline and intervals after initiation of CAB (92). Hemoglobin declined in all patients through 6 months and declined 25% or greater in 13% of patients who developed significant symptoms. Anemia usually resolved after discontinuation of therapy but was delayed in older men (older than 68 years) and those who had been treated for more than 1 year. For men older than 68 years treated for more than 1 year, recovery did not occur until 12 months after CAB was discontinued. The anemia was less significant when bicalutamide was used as the antiandrogen.

TABLE 41-5. MENTAL HEALTH INDEX TOTAL SCORE ASSESSED IN NATIONAL CANCER INSTITUTE 0105 COMBINED ANDROGEN BLOCKADE TRIAL

Assessment time	Flutamide		Placebo		
	Mdn	n	Mdn	n	*p*
Baseline	76	363	76	352	.71
1 mo	76	325	80	315	.004
3 mo	80	313	84	301	.001
6 mo	76	291	84	274	.002

Mdn, median scores; n, number of patients.
Note: Higher scores reflect better functioning.
From Moinpour CM, Savage MJ, Troxel M, et al. Quality of life in advanced prostate cancer: results of a randomized therapeutic trial. *J Natl Cancer Inst* 1998;90:1537–1544, with permission.

Critiques of the QOL assessment have noted that only half of the patients were included in the analysis, and the sampling method to capture the group studied was not clearly described. Furthermore, the QOL differences were studied at 1, 3, and 6 months but not beyond. By limiting evaluation to the first 6 months, short-term side effects are emphasized, and the long-term QOL benefits might be missed.

The morbidity associated with CAB has spawned a number of studies investigating intermittent androgen deprivation using the combination of medical or surgical castration with an antiandrogen. These trials are being conducted both in the setting of advanced disease, M1 SWOG (SWOG 9346, INT-0162) and the setting of minimal disease—namely, a rising PSA after external beam radiation (NCI Canada). These trials will assess end points of progression, survival, and QOL. QOL assessments are most important in view of the increasing awareness of androgen deprivation–related morbidity, both physical and psychological, that is associated with continuous therapy. Obviously, only medical castration lends itself to intermittent therapy protocols.

Metaanalysis

A methodology to investigate the overall conclusions that can be drawn from a number of trials addressing the same questions with disparate outcomes is termed *metaanalysis*. In addition, metaanalysis is a frequently used strategy to combine the results of a number of small trials to gain statistical power for determining differences that these small trials, individually, are not able to detect. The disparate outcomes in individual, prospectively randomized trials and the small number of patients included in some trials prompted several metaanalyses of the published and unpublished data. The merits of randomized trials and metaanalysis have been summarized by LeLorier (six in Fritz's) (93). Blumenstein (94) has published a discussion of the pros and cons of the metaanalysis of CAB trials. A metaanalysis should include studies comparable in design and conduct so that data can be pooled. Greater weight is given to those studies with larger patient numbers and longer follow-up periods. There are several metaanalyses initiatives dealing with CAB that warrant discussion. The largest and most inclusive was conducted by the Prostate Cancer Trialists collaborative group (95,96). Twenty-two of the 25 possible trials that could be included were subject to metaanalysis, and the results were published in 1995 (96). The NCI 0105 trial data were not included, as it was in the process of accrual. Individual data for 5,710 patients, 87% of whom had metastatic disease, were obtained. Castration was accomplished by LHRHa or orchiectomy, and the antiandrogens used were CPA, nilutamide, or flutamide. At the time of the study, 52.7% of patients had expired. No statistical benefit to CAB was recorded. The overall mortality among patients randomized to castration alone was 58.4%, compared to 56.3% among those randomized to CAB. When patients were grouped by the type of castration or antiandrogen therapy, the outcome was the same: No significant difference between subgroups was detected. Subgroup analysis by ages younger than 65, 65 to 74, and older than 75 years showed no significant difference between treatment, CAB, or monotherapy in these three age categories. Furthermore, a separate analysis of patients with M0 and M1 disease did not alter the results.

The 5-year survival estimates were 22.8% for castration alone versus 26.2% for CAB. This absolute difference of 3.5% was not statistically significant. However, the CI for absolute improvement in survival was 0% to 7%. The study concluded that there was no survival difference during the first 2 years after randomization but, interestingly, did note that there appeared to be a slight survival difference after the second year (Fig. 41-4). The observation was made that perhaps patients with less advanced disease who would not be expected to die within a 2-year follow-up interval might benefit from CAB with longer-term follow-up. Although a large improvement in survival among patients with advanced disease had been excluded by this study, the existence of a more moderate benefit was not. The Prostate Cancer Trialists also concluded that the absence of survival benefit did not preclude a potential palliative benefit and improved QOL. This study is open to several critiques. One objection of interest is based on the fact that patients in the analysis published to date were uniformly maintained on therapy until death. Was it possible that the benefit of CAB occurs during the hormone-dependent phase of the disease and that this preservation of survival benefit depends to some degree on the withdrawal of the antiandrogen on documentation of progression to eliminate the possible confound of antiandrogen stimulation? The Prostate Cancer Trialists Collaborative Group planned to update results in 1997 with inclusion of new studies and extended follow-up of existing studies. As of this writing, the updated analysis has not yet been published, but a preliminary evaluation has appeared (97). The sample for analysis now includes more than 8,000 patients with 6,000 deaths and includes the NCI 0105 study. No significant survival improvement among patients receiving CAB was confirmed. At 5 years, the survival improvement with androgen blockade was 2%, and this dropped to 1% at 10 years. CPA had a worse survival curve than flutamide and nilutamide, but even when it was excluded from analysis, the addition of antiandrogen improved 5-year survival from 24.7% to only 27.6%. Taking the widest confidence limits, the 5-year survival was improved by somewhere between 0% and 5% by the antiandrogen.

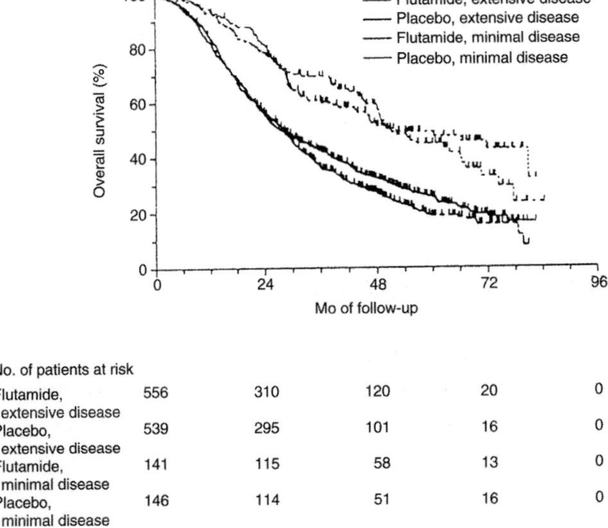

FIGURE 41-4. Overall survival among eligible patients with follow-up according to treatment assignment and extent of disease. (From Eisenberger MA, Blumenstein BA, Crawford ED, et al. Bilateral orchiectomy with or without flutamide for metastatic prostate cancer. *N Engl J Med* 1998;339:1040–1041, with permission.)

Although the first cycle of the analysis in 1995 found that CAB gave no survival advantage, with the caveat of larger confidence limits that did not exclude the possibility of a small improvement, the latest results effectively eliminate significant benefit from CAB.

Another metaanalysis evaluated the current outcome of nine clinical trials that had in common the use of flutamide as the antiandrogen (98). This study also included the NCI 0105 trial. The analysis of 4,128 patients demonstrated a 10% difference between monotherapy and combined therapy, and this effect size was statistically significant. It is of interest that the NCI 0105 trial indeed had found a 10% survival benefit with flutamide; however, the NCI 1015 trial had been sized to detect a larger difference, 25%, parallel to the difference of the first NCI study. However, with more subjects and more events, the same difference was statistically significant in the CAB with flutamide metaanalysis!

The Ontario Cancer Treatment Practice Guidelines Initiative suggested that the Prostate Cancer Collaborative Group metaanalysis had a series of methodologic weaknesses (99,100) in data collection and statistical decisions. The Canadian group conducted an analysis based only on published data (20 studies) and showed a clear benefit in 2-year survival with CAB over castration alone (99).

A recently updated European metaanalysis reanalyzed the metaanalysis of seven trials using CAB by orchiectomy with or without nilutamide, first reported in 1994

(101,102). With a follow-up of 52 to 78 months, the new metaanalysis showed that nilutamide added to orchidectomy significantly reduced the odds for disease progression by 17% and death from any cause by 16%, compared to orchidectomy alone. The reduction in the risk of death from cancer (16%) almost attained significance. Combination therapy also produced greater improvements in bone pain, tumor markers, and the response rate compared to orchidectomy alone (101). The authors commented that, in contrast to the Prostate Trialists (96) metaanalysis, they included only studies with similar methodology, inclusion and efficacy criteria, and follow-up period.

Another metaanalysis from the United States assessed the survival benefit associated with CAB (103). This analysis included only randomized controlled studies published as full articles and providing sufficient survival data; nine suitable studies were identified. CAB produced a significant overall and progression-free survival advantage compared to castration alone (16% to 22% and 23% to 26%, respectively) and also significantly increased the proportion of patients with objective tumor responses.

Last, an Agency for Health Care Policy and Research report completed in 1999 reached four conclusions and is reproduced verbatim (104):

1. There is no statistically significant difference in survival at 2 years between patients treated with CAB or monotherapy. Metaanalysis of the limited data available shows a statistically significant difference in survival at 5 years in favor of CAB. However, the magnitude of this difference is of questionable clinical significance. Eighteen trials (n = 5,485) reported no significant difference in overall survival, including the largest single trial (INT-0105), conducted by the SWOG, which included 1,382 patients. Three trials (n = 1,386) reported a statistically significant difference in overall survival favoring the CAB arm. The reported advantage in median survival ranged from 3.7 to 7.0 months; the advantage in the 5-year survival ranged from 3% to 9%. The metaanalysis found no difference between monotherapy and CAB in overall survival at 2 years (hazard ratio, 0.970; 95% CI, 0.866 to 1.087). There was an advantage in overall survival for CAB at 5 years (hazard ratio, 0.871; 95% CI, 0.805 to 0.942).
2. Only ten trials reporting 2-year survival also reported 5-year survival, which represents 66% of the patients in the metaanalysis. The results of sensitivity analyses suggest that if complete 5-year data were available, the magnitude of benefit from CAB would not be of greater clinical significance. The estimated combined hazard ratio for 5-year survival from all trials was 0.9146 for CAB compared to monotherapy (95% CI, 0.8461 to 0.9887).
3. For patients in a subgroup with good prognosis, there is no statistically significant difference in survival between CAB and monotherapy. Only six trials reported outcomes stratified by prognostic group. Two trials reported that CAB was of greater benefit than monotherapy for patients with good prognostic factors but did not report whether these results were statistically significant. Three other trials, which reported on both good and poor prognostic subgroups, found no statistically significant difference in outcome between treatment arms for either subgroup. The SWOG INT trial (INT-0105), the only trial prospectively designed and adequately powered to compare outcomes for good-risk patients, also found no significant difference in survival between CAB and monotherapy.
4. There is no statistically significant difference in survival among patients given CAB with different nonsteroidal antiandrogens. Of the three trials that reported a statistically significant difference in survival favoring CAB, two used flutamide and one used nilutamide. The metaanalysis found that CAB using flutamide or nilutamide appears to be equivalent. The hazard ratio is 0.878 (95% CI, 0.564 to 1.368) in trials using nilutamide and 0.945 (95% CI, 0.779 to 1.147) in trials using flutamide. In the only trial that directly compared two different regimens for CAB, there was no statistically significant difference in survival between men given flutamide or bicalutamide (hazard ratio, 0.87; 95% CI, 0.72 to 1.05) (17).
5. The evidence comparing adverse effects is limited but favors monotherapy over CAB. Evidence comparing QOL was available from only one study and also favored monotherapy. Patients randomized to CAB (10%) withdrew from treatment due to adverse effects more frequently than patients randomized to monotherapy (4%). The other evidence comparing adverse effects of these treatments is limited. The available evidence is inconsistent with respect to which adverse effects are reported and how these adverse effects are measured. In the recent SWOG trial (INT-0105) substudy, the only trial that compared QOL end points, patients randomized to CAB reported more problems with emotional functioning and diarrhea than those randomized to monotherapy.

TENTATIVE CONCLUSIONS

What is the urologist to make of all of this data and analytical and statistical gymnastics? It is clear that CAB has not been a major advance in the treatment of metastatic prostate cancer. It certainly has fallen short of any analogy to the "home run" that had originally been attributed to its benefits, when first applied clinically in a small select series of patients. Some would doubt that it could even be suitably described as a "base hit." However, there still lingers evidence that for some patients it might be useful: those patients receiving medical castration, those with minimal disease burden, and those with other, as yet unidentified, characteristics. Surgical castration monotherapy clearly does not benefit from the addition of flutamide by virtue of NCI 0105 results. Should combination androgen deprivation therapy be used when medical castration with an LHRHa is used, a conclusion consistent with NCI 0036 and EORTC 3085? Is medical castration identical to surgical castration such that the results of the NCI 0105 trial using surgical castration monotherapy can be extended to the use of medical castration monotherapy? As already noted, a castrate testosterone level may not universally follow LHRHa therapy, and response to surgical castration has been reported after LHRHa therapy (105). There may be a biologic difference between surgical and medical castration. LHRH and LH are decreased with LHRHa but increased after orchiectomy. Prostate cells display LH receptors, and cellular activity may be influenced (20,21,106). The question of whether surgical castration studies can be extended to LHRHa is critical, as LHRH analog administration is the preferred form of androgen deprivation (107). Patient preference studies and physician preference studies, which span the decade of the 1990s, have shown that medical castration is preferred to surgical castration. Is the blockade of potential miniflares with each LHRHa injection rationale for CAB? This may be especially pertinent when intermittent androgen blockade is being used where the initial exaggerated flair response with each resumption of LHRHa therapy might be expected.

The current information provides evidence that surgical castration and the antiandrogen flutamide are not better than castration monotherapy. Can this be extended to the use of other antiandrogens as well? Bicalutamide has not been used in combination versus monotherapy studies. However, nilutamide has been used in combination with surgical castration and has shown statistical advantages over monotherapy, as already discussed. However, nilutamide is infrequently used due to its side-effect profile. In the final analysis, one must conclude that, at best, CAB produces only a small improvement in survival or benefits significantly only a small proportion of those so treated. A small but statistically significant difference in a large group of patients in a clinical trial (or a metaanalysis) may well hide a few patients for whom the benefit is substantial. Nevertheless, identification of this favored subgroup is not possible by current prognostic parameters.

REFERENCES

1. Stephenson RA, Smart CH, Mineau GP, et al. The fall in incidence of prostate carcinoma. On the down side of a prostate specific antigen induced peak in incidence data from the Utah Cancer Registry. *Cancer* 1995;77:1342–1348.
2. Landis SH, Murray T, Bolden S, et al. Cancer statistics, 1999. *CA Cancer J Clin* 1999;49:8–31.
3. Scott R Jr., Mutchnik DL, Laskowski TZ, et al. Carcinoma of the prostate in elderly men: incidence, growth characteristics and clinical significance. *J Urol* 1969;101:602–607.
4. Sheldon CA, Williams RD, Fraley EE. Incidental carcinoma of the prostate: a review of the literature and critical reappraisal of classification. *J Urol* 1980;124:626–631.
5. Sakr WA, Haas GP, Cassin BP, et al. The frequency of carcinoma and intraepithelial neoplasia of the prostate in young male patients. *J Urol* 1993;150:379–385.
6. Mettlin C, Jones GW, Murphy GP. Trends in prostate cancer care in the United States 1974–1990: observations from the patient care evaluation studies of the American College of Surgeons Commission on Cancer. *CA Cancer J Clin* 1993; 43:83–91.
7. Harlan L, Brawley O, Pommerenke F, et al. Geographic, age, and racial variation in the treatment of local/regional carcinoma of the prostate. *J Clin Oncol* 1995;13:93–100.
8. Eastern Virginia Medical School Registry (unpublished data).
9. Schroder FH. Prostate cancer. *Cancer Screen Theory Pract* 1999;18:461–514.
10. Wasson JH, Fowler FJ, Barry MJ. Androgen deprivation therapy for asymptomatic advanced prostate cancer in the prostate specific antigen era: a national surgery of urologist's beliefs and practices. *J Urol* 1998;159:1993–1997.
11. Huggins C, Hodges CV. Studies in prostatic cancer. I. The effects of castration, of estrogen, and of androgen injection on serum phosphatases in metastatic carcinoma of the prostate. *Cancer Res* 1941;1:293–297.
12. Huggins C, Stevens RE, Hodges CV. Studies in prostatic cancer. II. The effects of castration on advanced cancer of the prostate gland. *Arch Surg* 1941;43:209–223.
13. Byar DP. The Veterans Administrative Cooperative Urological Research Group studies of cancer of the prostate. *Cancer* 1973;32:1126–1130.
14. Eisenberger MA, O'Dwyer PJ, Friedman MA. Gonadotropin-hormone-releasing hormone analogues: a new therapeutic approach for prostatic carcinoma. *J Clin Oncol* 1986;4:414–424.
15. Huggins C, Scott WW. Bilateral adrenalectomy in prostate cancer. Clinical features and urinary secretion of 17-ketosteroids and estrogen. *Ann Surg* 1945;122:1031–1041.
16. Robinson MR. Aminoglutethimide: medical adrenalectomy in the management of carcinoma of the prostate. A review after 6 years. *Br J Urol* 1980;52:328–329.
17. Schellhammer PF, Sharifi R, Block NL, et al. Clinical benefits of bicalutamide compared with flutamide in combined androgen blockade for patients with advanced prostatic carcinoma: final report of a double-blind randomized multicenter trial. *Urology* 1997;50:330–336.
18. Soloway M, Schellhammer P, Sharifi R, et al. Analysis by extent of disease and race comparing Casodex with Eulexin, each combined with luteinizing hormone releasing hormone analogue therapy, in 813 patients with advanced prostate cancer. Presented at American Urological Association Annual Meeting, 1996.
19. Labrie F, Auclair C, Cusan L, et al. Inhibitory effect of GnRH and its agonists on testicular gonadotropin receptors and spermatogenesis in the rat. *J Androl* 1978;2:303.
20. Dondi D, Limonta P, Moretti RM, et al. Antiproliferative effects of luteinizing hormone-releasing hormone (LHRH) agonists on human androgen-independent prostate cancer

cell line DU 145: evidence for an autocrine-inhibitory LHRH loop. *Cancer Res* 1994;54:4091–4095.

21. Pinski J, Reile H, Halmos G, et al. Inhibitory effects of analogs of luteinizing hormone-releasing hormone on the growth of the androgen-independent Dunning R-3327-AT-1 rat prostate cancer. *Int J Cancer* 1994;59:51–55.
22. Tolis G, Ackman D, Stellos A, et al. Tumor growth inhibition in patients with prostatic carcinoma treated with luteinizing hormone releasing hormone agonists. *Proc Natl Acad Sci U S A* 1982;79:1658–1662.
23. Debruyne FM, Dijkman GA, Lee DC, et al. A new long acting formulation of the luteinizing hormone-releasing hormone analogue goserelin: results of studies in prostate cancer. *J Urol* 1996;155:1352–1354.
24. Sharifi R, Soloway M. Clinical study of leuprolide depot formation in the treatment of advanced prostate cancer. The Leuprolide Study Group. *J Urol* 1990;143:68–71.
25. Soloway MS, Chodak G, Vogelzang NJ, et al. Zoladex versus orchiectomy in treatment of advanced prostate cancer: a randomized trial. Zoladex Prostate Study Group. *Urology* 1991;37:46–51.
26. Vogelzang NJ, Chodak GW, Soloway MS, et al. Goserelin versus orchiectomy in the treatment of advanced prostate cancer: final results of a randomized trial. Zoladex Prostate Study Group. *Urology* 1995;46:220–226.
27. Citrin DL, Resnick MI, Guinan P, et al. A comparison of Zoladex and DES in the treatment of advanced prostate cancer: results of a randomized, multicenter trial. *Prostate* 1991;18:139–146.
28. The Leuprolide Study Group. Leuprolide versus diethylstilbestrol for metastatic prostate cancer. *N Engl J Med* 1984;311:1281–1286.
29. Morsi A, Jamal S, Silverberg JD. Pituitary apoplexy after leuprolide administration for carcinoma of the prostate. *Clin Endocrinol (Oxf)* 1996;44:121–124.
30. Takezawa Y, Nakano K, Ohtake N, et al. Acute renal failure in a patient with chronic glomerulonephritis after the administration of LHRH analogue given for rectal obstruction due to prostate cancer. *Int J Urol* 1996;3:67–69.
31. Mahler C. Is disease flare a problem? *Cancer* 1993;72:3799–3802.
32. Thompson IM, Zeidman EJ, Rodriques FR. Sudden death due to disease flare with LHRH agonist therapy for carcinoma of the prostate. *J Urol* 1990;144:1479–1480.
33. Schulze H, Senge T. Influence of different types of antiandrogens on LHRH analogue induced testosterone surge in patients with metastatic carcinoma of the prostate. *J Urol* 1990;144:934–941.
34. Schellhammer P, Sharifi R, Block N, et al. Maximal androgen blockade for patients with metastatic prostate cancer: outcome of a controlled trial of bicalutamide versus flutamide, each in combination with luteinizing hormone-releasing hormone analogue therapy. Casodex Combination Study Group. *Urology* 1996;47:54–60.
35. Garnick MB, Cambridge MA, Campion MA, et al. PSA kinetics: rates of decline are significantly more rapid following therapy with the GnRH antagonist Abarelix-Depot (A-D), compared to superagonists Lupron (L) and Zoladex (Z) in prostate cancer (PrCA) patients (pts). *AUA* 1999: 367(abst).
36. Campion M, Garnick MB, Kuca B, et al. The magnitude of Lupron (L) or Zoladex (Z) testosterone (T) and luteinizing hormone (LH) surge is dependent on formulation: comparative results of L and Z vs. abarelix-depot (A-D), a GnRH antagonist devoid of androgen surge. *ASCO* 1999;B-11(abst).
37. Sharifi R, Bruskewitz RC, Gittleman MC, et al. Leuprolide acetate 22.5 mg 12-week depot formulation in the treatment of patients with advanced prostate cancer. *Clin Ther* 1996;18:647–657.
38. Soloway MS. Efficacy of goserelin in advanced prostate cancer and comparison with historical controls. *Am J Clin Oncol* 1988;11(Suppl 1):S29.
39. Beato M. Gene regulation by steroid hormones. *Cell* 1989;56:335–344.
40. Barradell LB, Faulds D. Cyproterone: a review of its pharmacology and therapeutic efficacy in prostate cancer. *Drugs Aging* 1994;5:59–80.
41. Neumann F, Furr BJ, Wakeling AE. Pharmacology and clinical uses of cyproterone acetate. In: *Pharmacology and clinical uses of inhibitors of hormone secretion and action*. London: Bailliere's Tindall, 1987;132–159.
42. Tveter KJ, Otnes B, Hannestad R. Treatment of prostatic carcinoma with cyproterone acetate. *Scand J Urol Nephrol* 1978;12:115–118.
43. Paisey RB, Kadow C, Bolton C, et al. Effects of cyproterone acetate and a long-acting LHRH analogue on serum lipoproteins in patients with carcinoma of the prostate. *J R Soc Med* 1986;79:210–211.
44. Pinganaud G, Chaslerie A, Marchasson IB, et al. Cyproterone-induced hepatotoxicity. *Ann Pharmacother* 1995;29:634.
45. Katchen B, Buxbaum S. Disposition of a new, nonsteroid, antiandrogen, xxx-trifluoro-2-methyl-4'-nitro-m-propionotoluidide (flutamide), in men following a single oral 20 mg dose. *J Clin Endrocrinol Metab* 1975;41:373–379.
46. Crawford ED, Eisenberger MA, McLeod DG, et al. A controlled trial of leuprolide with and without flutamide in prostatic carcinoma. *N Engl J Med* 1989;321:419–424.
47. Wysowski DK, Freiman JP, Tourtelot JB, et al. Fatal and nonfatal hepatotoxicity associated with Flutamide. *Ann Int Med* 1993;118:860–864.
48. Tremblay D, Dupont A, Meyer BJ, et al. The Kinetics of Antiandrogens in Humans. In: *Prostate cancer: a research into endocrine treatment and histopathology*. New York: Alan R. Liss, 1987:345–350.
49. Pfitzenmeyer P, Foucher P, Piard F, et al. Nilutamide pneumonitis: a report on eight patients. *Thorax* 1992;47:622–627.
50. Kennealey GT, Furr BJ. Use of nonsteroidal antiandrogen Casodex in advanced prostatic carcinoma. *Urol Clin North Am* 1991;18:99–110.
51. Furr BJA, Valcaccia B, Curry B, et al. ICI 176 (334). A novel nonsteroidal peripherally selective antiandrogen. *J Endocrinol* 1987;114:R7–R9.
52. Geller J, Albert JD. DHT in prostate cancer tissue: a guide to management and therapy. *Prostate* 1985;6:19–25.

52a. Labrie F, Belanger A, Dupont A, et al. Science behind total androgen blockade: from gene to combination therapy. *Clin Invest Med* 1993;16:475–492.

53. Labrie F, Dupont A, Belanger A. Complete androgen blockade for the treatment of prostate cancer. In: DeVita VT Jr.,

Hellman S, Rosenberg SA, eds. *Important advances in oncology*. Philadelphia: JB Lippincott Co, 1985:193–217.

54. Bracci U, Di Silverio F. Role of cyproterone acetate in urology. In: Martini L, Motta M, eds. *Androgens and antiandrogens*. New York: Raven Press, 1977:333–339.
55. Labrie F, Dupont A, Balanger A, et al. New approach in the treatment of prostate cancer: complete instead of partial withdrawal of androgens. *Prostate* 1983;4:579–594.
56. Labrie F, Dupont A, Belanger A. Complete androgen blockade for the treatment of prostate cancer. In: DeVita VT Jr., Hellman S, Rosenberg SA, eds. *Important advances in oncology*. Philadelphia: JB Lippincott Co, 1985:193–217.
57. Labrie F, Dupont A, Belanger A, et al. Combination therapy with Flutamide and castration (LHRH agonist or orchiectomy) in advanced prostate cancer: a marked improvement in response and survival. *J Steroid Biochem* 1985;23:833–841.
58. Schroder F, Van Steenbrugge GJ. Rationale against total androgen withdrawal. *Baillière's Clin Oncol* 1988;2:621.
59. Blumenstein BA. Some statistical considerations for the interpretation of trials of combined androgen therapy. *Cancer* 1993;72:3834–3840.
60. Suciu S, Sylvester R, Iverson P, et al. Comparability of prostate cancer trials. *Cancer* 1993;72:3841–3846.
61. Eisenberger MA, Crawford ED, Wolf M, et al. Prognostic factors in stage D2 prostate cancer: important implications for future trials: results of a cooperative intergroup study (INT. 0036). *Semin Oncol* 1994;21:613–619.
62. Denis L, Smith PH, Carnerio De Moura JL, et al. Orchiectomy vs Zoladex plus Flutamide in patients with metastatic prostate cancer. *Eur Urol* 1990;18(Suppl 3):34–40.
63. Keuppens F, Denis L, Smith P, et al. Zoladex and Flutamide versus bilateral orchiectomy: a randomized phase III EORTC 30853 study. *Cancer* 1990;6:1045–1057.
64. Denis LJ, Whelan P, Carneiro De Moura JL, et al. Goserelin acetate and Flutamide versus bilateral orchiectomy: a phase III EORTC trial (30853). *Urology* 1993;52:119–130.
65. Keuppens F, Whelan P, Carneiro De Moura JL, et al. Orchiectomy versus goserelin plus Flutamide in patients with metastatic prostate cancer (EORTC 30853). *Cancer* 1993;72:3863–3869.
66. Newling DW, Denis L, Vermeylen K, et al. Orchiectomy versus goserelin and Flutamide in the treatment of newly diagnosed metastatic prostate cancer. *Cancer* 1993;72:3793–3798.
67. Denis LJ, Keuppens F, Smith PH, et al. Maximal androgen blockade: final analysis of EORTC Phase III trial 30853. *Eur Urol* 1998;33:144–151.
68. Robinson MR, Smith PH, Richards B, et al. The final analysis of EORTC Genito-Urinary Tract Cancer Cooperative Group Phase III Clinical Trial (protocol 30805) comparing orchiectomy, orchiectomy plus cyproterone acetate and low dose stilboestrol in the management of metastatic carcinoma of the prostate. *Eur Urol* 1995;28:273–283.
69. De Voogt HJ, Studer U, Schroder FH, et al. Maximum androgen blockade using LHRH agonist buserelin in combination with short-term (two weeks) or long-term (continuous) cyproterone acetate is not superior to standard androgen deprivation in the treatment of advanced prostate cancer. *Eur Urol* 1998;33:152–158.
70. Sylvester R, Denis L, De Voogt H, et al. The importance of prognostic factors in the interpretation of two EORTC metastatic prostate cancer trials. *Eur Urol* 1998;33:134–143.
71. Janknegt RA, for the Anandron International Study Group. Total androgen blockade with the use of orchiectomy and nilutamide (Anandron) or placebo as treatment of metastatic prostate cancer. *Cancer* 1993;72:3874–3877.
72. Janknegt RA, Abbou CC, Bartoletti R, et al. Orchiectomy and nilutamide or placebo as treatment of metastatic prostatic cancer in a multinational double-blind randomized trial. *J Urol* 1993;149:77–83.
73. Dijkman GA, Janknegt RA, De Reijke TM, et al. Long-term efficacy and safety of nilutamide plus castration in advanced prostate cancer, and the significance of early prostate specific antigen normalization. International Anandron Study Group. *J Urol* 1997;158:160–163.
74. Eisenberger MA, Blumenstein BA, Crawford ED, et al. Bilateral orchiectomy with or without flutamide for metastatic prostate cancer. *N Engl J Med* 1998;339:1036–1042.
75. Dijkman GA, Fernandez Del Moral P, Debruyne FM, et al. Improved subjective responses to orchiectomy plus nilutamide (Anandron) in comparison to orchiectomy plus placebo in metastatic prostate cancer. *Eur Urol* 1995;27:196–201.
76. Moinpour CM, Savage MJ, Troxel M, et al. Quality of life in advanced prostate cancer: results of a randomized therapeutic trial. *J Natl Cancer Inst* 1998;90:1537–1544.
77. Tyrrell CJ, Altwein JE, Klippel F, et al. Multicenter randomized trial comparing Zoladex with Zoladex plus flutamide in the treatment of advanced prostate cancer. *Cancer* 1993;72: 3878–3879.
78. Tyrrell CJ, Altwein JE, Klippel F, et al. A multicenter randomized trial comparing the luteinizing hormone-releasing hormone analogue goserelin acetate along with flutamide in the treatment of advanced prostate cancer. *J Urol* 1991;146: 1321–1326.
79. Iversen P, Christensen MG, Friis E, et al. A phase III trial of Zoladex and flutamide versus orchiectomy in the treatment of patients with advanced carcinoma of the prostate. *Cancer* 1990;66:1058–1066.
80. Iversen P, Rasmussen F, Klarskov P, et al. Long-term results of Danish Prostatic Group Trial 86: goserelin acetate plus flutamide versus orchiectomy in advanced prostate cancer. *Cancer* 1993;72:3851–3854.
81. Iversen P, Danish Prostatic Cancer Group (DAP-ROCA). Zoladex plus flutamide vs. orchiectomy for advanced prostatic cancer. *Eur Urol* 1990;18(Suppl):41–44.
82. Denis L. Commentary on maximal androgen blockade in prostate cancer: a theory to put into practice? *Prostate* 1995; 27:233–240.
83. Boccardo F, Decensi A, Guarneri D, et al. Zoladex with or without flutamide in the treatment of locally advanced or metastatic prostate cancer: interim analysis of an ongoing PONCAP study. *Eur Urol* 1990;18(Suppl 2):48–52.
84. Fourcade RO, Cariou G, Coloby P, et al. Total androgen blockade with Zoladex plus flutamide vs Zoladex along in advanced prostatic carcinoma: interim report of a multicenter double-blind, placebo-controlled study. *Eur Urol* 1990;18(Suppl):45–47.
85. Di Silverio F, Serio M, D'Eramo G, et al. Zolodex vs. Zoladex plus cyproterone acetate in the treatment of advanced

prostatic cancer: a multicenter Italian study. *Eur Urol* 1990;18(Suppl 3):54–61.
86. Boccardo F, Rubagotti A, Barichello M, et al. Bicalutamide monotherapy versus flutamide plus goserelin in prostate cancer patients: results of an Italian prostate cancer project study. *J Clin Oncol* 1999;17:2027–2038.
87. Crawford ED, Smith JA, Soloway MS, et al. Treatment of stage D2 prostate cancer with leuprolide and Anandron compared to leuprolide and placebo. In: Murphy G, Khoury S, Chatelain C, et al., eds. *Recent advances in urological cancer diagnosis and treatment. Diagnostic and therapeutic progress in urological cancers.* Paris: FHS, 1990:61–62.
88. Beland G, Elhilali M, Fradet Y, et al. Total androgen ablation: Canadian experience. *Urol Clin North Am* 1991;18:75–82.
89. Schellhammer P, Cockett A, Boccon-Gibod L, et al. *Assessment of endpoints for clinical trials for localized prostate cancer.* New York: Elsevier Science, 1997.
90. Flemming TR. Surrogate markers in AIDS and cancer trials. *Stat Med* 1994;13:1423–1435.
91. Prentice RL. Surrogate endpoints in clinical trials: definition and operational criteria. *Stat Med* 1989;8:431–440.
92. Strum SB, McDermed JE, Scholz MC, et al. Anaemia associated with androgen deprivation in patients with prostate cancer receiving combined hormone blockade. *J Urol* 1997;79:933–941.
93. LeLorier J, Gregoire G, Benhaddad A, et al. Discrepancies between meta-analyses and subsequent large randomized controlled trials. *Eur Urol Update Series* 1995;4:186–194.
94. Blumenstein B. Overview analysis issues using the combined androgen deprivation overview analysis as an example. *Urol Oncol* 1995;1:95–100.
95. Dalesio O. Complete androgen blockade in prostate cancer: organizing an overview. *Cancer* 1990;66:1080–1082.
96. Prostate Cancer Trialists Collaborative Group. Maximum androgen blockade in advanced prostate cancer: an overview of 22 randomized trials with 3283 deaths in 5710 patients. *Lancet* 1995;346:265–269.
97. Key advances in the clinical management of prostatic cancer: androgen blockade makes little difference in survival. *Eur J Cancer* 1998;34:1822.
98. Bennett CL, Tosteson TD, Schmitt B, et al. Maximum androgen-blockade with medical or surgical castration in advanced prostate cancer: a meta-analysis of nine published randomized controlled trials and 4,128 patients using Flutamide. *Prostate Cancer Prostatic Disease* 1999;2:4–8.
99. Klotz LH, Newman T. Total androgen blockade for metastatic prostate cancer: history and analysis of the PCTCG overview. *Can J Urol* 1996;3(Suppl 2):102–105.
100. Trachtenberg J. Progress in complete androgen blockade. *Eur Urol* 1997;31(Suppl 2):8–10.
101. Bertagna C, DeGery A, Hicher M, et al. Efficacy of the combination of nilutamide plus orchiectomy in patients with metastatic prostate cancer. A meta-analysis of seven randomized double-blind trials (1056 patients). *Br J Urol* 1994;73:396–402.
102. Debruyne FM, De Gery A, Hucher M, et al. Maximum androgen blockade with Nilutamide combined with orchiectomy in advanced prostate cancer: an updated meta-analysis of 7 randomized, placebo-controlled trials (1191 patients). *Eur Urol* 1996;30(Suppl 2):264(abst).
103. Caubet J-F, Tosteson TD, Dong EW, et al. Maximum androgen blockade in advance prostate cancer: a meta-analysis of published randomized controlled trials using nonsteroidal antiandrogens. *Urology* 1997;49:71-78.
104. Submitted by AHCPR by the Evidence-Based Practice Center. *Testosterone suppression treatment for prostatic cancer.* AHCPR Publishers Clearinghouse, 1998.
105. Silver RI, Straus FH, Vogelzang NJ, et al. Response to orchiectomy following Zoladex therapy for metastatic prostate carcinoma. *Urology* 1991;37:17.
106. Sica G, Iacopino F, Settesoldi D, et al. Effect of Leuprorelin Acetate on cell growth and prostate-specific antigen gene expression in human prostatic cancer cells. *Eur Urol* 1999; 35(Suppl 1):2–8.
107. Cassileth BR, Seidmon EJ, Soloway MS, et al. Patients choice of the treatment in stage D prostate cancer. *Urology* 1989;33:57–62.

42

ALTERNATIVE HORMONE APPROACHES: INTERMITTENT, PERIPHERAL, TRIPLE

DAVID M. REESE
ERIC J. SMALL

For nearly six decades, the preferred primary treatment for advanced prostate cancer has been continuous suppression of testicular androgen production by medical or surgical castration (1,2). Although androgen deprivation is effective in inducing tumor regression in the large majority of cases, essentially all patients will develop progressive disease as indicated by rising prostate-specific antigen (PSA) levels, new lesions on radiologic studies, and, eventually, worsening symptoms. In addition, androgen deprivation may be associated with a variety of side effects, including hot flashes, fatigue, loss of lean muscle mass, sexual dysfunction (impotence and loss of libido), and cognitive changes or depression in some patients. Patients who have received long-term hormonal therapy may also develop anemia and, possibly, significant osteoporosis with the attendant risk of bone fracture (3,4). Finally, castration achieved by the use of luteinizing hormone releasing hormone (LHRH) agonists (with or without the addition of an antiandrogen) is very expensive. For these reasons, strategies that minimize the use of these agents could potentially lower the morbidity and cost associated with the treatment of advanced prostate cancer.

The observations that continuous androgen deprivation is not curative and may be associated with adverse effects, which compromise patient quality of life, have led to the search for alternative hormonal therapies. The general goals of these alternative approaches have been to increase the duration of effectiveness of hormonal intervention and to abrogate or eliminate common short- and long-term toxicities. The search for new methods of increasing the effectiveness of androgen deprivation has taken on particular urgency in the PSA era, because many patients are now being diagnosed with advanced or progressive prostate cancer on the basis of a rising PSA alone in the absence of objective evidence of recurrent disease or disease progression. Hormonal therapy is being used earlier in the course of the disease in many such patients, and these men may potentially be exposed to androgen deprivation for years. In the past, most patients receiving androgen deprivation had symptomatic metastatic disease and relatively short anticipated survival, but many patients now being treated with hormonal therapy are asymptomatic (or minimally symptomatic) and may survive for years. Thus, any long-term side effects of androgen deprivation may be particularly problematic in this patient population. It has been hoped that the development of alternative hormonal interventions might lead to enhanced antitumor efficacy as well as improvements in side effect profile.

INTERMITTENT ANDROGEN DEPRIVATION

Preclinical Observations

There is now accumulating experimental evidence to suggest that the progression of prostate cancer from an androgen-dependent to androgen-independent state represents an evolutionary process driven at least in part by androgen deprivation. A number of potential cellular and molecular mechanisms may mediate the progression of tumor cells to the androgen-independent state, including preferential expansion of clones of androgen-independent cells that already exist at the time that hormonal therapy is initiated, adaptation of tumor cells so that androgen-repressed proteins (i.e., growth factors or transcription factors) are up-regulated, or activation of alternative pathways involved in androgen receptor signaling (5). One or more of these mechanisms probably operates in any given case of progressive prostate cancer, and identifying the precise molecular alterations fundamental to the development of androgen-independent disease is a major focus of current research.

It has been suggested that the progression to androgen dependence may begin shortly after the initiation of androgen deprivation. In the 1970s, Noble reported that, in an androgen-dependent rat breast tumor model, intermittent endocrine therapy delayed the time to hormonal independence and postulated that intermittent androgen replacement (even in small amounts) could preserve the hormonal sensitivity of target tumor tissues (6). Subsequent studies in the Shionogi carcinoma cell line demonstrated that androgens are required for differentiation of parent stem cells (7). Once androgen-dependent tumor cells have undergone apoptosis (programmed cell death) in response to androgen deprivation, the remaining stem cells may rapidly evolve to an androgen-independent state. It therefore has been hypothesized that the reinstitution of androgen stimulation before this evolution may generate tumor cells still capable of responding to androgen deprivation (6). In fact, intermittent androgen deprivation (IAD) prolongs the time to evolution of androgen-independent Shionogi tumor cells, suggesting that this approach may have clinical use (7,8). Other studies in the LNCaP human prostate tumor cell model also demonstrate up to threefold prolongation of hormonal sensitivity through the use of IAD (9).

Another mechanism that tumor cells may use to escape androgen dependence is activation of autocrine or paracrine growth factor signaling pathways that provide a proliferative stimulus in the absence of androgen. For example, in the LAPC4 human prostate tumor model system, upregulated expression of the Her2/neu receptor tyrosine kinase occurs with serial passage of tumor cells in severe combined immunodeficiency mice (10). In these preclinical models, overexpression of Her2/neu appears to activate androgen receptor signaling pathways despite very low levels of androgen and also increases tumor cell proliferation *in vitro* and *in vivo*. The relevance of these observations to human prostate cancer requires confirmation.

Other growth factor receptor systems, such as epidermal growth factor and receptor, vitamin D3, transforming growth factor beta, and insulinlike growth factor 1, have been investigated in cell line and animal studies and may be altered in the evolution of androgen independence (11). Thus, prolonged androgen deprivation may provide the stimulus for activating signaling pathways otherwise dormant in prostate tumor cells, and intermittent replacement of androgen may, at least in theory, inhibit the biochemical switch leading to the activation of such pathways.

Clinical Studies

The previously mentioned preclinical data, coupled with a desire to minimize the side effects and cost of androgen deprivation therapy, have provided the impetus for a number of clinical trials exploring the use of IAD in men with advanced prostate cancer (12–21). Most of these studies have been single-institution phase II pilot trials, but they do provide valuable information regarding the timing, efficacy, and toxicity profile of IAD.

The first trial to examine the effects of IAD on patients with advanced prostate cancer was a retrospective review of 20 patients treated with intermittent diethylstilbestrol (DES) in the early 1980s (12). Patients were treated with DES until a clinical response occurred, and then the drug was discontinued until progressive disease became apparent. All patients responded to at least two cycles of therapy, and the median time off treatment was 8 months. In addition, the authors noted return of sexual function in many patients and suggested an improved quality of life.

Since this initial observation and the subsequent development of LHRH agonists, several studies have examined IAD in the PSA era (Table 42-1). Most of these trials have used a treatment scheme in which patients are treated with an LHRH agonist (with or without an antiandrogen) until serum PSA becomes undetectable or a nadir less than 4 ng per mL is reached, at which time androgen deprivation is stopped. In addition, patients usually receive androgen deprivation during the initial cycle for at least 6 to 9

TABLE 42-1. SELECTED TRIALS USING INTERMITTENT ANDROGEN DEPRIVATION

Author (reference)	Year	n	Initial median PSA (ng/mL)	Stage of disease (localized/ PSA relapse/metastatic)	Treatment (n)	Median off cycle duration (mo)
Klotz et al. (12)	1986	20	NR	12/0/8	DES	7.8
Goldenberg et al. (13)	1995	47	158	23/0/24	LHRH + AA	7.6
Higano et al. (14)	1996	22	20	2/10/10	LHRH + AA	6
Oliver et al. (15)	1997	20	NR	13/0/7	LHRH + AA (12) LHRH (6) DES (2)	24
Grossfeld et al. (16)	1998	47	8.4	47/0/0	LHRH + AA (33) LHRH (14)	7.5
Theyer et al. (17)	1998	52	31	15/0/37	LHRH + AA	16
Gleave et al. (18)	1998	70	110	41/0/29	LHRH + AA	9
Horwich et al. (19)	1998	16	164	0/0/16	LHRH	8
Crook et al. (20)	1999	54	37	11/4/39	LHRH + AA	8
Kurek et al. (21)	1999	44	6.3	15/29/0	LHRH + AA	11.6

AA, antiandrogen; DES, diethylstilbestrol; LHRH, luteinizing hormone releasing hormone agonist; NR, not reported; PSA, prostate-specific antigen.

months. Androgen deprivation is resumed once the PSA climbs to an arbitrarily fixed level (often 50% of the initial pretreatment value or an absolute value greater than 5 to 10 ng per mL) or clinical evidence of disease progression is noted.

As can be seen in Table 42-1, currently more than 300 patients treated with IAD have been reported, and a number of pertinent observations can be made. First, most studies have been comprised of a heterogeneous group of patients, including those with localized disease, metastatic disease, or biochemical relapse after primary therapy for localized prostate cancer. The precise method of androgen deprivation has also varied, although the majority of patients has received combined androgen blockade with an LHRH agonist and an antiandrogen. Finally, although time to disease progression and time spent in "off" cycles are commonly reported, few survival data are as yet available.

Despite the previously mentioned caveats, the reported trials of IAD have shown relatively uniform results with regard to treatment efficacy. First, most patients typically experience 6 to 9 months "off" therapy during the initial cycle, although the time "off" during subsequent cycles may decrease somewhat. However, there is wide variation in the amount of time patients spend without androgen deprivation, and some patients may experience holidays lasting 3 years or longer, particularly those who have localized disease or serologic (PSA) recurrence without objective evidence of metastases at the time therapy is initiated. It should be noted, however, that the amount of time spent in "off" cycles is directly dependent on the trigger (PSA level) used to resume androgen deprivation. On average, most patients appear to spend 40% to 60% of the total treatment time in "off" periods during the first cycle.

Importantly, the vast majority of patients (greater than 90%) will continue to respond to androgen deprivation when it is resumed after the first cycle. Initial data suggest that the time to hormone independence is comparable to or greater than that achieved in patients treated with continuous androgen deprivation, although more experience with IAD is required to ascertain this with certainty. Randomized trials currently in progress are directly comparing the efficacy of IAD and continuous androgen deprivation, and the time to hormonal independence will be an important end point in these studies.

Preliminary data are also available regarding quality of life in patients treated with IAD. Serum testosterone levels often return to the normal range after a median of 3 to 4 months, and, coincident with this, some patients report a reduction in symptoms associated with androgen deprivation during the off periods (12,14,19). Energy level and sense of well being were reported to improve in more than 50% of men during off periods in one trial, and more than 60% had resolution of hot flashes (22). Other troublesome side effects, such as weight gain, may also be ameliorated (14,22). Patients who are potent before initiating therapy, particularly younger patients, may recover libido and adequate sexual function during off cycles (12,14,22). Thus, at least a subset of patients appears to have enhanced quality of life with the use of IAD, although larger formal studies are required to determine the magnitude and duration of quality of life improvements achievable with this treatment modality.

IAD may also help to preserve bone mass in patients at risk of developing osteopenia. One study has reported bone density in abstract form in a cohort of patients treated with IAD. Bone density declined significantly during the first cycle of androgen deprivation, but there was partial recovery of bone mass or at least stabilization of bone loss during off cycles (23). If bone density can be preserved over multiple treatment cycles, then this could provide a significant advantage for IAD over continuous androgen deprivation, because emerging evidence indicates that many men will develop osteoporosis with standard hormonal therapy (4).

The most important unresolved clinical question regarding the use of IAD is its potential impact on survival (beneficial or adverse) in comparison with continuous androgen deprivation. One small nonrandomized trial has reported survival times of 5.1 years for patients with locally advanced tumors and 4.3 years for those with metastatic disease (24), data consistent or (perhaps) better than what one would expect with continuous androgen deprivation. Randomized multiinstitutional trials are currently under way in the United States and Europe to determine the comparative efficacy of IAD and continuous androgen deprivation. In North America and Europe, one international trial is comparing IAD with continuous androgen deprivation in men with metastatic prostate cancer, while in Europe a prospective randomized trial (the RELAPSE study) has been initiated in men with PSA relapse after radical prostatectomy. Both studies are comparing time to tumor progression, survival, and quality of life among treated patients, and the information from these trials will be crucial in determining the precise role of IAD in the future treatment of patients with advanced prostate cancer.

Another unresolved issue surrounding the use of IAD is the appropriate selection of patients for this modality. For example, initial extent of disease, Gleason score, PSA doubling time, and time to relapse after primary therapy may influence the use of IAD (19), and the importance of these factors in predicting the efficacy of IAD needs to be determined. In addition, it will be important to ascertain the fraction of men who recover normal testosterone levels during off cycles, because this will influence to a great extent the likelihood that quality of life will be improved. It is possible that age may play an important role in this regard, because older patients (older than 70 years) may be less likely to recover testicular function after 6 to 12 months of androgen deprivation (21).

In the absence of randomized data, IAD can be regarded as a reasonable treatment option in men with prostate cancer, provided patients are fully informed of the investiga-

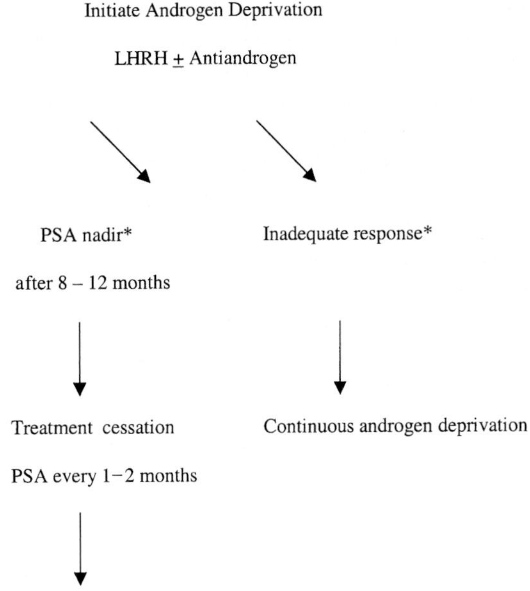

FIGURE 42-1. Algorithm for intermittent androgen deprivation in selected patients with prostate cancer. LHRH, luteinizing hormone releasing hormone agonist; PSA, prostate-specific antigen. *PSA nadir should be <1 ng/mL (and preferably undetectable) in those with PSA relapse after primary therapy, or <4 ng/mL in patients with metastatic disease.

tional nature of the therapy. We consider the use of IAD in patients who are not appropriate candidates for definitive local therapy because of age or co-morbid medical conditions but are at significant risk for disease progression, patients with localized disease who elect to receive androgen deprivation as their initial treatment strategy, patients with local or biochemical relapse after primary local therapy, and patients with metastatic disease who have a relatively low systemic tumor burden and a prompt response to initial androgen deprivation. In general, we follow a treatment algorithm similar to published strategies (Fig. 42-1). Patients receive initial androgen deprivation for at least 6 to 9 months if a PSA nadir of less than 1 ng per mL (PSA relapse) or 4 ng per mL (metastatic disease) is achieved and maintained cessation of therapy occurs. Patients have the serum PSA monitored once every 1 to 2 months, and androgen deprivation is resumed when the PSA reaches approximately 50% of its starting value or a level greater than 5 to 10 ng per mL. (Others have restarted hormonal therapy at a predetermined level, such as 4 ng per mL.) Patients receive bone scans or other appropriate imaging studies as clinically indicated. In our experience, this is a safe therapeutic strategy that can be easily implemented in the clinic setting, but we would again emphasize that the approach remains experimental until randomized data are available, and close clinical follow-up of patients is required.

PERIPHERAL ANDROGEN BLOCKADE

Peripheral androgen blockade, also sometimes termed *potency-sparing hormonal therapy,* refers to the use of agents that inhibit the action or production of testosterone or dihydrotestosterone (DHT) at the cellular level without lowering serum testosterone concentrations. Most commonly, peripheral androgen blockade involves the use of antiandrogen agents alone, finasteride alone, or a combination of an antiandrogen with finasteride. As with IAD, peripheral androgen blockade is an investigational approach that aims to effectively treat prostate cancer and at the same time avoid the potential side effects of standard androgen deprivation (medical or surgical castration). However, unlike IAD, peripheral androgen blockade has in general been associated with inferior clinical outcomes in patients with advanced prostate cancer when compared with continuous androgen deprivation, and its use cannot be recommended outside the investigational setting.

Antiandrogen Monotherapy

Nonsteroidal antiandrogens such as flutamide, bicalutamide, and nilutamide inhibit the binding of testosterone and DHT to the androgen receptor peripherally and centrally (25,26). In theory, nonsteroidal antiandrogens should be as effective as castration in the treatment of prostate cancer, although there is a risk that substantial elevations in serum testosterone may overcome their inhibitory effect. The published experience with antiandrogen monotherapy would suggest that this approach may be inferior to standard androgen deprivation in patients with advanced prostate cancer.

Several phase II studies have examined the use of antiandrogen monotherapy in patients with advanced prostate cancer (Table 42-2). In the late 1970s, soon after the development of flutamide, Sograni and Whitmore reported their experience using this agent alone in the treatment of metastatic prostate cancer (27). They noted that "favorable" clinical responses occurred in 19 of 21 patients treated with 250 mg of flutamide three times daily and concluded that flutamide monotherapy was worthy of further investigation. Additional studies by Lundgren (28), MacFarlane and Tolley (29), and Delaere and Van Thillo (30) also reported favorably on the use of flutamide monotherapy, although, in general, the number of patients responding to flutamide alone was less than would be expected with androgen deprivation. These reports do indicate that flutamide monotherapy is usually better tolerated than androgen deprivation, with the most common side effects being breast pain and enlargement as well as diarrhea. In addition, a majority of patients with potency before the initiation of therapy may preserve sexual function. Significant increases in serum testosterone level are commonly reported and, as noted earlier, may represent a mechanism of treatment resistance.

TABLE 42-2. SELECTED TRIALS USING ANTIANDROGEN MONOTHERAPY

Author (reference)	Year	Drug	n	Stage	Clinical response (%)[a]	PSA response (%)[b]	Duration of response (mo)
Jacobo et al. (33)	1976	Flutamide	8	Met	25	NR	7
Sograni et al. (27)	1979	Flutamide	21	Met	90	NR	10.5
MacFarlane et al. (29)	1985	Flutamide	3	Met	67	NR	NR
Lundgren (28)	1987	Flutamide	10	Met	20	NR	9
Lund (38)	1988	Flutamide	21	Met	65	NR	NR
Delaere et al. (30)	1991	Flutamide	35	Local or Met	86	NR	NR
Soloway et al. (31)	1995	Bicalutamide (50 mg/d)	151	Met	50	39	8
Chodak et al. (36)	1995	Bicalutamide (50 mg/d)	243	Met	58	16	9
Scher et al. (32)	1997	Bicalutamide (150 mg/d)	53	Local or Met	48	88[c]	14

Met, metastatic; NR, not reported; PSA, prostate-specific antigen.
[a]Defined as improvement in pain, other symptoms, or imaging studies.
[b]Defined as decline of the PSA to the normal range (0–4 ng/mL) or a >90% decline in PSA, or both.
[c]PSA decline >80%.

Bicalutamide has also been examined as a single agent. In one multicenter trial, 151 men with previously untreated metastatic prostate cancer received 50 mg of bicalutamide daily (31). Fifty percent of symptomatic patients (30 of 60) had subjective improvement, although only 39% of patients had a greater than 90% decline in serum PSA or declines of PSA into the normal range. In addition, the median duration of response was only 34 weeks, significantly less than anticipated with androgen deprivation. As expected, breast tenderness (76%) and gynecomastia (60%) were the most frequent adverse events.

More recently, Scher and colleagues used high-dose bicalutamide (150 mg daily) to treat 53 men with androgen-dependent prostate cancer (32). They found that 88% had significant reductions (more than 80%) in serum PSA, and 48% had improvements in bone scan with a median time to progression of 14 months. However, only one-third of patients responded to gonadal androgen suppression after disease progression occurred, and it is not clear whether the overall response rates and duration of response are comparable with castration. In addition, toxicity was perhaps higher than anticipated: Only 6% of patients with normal pretherapy sexual function reported the maintenance of normal libido, and only 17% reported normal erections. Hot flashes occurred in 40%, breast tenderness in 59%, and gynecomastia in 72%.

Some randomized comparisons of antiandrogen monotherapy and gonadal androgen deprivation have been performed (33–36). In the 1970s and 1980s, several European studies reported that flutamide had an equivalent response rate to 1 to 3 mg of DES daily (33,34). However, an Eastern Cooperative Oncology Group study found that overall and failure-free survival were inferior when flutamide was compared with 3 mg of DES daily (35). More recently, a large, randomized, multicenter trial compared 50 mg of bicalutamide alone (n = 243) to surgical castration or use of an LHRH agonist (n = 243) (36). Patients receiving castration had a significantly better PSA response proportion, with 47% achieving PSA normalization compared to 17% in the bicalutamide arm. More important, patients treated with bicalutamide had a higher likelihood of treatment failure during the follow-up period, although median survival had not been reached in either group at the time of publication. Patients in the bicalutamide group did have relatively improved quality of life in the areas of libido and sexual function, but at 1 year there were no significant differences between groups in terms of overall health, emotional well-being, and social functioning. In contrast, in a separate review of two high-dose bicalutamide trials performed in Europe, patient well-being as measured by subjective response to therapy was improved in those treated with bicalutamide, compared to those receiving standard androgen deprivation (37).

In aggregate, data on antiandrogen monotherapy indicate that this treatment modality can produce PSA responses and objective improvement in some patients with advanced prostate cancer. In addition, the side effect profile appears to be favorable, and preservation of sexual function occurs in a majority of men who are potent at the time therapy is initiated and who are treated with standard doses of antiandrogen. However, some evidence suggests that duration of response and perhaps survival may be compromised with this approach, especially in patients with metastatic disease, and it cannot be recommended outside of the setting of a clinical trial. Further investigation of antiandrogen monotherapy in patients with localized disease or PSA relapse after primary therapy may be warranted, however, because in this group of patients some might elect a therapy with reduced effectiveness if gains in quality of life were sufficient.

Finasteride Monotherapy

Finasteride is a 4-azasteroid competitive inhibitor of 5α-reductase that blocks the conversion of testosterone to the physiologically more potent androgen DHT (38). Finasteride monotherapy reduces intraprostatic concentrations of DHT and can induce regression of normal prostate epithelium in humans, dogs, and rats (39,40). Large randomized trials using finasteride to treat benign prostatic hyperplasia have shown that it is effective and well tolerated, with adverse events occurring in less than 5% of men (41). In particular, sexual potency is preserved in almost all men taking finasteride.

Because finasteride limits the intracellular concentration of DHT, it in theory may have efficacy as an antitumor agent in patients with advanced prostate cancer. Indeed, *in vitro* experiments with 5α-reductase inhibitors have demonstrated a growth-inhibitory effect in some prostate cancer cell lines (42,43), suggesting that these drugs may have clinical use.

These *in vitro* data, coupled with finasteride's favorable side effect profile, have led to its investigation in the treatment of prostate cancer. Unfortunately, the results of the few reported studies have been largely disappointing. In a small multicenter, randomized, double-blind placebo-controlled trial, Presti and colleagues compared finasteride and placebo for the treatment of men with asymptomatic metastatic prostate cancer (44). They found that finasteride produced minor decreases in serum PSA (15% decline) after 6 weeks of therapy, although there was no significant evidence for objective antitumor activity. In addition, those patients with a positive bone scan had no decrease in serum PSA. These results are much less than expected with medical or surgical castration and suggest that, in patients with advanced disease, finasteride monotherapy has minimal (if any) effectiveness.

Finasteride has also been investigated in patients with PSA recurrence after radical prostatectomy. Andriole and associates treated 120 men who had prior radical prostatectomy, serum PSA levels between 0.6 and 10.0 ng per mL, and no evidence of metastatic disease on imaging studies with finasteride or placebo for 1 year (45). Finasteride appeared to delay PSA progression for up to 9 months and slow the rate of PSA rise for 6 months thereafter, although there was not a statistically significant difference in the rates of objective tumor recurrence. Subset analysis did suggest that men with low initial PSA values derived the greatest benefit in terms of PSA decline or stabilization.

As with antiandrogen monotherapy, there is little evidence to support the routine use of finasteride alone, particularly in patients with metastatic disease. The use of finasteride may be considered in patients with PSA progression after primary therapy for localized prostate cancer who do not wish to pursue more aggressive or investigational therapies, but it is not clear whether finasteride in this setting provides a significant clinical benefit.

Combined Antiandrogen and Finasteride Therapy

In addition to their use as monotherapies, antiandrogens and finasteride have been used in combination to treat patients with hormone-dependent prostate cancer. It has been hypothesized that the combination of an antiandrogen with finasteride may be synergistic, with finasteride lowering DHT levels and the antiandrogen blocking the effects of any residual DHT. The combination should also spare potency, because serum testosterone levels should be unaffected or increased. In the Sprague-Dawley rat, in fact, treatment with finasteride and flutamide results in significantly less prostate growth than use of either agent alone, although combination therapy does not reduce prostate size as much as castration (46).

Combination finasteride and flutamide therapy has been investigated in patients with hormone-dependent prostate cancer (Table 42-3). Ornstein and colleagues treated 13 men with metastatic disease or PSA relapse after radiation therapy and noted PSA normalization in 85% of patients, with 46% achieving an undetectable level (47). These results were duplicated by Brufsky and colleagues in a similar patient population (48). In 22 patients with locally advanced or

TABLE 42-3. TRIALS OF FLUTAMIDE AND FINASTERIDE FOR ADVANCED PROSTATE CANCER

Author (reference)	Year	n	Stage (n)	Clinical response (%)[a]	PSA response (%)[b]	Median duration
Fleshner et al. (49)	1995	22	Local (6) D1 (16)	95	95	24+
Ornstein et al. (47)	1996	13	PSA relapse (7) D0 (1) D1 (1) D2 (4)	NR	85	11+
Brufsky et al. (48)	1997	20	PSA relapse (13) D1 (4) D2 (3)	95	72[c]	17+

D0, local disease with elevated prostatic acid phosphatase; D1, pelvic lymph node metastases; D2, bone metastases; NR, not reported; PSA, prostate-specific antigen.
[a]Defined as improvement in pain, other symptoms, or imaging studies.
[b]Defined as decline of PSA to the normal range (0–4 ng/mL) or >90% decline in PSA, or both.
[c]Decline of PSA to <1 ng/mL.

stage D1 disease, Fleshner and Trachtenberg reported that 95% had significant declines in PSA, and 86% maintained potency (49). In addition, 66% of patients had ongoing clinical and PSA responses 24 months after initiating therapy. Thus, the combination of flutamide and finasteride may have acceptable activity against hormone-dependent prostate cancer, although its use compared to standard androgen deprivation cannot be assessed in the absence of randomized clinical trials. The use of an antiandrogen and finasteride in patients with metastatic prostate cancer must be considered investigational and generally should be undertaken only in the context of a clinical trial or if the patient does not wish to pursue androgen deprivation and is aware that this therapy is not standard treatment.

TRIPLE ANDROGEN BLOCKADE

Triple androgen blockade refers to the concomitant use of medical or surgical castration, an antiandrogen, and finasteride for the treatment of advanced prostate cancer. Although the use of "triple" therapy may intuitively seem reasonable, there are in fact no preclinical data to suggest that this approach is superior to more standard androgen deprivation. In addition, no peer-reviewed publications exist to support this approach or even to describe its clinical impact. An uncontrolled, nonrandomized study reported in abstract form suggests that, in patients treated with IAD, those patients who received triple androgen blockade followed by maintenance finasteride during the off period had a significantly larger time "off" hormones before receiving androgen deprivation than patients treated with an LHRH agonist plus an antiandrogen alone (50). Whether this effect reflects true anticancer activity as opposed to suppression of PSA only is not known. Because the response proportion observed with standard combined androgen blockade is high and reasonably durable, the impact of adding finasteride, if any, is likely to be detected only in the context of a (prohibitively) large randomized clinical trial. Potential unproven benefits of such an approach must be weighed against increased cost and potential but as yet not reported toxicities.

REFERENCES

1. Huggins C, Hodges CV. Studies on prostatic cancer. I. The effect of castration, of estrogen, and of androgen injection on serum phosphatases in metastatic carcinoma of the prostate. *Cancer Res* 1941;1:293–297.
2. Huggins C, Stevens RF, Hodges CV. Studies on prostatic carcinoma. II. The effect of castration on advanced carcinoma of the prostate gland. *Arch Surg* 1941;43:209–223.
3. Strum SB, McDermed JE, Scholz MC, et al. Anaemia associated with androgen deprivation in patients with prostate cancer receiving combined hormonal blockade. *Br J Urol* 1997;79:933–941.
4. Daniell HW. Osteoporosis after orchiectomy for prostate cancer. *J Urol* 1997;157:439–444.
5. Galbraith SM, Duchesne GM. Androgens and prostate cancer: biology, pathology, and hormonal therapy. *Eur J Cancer* 1997;33:545–554.
6. Noble RL. Hormonal control of growth and progression in tumors of Nb rats and a theory of action. *Cancer Res* 1977; 37:82–94.
7. Bruchovsky N, Rennie PS, Goldman AJ, et al. Effects of androgen withdrawal on the stem cell composition of the Shionogi carcinoma. *Cancer Res* 1990;50:2275–2282.
8. Akakura K, Bruchovsky N, Goldenberg SL, et al. Effects of intermittent androgen suppression on androgen-dependent tumors: apoptosis and serum prostate specific antigen. *Cancer* 1993;71:2782–2790.
9. Sato N, Gleave ME, Bruchovsky N, et al. Intermittent androgen suppression delays time to non-androgen regulated prostate specific antigen gene expression in the human prostate LNCaP tumour model. *J Steroid Biochem Mol Biol* 1996;58:139–146.
10. Craft N, Shostak Y, Carey M, et al. A mechanism for hormone-independent prostate cancer through modulation of androgen receptor signaling by the HER-2/neu tyrosine kinase. *Nature Med* 1999;5:280–285.
11. Culig Z, Hobisch A, Cronauer MV, et al. Regulation of prostatic growth and function by peptide growth factors. *Prostate* 1996;28:392–395.
12. Klotz LH, Herr HW, Morse MJ, et al. Intermittent endocrine therapy for advanced prostate cancer. *Cancer* 1986;58: 2546–2550.
13. Goldenberg SL, Bruchovsky N, Gleave M, et al. Intermittent androgen suppression in the treatment of prostate cancer: a preliminary report. *Urology* 1995;45:839–844.
14. Higano CS, Ellis W, Russell K, et al. Intermittent androgen suppression with leuprolide and flutamide for prostate cancer: a pilot study. *Urology* 1996;48:800–804.
15. Oliver RTD, Williams G, Paris AMI, et al. Intermittent androgen deprivation after PSA-complete response as a strategy to reduce induction of hormone-resistant prostate cancer. *Urology* 1997;49:79–82.
16. Grossfeld G, Small EJ, Carroll PR. Intermittent androgen deprivation for clinically localized prostate cancer: initial experience. *Urology* 1998;51:137–144.
17. Theyer G, Hamilton G. Current status of intermittent androgen suppression in the treatment of prostate cancer. *Urology* 1998;52:353–359.
18. Gleave M, Bruchovsky N, Goldenberg SL, et al. Intermittent androgen suppression for prostate cancer: rationale and clinical experience. *Eur Urol* 1998;34(Suppl 3):37–41.
19. Horwich A, Huddart RA, Gadd J, et al. A pilot study of intermittent androgen deprivation in advanced prostate cancer. *Br J Urol* 1998;81:96–99.
20. Crook JM, Szumacher E, Malone S, et al. Intermittent androgen suppression in the management of prostate cancer. *Urology* 1999;53:530–534.
21. Kurek R, Renneberg H, Lübben G, et al. Intermittent complete androgen blockade in PSA relapse after radical prostatectomy and incidental prostate cancer. *Eur Urol* 1999; 35(Suppl 1):27–31.

22. Bales GT, Sinner M, Kim JH, et al. Impact of intermittent androgen deprivation on quality of life (QOL). *Proc Am Urol Assoc* 1996;155:578A.
23. Higano CS, Stephens C, Nelson P, et al. Prospective serial measurements of bone mineral density (BMD) in prostate cancer patients without bone metastases treated with intermittent androgen suppression (IAS). *Proc Am Soc Clin Oncol* 1999;18:314a.
24. Zerbib M, Conquy S, Gerbaud PF, et al. Efficacy and impact on quality of life (QOL) of intermittent androgen deprivation for prostate cancer treatment. *Eur Urol* 1998;33(Suppl 1):354(abst).
25. Simard J, Luthy I, Belanger A, et al. Characteristics of interaction of the antiandrogen flutamide with the androgen receptor in various target tissues. *Mol Cell Endocrinol* 1986; 44:261–270.
26. Mahler C, Denis L. Clinical profile of a new nonsteroidal antiandrogen. *J Steroid Biochem Mol Biol* 1990;37:921–924.
27. Sograni PC, Whitmore WF Jr. Experience with flutamide in previously untreated patients with advanced prostatic cancer. *J Urol* 1979;122:640–643.
28. Lundgren R. Flutamide as primary treatment for metastatic prostate cancer. *Br J Urol* 1987;59:156–158.
29. MacFarlane JR, Tolley DA. Flutamide therapy for advanced prostatic cancer: a phase II study. *Br J Urol* 1985;57:172–174.
30. Delaere KP, Van Thillo EL. Flutamide monotherapy as primary treatment in advanced prostatic carcinoma. *Semin Oncol* 1991;18(Suppl 6):13–18.
31. Soloway MS, Schellhammer PF, Smith JA Jr., et al. Bicalutamide in the treatment of advanced prostatic carcinoma: a phase II noncomparative multicenter trial evaluating safety, efficacy and long-term endocrine effects of monotherapy. *J Urol* 1995;154:2110–2114.
32. Scher HI, Liebertz C, Kelly WK, et al. Bicalutamide for advanced prostate cancer: the natural versus treated history of disease. *J Clin Oncol* 1997;15:2928–2938.
33. Jacobo E, Schmidt JD, Weinstein SH, et al. Comparison of flutamide (SCH-13521) and diethylstilbestrol in untreated advanced prostatic cancer. *Urology* 1976;8:231–233.
34. Lund F, Rasmussen F. Flutamide versus stilboestrol in the management of advanced prostatic cancer: a controlled prospective study. *Br J Urol* 1988;61:140–142.
35. Chang A, Yeap B, Blum R, et al. A double-blind study of primary treatment for stage D2 prostate cancer: diethylstilbestrol (DES) versus flutamide (F). *Proc Am Soc Clin Oncol* 1992;11:202.
36. Chodak G, Sharifi R, Kasimis B, et al. Single-agent therapy with bicalutamide: a comparison with medical or surgical castration in the treatment of advanced prostate carcinoma. *Urology* 1995;46:849–855.
37. Tyrrell CJ, Iversen P, Kaisary AV, et al. Improvements in subjective response in patients with advanced prostate cancer treated with "Casodex" (bicalutamide) 150mg monotherapy compared with castration. *Proc Am Soc Clin Oncol* 1998;17:315a.
38. Rittmaster RS. Finasteride. *N Engl J Med* 1994;330:120–125.
39. McConnell JD, Wilson JD, George FW, et al. Finasteride, an inhibitor of 5-alpha reductase, suppresses prostatic dihydrotestosterone in men with benign prostatic hyperplasia. *J Clin Endocrinol Metab* 1992;74:505–508.
40. Rittmaster RS, Norman RW, Thomas LN, et al. Evidence for atrophy and apoptosis in the prostates of men given finasteride. *J Clin Endocrinol Metab* 1996;81:814–819.
41. Gormley GL, Stoner E, Bruskewitz B, et al. The effect of finasteride in men with benign prostatic hyperplasia. *N Engl J Med* 1992;327:1185–1191.
42. Lamb JC, Levy MA, Johnson RK, et al. Response of rat and human prostatic cancers to the novel 5-alpha reductase inhibitor, SK&F 105657. *Prostate* 1992;21:15–34.
43. Bolona M, Muzi P, Biordi L, et al. Antiandrogens and 5-alpha-reductase inhibition of the proliferation rate in PC3 and DU145 human prostatic cancer cell lines. *Curr Ther Res* 1992;51:799–813.
44. Presti JC Jr., Fair WR, Andriole G, et al. Multicenter, randomized, double-blind, placebo controlled study to investigate the effect of finasteride (MK-906) on stage D prostate cancer. *J Urol* 1992;148:1201–1204.
45. Andriole G, Lieber M, Smith J, et al. Treatment with finasteride following radical prostatectomy for prostate cancer. *Urology* 1995;45:491–497.
46. Fleshner NE, Trachtenberg J. Sequential androgen blockade: a biological study in the inhibition of prostatic growth. *J Urol* 1992;148:1928–1931.
47. Ornstein DK, Rao G, Johnson B, et al. Combined finasteride and flutamide therapy in men with advanced prostate cancer. *Urology* 1996;48:901–905.
48. Brufsky A, Fontaine-Roth P, Berlane K, et al. Finasteride and flutamide as potency-sparing androgen-ablative therapy for advanced adenocarcinoma of the prostate. *Urology* 1997;49:913–920.
49. Fleshner NE, Trachtenberg J. Combination finasteride and flutamide in advanced carcinoma of the prostate: effective therapy with minimal side effects. *J Urol* 1995;154:1642–1646.
50. Strum S, McDermed J, Madsen L, et al. Intermittent androgen deprivation (IAD) with finasteride (F) given during the induction and maintenance periods results in prolonged time off IAD in patients with localized prostate cancer (LPC). *Proc Am Soc Clin Oncol* 1999;18:353a.

43

SECOND LINE HORMONE THERAPY

NANCY A. DAWSON

INTRODUCTION

Huggins and Hodges, in 1941, first reported the therapeutic efficacy of androgen deprivation in the treatment of advanced CaP (1). Although there is controversy over whether the addition of an antiandrogen to testicular androgen deprivation (total androgen blockade) improves outcome, it is not controversial that androgen deprivation is the primary approach to advanced disease (2–5). Unfortunately, despite response rates of 80% to 90%, nearly all men will develop progressive disease after an average of 18 to 24 months. It is at this point that second line hormone therapy should be considered. This chapter focuses on the growing number of options available to this patient population.

Changing Spectrum of Disease

Men with CaP who progress while on androgen deprivation are referred to as having *hormone-refractory* (HRPC) or *androgen-independent* CaP. This category encompasses a broad spectrum of disease as well as divergent response to second line therapy. In the 1970s, before the availability of prostate-specific antigen (PSA) testing and the early use of hormonal therapy, men with HR disease usually presented with widespread symptomatic metastatic disease. Today, most men are diagnosed as having progressive disease based on a rise in PSA. Consequently, it is common for the patient to be asymptomatic and often initially without evidence of progression on radiographic studies. Furthermore, with the common practice of initiating androgen deprivation in men with a rising PSA after curative intent prostatectomy or radiation therapy, an increasing number of men with HR disease have "PSA only" disease and no demonstrable distant disease. Furthermore, it is now apparent that men with progressive disease are not necessarily HR and that populations of tumor cells with androgen-dependent growth may persist. It is now appreciated that there is a variable transition from hormone-sensitive to hormone-responsive to truly HR disease and that during this transition hormone therapies aimed at alternate forms of androgen deprivation may be beneficial (6). Certainly the use of alternative hormonal therapies is especially attractive in the asymptomatic and "PSA only" patients in whom more toxic therapies might be undesirable.

Changing End Points

Assessment of response in CaP patients can be difficult owing to the nature of the disease. CaP most commonly metastasizes to bone, which is difficult to assess for response owing to the long lag time for bone lesions to heal, variability in interpretation of bone scans, and occasional "flare" responses, whereby a scan looks worse despite clinical or biochemical response (7,8). Bi-dimensionally measurable disease, although easy to assess for response, is only present in 10% to 20% of patients (9). On the other hand, PSA levels are elevated in 95% of men with advanced disease. Consequently, the use of posttherapy changes in the PSA has been adopted by most investigators as a surrogate end point for response, despite inadequate prospective validation (10). Justification for its use is derived from retrospective and prospective analyses of PSA changes in men treated in clinical trials that show improved survival in men whose PSA declines by more than 50% (11–13). Although for certain drugs there may be some discordance between PSA decline and tumor growth (14), it has now been generally adopted that in phase II trials in androgen-independent CaP, one end point to be reported is the percentage of men whose PSA declines at least 50%, confirmed by a second PSA value 4 or more weeks later (15). There has also been a heightened focus on palliation of pain as a clinically relevant end point irrespective of other disease parameters (10,16). As a consequence of these changes in disease assessment and a desire to more broadly assess a new therapy's efficacy, the standard classification of responses as complete or partial response, stable disease, and progressive disease are considered inadequate. Instead, there is a trend for investigators to report separately decline in PSA, measurable disease response, bone-scan response, and symptomatic response (10,17). Changes in how we report outcomes may make it difficult to assess the "true" value of certain drugs that have been in use for many years (i.e., prednisone) and occasionally justify the reassessment of an old drug using the newer response criteria (18).

CONTINUATION OF PRIMARY TESTICULAR ANDROGEN DEPRIVATION

The role of continued androgen suppression in the face of progressive disease remains controversial. Exogenous testosterone has been demonstrated to exacerbate disease in the setting of metastatic disease. Fowler and Whitmore (19) reported on 52 men with advanced disease treated with testosterone propionate. Of these men, objective and subjective unfavorable responses were documented in three of four with hormone-naïve disease, 9 of 14 were in symptomatic remission, and 33 of 34 in symptomatic relapse after endocrine therapy. All but two patients had prompt symptomatic improvement after stopping the androgen.

Chao and Harland (20) reported on three men progressing on endocrine therapy who, after an initial response to chemotherapy, had rising PSA that again declined when androgen deprivation was reinstituted and chemotherapy continued, suggesting that there may be persistent population of hormone-sensitive tumor cells despite overall progressive disease. Silver et al. (21) further demonstrated rises in serum testosterone and coinciding rises in PSA in three men progressing after 10, 16, and 30 months on goserelin acetate after discontinuation of the luteinizing hormone releasing hormone agonist (LHRHa). Orchiectomy resulted in reduction in PSA and testosterone in all three men, albeit short-lived decreases in two, suggesting a benefit to maintaining castrate levels of testosterone.

There are no prospective trials to assess the impact of discontinuation of testicular androgen deprivation. Two retrospective reviews showed conflicting results (22,23). Taylor et al. (22), in a retrospective multivariate analysis, reported on survival data on 341 patients with HRPC treated in four clinical trials. Factors included in the model were weight loss, age, performance status, disease site, prior radiotherapy, and continued androgen suppression. Controlling for the first three variables, which were all of prognostic importance, continued testicular androgen suppression was associated with a modest median survival benefit of 2 to 6 months. Hussain et al. (23), in a review of 205 men treated on five consecutive Southwest Oncology Group phase II trials, showed no obvious survival benefit to continued androgen suppression. However, only 33 patients (16%) had no prior orchiectomy.

Despite the lack of prospective clinical data, in a survey of 35 established investigators in HPRC clinical trials, 82% required continued testicular androgen suppression for patients enrolling on protocol (10). Furthermore, the 1999 published guidelines from the PSA Working Group for eligibility criteria for phase II trials in androgen-independent CaP (AICaP), recommended that all patients who have not undergone surgical castration should be continued on testicular androgen suppression (15).

ANTIANDROGEN WITHDRAWAL SYNDROME

In 1993, Kelly and Scher first reported on three men progressing on androgen deprivation who, after discontinuation of flutamide, had sustained PSA declines (24). They concluded that a trial of flutamide withdrawal is justified in an asymptomatic man with a rising PSA level before initiating alternate potentially toxic second line therapy. This phenomenon was named the *flutamide withdrawal syndrome* by these same investigators. In their follow-up report of 35 progressing men, 10 (29%) showed a greater than 50% decline in PSA from baseline (25). The response duration was 5+ months; range was 2 to 10+ months. Palliation of pain paralleled a decline in PSA; however, objective tumor regression was documented in only one patient. In this initial report, responses occurred only in the setting of initial combined androgen deprivation. Subsequently, Small et al. reported on a retrospective review of 107 consecutive patients with metastatic disease who had flutamide discontinued at the time of progression (26). A lower rate of PSA decline was noted in 14.6%. Additionally, a withdrawal response occurred in 4 of 25 men (16%) in whom flutamide had been prescribed as second line therapy at the time of initial progression. Scher et al., in an overview of the subsequently termed *antiandrogen withdrawal syndrome*, reported PSA declines in 47% (74 of 159; 95% confidence interval, 38% to 54%) of men after flutamide withdrawal (27).

Antiandrogen withdrawal responses also occur after discontinuation of bicalutamide or nilutamide (28–31). The smaller number of reported cases in the literature makes it difficult to determine whether this phenomenon occurs with equal frequency. Because the antiandrogens have different half-lives, there is variation in the time elapsed before PSA decline. With flutamide, which has a short half-life of 5 hours, withdrawal responses are seen in 1 to 2 weeks, whereas PSA declines may not occur for 3 to 6 weeks with nilutamide and bicalutamide, which have longer half-lives of 56 hours and 1 week, respectively.

Withdrawal responses also occur with discontinuation of steroidal antiandrogens. Significant PSA declines have occurred in patients with advanced CaP after discontinuation of megestrol acetate, chlormadinone acetate, and cyproterone acetate (32–36). The first reported case of megestrol acetate withdrawal response was in a patient who had been receiving 320 mg per day for 2 years for HRPC (32). His PSA level dramatically declined from greater than 100 to normal and remained in this range for more than 1 year. Subsequent reports have shown significant declines in

PSA after discontinuation of low-dose megestrol acetate (40 mg per day) administered to control hot flashes associated with androgen deprivation therapy (33,34). Akakura et al. reported two patients with significant declines in PSA levels after stopping chlormadinone acetate, a progestational steroid widely used in Japan for the treatment of CaP (35). Levels of testosterone, prolactin, dehydroepiandrosterone, dehydroepiandrosterone sulfate, and androstenedione were not elevated after chlormadinone acetate withdrawal to explain the antiandrogen withdrawal syndrome. Sella et al. reported on 12 men with progressive androgen-independent CaP in whom cyproterone acetate was discontinued at the time of progression (36). In 5 of 12 men, PSA levels declined. In four men (33%), the decrease exceeded 50%. All five men with decreased PSA levels had been receiving initial combined androgen deprivation. None of the four men receiving cyproterone acetate as a second line therapy had a decline in PSA level. One patient with a PSA decline had resolution of all pain. The median response duration was 24 weeks.

Responses to withdrawal of other hormones have also been reported. In one patient on diethylstilbestrol (DES), complete remission of disease persisted for 3 years after discontinuation of DES (37). It has now been accepted that the first therapeutic manipulation in a man with progressive advanced CaP is the discontinuation of his current antiandrogen or other secondary hormonal therapy. Furthermore, therapy should not be initiated until adequate time has elapsed to assess for a withdrawal response. This time interval is based on the half-life of the drug being stopped.

The mechanism of the antiandrogen withdrawal response is not known. The most popular hypothesis is that there is an acquired mutation in the androgen receptor (AR) that results in antiandrogens now having a stimulatory effect on prostate tumor cells. In support of this theory, *in vitro* experiments have documented that steroidal and nonsteroidal antiandrogens may stimulate the growth of LNCaP cells, a human prostate cell line with a known mutation in the hormone-binding domain of the AR. Cyproterone acetate, medroxyprogesterone acetate, flutamide, hydroxyflutamide, and nilutamide, as well as estradiol, have a proliferate effect on androgen-sensitive LNCaP cells in culture (38–41). Mutations in the AR have been demonstrated in bone marrow specimens and primary and metastatic tumor sites (42–47). Taplin et al. were able to demonstrate mutations in the AR gene in five of ten men with androgen-independent metastatic CaP (44). Functional studies in two of the mutant ARs showed activation by progesterone and estrogen. Fenton et al. further demonstrated that in CV-1 cells cotransfected with wild-type or mutant ARs and a luciferase receptor plasmid regulated by an androgen-responsive element, flutamide and nilutamide but not bicalutamide were agonistic to cells with the mutant receptor (45). Suzuki et al. demonstrated AR gene mutations in three of 22 men with endocrine therapy resistant disease (46). In all three cases, the mutation was at codon 877 (^{877}Thr → Ala). In the two patients for whom there was available clinical data, PSA levels fell by 95% and 72% after discontinuation of antiandrogen. It is apparent that not all antiandrogens react in the same way with the mutant AR. Bicalutamide has a decreased affinity for the receptor, increased transcript activation of the receptor, and a continued antagonist effect on prostate tumor cell growth (48).

Alternatively, this phenomenon may be due to previously unmasked agonistic properties of the antiandrogens or emergence of a hypersensitive clone of cells. Amplification of the AR gene has been shown to be common in recurrent CaP. This increased AR expression may allow tumor cells to be stimulated despite an androgen-deficient environment (49).

SECOND LINE ANTIANDROGENS

Antiandrogens were developed as an alternative form of endocrine ablation to avoid the adverse effects of hot flashes, loss of libido, and impotence associated with surgical or medical castration (50). There are two groups of antiandrogens: steroidal antiandrogens and nonsteroidal or "pure" antiandrogens.

The steroidal antiandrogens, which include cyproterone acetate and megestrol acetate, inhibit AR stimulation by interfering with AR binding. Second, they have progestational properties that inhibit gonadotropin secretion with resultant suppression of LH, testosterone, dihydrotestosterone, and estrogen. The nonsteroidal antiandrogens, which include flutamide, bicalutamide, and nilutamide, block binding to the AR but do not possess gestagenic properties. These drugs inhibit the negative diencephalic feedback system, and, therefore, in contrast to the steroidal antiandrogens, there is an associated increase in LHRH, LH, testosterone, dihydrotestosterone, and estradiol. Consequent to increases in estradiol, the normal diencephalic feedback system is progressively activated, halting the rise in testosterone.

Antiandrogens have been used clinically primarily in the setting of androgen-sensitive CaP. Currently, nonsteroidal antiandrogens have been U.S. Food and Drug Administration approved for use in combination with orchiectomy or an LHRHa as part of maximal androgen blockade (MAB) for treatment of hormone-sensitive metastatic disease and in combination with radiation for localized CaP. Ongoing clinical trials have also suggested their possible use as monotherapy for metastatic disease and as part of MAB to downstage inoperable (T3) localized disease. Antiandrogens are effective in preventing a flare of disease associated with the initial testosterone surge with a LHRHa. The use of antiandrogens as second line hormonal therapy can be supported based on the following currently available data.

Flutamide

Flutamide was the first of the "pure" antiandrogens. It is rapidly absorbed and metabolized to its active substance, 2-hydroxyflutamide. It has a short half-life of 5.5 hours and is almost completely secreted in the urine. Its primary toxicities are gynecomastia or breast tenderness in one-half of patients; liver dysfunction, which has been fatal on rare occasion; nausea; and diarrhea.

Using the objective criteria of the National Prostatic Cancer Project, Labrie et al. reported on the first large series of men treated with flutamide after failing initial hormonal therapy with orchiectomy, DES, or an LHRHa (51). Of 209 men, 13 had a complete response, 20 had a partial response, and 39 patients had a stable disease, yielding a total response rate of 34.5%. The mean duration of response was 24 months. The median survival was 8.1 months for nonresponders and more than 2.5 years for responders.

In a prospective, randomized, double-blind intergroup trial of leuprolide with or without flutamide in men with newly diagnosed metastatic CaP, men initially treated with placebo were offered the option of receiving flutamide at the time of progression (3). In an analysis of 261 men progressing on study, there was no survival difference between men who received flutamide at the time of progression and those treated at the investigator's discretion (52). The median survival times of these two respective groups, 12.3 and 11.9 months, were similar to other treatments for HRPC.

A third trial assessed the impact of deferred flutamide on the serum PSA level in men progressing on testicular androgen deprivation (53). Thirty-two of 40 (80%) evaluable men with localized disease and 27 of 50 (54%) men with metastatic cancer had a decline in PSA of 50% or more during flutamide treatment. The actuarial freedom from PSA elevation was significantly longer (p = .0054) for patients with localized disease whose PSA nadir was less than 50% of baseline compared to those who did not achieve this nadir. However, for men with metastatic disease, there was no difference in freedom from PSA progression based on this PSA nadir. Survival analyses were not done owing to too few deaths at the time of reporting.

Bicalutamide

Compared to flutamide, bicalutamide has a longer half-life of 1 week and is more potent with a binding affinity for the AR that is two to four times higher (54). It is well absorbed with a tenfold plasma concentration at all doses. The standard dose in hormone-sensitive disease is 50 mg orally once a day. Its toxicities include loss of libido, impotence, breast tenderness or gynecomastia, or both, in one-half of patients. Hot flashes occur in 10% to 20% of patients, and transient liver function abnormalities occur in less than 5%. Diarrhea occurring in 10% of men is half as frequent as reported with flutamide.

Bicalutamide is U.S. Food and Drug Administration approved as part of MAB in hormone-sensitive disease and has been approved in Europe for monotherapy in the same setting at a dose of 150 mg daily. Two clinical studies have evaluated the use of high-dose bicalutamide in men with HRPC. Scher et al. assessed a dose of 200 mg per day in 51 men with HRPC. PSA declines of more than 50% were documented in 12 of 51 (24%) men (55). None of the 12 men relapsing after two or more hormones responded to high-dose bicalutamide treatment. Of the 39 men with only one prior hormonal manipulation, 10 of 26 (38%) with prior flutamide and 2 of 13 (15%) without prior flutamide had a significant PSA decline. Responses were seen equally in men who had or had not experienced a response to flutamide withdrawal.

Joyce et al. assessed a 150 mg daily dose in this setting (56). Seven of 31 (22.5%) men had a greater than 50% decline in PSA. Clinically, there was significant improvement in performance status and decreased analgesic use. The median response duration was 4 months. Six of seven responses were in men on prior flutamide as a component of combined androgen deprivation for a response rate of 43% (6 of 14) in men failing flutamide.

The activity of bicalutamide in patients failing flutamide can be explained by some distinct differences between the two drugs. Bicalutamide has a longer half-life and a significantly increased affinity for the AR (54). Furthermore, unlike flutamide, bicalutamide retains its antagonistic properties for the mutant AR (44).

Nilutamide

Nilutamide, like the other nonsteroidal antiandrogens, blocks binding to the AR and, at high doses, may inhibit testosterone biosynthesis. The drug is nearly completely absorbed and has a long half-life of 56 hours. Toxicities include delayed adaptation to darkness in one-fourth of patients, nausea in 10%, reversible increases in hepatic transaminases in up to 8%, and alcohol intolerance in 5%. Interstitial pneumonitis, which can progress to fibrosis, has been reported in less than 2% of patients, primarily Japanese patients. A potential beneficial effect is an increase in the proportion of high-density lipoprotein cholesterol.

Nilutamide is approved in combination with testicular androgen deprivation for advanced CaP. In HR disease, a single case report of PSA decline in a patient progressing after initial responses to orchiectomy and subsequent flutamide has been published to date (57). However, biochemical responses have been noted by other investigators after flutamide and bicalutamide failure (P. Schultz, *personal communication*, June 1999). Clinical trials to assess the true response have been initiated.

ESTROGEN

Estrogens were first described as a palliative therapy for advanced CaP by Huggins and Hodges in 1941 (1). In hormone-sensitive disease, estrogens suppress LHRH stimulation of the pituitary with resultant inhibition of pituitary gonadotropins and, in turn, serum testosterone. Additionally, estrogens have been experimentally shown to be cytotoxic in human androgen-insensitive CaP cells (DU145, 1-LN, and PC3) and androgen-sensitive CaP cells (LNCaP) (3). This cytotoxic effect is estrogen receptor independent and involves induction of cell cycle arrest at the G2 interface and apoptosis at the G2/M transition (58).

Low-Dose Estrogen

DES is a nonsteroidal estrogen. It has been used for the treatment of advanced CaP from the 1950s to the 1980s. Clinical trials conducted by the Veterans Administration Cooperative Urological Research Group showed that DES was as effective as orchiectomy in treating metastatic disease but was associated with excess cardiovascular and thromboembolic complications (59). DES at 1 mg per day was as effective as 5 mg per day but did not lower testosterone to castrate levels in all men. (60) DES use declined after the availability of LHRHa as an alternative form of medical castration (61).

Smith et al. assessed the efficacy and toxicity of 1 mg per day of DES in 21 men failing first line androgen deprivation. Nine of 21 (43%; 95% confidence interval, 22% to 64%) had a decrease in two serial PSAs of greater than 50% from baseline (62). Eight of 13 men (62%) with only one prior hormonal manipulation had a PSA decline, compared to one of eight men (13%) with more than one hormone treatment (p = .07). The estimated survival rate at 2 years was 63%. Toxicity was minimal, consisting of nipple hypersensitivity in 19 patients, gynecomastia in three patients, and a deep vein thrombosis in one patient.

High-Dose Estrogen

DES diphosphate (DES-DP, DES-P, Stilphostrol, Honvan, fosfestrol) is a nonsteroidal estrogen with two hydroxyl radicals. The beneficial effects of high-dose estrogen therapy using conjugated estrogens and DES sulfate in men with androgen-resistant carcinoma were first reported in 1952 by Hertz (63). DES-DP is an inactive estrogen that is dephosphorylated *in vivo* to DES. In 1955, Flocks reported on 34 men who had failed to respond or had become refractory to low-dose estrogen treated with intravenous DES-DP in doses ranging from 250 mg to 1,250 mg per day (64). Palliation of symptoms was documented in 21 of 27 men with prior estrogen treatment and five of seven men with prior estrogen and orchiectomy. Acid phosphatase levels fell in seven of nine patients with a good response and an elevated level pretreatment; in one of two with a fair response; and in none of three patients with a poor response. Toxicity consisted of mild nausea and perineal burning if the drug was injected rapidly. There was no thrombosis or gynecomastia.

Droz et al. reported on composite data from six phase II clinical trials assessing the efficacy of DES-DP in progressive metastatic disease (65). The doses in these studies ranged from 0.5 to 4.0 g per day i.v. for 7 to 10 days. Oral daily DES was given between i.v. cycles in one of the trials. The results in 139 men showed no measurable tumor responses, a decrease in prostatic acid phosphatase by greater than 50% in 37 of 99 men, and palliative benefit in 74 men. Seven men experienced cardiovascular complications. The median survival was 5 months.

The apprehension to estrogen use is primarily concern for cardiovascular toxicity in an elderly population. In two trials by the European Organization for Research on Treatment of Cancer using oral DES at a standard dose of 3 mg per day, there was lethal cardiovascular toxicity in 11% of 185 men (66). Risk factors were identified and included older age, weight greater than 75 kg, and prior cardiovascular disease. The cardiovascular toxicity in the aforementioned phase II trials was 5%. Concomitant use of aspirin seems warranted as prophylaxis. Other common side effects include nausea, vomiting, weight gain, edema, and gynecomastia. Abnormal liver function tests are less common.

PC-SPES

PC-SPES is an unregulated herbal dietary supplement consisting of seven Chinese and one American herbal extract (67). They are *Isatis indigotica* (da quing ye), *Glycyrrhiza glabra* and *uralensis* (gan cao), panax pseudoginseng (san qi), *Ganoderma lucidum* (ling zhi), *Scutellaria baicalensis* (huang qin), Dendranthema *morifolium* (Chrysanthemum), *Rabdosia rubescens*, and *Serenoa repens* (saw palmetto). The name of the product emphasizes its intention: *PC* stands for "prostate cancer" and *spes* is Latin for "hope."

The eight herbs were selected for their immune-stimulating, cytotoxic, and cytostatic properties. *G. glabra* and *G. uralensis* contain saponin that, in addition to binding cholesterol and bile salts, has *in vitro* antitumor activity (68). *Glycyrrhiza* increases 17β-hydroxysteroid dehydrogenase and aromatase with resultant lowering of serum testosterone and increased estrogen levels (69). Panax pseudo-ginseng contains dammarane-type saponins that are believed to stimulate natural killer cell activity and have antitumor effects *in vivo* (70,71). Consumption of this herb has been associated with a lower incidence of cancer (72). *G. lucidum* has demonstrated *in vitro* activity against marine S-180 sarcoma cells and exhibited immunomodulatory activity (73,74). *S. baicalensis* contains *baicalein*, which has been shown to inhibit the growth of hepatoma and human T lymphoid leukemia cells *in vitro* (68,75). *R. rubescens* has demonstrated *in vitro* antitumor effects against multiple tumor cell lines, including HeLa cells, Ehrlich ascites cells, sarcoma 180 cells, hepatoma cells, cervical carcinoma U14 cells, Walker 256 carcinosarcoma cells, and reticular carcinoma cells. *S. repens* contains a phytoestrogen that lowers endogenous estrogens. (76) Extracts of *Serenoa* inhibit growth of benign and malignant prostate cells probably by preventing binding of dihydrotestosterone to the AR (77,78). Clinically, it is associated with prostate size reduction in men with benign prostatic hypertrophy (79,80).

Extracts of PC-SPES have been shown to have an inhibitory effect on PC3 and LNCaP CaP cells and MCF-7 breast tumor cells in culture (81). Inhibition of LNCaP cells was correlated with a reduction in the expression of the AR and decreased secretion of PSA (82). Additional studies demonstrated that PC-SPES induces apoptosis and down-regulation of bcl-2, the gene-protecting cells from apoptosis (83). In a Dunning R3327 rat CaP model, syngeneic Copenhagen rats intradermally injected with Mat-Ly Lu cells known to metastasize in lung and lymph nodes and then fed a PC-SPES diet showed a decreased tumor incidence and decreased rate of tumor growth compared to control animals (84). This inhibitory effect was dose dependent. Of note, animals fed a PC-SPES diet that showed no primary tumor growth also had no pulmonary metastases, whereas in those animals in which PC-SPES was not effective in inhibiting the primary tumor growth, the frequency of pulmonary metastases was equal to that demonstrated in control animals.

Additional studies have demonstrated that PC-SPES has estrogenic properties (85). Using two yeast strains, a 1:200 dilution of an ethanol extract of PC-SPES had estrogenic effect equivalent to 1 nm of estradiol. In ovariectomized CD1 mice, treatment with PC-SPES resulted in significant increase in uterine weight compared to untreated animals, similar to the effect seen with estrogen. In men with CaP treated with PC-SPES, six of six had decreased serum testosterone levels, and, in eight of eight men, PSA levels declined. Side effects were similar to those of estrogen, with all men having breast tenderness and impotence and one man having a superficial venous thrombosis. PC-SPES was shown to have estrogenic properties on high performance liquid chromatography, gas chromatography, and mass spectrometry. This compound, however, is distinct from DES, estrone, and estradiol.

In a preliminary report of a phase II trial in advanced disease, both hormone naïve and androgen independent, 34 of 60 planned patients were treated with nine capsules totaling 2,880 mg per day (86). Of the 24 evaluable men, nine of twelve men with androgen-independent disease progressing in the setting of anorchid levels of testosterone and after antiandrogen withdrawal demonstrated a greater than 50% PSA decline. Nine of twelve men with hormone-naïve disease demonstrated a similar PSA response. Testosterone levels fell to castrate in 7 of 21 hormone-naïve men with initial normal levels. Toxicity included tender gynecomastia in 71%, grade 1 diarrhea in 33%, and grade 1 nausea in 12%. One patient had a pulmonary embolism, and 60% of men with baseline normal testosterone and pretreatment potency had loss of libido.

P-450 ENZYME INHIBITORS

Ketoconazole

Ketoconazole (Nizoral) is an imidazole derivative that has antifungal property (87). The development of gynecomastia in some men treated with ketoconazole for mycosis led to an investigation of its effect on testosterone (88). Subsequent studies showed that this drug inhibits cytochrome P-450 enzyme–mediated synthesis of adrenal and gonadal steroids (89,90). Additionally, ketoconazole demonstrates a direct antitumor effect on prostatic cancer cells *in vitro* (91).

Ketoconazole has been assessed in multiple phase II trials in hormone-sensitive metastatic CaP (92–94). In one representative trial, Vanuytsel et al. reported antitumor effects in 15 of 17 evaluable men (1 complete and 8 partial responses and 6 with stable disease) (94). Although testosterone levels decreased rapidly to near castrate level, they rose steadily after 1 month, limiting this drug to short-term usage, not chronic androgen deprivation therapy.

Ketoconazole has found its role as a form of medical adrenalectomy in the treatment of HR disease. In a 1993 comprehensive review of second line therapies, an overall response rate of 46% was achieved in 171 patients treated in ten trials (95). These studies were conducted before the use of PSA decline as an end point. Using the then-current response criteria of the National Prostatic Cancer Project, 16% of men had objective responses and 30% had stable disease (96). The standard dose was 400 mg orally three times a day and the use of concomitant steroids was variable.

Two recent trials have reported the efficacy of ketoconazole using PSA decline as an end point (97,98). Small et al. first reported in 50 men with progressive disease after combined androgen blockade and antiandrogen withdrawal treated with ketoconazole and hydrocortisone therapy (97). Overall, 30 men (62%) had a greater than 50% decline in PSA maintained for at least 8 weeks. The median response duration was 3.5 months (range, 3.25 to 12.75+ months). Response was independent of prior response to antiandrogen withdrawal. In a second report, 20 men with HRPC were treated with simultaneous antiandrogen withdrawal and ketoconazole plus hydrocortisone (98). Eleven (55%) had a greater than 50% decline in PSA. The median response duration was 8.5 months with a median survival of 19 months in this mixed population of men with localized and distant HR disease.

Ketoconazole is a frequently used second line therapy in progressive metastatic disease (99). Its toxicities include nausea and vomiting in up to one-half of patients, rash or dry itchy skin in 10%, chemical hepatitis, fatigue, nail dystrophy, asthenia, and gynecomastia. Although recently prescribed in conjunction with steroids, adrenal insufficiency secondary to ketoconazole is relatively rare, and it is probably safe in men in whom there is a contraindication to steroid use (100). Ketoconazole should be taken on an empty stomach owing to its dependency on decreased gastric pH for maximum absorption (101). Additionally, antacids and histamine H2 receptor antagonists should be avoided if possible or at least maximally spaced temporally from ketoconazole ingestion. Vitamin C administration can increase bioavailability in men with atrophic gastritis.

Aminoglutethimide

Aminoglutethimide blocks several cytochrome P-450–mediated hydroxylation steps, including the formation of pregnenolone from cholesterol and the 18-hydroxylase, 11-hydroxylase, and 21-hydroxylase enzymes (102). This inhibition results in decreased production of adrenal glucocorticoids, mineralcorticoids, estrogens, and androgens. In a review of 13 clinical trials involving 583 men with HR disease, the overall response rate using the NPCP criteria was 32%, which was predominantly stable disease (23%) (95). In the largest trial of 119 patients, the 50% probability of survival was 21 months for responders and 9.2 months for nonresponders (103). The standard dose is 250 mg orally four times a day with replacement dose hydrocortisone due to associated adrenal insufficiency. Other toxicities include lethargy, nausea, skin rash, ataxia, hypothyroidism, abnormal liver function tests, and edema. In a more recent report, 17 patients progressing on leuprolide, flutamide, suramin, and hydrocortisone underwent simultaneous flutamide withdrawal and initiation of aminoglutethimide (104). Hydrocortisone and leuprolide were continued. Eleven of the 17 men (65%) had a decline in PSA of greater than 50% and in seven (41%) men, PSA normalized. Of the 11 patients with significant declines in PSA, seven had evaluable disease radiographically. Of these seven, one had complete resolution of disease, four had partial responses, and two had stable disease. The median duration of PSA response was 344 days (range, 30 to 1,393 days).

CORTICOSTEROIDS

The palliative benefit of glucocorticoids in men progressing after orchiectomy in the 1950s was first reported by Miller and Hinman in 1954 (105). They reported subjective benefits in eight of ten men treated with 50 to 100 mg of cortisone per day. Since that time, prednisone, hydrocortisone, and dexamethasone have been routinely used in symptomatic advanced disease. Glucocorticoids inhibit the hypothalamus pituitary axis leading to suppression of androgen synthesis.

Prednisone

Tannock et al., in 1989, reported improvement in pain in 14 of 37 men (38%) with symptomatic bone metastases treated with 7.5 to 10.0 mg prednisone daily (106). In a subsequent large phase III trial of mitoxantrone plus prednisone versus prednisone alone at a dose of 5 mg twice daily, decreased pain or decreased analgesic use, or both, occurred in 21% of the 81 men treated with prednisone alone (107). PSA declines of greater than 50% also occurred in 21% of men on the prednisone alone. Sartor et al., using PSA decline as a primary end point, reported PSA declines of greater than 50% in 10 of 29 men (34%) with a median progression-free survival of 2.8 months (18). Overall survival was 17.4 months versus 10.5 months (p = .027) for men whose PSA declined by 50% versus those who did not have this response. Toxicity was not inconsequential, with four patients having steroid myopathy, one having new onset diabetes, and one patient with dyspnea.

Hydrocortisone

Hydrocortisone has also been documented to be of palliative benefit in HRPC. It is also a potentially confounding variable in clinical trials in which it has been used in combination with other chemotherapy drugs or investigational agents. Harland and Duchesne, in an article addressing the role of hydrocortisone in the response rates reported with suramin, reported that in 15 men treated with 40 mg hydrocortisone daily, eight men (53%) had a greater than 50% decline in PSA on this treatment (108). In a subsequent phase III trial of suramin plus hydrocortisone versus placebo plus hydrocortisone, for the 230 patients receiving hydrocortisone alone, 28% had relief of bone pain for a median duration of 69 days, and 16% had a greater than 50% decline in PSA (109). Similarly, in another large phase III trial comparing mitoxantrone plus hydrocortisone versus hydrocortisone (40 mg per day), 25 of 116 men receiving hydrocortisone alone (21.5%) had a greater than 50% decline in serum PSA (110).

Dexamethasone

Dexamethasone has also been used in the treatment of HR CaP. Storlie et al. reported on a retrospective record review of 38 men who progressed after orchiectomy and were then treated with low-dose dexamethasone, 0.75 mg twice daily (111). Twenty-four men (63%) had symptomatic improvement and in 23 men (61%), PSA declined by greater than 50%. Of these latter patients, eight (35%) had radiographic evidence of regression, five (22%) were stable, seven (30%) had disease progression, and three (13%) did not have serial radiographic studies.

Dexamethasone may be a potentially confounding variable in clinical trials in which it is used as a premedication. However, in a recent study of 12 men treated with taxotere, a run-in assessment of dexamethasone alone using the same premedication dose and schedule (20 mg orally every 6 hours for three doses every 3 weeks) showed no decline in PSA with dexamethasone alone (112).

PROGESTERONES

Megestrol acetate is a synthetic progestin with expected activity in CaP based on its capacity to lower testosterone and luteinizing hormone, block binding of dihydrotestosterone to the AR, inhibit 5α-reductase conversion of testosterone to dihydrotestosterone, induce adrenal suppression, and, at high doses, inhibit CaP growth *in vitro* (113–116). In previously untreated metastatic disease, symptomatic improvement has been documented in up to 90% of men and objective regression in up to 45% (117,118). Common toxicities with megestrol acetate include edema, thrombosis, hypertension, hyperglycemia, and weight gain.

In HR CaP, Osborn et al. reported only a 14% response rate based on a greater than 50% decline in PSA in a retrospective review of 14 patients (119). In a larger trial, of 149 men randomized to 160 mg per day (low dose) or 640 mg per day (high dose) of megestrol acetate, the rate of PSA decline by greater than 50% was 13.8% and 8.8% in the low- and high-dose arms, respectively (120). Of concern in this trial was a suspected pain flare secondary to the megestrol acetate in 7% of men. Although the response rate to high-dose medroxyprogesterone acetate (1,000 mg per day) was slightly higher at 25% to 38% in two Swedish trials, it appears that the potential benefit of megestrol acetate is inadequate to justify its potential side effects (121,122).

CONCLUSION

Multiple potentially efficacious second line hormonal therapies are currently available for the treatment of men with HRPC. Overall response rates vary from 20% to 50%. For all men, it is recommended that they be continued on their primary testicular androgen deprivation. For patients on an antiandrogen, the antiandrogen should be discontinued and the patient should be observed for a withdrawal response. After subsequent documented progression, alternate hormonal therapy with a different antiandrogen, a P-450 enzyme inhibitor, or estrogenic compound may be beneficial. These therapies should be initiated sequentially. Lack of response to one hormonal therapy does not preclude response to a subsequent one. Appropriate patients should always be considered for inclusion in an investigational protocol if available.

REFERENCES

1. Huggins C, Hodges CV. Studies on prostate cancer, effects of castration, of estrogens and androgen injection on serum phosphatase in metastatic carcinoma of the prostate. *Cancer Res* 1941;1:293–297.
2. Eisenberger MA, Blumenstein BA, Crawford ED, et al. Bilateral orchiectomy with or without flutamide for metastatic prostate cancer. *N Engl J Med* 1998;339:1036–1042.
3. Crawford ED, Eisenberger MA, McLeod DG, et al. A controlled trial of leuprolide with and without flutamide in prostatic carcinoma. *N Engl J Med* 1989;321:419–424.
4. Caubet JF, Tosteson TD, Dong EW, et al. Maximum androgen blockade in advanced prostate cancer: a meta-analysis of published randomized trials using nonsteroidal antiandrogen. *Urology* 1997;49:71–78.
5. Prostate Cancer Trialists' Collaborative Group. Maximum androgen blockade in advanced prostate cancer: an overview of 22 randomized trials with 3,283 deaths in 5,710 patients. *Lancet* 1995;346:265–269.
6. Small EJ, Vogelzang NJ. Second-line hormonal therapy for advanced prostate cancer: a shifting paradigm. *J Clin Oncol* 1997;15:382–388.
7. Smith PH, Bono A, da Silva C, et al. Some limitations of the radioisotope bone scan in patients with metastatic prostatic cancer. *Cancer* 1990;66:1009–1016.
8. Pollen JJ, Witztum KF, Ashburn WL. The flare phenomenon on radionucleotide bone scan in metastatic prostate cancer. *AJR Am J Roentgenol* 1984;142:773–776.
9. Figg WD, Ammerman K, Patronas N, et al. Lack of correlation between prostate-specific antigen and the presence of measurable soft tissue metastases in hormone-refractory prostate cancer. *Cancer Invest* 1996;14:513–517.
10. Dawson NA. Apples and oranges: building a consensus for standardized eligibility criteria and end points in prostate cancer clinical trials. *J Clin Oncol* 1998;16:3398–3405.
11. Kelly WK, Scher HI, Mazumdar M, et al. Prostate-specific antigen as a measure of disease outcome in metastatic hormone-refractory prostate cancer. *J Clin Oncol* 1993;11:607–615.
12. Smith DC, Dunn RL, Strawderman MS, et al. Changes in serum prostate-specific antigen as a marker of response to cytotoxic therapy for hormone-refractory prostate cancer. *J Clin Oncol* 1998;16:1835–1843.
13. Dawson NA, Halabi S, Hars V, et al. Prostate specific antigen (PSA) decline as a predictor of survival: Cancer and Leukemia Group B (CALGB) 9181. *Proc Am Soc Clin Oncol* 1999;18:314a.
14. Thalmann GN, Sikes RA, Chang S, et al. Suramin-induced decrease in prostate-specific antigen expression with no effect on tumor growth in the LNCaP model of human prostate cancer. *J Natl Cancer Inst* 1996;88:794–801.
15. Bubley GJ, Carducci M, Dahut W, et al. Eligibility and response guidelines for clinical trials in androgen independent prostate cancer: recommendations from the Prostate-Specific Antigen Working Group. *J Clin Oncol* 1999;17: 3461–467.
16. Batel-Copel LM, Kornblith AB, Batel PC, et al. Do oncologists have an increasing interest in the quality of life of their patients? A literature review of the last 15 years. *Eur J Cancer* 1997;33:29–32.
17. Scher HI, Mazumdar M, Kelly WK. Clinical trials in relapsed prostate cancer: defining the target. *J Natl Cancer Inst* 1996;88:1623–1634.

18. Sartor O, Weinberger M, Moore A, et al. Effect of prednisone on prostate-specific antigen in patients with hormone-refractory prostate cancer. *Urology* 1998;52:252–256.
19. Fowler JE, Whitmore WF. The response of metastatic adenocarcinoma of the prostate to exogenous testosterone. *J Urol* 1981;126:372–375.
20. Chao D, Harland SJ. The importance of continued endocrine treatment during chemotherapy of hormone-refractory prostate cancer. *Eur Urol* 1997;31:7–10.
21. Silver RI, Straus FH, Vogelzang NJ, et al. Response to orchiectomy following Zoladex therapy for metastatic prostate carcinoma. *Urology* 1991;37:17–21.
22. Taylor CD, Elson P, Trump DL. Importance of continued testicular suppression in hormone-refractory prostate cancer. *J Clin Oncol* 1993;11:2167–2172.
23. Hussain M, Wolf M, Marshall E, et al. Effects of continued androgen-deprivation therapy and other prognostic factors on response and survival in phase II chemotherapy trials for hormone-refractory prostate cancer: a Southwest Oncology Group report. *J Clin Oncol* 1994;12:1868–1875.
24. Kelly WK, Scher HI. Prostate specific antigen decline after antiandrogen withdrawal: the flutamide withdrawal syndrome. *J Urol* 1993;149:607–609.
25. Scher HI, Kelly WK. Flutamide withdrawal syndrome: its impact on clinical trials in hormone-refractory prostate cancer. *J Clin Oncol* 1993;11:1566–1572.
26. Small EJ, Srinivas S. The antiandrogen withdrawal syndrome. *Cancer* 1995;76:1428–1434.
27. Scher HI, Zhang ZF, Nanus D, et al. Hormone and antihormone withdrawal: implications for the management of androgen-independent prostate cancer. *Urology* 1996; 47(Suppl 1A):61–69.
28. Small EJ, Carroll PR. Prostate-specific antigen decline after Casodex withdrawal: evidence for an antiandrogen withdrawal syndrome. *Urology* 1994;43:408–410.
29. Nieh PT. Withdrawal phenomenon with the antiandrogen bicalutamide. *J Urol* 1995;153:1070–1073.
30. Schelhammer P, Kolvenbag GJ. Serum PSA decline after bicalutamide withdrawal. *Urology* 1994;44:790–791.
31. Huan SD, Gerridzen RG, Yau JC, et al. Antiandrogen withdrawal syndrome with nilutamide. *Urology* 1997;49:632–634.
32. Dawson NA, McLeod DG. Dramatic PSA decline in response to discontinuation of megestrol acetate in advanced prostate cancer: expansion of the antiandrogen withdrawal syndrome. *J Urol* 1995;153:1946–1947.
33. Sartor O, Eastham JA. Progressive prostate cancer associated with use of megestrol acetate administered for control of hot flashes. *South Med J* 1999;92:415–416.
34. Burch PA, Loprinzi CL. Prostate-specific antigen decline after withdrawal of low-dose megestrol acetate. *J Clin Oncol* 1999;3:1087–1088.
35. Akakura K, Akimoto S, Ohki T, et al. Antiandrogen withdrawal syndrome in prostate cancer after treatment with steroidal antiandrogen chlormadinone acetate. *Urology* 1995;45:700–705.
36. Sella A, Flex D, Sulkes A, et al. Antiandrogen withdrawal syndrome with cyproterone acetate. *Urology* 1998;52:1091–1093.
37. Bassada NK, Kaczmarek AT. Complete remission of hormone refractory adenocarcinoma of the prostate in response to withdrawal of diethylstilbestrol. *J Urol* 1995;153:1944–1945.
38. Wilding G, Chen M, Gelmann EP. Aberrant response in *in vitro* hormone-responsive prostate cancer cells to antiandrogens. *Prostate* 1989;14:103–115.
39. Schuurmans ALG, Veldscholte BJ, Mulder E. Stimulatory effects of antiandrogens on LNCaP human prostate tumor cell growth, EGF-receptor level and acid phosphatase secretion. *J Steroid Biochem Mol Biol* 1990;37:849–853.
40. Olea N, Sakabe K, Soto AM, et al. The proliferative effect of "anti-androgens" on androgen-sensitive human prostate tumor cell line LNCaP. *Endocrinology* 1990;126:1457–1463.
41. Veldscholte J, Berrevoets CA, Ris-Stalper C, et al. The androgen receptor in LNCaP cells contains a mutation in the ligand binding domain which affects steroid binding characteristics and response to antiandrogens. *J Steroid Biochem Mol Biol* 1992;41:665–669.
42. Moul JW, Srivastava S, McLeod DG. Molecular implications of the antiandrogen withdrawal syndrome. *Semin Urol* 1995;13:157–163.
43. Gaddipati JP, McLeod DG, Heidenberg HB, et al. Frequent detection of codon 877 mutation in the androgen receptor gene in advanced prostate cancers. *Cancer Res* 1994;54: 2861–2864.
44. Taplin M-E, Bubley GJ, ShusterD, et al. Mutations of the androgen-receptor gene in metastatic androgen-independent prostate cancer. *N Engl J Med* 1995;332:1393–1398.
45. Fenton MA, Shuster TD, Fertig AM, et al. Functional characterization of mutant androgen receptors from androgen-independent prostate cancer. *Clin Cancer Res* 1997;3:1383–1388.
46. Suzuki H, Koichiro A, Komiya A, et al. Codon 877 mutation in the androgen receptor gene in advanced cancer: relation to antiandrogen withdrawal syndrome. *Prostate* 1996; 29:153–158.
47. Culig Z, Hobisch A, Cronauer MV, et al. Mutant androgen receptor detected in an advanced-stage prostatic carcinoma is activated by adrenal androgens and progesterone. *Mol Endocrinol* 1993;7:1541–1550.
48. Veldscholte J, Brevets CA, Brinkmann AO, et al. Antiandrogens and the mutated androgen receptor of LNCaP cells: differential effects on binding affinity, heat-shock protein interaction, and transcription activation. *Biochemistry* 1992;31:2393–2399.
49. Visakorpi T, Hyytinen E, Koivisto P, et al. *In vivo* amplification of the androgen receptor gene and progression of human prostate cancer. *Nat Genet* 1995;9:401–406.
50. Mahler C, Verhelst J, Denis L. Clinical pharmacokinetics of the antiandrogens and their efficacy in prostate cancer. *Clin Pharmacokinet* 1998;34:405–417.
51. Labrie F, Dupont A, Giguere M, et al. Benefits of combination therapy with flutamide in patients relapsing after castration. *Br J Urol* 1988;61:341–346.
52. McLeod DG, Benson RC, Eisenberger MA, et al. The use of flutamide in hormone-refractory metastatic prostate cancer. *Cancer* 1993;72:3870–3873.
53. Fowler JE, Pandey P, Seaver LE, et al. Prostate specific antigen after gonadal androgen withdrawal and deferred flutamide treatment. *J Urol* 1995;154:448–453.
54. Kolenbag GJ, Furr BJ, Blackledge GR. Receptor affinity and potency of non-steroidal antiandrogens: translation of preclinical findings into clinical activity. *Prostate Cancer and Prostatic Diseases* 1998;1:307–314.

55. Scher HI, Liebertz C, Kelly WK, et al. Bicalutamide for advanced prostate cancer: the natural versus treated history of disease. *J Clin Oncol* 1997;15:2928–2838.
56. Joyce R, Fenton MA, Rode P, et al. High dose bicalutamide for androgen independent prostate cancer: effect of prior hormonal therapy. *J Urol* 1997:159:149–153.
57. Eastham JA, Sartor O. Nilutamide response after flutamide failure in post-orchiectomy progressive prostate cancer. *J Urol* 1998;159:990.
58. Robertson CN, Roberson KM, Padilla GM, et al. Induction of apoptosis by diethylstilbestrol in hormone-insensitive prostate cancer cells. *J Natl Cancer Inst* 1996;88:908–917.
59. Byer DP. The Veteran's Administration Cooperative Urological Group's studies of carcinoma of the prostate. *Cancer* 1973;32:1126–1130.
60. Byer DP, Corle DK. Hormone therapy for prostate cancer: results of the Veteran's Administration Cooperative Urological Group's studies. *NCI Monogr* 1988;7:165–170.
61. Garnick MB, Globe IM, Leuprolide Study Group. Leuprolide versus diethylstilbestrol for metastatic prostate cancer. *N Engl J Med* 1984;311:1281–1286.
62. Smith DC, Redman BG, Flaherty LE, et al. A phase II trial of oral diethylstilbestrol as a second-line hormonal agent in advanced prostate cancer. *Urology* 1998;52:257–260.
63. Hertz R, Young JP, Tullner WW. Administration of massive dosage of estrogen to breast and prostatic cancer patients: blood levels attained. Philadelphia: Blakiston, Ciba Foundation. *Colloq Endocrinol* 1952;1:157–169.
64. Flocks RH, Marberger H, Begley BJ, et al. Prostatic carcinoma: treatment of advanced cases with intravenous diethylstilbestrol diphosphate. *J Urol* 1955;74:549–551.
65. Droz J, Kaftan J, Bonnay M, et al. High-dose continuous-infusion fosfestrol in hormone-resistant prostate cancer. *Cancer* 1993;71:1123–1130.
66. De Voogt HJ, Smith PH, Pavone-Macaluso M, et al. Cardiovascular side effects of diethylstilbestrol, cyproterone acetate, medroxyprogesterone acetate and estramustine phosphate used for the treatment of advanced prostatic cancer: results from the European Organization for Research on Treatment of Cancer trials 30761 and 30762. *J Urol* 1986;135:303–307.
67. Fan S, Wang X. Herbal composition for treating prostate cancer. PC-SPES. Pending United States patent number 08/697920.
68. Motoo Y, Sawabu N. Antitumor effects of saikosaponins, baicalin and baicalein on human hepatoma cells. *Cancer Lett* 1994;86:91–95.
69. Ghosh D, Wawrzak Z, Pletnev V, et al. Molecular mechanism of inhibition of steroid dehydrogenases by licorice-derived steroid analogs in modulation of steroid receptor function. *Ann N Y Acad Sci* 1995;761:341–343.
70. Tode T, Kikuchi Y, Kita T, et al. Inhibitory effects by oral administration of ginsenoside Rh2 on the growth of human ovarian cancer cells in nude mice. *J Cancer Res Clin Oncol* 1993;120:24–26.
71. Mochizuki M, Yoo YC, Matsuzawa K, et al. Inhibitory effect of tumor metastasis in mice by saponins, ginsenoside-Rb2, 20 (R) and 20 (S)-ginsenoside-Rg3 of red ginseng. *Biol Pharm Bull* 1995;18:1197–1202.
72. Yun TK, Choi SY. Preventive effect of ginseng intake against various human cancers: a case control study on 1987 pairs. *Cancer Epidemiol Biomarkers Prev* 1995:4: 401–408.
73. Maruyama H, Yamazaki K, Murofushi S, et al. Antitumor activity of *Sarccodn aspratus* (Berk.) S. Ito and *Ganderma lucidum* (Fr.) Karst. *J Pharmacobiodyn* 1989;12:118–123.
74. Tanaka S, Ko K, Kino K, et al Complete amino acid sequence of an immunomodulatory protein, ling zhi-8 (LZ-8). An immunomodulator from a fungus, *Ganoderma lucidium,* having similarity to immunoglobulin variable regions. *J Biol Chem* 1989;264:16372–16377.
75. Huang HC, Hsieh LM, Chen HW, et al. Effects of baicalcin and esculetin on transduction signals and growth factors expression in T-lymphoid leukemia cells. *Eur J Pharmacol* 1994;268:73–78.
76. Iehle C, Delos S, Guirou O, et al. Human prostatic steroid 5 alpha-reductase isoforms—a comparative study of selective inhibitors. *J Steroid Biochem Mol Biol* 1995;54:273–279.
77. Delos S, Carsol JL, Ghazarossian E, et al. Testosterone metabolism in primary culture of human prostate epithelial cell and fibroblasts. *J Steroid Biochem Molec Biol* 1995;55: 375–383.
78. Carilla E, Briley M, Fauran F, et al. Binding of Permixon, a new treatment for prostatic benign hyperplasia to the cytosolic androgen receptor in the rat prostate. *J Steroid Biochem* 1984;20:521–523.
79. Champault G, Patel JC, Bonnard AM. A double-blind trial of an extract of the plant *Serenoa repens* in benign prostatic hyperplasia to the cytosolic androgen receptor in the rat prostate. *J Steroid Biochem* 1984;20:521–523.
80. Grasso M, Montesano A, Buonaguidi A, et al. Comparative effects of alfuzosin versus *Serenoa repens* in the treatment of symptomatic benign prostatic hyperplasia. *Arch Esp Urol* 1995;48:97–103.
81. Halicka HD, Ardelt B, Juan G, et al. Apoptosis and cell cycle effects induced by extracts of the Chinese herbal preparation PC SPES. *Int J Oncol* 1997;11:437–438.
82. Hsieh T, Chen SS, Wang X, et al. Regulation of androgen receptor (AR) and prostate specific antigen (PSA) expression in the androgen-responsive human prostate LNCaP cells by ethanolic extracts of the Chinese herbal preparation PC-SPES. *Biochem Mol Biol Int* 1997;42:535–544.
83. Hsieh T, Ng C, Chang C, et al. Induction of apoptosis and downregulation of bcl-6 in Mutu I cells treated with ethanolic extracts of the Chinese herbal supplement PC-SPES. *Int J Oncol* 1998;13:1–4.
84. Tiwari RK, Geliebter J, Garikapaty VP, et al. Anti-tumor effects of PC-SPES, an herbal formulation in prostate cancer. *Int J Oncol* 1999;14:713–719.
85. DiPaola RS, Zhang H, Lambert GH, et al. Clinical and biologic activity of an estrogenic herbal combination (PC-SPES) in prostate cancer. *N Engl J Med* 1998;339:785–791.
86. Kameda H, Small EJ, Reese DM, et al. A phase II study of PC-SPES, an herbal compound for the treatment of advanced prostate cancer (Pca). *Proc Am Soc Clin Oncol* 1999;18:320a.
87. Graybill JR, Drutz DJ. Ketoconazole: a major innovation for treatment of fungal disease. *Ann Intern Med* 1980;93: 921–923.
88. DeFelice P, Johnson DG, Galgiani JN. Gynecomastia with ketoconazole. *Antimicrob Agents Chemother* 1981;19:1073–1074.

89. Pont A, Williams PL, Azhar S, et al. Ketoconazole blocks testosterone biosynthesis. *Arch Intern Med* 1982;142:2137–2140.
90. DeCoster R, Caers 1, Coene M-C, et al. Effects of high-dose ketoconazole therapy on the main plasma testicular and adrenal steroids in previously untreated prostatic cancer patients. *Clin Endocrinol* 1986;24:657–664.
91. Eichenberger T, Trachtenberg J, Toor P, et al. Ketoconazole: a possible direct cytotoxic effect on prostate carcinoma cells. *J Urol* 1989;14:190–191.
92. Pont A. Long-term experience with high dose ketoconazole therapy in patients with stage D2 prostatic carcinoma. *J Urol* 1987;137:902–904.
93. Percy LA. Ketoconazole in advanced prostate cancer. *Ann Pharmacother* 1992;26:1527–1529.
94. Vanuytsel L, Ang KK, Vantongelen K, et al. Ketoconazole therapy for advanced prostatic cancer: feasibility and treatment results. *J Urol* 1987;137:905–908.
95. Dawson NA. Treatment of progressive metastatic prostate cancer. *Oncology* 1993;7:17–27.
96. Murphy GP, Slack NH. Response criteria for the prostate of the USA National Prostatic Cancer Project. *Prostate* 1980;1:375–382.
97. Small EJ, Baron AD, Fippin L, et al. Ketoconazole retains activity in advanced prostate cancer patients with progression despite flutamide withdrawal. *J Urol* 1997;157:1204–1207.
98. Small EJ, Baron A, Bok R. Simultaneous antiandrogen withdrawal and ketoconazole and hydrocortisone in patients with advanced prostate cancer. *Cancer* 1997;80:1755–1759.
99. Dawson NA, Vogelzang NJ. Secondary hormonal therapy. In: Resnick MI, Thompson IM, eds. *Advanced therapy of prostate disease.* Ontario, Canada: B.C. Decker, 2000.
100. Tucker WS, Snell BB, Island DP, et al. Reversible adrenal insufficiency induced by ketoconazole. *JAMA* 1985;253: 2413–2414.
101. Blum RA, D'Andrea DT, Florentino BM, et al. Increased gastric pH and the bioavailability of fluconazole and ketoconazole. *Ann Int Med* 1991;114:755–757.
102. Haynes RC. Adrenocorticotropic hormone; adrenocortical steroids and their synthetic analogs; inhibitors or the synthesis and actions of adrenocortical hormones. In: Gillman AG, Rall TW, et al., eds. *Goodman and Gilman's the pharmacological basis of therapeutics.* New York: Pergamom Press, 1990;1458–1459.
103. Labrie F, Dupont A, Belanger A, et al. Anti-hormone treatment for prostate cancer relapsing after treatment with flutamide and castration. *Br J Urol* 1989;63:634–638.
104. Figg WD, Dawson N, Middleman MN, et al. Flutamide withdrawal and concomitant initiation of aminoglutethimide in patients with hormone refractory prostate cancer. *Acta Oncologica* 1996;35:763-765.
105. Miller GM, Hinman F. Cortisone treatment in advanced carcinoma of the prostate. *J Urol* 1954;72:485–496.
106. Tannock I, Gospodarowicz M, Meakin W, et al. Treatment of metastatic prostatic cancer with low-dose prednisone: evaluation of pain and quality of life as pragmatic indices of response. *J Clin Oncol* 1989;7:590–597.
107. Tannock IF, Osoba D, Stockler MR, et al. Chemotherapy with mitoxantrone plus prednisone or prednisone alone for symptomatic hormone-resistant prostate cancer: a Canadian randomized trial with palliative end points. *J Clin Oncol* 1996;14:1756–1764.
108. Harland SJ, Duchesne GM. Suramin and prostate cancer: the role of hydrocortisone. *Eur J Cancer* 1992;28A:1295.
109. Small EJ, Marshall ME, Reyno L, et al. Superiority of suramin + hydrocortisone (S+H) over placebo + hydrocortisone (P + H): results of a multi-center double-blind phase III study in patients with hormone refractory prostate cancer (HRPC). *Proc Am Soc Clin Oncol* 1998;17:308a.
110. Kantoff PW, Halabi S, Conaway MR, et al. Hydrocortisone with or without mitoxantrone in men with hormone-refractory prostate cancer: results of the cancer and leukemia group B 9182 study. *J Clin Oncol* 1999;17:2506–2513.
111. Storlie JA, Buckner JC, Wiseman GA, et al. Prostate specific antigen levels and clinical response to low dose dexamethasone for hormone-refractory metastatic prostate carcinoma. *Cancer* 1995;76:96–100.
112. Weitzman AL, Shelton G, Zuech N, et al. Dexamethasone does not contribute to the response rate of docetaxel and estramustine in androgen independent prostate cancer. *J Urol* 2000;163:834–847.
113. Geller J, Albert J, Geller S, et al. Effect of megestrol acetate (Megace) on steroid metabolism and steroid-protein binding in the human prostate. *J Clin Endocrinol Metabol* 1976;43:1000–1008.
114. Leinung MC, Liporace R, Miller CH. Induction of adrenal suppression by megestrol acetate in patients with AIDS. *Ann Intern Med* 1995;122:843–845.
115. Maltry E. Use of megestrol acetate (a new progestational agent) in the treatment of carcinoma of the prostate. In: *Proceedings of the Kimbrough Urological Seminar, 18th Annual Meeting, 1970.* Norwich: Eaton Laboratories, 1970: 135–137.
116. Anderson DG. The possible mechanisms of action of progestins on endometrial adenocarcinoma. *Am J Obstet Gynecol* 1972;113:195–211.
117. Johnson DE, Kaesler KE, Ayala AG. Megestrol acetate for treatment of advanced carcinoma of the prostate. *J Surg Oncol* 1975;7:9–15.
118. Bonomi P, Pessis D, Buntin N, et al. Megestrol acetate used as primary hormonal therapy in stage D prostate cancer. *Semin Oncol* 1985;12(Suppl 1):36–39.
119. Osborn JL, Smith DC, Trump DL. Megestrol acetate in the treatment of hormone refractory prostate cancer. *Am J Clin Oncol* 1997;20:308–310.
120. Dawson NA, Conaway M, Halabi S, et al. A randomized study comparing standard versus moderately high dose megestrol acetate in advanced prostate cancer: Cancer and Leukemia Group B (CALGB) study 9181. *Cancer* 2000;88: 825–834.
121. Johansson JE, Andersson SO, Holmberg. High-dose medroxyprogesterone acetate versus estramustine in therapy-resistant prostatic cancer: a randomized study. *Br J Urol* 1991;68:67–73.
122. Fossa SD, Jahnsen JU, Karlsen S, et al. High-dose medroxyprogesterone acetate versus prednisolone in hormone-resistant prostatic cancer. *Eur Urol* 1985;11:11–16.

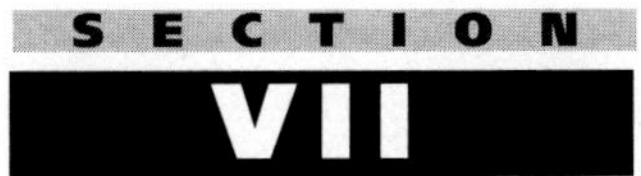

HORMONE-REFRACTORY DISEASE

44

PAIN AND SYMPTOM MANAGEMENT

NATHANIEL P. KATZ

Pain and other distressing symptoms have profound effects on the quality of life of individuals with prostate cancer (CaP) from the time of diagnosis to the terminal phases of illness. The old dichotomous concept of managing symptoms after "giving up" on cure is being replaced with a patient-oriented continuum of care, incorporating symptom management into cancer treatment at the outset.

The suffering of patients with CaP is thematic of cancer in general but also comprises issues specific for this particular malignancy. Patients experience general symptoms seen in cancer, such as fatigue, depression, anxiety, and pain. Symptoms seen especially in CaP include urinary and bowel symptoms, bone pain, and sexual dysfunction. Beyond specific symptoms, patients experience broader problems: emotional functioning, physical functioning, loss of social role, change of self-image, and the death and dying process. This model of suffering may be extended beyond the patient to the family.

Pain and symptom management programs have arisen to assist oncologists and other health care providers in the management of specific symptoms that arise in the oncologic setting. Palliative care programs provide more comprehensive support, particularly toward the terminal phases of illness. Palliative care includes social services, emotional and spiritual support, and bereavement counseling. Hospice programs have grown to allow terminal patients to pass through the dying process more comfortably at home without inappropriately aggressive care. Together, these services interdigitate to maximize the cancer patient's quality of life in all phases of the cancer experience.

This chapter focuses primarily on the management of pain and other symptoms in CaP.

SYMPTOMS IN PROSTATE CANCER

Symptoms of Disease

Symptoms in CaP may arise from the disease or from its treatment. Local disease, although often asymptomatic, may produce a characteristic set of symptoms including pain, hesitancy, urgency, poor stream, and dribbling. Metastatic disease produces a different constellation of characteristic symptoms (Table 44-1) dominated by bone pain. Other symptoms of metastatic disease include fatigue, nausea, anorexia, and depression. These symptoms are usually controlled by primary antineoplastic treatments, although treatments produce their own symptomatic complications, detailed later. Yet a third set of symptoms, similar across all malignancies, characterizes terminal illness (Table 44-1). Terminal symptoms include pain, delirium, restlessness, nausea, and vomiting. Management of issues that arise among family members assumes a greater role, including service issues, respite, and bereavement.

Symptoms of Treatment

Antiandrogen Therapy

Antiandrogenic therapy remains a mainstay of therapy for CaP. Reduction of androgens by any means—chemical or surgical—gives rise to a number of symptoms (1,2). These include depression, a belief of compromised well being, and emotional lability. *Orchiectomy* leads to overall improvement in quality of life in patients with metastatic CaP (3). However, a number of important side effects have been described including impotence, decreased libido, female body image, and cosmetic disturbance. Similar side effects have been described in patients receiving *antiandrogenic medications* compared to patients after orchiectomy without medications (3). These include diarrhea, body image disturbance, gynecomastia, fatigue, pain, overall symptom distress, emotional problems, and decreased physical functioning. These medication effects, reported primarily with flutamide, also may occur to a lesser extent with luteinizing hormone releasing hormone (LHRH) administration.

Radiotherapy

Overall quality of life appears similar in patients with CaP after prostatectomy, radiation therapy for localized disease, and age-matched "well" controls, despite specific treatment-

TABLE 44-1. SYMPTOMS IN PROSTATE CANCER

Related to disease			Related to treatment
Localized disease	**Metastatic disease**	**Terminal disease**	**Orchidectomy**
Urinary symptoms	Bone pain	Delirium	Impotence
Local pain	Fatigue		Fatigue
Sexual dysfunction	Nausea		Decreased concentration
Psychosocial adjustment	Depression		Hot flashes
	Anorexia		Body image problems
	Constipation		Cosmesis
	Sexual dysfunction		**Other antiandrogenic therapies**
	Lymphedema		Impotence, fatigue, concentration
			Hot flashes
			Diarrhea, gas pain
			Gynecomastia
			↓ Well-being
			Emotional lability
			Radiotherapy
			Proctitis: fecal leakage, gas, rectal discharge, cramps
			Erectile dysfunction
			Urinary tract symptoms: dysuria, hematuria, spasms
			Prostatectomy
			Sexual dysfunction
			Urinary incontinence

↓, decreased.

related morbidities. Primary predictors of quality of life in these patients remain the general cancer-related dimensions: physical and emotional functioning and fatigue. Specific side effects seen after radiation (4,5) include fecal leakage in 15% (6); erectile dysfunction, increasing with duration of follow-up (7,8) in 30% to 60% and causing psychological distress in 7%; and lower urinary tract symptoms including dysuria in 14%. Proctitis, consisting of gas, blood, or mucous discharge from the rectum; bowel cramps; and diarrhea occur in up to 14% (9).

Prostatectomy

The major symptom occurring after prostatectomy (5) has been sexual dysfunction (50% to 70%), which is more frequent with advanced patient age and causes psychological distress in 7% and urinary incontinence in 35%, despite nerve-sparing techniques.

PAIN MANAGEMENT

Barriers to Pain Relief

Guidelines for the treatment of cancer pain have been widely accepted and publicized (10). Validation studies of these guidelines have demonstrated that 75% to 90% of patients with cancer pain can enjoy satisfactory relief with the institution of these simple guidelines, using available medications. Yet survey studies continue to demonstrate success rates substantially less than this (11). Several critical barriers to the adoption of these guidelines have been identified (Table 44-2). These include barriers related to health care professionals, patients, and the health care system (11).

Pain Assessment

The major obstacle to adequate cancer pain management is underrecognition of pain, and the major obstacle to full recognition of pain is the lack of routine pain assessment. Health care providers should query patients about pain at every encounter: pain as the "fifth vital sign." Full assessment of pain should take place with every new report of pain and at suitable intervals after analgesic intervention (12). The primary goal of the initial assessment of a pain complaint is to arrive at a diagnosis. Too many patients have been inadequately treated because of the diagnosis of "cancer pain."

Example 1: A 49-year-old man with metastatic CaP was admitted to the hospital for intractable pain. He had been previously treated on multiple occasions for new pain complaints due to multiple bony metastases and had been successfully irradiated on several episodes. He was treated for worsening pain in the neck with maximal nonsteroidal antiinflammatory drugs (NSAIDs) and opioids, with dose-limiting sedation from opioids despite inadequate analgesia. Head and neck computed tomography (CT) scans were "negative." Terminal sedation was considered. The Pain Service was consulted. The medical history revealed recent onset of new pain at the top of the cervical spine on the left, with radiation to the top of the head, worsened by rotation. The exam revealed left occipital numbness. A CT

TABLE 44-2. BARRIERS TO EFFECTIVE PAIN MANAGEMENT

Problems related to health care professionals
- Inadequate knowledge of pain management
- Poor assessment of pain
- Lack of routine pain assessment
- Concern about regulation of controlled substances
- Fear of patient addiction
- Concern about side effects of analgesics
- Concern about patients becoming tolerant to analgesics

Problems related to patients
- Reluctance to report pain
- Concern about distracting physicians from treatment of underlying disease
- Fear that pain means disease is worse
- Concern about not being a "good" patient
- Reluctance to take pain medications
- Fear of addiction or of being thought of as an addict
- Worries about unmanageable side effects
- Concern about becoming tolerant to pain medications

Problems related to the health care system
- Low priority given to cancer pain treatment
- Inadequate reimbursement
- The most appropriate treatment may not be reimbursed or may be too costly for patients and families
- Restrictive regulations of controlled substances
- Problems of availability of treatment or access to it

Adapted from Agency for Health Care Policy and Research. *Management of cancer pain.* Clinical Practice Guideline Number 9. U.S. Department of Health and Human Services. AHCPR Pub. No. 94-0592, 1994.

scan of the C1-2 region, ordered to identify a spine lesion at that level compressing the C2 nerve root, was positive for such a lesion; this lesion had been missed on the previous "routine" head and neck studies, which did not incorporate the level of C2. Local irradiation resolved the pain.

Elements of the initial pain assessment include

- Medical history
  - Pain phenomenology: quality, intensity, location, time course, aggravating, and relieving factors
  - Previous treatments and results
  - Associated systemic or neurologic features
  - Psychosocial history, substance abuse history
  - Treatment goals (cure, palliation, terminal care)
- Physical examination
  - What provokes the pain
  - Relevant neurologic exam
- Appropriate diagnostic tests

Follow-up assessments focus on

- Evolution of symptom complex
- Changes in intensity
- Response to treatment, including side effects

Rational pain treatment requires setting appropriate goals and "managing expectations" of the patient, family, and health care team. Patients are often more willing and able to tolerate pain during some circumstances (e.g., procedure-related pain early in the illness) than others (terminal care). Patients may suffer from inappropriately pessimistic expectations ("I'm destined to die in pain.") or inappropriately optimistic expectations ("I deserve to be pain free at all times."). Patient education to minimize disparity between patient expectations and clinical reality may do more than analgesics to decrease suffering in the setting of painful illness.

A number of simple instruments have been validated for use in the cancer population (Fig. 44-1) and should be part of routine assessment.

Pain Syndromes in Prostate Cancer

Bone Pain

Bone pain is the most common symptom affecting those with metastatic CaP (13) and is the most common cause of cancer-related pain (14). Bone pain most often involves the spine and pelvis. Up to 25% of patients with bone metastases have no symptoms; in most cases, it is unclear what determines whether a metastasis is painful or not. Therefore, it is important to correlate radiologic signs with the clinical presentation to determine whether an individual metastasis is symptomatic. Pain may result from direct tumor involvement of bone, compression of adjacent nerves or the spinal cord, or involvement of soft tissue. Pain due to multiple metastases is common. In the setting of spine metastases, more than one metastasis is present in 85% of patients (15). The pain is usually described as dull or aching and is often aggravated by movement of the affected part or palpation. Bone lesions may cause referred pain in the absence of nerve compression. Lesions in the upper cervical spine may cause headache, referred to the occiput or frontal regions. Lesions in the lower cervical spine cause pain in the shoulder, arm, or interscapular region. Lesions in the thoracic spine may refer anteriorly to

Please describe your average pain:

Categorical scale:	None	Mild	Moderate		Severe	Excruciating
Numerical scale:	0	1	2	3	4	5

Visual Analog Scale:

No Pain ________________________________ Worst Pain

FIGURE 44-1. Pain assessment instruments.

the chest. Lumbosacral spine lesions may refer to the groin, buttocks, or proximal leg, and hip lesions may refer to pain down to the knee. Pathologic fractures and hypercalcemia may also occur, although these are less common than in metastases from cancers of the lung, breast, kidney, or myeloma.

The diagnosis is confirmed by radiologic studies, including plain x-rays, bone scans, magnetic resonance imaging (MRI), or CT. Bone scans and MRIs are the most sensitive of these modalities, often detecting abnormalities that are not visible on plain x-rays. Bone scans have the advantage of visualizing the entire skeleton with one imaging study. MRI of the spine has the advantage of detecting simultaneous lesions of any part of the spine; CT scans are typically limited to a segment of the spine. Plain x-rays are helpful in estimating the risk of pathologic fracture; CT scanning may be yet more helpful in this regard. Lesions considered to confer risk of pathologic fracture are those that

- Are painful,
- Are in weight-bearing bones,
- Involve more than 50% of the bony cortex, and
- Are greater than 2.5 cm in diameter.

Bone pain due to a metastatic tumor should be differentiated from nonmalignant causes of bone pain. Such causes include osteoporotic fractures, focal osteonecrosis (which may be due to steroids or radiation), and osteomalacia. Lesions of the cervical spine causing interscapular pain may be missed by imaging too low; upper cervical spine lesions causing headache may be missed by imaging only the head; low thoracic or upper lumbar lesions causing low back or hip pain may be missed by imaging only the lumbar spine or pelvis. "Routine" CT scans of the neck often do not include the upper cervical spine. CT or MRI scans of the "lumbosacral spine" and MRI scans of the "whole spine" often do not image the sacrum.

Spinal Cord Compression

Epidural compression of the spinal cord is a common complication of cancer, occurring in up to 10% of patients (16). Most cases of spinal cord compression are caused by extension of metastases from the vertebral body into the epidural space. Untreated spinal cord compression leads to the complete cord syndrome: paraplegia or quadriplegia. Because the success of treatment depends on the neurologic status at the time of its initiation, prompt diagnosis and institution of therapy is critical. Back pain is the initial symptom in almost all patients with spinal cord compression and, in 10%, it is the only symptom at the time of diagnosis. Characteristics of back pain in a cancer patient that increase the likelihood of epidural extension of tumor include rapid progression of pain (17), radicular pain (18), and worsening of pain by recumbency, cough, sneeze, or strain (19). Algorithms have been developed to assist in the cost-effective management of patients with cancer and back pain, starting with plain radiographs (20).

Incident Pain

Incident pain is defined as pain that occurs primarily with movement. The most common type is pain on standing or walking caused by metastases to the lumbar spine, sacrum, pelvis, or hip. Metastasis to any weight-bearing bone may cause incident pain, and lesions in the humerus or shoulder may cause incident pain on usage of the upper extremity. Pathologic fracture is a potential risk or causative entity in these situations. Recognition of incident pain is critical in the management of cancer pain, because this syndrome is often poorly controlled by systemic opioids. Incident pain may respond better to primary anticancer therapies, particularly radiation, and also to NSAIDs, bracing, intralesional steroid injections, spinal administration of local anesthetic/opioid combinations, and orthopedic fixation. The recognition of incident pain should therefore prompt early referral for pain management or orthopedic consultation in patients who do not respond promptly to appropriate analgesic interventions.

Luteinizing Hormone Releasing Hormone Tumor Flare

Initiation of LHRH hormonal therapy produces a transient symptom flare in 5% to 25% of patients (20). This flare may be caused by an initial stimulation of LH release before suppression is achieved. Presenting symptoms include increased bone pain or urinary retention; cord compression and sudden death have been reported. This syndrome typically begins within a week of initiation of therapy and persists for 1 to 3 weeks. Coadministration of an androgen antagonist during initiation of LHRH can prevent this tumor flare (21). Tumor flares have been observed with other hormonal agents as well, including androstenedione and medroxyprogesterone (20).

Radiation Proctitis

Radiotherapy is used to cure patients with local disease and to palliate pain in patients with noncurable local disease or metastases. Although effective in all these indications, radiotherapy may be followed by a number of complications that may adversely impact quality of life (4,5). Radiation proctitis occurs acutely in up to 50% of patients; symptoms persist in as many as 10% to 30% of patients (9,22). Symptoms include fecal leakage, cramps, gas, tenesmus, and discharge of blood or mucus per rectum. Chronic cases may progress to include strictures or fistula formation (23). The differential diagnosis includes infective proctitis and inflammatory bowel disease.

Radiation Cystitis

Radiation cystitis may follow pelvic radiotherapy and causes persistent symptoms in approximately 20% of patients (9). Symptoms include dysuria, impairment of urinary flow, incontinence, persistent hematuria, and bladder outlet obstruction. Chronic bleeding may cause significant morbidity.

Perineal Pain

Tumors of the prostate may produce perineal pain by local invasion, although cancers of the colon, rectum, and female reproductive tract are more common causes of cancer-related perineal pain (24). The pain is typically described as constant and aching, exacerbated by sitting or standing. Bladder spasms or tenesmus may be associated symptoms. In some patients, a similar pain syndrome may occur after pelvic surgery in the absence of concurrent neoplastic disease.

Neuropathic Pain

Neuropathic pain, defined as pain due to damage to the nervous system, is uncommon in CaP, compared to other cancers. Nevertheless, neuropathic syndromes do occur. Most important, recognition of a neuropathic pain syndrome requires identification of the neural structure involved (e.g., spinal cord, root, plexus, nerve) and etiology of the damage (tumor invasion, pathologic fracture with neural compression, radiation, postsurgical, infection, meningeal process, and others). Neuropathic pain usually presents with positive symptoms such as burning, tingling, and lancinations, as well as a neurologic deficit: loss of sensation, weakness, hyporeflexia, or loss of sphincter function. Contrary to popular belief, neuropathic pain is commonly described as aching, throbbing, or other descriptors usually ascribed to nonneuropathic causes. The pain may radiate in the distribution of the affected neural structure or may be perceived in only a portion of the territory.

The important neuropathic pain syndromes include

- Spinal cord compression (described earlier)
- Spinal nerve root compression: Pain is severe, and often radiates down the arm, around the trunk, or down the leg. This may be the presenting symptom of tumor invasion of the spine, compression fracture with root impingement, leptomeningeal metastases, or meningeal infections (uncommon in CaP).
- Lumbosacral plexopathies: This syndrome presents in the groin, sacral region, perineum, or leg. Lumbosacral plexopathy in the cancer population usually results from direct tumor invasion. In the setting of CaP, this syndrome is most likely to involve the sacral plexus, with involvement of the posterior thigh, leg, and foot, and perhaps the perineal region; sphincter disturbance may occur (25). Lymphedema of the leg is common. Radiation plexopathy is an uncommon complication of pelvic irradiation and may be delayed from 1 to 30 years after treatment (26). Patients typically present with neurologic deficits and leg swelling that may be bilateral; pain is less common than with tumor-induced plexopathies. Lumbosacral plexopathy may also result from surgical trauma or infections in the pelvis or psoas muscle.

Pain Treatment

General Principles

- Look for a specific diagnosis.
- The diagnosis should never be "cancer pain," but rather "bone pain due to metastatic disease," "incident pain," "nerve root compression due to pathologic fracture," "rectal pain due to radiation proctitis," and others.
- Treat the specific diagnosis with primary therapies (e.g., antibiotics); it is the best chance to cure.
- Start treating the pain while initiating the diagnostic work-up: Do not wait.
- Titrate medications to effect.
- Don't forget nonopioid analgesics.
- Never use a placebo.
- Patient self-report is the best measure of pain.
- Addiction is rare in this population.
- Treat analgesic-related side effects aggressively.
- Set reasonable goals for pain relief and strive to achieve them.
- Functional goals are achieved through analgesia combined with functional restoration (physical and occupational therapies, bracing, and others), not analgesics alone.

Primary Anticancer Treatment

The approach to cancer pain begins with maximizing primary anticancer therapies. In the case of CaP, these include radiotherapy, surgery, and hormonal therapies. Radiotherapy is highly successful in the treatment of painful bony metastases, with 80% to 90% of patients getting at least some relief. Unless bone pain is controlled by well-tolerated analgesics, radiotherapy is usually indicated. Other goals of radiotherapy are to prevent complications such as cord compression or pathologic fracture, decrease tumor growth, or decrease opioid requirement. Some patients may experience a pain flare for a few days, often followed by a prolonged reduction in pain. Radiation may be delivered by local treatment, hemibody treatment, or systemic radioisotopes. Factors to consider include life expectancy, functional status, bone marrow function, extent and volume of metastatic bone lesions, number of symptomatic sites, presence of visceral metastases, and previous treatment.

- Local radiation: Most appropriate for patients with only a few symptomatic lesions. Pain may flare for 2 to 3 days,

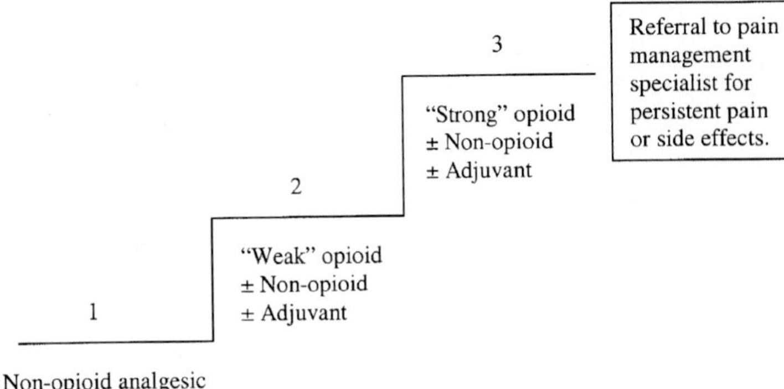

FIGURE 44-2. World Health Organization analgesic ladder. [Adapted from World Health Organization. Cancer pain relief and palliative care. Report of a WHO expert committee. (World Health Organization Technical Report Series, 804). Geneva, Switzerland: World Health Organization, 1990.]

which generally predicts good response. Relief begins 1 to 2 weeks after start of treatment and invariably is present within 1 to 3 months if it occurs. Imaging should correlate with symptoms. Generally well tolerated. Short course or single dose is as good as protracted treatment (13). Often indicated for debilitated patients.

- Hemibody radiation: Used for patients with many painful metastases and adequate bone marrow function. Main purpose is to avoid repeated trips to the hospital. Improves pain in 80%. Side effects include nausea, vomiting, and dehydration, which may require hospitalization or pretreatment.
- Systemic radionucleotides: Strontium 89 most commonly used in hormone-refractory CaP. Indicated for patients with multiple painful metastases for whom multiple single fields are impractical. Seventy percent get relief (13). Pain flares in a small percentage for 2 to 4 days. Relief begins in 2 to 3 weeks; maximal relief and nadir counts in 6 weeks. Main adverse effect is marrow toxicity. Poor candidates include patients with poor bone marrow or renal function or minimal uptake of main symptomatic lesions. Poor treatment for patients with fracture or pending fracture, cord, or root compression. Safety issues in incontinent men. Samarium 153 may be as effective with less toxicity (27); other agents in trials.

Other indications for radiation include hematuria, ureteric obstruction, perineal pain, leg edema or back discomfort due to pelvic or paraaortic adenopathy, and any symptoms related to tumor mass.

Pharmacologic Treatment

Fundamentals

The World Health Organization (WHO) has promoted a simple scheme for the treatment of cancer pain that has been shown in multiple validation studies to provide satisfactory pain relief in 75% to 90% of patients (10,28). This approach is based on an "analgesic ladder" (Fig. 44-2).

Step 1. The first step is to use acetaminophen, aspirin, or another NSAID for the management of mild to moderate pain. These drugs may be administered as needed or round the clock and titrated upwards to achieve optimal results. In addition, adjuvant analgesics may be added. An *adjuvant analgesic* is a medication that is not normally used to relieve pain but may relieve pain or enhance the effectiveness of other analgesics in certain circumstances [e.g., gabapentin (Neurontin) for neuropathic pain].

Step 2. For pain that persists or worsens, an opioid is *added* to (not substituted for) the NSAID. The so-called "weak opioids," (e.g., codeine or oxycodone) are usually used at this point, often in fixed combination preparations with aspirin or acetaminophen. The concept of a "weak opioid" has been largely discredited and relates in practice primarily to dosing limitations because of available preparations or dose-limiting side effects. However, the concept of adding an opioid on an as-needed basis to the NSAID in step 2 has remained useful. A major error in cancer pain management is dropping the NSAID when the opioid is introduced.

Step 3. For pain that persists, a *strong opioid*, or in practical terms a *round-the-clock opioid* is added. Morphine is the standard agent. At this stage, opioids are prescribed by the clock for background pain, with additional short-acting opioids available as needed for rescue pain. Long-acting opioids are particularly useful for the background pain. Patients with moderate to severe pain on presentation should begin with this step of the ladder. The same opioid should be used whenever possible for the background and breakthrough treatment.

Nonopioid Analgesics

General Considerations. The NSAIDs all have antiinflammatory, analgesic, and antipyretic properties. The analgesic approach to cancer pain management begins with this class of agents because they are effective for mild to moderate pain, generally well tolerated, usually inexpensive, readily available, sometimes over the counter, and they decrease opioid requirements in patients with moderate to severe pain (12). Because these agents act by a different mechanism than opioids and have different toxicities, the most effective analgesic approach generally involves combining opioids and NSAIDs for cancer pain. Although all types of pain may respond to NSAIDs, neuropathic pain is often unresponsive, and visceral pain is probably less than somatic pain. Bone pain and other inflammatory lesions may respond particularly well to NSAIDs, which may be more efficacious in these settings than opioids. Individual responses to particular NSAIDs may be idiosyncratic; therefore, it is logical to try more than one NSAID in an individual patient to seek optimal pain relief. These agents are limited by a "ceiling effect": increasing the dose beyond a maximal dose will not enhance analgesia, but will enhance side effects. The precise ceiling in an individual patient is never certain; therefore, it is sometimes appropriate to escalate beyond the recommended "maximum" dose. The NSAIDs do not produce tolerance, physical dependence, withdrawal phenomena, or addiction.

Mechanisms of Action. The mechanism of action of acetaminophen is not known, although acetaminophen does influence leukotriene metabolism and other aspects of the inflammatory process. The NSAIDs appear to reduce pain by decreasing peripheral production of prostaglandins from arachidonic acid by inhibiting the activity of the enzyme cyclooxygenase. Some studies have suggested a central action for NSAIDs as well. The analgesic effect of the NSAIDs appears to be independent of their antiinflammatory effects (29). Two forms of the enzyme cyclooxygenase designated COX-1 and COX-2 have been described (30). *COX-1* is a constitutive enzyme, present in normal tissues such as the gastrointestinal (GI) tract, kidney, and platelet. *COX-2* is an induced enzyme, present primarily in inflamed tissue. A tremendous amount of effort has resulted in the development of several NSAIDs that selectively block COX-2 (the so-called "COX-2 inhibitors"). It is hoped that these agents will confer the benefit of the NSAIDs without the toxicities.

Indications. All patients with cancer pain should be treated with an NSAID, with or without opioids, unless there is a specific contraindication. Bone pain or inflammatory pain may respond particularly well. NSAIDs may also work particularly well for incident pain.

Adverse Effects. *GI toxicity* is the most common side effect of NSAIDs. Nausea, dyspepsia, or vomiting occur in 10% to 20% of patients. Major GI tract injuries—ulcers, hemorrhagic gastritis, or perforation—may also occur. Estimates of this frequency range from 0.1% to 1.0% per year of exposure. Severe toxicity may occur without any warning signs. Patients at higher risk include those older than age 65 years with prior history of peptic ulcer disease, those on concomitant steroids or anticoagulants, and those with a history of substantial alcohol consumption. The traditional NSAIDs have been compared regarding their relative risk of producing GI toxicity (31). Ibuprofen appears to be safest, with most other agents falling into an intermediate category; piroxicam may produce somewhat more toxicity. The new COX-2 inhibitors celecoxib (Celebrex) and rofecoxib (Vioxx) appear to produce minimal GI toxicity but have not been studied in cancer pain. In the author's experience, both of these agents are approximately as effective for cancer pain as the traditional NSAIDs. The most appropriate strategy to minimize GI risks remains controversial. If patients require NSAID treatment, then misoprostol is probably the most effective agent for reducing GI risks (32); however, the selective COX-2 inhibitors may prove the safest approach.

Bleeding due to inhibition of platelet function by NSAIDs is a common concern in cancer patients. This is particularly the case in patients already thrombocytopenic from chemotherapy, those with marrow replacement by disease, patients receiving external beam radiation therapy or radioisotopes, or those who are on anticoagulant treatment. Many patients placed on NSAIDs for cancer pain subsequently undergo treatments that may be marrow toxic. The nonacetylated salicylates, choline-magnesium-trisalicylate and salsalate, appear not to alter platelet function significantly (33,34) and are often used in this situation. However, clinical experience suggests that these NSAIDs may not be as effective in relieving pain as other NSAIDs. The COX-2 inhibitors, which do not appear to influence platelet function or bleeding in anticoagulated patients, may offer a solution to this dilemma.

Renal failure or dysfunction induced by NSAIDs may be severe but is usually reversible after cessation of the NSAID. Several different subtypes have been identified, including interstitial nephritis and papillary necrosis. Patients with prostaglandin-dependent renal blood flow, such as those with cirrhosis, congestive cardiac failure, or other causes of impaired renal blood flow, are at highest risk. NSAIDs may also cause salt and water retention that may cause peripheral edema or antagonize the effects of diuretics or antihypertensive agents.

Liver dysfunction, which may be severe or fatal, may occur as a consequence of NSAID treatment. Patients on NSAIDs with a history of hepatic disease or on concomitant hepatotoxic medications should be followed carefully. NSAIDs may also precipitate bronchospasm, particularly in patients with a history of asthma. A variety of true allergic or allergic-type reactions may occur. Patients with a history of bronchospasm, laryngeal edema, or an urticarial rash from an NSAID in the past should not be prescribed an NSAID; in other types of rashes, repeat NSAID trials are probably safe.

Drug Selection. There are several points to bear in mind in selecting an NSAID for a patient with cancer pain (Table 44-3). The only NSAID available for parenteral use in the United States is ketorolac (Toradol). Ketorolac is a highly effective analgesic, similar in effectiveness to 10 mg mor-

TABLE 44-3. NONSTEROIDAL ANTIINFLAMMATORY AGENTS: AVAILABLE DOSING FORMS AND SELECTED COMMENTS

Drug	Available formulations	Dosing interval (h)	Max daily dose (mg)	Comments
Acetaminophen (Tylenol)	Elixir: 160 mg/5 mL Supp: 120, 325, 650 mg Tab: 325, 500 mg	4–6	4,000	< 2 g/d appears to be well tolerated in patients with cirrhosis, monitor closely; essentially no antiinflammatory activity; low risk of GI side effects; no effect on platelets
Aspirin	Supp: 125, 300, 600 mg Tab: 81, 300 mg EC Tab: 300, 600 mg	4–6	5,400	High risk of GI bleeding, use caution in preexisting liver disease and avoid in severe liver disease
Choline magnesium trisalicylate (Trilisate)	Tab: 500, 750, 1,000 mg (salicylate content) Liquid: 100 mg/mL	8–12	3,000	↓ GI bleeding vs. aspirin and perhaps NSAIDs as a class, possibly due to minimal antiplatelet activity
Choline salicylate (Arthropan)	Liquid: 870 mg/5 mL (= 600 mg ASA)	4–6	7,000	See choline magnesium trisalicylate
Diclofenac (Voltaren, Cataflam, Arthrotec)	Tab: 25, 50, 75 mg SR Tab: 100 mg (q.d. dosing)	12	200	↑ dizziness, ↓ GI side effects; possible ↑ nephrotoxicity
Diflunisal (Dolobid)	Tab: 250, 500 mg	8–12	1,500	↓ nephrotoxicity; related to salicylates, but may inhibit platelet function and prolong bleeding time
Etodolac (Lodine)	Cap: 200, 300, 500 mg	6–8	1,200	↓ nephrotoxicity and GI bleeding complications; may be safer than other NSAIDs in patients with cirrhosis
Fenoprofen (Nalfon)	Cap: 200, 300 mg Tab: 600 mg	4–8	3,200	↑ incidence of headache, somnolence, and dizziness; may cause genitourinary tract side effects
Flurbiprofen (Ansaid)	Tab: 50, 100 mg	6–12	300	↑ dizziness
Ibuprofen (Advil, Motrin)	Tab: 200, 400, 600, 800 mg Liquid: 160 mg/5 mL Chew tab: 50, 100 mg Drops: 40 mg/mL	4–8	3,200	Lowest risk of inducing serious GI complications among nonsalicylate NSAIDs (studies did not include etodolac or nabumetone), lower risk of hepatotoxicity
Indomethacin (Indocin)	Cap: 25, 50 mg Supp: 50 mg Inj: 1 mg SR Cap: 75 mg (b.i.d.) Susp: 5 mg/mL	8–12	200	High risk of nephrotoxicity vs. other NSAIDs; ↑ headache, tinnitus, dizziness, GI, CNS side effects
Ketorolac (Toradol)	Syr: 15, 30, 60 mg Tab: 10 mg	6–8	300	↑ headache, ↑ nephrotoxicity and GI complications; use max 5 d
Ketoprofen (Orudis, Oruvail)	Cap: 25, 50, 75 mg Tab: 12.5 mg SR Cap: 100, 150, 200 mg	6	120	↓ dose in hepatic dysfunction; SR cap allows for q.d. dosing
Nabumetone (Relafen)	Tab: 500, 750 mg Chew tab: 1,000 mg	12–24	2,000	↓ GI bleeding and side effects, reduce dose in hepatic dysfunction, q.d.–b.i.d. dosing
Naproxen (Naprosyn)	Tab: 250, 375, 500 mg EC Tab: 375, 500 mg SR Tab: 375, 500, 750 mg Susp: 25 mg/mL	8–12	1,500	↑ hepatotoxicity (↓ dose 50% in hepatic disease) and possible nephrotoxicity
Naproxen sodium (Aleve, Anaprox)	Tab: 220, 275, 550 mg	8–12	1,650	See naproxen; sodium content is approximately 10% (i.e., each 220-mg tab contains approximately 22 mg sodium)
Meclofenamate (Meclomen)	Cap: 50, 100 mg	4–6	400	High incidence of diarrhea, ↑ GI side effects; do not use for >1 continuous wk
Mefenamic acid (Ponstel)	Cap: 250 mg	6	1,000	↑ GI side effects
Oxaprozin (Daypro)	Tab: 600 mg	12–24	1,800	q.d.–b.i.d. dosing; use caution in severe hepatic impairment
Piroxicam (Feldene)	Cap: 10, 20 mg	12–24	20	High risk of serious GI adverse events vs. other NSAIDs; ↑ hepatotoxicity; q.d.–b.i.d. dosing
Salsalate (Disalcid)	Tab: 500, 750 mg Cap: 500 mg	8–12	4,000	See choline magnesium trisalicylate

(*continued*)

TABLE 44-3. (continued)

Drug	Available formulations	Dosing interval (h)	Max daily dose (mg)	Comments
Sulindac (Clinoril)	Tab: 150, 200 mg	12	400	High risk of hepatotoxicity vs. other NSAIDs, ↑ GI side effects, marketed as "renally sparing," but reports of renal failure exist
Tolmetin (Tolectin)	Tab: 200, 600 mg Cap: 400 mg	6–8	1,800	↑ incidence of auditory toxicity and GI adverse events
Celecoxib (Celebrex)	Tab:100, 200 mg	12	400	COX-2 inhibitors, ↓ incidence GI ulcerations, minimal to no inhibition platelet function
Rofecoxib (Vioxx)	Tab: 12.5, 25.0 mg Liquid:12.5 or 25.0 mg/ 5mL	24	25 chronic use, 50 acute (5 d max)	

↑, increased; ↓, decreased; ASA, acetylsalicylic acid; Cap, capsule; CNS, central nervous system; EC, enteric coated; GI, gastrointestinal; Inj, injection; max, maximum; NSAID, nonsteroidal antiinflammatory drug; SR, slow release; Supp, suppository; Susp, suspended; Syr, syrup; Tab, tablet.
Adapted from Briggs GR, Freeman RK, Yaffe SJ. *Drugs in pregnancy and lactation*, 4th ed. Baltimore: Williams & Wilkins, 1994; Conroy JM, Harvey SC. Management of cancer pain. *South Med J* 1996;89:744–760; Gelman CR, Rumack BH, Hutchinson TA, eds. *Nonsteroidal anti-inflammatory drug-induced gastrointestinal adverse events (drug consults)*. Englewood, CO: Micromedex, 1997; Imoto R, Reynolds MS, Eaton V. Nonsteroidal anti-inflammatory drug-induced hepatotoxicity (drug consults). In: Gelman CR, Rumack BH, Hutchinson TA, eds. *Nonsteroidal anti-inflammatory drug-induced gastrointestinal adverse events (drug consults)*. Englewood, CO: Micromedex, 1997; Levy MH. Pharmacologic management of cancer pain. *N Engl J Med* 1996;335:1124–1132; Levy MH. Pharmacologic management of cancer pain. *Semin Oncol* 1994;21:718–739; and Stancovich JE, Pugh MD. Nonsteroidal anti-inflammatory drug-induced nephrotoxicity (drug consults). In: Gelman CR, Rumack BH, Hutchinson TA, eds. *Nonsteroidal anti-inflammatory drug-induced gastrointestinal adverse events (drug consults)*. Englewood, CO: Micromedex, 1998.

phine intramuscular (i.m.). Ketorolac is therefore very useful in the rapid amelioration of severe pain in the hospitalized patient as an adjunct to opioid therapy. This agent should be used at a maximum dose of 30 mg intravenous (i.v.) every 6 hours for a maximum of 5 days; the dose should be halved for patients at risk for NSAID side effects. Ketorolac is not a useful drug for long-term oral treatment in view of its substantial GI toxicity and lack of analgesic advantages over the other NSAIDs when dosed orally. Several agents, such as nabumetone, can be dosed on a twice-daily basis and may therefore promote compliance. Ibuprofen is readily available, inexpensive, effective, and may have less GI toxicity than the other NSAIDs. Choline magnesium trisalicylate or salsalate can be considered for patients with platelet problems but may be less effective than other agents. The COX-2 inhibitors, celecoxib and rofecoxib, appear to have very limited side effects; these have been extensively used by the author in treating cancer pain with no significant toxicity. Their efficacy compared to traditional NSAIDs appears comparable but remains to be systematically studied.

Dosage and Administration. The NSAIDs may be dosed orally in tablets or elixirs, rectally, or topically. Table 44-3 gives details of dosing and administration of the NSAIDs. The usual route of administration is oral. However, for localized pain syndromes, topical administration of NSAIDs is as effective in relieving pain as systemic administration, with substantially fewer side effects (35). Although this has not been studied in the setting of cancer pain, in the case of a patient with a localized pain syndrome and relative contraindications to the use of systemic NSAIDs, the topical route may be a useful option. Topical formulations are only available in the United States if custom compounded; however, this service is widely available.

Opioids

The opioids are the mainstay of therapy for cancer pain. Millennia of anecdotal experience and decades of scientific research have confirmed that opioids are safe and effective in the treatment of cancer pain. It is worth emphasizing that the WHO guidelines call for adding opioids to a nonopioid analgesic, not substituting opioids for the nonopioid.

Pharmacology. Opioids produce analgesia by binding to receptors in the brain and spinal cord that decrease impulse conduction along nociceptive (pain-related) neural pathways. In the brain, this binding activates descending inhibitory pathways that travel down into the spinal cord and release inhibitory neurotransmitters in the spinal cord, inhibiting the nociceptive system. Opioids also bind to receptors in the spinal cord, directly inhibiting nociception. Several types of opioid receptors have been described. Opioids are classified according to the pattern of receptor binding (Table 44-4). Most opioids familiar to oncologists are classified as pure agonists, and act at the μ receptor. The pure μ agonists include morphine, methadone, hydromorphone, meperidine, oxycodone, fentanyl, and others. Buprenor-

TABLE 44-4. OPIOID ANALGESIC PHARMACOLOGY

	Pure agonists	Mixed agonist-antagonists	Partial agonists	Antagonists
	Morphine, meperidine, methadone, hydromorphone, fentanyl, oxycodone	Pentazocine, butorphanol, nalbuphine	Buprenorphine	Naloxone, naltrexone, nalmefene
Agonist at . . .	μ receptor	Kappa receptor	μ receptor	—
Antagonist at . . .	—	μ receptor	—	μ receptor
Causes withdrawal in patients on opioids	No	Yes	Yes	Yes
Ceiling effect for analgesia	No	Yes	Yes	NA
Available p.o.	Yes	Pentazocine	No	Naltrexone

NA, not applicable.

phine acts as a partial agonist at the μ receptor. Buprenorphine thus has a ceiling effect for analgesia after a certain dose; further dose escalation does not increase analgesia (but may increase side effects). Buprenorphine may also produce a withdrawal syndrome if prescribed to a patient dependent on pure μ agonists. The "agonist-antagonists" act as antagonists at the μ receptor but produce analgesia by binding the kappa receptor. These agents can also produce withdrawal if given to a patient on chronic μ agonists and also have a ceiling effect. The partial agonists include pentazocine (Talwin), nalbuphine (Nubain), and butorphanol (Stadol). *There is little, if any, role for the agonist-antagonists in the treatment of cancer pain.* Tramadol (Ultram) is an atypical opioid with μ agonist– and tricyclic antidepressant–type properties. It can be effective, but, due to its ceiling effect and reports of seizures at higher doses, it is not commonly used for cancer pain.

Addiction, Tolerance, and Physical Dependence. The most feared side effect of chronic opioid use is addiction. This fear has led to an "opioiphobia" that has in turn led to the underprescribing of opioids for cancer pain around the world, a problem that still exists in the United States (36). A confusion of terminology spanning centuries has impeded rational discourse on this subject. The phenomenon of *physical dependence* refers to the production of a withdrawal syndrome on abrupt discontinuation of the opioid, significant decrease in dose, or administration of an antagonist. Physical dependence on opioid analgesics typically occurs within days or weeks of initiation of treatment, is expected, rarely causes management difficulties, and bears no relationship to addiction (37). *Tolerance* refers to loss of effectiveness of the medication after prolonged use or the need to escalate the dose to maintain therapeutic effect. Large prospective and survey studies and tremendous accumulated experience with cancer pain suggest that tolerance is seldom a management issue in this population. Doses may escalate but typically plateau at stable levels for long periods of time. Dose escalations are often linked to disease progression rather than to loss of analgesic efficacy of the opioid. Patients appear to become more tolerant to the side effects of the opioid than to the benefit, such that the therapeutic window of the opioid over time—probably the relevant construct—appears to remain stable or widen with prolonged use.

Addiction refers to an aberrant psychiatric or behavioral condition characterized by loss of control over drug use, excessive preoccupation with drug use, or aberrant and destructive behavior surrounding the drug (37). This complication appears rare in the cancer population. Certainly patients with previous histories of substance abuse may develop cancer, and, in such cases, managing pain with opioids may require special considerations. These considerations have been recently reviewed (38). It must be emphasized that addiction is rarely an issue in managing cancer pain, and tolerance and physical dependence, which may occur, are rarely significant management issues and bear no relationship to addiction *per se.*

Opioid Side Effects. The most common side effects are nausea and vomiting, dizziness, sweating, itching, constipation, urinary retention, drowsiness, mental status changes, respiratory depression, and respiratory arrest. Patients become tolerant to these side effects with chronic use; nevertheless, these side effects may require management. Patients may develop these side effects differently with different opioids. Therefore, simply switching to an equianalgesic dose of a different opioid is often the best way to manage opioid side effects. When this strategy is unavailable or ineffective, specific treatment is warranted (Table 44-5). Antiemetics may be used for nausea and vomiting. Drowsiness often responds to the addition of a stimulant medication; there is some evidence that stimulant medications may synergistically improve opioid analgesia. Constipation must be prevented by dietary modification, fiber, adequate hydration, and prophylactic use of laxatives. Acute respiratory depression may require treatment with an opioid antagonist, for example, naloxone. The use of naloxone is generally ill advised in the terminal patient on opioid treatment and must be carefully considered and gently titrated when

TABLE 44-5. TREATMENT OF OPIOID SIDE EFFECTS

Adverse effect	Management considerations[a]
Allergic reaction	True allergic reactions are rare (i.e., IgE involvement). Symptoms are usually secondary to stem cell activation and subsequent histamine release. Selection of another opioid class[b] is usually necessary only if the patient has had a true allergic reaction and not simply sensitivity to histamine release.
Confusion/ delirium	Dose reduction, opioid rotation, neuroleptic therapy (haloperidol, 0.5–1.0 mg p.o./i.v. b.i.d.-t.i.d., or risperidone, 0.5 mg p.o. b.i.d.).
Constipation	Senokot daily, lactulose PRN, see Constipation.
Hallucinations	Dose reduction, opioid rotation, consider neuroleptics (see Delirium).
Myoclonic jerking	Dose reduction, opioid rotation, clonazepam, 0.25–0.50 mg p.o. t.i.d., baclofen, 5–10 mg t.i.d.
Nausea/ vomiting	Tolerance may develop. Consider an antiemetic on a fixed schedule for a few days; thereafter, PRN dosing is usually adequate; prochlorperazine, 10 mg p.o./i.v. q6–8h or 25 mg p.r. q12h or prochlorperazine Spansules, 10–30 mg p.o. q12h; metoclopramide, 10–30 mg p.o./i.v. q6h; droperidol, 1.25–5.0 mg i.v. q6h; ondansetron, 8 mg p.o./i.v. q8h.
Pruritus	Consider an antihistamine, such as diphenhydramine; long-acting antihistamines (e.g., loratadine, cetirizine, fexofenadine) may be effective; nalbuphine effective, but use cautiously to avoid withdrawal symptoms.
Respiratory depression	Hold opioid, supportive measures, consider naloxone with extreme caution.
Sedation	Tolerance typically develops; hold sedatives/anxiolytics; hold opioid; reduce dose; if persistent, consider CNS stimulants (e.g., caffeine, methylphenidate, or dextroamphetamine, 2.5–5.0 mg q.d. or b.i.d.).

CNS, central nervous system; IgE, immunoglobulin E; PRN, as needed.
[a]The above assumes that opioid therapy is a necessity. Non-opioid therapy options or alternative routes of administration should be considered.
[b]Opioids classified by chemical structure: Diphenylheptanes, methadone, propoxyphene; Phenylpiperidines, fentanyl, meperidine, sufentanil; Phenanthrenes, codeine, hydrocodone, hydromorphone, levorphanol, morphine, oxycodone.
Adapted from Jacox A, Carr DB, Payne R, et al. Management of cancer pain. *Clinical Practice Guideline No. 9.* AHCPR Publication No. 94-0593. Rockville, MD: Agency for Health Care Policy and Research, U.S. Department of Health and Human Services, Public Health Service, 1994; Levy MH. Pharmacologic treatment of cancer pain. *N Engl J Med* 1996;335:1124–1132; and Levy MH. Pharmacologic management of cancer pain. *Semin Oncol* 1994;21:718–739.

required. If satisfactory resolution of side effects cannot be achieved in the patient on systemic opioids, then alternative analgesic modalities must be considered, including spinal analgesia, neurolytic blockade, neurosurgical interventions, adjuvant analgesics, or primary anticancer therapies.

Route of Administration of Opioid Analgesics. The oral route is generally preferred: it is usually available, inexpensive, and effective. Nonoral routes are only indicated when the oral route is unavailable, has been ineffective, or under special circumstances when nonoral routes are preferred [e.g., i.v. patient-controlled analgesia (PCA)]. Because oral opioids undergo first-pass metabolism in the liver, higher doses are required, compared to the parenteral route. The ratio of oral to parenteral equianalgesic dose differs between opioids; conversion tables are required to accurately convert from parenteral to oral administration of an opioid and vice versa (Table 44-6). Opioids are available for oral administration in a variety of forms: rapid-release tablets, sustained-release tablets, liquids, and capsules. Liquids are useful for patients who have difficulty in swallowing, require very fine dosage titration, enterostomy tubes, or in using high-potency liquids for patients with high-dose requirements. Liquid formulations of morphine, oxycodone, methadone, and other opioids may be administered sublingually. A new transmucosally administered formulation of the potent opioid fentanyl called Actiq is available. This formulation provides rapid onset of analgesia and does not require oral administration, making it especially useful for breakthrough pain. When the oral route is unavailable, consideration should be given to the least invasive alternative routes: rectal and transdermal.

The rectal route is used commonly in the hospice and less in the acute care setting. The rectal route is generally chosen when the oral route is unavailable, either temporarily or long term, such as in the case of patients with oropharyngeal or upper digestive tract malignancies, or frequent nausea and vomiting. The rectal route is relatively contraindicated in patients with anorectal disease, impaction, or frequent diarrhea. Rectal formulations are available in the United States for morphine, hydromorphone, and oxymorphone. Controlled-release tablets are commonly administered rectally, although there is little information about the pharmacokinetics of controlled-release opioids delivered by this route. Custom suppositories may be compounded of nearly every opioid imaginable, in combination with adjuvant agents as well.

The transdermal route of administration has become popular since the introduction of the fentanyl transdermal delivery system (Duragesic patch). Analgesia begins in 12 to 24 hours and plateaus in approximately 3 days; each patch lasts 72 hours, after which it must be replaced. Thus, the fentanyl patch is neither effective nor safe when used for acute pain or for rapidly changing pain. The patch should be used as a "background" analgesic for chronic pain and supplemented with a breakthrough analgesic. With the availability of Actiq, the same opioid can be used for background and breakthrough medication. Although other opioids (e.g., morphine) have been compounded for transdermal use, there is little information available about this approach.

Parenteral opioid administration is selected when the oral route is unavailable and rectal administration is not possible

TABLE 44-6. OPIOID ANALGESICS

	Equianalgesic doses (mg)		Available strengths	
Drug	i.v./i.m.	Oral	Dosage forms	Comments
Morphine	10	30 (chronic) 60 (acute)	Liquid: 10 mg/5 mL, 20 mg/5 mL, 20 mg/1 mL SR Tab: 15, 30, 60, 100, 200 mg Tab: 15, 30 mg Injectable	Kadian marketed as 24-h formulation available as 20-, 50-, 100-mg caps
Hydromorphone	1.5	7.5	Supp: 3 mg Liquid: 5 mg/mL Tab: 2, 4, 8 mg Injectable	Controlled-release tablets in development
Oxycodone	NA	20	SR Tab: 10, 20, 40, 80 mg Tab: 5 mg Liquid: 5 mg/5 mL, 20 mg/mL	Percodan, Percocet[a]
Codeine	130	200	Elixir: 15 mg/mL Solution: 15 mg/mL Tab: 15, 30, 60 mg	High doses poorly tolerated
Fentanyl	0.1 (100 μg)	NA	Transdermal patch: 25, 50, 75, 100 μg/h Transmucosal lozenge: 200, 400, 600, 800, 1,200, 1,600 μg Injectable	Transdermal 25 μg/h patch is equianalgesic to 50-mg oral morphine
Oxymorphone	1	10 (rectal)	Supp: 5 mg Injectable	—
Meperidine[b]	75	300	Injectable Tab: 50, 100 mg Syrup: 50 mg/5 mL	Avoid oral dosing, CNS excitation from metabolite accumulation
Propoxyphene[b]	NA	130[c]–200[d]	Suspension: 50 mg/5 mL Darvocet-N 100[a]	Metabolite accumulation
Levorphanol	1 (chronic) 2 (acute)	1 (chronic) 4 (acute)	Tab: 2 mg Injectable	Long plasma half life, accumulates on day 2–3
Methadone[e]	10 (acute) 2–4 (chronic)	20 (acute) 2–4 (chronic)	Injectable Liquid: 1 mg/mL, 10 mg/5mL, 10 mg/1 mL Tab: 5, 10 mg	Long half-life, accumulates with repeated dosing, may require dose decrease day 2–5
Tramadol (Ultram)			Tab: 50 mg	Ceiling dose 400 mg/d, 50 mg tramadol equianalgesic to 60 mg oral codeine

caps, capsule; CNS, central nervous system; NA, not applicable; SR, slow release; supp, suppository; tab, tablet.
Adapted from Foley KM. The treatment of cancer pain. *N Engl J Med* 1985;313:84–95; Lacy C, Armstrong LL, Ingrim N, et al., eds. *Drug information handbook*, 1996–1997 ed. Cleveland, OH: American Pharmaceutical Association & Lexi-Comp, 1997; and American Pain Society. *Principles of analgesic use in the treatment of acute and cancer pain*, 4th ed. American Pain Society, 1999.
[a]Combination products containing either acetaminophen or aspirin.
[b]Routine or chronic use not recommended.
[c]HCl salt.
[d]Napsylate salt.
[e]Methadone begins to accumulate several days after initiation of therapy. To avoid excess sedation, a conversion ratio of approximately 8:1 should be used in converting oral morphine to methadone.

or preferred. Under several circumstances, parenteral administration may be required: rapid opioid titration for excruciating pain or postprocedural pain, inability to use simpler routes due to high-dose requirements, and patients unable to cooperate (e.g., mental status changes or terminal sedation). In general, parenteral administration refers to the i.v. or subcutaneous (s.q.) route. *Intramuscular injections are almost never indicated* in the cancer population: they are painful, erratically absorbed, may lead to complications (fibrosis or abscess formation), and are unnecessary. For patients with i.v. access, either short or long term, i.v. analgesia is relatively convenient and provides the flexibility of several different options for opioid administration: continuous infusion, intermittent boluses, both, or PCA.

PCA is generally the preferred modality, because patients tend to use the minimum opioid dose to achieve optimal analgesia. PCA is contraindicated in patients who are unable to understand or cooperate with the system or who are physically unable to activate the patient-controlled mechanism (e.g., severe rheumatoid arthritis). It is generally unsafe for family members or nursing staff to administer PCA boluses; however, this practice may be acceptable under certain circumstances. In considering prolonged i.v. analgesia, caregivers must consider the complications that may arise from prolonged i.v. catheterization (infection, clotting, need for trained personnel). Subcutaneous analgesia offers several advantages. Dosing is for all intents and purposes equivalent to that of the i.v. route. Needles may be inserted by personnel with minimal training, are changed approximately weekly, and do not cause the complications noted with the i.v. route. Small portable pumps are available for prolonged s.q. administration.

Intraspinal administration may result in improved pain control with fewer side effects than systemic administration, with a much smaller dose. Intraventricular opioid administration is rarely performed but, in select circumstances, such as intractable pain due to head and neck cancer, offer some of the same advantages as intraspinal opioids. These options are discussed in more detail under Interventional Techniques.

Selection of Opioid. For most clinical situations, opioids are all equally effective at relieving pain. It is important not to confuse milligram potency with effectiveness. Generally, one must consider which short-acting opioid to use for breakthrough pain and which long-acting opioid to use for background pain (Table 44-6). Among the long-acting opioids, cost is an important consideration: methadone is substantially less expensive than all the others. When patients do not have insurance coverage for prescriptions, methadone may be the only viable option. The transdermal route has advantages for patients who have compliance problems or for patients who intermittently are unable to tolerate the oral route. Morphine is available in a 24-hour formulation (Kadian) consisting of a capsule containing pellets; this may be opened and sprinkled on food or flushed down an enterostomy tube, maintaining the long duration of action. In general, long-acting formulations may not be cut or crushed. It is preferable to use the same short-acting opioid for breakthrough pain that has been chosen for the background regimen.

Dose and Titration. The key principle is titration to effect. Patients should be started at a standard dose, and the dose should then be increased until pain relief is achieved or until unacceptable side effects have ensued. Patients with moderate to severe pain generally require a round-the-clock opioid as well as a breakthrough medication. *Patients should not have unrelieved pain unless they have opioid side effects* because the absence of side effects suggests that the patient simply has been underdosed. Unrelieved pain should prompt rapid dose escalation; this is achieved safely by encouraging patients to take as much rescue medication as needed and, every 24 hours, simply calculating how much rescue medication has been consumed and adding it to the background dose. Patients should expect to take rescue medication one to three times daily; more frequent rescue medication usually implies a suboptimal background dose.

Example 2: A patient with metastatic CaP reports severe pain despite taking controlled-release morphine, 60 mg twice daily, and immediate-release morphine, 15 mg three times a day. How should his medications be prescribed?

After being encouraged to use as much immediate-release morphine as needed, the patient took 30 mg every 4 hours and achieved adequate analgesia. The patient's regimen was then changed to account for his morphine requirements as follows:

Background dose:	120 mg per day
Rescue requirements:	180 mg per day (30 mg × 6 doses per day)
Total:	300 mg per day
New background regimen:	150 mg twice daily

In practice, one may round down depending on what size tablets were available; in this case, 130 mg twice daily would be convenient. The size of the rescue dose typically must be 10% to 15% of the 24-hour dose requirement, in this case 30 to 45 mg.

Converting from One Opioid Regimen to Another. Conversions are frequently required in the management of cancer pain. Such circumstances include side effects, loss of a route of administration, loss of availability of an opioid for administrative reasons, need for a less expensive alternative, and opioid rotation to manage opioid metabolite accumulation. An equianalgesic conversion chart is indispensable for such conversion exercises to estimate what dose of the new opioid will be effective and safe for a patient on an established opioid (Table 44-6). The limitations of the available conversion charts, however, cannot be overstated. Cross-tolerance between opioids—that is, the degree to which a patient tolerant to one opioid will be tolerant to a second opioid—varies between opioids and between patients. Furthermore, most conversion charts are based on single-dose studies and may have little relevance to chronic opioid use. For example, it has been shown that methadone may be up to ten times more potent in chronic use than predicted by the conversion charts (39).

Example 3: A patient on fentanyl patch, 50 μg per hour, and i.v. morphine would like to convert completely to morphine, because it appears side effects may be due to the patch. He requires an all-oral regimen in preparation for discharge. His i.v. morphine consumption in the past 24 hours was 24 mg. What oral regimen should be prescribed?

- Step 1: Use the chart (Table 44-6) to convert all opioids to oral morphine equivalents:
  Fentanyl patch, 50 μg per hour = morphine, 100 mg per day by mouth
  Morphine, 24 mg i.v. = morphine, 72 mg per day by mouth
  Total opioid consumption = 172 mg per day oral morphine

- Step 2: Give half the total as background medication and allow the patient to make up the other half as rescue dosing. Each rescue dose must be 10% to 15% of the daily background dose:
  172 mg per day divided in half = 86 mg per day = 43 mg twice daily
  Round down based on available pill sizes: 30 mg twice daily plus 15 mg as needed for rescue.
- Step 3: Adjust the background dose as needed according to the patient's 24-hour use of rescue doses.

Adjuvant Analgesics

Corticosteroids. Corticosteroids remain among the most underused drug treatments in palliative care (Table 44-7). A number of important beneficial effects result from steroid treatment: decreased pain, improved appetite, weight gain, antiemetic action, and mood elevation (40,41). Steroids are particularly useful in the treatment of neuropathic pain due to cord compression, brachial or lumbosacral plexus invasion, or peripheral nerve infiltration. Other steroid-responsive pain syndromes include headache due to increased intracranial pressure, arthritic pains, and pain due to visceral obstruction (42). Dexamethasone, 12 to 24 mg per day, or prednisone, 30 to 100 mg per day, has been the most commonly prescribed chronic regimens, although benefits have been described for lower doses. Few systematic comparisons between different steroids or different doses have been conducted. Unfortunately, the beneficial effects of steroid use tend to wane after 2 to 3 months of treatment, at which time side effects (myopathy, edema, hyperglycemia, immune suppression, confusion, and others) may become relevant. Therefore, chronic palliative use of steroids is usually limited to patients with less than 2 to 3 months to live, or for short-term treatment while other palliative treatments are being instituted. Due to the risk of ulcers, steroids should generally not be used concomitantly with NSAIDs. In addition, abrupt dose reduction or discontinuation may result in a steroid withdrawal syndrome, which, among other symptoms, is often characterized by increased pain. Despite these concerns, low-dose steroid treatment is generally well tolerated even in the terminally ill.

Stimulants. Psychostimulant medications are used in the palliative care setting primarily to reverse opioid-induced sedation, although they also have analgesic properties independent of opioid effects. A number of randomized controlled trials have confirmed the antisedative and analgesic effects (43,44). Cognitive impairment has been shown to improve as well. As sedation reverses, the opioid therapeutic window opens, allowing further opioid dose escalation. The two most common regimens are methylphenidate (Ritalin), 5 to 10 mg by mouth twice a day, and dextroamphetamine (Dexedrine), 2.5 to 5.0 mg by mouth twice a day, with the second dose no later than midday to avoid insomnia. Both of these medications are also extremely useful as antidepressants in this population, with beneficial effects accruing within days [as opposed to weeks with the tricyclic or selective serotonin reuptake inhibitor (SSRI) antidepressants]. The doses are then escalated until the desired effect is achieved, with few patients requiring more than 40 mg per day of either drug. Occasional patients do best with a third dose. Significant side effects are uncommon, with mental status changes and cardiac arrhythmias being the chief concerns.

Antidepressants. Tricyclic antidepressants (TCAs) are useful agents in the treatment of neuropathic pain (Table 44-7). Although controlled studies demonstrating the benefit of TCAs have been demonstrated primarily in noncancer neuropathic pain states (45), a few studies and substantial anecdotal experience suggest their use in cancer-related pain as well, both neuropathic and nonneuropathic (46). The TCAs should be viewed as adjuvants, with opioids the mainstay of pharmacotherapy for cancer pain, including neuropathic pain. The most prudent indications for TCAs in cancer pain are neuropathic pain or nonneuropathic pain accompanied by other symptoms that might respond to a tricyclic (insomnia, depression, or visceral spasm). The most common side effects are anticholinergic: dry mouth, sedation, urinary retention, constipation, and orthostasis. Elderly and debilitated patients are at increased risk of falling. The commonly used tricyclics in order of most to least side effects are: amitriptyline (Elavil), doxepin (Sinequan), imipramine, nortriptyline (Pamelor), and desipramine (Norpramin). Efficacy of these agents is similar. Choice of agent depends primarily on side effects: in patients in whom nighttime sedation is desired, amitriptyline or doxepin is a reasonable choice. If avoidance of side effects is a high priority, desipramine or nortriptyline is best. Dosage of these agents is the same: Start with 10 to 25 mg by mouth every night and increase as tolerated until the desired effects are produced. The usual therapeutic doses for pain are 50 to 75 mg every night, but patients may require 150 mg per day or more. Serum levels are not clinically useful in adjusting doses to produce analgesia but have a role in toxicity monitoring. Analgesia takes 2 to 4 weeks to begin. These agents are not usually first choice antidepressants in this population, owing to the relatively high incidence of side effects at antidepressant doses. Of note, the SSRIs, although better tolerated as antidepressants, are not in general analgesic.

Anticonvulsants. Anticonvulsants are useful in some neuropathic pain states (Table 44-7) (47). Gabapentin has become popular in the management of neuropathic and other types of pain (48); other agents have some efficacy as well. Gabapentin is well tolerated, with the major dose-limiting side effects being dizziness, sedation, and nausea. Serious side effects or drug interactions are extremely rare. Gabapentin does not cause the common hematologic and hepatic side effects of the other anticonvulsants (although reversible leukopenia is rarely seen). No routine hematologic monitoring is required. Clinical experience has demonstrated a wide interpatient variability in the dose of gabapentin required to produce benefit (and

TABLE 44-7. ADJUVANT ANALGESICS

Drug	Indications	Usual starting dose and interval	Common dose range	Comments
Tricyclic antidepressants				
Amitriptyline (Elavil)	Neuropathic pain	25 mg p.o. HS (10 mg in frail, elderly)	50–150 mg p.o. HS	Titrate dose every few days to minimize side effects; allow 1–2 wk (up to 4) to see effect
Desipramine (Norpramin, Pertofrane)	Same	Same	50–200 mg p.o. HS	Side effects include: drowsiness, orthostatic hypotension, weight gain, arrhythmias, anticholinergic effects
Nortriptyline (Aventyl, Pamelor)	Same	Same	50–150 mg p.o. HS	Side effects greatest to least: amitriptyline > nortriptyline > desipramine
Anticonvulsants				
Gabapentin (Neurontin)	Same	100 mg t.i.d. increase by 100 mg t.i.d. q3d	300–4,800 mg/d in three divided doses	Adjust dose for renal dysfunction: (Clcr <60 mL/min); no documented drug-drug interactions First-choice anticonvulsant
Carbamazepine (Tegretol)	Neuropathic, tic-like, or lancinating pain	100 mg p.o. b.i.d.	200 mg p.o. b.i.d.–q.i.d.	Monitor serum levels (4–12 μg/mL), CBC, LFTs Multiple drug-drug interactions via enzyme induction, levels increased by enzyme inhibitors, highly PPB
Clonazepam (Klonopin)	Same	0.25–0.50 mg p.o. t.i.d.	0.5–1.0 mg p.o. t.i.d.	Starting dose should not exceed 1.5 mg/d, titrate every third d
Phenytoin (Dilantin)	Same	300 mg p.o. q.d. or 100 mg p.o. t.i.d.	300–400 mg/d	Monitor serum levels (10–20 μg/mL), lower efficacy versus other agents
Valproic acid (Depakene), Divalproex (Depakote)	Same	125 mg p.o. t.i.d.	500–1,000 mg p.o. t.i.d.	Monitor levels (50–100 μg/mL); potential ADRs: liver dysfunction, pancreatitis, thrombocytopenia, N/V; CYP-450 enzyme inhibitor; divalproex has ↓ GI side effects vs. valproic acid
Anxiolytics: benzodiazepines				
Alprazolam (Xanax)	Anxiety, skeletal muscle spasm	0.25–0.50 mg p.o. q.d.–t.i.d.	Minimum effective dose	$t^{1}/_{2}$ = 12–15 h, no active metabolite All benzodiazepines cause additive sedation with opioids
Chlordiazepoxide (Librium)	Panic, insomnia	10–25 mg p.o. q.d.–t.i.d.	Same	$t^{1}/_{2}$ = 5–30 h $t^{1}/_{2}$ (active metabolite) = 24–96 h
Diazepam (Valium)	Same	5–10 mg p.o. q.d.–b.i.d.	Same	$t^{1}/_{2}$ = 20–80 h $t^{1}/_{2}$ (active metabolite) = 50–100 h
Lorazepam (Ativan)	Same	0.5–2.0 mg p.o. q.d.–t.i.d.	Same	$t^{1}/_{2}$ = 10–20 h, no active metabolite
Oxazepam (Serax)	Same	10-15 mg p.o. q.d.–t.i.d.	Same	$t^{1}/_{2}$ = 5–20 h, no active metabolite
Flurazepam (Dalmane)	Insomnia	15–30 mg p.o. HS	Same	$t^{1}/_{2}$ (active metabolite) = 40–114 h
Midazolam (Versed)	Terminal crescendo pain	Doses vary depending on individual patient needs		$t^{1}/_{2}$ = 2–5 h, no active metabolite
Temazepam (Restoril)	Insomnia	15–30 mg p.o. HS	Minimum effective dose	$t^{1}/_{2}$ = 10–40 h, no active metabolite
Triazolam (Halcion)	Same	0.125–0.250 mg p.o. HS	Same	$t^{1}/_{2}$ = 2–3 h, no active metabolite
Anxiolytics: azapirones				
Buspirone (BuSpar)	Anxiety	5 mg p.o. t.i.d.	Max: 60 mg/d	Full effects not seen for 2–3 wk; allow adequate time for onset of action before titrating dose
Psychostimulants				
Dextroamphetamine (Dexedrine), Methylphenidate (Ritalin)	Opioid-induced sedation, opioid-induced sedation, depression	2.5–5.0 mg q.d. or b.i.d. Last dose before 2 p.m.	5–20 mg in divided doses. Last dose before 2 p.m.	For treatment of sedation; may increase delirium in confused patient

(*continued*)

TABLE 44-7. (continued)

Drug	Indications	Usual starting dose and interval	Common dose range	Comments
Corticosteroids				
Dexamethasone, methylprednisolone	Acute spinal cord compression, increased ICP	40–100 mg i.v. dexamethasone or equivalent as loading doses or q6h for first 24–72 h[a]	10–20 mg i.v. q6h dexamethasone or 40–80 mg i.v. q6h methylprednisolone	High-dose therapy should not exceed 72 h; if no benefit, dose can be rapidly tapered; if pain improves, the initial maintenance dose should be tapered to the lowest effective and least toxic dose Usefulness limited to 2–3 mo before steroid-induced side effects outweigh benefit
	Nerve compression, visceral distension, soft-tissue infiltration	Dexamethasone 4–8 mg p.o. q8–12h, prednisone 20–40 mg p.o. q8–12h	Use minimal effective dose	
	Alleviation of nausea, anorexia, pain in palliative care	Dexamethasone 4–12 mg/d, prednisone 5–10 mg t.i.d.		
Miscellaneous adjuvant analgesic agents				
Baclofen (Lioresal, Atrofen)	Neuropathic pain, spasticity	5–10 mg p.o. t.i.d.–q.i.d. intrathecal infusions	Max oral dose = 80–120 mg/d Intrathecal: 300–800 μg/d	Use with caution and at decreased doses in renal insufficiency
Clonidine (Duraclon)	Neuropathic pain	30 μg/h (epidural)	Doses >40 μg/h not well studied	FDA approved for epidural use, clinical experience supports intrathecal use
Mexiletine (Mexitil)	Neuropathic pain	150–300 mg p.o. t.i.d.	150–300 mg p.o. t.i.d.	Avoid in second- or third-degree AV block and S/P MI Third line therapy
Octreotide (Sandostatin)	Obstructed bowel spasm; diarrhea, VIPomas	50–100 μg s.q. b.i.d.–t.i.d.	Varies	Monitor for changes in glucose control, cholelithiasis Use caution in renal impairment
Pamidronate (Aredia)	Metastatic bone pain, delay of bone metastasis progression	90 mg i.v. q4wk	90 mg i.v. q4wk proven effective	Proven to decrease the impact of disease progression in patients with osteolytic lesions secondary to multiple myeloma, breast cancer, and prostate cancer; may lower serum calcium
Strontium chloride (^{89}Sr)	Metastatic bone pain	148 MBq, 4 mCi q3mo	148 MBq, 4 mCi q3mo	Typically reduces platelet count by ≈ 30%; nadir usually occurs 12–16 wk after administration; degree of neutropenia varies; 2–3 d after administration, pain may transiently increase for 2–3 d

ADR, adverse drug reaction; AV, arteriovenous; CBC, complete blood cell count; Clcr, creatine clearance; CYP-450, cytochrome P-450; FDA, U.S. Food and Drug Administration; GI, gastrointestinal; HS, at bedtime; ICP, intracranial pressure; LFTs, liver function tests; max, maximum; MBq, megabecquerel; mCi, millicurie; MI, myocardial infarction; N/V, nausea and vomiting; PPB, plasma protein binding; S/P, systolic pressure; ^{89}Sr, strontium-89; VIPomas, vasoactive intestinal polypeptide-secreting tumors.

Adapted from Conroy JM, Harvey SC. Management of cancer pain. *South Med J* 1996;89:744–760; Jacox A, Carr DB, Payne R, et al. *Management of cancer pain.* Clinical Practice Guideline No. 9. AHCPR Publication No. 94-0593. Rockville, MD: Agency for Health Care Policy and Research, U.S. Department of Health and Human Services, Public Health Service, 1994; Lacy C, Armstrong LL, Ingrim N, et al., eds. *Drug information handbook*, 1996–1997 ed. Cleveland, OH: American Pharmaceutical Association & Lexi-Comp, 1997; Levy MH. Pharmacologic treatment of cancer pain. *N Engl J Med* 1996;335:1124–1132; and Levy MH. Pharmacologic management of cancer pain. *Semin Oncol* 1994;21:718–739.

side effects), varying between as low as 50 mg three times a day and 3,600 mg three times a day. Therefore, one must start low (e.g., 100 mg three times a day) and titrate upwards as needed. Because efficacy is seen within approximately 2 days, upward titration may proceed every other day, if needed. Other choices have been carbamazepine (Tegretol) and phenytoin (Dilantin), but the hematologic and hepatic side effects of these drugs, as well as their limited efficacy, have made them less popular than the other available adjuvants. Lamotrigine and topiramate have been shown in small recent case series to have efficacy against neuropathic pain, but their potentially significant side effects and prolonged titration periods render them second-line agents at best at this time. It is worth reemphasizing that in the patient with neuropathic cancer pain, the adjuvant agents are just adjuvants. Opioids remain the mainstay of therapy except for a few patients whose pain can be well controlled with adjuvants alone.

Neuroleptics. Although neuroleptics have been used as adjuvant analgesics in the treatment of chronic pain for decades, their role is limited at best. The only neuroleptic with definite analgesic properties is methotrimeprazine (Levoprome) (49,50). Methotrimeprazine is occasionally used as an analgesic in patients with opioid tolerance or side effects; this drug also has antiemetic and anxiolytic properties. Sedation and hypotension are common side effects, which has led to its role in terminal sedation. Other phenothiazines have a role in the treatment of nausea and vomiting [especially haloperidol (Haldol)] and for anxiety, psychosis, hallucinations, or intractable insomnia.

Bisphosphonates. The bisphosphonates are a group of analogs of endogenous pyrophosphates that inhibit bone resorption *in vivo*. They are used for treatment of hypercalcemia of malignancy, prevention of pathologic fractures in malignancy (especially breast and multiple myeloma) and osteoporosis, and for the reduction of pain due to bony metastases (51). In the United States, pamidronate (Aredia) and etidronate are available; alendronate is used for the treatment of osteoporosis. Bisphosphonates may be less effective in osteoblastic bone tumors, such as CaP. However, even bony metastases from CaP have osteolytic components, and therapeutic responses to bisphosphonates have been demonstrated in CaP (52,53). An evidence-based review suggested that bisphosphonates should be part of routine treatment of patients with bone pain due to metastatic CaP. The usual regimen is pamidronate, 90 mg i.v. monthly.

Calcitonin. Calcitonin is also a potent osteoclast inhibitor used to treat hypercalcemia of malignancy and pain due to bony metastases. Although some studies have shown benefit (54,55), many patients fail to respond (56). Calcitonin is administered subcutaneously twice daily and causes nausea and vomiting in a substantial number of patients. Typical doses are in the range of 100 IU twice a day, although starting at lower doses may limit side effects. The optimal indications and administration guidelines are unknown.

Cannabinoids. The cannabinoids have analgesic properties in animal and human models of pain (46). However, side effects are common and analgesia inconsistent. Therefore, these drugs have not become widely used in the treatment of pain.

Nonpharmacologic Pain Management

Physical and psychosocial modalities are an important part of the overall approach to symptom management in cancer and to chronic illness in general (12). These approaches may be performed by professionals but also may be carried out by patients and their families, giving them the opportunity to participate in their self-care. Patients and families struggling with terminal illness often suffer from the sense of having no control. This may create anxiety, loss of coping skills, and leave them believing as if their fate lies entirely in the hands of health care providers. Patients should be taught psychosocial treatments for self application to not only feel better, but also to feel more in control, more able to function, and less reliant on the health care team. The physical modalities, especially exercise, focus on ability to function, which is often given inadequate attention in the health care setting. The psychosocial modalities focus on areas such as coping strategies and spiritual support, supplementing the disease focus of medical visits.

The physical modalities include heat and cold, massage, immobilization, transcutaneous electrical nerve stimulation, other physical therapy modalities, and acupuncture. These modalities should be introduced early in the disease process to help patients minimize the need for pharmacologic approaches and minimize the morbidity associated with the disease and its treatment. Exercise, in particular, is an important and frequently overlooked treatment for deconditioning and functional restoration. The guidance of a physical therapist experienced in treating cancer patients may be invaluable in maximizing function and quality of life in this population.

A variety of psychosocial techniques are available that help patients reduce pain and other symptoms, stabilize mood, and enhance the sense of coping, control, and participation that is so important in patients suffering from cancer. When introduced early in the illness when there is sufficient strength and ability to concentrate, these techniques may provide comfort to patients through the entirety of their disease course. Approaches include cognitive techniques, patient education, behavioral techniques (e.g., biofeedback, imagery), and psychotherapy.

Interventional Techniques

Spinal Analgesia

Background. The discovery in the late 1960s that opioids produce analgesia by binding to specific receptors in the brainstem and spinal cord led investigators to attempt to produce selective analgesia by directly infusing opioids onto the spinal cord. This approach has become widespread. In this chapter, the term *spinal* is used to refer to intrathecal (subarachnoid) and epidural use. In most anesthesia texts, spinal refers specifically to intrathecal use. Opioids injected intrathecally act by binding directly to receptors in the dorsal horn of the spinal cord. Opioids injected into the epidural space must traverse the dura, enter the subarachnoid space, and then bind to the spinal cord. Much of the medication is lost in transition; therefore, epidural doses of opioid analgesics are higher than subarachnoid doses. Systems are available for long-term administration by either route.

Drugs. A number of different opioid and nonopioid analgesics are available for long-term spinal administration (Table 44-8). The hydrophilic opioids, morphine and hydromorphone, are preferred, because their hydrophilicity

TABLE 44-8. SPINAL ANALGESICS

Class	Common agents	Advantages	Disadvantages
Opioids	Morphine, hydromorphone, fentanyl, sufentanil	Most experience with this class Good analgesia Hydrophilic agents (morphine, hydromorphone) spread well to cover widespread pain	Side effects: respiratory depression, nausea, vomiting, itching, sedation (high dose), urinary retention; tolerance in some
Local anesthetics	Bupivacaine	Synergism with opioids Excellent relief of movement-associated, incident pain Usually analgesia possible without numbness, weakness	Numbness, weakness, urinary retention, hypotension at higher doses Less experience with long-term intrathecal safety
α2 Agonists	Clonidine	At least as good as opioids for neuropathic pain Probable synergism with opioids No tolerance	Side effects: sedation, hypotension Limited experience with long-term infusions

confers the property of rostral spread in sufficient concentrations to produce analgesia along all dermatomes. Thus, a lumbar catheter may be used to treat pain arising from the feet to the head. The lipophilic opioids, such as fentanyl and sufentanil, are taken up rapidly into the systemic circulation. They are more useful for pain arising from a circumscribed dermatomal distribution, such as from pancreatic cancer or restricted chest wall pain. Opioids alone may provide better analgesia with fewer side effects than systemic (oral or i.v.) opioids, the addition of a dilute local anesthetic is usually much better, especially for neuropathic or incident pain. Clonidine (Duraclon), an α2 agonist, has been shown to have powerful analgesic properties when used epidurally. Dose-limiting side effects usually preclude using clonidine as a sole analgesic agent, and it is usually added to an opioid to boost analgesia.

Drug Side Effects. Side effects of spinal opioids are fairly common, although patients become rapidly tolerant to most. These include pruritus, nausea and vomiting, respiratory depression or arrest, confusion, sedation, and urinary retention. Side effects of spinal local anesthetics include hypotension, sensory loss, and motor weakness. These side effects are uncommon in clinical analgesic doses. The major side effects of clonidine are sedation and hypotension. The ideal agent or combination of agents is far from clear.

Devices. Several types of devices are available for implantation. A temporary epidural catheter is used for short-term pain relief (e.g., postoperatively). The advantage is ease of insertion, which can be done at the bedside. Disadvantages are the frequency of technical problems and infections with use lasting longer than 1 to 2 weeks. Several catheters are available for long-term use. The most commonly used is the Dupen epidural catheter, which is analogous to a Hickman catheter. Advantages are relative ease of implantation (a short operating room procedure) and relative durability, compared to temporary catheters. Disadvantages are the long-term costs of maintaining these catheters (related mainly to home care and pharmacy charges), cumulative risk of infection, and need for the patient to remain attached to an external pump. Epidural Port-A-Cath devices are available, analogous to the i.v. Port-A-Cath device. Advantages are durability and resistance to dislodgment and other technical complications. Disadvantages are cumulative risk of infection and the need, in general, to continuously access the port, with the patient attached to an external pump.

Completely implanted pumps are also available. These devices are approximately the size of a hockey puck, implanted in a s.q. pocket in the abdomen and connected via a tunneled catheter to the subarachnoid space. Advantages are that patients are not encumbered by attachments to an external pump and need only appear for pump refills every 1 to 3 months. Some of these pumps are programmable and may be programmed to give boluses at night, less medication during the day, and other indications. Disadvantages are that these pumps have no capacity for doses as needed, and patients usually still need to supplement with oral doses. The implantation procedure is more involved, but the long-term risks of infection is less than with the externalized catheters. These pumps are expensive, but the costs of externalized catheters exceed the costs of the implanted pump after approximately 3 to 6 months.

Several case series have demonstrated that a majority of patients who have failed conservative medical management for cancer pain do well with spinal analgesics (57–59). Patient selection criteria for these technologies are not completely defined and await randomized trials. In general, patients are candidates for spinal analgesia if they have failed comprehensive medical therapy, including all steps of the WHO ladder. This generally translates to inadequate analgesia from maximally tolerated doses of systemic opioids. The more caudad in the body the pain is, the greater the likelihood of success (i.e., leg pain responds better than head and neck). Contraindications to implantable devices include sepsis, uncontrolled coagulopathy, or poorly controlled psychiatric disorders. The main obstacle in optimal clinical application of spinal analgesic delivery systems is that patients are referred for implantation too late or not at all.

Nerve Blocks

General Considerations. Nerve blocks can be carried out with local anesthetics, steroids, or neurolytic agents (alcohol or phenol). Local anesthetics block nerve function for a few hours and are used to prognosticate whether a "permanent" neurolytic block would provide long-term pain relief. Lack of relief from a diagnostic local anesthetic block reliably indicates that a neurolytic block would fail; positive response to a diagnostic block, on the other hand, does not guarantee success. Affected body parts that can be denervated with greater or lesser success include the viscera (e.g., pancreas, liver, rectum, ovary), somatic structures (e.g., the chest wall and ribs), and nerves themselves (e.g., the brachial plexus). Some neurolytic blocks have the potential for the loss of normal function. These blocks are generally reserved for patients who have already lost function, or for whom conservative measures have failed. While the availability of nondestructive techniques has decreased the need for neurolytic procedures, overall, these procedures are probably underused owing to referral obstacles, limited expertise, and similar issues.

Patient Selection. Patients who fail to achieve pain relief from noninvasive modalities often face a choice between spinal analgesia and neural blockade. Advantages of spinal analgesia are its nondestructive and reversible nature. Disadvantages include the risk of infection of implanted systems, side effects of spinally administered medications, and the burden in many cases of being tied to an externalized pump and the relevant home care issues. Advantages of neurolytic blockade are that it is finished in one visit and either works or does not work, without any ongoing burden. The disadvantage is the risk of loss of neurologic function, but, for the commonly performed blocks, this risk is small and outweighed by the burden of the externalized pumps. In the author's experience, if a commonly performed neurolytic block is indicated, then it is preferable to start with the block and proceed to spinal analgesia, if needed. The most important blocks will be described briefly below. Readers interested in further information may consult a number of excellent references (11,60,61).

Celiac Plexus Block. The celiac plexus sits in front of the aorta at the T12-L1 level and innervates the upper abdominal viscera, including the pancreas, stomach, liver, spleen, lower esophagus, and intestine down to the transverse colon. This injection is classically performed for pancreatic cancer but may be performed for primary or metastatic disease of any of the previously mentioned visceral structures. In pancreatic cancer, 75% of patients achieve an average of 4 months of pain relief (range, weeks to a year). Complications are uncommon and include transient diarrhea (a blessing for most patients) and, rarely, genitofemoral neuritis or paraplegia.

Hypogastric Plexus Block. This plexus sits anterior to the iliac bifurcation at the L5-S1 level and innervates the pelvic viscera, including the uterus, ovaries, bladder (which also is innervated from sacral nerve roots), rectum, prostate, and, partially, the cervix. This block has primarily been used for gynecologic malignancies, with results similar to the celiac block (83). Serious complications have not been reported.

Subarachnoid Neurolysis. This is most widely used for chest wall pain, because there is little risk of loss of neurologic function. Subarachnoid alcohol may also be used to denervate the arm or leg in cases of intractable pain due to plexopathy, usually in which limb function has already been lost. In CaP, the most relevant application would be the neurolytic saddle block for perineal pain. For this block, patients are kept sitting, and a fine needle is placed in the subarachnoid space at L5-S1 as if to perform a lumbar puncture. Then, small aliquots of phenol are injected, producing a burning sensation in the perineum. In skilled hands, this block eliminates sensation in the saddle distribution of the perineum but does not alter leg function. Owing to the risk of bowel or bladder incontinence, this block is generally reserved for patients who have already lost these functions.

Sympathetic Blocks. Substantial evidence exists that blockade of the sympathetic chain (stellate ganglion, lumbar sympathetic ganglia) with local anesthetic reduces the pain of acute herpes zoster and may prevent postherpetic neuralgia. Neurolytic bilateral lumbar sympathetic blocks have been described for the treatment of tenesmus and pelvic visceral pain (62).

Intralesional and Intraarticular Steroid Injections. For patients with pain due primarily to a single bony metastasis, injection of a combination of local anesthetic and steroids may provide profound and long-lasting analgesia. Incident pain may respond completely to this technique. Injections may be performed into joints with juxtaarticular metastases or directly into metastatic lesions, such as in long bones or the pelvis. The author has performed approximately a dozen such procedures over several years and has observed analgesia lasting up to 6 months. Patients may benefit from repeated injections. No adverse effects have been seen. Sites have included the sternoclavicular, sacroiliac, glenohumeral, and knee joints, and the talus, scapula, and sternum. A clinical trial is in progress.

Neurosurgical Procedures

A variety of neurosurgical procedures have been performed over the years to provide relief from cancer pain. Potential benefits include reduction in pain and analgesic reliance; potential complications include return of pain, neurologic dysfunction, and new pain resulting from the procedure. Analogous comments to the neurolytic blocks apply: These procedures have in many cases been made unnecessary by the availability of nondestructive interventions but, due to referral obstacles, are still probably underused. Percutaneous anterolateral cordotomy is the most commonly performed procedure. Under local anesthesia, the surgeon directs a radiofrequency needle through the skin at C1-2 into the spinal cord under radiographic guidance. Small radiofrequency lesions are made in the spinothalamic tract. The result is loss of pain and thermal sensation on the opposite side of the body below the shoulder, with preservation of other functions. This procedure is useful for strictly unilateral pain involving mainly somatic structures. Bilateral percutaneous cordotomy is not done, owing to the risk of Ondine's curse (apnea) (63,64).

Hypophysectomy, or ablation of the pituitary gland, may produce profound pain relief in patients with pain due to metastatic cancer, whether the underlying tumor is hormone dependent or not. Ablation may be accomplished surgically or chemically and confers a 40% to 70% chance of pain relief (65). Hypopituitarism is an expected consequence of surgery and requires hormone replacement. Other complications include damage to the optic or oculomotor nerves and cerebrospinal fluid leakage. Clinical indications for hypophysectomy, as opposed to other interventional treatments for intractable cancer pain, are not clear. In general, procedures such as spinal analgesia are considered more conservative and reliable.

Intraventricular opioids may be delivered via an implanted Ommaya reservoir or by direct connection to an implanted pump. Results approach those of spinal opioids, with up to 90% of patients reporting successful pain relief (66). The major indication is pain due to head and neck cancer that is unresponsive to conservative modalities. Small doses of morphine (e.g., 1 mg) may last several days after a single injection. Major complications include infection of the device, nausea, pruritus, and drowsiness, and other typical opioid side effects may also occur (67).

SYMPTOM CONTROL

Nausea and Vomiting

General Considerations

Nausea and vomiting occur in approximately 15% of a palliative care population with advanced CaP (68) and may be much more common in the terminal phase. The approach to the patient with nausea and vomiting begins with a systematic diagnosis and treatment of underlying conditions that may be causing the symptoms (69). For patients with persistent symptoms, the next step is to determine the pathophysiologic category of the nausea and vomiting and to select an appropriate antiemetic or combination. Finally, patients require follow-up to monitor and modify treatment. In the CaP population, most cases are due to gastroparesis, cachexia, opioids, constipation, and metabolic abnormalities.

Pathophysiology

Much progress has been made in understanding the pathophysiology of nausea and vomiting (69). Nausea and vomiting are controlled by a loose collection of cells and tracts in the lateral medullary reticular formation called the *vomiting center* (VC). The VC integrates the various visceral, vestibular, cortical, respiratory, salivary, vasomotor, and somatic motor components into a complex coordinated reflex. The VC receives input from another center, the *chemoreceptor trigger zone* (CTZ), located in the floor of the fourth ventricle. The CTZ detects toxins in the blood or cerebrospinal fluid and gives input to the VC. Vagal afferents from the gut transmit information to the VC and possibly the CTZ as well. Multiple neurotransmitters and receptors have been identified in the CTZ and VC (70), including dopamine, serotonin, histamine, opioids, and cannabinoid receptors. Knowledge of this receptor pharmacology has driven the drug development process for antiemetics and guides their use (71).

Clinical Approach

The differential diagnosis of nausea and vomiting is presented in Table 44-9. As with all symptoms, the initial approach consists of a history and physical examination supplemented by laboratory examinations and radiologic tests, as indicated. Treatment-related nausea and vomiting are well described in oncologic patients; these syndromes are less common in CaP, owing to the lack of highly emetogenic chemotherapy regimens used in its treatment. Treatment-related nausea and vomiting are therefore not discussed in detail. The most effective treatment approaches have been combinations of a serotonin receptor antagonist [e.g., ondansetron (Zofran)] with a corticosteroid and a benzodiazepine.

Drug-induced nausea is among the most common causes. Common offenders include opioids, antibiotics, NSAIDs, digoxin, estrogens, and others. Most patients become tolerant to opioid-induced nausea, which can be managed meanwhile by dopamine antagonists [haloperidol, prochlorperazine, or metoclopramide (Reglan)]; otherwise, patients can be switched to another opioid. Metabolic causes include hypercalcemia, hyponatremia, and uremia [chlorpromazine (Thorazine) is said to be effective for the nausea of uremia]. Irritation or distention of the GI tract from pharynx to rectum may cause nausea or vomiting. Pharyngeal lesions may cause vomiting directly by stimulation of the VC or may cause persistent cough and cough-induced vomiting. Potential offenders include tenacious sputum or infectious lesions, such as candidiasis. Treatment of underlying causes, inhalational treatments to loosen sputum, and local anesthetic sprays are management options.

TABLE 44-9. DIFFERENTIAL DIAGNOSIS OF NAUSEA AND VOMITING

Syndrome	Etiology	Features	Pathways (transmitters)	Treatment
Toxic	Drugs: opioids, digoxin, anticonvulsants, antibiotics, cytotoxics Food poisoning Metabolic: hypercalcemia, organ failure, ketoacidosis	Constant nausea, variable vomiting, features of underlying illness	Stimulation of D2 in CTZ; 5-HT release in GIT (vagal stimulation)	Treat cause Remove offending drug haloperidol
Gastric stasis	Drug induced (opioids, anticholinergics) Ascites Hepatomegaly Autonomic failure	Epigastric pain, fullness, early satiety, reflux, hiccups, large volume vomitus	Gastric mechanoreceptors → vagal afferents → VC (Ach)	Treat underlying cause Prokinetic agents Reduce gastric secretions
Visceral distention	Steroids Constipation Intestinal obstruction Mesenteric mets Liver mets Ureteral distention	Colic, altered elimination, perhaps feculent vomiting	Visceral mechanoreceptors → vagal afferents → VC	Treat underlying cause Aggressive bowel regime
Gastrointestinal tract irritation	Infection Peptic ulceration Gastritis	Diarrhea, nausea, occasional vomiting	Vagal afferents → VC (anticholinergics)	—
Raised intracranial pressure	Cerebral tumor Brain mass Meningeal processes	Headache, nuchal rigidity, papilledema, decreased alertness	?Direct stimulation of cerebral H1 receptors Meningeal mechanoreceptors → VC (Ach)	Treat underlying cause High-dose steroids Anticholinergics
Motion sickness	Opioid induced Gut distortion Vestibular processes	Nausea/vomiting on sudden movement, turning	Sensitization of vestibular afferents Gut mechanoreceptors → vagal afferents → VC (H1, Ach)	Treat cause Anticholinergics
Anxiety	—	Triggers, distractible	Cortex → VC	Psychological techniques Benzodiazepines

Ach, acetylcholine; CTZ, chemoreceptor trigger zone; GIT, gastrointestinal tract; 5-HT, serotonin; mets, metastases; VC, vomiting center.

Distention of the stomach may result from mechanical pressure, known as the "squashed stomach syndrome"; possible causes include hepatomegaly, ascites, adjacent tumor, or gastroduodenal inflammatory lesions. Alternatively, gastric distention may result from physiologic stasis; possible causes include drugs (anticholinergics, opioids) or autonomic failure (e.g., due to diabetes). A syndrome in advanced cancer consisting of autonomic failure, including gastric distention, has been described. Patients must be evaluated for complete obstruction and treated appropriately, if needed, with curative or palliative measures. For a partial obstruction or physiologic stasis, prokinetic agents may be used. Metoclopramide increases peristalsis of the stomach and upper small bowel; cisapride (Propulsid) increases peristalsis of the entire bowel. Prokinetic agents may worsen colicky pain or produce esophageal spasm, which may create diagnostic difficulties. Gastric secretion may be decreased by adding H2 antagonists, omeprazole, or octreotide (Sandostatin). Anticholinergic agents may be used for otherwise unresponsive nausea, recognizing that their antiperistaltic effect may worsen constipation.

Constipation is a notorious and common cause of nausea and vomiting in cancer patients. Abdominal x-rays may be inconclusive; every patient evaluation for new or intractable nausea or vomiting should include a physical examination for constipation, including a rectal examination to rule out impaction. Increased intracranial pressure may present with nausea and vomiting; common causes include brain metastases or abscesses, cerebral edema, or intracranial hemorrhages. Treatment of the nausea consists of high-dose steroids plus antiemetics, if needed. Movement-associated nausea, akin to motion sickness, may occur in a variety of settings and may respond to anticholinergic antiemetics. Anxiety or pain commonly causes nausea and vomiting. *Anticipatory vomiting* is a well-known complication of chemotherapy; treatment may include benzodiazepines or psychological techniques.

For resistant cases of nausea and vomiting, several treatment options remain. Combinations of antiemetics acting at different receptors are often more effective than individual agents, regardless of the theoretically implicated receptor. Methotrimeprazine is a phenothiazine with antiemetic and analgesic properties that may be administered by continuous s.q. infusion. Propofol is an i.v. general anesthetic agent; anecdotal reports suggest that subanesthetic doses are antiemetic with a longer duration than their anesthetic effect. Psychological techniques (72) and acupuncture (73) have been effective in certain situations.

Pharmacology

Available antiemetic drugs are summarized in Table 44-10. They may be considered according to their receptor activity. Antagonists at the 5-HT_3 subtype of the serotonin receptor have achieved great importance in the treatment of nausea and vomiting (74). These receptors are present in the intestinal wall, vagal afferents in the intestine, and the CTZ and VC centrally. These agents are established for the treatment of treatment-induced nausea and vomiting and also appear to have a role in postoperative nausea and vomiting. Their role for other types of nausea is less clear, and they are expensive. Currently available agents in the United States are ondansetron and granisetron (Kytril). No clinically significant differences between them have been demonstrated, although several studies have shown greater patient preference for granisetron (75).

Constipation

Constipation is one of the most common and distressing symptoms suffered by cancer patients (76). Many patients choose to have pain rather than suffer the constipating effects of opioids. The vast majority of healthy individuals has bowel movements at least three times a week. Symptoms of constipation include decreased frequency of bowel movements, straining at stool, a sensation of incomplete evacuation, and small hard stools. Causes of constipation include

- Low fiber diet
- Dehydration, weakness, inactivity
- Drugs (opioids, anticholinergics, ondansetron, diuretics, iron)
- Reduced defecation (weakness, confusion, pain)
- Depression
- Hypercalcemia, hypothyroidism, hypokalemia
- Compression by extrinsic or intrinsic tumor
- Anal disorders: hemorrhoids, fissures, stenosis
- Autonomic neuropathy (diabetes, advanced cancer)

By far the most common cause of constipation in cancer patients is opioids given without laxatives. The author has seen many patients with abdominal pain due to constipation treated with morphine. Every patient on opioids should be started on prophylactic laxatives: Like pain, constipation is more easily prevented than treated. Patients often have alternating constipation and diarrhea due to intermittent use of laxatives. Patients who are not eating still produce feces and may become constipated. Constipation may produce anorexia, nausea, vomiting, abdominal pain, rectal pain, urinary retention or incontinence, confusion, and sometimes frank obstruction. The pain is usually colicky and can radiate to the back, chest, and proximal legs. Patients may present with liquid stools around a fecal obstruction.

The clinical approach begins with the history: When was the last bowel movement, the one before that, stool consistency, stool amount, laxatives, and associated symptoms (nausea, distention)? The physical examination may show abdominal distention, tenderness, and masses. The rectal examination may show fecal impaction, hemorrhoids, fissures, or an empty rectum if obstruction is higher up. Plain x-rays may show stool and may help rule out mechanical obstruction.

A reasonable goal of treatment is to have good bowel movements at least every 3 days. All patients on opioids should be on a stool softener, as well as a peristaltic agent (e.g., senna) on a daily basis, increased until treatment goals are reached. Once patients are on a stable prophylactic laxative regimen, if they fail to meet their bowel movement target, then a supplemental laxative (e.g., lactulose), suppository [e.g., bisacodyl (Dulcolax)], or enema should be used until a bowel movement occurs. Another option in the treatment of opioid-induced constipation is oral naloxone (77), which may soon be commercially available as a tablet. The starting dose is 1 mg twice daily, which may be increased as high as 16 mg twice daily. The major side effects of oral naloxone are occasional abdominal cramping, reversal of analgesia, or frank withdrawal. Patients with an empty rectum due to high impaction may need high enemas. Patients with multiple palpable fecal masses may need oil retention or soap suds enemas to soften the feces, followed by phosphate enemas or other prokinetic agents to stimulate the bowel. Manual disimpaction may be required. This is often painful and should be preceded by analgesics.

General measures include maximizing the patient's physical activity levels, adequate oral hydration when possible, having the patient sit for bowel movements rather than lie on a bedpan, maximize fiber content of the diet, and avoiding constipating drugs when possible. Despite these measures, most patients with advanced cancer, whether on opioids or not, will require laxatives. Approximately half of patients in hospice will require rectal measures on a regular basis (78). *Bulk forming laxatives* are high-fiber foods that contain polysaccharides or cellulose compounds that resist digestion and contribute to higher volume, softer stools. If not taken with adequate quantities of fluid, then they may make matters worse. Bulk-forming agents have a limited role in the cancer population. *Emollient laxatives* act as detergents, allowing water to enter fat in the stool, producing a softening effect. Docusate (Colace) at a dose of 100 mg three times a day alone or combined with an antiperistaltic agent

TABLE 44-10. ANTIEMETIC DOSING GUIDELINES

Drug	Route/dose	Comments
Dopamine antagonists		
Phenothiazines		Good general antiemetics
Prochlorperazine (Compazine)	p.o.: tablets, 5–10 mg q6h PRN; Spansules, 10–15 mg q8–12h p.r.: 25 mg q8h PRN i.v.: 10 mg q6h PRN	Side effects: sedation, EPS May potentiate CNS depressant effect of other medications Hypotension possible with i.v. dosing
Thiethylperazine (Torecan)	p.o.: 10 mg q4–6h p.r.: 10 mg q4–6h	—
Perphenazine (Trilafon)	p.o.: 2–4 mg q6h i.v.: 2–4 mg q6h	—
Substituted benzamide		
Metoclopramide (Reglan)	p.o.: 10–20 mg q6h i.v.: up to 1–2 mg/kg q6h	Weak 5-HT_3 antagonist in high doses Promotility agent Side effects: EPS (higher incidence in <30 yr age group)
Butyrophenones		
Droperidol	i.v.: 1.25–5.0 mg q6h	Helpful when anxiety aggravates nausea and vomiting symptoms Side effects: sedation
Haloperidol (Haldol)	p.o.: 0.5–2.0 mg q6h	EPS can be severe
Serotonin antagonists		
Ondansetron (Zofran)	p.o.: 8 mg q8–12h or 8–24 mg q.d. i.v.: 0.15 mg/kg q8–12h or 8–24 mg q.d.	Best protection against moderately to highly emetogenic agents p.o./q.d. dosing supported by newest research Expensive
Granisetron (Kytril)	p.o.: 1 mg b.i.d. or 2 mg q.d. i.v.: 1 mg b.i.d. or 2 mg q.d.	Combine with dexamethasone for best effect Side effects: headache, constipation, minimal sedation
Dolasetron (Anzemet)	p.o.: 100 mg q.d. i.v.: 100 mg q.d. or 1.8 mg/kg q.d.	—
Corticosteroids		
Dexamethasone (Decadron)	p.o.: 2–4 mg b.i.d.–q.i.d. i.v.: 10–20 mg q.d.	Helpful with delayed and acute nausea and vomiting Side effects: euphoria/dysphoria, insomnia
Benzodiazepine		
Lorazepam (Ativan)	p.o./s.l.: 0.5–1.0 mg q6h i.v.: 0.5–1.0 mg q6h	Help with anticipatory symptoms Side effects: sedation, amnesia Not true antiemetic Cumulative effect if renal, hepatic impairment
Cannabinoids		
Dronabinol (Marinol)	p.o.: 2.5–10.0 mg q4–6h	Not first line Side effects: sedation, dizziness, disorientation, dysphoria, orthostatic hypotension Consider cost
Antihistamine		
Diphenhydramine (Benadryl)	p.o.: 12.5–50.0 mg q6h i.v.: 12.5–50 mg q6h	Prevent/treat EPS Side effects: sedation, hypotension, dry mouth
Anticholinergics		
Scopolamine (Transderm scop)	TD: 1.5 mg q72h	Anticholinergic effects: dry mouth, constipation, urinary retention, palpitations
Miscellaneous		
Cisapride (Propulsid)	p.o.: 10 mg q.i.d.	Promotility agent May help with delayed nausea and vomiting Minimal EPS Multiple drug-drug interactions May come off market due to ECG changes

CNS, central nervous system; ECG, electrocardiogram; EPS, extrapyramidal symptoms; 5-HT_3, serotonin; mg, milligrams; PRN, as needed; s.l., sublingual; TD, transdermal.

[casanthranol (Peri-Colace)] is commonly used. The efficacy of docusate alone is questionable. *Lubricant laxatives* include mineral oil and paraffin. These agents lubricate the stool surface, allowing easier colonic passage. Paraffin alone has been associated with complications and is not popular. *Saline laxatives* include magnesium citrate or sulfate and sodium phosphate or sulfate. These agents exert an osmotic effect throughout the intestine. In sick patients, these agents may cause undesirably strong cathartic effects or electrolyte imbalances and are therefore used when standard agents have failed. *Stimulant laxatives* are the most popular agents for constipation. These include anthraquinone derivatives (senna, cascara, and danthron) and diphenylmethane derivatives (bisacodyl and phenolphthalein). Some patients may develop cramping. Starting doses are senna, 15 mg per day; danthron, 50 mg per day; or bisacodyl, 10 mg per day. Bisacodyl is also effective as a rectal suppository. *Osmotic laxatives* are not broken down in the intestine and act as osmotic agents to draw water intraluminally. Options include lactulose, mannitol, and sorbitol. Lactulose is effective and popular but expensive. Some patients may experience bloating, colic, or flatulence, and the sickly sweet taste is intolerable to some patients. *Prokinetic agents* may be considered as well. These include metoclopramide, which enhances motility of the stomach and upper small bowel, and cisapride, which enhances motility of the entire bowel. These agents may help in constipation, nausea, early satiety, and vomiting caused by functional disorders of bowel motility. Contraindications to the use of these agents include partial or complete bowel obstruction. Metoclopramide may cause dystonic reactions or akathisia; cisapride is contraindicated in patients with a prolonged QT interval and a pretreatment electrocardiogram is required.

Our regimen at Brigham and Women's Hospital calls for senna, two tablets nightly, which is increased up to eight tablets a day, if needed. In addition, patients take docusate, 100 mg twice a day to three times a day. If the patient fails to have a bowel movement for 3 days, lactulose, 30 mL, is taken every 4 hours until a bowel movement occurs.

Bowel and Bladder Symptoms

Bladder spasms are caused by hyperactivity of the detrusor muscle and cause intermittent suprapubic pain and urinary urgency. Spasms occur from radiation cystitis, tumors of the bladder or prostate, bleeding, or indwelling catheters. Urinary infection and fecal impaction must be excluded. Bladder spasms (e.g., with catheters) may be treated with belladonna and opium suppositories per rectum every 4 hours, low-dose oxybutynin, 2.5 to 5.0 mg orally two times per day, up to 10 mg three times a day (79), or hyoscine butylbromide, 10 mg orally once or twice per day. Oxybutynin and other agents may be administered directly into the bladder (80,81). TCAs also reduce bladder spasms (e.g., imipramine, 25 to 50 mg at bedtime). NSAIDs can sometimes reduce detrusor activity (e.g., naproxen, 500 mg twice a day) (82). Bromocriptine starting at 1.25 mg per day and increasing up to 2.5 mg twice a day may reduce urgency and frequency but may cause nausea, headache, and postural hypotension. Constant bladder pain may arise from a tumor of the bladder, prostate, or rectum and infection or blood clot. The primary cause should be addressed when possible. A conventional analgesic approach beginning with NSAIDs and opioids should begin the process. Pyridium is often taken orally to provide a local anesthetic effect on the bladder but is seldom effective. Interventional procedures may be appropriate for intractable pain from the bladder. The procedures used include superior hypogastric plexus block, bilateral lumbar sympathetic block (62), intrathecal alcohol or phenol neurolysis, and neurolytic sacral root block. Spinal administration of analgesics may also be effective (84).

Urinary frequency can be caused by infections, fecal impaction, diuretics, atrophic vaginitis, diabetes insipidus, diabetes mellitus, hypercalcemia, and bladder spasms. Dysuria tends to be relatively opioid insensitive. Other options for dysuria include potassium citrate, 10 mL four times a day; sodium bicarbonate, 2 to 4 g per day; and phenazopyridine, 200 mg four times a day (76).

Bowel symptoms in the setting of CaP are usually consequences of radiotherapy. Corticosteroid enemas or sulfasalazine have been effective in some patients (85). Laser treatment may be useful for bleeding. The successful use of sucralfate enemas has been reported, but studies have only described short-term follow-up (23).

Diarrhea may occur in the palliative care setting. Common causes include fecal impaction, partial mechanical bowel obstruction, steatorrhea (malabsorption), laxatives, drugs (antibiotics, antacids, NSAIDs, oral phosphate, chemotherapy, and antifibrinolytics), rectal tumors, and fecal incontinence. Beyond removing the offending cause when possible, symptomatic treatments include loperamide, 2 to 4 mg every 6 hours, and octreotide for secretory diarrheas.

Rectal pain may be of several different types. Constant pain in the rectal area may arise from local tumor. Such pain may persist even after the rectum is removed, so-called phantom rectal pain. *Tenesmus* refers to a frequent painful sensation of having to move the bowels. It is usually caused by rectal or pelvic tumor but may also arise from radiation proctitis or fecal impaction. Conventional analgesic approaches, including NSAIDs and opioids, should be used but are often unsatisfactory. Medications that reduce smooth muscle spasm, such as dicyclomine (Bentyl), are often used for rectal spasm or tenesmus; unfortunately, doses that reduce spasms often produce intolerable anticholinergic side effects. Anecdotal reports describe the use of calcium channel blocking agents (86). Radiation for rectal tumor or systemic steroids may help. Interventional treatments have been used successfully, including ganglion of impar blocks (87), bilateral lumbar sympathetic blocks (63), intrathecal neurolysis (88), and spinal analgesic infusions.

Anorexia

Anorexia occurs in approximately 65% of patients in hospice and approximately 33% of patients with advanced CaP in a palliative care setting (68). Specific causes of anorexia include oral thrush, nausea, constipation, hypercalcemia, chemotherapy, radiation, and drugs. Often no specific cause is found. Psychological factors may be important, and depression should be assessed and treated. Pharmacologic approaches that have been shown to be effective include steroids (dexamethasone, 4 mg or prednisone, 10 mg three times a day) and megestrol acetate (Megace) (480 to 1,600 mg per day). Megestrol additionally improves food intake, reduces fatigue, and improves sense of well-being (13). Steroids also help nausea and pain and also improve sense of well-being but do not increase food intake or promote weight gain, and the effects often decline after a few months. It is often most appropriate to use megestrol in relatively well patients and steroids for patients in their last few months. For patients with small stomach syndrome or delayed gastric emptying, metoclopramide, 10 mg four times daily (before meals), plus frequent small feedings may help. Making meals attractive to the individual patient, sometimes strongly flavored food, and eating in a room other than the sickroom may help (76). Consultation from a dietitian may also be helpful.

Fatigue

Fatigue is a common and distressing symptom in cancer patients that as yet has not been clearly characterized or well studied. A variety of studies of fatigue using different criteria have found this symptom to be present in approximately 75% of cancer patients (89), even higher after treatment (90,91), and to be distressing on one-third to one-half of these (92). In CaP patients, fatigue has been associated with hormonal treatments, especially after orchidectomy (93). The differential diagnosis of fatigue is broad and not well defined. The underlying disease or its treatments (chemotherapy, radiotherapy, surgery, or biologic response modifiers) may be implicated. Other medical causes include anemia, infection, organ failure, malnutrition, neuromuscular disorders, dehydration, electrolyte disturbances, hypothyroidism, adrenal insufficiency or steroid withdrawal, and drugs (e.g., opioids, sedatives, antiemetics, antihistamines). Miscellaneous causes include sleep disorders, deconditioning, and chronic pain. Psychosocial factors are important and may include anxiety and depression. Anemia appears to be an important factor in producing fatigue in the cancer patient. Several studies (94,95) have demonstrated that administration of erythropoietin can increase hematocrit in anemic cancer patients and improve fatigue and overall quality of life.

The management of fatigue begins with a comprehensive assessment, including identification of potential causative factors. There must be an overall sense of goals of treatment set by the health care team in collaboration with patient and family. There may be multiple potential predisposing factors; some may be easily treatable (e.g., polypharmacy or depression), some may be treatable only with difficulty or by excessively burdening the patient (e.g., decreasing analgesics, obtaining multiple tests), and some may not be treatable (e.g., renal failure or advancing malignant disease). Pharmacologic options for the treatment of fatigue have not been well studied, but several reasonable options exist. The psychostimulant class of medications may be applicable (96). Corticosteroids have been shown to be useful for fatigue (40). Amantadine has been used for fatigue related to multiple sclerosis but has not been reported in cancer-related fatigue. An antidepressant is warranted in any fatigued patient with depression; a minimally sedating antidepressant, such as an SSRI, would be appropriate. Nonpharmacologic interventions—exercise, sleep hygiene, appropriate pacing of activities, judicious use of naps and rest periods, patient education, and stress management techniques—may also be effective.

Sexual Dysfunction

Many patients diagnosed with CaP are already older and have decreases in sexual function due to age and to diseases of aging (e.g., hypertension, diabetes, and their treatment) (97). The prevalence of precancer sexual dysfunction in patients developing CaP has ranged from 20% to 60% (98). Nerve-sparing techniques have significantly decreased the incidence of posttreatment sexual dysfunction (99), but recovery of sexual function may take many months. Long-term erectile dysfunction after radiotherapy ranges from 14% to 46% (100). All of the antiandrogen treatments for CaP can produce sexual dysfunction as a side effect.

Increasing awareness has led to the introduction of new approaches to the preservation of sexual function and fertility in cancer patients. Radiation exposure to the gonads in men undergoing pelvic radiotherapy may be reduced by the use of special testicular shields. For men in their reproductive years about to undergo therapy, cryo-banking of sperm is an option. For men with erectile dysfunction, agents are available for injection into the corpus cavernosum. Multiple recent studies (101,102) found sildenafil (Viagra) effective in restoring erections in men with CaP suffering postradiation erectile dysfunction. Full response took 6 weeks in one study. Concomitant hormonal therapy may reduce the effectiveness of sildenafil.

Nonmedical factors impact on sexuality during the experience of cancer and its treatment. Such issues include pre-illness sexual functioning, mood alterations, emotional and physical stresses, pain, altered body image, response of the partner, and cancer myths. If these issues are not identified, then no opportunity will arise for addressing them. A majority of cancer patients want information about sexuality, but most do not bring it up with their doctors (103). If patients are elderly, young, single, widowed, or homosexual, then these discussions may be more difficult. Sexuality should be discussed routinely at appropriate times in the context of potential side effects of treatments and as a legitimate quality of life issue. For patients with persistent sexual difficulties, referral to a sex therapist should be considered. A useful booklet on sexuality and cancer is also available (104).

Delirium

Delirium is a syndrome of acute onset of disordered attention and cognition accompanied by disturbances of psychomotor behavior and perception (105). Delirium affects approximately 30% of cancer patients at some point in their illness. More than 85% of patients with CaP will experience progressive confusion before death (106). The occurrence of delirium increases hospital stay, morbidity, and mortality (107). The differential diagnosis includes drugs, pain, urinary retention, fecal impaction, dehydration, brain metastases (rare in CaP), the postictal state, infection, renal failure, hypoxia, metabolic causes, severe depression or anxiety, sleep deprivation, and withdrawal syndromes. Drugs are probably the most common cause and include opioids, benzodiazepines, NSAIDs (less commonly), beta blockers, diuretics, and anticholinergics. Commonly missed metabolic derangements in confused patients include hypo- or hypercalcemia and hypomagnesemia. Signs of infection may be absent in patients on steroids, NSAIDs, or in the elderly. Postictal confusion or sedation may follow unwitnessed seizures. Delirium is often multifactorial. Approximately one-third of episodes of delirium are reversible with simple measures. Delirium is difficult and stressful to manage at home.

Management begins with addressing potential causes in the context of the overall plan of care of the patient (108). Unnecessary medications should be eliminated. Explanation and reassurance should be provided to the patient and family. The patient should be in a calm, well-lit, familiar environment, and should be frequently reoriented by attendants. Patients with suspected opioid metabolite accumulation syndrome, who often have irritability, myoclonus, and hyperalgesia, should undergo opioid rotation. Symptomatic drug treatment should be used when necessary but not reflexively. Neuroleptics are preferred over benzodiazepines, owing to the potential for paradoxic increases in agitation or confusion with the latter, and haloperidol is the drug of choice (109). Haloperidol may be administered orally, intramuscularly, subcutaneously, or intravenously. Starting doses are 1 to 2 mg two to four times a day; for frail patients, 0.5 mg may be sufficient. Severely agitated patients may require 10 mg haloperidol hourly until calmness is achieved. Chlorpromazine is a more sedating alternative and may be dosed at 10 to 50 mg three times a day; for severe agitation, 100 mg hourly may rarely be necessary. The major concern with use of neuroleptics is the development of movement disorders that range from acute dystonia to restlessness and akathisia. These syndromes respond to diphenhydramine, benztropine, and trihexyphenidyl. If a benzodiazepine must be added, then the most common choice is lorazepam (Ativan). Midazolam has the advantage of being appropriate for s.q. administration; owing to its short duration of action, continuous infusions are often required, which may lead to accumulation and delayed recovery. The use of physical restraints should be minimized and used only acutely to prevent harm to the patient or others. Many patients require more than one agent for control of delirium.

A common situation of escalating delirium is the patient with anxiety treated with benzodiazepines who then develops delirium due to benzodiazepine accumulation. The delirium is then treated with escalating doses of benzodiazepines, creating a vicious cycle. This situation is managed by instituting a fixed benzodiazepine taper (to avoid withdrawal) and treating delirium, if necessary, with neuroleptic agents. Useful agents for the treatment of terminal agitation include morphine, scopolamine, chlorpromazine, and methotrimeprazine.

Lymphedema

Lymphedema is sometimes seen in advanced CaP due to involvement of pelvic lymphatics. Cardiac disease, diabetes, renal or hepatic failure, or malnutrition may compound matters (110). Patient assessment includes evaluation for the previously mentioned factors, assessment of motor and sensory function, assessment of the degree of edema and chronic skin changes, pulses, and measurement of the limb at standard sites in comparison to the contralateral limb. Venous obstruction must be ruled out. Treatment is multifactorial (111). Radiotherapy, high-dose steroids, and diuretics are used but are usually of little help. The components of management (76) include

- Bandaging: initial treatment of moderate to severe edema
- Compression stockings: may need to be worn continuously
- Sequential compression pumps: speed initial rate of edema reduction
- Massage and exercise: should be done daily by patients and family
- Skin care: daily application of hydrating lotions, inspection for early damage, ulceration, or infection
- Prophylactic antibiotics: for patients with recurrent cellulitis

Hot Flashes

Hot flashes occur in 58% to 76% of patients after orchiectomy and 75% of patients after medical castration with gonadotropin-releasing hormone (GnRH) analogs (112). Of these, approximately one-fourth find the hot flashes distressing. Although similar to the hot flashes experienced by menopausal women, the hot flashes in women disappear in 2 to 5 years; in patients with CaP, the hot flashes usually do not disappear at all. The pathophysiology of hot flashes remains uncertain (113). Hot flashes may thus be caused by instability of negative feedback by estradiol on GnRH release, mediated by endogenous opioids (114).

Several treatments have been studied for hot flashes. The most useful appears to be megestrol acetate. A recent randomized placebo-controlled trial (115) demonstrated low doses of 20 mg twice daily reduced hot flashes in 85% of patients (men with a history of CaP and women with breast cancer), compared to 21% from placebo, with no significant side effects. Clonidine and belladonna with phenobarbital preparations have been shown to be only minimally effective, with side effects (116,117). The efficacy of diethylstilbestrol has been demonstrated in two studies (117,118). One study demonstrated the efficacy of acupuncture (119), which was maintained at 3 months after treatment.

Psychosocial Symptoms

Depression

The diagnosis of cancer is stressful. A number of fears are engendered, including fear of a painful death, becoming disabled and dependent, alteration of appearance or function, and missing loved ones (120). The level of psychological distress generated depends on the intensity of the medical situation, premorbid psychological factors, and the patient's social situation. The normal response to such stress includes initial shock, a period of anxiety and depression, disruption of appetite and sleep, and decreased ability to concentrate and carry out usual activities that usually resolve in 7 to 10 days. If these symptoms are prolonged, intolerable, or compromise the ability of the patient to function for prolonged periods, further investigation and intervention may be indicated. The most common psychiatric disorders diagnosed in cancer patients are adjustment disorders with anxious or depressed mood (121). Suicidality is another common reason for psychiatric consultation (122). The diagnosis of depression in cancer relies primarily on psychological, rather than somatic symptoms, because the latter (e.g., anorexia, fatigue) are common in cancer. The characteristic psychological symptoms are dysphoria, anhedonia, helplessness, hopelessness, feelings of worthlessness or guilt, and preoccupation with death or suicide. In the elderly, the salient manifestations of depression may be cognitive ("depressive pseudodementia").

Organic causes of depression must be ruled out. These include electrolyte disturbances (e.g., hypercalcemia), endocrinopathies (e.g., hypothyroidism, hypotestosteronism), nutritional deficiencies (e.g., B_{12}), infections, and drugs (e.g., beta blockers, steroids, chemotherapy, opioids, NSAIDs). It must be noted that chronic use of opioids may cause hypothyroidism or hypotestosteronism. Risk factors for suicide in the cancer population include mild encephalopathy, uncontrolled pain, hopelessness, and previous history of psychiatric disorders or suicide attempts.

A course of crisis-oriented supportive psychotherapy is often indicated. Antidepressant medications are often indicated and need not await resolution of organic factors or completion of psychotherapy. SSRIs are often chosen first because they are better tolerated than the TCAs. Fluoxetine (Prozac), sertraline (Zoloft), and paroxetine (Paxil) are the most common choices, at starting doses of 20, 50, and 10 mg per day, respectively. Potential downsides of SSRIs in patients with cancer include decreased appetite and transiently increased anxiety, agitation, or insomnia. The TCAs are often used when insomnia, anxiety, or anorexia dominates the picture, because these drugs, dosed at night, often improve these symptoms. Therapeutic doses for depression in cancer patients appear to be lower than in noncancer patients, in the range of 75 to 125 mg per day (120). Patients with prominent insomnia are usually prescribed amitriptyline or doxepin. To avoid the anticholinergic TCA side effects (sedation, urinary retention, tachycardia, and constipation), use desipramine or nortriptyline. Typical starting doses of TCAs are 10 to 25 mg nightly, increased as needed and tolerated.

Psychostimulants are probably the drugs of choice in the treatment of the depressed patient with cancer (44,123–125). Onset of action is more rapid than with TCAs or SSRIs. Psychostimulants are also effective for opioid-induced sedation and potentiate the analgesic effects of opioids. Options are methylphenidate, dextroamphetamine, and pemoline (Cylert) starting at 5 mg twice a day, 2.5 mg twice a day, and 18.75 mg twice a day, respectively.

Anxiety

Anxiety may present with psychological symptoms, such as tension, fear, worry, rumination, or apprehension, or physical symptoms, such as restlessness, autonomic hyperactivity, insomnia, dyspnea, or sensory disturbances (126). Anxiety may occur as a manifestation of a variety of psychiatric disorders, including adjustment disorders, generalized anxiety disorders, panic disorder, or agitated depression. The differential diagnosis of these disorders in the terminally ill patient includes organic delirium, other organic mental disorders, hypoxia, pain, sepsis, akathisia (from drugs), or withdrawal. Once underlying medical disorders are excluded or dealt with, the need for treatment depends on the level of patient distress or interference with patient function.

Physicians should not discount the value of empathetic listening even when there is little consolation to offer. Pharmacologic treatment relies on benzodiazepines, neuroleptics, antihistamines, antidepressants, and opioids. The benzodiazepines are generally most effective and well tolerated. It is commonly stated that short-acting agents such as lorazepam, alprazolam (Xanax), and oxazepam (Serax) are safest; however, these agents have disadvantages of peak-dose sedation and end-of-dose breakthrough symptoms (127). In the author's experience, lorazepam is greatly overused and a common cause of delirium in the hospitalized patient with terminal illness. Small, infrequent doses of longer-acting agents,

TABLE 44-11. MEDICATIONS FOR ANXIETY

Agent	Trade name	Dose range (mg)	Route
Benzodiazepines[a]			
Very short acting			
Midazolam	Versed	10–60/24 h	i.v., s.q.
Short-acting			
Alprazolam	Xanax	0.25–2.0 t.i.d.–q.i.d.	p.o., s.l.
Oxazepam	Serax	10–15 t.i.d.–q.i.d.	p.o.
Lorazepam	Ativan	0.5–2.0 t.i.d.–q.i.d.	p.o., s.l., i.v., i.m.
Intermediate acting			
Chlordiazepoxide	Librium	10–50 t.i.d.–q.i.d.	p.o., i.m.
Long acting			
Diazepam	Valium	5–10 b.i.d.–q.i.d.	p.o., i.v., i.m., p.r.
Clonazepam	Klonopin	0.5–2.0 b.i.d.–q.i.d.	p.o.
Non-benzodiazepines			
Buspirone	BuSpar	5–20 t.i.d.	p.o.
Neuroleptics			
Haloperidol	Haldol	0.5–5.0 q2–12h	p.o., i.v., s.q., i.m.
Methotrimeprazine	Levoprome	10–20 q4–8h	i.v., s.q., p.o.
Chlorpromazine	Thorazine	12.5–50.0 q4–12h	p.o., i.v., i.m.
Antihistamines			
Hydroxyzine	Vistaril, Atarax	25–50 q4–6h	p.o., i.v., s.q.
TCAs			
Imipramine	Tofranil	10–150 qHS	p.o., i.m.
Amitriptyline	Elavil	10–150 qHS	p.o.
Nortriptyline	Pamelor	10–150 qHS	p.o.

HS, at bedtime; TCAs, tricyclic antidepressants.
[a]In practice, distinctions between short, intermediate, and long may be indistinct and depend more on the patient and duration of administration than the specific agent.
Modified from Breitbart W, Chochinow HM, Passik S. Psychiatric aspects of palliative care. In: Doyle D, Hanks GWC, MacDonald N, eds. *Oxford textbook of palliative medicine*, 2nd ed. Oxford: Oxford Medical Publications, 1998:933–954.

such as clonazepam or diazepam, are often most effective and well tolerated. Common dose regimens are summarized in Table 44-11. Rectal diazepam may be administered in terminal patients. Midazolam can be administered by continuous i.v. or s.q. infusion to control agitation or provide terminal sedation. Clonazepam appears to have analgesic properties in neuropathic pain. Benzodiazepines are generally not appropriate in patients with anxiety or agitation in the context of delirium or with psychotic features.

Neuroleptics are useful when symptoms are too severe to be controlled by benzodiazepines alone, when anxiety is a symptom of organic conditions, for psychotic features, and when respiratory depression is a concern. The high-potency neuroleptics (e.g., haloperidol) are especially useful because sedation, anticholinergic effects, and hypotension are minimal. Conversely, if sedation is desired, then low-potency neuroleptics, such as chlorpromazine, are useful. Methotrimeprazine is the only neuroleptic with analgesic properties. All the neuroleptics confer increased risk of extrapyramidal symptoms in patients who are also on neuroleptic antiemetics for nausea.

Hydroxyzine is an antihistamine with mild anxiolytic and sedative properties. Its analgesic properties are often cited but rarely seen. The TCAs are useful for anxiety in the context of depression and for the treatment of panic disorder (128). They may help with insomnia immediately, but relief of depression and anxiety may take weeks once titration is complete, which may take a few more weeks. Opioids are most useful for anxiety in the context of pain or respiratory distress or for terminal sedation. Buspirone, a nonbenzodiazepine anxiolytic, is mainly useful for chronic anxiety in the nonterminally ill population.

TERMINAL CARE

Symptom profiles often change in the last hours to days of life (76). Most patients become unconscious, but some patients develop terminal agitation. This syndrome consists of restlessness; confusion; increasing distress; and, in some patients, agitated behavior, including thrashing in bed or walking around. Patients with premorbid psychological issues may be more at risk, although other issues (hypoxia, pain, bladder fullness) may contribute as well. Generally, powerful sedatives are required (e.g., morphine, chlorpromazine, scopolamine, and diazepam or midazolam), given separately or in combination by injection or continuous s.q. infusion (Table 44-12). If a patient needed morphine, then he will continue to need it during the terminal phase; otherwise, opioid withdrawal will be added to his woes. Generally, half of the oral dose given s.q. or by continuous infusion is sufficient; more can be given, if needed.

TABLE 44-12. DRUGS USED FOR TERMINAL SEDATION

Drug	q4h i.m. dose	Continuous s.q. dose/24 h
Morphine	1/2 the q4h p.o. dose	1/2 the q24h p.o. dose
Chlorpromazine	25–75 mg	—
Methotrimeprazine	25–75 mg	75–150 mg
Scopolamine	0.4 mg	1.2–2.4 mg
Diazepam	10 mg (i.m. or p.r.)	—
Midazolam	—	20–80 mg

Adapted from Kaye P. *Notes on symptom control in hospice and palliative care*. Essex, CT: Hospice Education Institution, 1995.

Indomethacin suppositories can be useful for bony pain in patients who benefited from NSAIDs. For sedation, chlorpromazine is useful (e.g., 25 to 50 mg every 4 hours). Methotrimeprazine is approximately twice as potent as chlorpromazine and has analgesic properties as well. Scopolamine is a very useful drug in the terminal phase: It dries up secretions, decreases respiratory bubbling, is sedating, and decreases nausea and vomiting. Typical doses are 0.4 mg s.q. or i.m. every 4 hours or continuous s.q. infusion 0.8 to 2.4 mg per 24 hours. Diazepam, 10 mg rectally by an enema, i.m., or i.v., can be helpful for terminal muscle twitching or seizures or for sedation.

Obtunded or bed-confined patients require standard care procedures. Urinary retention is common and may contribute to agitation. Indwelling bladder catheters can be inserted if physical exam indicates a full bladder. Mouth care is needed hourly. Artificial tears are used up to every 2 hours as needed. Warfarin (Coumadin) should be stopped in the terminal phase; otherwise, terminal GI bleeding can occur.

Family support is a critical goal of the terminal period (76). All of the previously mentioned medical procedures should be explained; some family members may find solace in participating in these terminal care procedures. Often family members find it difficult to concentrate or think clearly, and they may need guidance as to what is appropriate behavior. There may be simple questions about death, asked or unasked, that can be explained—for example, How long will it take? Is he suffering? Can he hear us? Why has his skin color changed? and Should we stay? Patients often feel guilty about wishing the patient would die to end his suffering. Family members may need guidance about taking shifts in the vigil or permission to leave if they are distressed. After death, family members should be allowed to stay for a period to achieve closure, pray, say goodbye, or for other procedures that may bring comfort.

REFERENCES

1. McFarlane JR, Rolley DA. Flutamide therapy for advanced prostatic cancer: a phase II study. *Br J Urol* 1985:57:172–174.
2. Higano CS, Ellis W, Russell K, et al. Intermittent androgen suppression with leuprolide and flutamide for prostate cancer: a pilot study. *Urology* 1996:48;800–804.
3. Moinpour CM, Savage MJ, Troxel A, et al. Quality of life in advanced prostate cancer: results of a randomized therapeutic trial. *J Natl Cancer Inst* 1998;90:1537–1544.
4. Caffo O, Fellin G, Graffer U. Assessment of quality of life after radical radiotherapy for prostate cancer. *Br J Urol* 1996;78:557–553.
5. Lim AJ, Brandon AH, Fiedler J, et al. Quality of life: radical prostatectomy versus radiation therapy for prostate cancer. *J Urol* 1995;154:1420–1425.
6. Widmark A, Fransson P, Tavelin B. Self-assessment questionnaire for evaluating urinary and intestinal late side effects after pelvic radiotherapy in patients with prostate cancer compared with an age-matched control population. *Cancer* 1994;74: 2520–2532.
7. Beard CJ, Propert KJ, Rieker PP, et al. Complications after treatment with external-beam irradiation in early-stage prostate cancer patients: a prospective multiinstitutional outcomes study. *J Clin Oncol* 1997;1:223–229.
8. Helgason AR, Fredrikson M, Adolfsson J, et al. Decreased sexual capacity after external radiation therapy for prostate cancer impairs quality of life. *Int J Radiat Oncol Biol Phys* 1995;32:33–39.
9. Lilleby W, Fossa SD, Waehre HR, et al. Long-term morbidity and quality of life in patients with localized prostate cancer undergoing definitive radiotherapy or radical prostatectomy. *Int J Radiat Oncol Biol Phys* 1999;43:735–743.
10. World Health Organization. Cancer pain relief and palliative care. Report of a WHO expert committee [World Health Organization Technical Report Series, 804]. Geneva, Switzerland: World Health Organization, 1990.
11. Bonica JJ, ed. *The management of pain.* Philadelphia: Lea & Febiger, 1990.
12. Agency for Health Care Policy and Research. *Management of cancer pain.* Clinical Practice Guideline Number 9. U.S. Department of Health and Human Services. AHCPR Pub. No. 94-0592, 1994.
13. Iscoe NA, Bruera E, Choo RC. Prostate cancer: 10. Palliative care. *CMAJ* 1999;160:365–371.
14. Foley KM. The treatment of cancer pain. *N Engl J Med* 1985;313:84–95.
15. Constans JP, DeVitis E, Donzelli R, et al. Spinal metastases with neurological manifestations: review of 600 cases. *J Neurosurg* 1983;59:111–118.
16. Posner JB. Back pain and epidural spinal cord compression. *Med Clin North Am* 1987;71:185–206.
17. Rosenthal MA, Rosen D, Raghavan D, et al. Spinal cord compression in prostate cancer. A 10-year experience. *Br J Urol* 1992;69:530–533.
18. Helweg-Larsen S, Srensen PS. Symptoms and signs in metastatic spinal cord compression: a study of progression from first symptom until diagnosis in 153 patients. *Eur J Cancer* 1994;30a:396–398.
19. Ruff RL, Lanska DJ. Epidural metastases in prospectively evaluated veterans with cancer and back pain. *Cancer* 1989;63:2234–2241.
20. Cherny NI. Cancer pain: principles of assessment and syndromes. In: Berger A, Portenoy R, Weissman D, eds. *Princi-*

ples and practice of supportive oncology. Philadelphia: Lippincott–Raven Publishers, 1998.

21. Labrie F, Dupont A, Belanger A, et al. Flutamide eliminates the risk of disease flare in prostatic cancer patients treated with a luteinizing hormone-releasing hormone agonist. *J Urol* 1987;138:804–806.
22. Buchi K. Radiation proctitis: therapy and prognosis. *JAMA* 1991;265:1180.
23. Babb RR. Radiation proctitis: a review. *Am J Gastroenterol* 1996;91:1309–1311.
24. Stillman M. Perineal pain: diagnosis and management, with particular attention to perineal pain of cancer. In: Foley KM, Bonica JJ, Ventafridda V, eds. *Second international congress on cancer pain. Advances in pain research and therapy,* vol. 16. New York: Raven Press, 1990;359–377.
25. Jaeckle KA, Young DR, Foley DM. The natural history of lumbosacral plexopathy in cancer. *Neurology* 1985;35:8–15.
26. Glass JP, Pettigrew LC, Maor M. Plexopathy induced by radiation therapy. *Neurology* 1985:35:1261.
27. Serafini AN, Houston SJ, Resche I, et al. Palliation of pain associated with metastatic bone cancer using samarium-153 lexidronam: a double-blind placebo-controlled clinical trial. *J Clin Oncol* 1998;16:1574–1581.
28. Ventafridda V, Caraceni A, Gamba A. Field-testing of the WHO Guidelines for Cancer Pain Relief: summary report of demonstration projects. In: Foley KM, Bonica JJ, Ventafridda V, eds. *Proceedings of the second international congress of pain. Advances in pain research and therapy,* vol. 16. New York: Raven Press, 1990:451–464.
29. Brodgen RN. Non-steroidal anti-inflammatory analgesics other than salicylates. *Drugs* 1986;32(Suppl 4):27–45.
30. Mitchell JA, Akaarasereenot P, Thierermann C, et al. Selectivity of non-steroidal anti-inflammatory drugs as inhibitors of constitutive and inducing cyclo-oxygenases. *Proc Natl Acad Sci U S A* 1993;80:11693–11697.
31. Rawlins MD. Non-opioid analgesics. In: Doyle D, Hanks GW, MacDonald N, eds. *Oxford textbook of palliative medicine,* 2nd ed. Oxford: Oxford University Press, 1998.
32. American College of Rheumatology Ad Hoc Committee on Clinical Guidelines. Guidelines for monitoring drug therapy in rheumatoid arthritis. *Arthritis Rheum* 1996;39:723–731.
33. Estes D, Kaplan K. Lack of platelet effect with the aspirin analog salsalate. *Arthritis Rheum* 1980;23:1303–1307.
34. Stuart JJ, Pisko EJ. Choline magnesium trisalicylate does not impair platelet aggregation. *Pharmacotherapeutica* 1981;2: 547–551.
35. Moore RA, Tramer MR, Carroll D, et al. Quantitative systematic review of topically applied non-steroidal anti-inflammatory drugs. *BMJ* 1998;316:333–338.
36. Portenoy RK. Chronic opioid therapy for persistent non-cancer pain: can we get past the bias? *Am Pain Soc Bull* 1991;1:4–5.
37. Portenoy RK. Chronic opioid therapy in nonmalignant pain. *J Pain Symptom Manage* 1990;5:S46–S62.
38. Passik SD, Portenoy RK, Ricketts PL. Substance abuse issues in cancer patients. Part 1: Prevalence and diagnosis. *Oncology (Huntingt)* 1998;12:517–521.
39. Bruera E, Neumann CM. Role of methadone in the management of pain in cancer patients. *Oncology (Huntingt)* 1999;13:1275–1282.
40. Bruera E, Roca E, Cedaro L, et al. Action of oral methylprednisolone in terminal cancer patients: a prospective randomized double-blind study. *Cancer Treat Rep* 1985;69:751–754.
41. Della Cuna GR, Pellegrini A, Piazzi M. Effect of methylprednisolone sodium succinate on quality of life in preterminal cancer patients. A placebo-controlled multicenter study. The Methylprednisolone Preterminal Cancer Study Group. *Eur J Clin Oncol* 1989;25:1817–1821.
42. Fainsinger RL, Spanchynski K, Hanson J, et al. Symptom control in terminally ill patients with malignant bowel obstruction. *J Pain Sympt Manage* 1994;9:12.
43. Bruera E, Chadwich S, Brenneis C, et al. Methylphenidate associated with narcotics for the treatment of cancer pain. *Cancer Treat Rep* 1987;71:67–70.
44. Bruera E, Miller MJ, Macmillan K, et al. Neuropsychological effects of methylphenidate in patients receiving a continuous infusion of narcotics for cancer pain. *Pain* 1992;48:163–166.
45. McQuay HJ, Tramer M, Nye BA, et al. A systematic review of antidepressants in neuropathic pain. *Pain* 1996;68:217–227.
46. Portenoy RK. Adjuvant analgesics in pain management. In: Doyle D, Hanks GWC, MacDonald N, eds. *Oxford textbook of palliative medicine,* 2nd ed. Oxford: Oxford University Press, 1998:361–389.
47. McQuay H, Carroll D, Jadad AR, et al. Anticonvulsant drugs for management of pain: a systematic review. *BMJ* 1995;311:1047–1052.
48. Rowbotham M, Harden N, Stacey B, et al. Gabapentin for the treatment of postherpetic neuralgia: a randomized controlled trial. *JAMA* 1998;280:1837–1842.
49. Lasagna L, DeKornfeld RJ. Methotrimeprazine: a new phenothiazine derivative with analgesic properties. *JAMA* 1961;178:887–890.
50. Beaver WT, Wallenstein SL, Houde RW, et al. A comparison of the analgesic effects of methotrimeprazine and morphine in patients with cancer. *Clin Pharmacol Ther* 1966;7: 436–446.
51. Ernst DS, MacDonald N, Paterson AH, et al. A double-blind, cross-over trial of intravenous clodronate in metastatic bone pain. *J Pain Sympt Manage* 1992;7:4.
52. Pelger RC, Hamdy NA, Zwinderman AH, et al. Effects of the bisphosphonate olpadronate in patients with carcinoma of the prostate metastatic to the skeleton. *Bone* 1998; 22:403–408.
53. Adami S. Bisphosphonates in prostate carcinoma. *Cancer* 1997;80:1674–1679.
54. Roth A, Kolaric K. Analgetic activity of calcitonin in patients with painful osteolytic metastases of breast cancer. *Oncology* 1986;43:283–287.
55. Hindley AC, Hill AB, Leyland MJ, et al. A double-blind controlled trial of salmon calcitonin in pain due to malignancy. *Cancer Chemother Pharmacol* 1982;9:71–74.
56. Blomquist C, Elomaa I, Porkka L, et al. Evaluation of salmon calcitonin treatment in bone metastases from breast cancer—a controlled trial. *Bone* 1988;9:45–51.
57. Devulder J, Ghys L, Dhondt W, et al. Spinal analgesia in terminal care: risk versus benefit. *J Pain Symptom Manage* 1994;9:75–81.
58. Hassenbusch SJ, Pillay PK, Magdinec M, et al. Constant infusion of morphine for intractable cancer pain using an implanted pump. *J Neurosurg* 1990;73:405–409.

59. Onofrio BM, Yaksh TL. Long-term pain relief produced by intrathecal morphine infusion in 53 patients. *J Neurosurg* 1990;72:200–209.
60. Cousins MJ, Bridenbaugh PO, eds. *Neural blockade in clinical anesthesia and management of pain*, 3rd ed. Philadelphia: Lippincott–Raven Publishers, 1998.
61. Patt RB. *Cancer pain*. Philadelphia: JB Lippincott Co, 1993.
62. Bristow A, Foster JM. Lumbar sympathectomy in the management of rectal tenesmoid pain. *Ann Roy Coll Surg Engl* 1988;70:38–39.
63. Ischia S, Ischia A, Luzzani A, et al. Results up to death in the treatment of persistent cervico-thoracic (Pancoast) and thoracic malignant pain by unilateral percutaneous cervical cordotomy. *Pain* 1985;21:339–355.
64. Lahuerta J, Bowsher D, Lipton S, et al. Percutaneous cervical cordotomy: a review of 181 operations on 146 patients with a study on the location of "pain fibers" in the C-2 spinal cord segment of 29 cases. *J Neurosurg* 1994;80:975–985.
65. Ramirez LF, Levin AB. Pain relief after hypophysectomy. *Neurosurgery* 1984;14:499–504.
66. Choi CR, Ha YS, Ahn MS, et al. Intraventricular or epidural injection of morphine for severe pain. *Neurochirurgia (Stuttg)* 1989;32:180–183.
67. Lazorthes YR, Sallerin BA, Verdie JC. Intracerebroventricular administration of morphine for control of irreducible cancer pain. *Neurosurgery* 1995;37:422–428.
68. Vainio A, Auvinen A. Prevalence of symptoms among patients with advanced cancer: an international collaborative study. Symptom Prevalence Group. *J Pain Symptom Manage* 1996;12:3–10.
69. Mannix KA. Palliation of nausea and vomiting. In: Doyle D, Hanks GW, MacDonald N, eds. *Oxford textbook of palliative care*, 2nd ed. Oxford: Oxford Medical Publications, 1998:489–498.
70. Borison HL, Wang SC. Physiology and pharmacology of vomiting. *Pharmacol Rev* 1953;5:192–230.
71. Peroutka SJ, Snyder SH. Antiemetics: neurotransmitter binding predicts therapeutic actions. *Lancet* 1982;2:658–659.
72. Burish TG, Tope DM. Psychological techniques for controlling the adverse effects of cancer chemotherapy: findings from a decade of research. *J Pain Symptom Manage* 1992;7:287–301.
73. Dundee JW, Yang J. Prolongation of the effect of P6 acupuncture by acupressure in patients having cancer chemotherapy. *J Roy Soc Med* 1991;83;360–362.
74. Kris MG, Baltzer I, Pisters KM, et al. Enhancing the effectiveness of the specific serotonin antagonists. *Cancer* 1993;72:3436–3442.
75. Yarker YE, McTavish D. Granisetron: an update of its therapeutic use in nausea and vomiting induced by antineoplastic therapy. *Drugs* 1994;48:761–93.
76. Kaye P. *Notes on symptom control in hospice and palliative care*. Essex, CT: Hospice Education Institution, 1995.
77. Meissner W, Schmidt U, Hartmann M, et al. Oral naloxone reverses opioid-associated constipation. *Pain* 2000;84:105–109.
78. Twycross RG, Lack SA. Constipation. In: *Control of alimentary symptoms in far advanced cancer*. London: Churchill Livingstone, 1986:166–207.
79. Kirkali Z, Whitaker RH. The use of oxybutynin in urological practice. *Int Urol Nephrol* 1987;19:385–391.
80. Brendler CB, Radebaugh LC, Mohler JL. Topical oxybutynin chloride for relaxation of dysfunctional bladders. *J Urol* 1989;141:1350–1352.
81. Ekstrom B, Andersson K-E, Mattiasson A. Urodynamic effects of intravesical instillation of atropine and phentolamine in patients with detrusor hyperactivity. *J Urol* 1993; 149:135–138.
82. Cardozo LD, Stanton SL. A comparison between bromocriptine and indomethacin in the treatment of detrusor instability. *J Urol* 1980;123:399–401.
83. Plancarte R, de Leon-Casasola OA, El-Helaly M, et al. Neurolytic superior hypogastric plexus block for chronic pelvic pain associated with cancer. *Reg Anesth* 1997;22:562–568.
84. Olshwang D, Shapiro A, Perlberg S, et al. The effect of epidural morphine on ureteral colic and spasm of the bladder. *Pain* 1984;18:97–101.
85. Goldstein F, Khoury J, Thornton JJ. Treatment of chronic radiation enteritis and colitis with salicylazosulfapyridine and systemic corticosteroids. *Am J Gastroenterol* 1976;65:201–208.
86. Castell DO. Calcium channel blocking agents for gastrointestinal disorders. *Am J Cardiol* 1985;55:210B–213B.
87. Plancarte R, Amescua C, Patt RB, et al. Presacral blockade of the ganglion of Walther (ganglion impar). *Anesthesiology* 1990;73:A751.
88. Lynch J, Zech D, Grond S. The role of intrathecal neurolysis in the treatment of cancer-related perianal and perineal pain. *Palliat Med* 1992;6:140–145.
89. Curtis EB, Kretch R, Walsh TD. Common symptoms in patients with advanced cancer. *J Palliat Care* 1991;7;25–29.
90. Irvine D, Vincent L, Graydon JE, et al. The prevalence and correlates of fatigue in patients receiving treatment with chemotherapy and radiotherapy. *Cancer Nurs* 1994;17:367–378.
91. Pickard-Holley S. Fatigue in the cancer patient. *Cancer Nurs* 1991;14:13–19.
92. Vogelzang NJ, Breitbart W, Cella D, et al. Patient, caregiver, and oncologist perceptions of cancer-related fatigue: results of a tripart assessment survey. The Fatigue Coalition. *Semin Hematol* 1997;34(Suppl 2):4–12.
93. Newling DW. The palliative therapy of advanced prostate cancer, with particular reference to the results of recent European clinical trials. *Br J Urol* 1997;79(Suppl 1):72–81.
94. Abels RI, Larholt DM, Drantz KD, et al. Recombinant human erythropoietin (r-HuEPO) for the treatment of the anemia of cancer. In: Murphy MJ, ed. *Blood cell growth factors: their present and future use in hematology and oncology*. Dayton, OH: AlphaMed Press.
95. Glaspy J, Bukowski R, Steinberg D, et al. The impact of therapy with epoetin alfa on clinical outcomes in patients with nonmyeloid malignancies during cancer chemotherapy in community oncology practice. *J Clin Oncol* 1997;15:1218–1234.
96. Krupp LB, Coyle PK, Doscher C, et al. Fatigue therapy in multiple sclerosis: a double-blind, randomized, parallel trial of amantadine, pemoline and placebo. *Neurology* 1995;45:1956–1961.
97. Ofman US. Disorders of sexuality and reproduction. In: Berger A, Portenoy R, Weissman D, eds. *Principles and practice of supportive oncology*. Philadelphia: Lippincott–Raven Publishers, 1998.

98. Zinreich ES, Derogatis LR, Herpst J, et al. Pretreatment evaluation of sexual function in patients with adenocarcinoma of the prostate. *Int J Radiat Oncol Biol Phys* 1990;19: 1001–1004.
99. Quinlan DM, Epstein JI, Carter S, et al. Sexual function following radical prostatectomy: influence of preservation of neurovascular bundles. *J Urol* 1991;145:998–1002.
100. Schover LR, Von Eschenbach AC. Sexual and marital relationships after treatment for prostate cancer. *Cancer* 1993;71(Suppl):1024.
101. Kedia S, Zippe CD, Agarwal A, et al. Treatment of erectile dysfunction with sildenafil citrate (Viagra) after radiation therapy for prostate cancer. *Urology* 1999;54:308–312.
102. Weber DC, Bieri S, Kurtz JM, et al. Prospective pilot study of sildenafil for treatment of postradiotherapy erectile dysfunction in patients with prostate cancer. *J Clin Oncol* 1999;17:3444–3449.
103. Vincent CE, Vincent B, Greiss FC, et al. Some marital-sexual concomitants of carcinoma of the cervix. *South Med J* 1975;68:52.
104. Schover LR, Randers-Pehrson M. *Sexuality and cancer for the man who has cancer and his partner*. New York: American Cancer Society, 1988.
105. Lipowski ZJ. Delirium (acute confusional states). *JAMA* 1987;258:1789–1792.
106. Pereira J, Hanson J, Bruera E. The frequency and clinical course of cognitive impairment in patients with terminal cancer. *Cancer* 1997;79:835–842.
107. Marcantonio ER, Juarez G, Goldman L, et al. The relationship of postoperative delirium with psychoactive medications. *JAMA* 1994;272:1518–1522.
108. Fainsinger RL, Tapper M, Bruera E. A perspective on the management of delirium in terminally ill patients on a palliative care unit. *J Palliat Care* 1993;9:4–8.
109. Breitbart W, Marotta R, Platt MM, et al. A double-blind trial of haloperidol, chlorpromazine, and lorazepam in the treatment of delirium in hospitalized AIDS patients. *Am J Psychiatry* 1996;153:231–237.
110. Brennan M. Lymphedema following the surgical treatment of breast cancer: a review of pathophysiology and treatment. *J Pain Sympt Manage* 1992;7:110–116.
111. Boris M, Weibdorf S, Lasinski PT, et al. Lymphedema reduction by noninvasive complex lymphedema therapy. *Oncology* 1994;8:95–106.
112. Karling P, Hammar M, Varenhorst E. Prevalence and duration of vasomotor symptoms after surgical or medical castration in men with prostatic carcinoma. *J Urol* 1994;152:1170–1173.
113. Kronenberg F. Hot flushes: epidemiology and physiology. *Ann N Y Acad Sci* 1990;592:52–86.
114. Cagnacci A, Melis GB, Soldani R, et al. Effect of sex steroids on body temperature in postmenopausal women. Role of endogenous opioids. *Life Sci* 1992;50:515–521.
115. Loprinzi CL, Michalak JC, Quella SK, et al. Megestrol acetate for the prevention of hot flushes. *N Engl J Med* 1994;331:347–352.
116. Goldberg RM, Loprinzi CL, O'Fallon JR, et al. Transdermal clonidine for ameliorating tamoxifen-induced hot flushes. *J Clin Oncol* 1994;12:155–158.
117. Smith JA Jr. A prospective comparison of treatments for symptomatic hot flushes following endocrine therapy for carcinoma of the prostate. *J Urol* 1994;152:132–134.
118. Atala A, Amin M, Harty JI. Diethylstilbestrol in treatment of postorchiectomy vasomotor symptoms and its relationship with serum follicle-stimulating hormone, luteinizing hormone, and testosterone. *Urology* 1992;39:108–110.
119. Hammar M, Frisk J, Grimas O, et al. Acupuncture treatment of vasomotor symptoms in men with prostatic carcinoma: a pilot study. *J Urol* 1999;161:852–856.
120. Payne DK, Massie MJ. Depression and anxiety. In: Merger A, Portenoy RK, Weissman DE, eds. *Principles and practice of supportive oncology*. Philadelphia: Lippincott–Raven Publishers, 1998:497–511.
121. Derogatis LR, Morrow GR, Fetting J, et al. The prevalence of psychiatric disorders among cancer patients. *JAMA* 1983;249:751.
122. Breitbart W. Suicide in cancer patients. *Oncology* 1987;1:49.
123. Woods SW, Tesar GE, Murray GB, et al. Psychostimulant treatment of depressive disorders secondary to medical illness. *J Clin Psychiatry* 1986;47:12.
124. Fernandez F, Adams F, Holmes VF, et al. Methylphenidate for depressive disorders in cancer patients. *Psychosomatics* 1987;28:455.
125. Chiarello RJ, Cole JO. The use of psychostimulants in general psychiatry: a reconsideration. *Arch Gen Psychiatry* 1987;44:286.
126. Holland JC. Anxiety and cancer: the patient and family. *J Clin Psychiatry* 1989;50:20–25.
127. Breitbart W, Chochinow HM, Passik S. Psychiatric aspects of palliative care. In: Doyle D, Hanks GWC, MacDonald N, eds. *Oxford textbook of palliative medicine*, 2nd ed. Oxford: Oxford Medical Publications, 1998:933–954.
128. Popkin MK, Callies AL, Mackenzie TB. The outcome of antidepressant use in the medically ill. *Arch General Psychiatry* 1985;42:1160–1163.

45

MANAGEMENT OF BONE METASTASES: EXTERNAL BEAM RADIATION THERAPY, RADIOPHARMACEUTICALS, AND BISPHOSPHONATES

MATTHEW R. SMITH
DONALD S. KAUFMAN

Skeletal complications are a major cause of morbidity for men with advanced prostate cancer. More than 80% of men with metastatic prostate cancer have radiographic evidence of bone involvement (1). A similar majority of men who die from prostate cancer has bone metastases at autopsy (2). The clinical manifestations of bone metastases include pain, spinal cord compression, fracture, and myelophthisis (3).

Prostate cancer is the only malignancy to form predominantly osteoblastic metastases (4,5). Bone metastases are categorized as osteolytic or osteoblastic based on their radiographic appearance. Both osteolytic and osteoblastic metastases, however, are characterized by increased bone resorption. Biochemical markers of bone resorption are increased in most men with osteoblastic metastases from prostate cancer (6–9). Bone biopsies from men with osteoblastic metastases demonstrate increased bone resorption in tumor-infiltrated bone, bone adjacent to bone metastases, and distant uninvolved bone (7,8). Androgen deprivation, the mainstay of treatment for metastatic prostate cancer, increases bone resorption and accelerates bone loss (10).

Reciprocal interactions between prostate cancer cells and bone stroma appear to account for the predominant skeletal localization of prostate cancer metastases and typical osteoblastic response (1,11). The bone extracellular matrix supports the adhesion of prostate cancer cells, and several bone-derived growth factors modulate prostate cancer growth and differentiation, including epidermal growth factor, transforming growth factor beta, and basic fibroblast growth factor. Prostate cancer cells produce growth factors that promote osteoblast growth, including insulinlike growth factors, bone morphogenic proteins, and endothelin-1 (12–14).

The primary clinical manifestation of bone metastases is pain. Pain may result from compression of the spinal cord or peripheral nerves, fracture, release of cytokines at the site of metastases, local action of neuropeptides on bone-associated nerves, and mechanical stretching of the periosteum (15,16). The major objectives of treatment for men with androgen-independent prostate cancer and symptomatic bone metastases are pain relief and improved quality of life. This chapter reviews the palliative management of bone metastases with radiation therapy, radiopharmaceuticals, and bisphosphonates.

EXTERNAL BEAM RADIATION THERAPY

Local Field Radiation

Retrospective studies have reported that local radiation therapy results in pain relief in approximately 80% of patients with bone metastases from various primary sites (15). The probability of pain relief for an individual patient appears to be influenced by baseline patient characteristics, primary site, methods of pain evaluation, and concurrent treatment.

The optimum dose and fractionation schedule for palliative radiation therapy have not been defined. Several prospective randomized studies of bone metastases from various primary sites have reached different conclusions about the relative benefit of high-dose fractionated therapy compared to single-dose or low-dose treatment (17–19).

In the Radiation Therapy Oncology Group study 74-02, 1,016 patients with painful bone metastases were randomized into various dose fractionation schedules (17). Patients with solitary bone metastases (26%) were randomized to 40.5 Gy in 15 fractions or 20 Gy in 5 fractions. Patients with multiple bone metastases (74%) were randomized to 30 Gy in 10 fractions, 15 Gy in 5 fractions, 20 Gy in 5 fractions, or 25 Gy in 5 fractions. Radiation therapy resulted in some pain relief in 90% of patients and complete pain relief in 54% of patients. The initial report concluded that all dose fractionation schedules resulted in equivalent palliative outcomes. The study was later reanalyzed by combining the solitary and multiple metastases groups and redefining benefits, based on pain scores, narcotic usage, and need for retreatment (18). In the reanalysis, high-dose–protracted treatment schedules were associated with higher response rates and lower rates of retreatment.

In a randomized prospective study at the Royal Marsden Hospital, 288 patients with painful bone metastases were randomized to a single fraction of 8 Gy or 30 Gy in 10 daily fractions (19). Primary tumor sites included breast (37%), lung (20%), and prostate (8%). Response was evaluated using pain questionnaires. There were no differences in survival, onset of pain relief, or duration of pain relief between the two treatment groups. Pain relief was independent of tumor histology.

In a retrospective review of 281 patients with painful bone metastases from various primary sites, local radiation therapy resulted in a 67% rate of complete pain relief (20). Complete pain relief was less common for metastases from renal cell carcinoma (p <.05) or non–small cell lung cancer (p = .06). Complete pain relief rates were otherwise independent of primary histology. Pain relief and duration of response were correlated with total radiation dose (p <.001). Among 47 men with metastatic prostate cancer, treatment with 40 Gy or greater resulted in 75% rate of complete pain relief, compared to 62% rate of complete pain relief for men treated with less than 40 Gy.

The dose and schedule of treatment should be influenced by the anticipated patient survival. Large (4 to 8 Gy) single fraction treatments are more convenient but associated with higher rates of retreatment. Accordingly, single fraction treatments may be appropriate for patients with relatively short life expectancies.

Wide-Field Radiation

Patients with multiple sites of painful bone metastases can be palliated with external beam radiation therapy to multiple local fields, wide-field radiation, or treatment with radiopharmaceuticals. Wide-field or hemibody radiation is administered in single or multiple fractions to the upper half, lower half, or middle segment of the body using a megavoltage radiation beam. Wide-field radiation results in pain relief in 60% to 80% of patients and complete pain relief in 20% to 25% of patients (21). The majority of patients report pain relief within 48 hours of treatment. Retreatment with wide-field radiation results in similar rates of pain relief and toxicity as the first course of treatment.

The optimum dose and fractionation schedule for palliative hemibody radiation are undefined. In a retrospective review of 26 men with androgen-independent prostate cancer, fractionated wide-field radiation therapy (25 to 30 Gy in 8 to 10 fractions) was associated with better palliation than single fraction wide-field radiation (6 Gy for the upper hemibody or 8 Gy for the lower hemibody segment) (22). Compared to single fraction treatment, fractionated wide-field radiation resulted in a longer median duration of pain relief (8.5 months vs. 2.8 months) and lower rates of retreatment within the targeted hemibody (13% vs. 71%). Treatment-related side effects were similar for both groups.

Adjuvant hemibody radiation reduces the requirement for retreatment within the targeted hemibody segment. In the Radiation Therapy Oncology Group study 82-06, 499 patients with various malignancies and painful bone metastases limited to one hemibody area were randomized to treatment with local radiation therapy (30 Gy in 10 daily fractions) with or without a single adjuvant 8-Gy fraction of hemibody radiation (23). Compared to local radiation therapy alone, treatment with local plus hemibody radiation resulted in improved time to disease progression and time to retreatment within the radiated hemibody segment. Among the 146 study participants with prostate cancer, treatment with local plus hemibody radiation resulted in a 31% reduction in the requirement for retreatment within the targeted hemibody (78% vs. 54%, p = .001) (24). Prostate cancer patients treated with local plus hemibody radiation had a better 1-year survival rate than patients treated with local radiation therapy without adjuvant hemibody radiation (44% vs. 33%, p = .165).

The side effects of wide-field radiation include nausea, vomiting, diarrhea, pancytopenia, and pulmonary toxicity. Severe complications have been reported in 2% to 8% of patients treated with wide-field radiation to the lower half of the body. Severe complications, including fatal pneumonitis, have been reported in 4% to 32% of patients treated with wide-field radiation to the upper body. Methods to reduce the toxicity of wide-field radiation include careful patient selection, limitation of lung dose, shielding previously radiated sites, and use of shaped fields to protect the viscera (15,24).

RADIOPHARMACEUTICALS

Background

Three radioisotopes are approved for the treatment of symptomatic bone metastases: phosphorus-32 (^{32}P), strontium-89 (^{89}St) chloride, and samarium-153 (^{153}Sm). These radioisotopes share three important characteristics (Table 45-1). First, they are preferentially incorporated into bone. Second, therapeutic activity results from emission of low-energy electrons (beta emission). Third, they accumulate in bone metastases and other sites of active bone turnover. In contrast to the other approved agents, ^{153}Sm has a relatively short beta emission half-life (46 hours), and gamma emission is appropriate for imaging and prospective dose estimation.

TABLE 45-1. PROPERTIES OF SELECTED RADIONUCLIDES

Radionuclide	Emission	Decay energy (MeV)	Half-life (days)
Phosphorus-32	Beta	1.71	14.2
Strontium-89	Beta	1.49	50.6
Samarium-153	Beta	0.81	1.93
	Gamma	0.10	
Rhenium-186	Beta	1.07	3.88
	Gamma	0.14	
Rhenium-188	Beta	2.12	0.70

MeV, megavolt.

Rhenium-186 (^{186}Re) and rhenium-188 (^{188}Re) are investigational radioisotopes. ^{186}Re is similar to ^{153}Sm, with a relatively short beta emission half-life (91 hours) and gamma emission suitable for imaging and dose estimation. ^{188}Re is distinguished by a very short beta emission half-life (17 hours).

^{32}P orthophosphates enter all metabolic pathways. Because the skeleton contains the largest phosphate pool, more ^{32}P orthophosphates are incorporated in the skeleton than other metabolically active sites, including the bone marrow and liver. Newer radioisotopes are selectively incorporated into bone, and approximately one-half of an intravenously administered dose accumulates in the skeleton. Because calcium competes with radioisotopes for skeletal uptake, calcium-containing medications should be discontinued before treatment. Unincorporated radioisotopes are cleared in the urine, and treatment for patients with urinary incontinence requires special precautions.

There have been no comparative studies with different radioisotopes, although the pain response rates and patterns of pain relief with different radioisotopes appear similar (25). The major toxicity of radioisotope treatment is myelosuppression. Because newer radioisotopes are not incorporated into hematopoietic stem cells, they may have less hematologic toxicity than ^{32}P.

The mechanisms of pain relief after radioisotope treatment are poorly understood. Objective biochemical or radiographic responses are rare (25). Patients often experience marked pain relief within several days of treatment, further suggesting that symptomatic responses are mediated by an indirect mechanism.

Clinical Experience

^{32}P-labeled orthophosphates have been used to treat bone metastases from prostate cancer for several decades (26,27). Most patients have been treated with multiple daily injections and concurrent parathyroid hormone or testosterone to increase bone uptake. Most studies reported pain relief for the majority of patients, although small sample size and problems with methodology complicate interpretation. The efficacy of treatment with ^{32}P-labeled phosphates has never been evaluated in a randomized study. The dose-limiting toxicity of ^{32}P treatment is myelosuppression. Concerns about toxicity have limited the clinical use of ^{32}P-labeled orthophosphates.

The palliative effects of ^{89}St have been extensively evaluated in phase II studies of men with androgen-independent prostate cancer and symptomatic bone metastases. The primary outcome measure in most of these studies was pain relief. The reported rates of complete or partial pain relief vary from 0% to 82% (25). The wide range of clinical responses may be related to the small sample sizes and variable response definitions for individual studies. In addition, the variability in response rates may be related to differences in the volume of metastatic disease among different study populations. In a multicentered study of 83 men with prostate cancer, response rates were reported according to estimated volume of metastatic disease on pretreatment bone scan (28). Symptomatic responses were observed in 78% of men with minimal metastatic disease, compared to only 42% of men with extensive bone metastases.

Three randomized studies of ^{89}St have been reported (29–31). In a small, double-blind study, 32 men with androgen-independent prostate cancer and painful bone metastases were randomized to ^{89}St [150 megabecquerel (MBq)] or nonradioactive strontium chloride (29). Twenty-six men were evaluable. Treatment with ^{89}St resulted in significantly higher pain response rates. Complete pain responses were observed only in men treated with ^{89}St.

The United Kingdom study directly compared the palliative effects of ^{89}St to external beam radiation therapy (30). Men with androgen-independent prostate cancer and painful bone metastases were stratified as appropriate candidates for local field radiotherapy (148 patients) or hemibody radiotherapy (157 patients). Men were then randomized to radiotherapy or ^{89}St (200 MBq). Study end points included pain at the index skeletal site, appearance of new painful sites, requirement for additional palliative radiotherapy, and survival. Both comparisons (local field radiotherapy vs. ^{89}St and hemibody radiotherapy vs. ^{89}St) demonstrated that radiotherapy and ^{89}St were equally effective for controlling pain at index sites, although significantly fewer ^{89}St-treated men developed new painful sites ($p < .05$). Compared to local radiotherapy, significantly fewer ^{89}St-treated men required radiotherapy to painful bone metastases ($p < .01$). ^{89}St treatment was associated with less gastrointestinal toxicity and more hematologic toxicity than radiotherapy. There were no differences in survival.

The TransCanada study evaluated the role of adjuvant ^{89}St after local external beam radiotherapy (31). One hundred twenty-six men with androgen-independent prostate cancer and painful bony metastases were treated with local external beam radiotherapy and then randomized to adjuvant ^{89}St (400 MBq) or placebo. Study end points included pain at the index skeletal site, appearance of new painful sites, need for additional palliative therapy, prostate-specific antigen response, survival, and quality of life. Both treatment groups had similar pain control at the irradiated index site. More ^{89}St-treated men were pain free (40% vs. 23%), and fewer required analgesics (2.4% vs. 17.1%). ^{89}St treatment resulted in significantly fewer new sites of bone pain (0.59 vs. 1.21, $p < .002$) and prolonged time to next external beam radiotherapy treatment by a median of 15 weeks. There was no difference in survival.

^{153}Sm chelated to ethylenediamine tetramethylene phosphonic acid, termed *^{153}Sm lexidronam*, is approved for the treatment of osteoblastic bone metastases. Phase I/II studies of men with androgen-independent prostate cancer have reported complete or partial relief of pain in the majority of patients (25). As with other radioisotopes, the dose-limiting toxicity of ^{153}Sm is myelosuppression (32,33). Platelet counts decline starting 2 weeks after administration, and the platelet nadir occurs at 3 to 4 weeks after administration.

^{153}Sm lexidronam has been compared to placebo in two unpublished randomized studies (34). In the first study, 118 patients with androgen-independent prostate cancer (n = 80) or other primary tumor (n = 38) and symptomatic osteoblastic metastases were randomized to a single intravenous dose of ^{153}Sm lexidronam (0.5 or 1.0 mCi per kg) or placebo. Compared to placebo, treatment with the higher dose of ^{153}Sm lexidronam (1 mCi per kg) resulted in statistically significant decreases in pain scores in the third and fourth weeks after treatment. In the second study, 152 men with androgen-independent prostate cancer were randomized to ^{153}Sm lexidronam (1.0 mCi per kg) or placebo. Treatment with ^{153}Sm lexidronam resulted in statistically significant decreases in pain scores in the second, third, and fourth weeks. No study has compared ^{153}Sm to external beam radiation therapy or other radioisotopes.

^{186}Re was compared with placebo in a double-blind crossover study (35). Treatment with ^{186}Re resulted in significantly greater decreases in pain scores than placebo. ^{186}Re has not undergone further development because of similarity to other marketed radioisotopes. In contrast, with a very short beta emission half-life (17 hours), ^{188}Re is an attractive candidate for evaluation in combination and dose intense therapy. In a phase I study, treatment with ^{188}Re resulted in decreased pain in five of eight men with androgen-independent prostate cancer (36).

BISPHOSPHONATES

Background

Bisphosphonates are a major therapeutic advance in the management of osteolytic bone disease (37). Treatment with bisphosphonates reduces skeletal morbidity from multiple myeloma and breast cancer with osteolytic bone metastases.

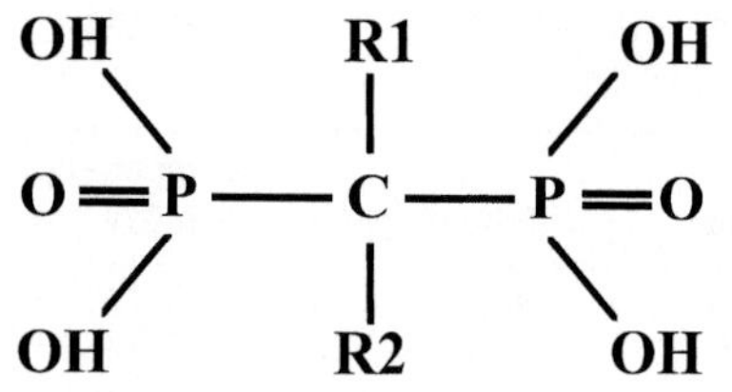

```
OH          R1         OH
  \         |         /
O=P ------- C ------- P=O
  /         |         \
OH          R2         OH
```

FIGURE 45-1. General chemical structure of a bisphosphonate.

For women with high-risk localized breast cancer, adjuvant treatment with bisphosphonates appears to prevent the development of bone metastases and improve survival (38). This section reviews the potential role of bisphosphonates in the management of osteoblastic metastases from prostate cancer.

Bisphosphonates are synthetic analogs of pyrophosphate, characterized by a phosphorus-carbon-phosphorus backbone that renders them resistant to hydrolysis (Fig. 45-1). The properties of bisphosphonates are determined by the R1 and R2 carbon side chains (39). Most bisphosphonates contain a hydroxyl group at the R1 position that confers high-affinity binding to calcium phosphate. The R2 side chain is the critical determinant of antiresorptive potency (Table 45-2).

Bisphosphonates inhibit normal and pathologic bone resorption by multiple mechanisms. They directly inhibit osteoclast activity by cellular mechanisms that affect osteoclast attachment to bone, osteoclast precursor differentiation, and osteoclast survival (39). Bisphosphonates also reduce osteoclast activity indirectly through effects on osteoblasts. Bisphosphonates increase osteoblast secretion of an inhibitor of osteoclast recruitment (40). They also increase osteoblast secretion of transforming growth factor beta, a signal for osteoclast apoptosis (41).

The growth of bone metastases involves reciprocal interactions between tumor cells and metabolically active bone (3,42). Bisphosphonates may interrupt these interactions by inhibiting local production of bone-derived growth factors. The anticancer activity of bisphosphonates may also involve modification of the bone surface, inhibition of specific enzymatic pathways, and induction of tumor cell apoptosis (42).

Bisphosphonate treatment decreases bone resorption in men with prostate cancer. Serial histomorphometry of bone and measurement of biochemical markers of osteoclast activity indicate that treatment with intravenous pamidronate mark-

TABLE 45-2. PROPERTIES OF SELECTED BISPHOSPHONATES

Drug	Trade name	R1 side chain	R2 side chain	Relative potency
Etidronate	Didronel	–OH	$-CH_3$	1
Clodronate	Ostac	$-C1_2$	$-C1_2$	10
Pamidronate	Aredia	–OH	$-(CH_2)_2NH_2$	100
Zoledronate	Zometa	–OH	$-CH_2N$–(ring, N)	10,000

TABLE 45-3. PROSPECTIVE STUDIES OF BISPHOSPHONATES FOR METASTATIC PROSTATE CANCER

Study (reference)	Study design	n	Treatment	Results
Italy (51)	Phase II	17	Intravenous clodronate followed by oral maintenance	Decreased pain and analgesic use in 10 of 17 men
United States (52)	Phase II	12	Intravenous etidronate followed by oral maintenance	Decreased pain and analgesic use in 10 of 12 men
United Kingdom (44)	Phase II	25	Intravenous pamidronate	Ten of 17 men pain free at study completion
Netherlands (51)	Phase II	28	Intravenous olpodronate followed by oral maintenance	Decreased pain and analgesic use in 21 of 28 men
Finland (53)	Phase II	16	Intravenous clodronate followed by oral maintenance	Decreased pain in 9 of 16 men
Italy (54)	Sequential phase III	56	Intravenous clodronate, placebo, oral clodronate, intravenous clodronate with or without oral maintenance	Men treated with intravenous clodronate had better pain relief and decreased analgesic usage, oral maintenance associated with more durable responses
Finland (55)	Phase III	75	Estramustine plus oral clodronate vs. estramustine alone	Greater proportion of clodronate-treated men discontinued analgesics, 38% vs. 18%
United States (56)	Phase III double-blind	57	Intravenous etidronate followed by oral maintenance vs. placebo	No differences in pain or analgesic use

edly inhibits bone resorption (43,44). Similar results have been reported with oral clodronate and olpadronate (45,46).

Bisphosphonates have potent anticancer activity in preclinical models of prostate cancer. Bisphosphonates inhibit adhesion of prostate cancer cells to mineralized and unmineralized bone extracellular matrix *in vitro* (47). In rat models of prostate cancer, treatment with bisphosphonates prevents or delays the development of bone metastases (48–50).

Clinical Experience

Several phase II clinical trials of bisphosphonates for men with prostate cancer and symptomatic bone metastases have been reported (44,46,51–53) (Table 45-3). In each study, pain or analgesic use, or both, decreased in the majority of patients. Markers of bone resorption were elevated in 50% to 80% of men at study entry (44,46,53). Bisphosphonate treatment resulted in significant decreases in bone resorption markers.

Three randomized phase III clinical studies of bisphosphonates for men with androgen-independent prostate cancer and symptomatic bone metastases have been reported (54–56) (Table 45-3). In an Italian study, a total of 56 men were treated in a series of small single-blind randomized comparisons (54). Bone pain was evaluated using a visual analog scale and daily analgesic consumption. In the first comparison, 13 men were randomly assigned to daily intravenous clodronate or placebo for 2 weeks. Pain scores and daily analgesic use were markedly decreased in the clodronate-treated group. In a second comparison, 24 men were assigned to oral daily clodronate (1,200 mg) for 2 weeks or daily intravenous clodronate (300 mg) for 2 weeks. Oral clodronate was ineffective. Intravenous clodronate resulted in transient improvements in pain scores and daily analgesic use. In a subsequent comparison, men were randomly assigned to daily intravenous clodronate (300 mg) for 2 weeks with or without oral daily clodronate (1,200 mg) as maintenance therapy. Bone pain and analgesic use were equivalent in both groups.

In a Finnish study, 75 men were randomly assigned to oral clodronate (3,200 mg daily for 1 month followed by 1,600 mg daily) or placebo (55). All men were treated with daily oral estramustine phosphate. Primary study end points were pain score and analgesic usage. Decreased pain was observed in both treatment groups. More clodronate-treated men discontinued analgesic use (38% vs. 18%), although this difference was not significant. Side effects were uncommon and equivalent between the treatment groups. There was no difference in median survival. Small sample size and poor bioavailability of oral clodronate flawed the study.

In an American study, 57 men with prostate cancer and bone pain requiring analgesics were randomly assigned to placebo or etidronate (7.5 mg intravenously daily for 3 days, then 400 mg by mouth daily) (56). There were no significant differences in pain scores or analgesic use between the two treatment groups. Etidronate is now considered pharmacologically unsuitable for the treatment of bone metastases because of its low antiresorptive potency and inhibition of normal bone mineralization (57).

Several ongoing, large randomized studies will evaluate the effect of intravenous bisphosphonates on pain, analgesic use, skeletal-related events, and quality of life. National Cancer Institute of Canada-Protocol 6 is a randomized comparison of mitoxantrone and prednisone with or without intravenous clodronate for men with symptomatic bone metastases. Primary study end points include bone pain, quality of life, and survival. Novartis 032 is a multicentered randomized comparison of pamidronate (90 mg intravenously every 3 weeks) or placebo for men with androgen-independent prostate cancer and bone metastases requiring narcotic analgesics. Primary study end points are pain, daily analgesic use, and skeletal-related events. Novartis 039 is a multicentered randomized comparison of zoledronate (4 or 8 mg intravenously every 3 weeks) or placebo for men with androgen-independent prostate cancer and asymptomatic or minimally symptomatic bone metastases. The primary study end point is the proportion of men with any skeletal-related events during the first 15 months of study.

CONCLUSION

Local field radiation therapy results in palliative benefit for most patients with symptomatic bone metastases. The optimum dose and fractionation schedule are undefined, although high-dose protracted treatment schedules appear to result in higher response rates and lower rates of retreatment. Wide-field radiation also provides palliative benefit for most men with symptomatic bone metastases and reduces the need for subsequent palliative radiation within the treated hemibody segment. Wide-field radiation therapy is rarely used because of high toxicity rates and availability of other options for managing multiple bone metastases, including radiopharmaceuticals and conventional radiation therapy to multiple fields.

Treatment with radioisotopes decreases pain in most men with androgen-independent prostate cancer and symptomatic bone metastases. Pain response rates and patterns of pain relief with different radioisotopes appear similar. Optimal criteria for patient selection and timing of treatment remain undefined. Radioisotope therapy in combination with other treatment modalities has not been adequately evaluated.

Available evidence suggests that bisphosphonate treatment may decrease bone pain for most men with symptomatic bone metastases. Ongoing large randomized studies will evaluate the effect of newer and more potent bisphosphonates on pain, analgesic use, and skeletal-related events in men with androgen-independent prostate cancer. Future clinical trials are needed to evaluate adjuvant bisphosphonate treatment for prevention of bone metastases among men with high-risk nonmetastatic prostate cancer.

REFERENCES

1. Stamey TA, McNeal JE. In: Walsh PC, Retik AB, Stamey TA, et al., eds. *Campbell's urology*, 6th ed. Philadelphia: Saunders, 1992:1159–1199.
2. Harada M, Iida M, Yamaguchi M, et al. Analysis of bone metastasis of prostatic adenocarcinoma in 137 autopsy cases. *Adv Exp Med Biol* 1992;324:173–182.
3. Scher HI, Chung WK. Bone metastasis: improving the therapeutic index. *Semin Oncol* 1994;21:630–656.
4. Jacobs SC. Spread of prostatic carcinoma to the bone. *Urology* 1983;21:337–344.
5. Zetter BR. The cellular basis for site-specific tumor metastases. *N Engl J Med* 1990;322:605–612.
6. Percival RC, Urwin GH, Watson ME. Biochemical and histological evidence that carcinoma of the prostate is associated with increased bone resorption. *Eur J Surg Oncol* 1987;113:41–49.
7. Clarke NW, McClure J, George NJ. Morphometric evidence for bone resorption and replacement in prostate cancer. *Br J Urol* 1991;68:74–80.
8. Clarke NW, McClure J, George NJ. Osteoblast function and osteomalacia in metastatic prostate cancer. *Eur Urol* 1993;24:286–290.
9. Coleman RE, Houston S, James I, et al. Preliminary results of use of urinary excretion of Pyridium cross-links for monitoring bone disease. *Br J Cancer* 1992;73:1089–1095.
10. Smith MR. Androgen deprivation and osteoporosis. *Prostate J* 1999;1:161–164.
11. Mundy GR. Mechanisms of bone metastasis. *Cancer* 1997; 80(8 Suppl):1546–1556.
12. Ware J. Growth factors and their receptors as determinants in the proliferation and metastasis human prostate cancer. *Cancer Metastasis Rev* 1993;12:287–301.
13. Battistini B, Chailler P, D'Orleans-Juste P, et al. Growth regulatory properties of the endothelins. *Peptides* 1993;14:385–399.
14. Peehl DM, Cohen P, Rosenfeld RG. The insulin-like growth factor system in the prostate. *World J Urol* 1995;13:306–311.
15. Nielsen OS, Munro AJ, Tannock IF. Bone metastases: pathophysiology and management policy. *J Clin Oncol* 1991; 9:509–524.
16. Mertens WC, Filipczak LA, Ben-Josef E, et al. Systemic bone-seeking radionuclides for palliation of painful osseous metastases: current concepts. *CA Cancer J Clin* 1998;48: 361–374.
17. Tong D, Gillick L, Hendrickson FR. The palliation of symptomatic osseous metastases: final results of the Study by the Radiation Therapy Oncology Group. *Cancer* 1982; 50:893–899.
18. Blitzer PH. Reanalysis of the RTOG study of the palliation of symptomatic osseous metastasis. *Cancer* 1985;55:1468–1472.
19. Price P, Hoskin PJ, Easton D, et al. Prospective randomised trial of single and multifraction radiotherapy schedules in the treatment of painful bony metastases. *Radiother Oncol* 1986;6:247–255.
20. Arcangeli G, Micheli A, Arcangeli G, et al. The responsiveness of bone metastases to radiotherapy: the effect of site, histology and radiation dose on pain relief. *Radiother Oncol* 1989;14:95–101.
21. Ciezki J, Macklis RM. The palliative role of radiotherapy in the management of the cancer patient. *Semin Oncol* 1995; 22(Suppl 3):82–90.
22. Zelefsky MJ, Scher HI, Forman JD, et al. Palliative hemiskeletal irradiation for widespread metastatic prostate cancer: a comparison of single dose and fractionated regimens. *Int J Radiat Oncol Biol Phys* 1989;17:1281–1285.
23. Poulter CA, Cosmatos D, Rubin P, et al. A report of RTOG 8206: a phase III study of whether the addition of single

dose hemibody irradiation to standard fractionated local field irradiation is more effective than local field irradiation alone in the treatment of symptomatic osseous metastases. *Int J Radiat Oncol Biol Phys* 1992;23:207–214.

24. Ratanatharathorn V, Powers WE. Role of radiation therapy in the management of hormone-refractory metastatic prostate cancer. In: Vogelzang NJ, Scardino PT, Shipley WU, et al., eds. *Comprehensive textbook of genitourinary oncology.* Baltimore, MD: Williams & Wilkins, 1996:891–897.
25. Mertens WC, Filipczak LA, Ben-Josef E, et al. Systemic bone-seeking radionuclides for palliation of painful osseous metastases: current concepts. *CA Cancer J Clin* 1998;48: 361–374.
26. Van Norstrand D, Silberstein EB. Therapeutic uses of 32P. In: Freeman LM, Weissman HS, eds. *Nuclear medicine annual 1985.* New York: Raven Press, 1985:289–344.
27. Silberstein EB. The treatment of painful osseous metastases with phosphorus-32-labeled phosphates. *Semin Oncol* 1993;20(Suppl 2):10–21.
28. Laing AH, Ackery DM, Bayly RJ, et al. Strontium-89 chloride for pain palliation in prostatic skeletal malignancy. *Br J Radiol* 1991;64:816–822.
29. Lewington VJ, McEwan AJ, Ackery DM, et al. A prospective, randomised double-blind crossover study to examine the efficacy of strontium-89 in pain palliation in patients with advanced prostate cancer metastatic to bone. *Eur J Cancer* 1991;27:954–958.
30. Quilty PM, Kirk D, Bolger JJ, et al. A comparison of the palliative effects of strontium-89 and external beam radiotherapy in metastatic prostate cancer. *Radiother Oncol* 1994;31:33–40.
31. Porter AT, McEwan AJ, Powe JE, et al. Results of a randomized phase-III trial to evaluate the efficacy of strontium-89 adjuvant to local field external beam irradiation in the management of endocrine resistant metastatic prostate cancer. *Int J Radiat Oncol Biol Phys* 1993;25:805–813.
32. Turner JH, Claringbold PG, Hetherington EL, et al. A phase I study of samarium-153 ethylenediaminetetramethylene phosphonate therapy for disseminated skeletal metastases. *J Clin Oncol* 1989;7:1926–1931.
33. Bayouth JE, Macey DJ, Kasi LP, et al. Dosimetry and toxicity of samarium-153-EDTMP administered for bone pain due to skeletal metastases. *J Nucl Med* 1994;35:63–69.
34. Anonymous. Samarium-153 lexidronam for painful bone metastases. *Med Lett Drugs Ther* 1997;39:83–84.
35. Maxon HR 3rd, Schroder LE, Hertzberg VS, et al. Rhenium-186(Sn)HEDP for treatment of painful osseous metastases: results of a double-blind crossover comparison with placebo. *J Nucl Med* 1991;32:1877–1881.
36. Maxon HR 3rd, Schroder LE, Washburn LC, et al. Rhenium-188(Sn)HEDP for treatment of osseous metastases. *J Nucl Med* 1998;39:659–663.
37. Body JJ, Bard P, Burckhardt P, et al. Current use of bisphosphonates in oncology. *J Clin Oncol* 1998;16:3890–3899.
38. Diel IJ, Solomayer EF, Costa SD, et al. Reduction in new metastases in breast cancer with adjuvant clodronate treatment. *N Engl J Med* 1998;339:357–363.
39. Rogers MJ, Watts DJ, Russell RG. Overview of bisphosphonates. *Cancer* 1997;80(8 Suppl):1652–1660.
40. Vitte C, Fleisch H, Guenther HL. Bisphosphonates induce osteoblasts to secrete an inhibitor of osteoclast-mediated resorption. *Endocrinology* 1996;137:2324–2333.
41. Hughes DE, Wright KR, Uy HL, et al. Bisphosphonates promote apoptosis in murine osteoclasts in vitro and in vivo. *J Bone Miner Res* 1995;10:1478–1487.
42. Mundy GR, Yoneda T. Bisphosphonates as anticancer drugs. *N Engl J Med* 1998;339:398–400.
43. Clarke NW, Holbrook IB, McClure J, et al. Osteoclast inhibition by pamidronate in metastatic prostate cancer: a preliminary study. *Br J Cancer* 1991;63:420–423.
44. Clarke NW, McClure J, George NJ. Disodium pamidronate identifies differential osteoclastic bone resorption in metastatic prostate cancer. *Br J Urol* 1992;69:64–70.
45. Kylmala T, Tammela T, Risteli L, et al. Evaluation of the effect of oral clodronate on skeletal metastases with type 1 collagen metabolites. A controlled trial of the Finnish Prostate Cancer Group. *Eur J Cancer* 1993;29A:821–825.
46. Pelger RC, Hamdy NA, Zwinderman AH, et al. Effects of the bisphosphonate olpadronate in patients with carcinoma of the prostate metastatic to the skeleton. *Bone* 1998;22:403–408.
47. Boissier S, Magnetto S, Frappart L, et al. Bisphosphonates inhibit prostate and breast carcinoma cell adhesion to unmineralized and mineralized bone extracellular matrices. *Cancer Res* 1997;57:3890–3894.
48. Pollard M, Luckert PH. Effect of dichloromethylene diphosphonate on the osteolytic and osteoplastic effects of rat prostate adenocarcinoma cells. *J Natl Cancer Inst* 1985; 75:949–954.
49. Sun YC, Geldof AA, Newling DW, et al. Progression delay of prostate tumor skeletal metastasis effects by bisphosphonates. *J Urol* 1992;148:1270–1273.
50. Stearns ME, Wang M. Effects of alendronate and Taxol on PC-3 ML cell bone metastases in SCID mice. *Invasion Metastasis* 1996;16:116–131.
51. Adami S, Salvagno G, Guarrera G, et al. Dichloromethylene-diphosphonate in patients with prostatic carcinoma metastatic to the skeleton. *J Urol* 1985;134:1152–1154.
52. Carey PO, Lippert MC. Treatment of painful prostatic bone metastases with oral etidronate disodium. *Urology* 1998; 32:403–407.
53. Kylmala T, Tammela TL, Lindholm TS, et al. The effect of combined intravenous and oral clodronate treatment on bone pain in patients with metastatic prostate cancer. *Ann Chir Gynaecol* 1994;83:316–319.
54. Adami S, Mian M. Clodronate therapy of metastatic bone disease in patients with prostatic carcinoma. *Recent Results Cancer Res* 1989;116:67–72.
55. Elomaa I, Kylmala T, Tammela T, et al. Effect of oral clodronate on bone pain. A controlled study in patients with metastatic prostatic cancer. *Int Urol Nephrol* 1992;24:159–166.
56. Smith JA Jr. Palliation of painful bone metastases from prostate cancer using sodium etidronate: results of a randomized, prospective, double-blind, placebo-controlled study. *J Urol* 1989;141:85–87.
57. Bloomfield DJ. Should bisphosphonates be part of standard therapy of patients with multiple myeloma or bone metastases from other cancers? An evidence-based review. *J Clin Oncol* 1998;16:1218–1225.

46

HEMATOLOGIC COMPLICATIONS OF PROSTATE CANCER

WILLIAM K. OH

Patients with advanced prostate cancer often experience hematologic complications that can have clinical as well as prognostic significance. In spite of a long-standing recognition of its existence, this relationship between blood and coagulation disorders and prostate cancer has been relatively neglected, despite important strides in other areas of prostate cancer research. Anemia is the most common hematologic abnormality in this group. Many causes of anemia can be seen in association with prostate cancer and need to be clearly distinguished so that appropriate management can be instituted. In particular, anemia associated with androgen withdrawal is unique to patients with advanced prostate cancer. Treatment options for anemia generally are directed at the underlying etiology but may also include blood transfusions or recombinant human erythropoietin. Leukopenia and thrombocytopenia are often related to therapy for advanced prostate cancer and can have profound implications for the patient. Finally, coagulation disorders and, in particular, disseminated intravascular coagulation (DIC) have been associated with prostate cancer for many years, although questions remain about the prevalence of this problem and its underlying mechanism.

ANEMIA

Anemia is a frequent complication of advanced prostate cancer (1). As is the case with cancer-related anemia in general, few studies have evaluated the impact of anemia on the clinical course of patients with hormone-refractory prostate cancer. It is a generally accepted practice that transfusions are given to cancer patients whose hemoglobin or hematocrit values fall below an institutionally defined point. Guidelines have been issued by several groups that generally recommend a threshold hemoglobin of 8 g per dL for transfusion, although a higher threshold of 10 g per dL has been advocated for patients with a history of ischemic heart disease (2). Although exceptions are made to this rule in individual circumstances, the rationale for transfusion of packed red blood cells had followed this paradigm independent of how the patient feels and in the absence of sufficient data to support such an approach. More recently, the availability of a new therapeutic option for cancer patients with anemia—erythropoietin—has opened the door to reconsideration of the parameters by which clinicians treat anemia (3).

Causes of Anemia in Prostate Cancer Patients

Anemia may be secondary to the cancer itself, therapy for the cancer, or an unrelated cause (4) (Table 46-1). Therefore, an investigation into the cause of anemia in a prostate cancer patient should be the same as for any patient. Various methods have been proposed to classify anemias to arrive at the correct diagnosis. A modern approach to classify anemia first distinguishes between patients with decreased red cell production (bone marrow failure) and increased red cell production (acute blood loss and hemolysis) (5). Patients with bone marrow failure constitute the majority of patients with anemia, have a low reticulocyte count, and are further classified based on red cell size. Microcytic anemias (mean corpuscular volume less than 80 fL) include iron deficiency and thalassemias, and macrocytic anemias (mean corpuscular volume greater than 100 fL) include vitamin B_{12} and folate deficiency, myelodysplasia, hypothyroidism, and liver disease. Normocytic anemias may include anemia of chronic disease, liver and renal disease, and primary diseases of the bone marrow. Anemia associated with increased red cell production includes the hemolytic anemias and anemia due to acute blood loss. Evaluation of the peripheral smear in the diagnosis of anemia is a simple procedure that can sometimes yield a diagnosis. Although any possible etiology for anemia may exist in prostate cancer patients, the most common are discussed below.

Iron Deficiency Anemia

Iron deficiency anemia in cancer patients may be related to inadequate iron absorption but more often is associated

TABLE 46-1. POTENTIAL CAUSES OF ANEMIA IN PROSTATE CANCER

Iron deficiency anemia
Bleeding
Malnutrition
Anemia of chronic disease
Anemia related to hormonal therapy
Megaloblastic anemia
B_{12} or folate deficiency
Leukoerythroblastic anemia
Pure red cell aplasia
Hemolytic anemia
Autoimmune
Microangiopathy

with chronic blood loss from the gastrointestinal and genitourinary tracts. In patients with prostate cancer, sources of bleeding include those directly related to the cancer, as well as those related to therapies directed at cancer. For instance, gastritis or peptic ulcer disease may cause occult upper gastrointestinal bleeding in patients treated for pain with aspirin or nonsteroidal antiinflammatory drugs. Direct extension of prostate cancer into the colon or rectum occurs on occasion and may be associated with bright red blood per rectum. Another possible source of bleeding is the bladder, although significant bleeding is seldom occult. Hematuria is rare as a presenting sign for prostate cancer but can be seen in some patients with locally advanced cancers. Other causes of iron deficiency should be considered as well, even in prostate cancer patients. Unrelated etiologies, including second cancers in the colon or kidney and malabsorption disorders, should be ruled out in the appropriate clinical setting (6).

The diagnosis of iron deficiency anemia can be confirmed in several ways. The peripheral blood smear generally shows hypochromic microcytes as well as pencil-shaped red blood cells. A low serum iron and total iron-binding capacity is characteristic of the diagnosis, as is a low serum ferritin (i.e., less than 10 µg per L). A bone marrow biopsy is pathognomonic in patients with anemia if iron stains are negative. In anemia of chronic disease and beta thalassemia, both of which are in the differential diagnosis for iron deficiency anemia, a bone marrow biopsy demonstrates normal staining for iron stores.

Treatment of iron deficiency must initially be directed toward the underlying cause of the anemia. Replacement of iron without further investigation of the source of iron loss can be potentially dangerous. Oral iron replacement is generally the most acceptable means to replenish iron stores. Ferrous sulfate at a dose of 325 mg given from one to three times a day is recommended (7). The most common side effects of this preparation include nausea and constipation. Parenteral forms of iron are available but are rarely needed in cancer patients. Blood transfusions are also a good source of iron and can be used in advanced prostate cancer patients who are iron deficient (2).

Anemia of Chronic Disease

Many chronic disorders have been associated with this anemia (8). Inflammatory diseases, such as rheumatoid arthritis and inflammatory bowel disease, were originally described in association with this anemia, but it was later appreciated that cancer and chemotherapy can lead to anemia of chronic disease. It has since been discovered that a defining characteristic of these disparate disease processes is a disproportionately low serum erythropoietin level for a given level of hemoglobin (9).

Usually characterized by a mild to moderate decrease in hemoglobin, anemia of chronic disease can be microcytic or normocytic. In addition, bone marrow iron stores usually are normal or high. The underlying mechanism is believed to be abnormal iron metabolism, which is associated with a shortened red-cell life span (8). There is rapid turnover of iron, with low serum iron and total iron-binding capacity levels. Ferritin levels typically are normal or elevated.

The diagnosis of anemia of chronic disease is often made by the exclusion of other disorders. Bone marrow biopsies are rarely necessary but can rule out iron deficiency. Determining serum erythropoietin levels is not of clinical benefit in cancer patients, because these values are not predictive of the efficacy of treatment. Cisplatin chemotherapy is classically associated with a normocytic normochromic anemia and is also associated with a relative lack of erythropoietin (10). Anemia related to hormonal ablation therapy is discussed in greater detail later. Therapy for anemia of chronic disease is generally directed toward the underlying chronic disorder. Red blood cell transfusions and recombinant human erythropoietin can both be considered in this setting.

Anemia Related to Hormonal Therapy for Prostate Cancer

Androgens have been known for many years to stimulate erythropoiesis. In fact, androgens have been used to treat aplastic anemia and anemia of end-stage renal disease. The mechanism for this effect may be through direct activation of erythroid precursors in the bone marrow or through activation of erythropoietin (11). Although anemia has been a well-described negative prognostic factor for survival in advanced prostate cancer (12), the reason for such an association has never been fully understood. One important association, which is unique to prostate cancer patients, is the effect of hormonal therapy on hemoglobin, a subject only recently explored in greater detail.

Bilateral orchiectomy has been used as a therapeutic maneuver for metastatic prostate cancer since 1941. A report from 1948 described hormonal effects in six imprisoned men castrated involuntarily for their crimes. Serum testosterone levels fell to castrate levels within 10 days, while mean hemoglobin concentrations fell by 1 g per dL within 40 days (13) (Table 46-2). More recently, 187 patients who had bilateral orchiectomy for prostate cancer

TABLE 46-2. EFFECT OF HORMONAL THERAPY ON HEMOGLOBIN

Type of hormone therapy	n	Drugs	Duration	Mean drop in hemoglobin (g/dL)	Reference
Orchiectomy	6	None	40 d	1	13
Orchiectomy	64	None	60 d	1.2	14
LHRH agonist	7	Nafarelin	6 mo	1.1	16
LHRH agonist	25	Leuprolide, 3.75 mg q mo	6 mo	0.8	17
CAB plus XRT	131	Goserelin, 3.6 mg q mo	2 mo	1.6	18
		Flutamide, 250 mg t.i.d.	4 mo	2.8	
CAB	133	Mixed, most had leuprolide, 7.5 mg q mo	3 mo	1.8	1
		Flutamide, 250 t.i.d.	5.6 mo	2.5 (maximum decline)	
CAB vs. antiandrogen monotherapy	112	Goserelin, 3.6 mg; flutamide, 250 mg t.i.d.	6 mo	0.8	19
	108	Bicalutamide, 150 mg q.d.	6 mo	None	
Peripheral androgen blockade	19	Finasteride, 5 mg q.d.; bicalutamide, 150 mg q.d.	6 mo	1.6	20

CAB, combined androgen blockade; LHRH, luteinizing hormone releasing hormone; XRT, radiation therapy.

were retrospectively reviewed. Patients were included for further analysis if they had normal preoperative hemoglobin and creatinine levels, no evidence of clinical disease progression, and no other causes of anemia. Of the 64 patients included in the analysis, the median decrease in hemoglobin concentration was 1.2 g per dL after orchiectomy. This difference was seen within 90 days postoperatively and was maintained at the same level through all the intervals studied (14).

In a clinical trial of more than 1,300 metastatic prostate cancer patients randomized to bilateral orchiectomy with or without flutamide, the Southwest Oncology Group found no difference in overall survival between the two groups (15). In a toxicity analysis, anemia of grade 2 or higher (i.e., less than 8 g per dL) was seen in 5.4% of the orchiectomy alone group and 8.5% in the orchiectomy plus flutamide group (p = .024). This minimal difference, although statistically significant, was not associated with any discernible difference in symptoms between the groups. In conclusion, bilateral orchiectomy alone frequently leads to a mild, clinically silent anemia in many patients and rarely produces hemoglobin levels less than 8 g per dL. The addition of flutamide to orchiectomy causes a small, statistically significant increase in serious anemia but is generally of no clinical importance.

Luteinizing hormone releasing hormone (LHRH) agonists, such as leuprolide and goserelin, similarly are associated with a normocytic normochromic anemia. This is particularly the case when LHRH agonists are combined with antiandrogens to achieve "total" or "combined" androgen blockade. Although anemia is seen frequently in advanced prostate cancer patients, multiple factors make it difficult to clarify the individual contribution of LHRH agonist versus the antiandrogen being used. The relative contributions of the disease itself, prior treatments such as pelvic radiotherapy, anemia related to progression of disease, and the side effects of medication are difficult to tease apart.

The purest method to judge anemia related to LHRH agonists alone is seen in studies of these drugs in benign prostatic hypertrophy (BPH), because it is used alone in such trials, and progressive bone metastases and prior radiotherapy are not concerns. A small pilot trial evaluated the effects of the LHRH agonist nafarelin in seven men with BPH. Hemoglobin levels declined a mean of 1.1 g per dL after 6 months of treatment, interestingly, with no associated change in serum erythropoietin levels during that time (16). A subsequent randomized double-blind placebo-controlled trial of 50 patients with BPH symptoms was reported. Half of the patients received depot leuprolide, 3.75 mg intramuscularly every 28 days for 6 months. Hemoglobin levels dropped by 0.8 g per dL at 6 months in the leuprolide group, compared with no change in the placebo group (p = .0052). This effect was reversed within 6 months of stopping therapy. Thus, in this group of men without cancer, leuprolide therapy alone (at half the doses used for prostate cancer) caused a reversible drop in hemoglobin similar to orchiectomy (17).

Combined androgen blockade (CAB) may increase the level of anemia even further, although controlled data are lacking. A study addressing this question evaluated the incidence of anemia in 131 patients with locally advanced prostate cancer treated with 2 months of goserelin acetate (Zoladex) plus flutamide, followed by another 2 months of goserelin acetate plus flutamide with concurrent prostate radiotherapy. After 2 months of CAB, hemoglobin levels in all patients decreased an average of 1.6 g per dL (range, 0 to 4.5 g per dL). After 2 more months of CAB and concurrent radiotherapy, hemoglobin levels decreased 2.8 g per dL (range, 0.1 to 6.8 g per dL). This decrease in hemoglobin paralleled a decrease in testosterone levels, and no evidence of blood loss or hemolysis was noted, even in men whose hemoglobin levels dropped more than 4 g per dL. Although not a controlled trial, the investigators compared these results to their historical experience with prostate radiotherapy alone, with which they reported minor drops in hemoglobin of less than 0.5 g per dL. Interestingly, they also found racial differences in recovery rates of anemia, with African-American patients having delayed recovery compared to white patients (18).

The largest descriptive analysis of anemia associated with CAB was reported in 1997. One hundred and thirty-three evaluable patients were analyzed, although they were treated with various combinations of hormonal ablation medications. Most received leuprolide monthly and flutamide in standard doses, but approximately 10% of patients received some other type of LHRH agonist or antiandrogen, or both. More than one-third also received finasteride as additional hormone therapy. Hemoglobin levels fell significantly from 14.9 to 13.1 g per dL after 3 months of therapy (p <.001). The average nadir hemoglobin value of 12.3 g per dL, representing a 17% decline compared to baseline, was achieved after an average of 5.6 months. Ninety percent of patients had a decline in hemoglobin levels of 10% or greater, whereas 13% had a 25% or greater decrease, which was equivalent to a mean decline of 4.3 g per dL. Subset analyses of these patients also suggested that finasteride did not contribute further to anemia and that bicalutamide was less likely to cause anemia than flutamide. Thirteen percent of patients had symptoms attributed to anemia and were treated with recombinant human erythropoietin, to which all the patients responded (1).

Antiandrogen monotherapy has been advocated as one means to minimize side effects related to hormonal therapy while maintaining control of prostate cancer. In a randomized comparison of bicalutamide monotherapy with CAB (goserelin plus flutamide), the Italian Prostate Cancer Project study reported equivalent progression-free and overall survival in stage C and D patients, although median follow-up was only 38 months. Of note, however, mean hemoglobin levels decreased significantly in the group treated with goserelin plus flutamide, compared with bicalutamide. At the start of treatment, hemoglobin levels were 13.6 and 13.5 g per dL, respectively (p = not significant). After 3 months, mean hemoglobin had dropped in the goserelin plus flutamide patients to 12.8 g per dL, compared to 13.6 g per dL in the bicalutamide group (p = .008). This difference was maintained at 6 months (19).

However, another trial did demonstrate anemia in men receiving finasteride and flutamide as primary hormonal therapy for advanced prostate cancer. Of 19 men treated for 6 months with this regimen, hemoglobin levels decreased an average of 1.6 g per dL. No specific data were collected on symptoms associated with this anemia (20).

In summary, several recent studies have examined the anemia associated with hormonal ablation therapy and concluded similar results (Table 46-2). Whether treatment consists of bilateral orchiectomy, LHRH agonist, antiandrogen therapy, or some combination of these, a mild normocytic anemia is common, with decrease in hemoglobin levels of 1 to 2 g per dL after approximately 6 months. What remains unclear from the available data is the clinical sequelae of these findings, if any, and the differences between monotherapy and CAB in causing anemia. The guidelines for treating patients on hormonal therapy for prostate cancer are generally similar to those for any anemia of chronic disease. Blood transfusions and erythropoietin can be considered. Continued studies are evaluating the role of hormonal strategies that are alternatives to standard CAB and, in particular, its relative effects on anemia. For instance, intermittent androgen ablation therapy may provide similar levels of prostate cancer control with fewer symptomatic complications (21). It is unknown whether one mechanism mediating this improvement is a decreased incidence of anemia.

Leukoerythroblastic Anemia

Bone marrow replacement by neoplastic cells is a significant clinical problem in advanced prostate cancer. Because bone is involved in more 90% of patients with metastatic disease, patients frequently develop complications related to growth of cancer into bone marrow. This process is often associated with inflammation that leads to fibrosis. The resulting clinical syndrome has been referred to as leukoerythroblastic anemia (LKEA) (22). Leukoerythroblastic features are diagnosed when nucleated erythrocytes and immature myeloid cells are present in peripheral blood. It is usually, but not always, associated with anemia, and peripheral white blood cell and platelet counts also may be concomitantly decreased.

LKEA was first described in relation to prostate cancer more than 50 years ago. The largest contemporary series to evaluate the clinical and prognostic significance of LKEA in hormone-refractory prostate cancer patients was reported in 1993. One hundred and six patient records were retrospectively reviewed and peripheral blood smears analyzed for the presence of leukoerythroblastic changes. Twenty-six of 91 evaluable patients (29%) had evidence of LKEA. As might have been expected, patients with LKEA had significantly greater transfusion requirements (p <.00001), but median survival length was no different between those with or without LKEA (9 months vs. 11 months) (23). Treatment clearly needs to be directed toward the underlying cancer in this circumstance.

Pure Red Cell Aplasia

Pure red cell aplasia is a rare clinical entity characterized by anemia, reticulocytopenia, and an absence of erythrocyte precursors in the bone marrow. Although classically associated with thymomas, other cancers, as well as nonmalignant diseases, have been complicated by this syndrome. In addition, a large number of drugs have been associated with pure red cell aplasia, including anti-seizure medications and sulfa antibiotics. Chlormadinone, a progestational agent with antiandrogen properties used in Europe, was reported to induce pure red cell aplasia (24). More recently, a case was reported of leuprolide-induced pure red cell aplasia. A 67-year-old man with locally advanced prostate cancer was started on monthly leuprolide and developed a decrease in hemoglobin from normal to 7.6 g per dL within 4 months. Reticulocyte count was 0.9%, and his white blood cell and platelet counts were normal. A bone marrow evaluation showed severe erythroid hypoplasia. He was taken off leuprolide, had a bilateral orchiectomy, and was treated with prednisone with return of his hemoglobin to 11.9 g per dL within 5 months (25).

Hemolytic Anemia

Hemolytic anemia includes a wide spectrum of pathophysiologic processes that share the final common pathway of hemolyzed erythrocytes (5). Two major categories of hemolyses are seen more frequently than others in prostate cancer patients: autoimmune and microangiopathic hemolytic anemias. Obviously, other causes of hemolysis can be seen in the general population, including rare red cell membrane disorders, hemoglobinopathies, glucose-6-phosphate dehydrogenase deficiency, and hemolysis associated with certain chemicals or infections.

Hemolysis is evident when increased red cell destruction and production occur. Indirect serum bilirubin and lactate dehydrogenase levels generally rise, serum haptoglobin levels fall, and reticulocytosis is generally seen. A Coombs' antibody test can often separate immune hemolytic anemias from nonimmune causes. Red cell morphology can also be helpful in distinguishing specific types of hemolysis, with spherocytes or schistocytes signifying immune or red cell fragmentation syndromes, respectively.

Autoimmune hemolysis directly associated with cancer is a rare event. In the largest analysis of its kind, the Trent Regional Blood Transfusion Center reviewed the records of patients with erythrocyte autoantibodies and a confirmed cancer diagnosis seen during a 10-year period. There was a highly significant association between the presence of autoantibodies and carcinoma, occurring together 12 to 13 times more frequently than expected. Fourteen of 160 patients in this cohort had prostate cancer, ten with warm autoantibodies, three with cold, and one mixed. Half of these patients had clinical evidence of hemolysis. Other potential causes of autoimmune hemolytic anemia were detected in two of these patients. The investigators concluded that erythrocyte autoimmune antibodies are seen more frequently associated with cancer than expected in this observational database, and these autoantibodies can be associated with clinical sequelae. Unfortunately, this retrospective analysis was unable to clearly elucidate whether confounders such as concurrent treatments may have contributed to the autoimmune hemolysis (26).

Microangiopathic hemolytic anemia has been described as a complication of certain metastatic cancers, including gastric, breast, and lung cancer (27). The primary location for this pathologic process is thought to be small blood vessels in the lung, in which deposits of fibrin thrombi cause shearing of red cells. Hemolytic uremic syndrome (HUS) has an identical component of microangiopathic hemolysis with associated thrombocytopenia and renal failure. Renal biopsies typically demonstrate deposition of fibrin and platelet thrombi in arterioles and glomeruli.

HUS has been described in several case reports of advanced prostate cancer. In a summary of the seven published cases of HUS in prostate cancer, patient characteristics were more clearly outlined (28). Most patients presented with HUS before a diagnosis of metastatic prostate cancer, generally within a year. All seven patients required dialysis and four were treated with plasmapheresis. Three developed relapses of HUS in the follow-up period, and three developed DIC during follow-up. DIC, which likely shares a pathogenic mechanism with HUS, is discussed separately in Coagulation Disorders.

Several drugs used in prostate cancer treatment have also been implicated as a cause of HUS. Mitomycin C is the most common cancer drug associated with this disorder, but others, including cisplatin, have been implicated. Tamoxifen (29) and estramustine (30) may also cause HUS. Generally, the disease improves after discontinuing the causative agent, along with the necessary supportive care for anemia and renal failure.

Treatment of Anemia

The first therapeutic maneuver to consider in the management of anemia is to address the underlying cause. For example, gastritis from the use of nonsteroidal antiinflammatory drugs can lead to chronic blood loss that may require a change in pain medication, initiation of H2 blockers such as ranitidine, and the use of oral iron. Alternatively, an autoimmune hemolytic anemia requires investigation of underlying potential causes, including certain drugs, and subsequent steroid therapy. Anemia that is the direct result of the cancer, such as LKEA or microangiopathic hemolytic anemia, generally responds only to effective treatment of the underlying disease itself.

Transfusions represent the fastest and most effective means to treat symptomatic anemia. With rare exception, transfusion of a unit of packed red blood cells will increase the patient's hemoglobin 1 g per dL and hematocrit approximately 3 percentage points. The risks of blood transfusion are minimal with modern screening and administration methods. The greatest infectious risk remains hepatitis C, which occurs in one of 30,000 to 150,000 transfusions, and hepatitis B, which occurs in one of 30,000 to 250,000 transfusions (31). Human immunodeficiency virus infection is even less likely, occurring in 1 of 225,000 to 2,000,000 transfusions (32). Other rare risks of transfusion include acute and delayed

TABLE 46-3. TRIALS OF RECOMBINANT HUMAN ERYTHROPOIETIN IN CANCER PATIENTS

Study type	n	Dose and schedule	Outcome	Reference
Non-cisplatin chemotherapy, phase I/II	30	25–300 U/kg i.v. × 5 d/wk for 4 wk	↑ Hb >10% in 15 of 30 patients; in 15 responders, mean ↑ Hb of 1.7 g/dL	37
Non-cisplatin chemotherapy, RCT	153	150 U/kg s.c. t.i.w. or placebo for 12 wk	Mean, ↑ Hct 6.9% in Epo arm vs. 1% placebo arm (p = .0001); also, ↑ energy and fewer transfusions with Epo	36
Cisplatin chemotherapy, phase I/II	20	50–100 U/kg s.c. t.i.w. for >3 wk	15/20 Hb levels from median 8.6 g/dL to >10 mg/dL	10
Cisplatin chemotherapy, phase I/II	21	25–200 U/kg i.v. × 5d/wk for 4 wk	At 100 and 200 U/kg doses, significant ↑ in Hb of 1.9 and 2.4 g/dL, respectively	65
Cisplatin chemotherapy, phase II	103	150–300 U/kg s.c. t.i.w. titrated to Hct 38%	58% had ↑ Hct ≥6% with a mean Epo dose of 488 U/kg/wk	34
Cisplatin chemotherapy, RCT	99	100 U/kg s.c. t.i.w. or placebo × 9 wk	Mean Hb with Epo, 10.5 vs. placebo, 8.1 g/dL (p ≤.01); transfusions in 20% vs. 56%, respectively (p = .01)	35
Any chemotherapy, open label community patients	2,030	150–300 U/kg s.c. t.i.w. × 4 mo	Mean ↑ Hb of 1.8 g/dL over baseline (p <.001); significant improvement in QOL score (p = .037); Epo caused ~50% decrease in proportion, requiring transfusion and number of units transfused/patient/mo	38

Epo, erythropoietin; Hb, hemoglobin; Hct, hematocrit; QOL, quality of life; RCT, randomized clinical trial.

hemolytic reactions and transfusion-related acute lung injury (2).

Recombinant human erythropoietin (epoetin alfa) was first evaluated in chronic renal failure patients in the 1980s and produced clinically meaningful levels of erythropoiesis in the majority of patients, such that most patients were rendered transfusion independent (33). A series of trials have explored the use of epoetin alfa in the treatment of cancer patients (Table 46-3). Because cisplatin-based chemotherapy may induce a greater suppression of endogenous erythropoietin levels than non-cisplatin–based regimens, initial clinical trials analyzed the effects of epoetin alfa separately in these two populations. Phase I/II studies established that various parenteral routes (intravenous or subcutaneous), doses (25 to 300 U per kg), and schedules (3 to 5 days per week) could induce clinically significant increases in hemoglobin, hematocrit, and quality of life in cancer patients receiving chemotherapy (34–37).

Two randomized clinical trials have compared epoetin alfa to placebo in cancer patients receiving chemotherapy. Case et al. performed a randomized double-blind placebo-controlled trial of epoetin alfa (150 U per kg) versus placebo in 153 anemic cancer patients (6% with prostate cancer) receiving non-cisplatin–based chemotherapy (36). Three separate measures of response demonstrated benefit with epoetin alfa, compared to placebo: rise in hematocrit greater than 38% (41% vs. 4%, p = .0001), 6 percentage points or more rise in hematocrit from baseline (58% vs. 13.5%, p = .0001), and mean percentage point change in hematocrit after 12 weeks (6.9 vs. 1.0, p = .0001). There was a trend toward fewer transfusions with epoetin alfa, compared to placebo (29% vs. 37%, p = .056). Finally, quality of life assessments in 124 patients demonstrated significant improvements in energy level and ability to perform the activities of daily living in treated patients (p <.05) (36). A similar randomized controlled trial of 99 patients treated with cisplatin-based chemotherapy, none of whom had prostate cancer, showed similar favorable outcomes (35).

An open label trial of 2,342 patients treated in the community by more than 500 oncologists was reported in 1997 (38). All anemic patients with nonmyeloid malignancies receiving chemotherapy were eligible, but only 4% had prostate cancer. Epoetin alfa was scheduled to be given subcutaneously, 150 U per kg three times a week for 4 months, but only 1,047 patients completed the prescribed course. Even in this mixed population, however, epoetin alfa demonstrated a significant increase in hemoglobin over baseline, improvements in quality of life, and decreased transfusion requirements, all of which were statistically significant. However, no correlation was seen between baseline serum erythropoietin levels and hemoglobin response (38).

Only a single small clinical trial specifically evaluated the effect of epoetin alfa in anemic prostate cancer patients. Beshara et al. treated nine men with hormone-refractory disease with epoitin alfa, 150 U per kg subcutaneous three times a week. Seven patients had a significant increase in hemoglobin, 1.7 g per dL or greater. Only two patients had low serum erythropoietin levels (39). A larger multicenter randomized trial is currently evaluating the use of epoetin alfa therapy in advanced prostate cancer patients.

Epoetin alfa is extremely well tolerated. Although thrombotic complications have been reported (primarily in renal failure patients), the incidence is very low and may be similar to the general cancer population. Hypertension and neurologic symptoms have also been reported. Unfortunately, epoetin alfa is expensive therapy, costing approximately $300 to $400 per week. The cost effectiveness of this therapy in cancer patients remains an unresolved issue (40). Thus, appropriate patient selection and optimal dosing schedules continue to be explored. Although the ability of epoetin alfa therapy to improve anemia in cancer patients receiving chemotherapy has been well demonstrated, there are important concerns about the relative clinical benefit that such therapy provides. In addition, although new approaches such as weekly subcutaneous dosing have been shown to produce equally good results as daily or thrice weekly dosing in presurgical (41) and end-stage renal disease patients (42), it has yet to be adequately studied in cancer patients.

In summary, treatment of anemia in prostate cancer patients should focus on reversible underlying causes first. Transfusions of red cells can be a quick and effective means to relieve symptoms of severe anemia with relative safety. Erythropoietin may play a role in cancer-related anemia, particularly in those patients being treated with chemotherapy. Serum erythropoietin levels are generally not of value in distinguishing those most likely to benefit. Treatment should be individualized depending on the patient and the goals of therapy, but ongoing randomized trials in prostate cancer should more clearly define the role of epoetin alfa in the future.

Hemoglobin Levels and Prognosis

Hemoglobin has been shown in many studies to be an independent significant factor for predicting survival in hormone-refractory prostate cancer. Of at least eight trials that have done a multivariable analysis of hemoglobin as a predictor for survival, four demonstrated independent negative prognostic value to a low hemoglobin level (12).

The exact mechanism for this association is poorly understood. Presumably, hemoglobin represents an indirect measure of tumor volume, particularly in the bone marrow in which, by direct metastases (e.g., LKEA) or some other means, cancer cells exert an effect on erythropoiesis that is important. This is an important topic for further basic and clinical research.

LEUKOPENIA AND THROMBOCYTOPENIA

Generally, leukopenia and thrombocytopenia in prostate cancer patients are a result of treatment. In particular, cytotoxic chemotherapy is well-known to cause myelosuppression, but hormonal therapy, radiopharmaceuticals, and other agents also may be associated with decreased white blood cell and platelet counts. Thrombocytopenia that is related to DIC is discussed further in the following section.

Secondary hormonal therapies have rarely been associated with severe hematologic toxicities. In one study, aminoglutethimide at a dose of 500 to 1,000 mg per day induced marked leukopenia (defined as a white blood count of less than 1,500 per mm^3) or thrombocytopenia (platelet count of less than 50,000 per mm^3), or both, in 12 of 1,333 (0.9%) patients treated for metastatic breast or prostate cancer. Depression of blood counts was noted within 7 weeks of starting therapy and recovered after stopping treatment in all except one patient who died from marrow aplasia and subsequent sepsis (43). Another trial noted transient mild thrombocytopenia during diethylstilbestrol infusion in 10 of 13 patients (44).

The dose-limiting toxicity of radiopharmaceutical agents, including strontium-89, samarium, and rhenium-186-HEDP, remains myelosuppression and, in particular, thrombocytopenia. The mechanism for this effect is based on the absorbed dose by the bone marrow, which correlates well with the degree of thrombocytopenia (45). Some groups have advocated a dosing strategy for such drugs on the basis of a pretreatment bone scan with subsequent dose adjustment to avoid unacceptable levels of thrombocytopenia (46). In addition, when administered to the pelvis, a common site for bony metastases, external beam radiotherapy can cause myelosuppression and, in particular, thrombocytopenia. Because many of these patients also have had prostate irradiation, the cumulative dose to the pelvis can be significant.

Chemotherapy for prostate cancer has had a checkered past. Initial studies in the 1970s suggested that traditional drugs, such as cyclophosphamide and hydroxyurea, might have some efficacy in treating hormone-refractory disease. However, by the 1980s, the tide of opinion shifted, and cytotoxic chemotherapy fell out of favor for any stage of prostate cancer. In the past several years, the tide has shifted again, as phase II and III studies are demonstrating subjective and objective evidence of benefit in advanced prostate cancer patients (47).

Many recent trials of combination chemotherapy in hormone-refractory prostate cancer have demonstrated meaningful improvements in pain and evidence of tumor response. Active regimens include mitoxantrone plus prednisone and estramustine combined with vinblastine, paclitaxel, docetaxel, etoposide or carboplatin, or both. The most promising regimens appear to combine drugs that have antimitotic effects. Response rates in these clinical trials range from 40% to 60% when using PSA declines of 50% or greater, with objective measurable responses or symptomatic improvements in pain as primary end points (47).

Mitoxantrone, which has been approved for this use by the U.S. Food and Drug Administration, caused mild myelosuppression in two phase III trials in prostate cancer (48,49). This was despite the fact that many of these patients had received prior pelvic radiotherapy. Estramustine causes no myelosuppression but, in fact, has been shown to ameliorate the leukopenia associated with vinblastine in a randomized trial of the combination compared to vinblastine alone (50). Taxanes are among the more active drugs currently being evaluated in prostate cancer and clearly can be associated with myelosuppression (47). However, new regimens currently under study include weekly dosing strategies that have much less effect on white blood cell and platelet counts.

In summary, many therapies in common use for advanced metastatic prostate cancer can be associated with significant thrombocytopenia or leukopenia. Culprits may include hormonal therapies, cytotoxic chemotherapy, external beam radiotherapy, radiopharmaceutical injections, and other drugs. Drugs such as filgrastim (Neupogen) have been used as a component of some combination chemotherapy regimens. Platelet transfusions may be given for a platelet count of less than 50,000 per mm^3 associated with bleeding or platelet counts of less than 10,000 to 20,000 per mm^3 in an asymptomatic patient.

COAGULATION DISORDERS

Bleeding diathesis had been recognized as a complication of advanced prostate cancer as early as 1930 (51). Since that time, reports based on several small case series suggested the existence of a strong association between prostate cancer and coagulation disorders. In 1953, Tagnon and colleagues noted that prostate cancer patients with bleeding difficulties had low levels of serum fibrinogen and displayed marked fibrinolysis that the researchers theorized was from a plasminlike enzyme secreted directly from prostate tumor cells. This concept held sway into the 1970s, when increasing experimental and clinical evidence suggested that fibrinolysis was secondary to systemic intravascular coagulation and not a primary phenomenon (51).

DIC is characterized by widespread activation of the coagulation pathways, leading ultimately to thrombus formation in small- and medium-sized blood vessels and subsequent organ failure (52). The current model of the pathogenesis of DIC in prostate cancer is not well understood. Some tumor cell factors are able to activate various cytokines (primarily interleukin-6) to trigger thrombin and, therefore, fibrin formation. In addition, plasminogen activator inhibitor type 1 suppresses fibrinolysis, which inhibits fibrin degradation, resulting in systemic intravascular coagulation.

Traditionally, the incidence of DIC in prostate cancer has been reported to be as high as 25% (53). In fact, a prominent review published in 1999 lists pancreatic and prostate cancers as examples of solid tumors that cause DIC. However, several groups have reported that the incidence of coagulation disorders in untreated prostate cancer is actually much lower (54). In a retrospective analysis of more than 1,600 patients with prostate cancer seen at M. D. Anderson Cancer Center (MDACC) over 5 years, only 60 patients were evaluable who had surgery at MDACC and available clinical follow-up. Of these, only one patient had low-grade DIC and another had deep venous thrombosis (54). In another retrospective evaluation of 35 patients with metastatic prostate cancer, three patients (9%) were reported in one series to have "abnormal clotting" (55). In one series of 80 patients diagnosed with prostate cancer in the Phoenix Veterans Administration Hospital from 1982 to 1984, four (5%) presented with acute gastrointestinal bleeding. Three patients had evidence of DIC, two of whom had dramatic resolution of DIC after hormone therapy (56).

Other groups have prospectively evaluated coagulation laboratory parameters to assess the risk of bleeding. Thirty patients with metastatic prostate cancer were found to have statistically significant lower levels of antithrombin III compared to healthy controls (57). In another study, 165 prostate cancer patients were screened preoperatively, with only 3.7% having a significant coagulation laboratory abnormality. Only one patient experienced postoperative DIC (58). In the MDACC series noted earlier, 16 patients were prospectively evaluated and only one patient had an abnormal coagulation test, an elevated fibrinopeptide A level (54).

Although individual case reports have described DIC after transrectal prostate biopsy (59), at the time of surgery and in advanced metastatic disease, the largest series have evaluated patients with localized disease. Although it seems reasonable to assume that the prevalence of DIC would increase with stage or progression of disease, such data are unavailable. There are also no data regarding DIC in hormone-refractory prostate cancer.

DIC diagnosed concurrently with advanced prostate cancer has been treated with various hormonal ablation therapies, including estrogen (60) and ketoconazole (61,62). One patient with DIC and excessive fibrinolysis responded to epsilon aminocaproic acid (63). Other measures that have been used to treat acute effects of DIC are generally ineffective unless the underlying cause is addressed first. Heparin in low doses, platelet and plasma transfusions, concentrates of coagulation inhibitors such as antithrombin III, and antifibrinolytic agents have all been used with mixed results (52).

Thrombocytopenic thrombotic purpura represents another end of a clinicopathologic spectrum of coagulation disorders that include HUS and DIC. It rarely has been reported in association with cancer, and only a single case report has been reported in a patient with prostate cancer (64).

In summary, coagulation disorders are associated with prostate cancer, usually DIC, in a modest proportion of cases. Although the exact incidence is difficult to specify, it is likely much lower than the 25% that was reported 30 years ago. Treatment of the underlying malignancy with hormonal therapy frequently can reverse the disorder, although other supportive measures may need to be considered.

CONCLUSION

In summary, prostate cancer is associated with clinically significant hematologic abnormalities that may be caused by the cancer or treatment directed at the cancer. Anemia is a common complication of advanced prostate cancer and may be related to iron deficiency anemia, anemia of chronic disease, hemolytic anemias, LKEA, or other causes. Anemia related to hormonal ablation therapy is an important etiology of normocytic anemia in this population, generally decreasing hemoglobin by 1 to 2 g per dL. Treatment for anemia is directed at the underlying cause but may also include blood transfusions and recombinant human erythropoietin. Epoetin is being studied in a large randomized multicenter clinical trial in patients with hormone-refractory prostate cancer that should address its value for such patients. Leukopenia is a potential complication of cytotoxic chemotherapy for prostate cancer. Thrombocytopenia may be related to treatment as well, including chemotherapy, external beam radiation, and radiopharmaceuticals. Thrombocytopenia can also be associated with coagulation disorders such as DIC. Coagulation disorders have been associated with all stages of prostate cancer, although patients usually have advanced disease. Hematologic complications of prostate cancer deserve a renewed evaluation, particularly as new treatments are evolving.

REFERENCES

1. Strum SB, McDermed JE, Scholz MC, et al. Anaemia associated with androgen deprivation in patients with prostate cancer receiving combined hormone blockade. *Br J Urol* 1997;79:933–941.
2. Goodnough LT, Brecher ME, Kanter MH, et al. Transfusion medicine. First of two parts—blood transfusion [see comments]. *N Engl J Med* 1999;340:438–447.
3. Demetri GD, Kris M, Wade J, et al. Quality-of-life benefit in chemotherapy patients treated with epoetin alfa is independent of disease response or tumor type: results from a prospective community oncology study. Procrit Study Group. *J Clin Oncol* 1998;16:3412–3425.
4. Spivak JL. Cancer-related anemia: its causes and characteristics. *Semin Oncol* 1994;21(2 Suppl 3):3–8.
5. Lindenbaum J. An approach to anemias. In: Plum F, Bennett JC, eds. *Cecil textbook of medicine*, 20th ed. Philadelphia: WB Saunders, 1996.
6. Joosten E, Ghesquiere B, Linthoudt H, et al. Upper and lower gastrointestinal evaluation of elderly inpatients who are iron deficient. *Am J Med* 1999;107:24–29.
7. Provan D. Mechanisms and management of iron deficiency anaemia. *Br J Haematol* 1999;105(Suppl 1):19–26.
8. Krantz SB. Pathogenesis and treatment of the anemia of chronic disease. *Am J Med Sci* 1994;307:353–359.
9. Miller CB, Jones RJ, Piantadosi S, et al. Decreased erythropoietin response in patients with the anemia of cancer. *N Engl J Med* 1990;322:1689–1692.
10. Cascinu S, Fedeli A, Fedeli SL, et al. Cisplatin-associated anaemia treated with subcutaneous erythropoietin. A pilot study. *Br J Cancer* 1993;67:156–158.
11. Besa EC. Hematologic effects of androgens revisited: an alternative therapy in various hematologic conditions. *Semin Hematol* 1994;31:134–145.
12. George DJ, Kantoff PW. Prognostic indicators in hormone refractory prostate cancer. *Urol Clin North Am* 1999;26: 303–310.
13. Hamilton JB. Role of testicular secretions as indicated by effects of castration in man and by studies of pathological conditions and short lifespan associated with maleness. *Recent Prog Horm Res* 1948;3:257–289.
14. Fonseca R, Rajkumar SV, White WL, et al. Anemia after orchiectomy. *Am J Hematol* 1998;59:230–233.
15. Eisenberger MA, Blumenstein BA, Crawford ED, et al. Bilateral orchiectomy with or without flutamide for metastatic prostate cancer [see comments]. *N Engl J Med* 1998; 339:1036–1042.
16. Weber JP, Walsh PC, Peters CA, et al. Effect of reversible androgen deprivation on hemoglobin and serum immunoreactive erythropoietin in men. *Am J Hematol* 1991;36:190–194.
17. Eri LM, Tveter KJ. Safety, side effects and patient acceptance of the luteinizing hormone releasing hormone agonist leuprolide in treatment of benign prostatic hyperplasia. *J Urol* 1994;152:448–452.
18. Asbell SO, Leon SA, Tester WJ, et al. Development of anemia and recovery in prostate cancer patients treated with combined androgen blockade and radiotherapy. *Prostate* 1996;29:243–248.
19. Boccardo F, Rubagotti A, Barichello M, et al. Bicalutamide monotherapy versus flutamide plus goserelin in prostate cancer patients: results of an Italian Prostate Cancer Project study. *J Clin Oncol* 1999;17:2027–2038.
20. Ornstein DK, Beiser JA, Andriole GL. Anaemia in men receiving combined finasteride and flutamide therapy for advanced prostate cancer. *BJU Int* 1999;83:43–46.
21. Gleave M, Bruchovsky N, Goldenberg SL, et al. Intermittent androgen suppression for prostate cancer: rationale and clinical experience. *Eur Urol* 1998;34(Suppl 3):37–41.
22. Eriksson S, Killander J, Wadman B. Leuco-erythroblastic anaemia in prostatic cancer. *Scand J Haemat* 1972;9:648–653.
23. Shamdas GJ, Ahmann FR, Matzner MB, et al. Leukoerythroblastic anemia in metastatic prostate cancer. Clinical and prognostic significance in patients with hormone refractory disease. *Cancer* 1993;71:3594–3600.
24. Tsuda H, Kuniyasu W, Fukuda K, et al. Pure red cell aplasia caused by chlormadinone [letter]. *Lancet* 1994;344:1370–1371.
25. Maeda H, Arai Y, Aoki Y, et al. Leuprolide causes pure red cell aplasia. *J Urol* 1998;160:501.
26. Sokol RJ, Booker DJ, Stamps R. Erythrocyte autoantibodies, autoimmune haemolysis, and carcinoma. *J Clin Pathol* 1994;47:340–343.
27. Antman KH, Skarin AT, Mayer RJ, et al. Microangiopathic hemolytic anemia and cancer: a review. *Medicine (Baltimore)* 1979;58:377–384.
28. Muller NJ, Pestalozzi BC. Hemolytic uremic syndrome in prostatic carcinoma. *Oncology* 1998;55:174–176.
29. Montes A, Powles TJ, O'Brien ME, et al. A toxic interaction between mitomycin C and tamoxifen causing the haemolytic uraemic syndrome. *Eur J Cancer* 1993;29A:1854–1857.
30. Tassinari D, Sartori S, Panzini I, et al. Hemolytic-uremic syndrome during therapy with estramustine phosphate for advanced prostatic cancer. *Oncology* 1999;56:112–113.
31. Schreiber GB, Busch MP, Kleinman SH, et al. The risk of transfusion transmitted viral infections. *N Engl J Med* 1996; 334:1685–1690.

32. Lackritz EM, Satten GA, Aberle-Grasse J, et al. Estimated risk of transmission of the human immunodeficiency virus by screened blood in the United States [see comments]. *N Engl J Med* 1995;333:1721–1725.
33. Eschbach JW, Abdulhadi MH, Browne JK, et al. Recombinant human erythropoietin in anemic patients with end-stage renal disease. Results of a phase III multicenter clinical trial. *Ann Intern Med* 1989;111:992–1000.
34. Henry DH, Abels RI. Recombinant human erythropoietin in the treatment of cancer and chemotherapy-induced anemia: results of double-blind and open-label follow-up studies. *Semin Oncol* 1994;21(2 Suppl 3):21–28.
35. Cascinu S, Fedeli A, Del Ferro E, et al. Recombinant human erythropoietin treatment in cisplatin-associated anemia: a randomized, double-blind trial with placebo. *J Clin Oncol* 1994;12:1058–1062.
36. Case DC Jr., Bukowski RM, Carey RW, et al. Recombinant human erythropoietin therapy for anemic cancer patients on combination chemotherapy. *J Natl Cancer Inst* 1993;85: 801–806.
37. Platanias LC, Miller CB, Mick R, et al. Treatment of chemotherapy-induced anemia with recombinant human erythropoietin in cancer patients. *J Clin Oncol* 1991;9: 2021–2026.
38. Glaspy J, Bukowski R, Steinberg D, et al. Impact of therapy with epoetin alfa on clinical outcomes in patients with nonmyeloid malignancies during cancer chemotherapy in community oncology practice. Procrit Study Group. *J Clin Oncol* 1997;15:1218–1234.
39. Beshara S, Letocha H, Linde T, et al. Anemia associated with advanced prostatic adenocarcinoma: effects of recombinant human erythropoietin. *Prostate* 1997;31:153–160.
40. Ortega A, Dranitsaris G, Puodziunas AL. What are cancer patients willing to pay for prophylactic epoetin alfa? A cost-benefit analysis [see comments]. *Cancer* 1998;83: 2588–2596.
41. Goldberg MA, McCutchen JW, Jove M, et al. A safety and efficacy comparison study of two dosing regimens of epoetin alfa in patients undergoing major orthopedic surgery. *Am J Orthop* 1996;25:544–552.
42. Zappacosta AR, Perras ST, Bell A. Weekly subcutaneous recombinant human erythropoietin corrects anemia of progressive renal failure. *Am J Med* 1991;91:229–232.
43. Messeih AA, Lipton A, Santen RJ, et al. Aminoglutethimide-induced hematologic toxicity: worldwide experience. *Cancer Treat Rep* 1985;69:1003–1004.
44. Nachtsheim DA, McPherson RA, Pollen JJ, et al. Thrombocytopenia during diethylstilbestrol diphosphate (Stilphostrol) infusion for carcinoma of the prostate. *Prostate* 1980;1:105–109.
45. de Klerk JM, van Dieren EB, van het Schip AD, et al. Bone marrow absorbed dose of rhenium-186-HEDP and the relationship with decreased platelet counts. *J Nucl Med* 1996; 37:38–41.
46. de Klerk JM, van het Schip AD, Zonnenberg BA, et al. Evaluation of thrombocytopenia in patients treated with rhenium-186-HEDP: guidelines for individual dosage recommendations. *J Nucl Med* 1994;35:1423–1428.
47. Oh WK, Kantoff PW. Management of hormone refractory prostate cancer: current standards and future prospects [see comments]. *J Urol* 1998;160:1220–1229.
48. Kantoff PW, Halabi S, Conaway M, et al. Hydrocortisone with or without mitoxantrone in men with hormone-refractory prostate cancer: results of the Cancer and Leukemia Group B 9182 study. *J Clin Oncol* 1999;17:2506–2513.
49. Tannock IF, Osoba D, Stockler MR, et al. Chemotherapy with mitoxantrone plus prednisone or prednisone alone for symptomatic hormone-resistant prostate cancer: a Canadian randomized trial with palliative end points [see comments]. *J Clin Oncol* 1996;14:1756–1764.
50. Hudes G, Einhorn L, Ross E, et al. Vinblastine versus vinblastine plus oral estramustine phosphate for patients with hormone-refractory prostate cancer: a Hoosier Oncology Group and Fox Chase Network phase III trial. *J Clin Oncol* 1999;17:3160–3166.
51. Pergament ML, Swaim WR, Blackard CE. Disseminated intravascular coagulation in the urologic patient. *J Urol* 1976;116:1–7.

51a. Tagnon HJ, Whitmore WF, Schulman P, et al. The significance of fibrinolysis occurring in patients with metastatic cancer of the prostate. *Cancer* 1953;6:63–70.

52. Levi M, Ten Cate H. Disseminated intravascular coagulation. *N Engl J Med* 1999;341:586–592.
53. Straub PW. Chronic intravascular coagulation. Clinical spectrum and diagnostic criteria, with special emphasis on metabolism, distribution and localization of I 131-fibrinogen. *Acta Med Scand (Suppl)* 1971;526:1–95.
54. Drewinko B, Cobb P, Guinee V, et al. Untreated prostatic carcinoma is not associated with frequent thrombohemorrhagic disorders. *Urology* 1987;30:11–17.
55. Burgess NA, Hudd C, Rees RW. Haemostatic pitfalls in advanced prostatic cancer. *Br J Urol* 1993;71:231–233.
56. Doll DC, Kerr DM, Greenberg BR. Acute gastrointestinal bleeding as the presenting manifestation of prostate cancer. *Cancer* 1986;58:1374–1377.
57. Dobbs RM, Barber JA, Weigel JW, et al. Clotting predisposition in carcinoma of the prostate. *J Urol* 1980;123:706–709.
58. Rader ES. Hematologic screening tests in patients with operative prostatic disease. *Urology* 1978;11:243–246.
59. Harvey MH, Osborn DE, Hutchinson RM. Disseminated intravascular coagulation following transrectal prostatic biopsy. *Br J Urol* 1987;59:363–364.
60. Goldenberg SL, Fenster HN, Perler Z, et al. Disseminated intravascular coagulation in carcinoma of prostate: role of estrogen therapy. *Urology* 1983;22:130–132.
61. Litt MR, Bell WR, Lepor HA. Disseminated intravascular coagulation in prostatic carcinoma reversed by ketoconazole. *JAMA* 1987;258:1361–1362.
62. Lowe FC, Somers WJ. The use of ketoconazole in the emergency management of disseminated intravascular coagulation due to metastatic prostatic cancer. *J Urol* 1987;137: 1000–1002.
63. Cooper DL, Sandler AB, Wilson LD, et al. Disseminated intravascular coagulation and excessive fibrinolysis in a patient with metastatic prostate cancer. Response to epsilon-aminocaproic acid. *Cancer* 1992;70:656–658.
64. Cherin P, Brivet F, Tertian G, et al. [Recurrent thrombocytopenic thrombotic purpura associated to prostatic cancer. A case]. *Presse Med* 1991;20:1073–1077.
65. Miller CB, Platanias LC, Mills SR, et al. Phase I-II trial of erythropoietin in the treatment of cisplatin-associated anemia. *J Natl Cancer Inst* 1992;84:98–103.

47

NEUROLOGIC COMPLICATIONS OF PROSTATE CANCER

PATRICK Y. WEN
DAVID SCHIFF

Prostate cancer is the most frequently diagnosed cancer and the second leading cause of cancer death in men in the United States (1). An early study found that neurologic complications occurred in 21% of prostate cancer patients, especially those with advanced disease (2). Today, the incidence of neurologic complications in patients with prostate cancer is likely to be significantly lower, as patients are diagnosed increasingly earlier in the course of their disease. The most common neurologic complications are epidural spinal cord compression (ESCC) and toxic metabolic encephalopathies, which are usually caused by medications and infections (2). Other neurologic complications are relatively uncommon. This chapter reviews the neurologic complications of prostate cancer and its therapies. Toxic metabolic encephalopathies and pain from bony metastases without associated neurologic dysfunction are not discussed.

EPIDURAL SPINAL CORD COMPRESSION

Background

ESCC refers to compression of the thecal sac from tumor in the epidural space at the level of the spinal cord or cauda equina. This is the most common neurologic complication in patients with prostate cancer and is associated with significant morbidity (2). ESCC tends to occur in patients with advanced-stage disease and poorly differentiated tumors (3,4). Prostate cancer accounts for approximately 15% to 20% of all cases of ESCC (5) and is the second most common cause of cord compression in men after lung cancer (3,4,6–9). In older series, ESCC affected up to 7% of patients with prostate cancer and was the presenting symptom in 10% to 25% of these patients (3,4,7,8). The introduction of screening tests such as prostate-specific antigen has resulted in patients being diagnosed increasingly at an earlier stage, and it is likely that the incidence of ESCC in prostate cancer patients is now lower. Nonetheless, ESCC remains a common problem in patients with prostate cancer, and it is important to have a high index of suspicion, because it is treatable when diagnosed early but is associated with a poor outcome once neurologic function is affected (7,10).

Pathogenesis

The spine is one of the most common sites of bony metastases in patients with prostate cancer and may be involved in up to 80% of patients with advanced disease (9). Most cases of ESCC arise from seeding of vertebral body bone marrow by tumor cells travelling in the paravertebral blood vessels or Batson's plexus (9). The tumor within the vertebral body grows posteriorly, compressing the spinal cord directly or indirectly by producing collapse of the bone. Less commonly, ESCC results from tumors arising from the posterior spinal elements or growth of a paraspinal mass through the neuroforamen. Direct vascular seeding of the epidural space is extremely uncommon. The enlarging epidural tumor initially causes obstruction of the epidural venous plexus, resulting in vasogenic edema. The beneficial effects of steroids may be due to its effects on this edema (10). Prostaglandin and serotonin levels are increased at the site of compression, and, in animal studies, indomethacin and serotonin receptor blockers have been effective (10,11). Eventually, blood flow is compromised and spinal cord infarction results (11). The rate at which spinal cord compression develops is an important determinant of potential reversibility of pathologic changes and clinical dysfunction, with slowly progressive lesions much more likely to be reversible than rapidly progressive ones (10).

The distribution of ESCC in the spine is roughly in proportion to the combined volumes of the vertebral bodies in each region. Approximately 60% of cases occur in the thoracic spine, 30% in the lumbosacral spine, and 10% in the cervical spine (3,4,7,9,12). Up to one-third of patients will have multiple epidural metastases (13,14).

Clinical Features

Pain is present in 95% of ESCC patients and is generally the initial symptom. Pain typically precedes other symptoms of ESCC by 1 to 2 months (5,15,16). Certain features of the pain increase the likelihood of ESCC. These include pain that worsens with recumbency (due to distension of the epidural venous plexus), thoracic localization, and percussion tenderness. Acute worsening of pain suggests a pathologic compression fracture. Radicular symptoms may develop when epidural disease is located laterally and tend to be more common with lumbar and cervical ESCC (16). Pain in these areas tends to produce unilateral pain, whereas thoracic radicular pain is almost always bilateral. Unfortunately, weakness is present in approximately 75% of patients with ESCC by the time of diagnosis (16,17), and, in most large series, a majority of patients are no longer ambulatory (3,5,7,8,12,15). When the site of compression is above the level of the conus medullaris, the corticospinal tracts are involved, producing pyramidal weakness in which the flexors are affected more than the extensors. This weakness may be associated with spasticity, hyperreflexia, and extensor plantar responses. In general, the weakness tends to be symmetrical and hemicord syndromes are uncommon. Lesions below the conus involve the cauda equina, producing a polyradiculopathy with weakness and depressed reflexes. Sensory complaints occur less frequently than weakness but are still present in the majority of patients at presentation (10) and usually take the form of ascending numbness and paresthesias. Although a spinal sensory level may be present, the lesion is often several spinal segments rostral to the clinical level. Cauda equina lesions often produce saddle sensory loss, whereas lesions above the cauda equina frequently spare the sacral dermatomes. Lateral lesions may produce radicular pain and sensory loss in a dermatomal distribution. Radiculopathies occur more commonly in the lumbosacral spine and have greater localizing value. Autonomic dysfunction, especially urinary retention, is common (8,7,12,18) but is generally a late finding in ESCC.

Neuroimaging

The diagnosis of ESCC has been revolutionized by the introduction of magnetic resonance imaging (MRI) (Fig. 47-1). Careful imaging of the spine is necessary not only to establish the diagnosis of ESCC but also to determine the extent of the lesion and the presence of other sites of ESCC. Clinical localization of the level of spinal cord compression is often inaccurate. Even neurooncologists "miss"

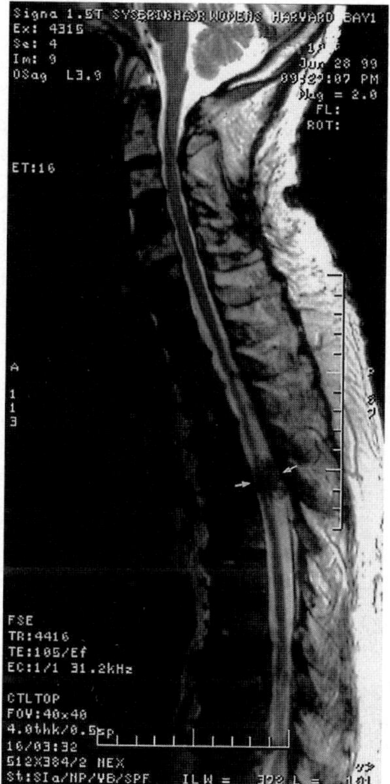

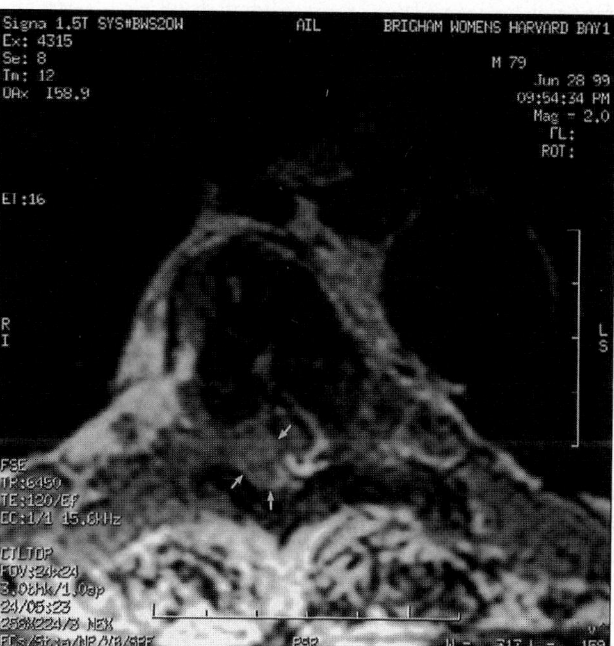

FIGURE 47-1. A: Sagittal and **(B)** axial T1-weighted magnetic resonance imaging scan of the thoracic spine showing compression of the spinal cord by prostate cancer. Arrows point to the tumor.

the localization of symptomatic ESCC by more than one spinal level more than 25% of the time (13,19).

Plain spinal radiographs are useful, if abnormal. Unfortunately, false negatives occur in 10% to 17% of patients (5,20) owing to paraspinal tumor invasion through the neuroforamen, involvement of multiple vertebrae obscuring the relevant lesion, and the fact that 30% to 50% of bone must be destroyed before the radiograph is positive. The usefulness of plain films is highlighted by the fact that, in cancer patients with back pain, major vertebral body collapse on radiograph regardless of clinical state and pedicle erosion with associated radiculopathy predict a more than 75% chance of ESCC (21). Algorithms combining the use of plain radiographs with bone scanning suggest that if both studies are negative in a cancer patient with spinal symptoms, then the risk of ESCC may be as low as 2% (22). Such an approach may be reasonable in cancer patients with back pain alone; however, radiculopathy, myelopathy, and severe or progressive pain should lead to more definitive studies.

MR scanning and myelography (particularly when combined with computed tomography) are capable of delineating extradural compression of the thecal sac. Several studies dating from MR scanning's early years yielded conflicting results but demonstrated no major superiority for MR (23,24). MR scanning's recent technical improvements, in addition to its convenience, ability to screen the entire spine, and superiority to myelography in demonstrating bone and intramedullary lesions, make it the study of choice for most patients. Computed tomography myelography may be used in patients who cannot have MRI (e.g., patients with pacemakers). It may occasionally display laterally placed lesions not seen on MR scanning and allows for simultaneous cerebrospinal fluid (CSF) collection.

Differential Diagnosis

Epidural metastasis must be differentiated from nonmalignant conditions that can produce back pain and neurologic dysfunction, as well as malignant, non-ESCC causes of these symptoms. Benign conditions that can compress the thecal sac include disc herniation, spinal stenosis, suppurative bacterial infections, tuberculosis, vascular malformations, epidural hematoma, and compression fractures. Tumors, such as chordoma, may involve the cauda equina, whereas meningiomas and neurofibromas can compress the spinal cord and produce radicular and myelopathic syndromes.

Among the malignant conditions that must be differentiated from ESCC are vertebral metastases without epidural extension; tumor infiltration of the lumbosacral plexus (leading to severe local or radicular pain, followed by weakness and numbness); and, very rarely, leptomeningeal and intramedullary metastases. Radiation myelopathy must also be considered if the spinal cord has been previously irradiated (25). The total previous radiation dose and fraction size are important risk factors, as is the length of cord irradiated. The latency after radiotherapy (RT) is typically 9 to 15 months but can be shorter or longer. Radiation myelopathy usually presents as a progressive myelopathy, beginning with ascending sensory symptoms followed by upper motor neuron signs. Pain is common, and the frequent presence of a Brown-Sequard syndrome (with ipsilateral weakness, dorsal column sensory loss, contralateral pain, and temperature loss) may be diagnostically helpful.

Management of Epidural Spinal Cord Compression

Supportive Care

Patients with ESCC are frequently in considerable pain. Corticosteroids usually improve pain within a few hours, but patients frequently will also require opiate analgesics. The autonomic dysfunction, analgesics, and reduced mobility in patients with ESCC often result in constipation and occasionally ileus and perforation of abdominal viscus. The symptoms of bowel perforation may be masked in patients receiving steroids. To avoid these complications, ESCC patients require an aggressive bowel regimen. Prophylaxis against venous thromboembolism should be strongly considered in nonambulatory patients. External spinal bracing is sometimes used but unproven and may be poorly tolerated. There is generally no need to confine patients to bed if they are ambulatory.

Corticosteroids

The beneficial effects of corticosteroids in patients with ESCC were initially noted empirically in the 1960s (26) and subsequently supported by animal studies (27,28). To date, there has been only one randomized clinical trial addressing the usefulness of corticosteroids in ESCC (29). In this trial, 57 patients with carcinoma and myelographically confirmed ESCC, all of whom underwent standardized RT, received either no dexamethasone or 96 mg followed by 24 mg four times daily, tapering over 10 days. Patients were stratified according to primary tumor type and neurologic function. A significantly higher percentage of patients receiving steroids remained ambulatory over time (81% vs. 63%). However, these high doses of dexamethasone were associated with serious side effects in 11% of patients. Heimdal et al. (30) similarly noted a 14% serious complication rate in 28 patients with ESCC undergoing RT using this high dose of dexamethasone. In contrast, no serious side effects were seen in 38 patients receiving 16 mg of dexamethasone daily tapered over 2 weeks. There was no difference in ambulatory outcome between the two groups.

In summary, there is good evidence that "high-dose" dexamethasone is an effective adjunct to RT but is associated with a moderate probability of serious toxicity, whereas "low-dose" dexamethasone is associated with fewer side effects but is not supported by randomized, controlled data (31). In general, we reserve the use of high-dose dexamethasone for patients with paraplegia or paraparesis and treat all other patients with 16 mg of dexamethasone daily in divided doses. When high-dose dexamethasone is used, it is important to taper the dose fairly rapidly to diminish the risk of complications, such as steroid myopathy and infection. One approach is to halve the total daily dexamethasone dose every 3 days as long as the patient has not neurologically deteriorated (10). There is some evidence that patients with back pain but no evidence of myelopathy and less than 50% narrowing of the spinal canal with epidural disease can safely undergo RT without corticosteroids (32).

Radiotherapy

For most patients, fractionated external beam radiation therapy is the treatment of choice for ESCC. No dose-fractionation schema has proven superior to others. Most patients receive 2,500 to 4,000 cGy in 10 to 20 fractions over 2 to 4 weeks, with 3,000 cGy in 10 fractions being a particularly popular regimen (10,31,33). In general, only symptomatic regions or asymptomatic sites with significant epidural disease are treated, with a margin of one to two vertebral bodies above and below the site. For prostate cancer patients with poor performance status and a short life expectancy, an RT regimen of two fractions of 800 cGy given 1 week apart produces comparable outcomes to more conventional fractionation schedules (34).

Many series have demonstrated that 80% to 100% of patients who are ambulatory at the onset of treatment will remain ambulatory at the conclusion of therapy. In contrast, only one-third of paraparetic patients and 2% to 6% of paraplegic patients will regain the ability to walk (5,32,33,35,36). These outcomes highlight the fact that pretreatment neurologic function is the strongest predictor of posttreatment neurologic function and the importance of early diagnosis of this condition. The second strongest predictor of outcome is the radiosensitivity of the tumor. Patients with a radiosensitive tumor, such as prostate cancer, have a much higher chance of regaining neurologic function than other histologies (33). Similarly, patients with favorable histologies appear less likely to suffer eventual local relapse of their epidural disease (15). The degree of thecal sac compression is also a weak prognostic factor for outcome (37,38).

Surgery

Laminectomy

For many years, decompressive laminectomy was the standard treatment of patients presenting with ESCC and neurologic deficits. However, outcomes were often disappointing, probably due in part to poor access to anteriorly located tumor and in part from further destabilization of the spine. Retrospective case series comparisons (39) and one small randomized trial (40) found no difference in outcome between patients receiving laminectomy and RT compared to RT alone. Consequently, decompressive laminectomy has fallen out of favor for the treatment of ESCC (31).

Vertebrectomy

Improvements in spinal instrumentation led some surgeons to investigate more aggressive tumor resections, often consisting of vertebral corpectomy, for patients with ESCC (41–43). The goal of such procedures is gross total tumor resection followed by spinal reconstruction, if necessary. These investigators reported promising results by curetting out the tumor from the vertebral body and epidural space, followed by bone grafting or the use of methylmethacrylate and instrumentation to achieve stabilization. Patients frequently experienced improvement over preoperative neurologic status, and some paraplegic patients regained the ability to walk. One series suggested that 82% of operated patients improved after the procedure, and two-thirds of patients who were nonambulatory preoperatively were able to walk after the surgery (43). However, another study found that the inability to ambulate preoperatively prognosticated a poor outcome (44). Although the promising results from aggressive surgical resection have not yet been confirmed in a randomized controlled trial (such a trial is ongoing), this option should be strongly considered in cases of spinal instability, bony compression, local recurrence after spinal RT or deterioration during RT, and minimal or controllable malignancy elsewhere (10,31). Patients who have not previously received spinal RT generally do so after postsurgical healing has occurred. Aggressive resection carries a significant morbidity and mortality rate. Mortality ranges between 6% and 10%, and the complication rate is as high as 48%, with wound breakdown (probably related to corticosteroids and, in some cases, prior RT), stabilization failure, infection, and hemorrhage occurring fairly commonly (43).

Chemotherapy

Chemotherapy does not have a role in the standard treatment of ESCC in patients with prostate cancer, although it can be useful for ESCC from more chemosensitive tumors, such as non-Hodgkin's lymphoma (45).

Hormonal Therapy

There are several anecdotal reports of ESCC from prostate cancer responding to hormonal manipulation alone (3,46,47). Hormonal manipulation may also have a role in the treatment of ESCC in combination with other therapies (48). In one study, 37 men with prostate cancer and ESCC were treated with laminectomies. Fifteen of these men were also treated with hormonal manipulation. Of these patients, 80% were ambulatory after therapy, compared to only 42%

of patients who had received prior hormonal therapy and were treated only with surgery (9,48). Unfortunately, 57% to 82% of prostate cancer patients who develop ESCC have already had prior hormonal therapy (3,9,12,48), limiting the usefulness of this approach.

Bisphosphonates such as clodronate and pamidronate are of proven benefit in reducing bone pain in patients with prostate cancer (49,50), but they have not yet been shown to decrease the incidence of ESCC.

Recurrent Epidural Spinal Cord Compression

Because the prognosis for patients with ESCC from prostate cancer is poor after treatment for ESCC (8), locally recurrent epidural disease is a relatively infrequent problem. However, for those patients who recover from the initial episode of ESCC, there is a 45% risk of developing a further episode of ESCC at the same site or at a different site within the next 2 years (8). Further treatment with RT can be given if the recurrent disease occurs outside the previous radiation field. If the relapse occurs within the previous radiation field, then surgery should be considered. A second course of RT has generally been avoided in the past because of concerns about radiation injury. However, there is some evidence suggesting that a second course of spinal radiation can be given reasonably safely to patients in whom there are no other satisfactory options (10). Although re-irradiation may result in a cumulative dose exceeding the spinal cord's reported radiation tolerance, radiation myelopathy in this setting is uncommon. This may be attributable to repair of radiation damage between courses, the generally short survival of patients receiving re-irradiation compared to the latency of radiation myelopathy, or a combination of these factors. Radiosurgery delivered with a linear accelerator is another modality in the early stages of investigation for such patients (51).

Prognosis

The prognosis of prostate cancer patients with ESCC is generally poor, with a median survival of approximately 4 to 9 months and 13% to 25% of patients surviving 2 years (3,7,8,33). The prognosis is significantly better for those patients with no prior hormone therapy (median survival of 16 to 21 months) (3,8). Other favorable prognostic factors include a single level of compression and a young age (younger than 65 years) (8). One study found that patients with poorly differentiated tumors had a worse prognosis (4), but another study could not confirm this association (7).

INTRACRANIAL METASTASES

Intracranial metastases occur in less than 5% of patients with prostate cancer (52–55). Many of these are asymptomatic and detected only at postmortem (52,55). The majority of these intracranial metastases are usually located in the dura, and metastases to the brain parenchyma are relatively uncommon (54–59).

Brain Metastases

Brain metastases occur in fewer than 1% of patients with prostate cancer in most autopsy series (54,56,57). These metastases are thought to reach the brain via the Batson's plexus or through the systemic circulation. The majority of these metastases are asymptomatic (54). The precise clinical features of symptomatic lesions vary depending on their location and include headaches, seizures, and focal neurologic deficits. The management is similar to other brain metastases and includes corticosteroids, surgery for single or symptomatic lesions, and whole brain RT (60). Radiosurgery may be useful for recurrent metastases. There has also been a report of a patient with a brain metastasis who responded to estramustine (61).

Calvarial Metastases

Prostate metastases probably reach the skull vault via Batson's plexus. Calvarial metastases are common and often asymptomatic, although they may occasionally cause pain or present as a palpable mass (Fig. 47-2). Less often, they may compress the underlying brain and produce neurologic symptoms. Rarely, calvarial metastases may compress the sagittal or lateral sinus (62). This may lead to increased intracranial pressure with headaches and papilledema. Occa-

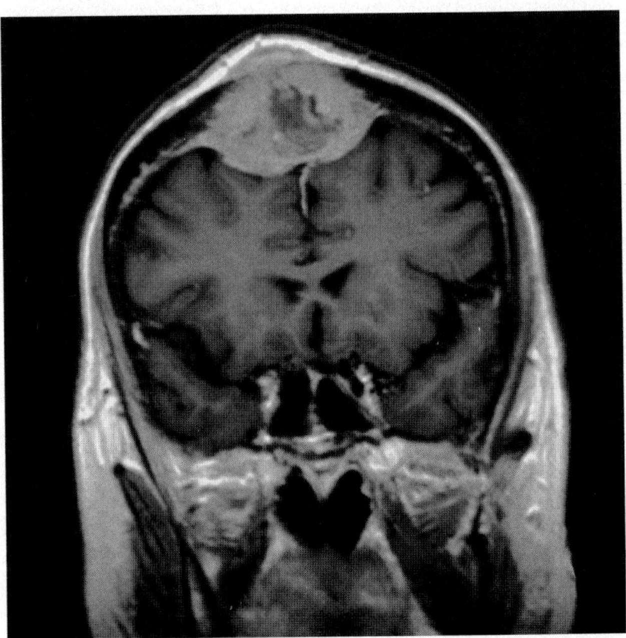

FIGURE 47-2. Coronal T1-weighted magnetic resonance imaging of brain showing a large calvarial metastasis from prostate cancer.

sionally, the sinuses become occluded and venous infarction of the brain results with headaches, seizures, and focal neurologic deficits. There has been a report of a patient with prostate cancer and venous sinus thrombosis who subsequently developed dural arteriovenous malformations (63).

Asymptomatic calvarial metastases may not require treatment. Symptomatic lesions usually respond to RT. Surgery may occasionally be necessary to remove a large lesion, especially if it is compressing the underlying brain.

Dural Metastases

Metastases to the dura usually arise by direct extension from the adjacent skull or hematogenous spread. Carcinoma of the prostate is one of the most common causes of dural metastases, together with lung and breast cancer (64,65).

Dural metastases may act as a mass lesion, compressing the underlying brain, producing seizures, headaches, and focal neurologic deficits. The adjacent bone may or may not be involved. When these metastases are located at the base of the skull, a number of characteristic syndromes can be produced, depending on the location of the lesion (66,67).

Jugular Foramen Syndrome

Metastases to the region of the jugular foramen produce a dull constant pain that typically radiates to the occiput or postauricular region or occasionally to one or both shoulders. Involvement of the glossopharyngeal nerve may produce a sharp lancinating pain in the throat or ear that may be exacerbated by neck flexion or swallowing (glossopharyngeal neuralgia). Rarely, syncope may occur. There may be deficits involving cranial nerves IX to XI.

Clivus Syndrome

Involvement of the clivus produces a headache in the region of the vertex, which is exacerbated by neck flexion. Depending on the location of the metastases, any of the cranial nerves that pass through the dura in the region of the clivus (cranial nerves VI to XII) may be affected.

Parasellar and Middle Cranial Nerve Fossa Syndrome

Metastases to the cavernous sinus may produce ipsilateral facial pain in the periorbital or maxillary region. Cranial nerve involvement (III to VI) is common, resulting in ophthalmoplegia and facial numbness (Fig. 47-3). Less often there is proptosis and vision loss.

Orbital Syndrome

Metastases to the orbit produces pain behind the eye or supraorbital or periorbital pain. The pain is dull and constant and worse with eye movement or when the patient

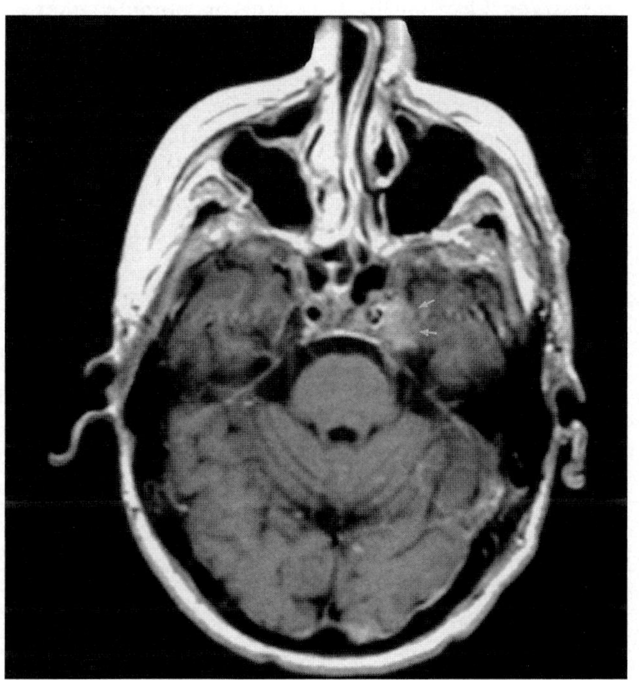

A

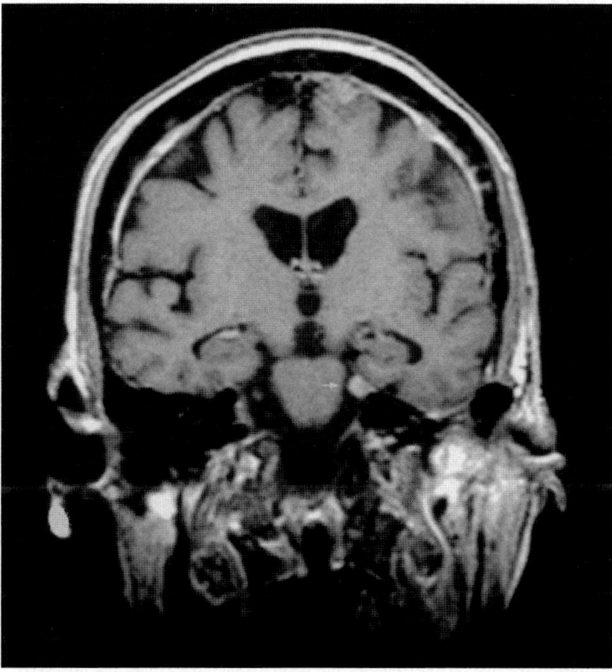

B

FIGURE 47-3. **A:** Axial T1-weighted magnetic resonance imaging of the brain with gadolinium showing an irregular enhancing metastasis in the left trigeminal ganglion and extending anteriorly into the cavernous sinus. This patient had symptoms of left facial numbness. **B:** Coronal T1-weighted magnetic resonance imaging of the brain with gadolinium showing the same lesion.

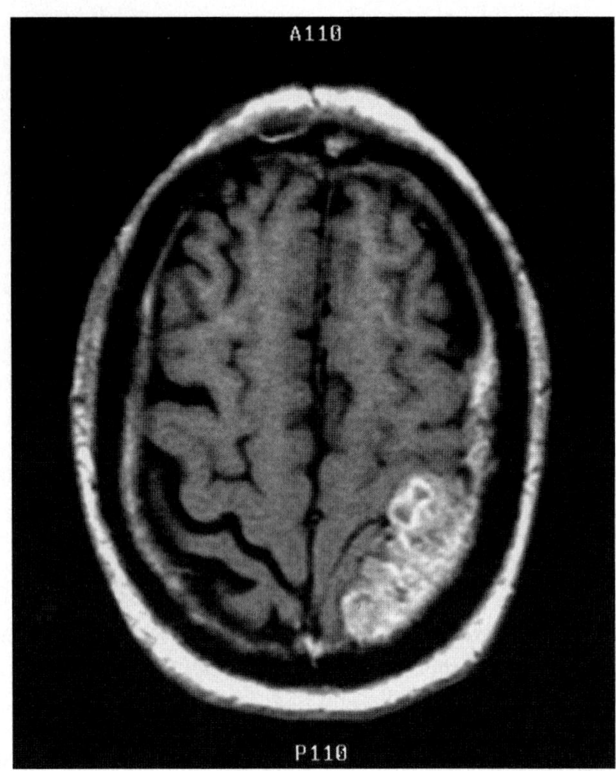

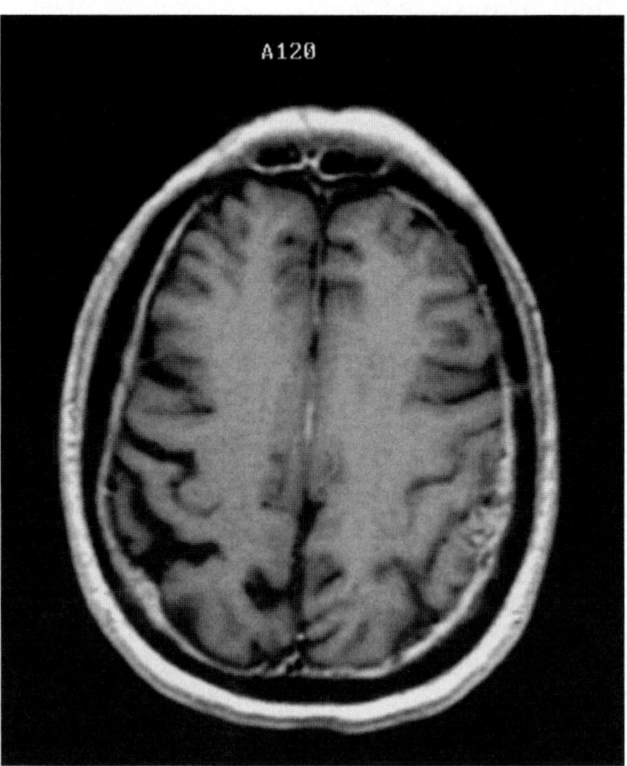

FIGURE 47-4. Axial T1-weighted magnetic resonance imaging of the brain with gadolinium showing a large dural-based metastasis from prostate cancer in the left frontal parietal region before **(A)** and after radiotherapy **(B)**, showing the radiosensitive nature of many of these metastases.

lies down. Proptosis, vision loss, and disorders or cranial nerves II, IV, V1, V2, and VI may occur.

Occipital Condyle Syndrome

Metastases to the occipital condyle produces a dull, constant pain in the occipital region exacerbated by neck movements. There may be tenderness to palpation in the occiput and neck stiffness. Involvement of the hypoglossal nerve in the hypoglossal canal results in ipsilateral wasting, fasciculations, and tongue weakness. Occasionally, sternocleidomastoid weakness may result from XI nerve involvement.

Mental Neuropathy

Metastases to the dura or leptomeninges may partially affect the mandibular division of the trigeminal nerve in the foramen ovale and result in numbness over the ipsilateral chin ("numb chin syndrome"). However, this syndrome is more commonly caused by metastases to the jaw involving the mental or inferior alveolar branch of the mandibular nerve (68,69). There may be associated pain and swelling, but painless involvement of the mental nerve can also occur. Plain x-rays or bone scans may be helpful in making the diagnosis, but often these tests are negative.

MRI is the most sensitive test for detecting dural metastases. Occasionally, bone scans or computed tomography scans with bone windows may help with skull-base lesions. Most patients can be treated with corticosteroids and standard external beam radiation therapy (Fig. 47-4). Surgery is rarely feasible or necessary. For single isolated dural metastases, or a tumor that has recurred after standard external beam radiation therapy, stereotactic radiosurgery may have a role. In general, cranial neuropathies tend to respond poorly to treatment (65,70). Treatment of symptoms within 1 month of onset and higher doses of RT (36 Gy) are associated with slightly better outcome (65).

Rarely, dural metastases may cause symptoms by exuding fluid into the subdural space, producing a subdural hematoma or effusion (71–73). Patients may be asymptomatic, but, as the fluid or blood collection increases in size, they may experience headaches, lethargy, and focal neurologic deficits. Rarely, patients may present acutely as a result of the subdural hematoma (72).

The diagnosis of multiple dural metastases in a patient with metastatic prostate cancer is usually straightforward. However, it can be difficult to differentiate dural-based metastases from meningiomas if there are only one or two lesions. Dural metastases usually respond to RT, but surgery may be needed for large symptomatic lesions or if the diagnosis of meningioma cannot be excluded by neuroimaging.

LEPTOMENINGEAL METASTASES (CARCINOMATOUS MENINGITIS)

Leptomeningeal metastases from prostate cancer are extremely uncommon with only a few reported cases (74,75). The response to treatment is generally poor.

PERIPHERAL NEUROMUSCULAR DISORDERS

Lumbosacral Plexus Lesions

Prostate cancer tends to metastasize to the spine and produce neurologic symptoms in the lower extremities by compressing the cauda equina or the lumbosacral nerve roots. Rarely, the tumor will infiltrate the lumbosacral plexus directly, producing pain, weakness, and paresthesias in the legs (76).

Peroneal Neuropathies

Prostate cancer patients are at increased risk of developing peroneal neuropathies, characterized by foot drop and numbness over the anterolateral aspect of the shin and the dorsum of the foot. This condition results from compression of the common peroneal nerve at the level of the fibular head. Predisposing factors include weight loss, prolonged bed rest, leg crossing, and chemotherapy. In general, the prognosis is good and the neuropathy improves in the majority of patients (77).

Paraneoplastic Neuromuscular Disorders

Sensory neuronopathy, Lambert-Eaton myasthenic syndrome (LEMS), and inflammatory myopathies may occur in prostate cancer patients as paraneoplastic syndromes. These are discussed in Paraneoplastic Syndromes.

CEREBROVASCULAR DISORDERS

Cerebral Infarction

The majority of strokes in patients with prostate cancer are due to atherosclerosis and unrelated to the neoplasm (78,79). However, some of these strokes may be caused by the hypercoagulable state present in many patients with metastatic prostate cancer. These patients may develop nonbacterial thrombotic endocarditis characterized by the formation of platelet fibrin vegetations on heart valves. These vegetations can embolize to cerebral vessels of any size, typically producing focal deficits, although occasionally patients may develop an encephalopathy without focal features. Echocardiography sometimes demonstrates the vegetations, but these vegetations are usually small and may not be detected. Some of these patients experience concomitant systemic venous or arterial thromboembolic disease. The absence of controlled studies makes treatment recommendations problematic. When feasible, treatment directed at the underlying tumor is indicated. Heparin has been of anecdotal benefit in this setting (80).

Chronic disseminated intravascular coagulation (DIC) may coexist with nonbacterial thrombotic endocarditis or can occur in its absence. Typically, it produces an encephalopathy with little in the way of focal findings (79). Chronic DIC may be very difficult to diagnose, as the usual hematologic parameters, such as prothrombin time, partial thromboplastin time, and platelet count (which are abnormal in acute DIC), are usually normal, although fibrin degradation products and D-dimer should be positive. However, these laboratory abnormalities are also frequently present in cancer patients without central nervous system (CNS) complications from DIC. Heparin has occasionally been of anecdotal benefit.

Rarely, prostate metastases to the dura will cause venous sinus thrombosis and hemorrhagic infarction of the brain (71,72).

Cerebral Hemorrhage

Cerebral hemorrhage is very uncommon in patients with prostate cancer. As discussed earlier, metastases to the dura may result in subdural hematomas (71,73). Rarely, patients may present after hemorrhage into a cerebral metastasis (81). The treatment for dural and parenchymal metastases is RT, but, if the hematoma is large, surgical evacuation may be necessary.

PARANEOPLASTIC SYNDROMES

Paraneoplastic syndromes are a group of neurologic disorders occurring in cancer patients that are not caused by the direct effect of the cancer itself or its metastases or other nonmetastatic effects of cancer, such as opportunistic infections, side effects of therapy, nutritional, metabolic, or vascular disorders. These disorders are rare, affecting fewer than 1% of patients with cancer. Paraneoplastic neurologic disorders are most commonly associated with small cell lung cancer. Nonetheless, they occasionally occur in conjunction with prostate cancer and are probably most common in patients with a small cell component (82–84) (Table 47-1).

The pathogenesis of most paraneoplastic syndromes is unknown, but there is increasing evidence that an autoimmune process is frequently involved (81–83). A number of autoantibodies has been identified that react with tumor and neuronal antigens (onconeural antigens) (85). The antibodies directed against tumor antigens presumably cross-react with antigens in neurons, resulting in paraneoplastic syndromes. These antibodies may be present in the serum and CSF and may help in the diagnosis of these disorders.

TABLE 47-1. PARANEOPLASTIC SYNDROMES ASSOCIATED WITH PROSTATE CANCER

Syndrome (ref)	Antibody	Clinical features	Course
Encephalomyelitis (87,88)	Anti-Hu (ANNA-1)	Variable, may include: sensory neuronopathy, limbic encephalitis, cerebellar degeneration, brainstem encephalitis, myelitis, autonomic dysfunction	Rarely may respond to treatment of tumor or immunosuppression
Brainstem encephalitis (83)	None	Loss of horizontal eye movements, facial and pharyngeal spasms, mild gait unsteadiness	No response to treatment
Cerebellar degeneration (82,87,90)	Anti-Hu	Progressive ataxia	Usually no improvement
Lambert-Eaton myasthenic syndrome (92,93)	Anti-VGCC	Weakness, fatigability, limb pain, autonomic dysfunction	Responds to treatment of tumor, immunosuppression, 3,4-aminopyridine, pyridostigmine (Mestinon)
Polymyositis and dermatomyositis (94–96)	None	Proximal and bulbar weakness, rash (dermatomyositis)	Responds to immunosuppression
Paraneoplastic retinal degeneration (98)	Anti-recoverin	Vision loss, photosensitivity	May respond to steroids

ANNA-1, antineuronal nuclear antibody type 1; Anti-Hu, antihuman antibody; Anti-VGCC, antibody to voltage-gated calcium channels.

Paraneoplastic Encephalomyelitis

One of the most common paraneoplastic syndromes associated with prostate cancer is defined by the presence of an antibody that binds to neuronal nuclei in the central and peripheral nervous system. This antibody is variously known as anti-Hu or antineuronal nuclear antibody type 1. Laboratory tests for the presence of this antibody are commercially available. Approximately 80% of patients with neurologic symptoms associated with the anti-Hu antibody have small cell lung cancer, but 2% to 3% have prostate cancer (86,87).

The patient with anti-Hu antibodies may present with varied neurologic symptoms and signs. The most common clinical presentation is a rapidly progressive sensory neuronopathy over days to weeks causing paresthesias, numbness, and sensory ataxia. The pathologic concomitant is a dorsal root ganglionitis. However, patients may also present with severe amnestic syndromes and seizures characteristic of limbic encephalitis. MR scans in these patients may show mesial temporal lobe abnormalities. Patients may present with cerebellar degeneration characterized by rapidly developing ataxia, dysarthria, nystagmus, and oscillopsia. Patients with anti-Hu may also develop brainstem signs, myelopathy, constipation, and anterior horn-cell dysfunction, producing neurogenic atrophy. Mixtures of findings are common (85,86,88,89). The CSF may show a lymphocytic pleocytosis, mild protein elevation, and oligoclonal bands. The anti-Hu antibody is present in the serum and CSF. No therapy specifically directed at the neurologic symptoms is of proven benefit, although various forms of immunosuppression have been tried (85,86,88,89).

Two patients have been reported with a unique paraneoplastic syndrome thus far exclusively associated with prostate carcinoma (83). These patients developed loss of horizontal eye movements, facial and pharyngeal spasms, and mild gait unsteadiness. Although no antineuronal antibodies were detected, both patients had evidence of chronic brainstem inflammation on postmortem.

Paraneoplastic Cerebellar Degeneration

Prostate cancer is a rare cause of paraneoplastic cerebellar degeneration (82,89,90). In one large series, 3 of 199 cases of cerebellar degeneration were associated with prostate cancer (89). Cerebellar degeneration is characterized by a subacute cerebellar syndrome that progresses over weeks or months, resulting in severe truncal and appendicular ataxia, dysarthria, and, frequently, down-beating nystagmus, vertigo, and diplopia (85,86,88,89). The cerebellar deficits usually stabilize, but the patient is frequently severely incapacitated by then. Cerebellar degeneration tends to occur with small cell prostate cancer and may be associated with the anti-Hu antibody, as discussed earlier (82). Pathologically, there is loss of Purkinje cells in the cerebellum. The prognosis is generally poor and most patients do not recover despite treatment of the prostate cancer or immunosuppressive therapy.

Motor Neuron Disease

There have been rare reports of amyotrophic lateral sclerosis in patients with prostate cancer, but it is likely that these associations are fortuitous (91).

Lambert-Eaton Myasthenic Syndrome

LEMS is characterized by weakness and fatigability, especially of proximal muscles in the lower extremities. Muscle aching and limb pain are common. Autonomic involvement occurs in 80% of patients (85,88,89) and typically manifests as dry mouth and impotence. Cranial nerve symptoms, such as diplopia, ptosis, and dysphagia, are usually mild and transient but may lead to an incorrect diagnosis of myasthenia gravis. On examination, there is usually proximal muscle weakness and reduced or absent deep tendon reflexes. With repeated muscle contractions, there may be improvement in muscle strength and potentiation of reflexes (89). LEMS is typically associated with small cell lung cancer, but it has been reported with adenocarcinoma (92) and small cell carcinoma of the prostate (93).

Neurophysiologic studies are helpful in making the diagnosis. Nerve conduction studies show normal conduction velocities but very low amplitude compound muscle action potentials (less than 10% of normal). After exercising the muscle for 10 to 15 seconds, the compound muscle action potentials may increase more than 200%. Repetitive stimulation produces a decrement at low rates of stimulation (2 to 5 Hz), but at high rates (20 to 50 Hz), a marked increment (200% to 1,000%) may occur (89). Electromyography shows variation in the amplitude of voluntary muscle potentials, indicating presynaptic dysfunction (89).

LEMS is an autoimmune disorder in which antibodies react with the N and P/Q types of voltage-gated calcium channels (VGCCs) on presynaptic nerve terminals (85,89). The beta subunit of the calcium channel and synaptotagmin are thought to be the specific targets of the immune response. It is postulated that the VGCCs expressed on tumor cells trigger an antibody response in which immunoglobulin G cross reacts with presynaptic VGCCs (85,88,89). Loss of VGCCs leads to reduced calcium entry during nerve terminal depolarization and concomitant decrease in neurotransmitter release (85,89). The transient beneficial effect of muscle contraction is owed to an increase in calcium concentration in the axon terminal, temporarily increasing acetylcholine release (85,89). These autoantibodies have been used as a diagnostic test for LEMS (85,88,89).

Effective treatment of the tumor usually results in improvement of the condition. Steroids, plasmapheresis, and intravenous gamma globulins have all been reported to produce symptomatic improvement in some patients (85,88,89). 3,4-Diaminopyridine, which promotes the release of acetylcholine through its effects on potassium channels, is useful in patients with LEMS and may be used alone or in combination with other therapies. Anticholinesterases may also improve muscle strength slightly, especially when used with 3,4-diaminopyridine (85,88,89).

Polymyositis and Dermatomyositis

Perhaps 10% of cases of inflammatory myopathies, such as dermatomyositis and polymyositis, are associated with systemic cancer. This association appears strongest with dermatomyositis and increases with age. There are case reports of dermatomyositis and polymyositis associated with prostate cancer (94–96). Patients with dermatomyositis and polymyositis develop proximal muscle weakness, whereas those with dermatomyositis also have characteristic skin changes. Serum creatine kinase and aldolase levels are elevated. Electromyography shows characteristic myopathic changes (short-duration, low-amplitude polyphasic units on voluntary contraction, increased spontaneous activity with fibrillations, complex repetitive discharges, and positive sharp waves), and muscle biopsy confirms the presence of an inflammatory myopathy (97). The muscle disorder responds to conventional immunosuppressive treatment. There have been anecdotal reports of improvement after treatment of the underlying tumor.

Paraneoplastic Retinal Degeneration

Paraneoplastic retinal degeneration or cancer-associated retinopathy is usually associated with small cell lung cancer but has been reported with prostate cancer (98). These patients have a clinical triad of severe photosensitivity, scotomatous vision loss, and attenuation of retinal arteriole caliber (85,88,89). In addition, there may be light-induced glare, impaired color vision, night blindness, and bizarre visual obscurations. Pathologically, there is widespread degeneration of photoreceptors, loss of nuclei from the outer nuclear layer of the retina, and infiltration of macrophages in the outer layers and retinal pigment epithelium. This syndrome is thought to be immune mediated, and autoantibodies recognizing antigens in the retina have been characterized. One antibody to a 23-kd cancer-associated retinopathy antigen located within photoreceptors (recoverin) has been used to diagnose this syndrome (85,88,89).

NEUROLOGIC COMPLICATIONS OF PROSTATE CANCER THERAPY

Hormonal Therapy

Bicalutamide (Casodex)

Bicalutamide is a nonsteroidal antiandrogen that occasionally causes confusion, somnolence, and nervousness (99).

Estramustine (Emcyt)

Estramustine has estrogenic effects on tissues, as well as inhibiting microtubules and producing metaphase arrest. It is often used in combination with vinblastine. Estramustine occasionally causes headaches and has been associated with cerebrovascular events (100).

Flutamide (Eulexin)

Neurologic symptoms are uncommon with flutamide. Very rarely, patients may complain of drowsiness and confusion (99).

Goserelin (Zoladex)

Goserelin is an analogue of luteinizing hormone releasing hormone that inhibits gonadotropin release from the pituitary gland. Neurologic complications are uncommon, but, like leuprolide, it can result in bone pain during the first week of therapy in patients as a result of tumor flare. This can be blocked with concurrent use of flutamide (99).

Ketoconazole (Nizoral)

Ketoconazole is an antifungal agent that has antiandrogen activity and is occasionally used in patients with prostate cancer. Rarely, it can cause confusion, apathy, and confabulation. These symptoms resolve when the medication is withdrawn (101).

Leuprolide Acetate (Lupron)

Neurologic complications are uncommon with leuprolide, a gonadotropin-releasing hormone analogue, but it can cause headaches, dizziness, and paresthesias. It can also produce bone pain during the first weak of treatment as a result of tumor flare (99).

Pamidronate (Aredia)

Pamidronate is a biphosphate used to treat hypercalcemia and bony metastases. Approximately 2% of patients experience insomnia, sleepiness, or abnormal vision (99).

Chemotherapy

Carboplatin

Unlike cisplatin, peripheral neuropathy and CNS toxicity occur only rarely at conventional doses with carboplatin. However, a severe neuropathy can develop after high-dose carboplatin (102).

Cisplatin

The main neurologic complication of cisplatin is an axonal neuropathy affecting predominantly large myelinated sensory fibers (100,102,103). The primary site of damage is the dorsal root ganglion, but the peripheral nerve may also be affected. The neuropathy is characterized by subacute development of numbness; paresthesias; and, occasionally, pain in the extremities. Proprioception is impaired and reflexes are lost, but pin prick, temperature sensation, and power are often spared. Nerve conduction studies show decreased amplitude of sensory action potentials and prolonged sensory latencies compatible with a sensory axonopathy. Sural nerve biopsy shows demyelination and axonal loss. Typically, neuropathies develop in patients after cumulative doses of cisplatin greater than 400 mg per m^2 (100,102,104), although there is marked individual variability. Patients with mild neuropathies can continue to receive full doses of cisplatin, but those with more severe neuropathies may require dose reduction or discontinuation of the drug. After cessation of chemotherapy, the neuropathy continues to deteriorate for several months in 30% of patients (105). Most patients eventually improve, although the recovery is often incomplete. There is no effective treatment for cisplatin neurotoxicity, although agents, such as amifostine (106) and the adrenocorticotropic hormone (4–9) analogue Org 2766 (107), provide partial protection.

Cisplatin may cause ototoxicity, leading to high-frequency sensorineural hearing loss and tinnitus or a vestibulopathy, resulting in ataxia and vertigo. Rare neurologic complications associated with cisplatin include Lhermitte's sign (paresthesias in the back and extremities with neck flexion due to transient demyelination of the cord), autonomic neuropathy, encephalopathy, seizures, and stroke (100,102).

Etoposide

Etoposide is a topoisomerase II inhibitor used occasionally for prostate cancer in combination with other drugs. It generally has little neurotoxicity, even in high doses. Rarely, it can cause a peripheral neuropathy, mild disorientation, seizures, transient cortical blindness, and optic neuritis (108).

5-Fluorouracil

5-Fluorouracil is a fluorinated pyrimidine that disrupts DNA synthesis by inhibiting thymidylate synthetase. An acute cerebellar syndrome occurs in approximately 5% of patients (100,108). This usually begins weeks or months after treatment and is characterized by the acute onset of ataxia, dysmetria, dysarthria, and nystagmus. The drug should be discontinued in any patient who develops a cerebellar syndrome, and, with time, these symptoms usually resolve completely. Rarely, 5-fluorouracil may cause encephalopathies, optic neuropathies, eye movement abnormalities, focal dystonias, cerebrovascular disorders, parkinsonian syndromes, or peripheral neuropathies (100,102).

Suramin

Suramin inhibits the binding of a number of growth factors to their receptors, including platelet-derived growth factor, basic fibroblast growth factor, and transforming growth factor beta. It also inhibits DNA polymerases and glycosaminoglycan catabolism. Suramin causes a severe peripheral neuropathy in 10% of patients (109). There are two patterns of neuropathy, an inflammatory demyelinating neuropathy resembling Guillain-Barré syndrome clinically, which may improve after the drug is discontinued, and a distal axonal sensorimotor polyneuropathy (110). Because the development of neuropathy correlates with blood levels of suramin, it can be prevented by monitoring blood levels of the drug (serious complications are uncommon at plasma levels less than 350 μg per mL) (102).

Taxanes: Paclitaxel (Taxol) and Taxotere (Docetaxel)

The taxanes, paclitaxel and taxotere, are plant alkaloids that inhibit microtubule function, leading to mitotic arrest (100,103). Paclitaxel produces a dose-limiting peripheral neuropathy, which occurs in 60% of patients receiving 250 mg per m^2 (111). The neuropathy is predominantly sensory and affects large and small fibers. Symptoms usually begin after 1 to 3 weeks of treatment. Patients develop burning paresthesias of the hands and feet and loss of reflexes. The neuropathy often does not progress despite continued treatment, and there have even been reports of patients improving with continuing therapy. Some patients develop arthralgias and myalgias beginning 2 to 3 days after a course of paclitaxel and lasting 2 to 4 days. Less commonly, paclitaxel can result in motor neuropathies that predominantly affect proximal muscles, perioral numbness, and autonomic neuropathies (102,103,112). Rarely, paclitaxel causes seizures or transient encephalopathies (102,103). Neuropathies are less common with taxotere but some patients develop sensory and motor neuropathies similar to paclitaxel (112,113).

Vinca Alkaloids

The main toxicity of vinca alkaloids is an axonal neuropathy resulting from disruption of the microtubules within axons and interference with axonal transport (103). The neuropathy involves sensory and motor fibers, although small sensory fibers are especially affected. Virtually all patients have some degree of neuropathy, which is the dose-limiting toxicity. The earliest symptoms are usually paresthesias in the fingertips and feet and muscle cramps. These symptoms may occur after several weeks of treatment or even after the drug has been discontinued and progress for several months before improving. Initially, objective sensory findings tend to be mild compared to the symptoms, but loss of ankle jerks is common. Occasionally, there may be profound weakness, with bilateral foot drop and wrist drop and loss of all sensory modalities. Severe neuropathies are particularly likely to develop in older patients who are cachectic, patients who have received prior radiation to the peripheral nerves, and those who have preexisting neurologic conditions, such as Charcot-Marie-Tooth disease (114). Patients with mild neuropathies can receive full doses of the drugs, but when the neuropathies interfere with neurologic function, reduction in dose or discontinuation of the drug may be necessary. Neurophysiologic studies show a primarily axonal neuropathy (102). Although there are anecdotal reports that glutamine may help some patients with vincristine neuropathy, there is generally no effective treatment (108).

Autonomic neuropathy is common in patients receiving vinca alkaloids. Colicky abdominal pain and constipation occur in almost 50% of patients and, rarely, paralytic ileus results. Because of this, patients should take prophylactic stool softeners and laxatives. Less commonly, patients may develop impotence, postural hypotension, and atonic bladders. Rarely, focal neuropathies and cranial neuropathies can occur (102,108). Other rare CNS complications include the syndrome of inappropriate secretion of antidiuretic hormone, seizures, encephalopathy, transient cortical blindness, ataxia, athetosis, and parkinsonism (100,102,108).

The vinca alkaloids vinblastine and vinorelbine, which are used most frequently in patients with prostate cancer, tend to have less neurotoxicity than vincristine.

Other Chemotherapeutic Agents

Other chemotherapeutic agents that may be used in patients with hormone-refractory prostate cancer, such as mitoxantrone and doxorubicin, have negligible neurotoxicity. Methotrexate is often associated with neurologic complications when administered intrathecally or at high doses, but the doses of intravenous methotrexate used in treatment regimens for prostate cancer usually have few neurologic complications.

Radiation Therapy

External beam radiation therapy for prostate cancer is frequently associated with bowel and genitourinary complications, including a high incidence of impotence, but more extensive injury to the lumbosacral plexus is extremely uncommon (115). Rarely, radiation therapy for epidural spinal cord compression may result in radiation myelopathy (10).

REFERENCES

1. Landis SH, Murray T, Bolden S, et al. Cancer Statistics, 1999. *CA Cancer J Clin* 1999;49:8–31.
2. Campbell JR, Godsall JW, Bloch S. Neurologic complications in prostate cancer. *Prostate* 1981;2:417–423.
3. Flynn DF, Shipley WU. Management of spinal cord compression secondary to metastatic prostatic carcinoma. *Urol Clin North Am* 1991;18:145–152.
4. Kuban DA, El-Mahdi AM, Sigfred SV, et al. Characteristics of cord compression in adenocarcinoma of prostate. *Urology* 1986;28:364–369.
5. Bach F, Larsen BH, Rohde K, et al. Metastatic spinal cord compression. Occurrences, symptoms, clinical presentations, and prognosis in 398 patients with spinal cord compression. *Acta Neurochir* 1990;107:37–43.
6. Liskow A, Chang CH, DeSanctis P, et al. Epidural cord compression in association with genitourinary neoplasms. *Cancer* 1986;58:949–954.

7. Rosenthal MA, Rosen D, Raghavan D, et al. Spinal cord compression in prostate cancer: a 10-year experience. *Br J Urol* 1992;69:530–533.
8. Huddart RA, Rajan B, Law M, et al. Spinal cord compression in prostate cancer: treatment outcome and prognostic factors. *Radiother Oncol* 1997;44:229–236.
9. Osborn JL, Getzenberg RH, Trump DL. Spinal cord compression in prostate cancer. *J Neurooncol* 1995;23:135–147.
10. Schiff D. Epidural spinal cord compression. UpToDate 2001.
11. Siegal T. Spinal cord compression: from laboratory to clinic. *Eur J Cancer* 1995;31A:1748–1753.
12. Smith EM, Hampel N, Ruff RL, et al. Spinal cord compression secondary to prostate carcinoma: treatment and prognosis. *J Urol* 1993;149:330–333.
13. van der Sande JJ, Kroger R, Boogerd W. Multiple spinal epidural metastases: an unexpectedly frequent finding. *J Neurol Neurosurg Psychiatry* 1990;53:1001–1003.
14. Helweg-Larsen S, Hansen SW, Sorensen PS. Second occurrence of symptomatic metastatic spinal cord compression and findings of multiple spinal epidural metastases. *Int J Radiat Oncol Biol Phys* 1995;33:595–598.
15. Gilbert RW, Kim JH, Posner JB. Epidural spinal cord compression from metastatic tumor: diagnosis and treatment. *Ann Neurol* 1978;3:40–51.
16. Helweg-Larsen S, Sorensen PS. Symptoms and signs in metastatic spinal cord compression: a study of progression from first symptoms until diagnosis in 153 patients. *Eur J Cancer* 1994;30A:396–398.
17. Posner JB. Spinal metastases. In: *Neurologic complications of cancer*. Philadelphia: F. A. Davis, 1995:111–141.
18. Zelefsky MJ, Scher HI, Krol G, et al. Spinal epidural tumor in patients with prostate cancer. *Cancer* 1992;70:2319–2325.
19. Boogerd W, van der Sande JJ. Diagnosis and treatment of spinal cord compression in malignant disease. *Cancer Treat Rev* 1993;19:129–150.
20. Schiff D, Batchelor T, Wen PY. Neurologic emergencies in cancer patients. *Neurol Clin* 1998;16:449–483.
21. Graus F, Krol G, Foley KM. Early diagnosis of spinal epidural metastasis (SEM): correlation with clinical and radiological findings. *Proc Am Soc Clin Oncol* 1985;4:269.
22. Portenoy RK, Galer BS, Salamon O, et al. Identification of epidural neoplasm: radiography and bone scintography in the symptomatic and asymptomatic spine. *Cancer* 1989;64: 2707–2713.
23. Helweg-Larsen S, Wagner A, Kjaer L, et al. Comparison of myelography combined with post-myelographic spinal CT and MRI in suspected metastatic disease of the spinal canal. *J Neurooncol* 1992;13:231–237.
24. Hagenau C, Grosh W, Currie M, et al. Comparison of spinal magnetic resonance imaging and myelography in cancer patients. *J Clin Oncol* 1987;5:1663–1669.
25. Schultheiss TE, Stephens LC. Invited review: permanent radiation myelopathy. *Br J Radiol* 1992;65;737–753.
26. Cantu RC. Corticosteroids for spinal metastases [Letter]. *Lancet* 1968;2:912.
27. Ushio Y, Posner R, Kim J-H, et al. Treatment of experimental spinal cord compression by extradural neoplasms. *J Neurosurg* 1977;47:380–390.
28. Delattre J-Y, Arbit E, Thaler HT, et al. A dose-response study of dexamethasone in a model of spinal cord compression caused by epidural tumor. *J Neurosurg* 1989;70:920–925.
29. Sorensen PS, Helweg-Larsen S, Mouridsen H, et al. Effect of high-dose dexamethasone in carcinomatous metastatic spinal cord compression treated with radiotherapy: a randomised trial. *Eur J Cancer* 1994;30A:22–27.
30. Heimdal K, Hirschberg H, Slettebo H, et al. High incidence of serious side effects of high-dose dexamethasone treatment in patients with epidural spinal cord compression. *J Neurooncol* 1992;12:141–144.
31. Loblaw DA, Laperriere NJ. Emergency treatment of malignant extradural spinal cord compression: an evidence based guideline. *J Clin Oncol* 1998;16:1613–1624.
32. Maranzano E, Latini P, Beneventi S, et al. Radiotherapy without steroids in selected metastatic spinal cord compression patients. A phase II trial. *Am J Clin Oncol* 1996;19:179–183.
33. Maranzano E, Latini P. Effectiveness of radiation therapy without surgery in metastatic spinal cord compression. Final results from a prospective trial. *Int J Radiat Oncol Phys* 1995;32:959–967.
34. Maranzano E, Latini P, Beneventi S, et al. Comparison of two different radiotherapy schedules for spinal cord compression in prostate cancer. *Tumori* 1998;84:472–477.
35. Greenberg HS, Kim JH, Posner JB. Epidural spinal cord compression from metastatic tumor: results with a new treatment protocol. *Ann Neurol* 1980;8:361–366.
36. Martenson JA Jr., Evans RG, Lie MR, et al. Treatment outcome and complications in patients treated for malignant epidural spinal cord compression (SCC). *J Neurooncol* 1985;3:77–84.
37. Maranzano E, Latini P, Checcaglini F, et al. Radiation therapy in metastatic spinal cord compression. A prospective analysis of 105 consecutive patients. *Cancer* 1991;67;1311–1317.
38. Kim RY, Spencer SA, Meredith RF, et al. Extradural spinal cord compression: Analysis of factors determining functional prognosis—prospective study. *Radiology* 1990;176:279–282.
39. Findlay GF. Adverse effects of the management of malignant spinal cord compression. *J Neurol Neurosurg Psychiatry* 1984;47:761–768.
40. Young RF, Post EM, King GA. Treatment of spinal epidural metastases. Randomized prospective comparison of laminectomy and radiotherapy. *J Neurosurg* 1980;53:741–748.
41. Siegal T, Siegal T, Robin G, et al. Anterior decompression of the spine for metastatic epidural cord compression: a promising avenue of therapy? *Ann Neurol* 1982;11:28–34.
42. Harrington KD. Anterior decompression and stabilization of the spine as a treatment for vertebral collapse and spinal cord compression from metastatic malignancy. *Clin Orthop* 1988;233:177–197.
43. Sundaresan N, Sachdev VP, Holland JF, et al. Surgical treatment of spinal cord compression from epidural metastasis. *J Clin Oncol* 1995;13:2330–2335.
44. Sioutos PJ, Arbit E, Meshulam CF, et al. Spinal metastases from solid tumors. *Cancer* 1995;76:1453–1459.
45. Wong ET, Portlock CS, O'Brien JP, et al. Chemosensitive epidural spinal cord disease in non-Hodgkin's lymphoma. *Neurology* 1996;46:1543–1547.
46. Sasagawa I, Gotoh H, Miyabayashi H, et al. Hormonal treatment of symptomatic spinal cord compression in advanced prostate cancer. *Int Urol Nohrol* 1991;23:351–356.

47. Gonzalez-Barcena D, Vadillo-Buenfil M, Cortez-Morales A, et al. Luteinizing hormone-releasing hormone antagonist cetrorelix as primary single therapy in patients with advanced prostatic cancer and paraplegia due to metastatic invasion of the spinal cord. *Urology* 1995;45:275–281.
48. Iacovou JW, Marks JC, Abrams PH, et al. Cord compression and carcinoma of the prostate: is laminectomy justified? *Br J Urol* 1985;57:733–736.
49. Bloomfield DJ. Should bisphonates be part of the standard therapy of patients with multiple myeloma or bone metastases from other cancers? An evidence-based review. *J Clin Oncol* 1998;16:1218–1225.
50. Coleman RE, Purohit OP, Vinholes JJ, et al. High dose pamidronate: clinical and biochemical effects in metastatic bone disease. *Cancer* 1997;80:1686–1690.
51. Hamilton AJ, Lulu BA, Fosmire H, et al. Preliminary clinical experience with linear accelerator-based spinal stereotactic radiosurgery. *Neurosurgery* 1995;36:311–319.
52. Taylor HG, Lefkowitz M, Skoog SJ, et al. Intracranial metastases in prostate cancer. *Cancer* 1984;53:2728–2730.
53. Castaldo JE, Bernat JL, Meier FA, et al. Intracranial metastases due to prostatic carcinoma. *Cancer* 1983;52:1739–1747.
54. Sutton MA, Watkins HL, Green LK, et al. Intracranial metastases as the first manifestation of prostate cancer. *Urology* 1996;48:789–793.
55. Kankonde M, Arcenas A, Long J, et al. Intracranial metastases from prostate cancer. *Proc Ann Meet Am Soc Clin Oncol* 1996;15:A663.
56. Zachariah B, Casey L, Zachariah SB, et al. Case report: brain metastases from primary small cell carcinoma of the prostate. *Am J Med Sci* 1994;308:177–179.
57. Catane R, Kaufman J, West C, et al. Brain metastases from prostatic carcinoma. *Cancer* 1976;38:2583–2587.
58. Kasabain NG, Previte SR, Kaloustian HD, et al. Adenocarcinoma of the prostate presenting initially as an intracerebral tumor. *Cancer* 1992;70:2149–2151.
59. Zhang X, Tsukuda F, Yamamoto N, et al. Brain metastasis from prostate cancer: a case report. *Int J Urol* 1997;4:519–521.
60. Wen PY, Loeffler JS. Management of brain metastases. *Oncology* 1999;13:941–961.
61. Kohri K, Yamate T, Tsujihashi H, et al. Effect of endocrine therapy on a brain metastatic lesion of prostatic carcinoma. *Urol Int* 1991;47:100–102.
62. Raizer JJ, DeAngelis LM. Cerebral vein thrombosis in patients with cancer. *Neurology* 1998;50;A189.
63. Sakurai N, Koike Y, Hashizume Y, et al. Dural arteriovenous malformation and sinus thrombosis in a patient with prostate cancer: an autopsy case. *Intern Med* 1992;31:1032–1037.
64. Ransom DT, Dinapoli RP, Richardson RL. Cranial nerve lesions due to base of the skull metastases in prostate carcinoma. *Cancer* 1990;65:586–589.
65. Gupta SR, Zdonczyk DE, Rubino FA. Cranial neuropathy in systemic malignancy in a VA population. *Neurology* 1990;40:997–999.
66. Hammack JE. Neurologic pain syndromes in cancer patients. In: Samuels MA, Feske S, eds. *Office practice of neurology.* New York: Churchill Livingstone, 1996;934–944.
67. Svare A, Fossa SD, Heier MS. Cranial nerve dysfunction in metastatic cancer of the prostate. *Br J Urol* 1998;61:441–444.
68. Burt RK, Sharfman WH, Karp BI, et al. Mental neuropathy (numb chin syndrome). A harbinger of tumor progression or relapse. *Cancer* 1992;70:877–881.
69. Cousin GC, Llankovan V. Mental nerve anaesthesia as a result of mandibular metastases of prostatic adenocarcinoma. *Br Dent J* 1994;177:383–384.
70. Seymore CH, Peeples WJ. Cranial nerve involvement with carcinoma of prostate. *Urology* 1988;31:211–213.
71. Posner JB. Vascular disorders. In: *Neurologic complications of cancer.* Philadelphia: F. A. Davis, 1995:199–229.
72. Barolat-Romana G, Maiman D, Dernbach P, et al. Prostate carcinoma presenting as intracranial hemorrhage. Case report. *J Neurosurg* 1984;60:414–416.
73. Minette SE, Kimmel DW. Subdural hematoma in patients with systemic cancer. *Mayo Clin Proc* 1989;64:637–642.
74. Schaller B, Merlo A, Kirsch E, et al. Prostate-specific antigen in the cerebrospinal fluid leads to diagnosis of solitary cauda equina metastasis: a unique case report and review of the literature. *Br J Cancer* 1998;77:2386–2389.
75. Lee JY, Bergmann M, Kuchelmeister K, et al. Metastasizing extraneural tumors along the CSF pathway. *Clin Neuropathol* 1997;16:117–121.
76. Aguilera Navarro JM, Lopez Dominguez JM, Gil Neciga E, et al. [Neoplastic lumbosacral plexopathy and "hot foot"]. *Neurologia* 1993;8:271–273.
77. Rubin DI, Kimmel DW, Cascino TL. Outcome of peroneal neuropathies in patients with systemic malignant disease. *Cancer* 1998;83:1602–1606.
78. Graus F, Rogers LR, Posner JB. Cerebrovascular complications in patients with cancer. *Medicine* 1985;64:16–35.
79. Chaturvedi S, Ansell J, Recht L. Should cerebral ischemic events in cancer patients be considered a manifestation of hypercoagulability? *Stroke* 1994;25:1215–1218.
80. Rogers LR, Cho E-S, Kempin S, et al. Cerebral infarction from nonbacterial thrombotic endocarditis. Clinical and pathological study including the effects of anticoagulation. *Am J Med* 1987;83:746–756.
81. Chang DS, Hwang SL, Hwong SL, et al. Prostatic carcinoma with brain metastasis presenting as a tumor hemorrhage. *Kaohsiung J Med Sci* 1998;14:247–250.
82. Greenlee JE, Jaeckle KA, Bashear HR, et al. Type II (Anti-Hu) antibody in suspected paraneoplastic syndromes: association with conditions other than small-cell lung cancer and initial detection of antibody at very low titer. *Ann Neurol* 1991;30:308(abst).
83. Baloh RW, DeRossett SE, Cloughesy TF, et al. Novel brainstem syndrome associated with prostate carcinoma. *Neurology* 1993;43:2591–2596.
84. Matzkin H, Braf Z. Paraneoplastic syndromes associated with prostatic carcinoma. *J Urol* 1987;138:1129–1133.
85. Dalmau JO, Rosenfeld MR. Paraneoplastic syndromes. *Oncology* (in press).
86. Dalmau J, Graus F, Rosenblum MK, et al. Anti-Hu–associated paraneoplastic encephalomyelitis/sensory neuronopathy. A clinical study of 71 patients. *Medicine* 1992;71:59–72.
87. Lucchinetti CF, Kimmel DW, Lennon VA. Paraneoplastic and oncologic profiles of patients seropositive for type 1

antineuronal nuclear autoantibodies. *Neurology* 1998;50: 652–657.

88. Dalmau JO, Posner JB. Neurological paraneoplastic syndromes. *Neuroscientist* 1998;4:443–453.
89. Posner JB. Paraneoplastic syndromes. In: *Neurologic complications of cancer*. Philadelphia: F. A. Davis, 1995:353–386.
90. McLaughlin J, Gingell JC, Harper G, et al. Cerebellar manifestations of prostatic carcinoma. *Postgrad Med J* 1992;68: 584–586.
91. Boninsegna C, Lovaste MG, Ferrari G. Carcinoma of the prostate and motor neuron disease. *Ital J Neurol Sci* 1985;6: 101–105.
92. Agarawal SK, Birch BR, Abercrombie GF. Adenocarcinoma of the prostate and Eaton-Lambert syndrome. A previously unreported association. *Scand J Urol Nephrol* 1995;29:351–353.
93. Tetu B, Ro JY, Ayala AG, et al. Small cell carcinoma of the prostate associated with myasthenic (Eaton-Lambert) syndrome. *Urology* 1989;32:148–152.
94. Machtey I. Polymyositis associated with carcinoma of the prostate. *J Am Geriatr Soc* 1970;18:250–255.
95. Ansai S, Koseki S, Takeda H, et al. Dermatomyositis accompanied by prostatic cancer and elevated serum CA 19.9. *Int J Dermatol* 1996;35:570–571.
96. Park Y, Oster MW, Olarte MR. Prostatic cancer with an unusual presentation: polymyositis and mediastinal adenopathy. *Cancer* 1981;48:1262–1264.
97. Dalakas MC. Polymyositis, dermatomyositis, and inclusion-body myositis. *N Engl J Med* 1991;325:1487–1498.
98. Lafeuillade A, Quilichim R, Chiozza R, et al. Paraneoplastic retinopathy (CAR syndrome) revealing prostatic cancer. *Presse Med* 1993;22:35.
99. *Physicians' desk reference*, 53rd ed. Montvale, NJ: Medical Economics Company, 1999.
100. Paleologos N. Complications of chemotherapy. In: Biller J, ed. *Iatrogenic neurology*. Boston: Butterworth–Heinemann, 1998:439–460.
101. Hanash KA. Neurologic complications of ketoconazole therapy for advanced prostate cancer. *Urology* 1989;39:368–373.
102. Wen PY. Neurologic complications of chemotherapy. In: Gilman S, ed. *Neurobase*. San Diego: Arbor Publishing, 1999.
103. Postma TJ, Heimans JJ. Chemotherapy-induced peripheral neuropathy. In: Vecht CJ, ed. *Handbook of clinical neurology*. Amsterdam: Elsevier Science, 1998:459–479.
104. van der Hoop RG, van der Berg ME, ten Bokkel Huinink WW, et al. Incidence of neuropathy in 395 patients with ovarian cancer treated with or without cisplatin. *Cancer* 1990;66:1697–1702.
105. Siegal T, Haim N. Cisplatin-induced peripheral neuropathy. Frequent off-therapy deterioration, demyelinating syndromes, and muscle cramps. *Cancer* 1990;66:1117–1123.
106. Kemp G, Rose P, Lurain J, et al. Amifostine pretreatment for protection against cyclophosphamide-induced and cisplatin-induced toxicities: results of a randomized control trial in patients with advanced ovarian cancer. *J Clin Oncol* 1996;14:2101–2112.
107. van der Hoop GR, Vecht CJ, van der Burg ME, et al. Prevention of cisplatin neurotoxicity with an ACTH(4-9) analogue in patients with ovarian cancer. *N Engl J Med* 1990;322:89–94.
108. Forsyth PA, Cascino TL. Neurologic complications of chemotherapy. In: Wiley RG, ed. *Neurologic complications of cancer*. New York: Marcel Dekker Inc, 1995:241–266.
109. La Rocca RV, Meer J, Gilliatt RW, et al. Suramin-induced polyneuropathy. *Neurology* 1990;40:954–960.
110. Chaudhry V, Eisenberger MA, Sinibaldi VJ, et al. A prospective study of suramin-induced peripheral neuropathy. *Brain* 1996;119:2039–2052.
111. Lipton RB, Apfel SC, Dutcher JP, et al. Taxol produces a predominantly sensory neuropathy. *Neurology* 1989;39:368–373.
112. Freilich RJ, Balmaceda C, Seidman AD, et al. Motor neuropathy due to docetaxel and paclitaxel. *Neurology* 1996;47: 115–118.
113. New PZ, Jackson CE, Rinaldi D, et al. Peripheral neuropathy secondary to docetaxel (Taxotere). *Neurology* 1996;46:108–111.
114. Hogan-Dann CM, Fellmeth WG, McGuire SA, et al. Polyneuropathy following vincristine therapy in two patients with Charcot-Marie-Tooth syndrome. *JAMA* 1984;252:2862–2863.
115. Beard CJ, Lamb C, Buswell L, et al. Radiation-associated morbidity in patients undergoing small-field external beam irradiation for prostate cancer. *Int J Radiat Oncol Biol Phys* 1998;41:257–262.

48

ORTHOPEDIC CONSIDERATIONS: IMPLICATIONS AND MANAGEMENT OF METASTATIC PROSTATE CANCER

BRENT ANDREW PONCE
JOHN E. READY

Prostate cancer is the most common diagnosed internal cancer and has the second highest number of cancer-related deaths in men, with more than 200,000 new diagnoses of prostate cancer in the United States and nearly 40,000 deaths anticipated in 1998 (1,2). There are several potential orthopedic consequences of metastatic prostate cancer, including skeletal pain, spinal cord compression, and impending or pathologic fracture. With a one in six lifetime incidence for men to be diagnosed with prostate cancer, the orthopedic management of metastatic prostate cancer is a frequent medical and surgical challenge (3). The goal of this chapter is to discuss the musculoskeletal implications and management of metastatic prostate cancer to bone.

Each year in the United States approximately 1.2 million new cases of cancer are diagnosed (2). Of this, only a fraction of 1%, roughly 2,000 cases, are primary bone sarcomas. In comparison, each year more than 600,000 bone metastases are diagnosed (2). The majority of skeletal metastases, up to 85%, are metastases from breast, lung, and prostate cancer (4). Bone is the third most frequent organ for metastatic carcinoma spread after the lung and liver. At the time of death, it is estimated that more than 50% of individuals with breast, lung, and prostate cancer will have skeletal metastases (2). Impending or pathologic fractures account for the majority of orthopedic procedures in patients with skeletal metastases (5).

The treatment goals for patients with prostatic skeletal metastases are to improve pain, control local tumor growth, and preserve or restore skeletal stability and clinical function. The goal is not to cure the patient of cancer. These goals are realized in controlling the foci of metastases and therefore reducing skeletal pain; preventing spinal cord compromise; and preventing, delaying, or prophylactically stabilizing impending pathologic fractures before they become orthopedic emergencies. In the event of spinal cord impingement or pathologic fracture, the goals become preservation of neurologic and ambulatory status in addition to pain control.

It is well known that prostate cancer has a predilection for skeletal metastases. In 1854, Thompson reported a case of paraplegia secondary to metastatic prostate cancer (6). Since then, the medical literature has documented the difficulties in managing osseous metastases from prostate cancer.

Over the past century, there have been significant medical and surgical advances in the management of skeletal metastases. In 1905, after reviewing more than 15 years of literature, Grunert wrote, "union of (pathologic fracture) fragments can never occur" (7). The espoused view was that pathologic fractures were untreatable and synonymous with terminal complications. Thirty years later, in the 1930s, this view began to change. However, standard treatment then included amputation, immobilization with traction, bracing or casting, and radiation (8). By the 1950s, surgical use of allografts and internal fixation was increasing (9). In the mid-1970s, favorable results were reported with methylmethacrylate augmentation of internal fixation (5). Over the past decade, improved internal fixation devices and modular arthroplasty prostheses have become increasingly available. In the past 60 years, several medical advancements have been made. These include hormonal therapy, chemotherapy, bisphosphonate treatment, radiation therapy, and systemic radionuclide administration. Overall, increased aggressiveness and capacity to manage metastatic prostate cancer has improved life expectancy and function while reducing pain (10–12).

EPIDEMIOLOGY

By definition, metastatic prostate cancer is considered stage M1 disease by the tumor-node-metastasis staging classification (13). The lymph nodes are the most frequent site of metastatic disease for prostate cancer followed by skeletal metastases (14). Metastases to the lungs, liver, pleura, and adrenals follow in descending frequency behind lymph node and skeletal metastases (15). Skeletal complaints secondary to metastases may be the initial presentation of prostate cancer in 10% to 20% of patients (4).

The pattern of skeletal metastases can vary considerably from an isolated axial or appendicular site to multiple regional areas or diffuse dissemination. The distribution of skeletal metastases within these sites can also vary. For example, spinal metastases rarely involve the transverse and spinous processes or the posterior arch and are typically concentrated in the vertebral bodies. Another example is found in the skull, in which metastatic lesions predominate in the calvaria as opposed to the mandible (16).

The likelihood of skeletal metastases from prostate cancer is dependent on the time of diagnosis and method of diagnosis. The frequency of skeletal metastases on being first diagnosed with prostate cancer ranges from 8% to 62% (4,17). Greater numbers of patients will eventually develop skeletal metastases, even after initial treatment. The sites with the greatest frequency of skeletal metastases determined by bone scan on initial diagnosis of prostate cancer are spine, pelvis, rib cage, skull, femur, shoulder, humerus, distal leg, and arm (18–20).

The frequency of skeletal metastases by the time of death increases dramatically. Autopsy evaluations have shown rates of osseous metastatic involvement ranging from 58% to 90% (15,21–24). The order of frequency for skeletal metastases also changes slightly with autopsy evaluation. The sites of greatest frequency include spine, femur, pelvis, ribs, sternum, skull, and humerus (25). Of interest, radiographic evidence of skeletal metastases at the time of death from metastatic prostate cancer was generally less than autopsy evaluation, with only 30% to 77% of patients having plain radiographic evidence of metastases (26,27).

Although the prevalence of prostate cancer is high and the occurrence of skeletal metastases is common, the frequency of orthopedic complaints varies. The frequency of impending or pathologic fractures appears to be only 3% to 4% of all impending or pathologic fractures (28,29). This is less than one-tenth of the number of pathologic fractures caused by breast cancer (29,30). The difference is believed to be secondary to prostate cancer primarily forming blastic and not lytic skeletal lesions. The frequency of neurologic deficits from spinal cord or nerve root compression is roughly 5% in patients with diffuse metastatic cancer (31). With spinal metastases, only a minority will eventually require surgical intervention. Although not specific to prostate cancer, the complaint of pain is present in nearly 80% of patients diagnosed with cancer (32).

The outcome of prostate cancer is determined primarily by the metastatic load (33,34). Although skeletal involvement is staged as M1, not all patients with skeletal metastases have equivalent life expectancies. The life expectancy of patients with a lower metastatic tumor load, such as an isolated thoracic vertebra or pelvis metastasis (median survival of 1,250 or 1,570 days, respectively), is significantly greater compared to patients with higher metastatic loads, such as in diffuse disease or metastases in distal sites (median survival 675 days or less) (19).

Once diagnosed with skeletal metastases, the average life expectancy is 30 to 35 months. (35). However, in 20% of patients with prostatic metastases, survival has averaged beyond 60 months in two study groups (36,37). The median survival after prostate cancer becomes hormonally refractive is approximately 1 year (38). Although not exclusive to prostate cancer, the life expectancies after sustaining a pathologic fracture are 40% survival at 6 months and 30% at 1 year (39).

BIOLOGY OF METASTATIC SPREAD

Several theories have been proposed to explain why and where metastatic foci are established. Ewing proposed a mechanical phenomenon of filtration related to vascular anatomy and hemodynamic factors (40). Paget's hypothesis, often referred to as the "seed and soil" theory, focuses on multifactorial host and cell factor interactions that determine nonrandom sites of metastatic survival from randomly distributed tumor emboli (41). Further "soil" support for a site-specific metastatic survival pattern came from Baston. He described a valveless paravertebral venous plexus and demonstrated connection with prostate veins (42). Through this network of veins, he and others hypothesize that prostate cancer cells could metastasize to the axial skeleton without entering the inferior vena cava or pelvic veins and, therefore, bypass the liver and lungs (18). Once established, a vicious cycle begins, in which metastases produce factors that facilitate growth and future skeletal metastases (43).

The mechanism of bony destruction by cancer metastases has been extensively studied. The determinant between lytic, sclerotic, and mixed radiographic appearances of skeletal metastases is in the balance between bone destruction by osteoclasts and bone production by osteoblasts. Some tumor metastases increase osteoclast bone-binding capacity and increase osteoclast formation and activity (44). Although prostate cancer primarily produces sclerotic metastases, there is evidence that microscopic lytic lesions may be required before the formation of blastic lesions (45,46).

RECURRENCE RISK

A critical issue for a patient diagnosed with prostate cancer is the rate of recurrence after treatment. Identification of patients at greatest risk for recurrence may assist early diagnosis of skeletal metastases and lessen potential musculoskeletal complications.

The risk of treatment failure after radical prostatectomy is related to the biologic aggressiveness of the tumor. Treatment failure is defined by increasing serum prostate-specific antigen (PSA) levels or clinical evidence of recurrence. Preoperative and postoperative nomograms have helped to identify patients at increased risk. Preoperative nomograms, frequently called Partin tables, include clinical stage of cancer, Gleason grade, and serum PSA level (47). Postradical prostatectomy nomograms have increased accuracy and include preoperative serum PSA level, Gleason sum, spread beyond the prostate into the seminal vesicles and lymph nodes, and the size of the largest nodal metastasis (48,49). In pre- and postoperative nomograms, higher values and more distant spread correlate with increased risk of recurrence. Recurrence beyond 7 years after radical prostatectomy is rare (49).

There are several markers that may reflect metastatic spread of prostate cancer. Some are not specific enough and others are not readily available for physicians to routinely follow. These include serum alkaline phosphates; serum acid phosphatase; osteoblastic markers, such as bone 4-carboxyglutamic acid protein and procollagen-I carboxyterminal peptide; biomarkers p27, p53, bcl-2, and Ki-67; and increased apoptotic index (50–54).

EVALUATION

The evaluation of all patients with metastatic disease begins with a thorough history and physical examination. Skeletal pain is often the harbinger for skeletal metastases and is the most common clinical complaint of osseous spread (55). In the patient interview, the clinician must identify prior history of any cancer, risk factors for cancer, and any constitutional symptoms, such as fatigue, a decrease in activity level, or unexplained weight loss.

The characterization of skeletal pain is an important feature of the history. The presentation can vary from mild discomfort to sharp, severe, intermittent, or constant pain. Increasing pain and weight-bearing pain may reflect an impending pathologic fracture, whereas constant pain may be evidence of a pathologic fracture. Constant, increasing, and night pain may also represent infection. With the complaint of skeletal pain, further evaluation is frequently delayed, because pain is often attributed to osteoarthritis or other benign conditions.

Patients with skeletal metastases from prostate cancer typically have one of three presentations. A large segment of patients have a known diagnosis of prostate cancer with a bone scan suggestive of skeletal metastases. Patients may or may not have skeletal complaints. Another common presentation is skeletal pain with abnormal plain radiographs, concerning for metastatic disease with or without a diagnosis of prostate cancer. A third presentation includes patients seen in the emergency room with a pathologic fracture or spinal cord compression. They also may or may not have a diagnosis of prostate cancer.

The details of each presentation are important. For example, it is helpful for the clinician to know that, in patients with prostate cancer, 85% with skeletal metastases at the time of initial diagnosis have serum PSA levels of 20 or greater (56). Skeletal metastases are rare (less than 3%) in patients with prostate cancer and a positive bone scan when their PSA level is 8 ng per mL or lower (57). Also, it is important to know that not all positive bone scans reflect skeletal metastases. Forty-five percent of bone scans in patients with a known primary cancer may be false positives (58).

Patients with skeletal pain and abnormal plain films are often referred to orthopedic surgeons for impending fracture evaluation. Frequently, a workup has been initiated to identify a primary source, supposing the lesion to be metastatic foci if the patient is more than 40 years old. The primary cancer may be identified nearly 80% of the time through a complete history, physical examination, and imaging with a chest x-ray, a chest computed tomography (CT) when indicated, abdominal and pelvis CT, and bone scan (59). The standard workup for patients with metastatic disease at our institution includes a chest x-ray, CT of the chest, abdomen and pelvis, and a bone scan in addition to the appropriate labs (we order a complete blood count, serum alkaline phosphatase, phosphorous, calcium, erythrocyte sedimentation rate, urine and serum immunoelectrophoresis, thyroid screen, blood urea nitrogen, and liver function tests). Even with a known diagnosis of prostate cancer, the isolated complaint of skeletal pain does not mandate the presence of skeletal metastases. More than one-third of patients with prostate cancer has bone pain without osseous metastases (60). It is also important to know that plain radiographs have high false-negative rates. X-ray findings can lag behind bone scan identification of metastatic spread by up to 18 months (61). Owing to the high false-negative rates of plain films, patients with skeletal complaints are often not referred for evaluation or do not receive a bone scan.

The history of patients presenting with spinal cord compromise is critical and directly correlates with outcome. With the acute onset of motor deficits, defined by a clinical course of less than 48 hours between onset and maximum deficit, the prognosis is significantly worse, compared with slowly evolving deficits (62). Frequently, radicular symptoms are present before the development of cord compression (63).

IMAGING

Several imaging modalities may be used in the workup of metastatic cancer. They include plain radiographs, bone scan, CT, magnetic resonance imaging (MRI), and positron emission tomography (PET).

Routine plain radiographs are the most readily attainable imaging study for skeletal complaints. As an initial screening study, they provide important information when abnormalities are detected. Appreciation of location, size, and type (lytic,

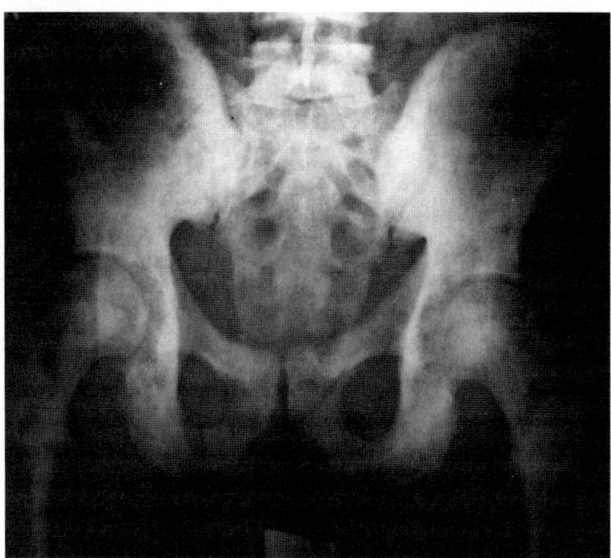

FIGURE 48-1. X-ray of pelvis and hips displaying extensive sclerotic lesions consistent with widespread prostatic disease.

blastic, or mixed) of lesion can be made from plain radiographs. It is essential to obtain radiographs of the entire length of the bone under investigation to avoid missing skip lesions.

Metastatic prostate cancer is suggested when plain radiographs demonstrate sclerotic skeletal lesions in a patient with a known diagnosis of prostate cancer with a rising serum PSA level (Fig. 48-1). Although unusual, some benign conditions, such as osteoarthritis, trauma, Paget's disease, or even metastatic foci from different undiagnosed cancers, may be confused with metastatic prostate lesions.

Even with metastatic skeletal pain, plain radiographs often have little or no detectable abnormalities. Although radiographically visible lesions direct the diagnosis, the absence of identifiable lesions does not exclude metastatic disease. More than 20% of patients that are considered to have no skeletal metastases by plain radiographic evaluation are found to have metastases by bone scan (64). Plain radiographs are notoriously poor in identifying skeletal metastases. For example, on an anteroposterior and lateral radiograph of the spine, 50% to 60% of cancellous destruction may be necessary before lesion identification (65). For long bones, more than half of the medullary canal needs to be destroyed before radiographic identification (65). In cases in which patients with prostate cancer continue to have pain, a bone scan and CT or MRI are indicated.

More than 90% of skeletal metastases from prostate cancer are blastic or sclerotic, appearing on plain radiographs (66). Other lesions may be lytic or mixed in appearance. Outside of their opaque radiographic appearance, the presentation may mirror any metastatic cancer foci. For example, in the spine there are two gross radiographic appearances of metastatic carcinoma: anterior compression fracture with resultant kyphosis or a uniform vertebral collapse with destruction of the posterior column and evidence of focal instability (31). In addition to the cancellous bony destruction of vertebral bodies, other findings of metastatic prostate cancer to the spine include the disappearance of pedicles, obscuring of trabecular margins, and ossification of the anterior longitudinal ligament or vertebral body (ivory body).

Technetium bone scans provide valuable information in the workup. Active areas on the bone scan reflect osteoblastic activity and may suggest sites of skeletal metastases. Solitary lesions on the bone scan may also represent a primary bone tumor (sarcoma, lymphoma, or plasmacytoma). There is approximately an 8% false-negative rate with bone scans from metastases that do not cause an osteoblastic response (67).

Imaging with CT helps to further clarify the size and location of lesions. In the future, it is hoped that CT quantification of lesion size will better help to assess fracture risk. CTs are also particularly helpful in understanding complex lesions or fracture patterns such as those found in acetabular or spinal metastases.

The use of MRI has increased over the past several years and is the imaging study of choice in spinal metastases. MRI is particularly helpful in identifying cord and root compression and metastatic margins from the extent of marrow involvement. Often, the treatment of prostate cancer renders bone vulnerable to osteopenic fractures or osteomyelitis from long-term hormonal therapy or chemotherapy-induced neutropenia. MRI assists in identifying nonmalignant compression fractures and osteomyelitis from metastatic disease (31).

PET is a nuclear medicine technique that provides improved spatial resolution, decreased scatter, and superior quantification, leading to increased sensitivity and specificity over traditional bone scans. The future use of PET is promising, but the parameters for using this technology in evaluating skeletal metastases are still being defined (68).

BIOPSY

It is normal to presume that patients with known prostate cancer who present with skeletal pain and abnormal imaging studies have metastatic prostate disease. Yet it is not uncommon for patients to have a primary bone sarcoma or metastatic disease from a previously undiagnosed second cancer. Regardless of a previous diagnosis of prostate cancer, an isolated lesion requires a thorough workup with a tissue diagnosis before definitive treatment with stabilization. Fine-needle aspiration (FNA) and core needle biopsies represent the two types of closed tissue biopsies. FNA has proved to be reliable in diagnosing metastatic tumors but has poor accuracy (as low as 54%) in diagnosing primary malignant bone tumors (69,70). Core needle biopsies are different from FNA biopsies in that they use a trocar-cannula apparatus to extract a core of tissue, which helps to preserve the tissue architecture. The reported diagnostic accuracy of core biopsies is 76% to 96% (71,72). Open biopsies offer slightly higher accuracy rates at the expense of time, cost, and convenience (73). At our institution, our initial biopsy is a core needle biopsy with ultrasound or CT guidance, if necessary. If the specimen is nondiagnostic, then we repeat a core needle biopsy or perform an open biopsy. Internal fixation or reconstruction is only performed after the pathologic diagnosis has been verified. Owing to the significant increase in biopsy complications when performed by referring hospitals, the Musculoskeletal Tumor Society in 1982 recommended that treating institutions should perform biopsies whenever possible (74).

FRACTURE RISK EVALUATION

In skeletal metastases, the dilemma is over which lesions to observe, irradiate, or prophylactically stabilize. Several frequently referenced recommendations for prophylactic stabilization, including the complaint of increasing skeletal pain and the findings of cortical defects more than 2.5 cm and lesions with 50% or greater cortical destruction, were first suggested in the early 1970s (75–78). Other criteria such as location around the lesser trochanter or failure of radiation therapy treatment have been included in the criteria for lesions at risk for fracture (5). Although these recommendations are helpful, it has been suggested that there is no reliable relationship between lesion size, pattern, or degree of pain and the risk of fracture (79–81).

In 1989, Mirels presented a scoring system for assessing pathologic fractures of long bones (82). Four findings are assessed, including the location of the lesions (1 point, upper extremity; 2 points, lower extremity; or 3 points, peritrochanteric), degree of pain (1 point, mild; 2 points, moderate; or 3 points, severe), type of lesion (1 point, blastic; 2 points, mixed; or 3 points, lytic), and size (the shaft diameter proportion: 1 point, less than 1/3; 2 points, 1/3 to 2/3; or 3 points, greater than 2/3). A maximum score of 12 results from the combination of a lytic, peritrochanteric lesion with severe pain involving more than 2/3 of the shaft diameter proportion. It is suggested that combined scores greater than or equal to nine have a high risk (33%) for future fracture and merit prophylactic stabilization.

However, despite the simplicity of the Mirels scoring system and its small interobserver error rate, greater prediction accuracy and lower reliance on the scoring system is found among experienced physicians (83). Even with improved imaging technology, the inaccuracy of evaluating impending pathologic fractures remains. Three orthopedic oncology surgeons had only modest agreement in judging lesion size from plain radiographs and CTs (84). Within this group, there was no relationship between actual femoral load-bearing capacity and their estimates.

Although the standard assessment of impending fractures relies primarily on geometric measurements, the mechanical behavior—that is, its rigidity—depends on the material itself, in addition to its geometric properties. Recently, Whealan et al. have shown noninvasive measurements of structural rigidity from composite beam theory analysis and quantitative CT to correlate well with measured yield loads (81). Identification of a 35% loss of bending rigidity with this technique has provided the highest specificity and sensitivity criteria (94% and 100%, respectively) for predicting pathologic fractures to date (85). Although the study predicted fractures of benign pediatric tumors, the principles are applicable to metastatic lesions, with a study presently under way for predicting fractures in skeletal metastases (B. D. Snyder, *personal communication*, 2001).

MEDICAL MANAGEMENT

It is important for physicians to tailor treatment through understanding the patient's cancer stage, desires and expectations, and the potential for treatment complications. The well-known relationship between age and prevalence of prostate cancer biases the treatment population toward additional medical issues and reinforces the importance of communication between the treating specialties (medicine, oncology, physiatry, urology, radiation oncology, and orthopedics).

Not all patients with prostate-contained cancer require radical prostatectomy. A select group of patients older than 65 years of age with stage T1c disease may be conservatively managed. The identified criteria for "watchful waiting" includes PSA density (serum PSA divided by prostate size by ultrasound determination), 0.15 mg per mL per g or less, Gleason score of 6 or less, less than or equal to two biopsy cores with cancer, and maximum 50% biopsy core involvement with cancer (86). In this group, conservative management is defined by yearly prostate biopsies and twice-yearly digital rectal examinations and serum PSA testing.

For the majority of patients with prostate-contained cancer, the recommended treatment is a prostatectomy. Yet, roughly 50% of prostatectomy pathology specimens have disease extending beyond the prostate (87). Although hormonal therapy remains the keystone treatment for metastatic spread, several other medical modalities, including chemotherapy, bisphosphonates, irradiation, and radioisotopes, may also be used. As with many pain-producing conditions, analgesics are also frequently prescribed. First-line treatment typically begins with nonsteroidal antiinflammatory drugs with progression to opioid analgesics when pain increases.

It has been nearly 60 years since Huggins and Hodges published their Nobel Prize–winning research on the influence of testosterone on metastatic prostate cancer (88). Early hormonal therapy in metastatic prostate cancer has reduced the frequency and severity of ureteral obstruction, spinal cord compression, pathologic fractures, and extraskeletal metastases (12). Yet, patients receiving long-term hormonal therapy are more likely to have an osteoporotic fracture than a malignant fracture (89). Hormonal treatment remains beneficial once skeletal metastases are identified. Forty percent to 70% of patients with metastases report reduction in pain and improved ambulation with hormonal treatment (90). Potential complications from hormonal therapy include impotence and decreased libido, decreased bone density, feminization, hot flashes, decrease in energy, osteoporosis, and osteoporotic fractures.

Long-term treatment of prostate cancer treated with hormonal therapy eventually induces hormonal resistance. Elevating serum PSA levels while on hormonal therapy signals resistance. When prostate cancer becomes hormone resistant, various chemotherapy regimens may be used. The principal guiding chemotherapy is based on chemotactic agents acting on dividing cells. It has been estimated that only 2% to 3% of prostate cancer cells are dividing at any one time (91). Although agents may have some early efficacy, they have not significantly increased survival (86). Agents used individually or in combination include suramin, doxorubicin (Adriamycin), paclitaxel (Taxol), liarozole, and estramustine. Potential complications from the treatment with chemotherapy agents include cytopenia, neurotoxicity, skin rashes, nausea, and vomiting.

Bisphosphonates are increasingly being used in the treatment of skeletal metastases. Bisphosphonates are synthetic derivatives of naturally occurring pyrophosphates that are preferentially absorbed by the skeleton and reduce bone resorption. Treatment with bisphosphonates in breast cancer and multiple myeloma patients has significantly reduced the development of skeletal complications (92). Bisphosphonates are also effective in treating tumor-induced hypercalcemia (93). There are relatively few prostate cancer studies with bisphosphonates, compared to the use of bisphosphonates with lytic lesion–producing cancers. In spite of this, some studies suggest clinical benefits from bisphosphonates in treating prostatic skeletal metastases. One of the earliest studies with intravenous clodronate and its role in decreasing skeletal pain was ethically stopped early, owing to significant pain improvements compared to placebo (94). An *in vivo* study has shown that bisphosphonates may help prevent prostate cancer metastatic adhesions to bone and, therefore, reduce the number of bony metastases (95,96). Charhon et al. have shown that bone resorption before osteoblastic bone formation may be necessary. This finding would further anticipate clinical benefits from bisphosphonate therapy (97). The common side effects of bisphosphonate treatment are nausea and vomiting.

External beam radiation therapy is typically reserved for symptomatic skeletal metastases. Significant pain relief is consistently found in 80% or greater of patients after radiation treatment (98). It is important to differentiate whether the painful skeletal lesion is an isolated metastasis or a site of diffuse metastases. Patients with painful regional disease may receive wide-field irradiation but usually have poorer and shorter relief rates (99). After radiation therapy, radiographic evidence of healing is typically present by 3 to 4 months, with near normal bone imaging frequently restored by 6 months (100). If surgical stabilization is not needed, then it is important to consider protecting a patient's weight-bearing status in lower extremity lesions during the initial period of bony resorption and healing. If operative intervention is required, then postoperative radiation is required to prevent tumor growth, which would jeopardize stabilization. Potential side effects from radiation therapy include nausea, vomiting, skin irritation, and bone marrow suppression.

Radioactive isotopes are able to systemically deliver radiation to multiple osteoblastic lesions with a single injection. Studies with phosphorus-32, strontium-89, and samarium-153 reduced pain in 60% to 75% of patients (101–104). Pain relief typically begins within weeks and lasts for months. Unlike external beam radiation, radionuclide therapy can be given multiple times due to its low toxicity to surrounding healthy tissue and bone. Potential complications include pain exacerbation before pain relief, nausea, vomiting, and transient bone marrow suppression.

Early medical treatment of metastatic prostate cancer helps to prevent or delay complications. Frequently, after patients with metastatic disease are identified, consultation is made for treatment recommendations. After reviewing the patient's history and imaging studies, if the concern for a pathologic fracture is low, then irradiation, initiation, or continuation of hormonal therapy and possible treatment with bisphosphonates or radioisotopes should be considered. With many lesions, early treatment is able to delay operative intervention. With spine lesions, the majority does not progress to neurologic deficits or instability and are able to be treated with irradiation and bracing. Even pathologic compression fractures without neurologic deficits can be approached nonoperatively with rest and bracing. In Harrington's experience, nearly 80% of patients with spinal metastases are nonoperatively managed (63,105).

SURGICAL MANAGEMENT

Until future research provides an accurate, easily reproducible model to predict the risk of pathologic fracture, the decision to surgically intervene on "impending fractures" will remain more of an art rather than a science. Lesion size, location, type, and response to prior treatment, along with degree of pain, are only a part of the guiding criteria a surgeon should consider. Even with pathologic fractures, two principles must guide the decision process. First is patient selection. Life expectancy should be greater than the convalescent period from surgery to have the adequate benefits of improved function, pain, and ease of care (106,107). This varies for different operations. Load-sharing fixation devices, such as intramedullary rods for long bone stabilization, result in shorter recovery than a large megaprosthesis with a complex acetabular reconstruction or multilevel anterior and posterior spine stabilization. Relative contraindications to surgery include medically unstable patients and those with life expectancies less than a month (63). Good to excellent pain relief and regaining the ability to walk have been 90% or higher in patients after surgical stabilization with arthroplasty or internal fixation (5,28).

The second surgical principle after patient selection is the choice of surgical fixation. Hopes for a rapid postoperative recovery are dependent on immediate operative stabilization. The goal after surgery must be immediate full-weight bearing. With limited life expectancies, multiple surgeries are not acceptable and carry increased risk of complications. The fixation must be stable, because the mechanical demands across a joint are high even with normal activities. This is in addition to working with a population of patients whose healing process is slower (108,109). Methylmethacrylate assists immediate stabilization and has the benefit of not being negatively affected by radiation (110). Another surgical decision caveat is consideration of future disease spread. This would make a load-sharing device, such as a long-stemmed prosthesis or intramedullary rod, a more attractive choice over a load-sparing internal fixation device, such as a dynamic hip screw and side plate. Disease recurrence or local spread could lead to failure of the load-sharing device (111). However, load-sharing devices may be difficult to use if the medullary canal is obliterated by osteoblastic lesions.

Spine

The operative indications for surgical intervention with metastatic spinal lesions include progressive neurologic deficits attributable to metastatic foci, pain unresponsive to treatment, and instability or impending instability related to pathologic fracture. Until the advent of routine anterior decompression with stabilization, the natural history for surgical intervention with laminectomy and decompression without stabilization did not return neurologic function and allowed progressive spinal deformity and instability. The results from treatment with radiation alone were identical to early surgical intervention (112). Less than one-half of these patients regained the ability to walk. The current recommended surgical intervention for cervical or thoracic disease is an anterior approach with decompression and stabilization. If additional stabilization is required, a posterior approach with stabilization may be included. In lumbar disease or in cervical and thoracic situations with circumferential cord compression (a "napkin-ring" constriction), anterior and posterior approaches are necessary for decompression with stabilization. Due to poor graft incorporation after postoperative irradiation, methylmethacrylate with a fixation device is frequently used for anterior fixation. When posterior fixation is required, Luque rods with sublaminar wire fixation three levels above and below the laminectomy decompression levels or any segmental hook and pedicle screw system is advised. In cases with advanced tumor involvement of the pedicles, stable fixation with pedicle screws and rods is precluded.

Pelvis and Acetabulum

Lesions involving the acetabulum and the weight-bearing portions of the pelvis that require operative stabilization are technically challenging. Imaging with CT and MRI is necessary to evaluate the extent of the involvement and to plan for adequate stabilization. In 1981, Harrington classified metastatic involvement of the acetabulum by location, amount of involvement, and reconstruction technique required (113). In class I and II lesions, conventional total hip arthroplasty with possible use of a protrusio ring, jumbo cup, or cage provides stable reconstruction (Fig. 48-2). For class III and IV lesions, reconstruction is more difficult, requiring additional use of Steinmann pins and methylmethacrylate or complete *en bloc* resection and reconstruction. Although historically associated with poor functional results, Girdlestone resection arthroplasty or nonoperative treatment infrequently may be recommended for cases with extensive skeletal involvement precluding stable fixation (114).

Femoral Head and Neck

The femur is involved in 60% of long-bone pathologic fractures (107). Fifty percent of femur fractures involve the neck, 15% are intertrochanteric, and 30% are subtrochanteric. For pathologic subcapital fractures, the recommended treatment is prosthetic replacement secondary to an unacceptably high risk of failure with internal fixation (115). The length of prosthetic stem needs to span the distal lesion by at least two bone diameter lengths or the anticipated areas of future spread. With isolated femoral head and neck disease, the treatment of the acetabulum is controversial. Debate remains whether to perform a hemiarthroplasty or total arthroplasty. One study shows that more than 80% of patients undergoing arthroplasty for metastatic disease of the hip had occult acetabular metastases on biopsy. Based on this finding, this group's recommendation is to perform a total hip arthroplasty rather than hemiarthroplasty (28). This view is contrasted with the concern of a larger and longer operation without evidence supporting occult acetabular disease clinically progressing to future instability or pain (115).

Our experience supports using third generation intramedullary reconstruction nails for impending fractures without involvement of the tumor into the head. This intramedullary device spans the entire femur, has proximal fixation into the femoral head, and is locked distally. When proximally based intramedullary fixation devices fail, it is typically due to screw cutout in the femoral neck (116,117). This emphasizes the importance of assessing proximal bone involvement and, therefore, bone strength before using this device. When disease involvement of the femoral head is too great to obtain immediate stability from the third generation intramedullary reconstruction

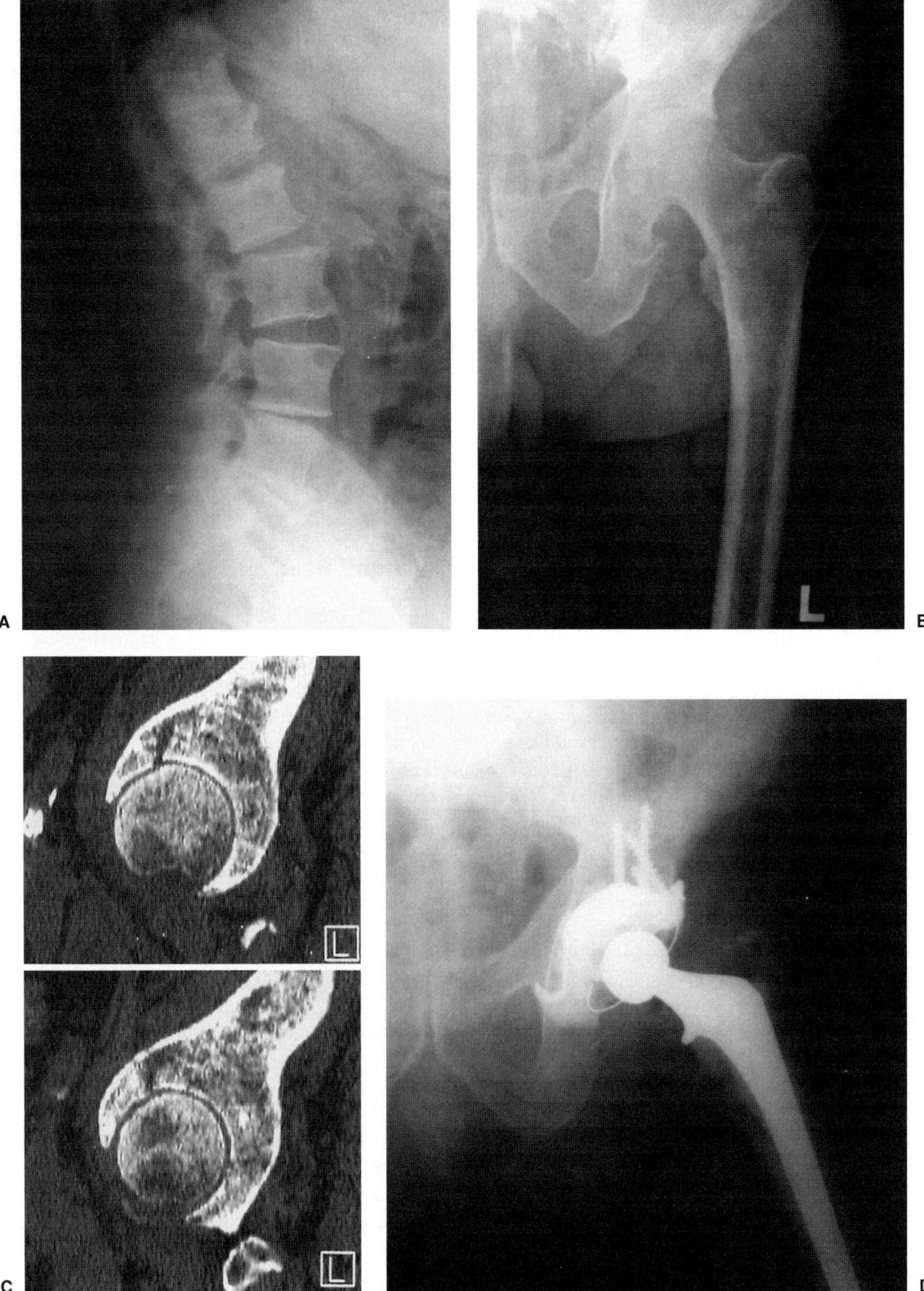

FIGURE 48-2. **A:** Pathologic fracture of first lumbar vertebra in patient with metastatic prostate carcinoma. **B:** The patient developed hip pain, and hip x-ray demonstrates mixed lytic and sclerotic periacetabular lesions. **C:** The computed tomography scan shows extensive disease and fracture of dome of acetabulum. **D:** Despite radiation therapy and crutches, the patient continued to experience pain, necessitating total hip replacement with an antiprotrusion cage.

device, we recommend using a long-stemmed hemiarthroplasty prothesis.

Intertrochanteric and Subtrochanteric Femur

The dynamic hip screw, a sliding compression screw and plate device, is frequently used with methylmethacrylate packing for intertrochanteric femur lesions. The familiarity of the dynamic hip screw technique by orthopedists makes this a favored treatment choice. There is a concern, however, for higher failure secondary to increased survival times, disease progression, delayed union or nonunion, lack of load-sharing, and inexperience with cement packing. Third-generation reconstruction-type intramedullary nails are increasingly being used for these lesions (118,119). Although a more extensive procedure, calcar-replacing arthroplasty with long-stemmed prosthesis is an excellent option. It allows immediate stability because diseased bone is resected, thus removing the concern for fixation failure secondary to slower healing by the diseased bone or local disease progression.

Subtrochanteric fractures are the second most common pathologic femur fracture. The surgical management decision with subtrochanteric femur fractures is also based on the proximal bone stock in the head and neck. When the head and neck are not involved with metastatic disease, fixation with a reconstruction intramedullary nail provides adequate fixation. Two types of third generation nails also offer acceptable options—spiral blade plate and large single bone hip screw (120). Again, if metastatic involvement extends proximally, then use of these internal fixation devices will fail. In these situations, proximal femoral calcar replacement arthroplasty is recommended. Use of megaprosthesis is a more extensive surgery than a standard arthroplasty or use of a reconstruction intramedullary nail, with higher blood loss, potential neurologic injury, and difficulties with abductor mechanism attachment (121).

For impending intertrochanteric and subtrochanteric fractures, our recommendation is to use third-generation intramedullary reconstruction nail devices. However, when a fracture has occurred in the intertrochanteric area, we use a calcar-replacing, long-stemmed hemiarthroplasty prothesis. For pathologic subtrochanteric fractures, we recommend third-generation intramedullary reconstruction nail devices, when possible. Otherwise, we use long-stemmed hemiarthroplasty prostheses. If using intramedullary reconstruction nails, then the medullary canal may need to be recreated owing to blastic filling by the osseous metastases. This does not preclude nail insertion but highlights the care required when using this form of fixation and the complications that may arise.

Shaft and Distal Femur

For femoral shaft lesions and fractures, the recommended treatment is use of a closed, reamed, statically locked intramedullary nail (122). Use of a proximally and distally locked load-sharing device prevents telescoping of the fracture and proximal migration of the rod. In severely comminuted fractures, large lesions requiring methylmethacrylate augmentation, or circumstances in which blastic tumor fills the canal (Fig. 48-3), it may be necessary to open the lesion or fracture site and use a compression plate and screw device.

Fixation of impending lesions or fractures of the femoral condyles and supracondylar region depends on bone stock. If adequate bone is present, then dynamic compression screw augmented with methylmethacrylate or supracondylar nail can be used (123). If poor bone is present, then the fixation device can be augmented with methylmethacrylate or reconstructed with a modular long-stemmed knee arthroplasty prosthesis.

Upper Extremity

Metastases to the upper extremity are infrequent. The upper extremities are typically not weight-bearing limbs and lesions can frequently be treated with radiation and functional bracing. However, surgical stabilization is appropriate when the limb is weight bearing or there is persistent pain or a pathologic fracture. The choice of fixation includes intramedullary rod, long-stemmed shoulder hemiarthroplasty, or plates and screws with or without methylmethacrylate. Nonoperative management of pathologic fractures is typically unsatisfactory (124,125). As noted earlier, the decision as to which fixation device to use is based on bone stock, quality, and extent of disease. In cases in which tumor involvement of the proximal humerus would prevent fixation stability, a long-stemmed hemiarthroplasty is required.

PERIOPERATIVE CARE

With any invasive procedure, the risks of infection, bleeding, injury to important anatomy, persistent pain, hardware failure, instability, and potential for future surgery remain. Patients with metastatic cancer tend to be more susceptible to complications. Often, surgery is urgently performed owing to a pathologic fracture. Frequently, patients are malnourished, immunosuppressed, osteopenic, bedridden, and have coagulopathies and electrolyte imbalances. In a report from the Mayo Clinic on proximal femoral replacement prostheses secondary to metastatic disease and multiple myeloma, there was nearly a 50% complication rate (121).

Surgical stabilization allowing immediate weight bearing and ambulation to reduce the potential for pulmonary, thrombotic, and disuse hypercalcemia is only one aspect of the patient's care that may reduce complications. Aggressive anticoagulation along with judicious use of perioperative antibiotics is critical. If a patient is bedridden and undergoing a workup before surgery, then we recommend short-term,

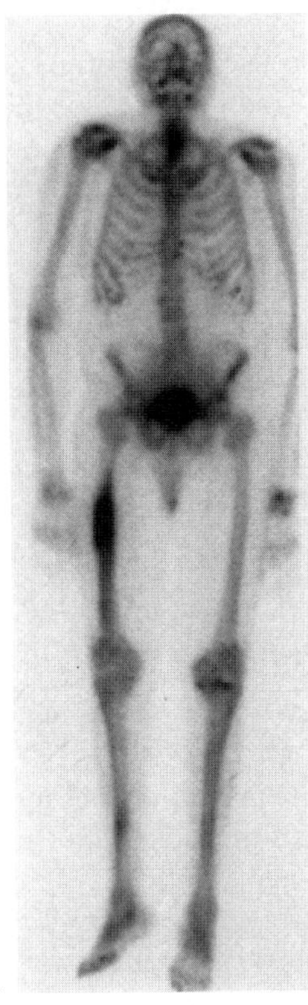

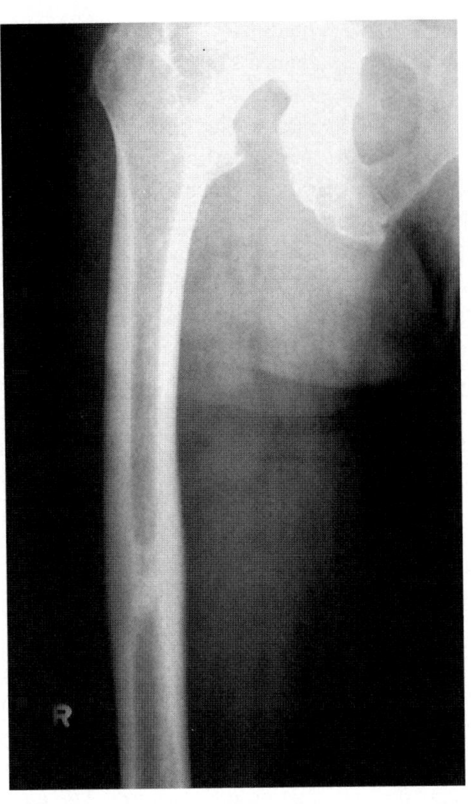

FIGURE 48-3. **A:** Patient with thigh pain and solitary "hot spot" on bone scan. This required biopsy for diagnosis and later an intermedullary rod for continued pain with risk of impending fracture. **B:** The sclerotic metastases tend to obliterate the medullary canal and make it difficult to insert an intramedullary nail.

quickly reversible anticoagulation. After surgery, our anticoagulation protocol for lower extremity surgery is warfarin (Coumadin) for 6 weeks with a target international normalized ratio range of 1.5 to 2.0. In keeping with standard surgical practice, a single dose of antibiotics is given before surgery, with coverage extending for 24 hours after surgery.

Postoperative radiation to the entire operative field and the entire length of the fixation device is an important treatment modality. Radiation treatment improves function, and reduces postoperative disease recurrence and progression and the need for future surgery (126). The timing for radiation treatment varies depending on the expected time needed to prevent wound complications or allow for healing of spinal fusions. For long-bone intramedullary fixation, the typical period we wait is 1 to 2 weeks. After arthroplasty, we wait 4 weeks. With spinal fusions, we wait 6 to 8 weeks to allow for healing of fusion before radiation treatment.

CONCLUSION

Prostate cancer is a common cancer in men with frequent skeletal metastases. The orthopedic sequelae of osseous metastases include pain, impending or pathologic fractures, and spinal cord and root compression. Before and after surgery, medical management with hormonal therapy, chemotherapy, bisphosphonate treatment, radiation therapy, and radionuclide administration seeks to prevent or reduce these sequelae. The majority of skeletal lesions can be treated nonoperatively. The criteria for predicting a pathologic fracture remain elusive, with the hope that future research and imaging techniques will improve prediction accuracy. Success of surgical stabilization rests on rigid fixation allowing early weight bearing. There are many surgical implants; implant selection must be performed on a case by case basis. The greatest hope for achieving the treatment goals is found in a multidisciplinary approach with high levels of communication between the treating specialties.

REFERENCES

1. Wingo PA, Landis S, Ries L. An adjustment to the 1997 estimate for new prostate cancer cases. *Cancer* 1997;80:1810–1813.
2. Landis SH, Murray T, Bolden S, et al. Cancer statistics 1998. *Cancer J Clin* 1998;48:6–29.
3. Pienta KJ. Etiology, epidemiology, and prevention of carcinoma of the prostate. In: Walsh PC, Retic AB, Vaughan ED Jr., et al., eds. *Campbell's urology*, 7th ed. Philadelphia: WB Saunders, 1997:2489–2496.
4. Tofe AJ, Francis MD, Harvey WJ. Correlation of neoplasms with incidence and localization of skeletal metastasis: an analysis of 1,355 diphosphonate bone scans. *J Nucl Med* 1975;16:986–989.
5. Harrington KD, Sim FH, Enis JE, et al. Methylmethacrylate as an adjunct in internal fixation of pathological fractures: experience with three hundred and seventy-five cases. *J Bone Joint Surg* 1976;58:1047–1055.

6. Thompson H. Comments. *Trans Path Soc London* 1854;5: 204.
7. Grunert D. Über pathologische Frakturen (Spontan-Frakturen). *Dtsch Z Chir* 1905;76:254–289.
8. Welch CE. Pathological fractures due to malignant disease. *Surg Gynecol Obstet* 1936;62:735–744.
9. Berman AT, Hermantin FU, Horowitz SM. Metastatic disease of the hip: evaluation and treatment. *J Am Acad Orthop Surg* 1997;5:79–86.
10. Bolla M, Gonzalez D, Warde P, et al. Improved survival in patients with locally advanced prostate cancer treated with radiotherapy and goserelin. *N Engl J Med* 1997;337:295–300.
11. Messing EM, Manola J, Sarosdy M, et al. Immediate hormonal therapy compared with observation after radical prostatectomy and pelvic lymphadenectomy in men with node-positive prostate cancer. *N Engl J Med* 1999;341:1781–1788.
12. Immediate versus deferred treatment for advanced prostate cancer: initial results of the Medical Research Council Trial. The Medical Research Council Prostate Cancer Working Party Investigators Group. *Br J Urol* 1997;79:235–246.
13. Wallace DM, Chisholm GD, Hendry WF. TNM classification for urological tumours. *Br J Urol* 1975;47:1–12.
14. Franks LM. The spread of prostatic carcinoma. *J Pathol* 1956;72:603.
15. Bubendorf L, Schopfer A, Wagner U, et al. Metastatic patterns of prostate cancer: an autopsy study of 1,589 patients. *Hum Pathol* 2000;31:578–583.
16. Jacobs SC. Spread of prostatic cancer to bone. *Urology* 1983; 21:337–344.
17. Whitmore WJ Jr. Natural history and staging of prostate cancer. *Urol Clin North Am* 1984;11:209–220.
18. Morgan JW, Adcock KA, Donohue RE. Distribution of skeletal metastases in prostatic and lung cancer. *Urology* 1990; 36:31–34.
19. Rana A, Chisholm GD, Khan M, et al. Patterns of bone metastasis and their prognostic significance in patients with carcinoma of the prostate. *Br J Urol* 1993;72:933–936.
20. Dodds PR, Caeide JV, Lytton B. The role of vertebral veins in the dissemination of prostatic cancer. *J Urol* 1981;126: 753–755.
21. Turner JW, Jaffe HL. Metastatic neoplasms: a clinical and roentgenological study of involvement of skeleton and lungs. *AJR Am J Roentgenol* 1940;43:479–492.
22. Ewing J. *Neoplastic diseases*, 3rd ed. Philadelphia: WB Saunders, 1928:827.
23. Brage ME, Simon MA. Metastatic bone disease: evaluation, prognosis, and medical treatment considerations of metastatic bone tumors. *Orthopedics* 1992;15:589–596.
24. McCrea LE, Karafin L. Carcinoma of the prostate: metastases, therapy, and survival. A statistical analysis of 500 cases. *Int Coll Surg J* 1958;29:723–728.
25. Willis RA. Secondary tumors of bones. In: Willis RA, ed. *The spread of tumours in the human body*, 3rd ed. London: Butterworth & Co., 1973;3:229–250.
26. Bumpus HC. Carcinoma of prostate: clinical study. *Surg Gynec Obst* 1921;32:31.
27. Elkin M, Mueller HP. Metastases from cancer of the prostate: autopsy and roentgenological findings. *Cancer* 1954; 7:1246–1248.
28. Habermann ET, Sachs R, Stern RE, et al. The pathology and treatment of metastatic disease of the femur. *Clin Orthop* 1982;169:70–82.
29. Higinbotham NL, Marcove RC. The management of pathological fractures. *J Trauma* 1965;5:792–798.
30. Oda MAS, Shurman DJ. Monitoring of pathological fracture. In: Stoll BA, Parbhoo S, eds. *Bone metastasis: monitoring and treatment*. New York: Raven Press, 1983:271–287.
31. Harrington KD. Metastatic tumors of the spine: diagnosis and treatment. *J Am Acad Orthop Surg* 1993;1:76–86.
32. Bonica JJ, Ventafridda V, Twycross RG. Cancer pain. In: Bonica JJ, ed. *The management of pain*. Philadelphia: Lea & Febiger, 1990:400–460.
33. McNeal J, Kindrachuck R, Freiha F, et al. Patterns of progression in prostrate cancer. *Lancet* 1986;1:60.
34. Stamey T, McNeal J, Freiha F, et al. Morphometric and clinical studies on 68 consecutive radical prostatectomies. *J Urol* 1988;139:1235–1241.
35. Prostate Cancer Trialists' Collaborative Group. Maximum androgen blockade in advanced prostate cancer: an overview of 22 randomized trials with 3,283 deaths in 5,710 patients. *Lancet* 1995;346:265–269.
36. Bayard S, Greenberg R, Showalter D, et al. Comparison of treatments for prostatic cancer using an exponential-type life model relating survival to concomitant information. *Cancer Chemother Rep* 1974;58:845–859.
37. Nesbit RM, Baum WC. Endocrine control of prostatic carcinoma: clinical and statistical survey of 1,818 cases. *JAMA* 1984;143:471–482.
38. Kantoff PW, Halabi S, Conaway M, et al. Hydrocortisone with or without mitoxantrone in men with hormone-refractory prostate cancer: results of the Cancer and Leukemia Group B9182 study. *J Clin Oncol* 1999;17:2506–2513.
39. Marcove RC, Yang DJ. Survival times after treatment of pathologic fractures. *Cancer* 1967;20:2154–2158.
40. DeVita VT, Hellman S, Rosenberg S. *Cancer principles and practice of oncology*. Philadelphia: JB Lippincott Co, 1982;113–125.
41. Paget J. The distribution of secondary growth in cancer of the breast. *Lancet* 1889;1:571.
42. Baston O. The function of the vertebral veins and their role in the spread of metastases. *Ann Surg* 1940;112:138.
43. Fair WR, Heston WD, Coron-Cardo C. An overview of cancer biology. In: Walsh PC, Retic AB, Vaughan ED Jr., et al., eds. *Campbell's urology*, 7th ed. Philadelphia: WB Saunders, 1997:2259–2282.
44. Charhon SA, Chapuy MC, Delvin EE, et al. Histomorphometric analysis of sclerotic bone metastases from prostatic carcinoma with special reference to osteomalacia. *Cancer* 1983;51:918–924.
45. Goltzman D. Mechanisms of the development of osteoblastic metastases. *Cancer* 1997;80:1546–1556.
46. Clohisy DR, Perkins SL, Ramnaraine ML. Review of cellular mechanisms of tumor osteolysis. *Clin Ortho Research* 2000;373:104–114.
47. Kattan MW, Eastman JA, Stapleton AM, et al. A preoperative nomogram for disease recurrence following radical prostatectomy for prostate cancer. *J Natl Cancer Inst* 1998; 90:766–771.

48. Cheng L, Bergstralh DJ, Cheville JC, et al. Cancer volume of lymph node metastasis predicts progression in prostate cancer. *Am J Surg Pathol* 1998;22:1491–1500.
49. Kattan MW, Wheeler TM, Scardino PT. Postoperative nomogram for disease recurrence after radical prostatectomy for prostate cancer. *J Clin Oncol* 1999;17:1499–1507.
50. Schaffer DL, Pendergrass HP. Comparison of enzyme, clinical, radiographic, and radionuclide methods of detecting bone metastases from carcinoma of the prostate. *Radiology* 1976;121:431–434.
51. Twycross RG. Management of pain in skeletal metastases. *Clin Orthop* 1995;312:187–196.
52. Koiaumi M, Yamada Y, Takiguchi T, et al. Bone metabolic markers in bone metastases. *J Cancer Res Clin Oncol* 1995;121:542–548.
53. Bauer JJ, Connelly RR, Seterhenn IA, et al. Biostatistical modeling using traditional variables and genetic biomarkers for predicting the risk of prostate carcinoma recurrence after radical prostatectomy. *Cancer* 1997;79:952–962.
54. Stapleton AM, Zbell P, Kattan MW, et al. Assessment of the biological markers p53, Ki-67, and apoptotic index as predictive indicators of prostate cancer recurrence following surgery. *Cancer* 1998;82:168–175.
55. Tursky B. The development of a pain perception profile: a psychophysical approach. In: Weisenberg M, Tursky B, eds. *Pain: new perspectives in therapy and research.* New York: Plenum Publishing, 1976:171–194.
56. Miller PD, Eardley I, Kirby RS. Prostate specific antigen and bone scan correlation in the staging and monitoring of patients with prostatic cancer. *Br J Urol* 1992;70:295–298.
57. Freitas JE, Gilvydas R, Ferry JD, et al. The clinical utility of prostate-specific antigen and bone scintigraphy in prostate cancer follow-up. *J Nucl Med* 1991;32:1387–1390.
58. McNeil BJ. Value of bone scanning in neoplastic disease. *Sem Nucl Med* 1984;14:277–286.
59. Roughgraff BT, Kneisl JS, Simon MA. Skeletal metastases of unknown origin. A prospective study of a diagnostic strategy. *J Bone Joint Surg* 1993;75A:1276–1281.
60. Heim HM, Oei TP. Comparison of the prostate cancer patients with and without pain. *Pain* 1993;53:159–162.
61. Galasko CS. Skeletal metastases and mammary cancer. *Ann R Coll Surg Engl* 1972;50:3–28.
62. Tarlov IM, Herz E. Spinal cord compression studies. IV. Outlook with complete paralysis in man. *AMA Arch Neurol Psychiatry* 1954;72:43–59.
63. Harrington KD. *Orthopaedic management of metastatic bone disease.* St. Louis: Mosby, 1988.
64. Paulson DF. The impact of current staging procedures in assessing the disease extent of prostatic adenocarcinoma. *J Urol* 1979;121:300–302.
65. Edelsyn GA, Gillespie PJ, Grebbell FS. The radiological demonstration of osseous metastases: experimentation and observations. *Clin Radiol* 1967;18:158–162.
66. Cook GB, Watson FR. Events in the natural history of prostate cancer, using salvage curve, mean age distributions and contingency coefficients. *J Urol* 1968;99:87–96.
67. Hricak H, Theoni RF. Neoplasms of the prostate gland. In: Pollack HM, ed. *Clinical urography.* Philadelphia: WB Saunders, 1990.
68. Cook GJ, Fogelman I. The role of positron emission tomography in the management of bone metastases. *Cancer Supp* 2000;88:2927–2933.
69. El-Khoury GY, Terepka RH, Mickelson MR, et al. Fine-needle aspiration biopsy of bone. *J Bone Joint Surg* 1983; 65A:533–525.
70. Kreicbergs A, Bauer HC, Brosjo O, et al. Cytologic diagnosis of bone tumors. *Orthop Trans* 1995;18:1131.
71. Barth RJ Jr., Merino MJ, Solomon D, et al. A prospective study of the value of core needle biopsy and fine needle aspiration in the diagnosis of soft tissue masses. *Surgery* 1992;112:536–543.
72. Moore TM, Meyers MH, Patzakis MJ, et al. Closed biopsy of musculoskeletal lesions. *J Bone Joint Surg* 1979;61A:375–380.
73. Skrzynski MC, Biermann JS, Montag A, et al. Diagnostic accuracy and charge-savings of outpatient core needle biopsy compared with open biopsy of musculoskeletal tumors. *J Bone Joint Surg* 1996;76A:644–649.
74. Mankin HJ, Lange TA, Spainer SS. The hazards of biopsy in patients with malignant primary bone and soft-tissue tumors. *J Bone Joint Surg* 1982;64A:1121–1127.
75. Beals RK, Lawton GD, Snell WE. Prophylactic internal fixation of the femur in metastatic breast cancer. *Cancer* 1971;28:1350–1354.
76. Fidler M. Prophylactic internal fixation of secondary neoplastic deposits in long bones. *BMJ* 1973;10:341–343.
77. Parrish FF, Murray JA. Surgical treatment for secondary neoplastic fractures. A retrospective study of ninety-six patients. *J Bone Joint Surg* 1970;52A:665–686.
78. Schurman DJ, Amstutz HC. Orthopedic management of patients with metastatic carcinoma of the breast. *Surg Gynecol Obstet* 1973;137:831–836.
79. Cheng DS, Seitz CB, Eyre HJ. Nonoperative management of femoral, humeral, and acetabular metastases in patients with breast carcinoma. *Cancer* 1980;45:1533–1537.
80. Keene JS, Sellinger DS, McBeath AA, et al. Metastatic breast cancer in the femur. A search for the lesion a risk of fracture. *Clin Orthop* 1986;203:282–288.
81. Whealan KM, Kwak SD, Tedrow JR, et al. Noninvasive imaging predicts failure load of the spine with simulated osteolytic defects. *J Bone Joint Surg* 2000;82A:1240–1251.
82. Mirels H. Metastatic disease in long bones. A proposed scoring system for diagnosing impending pathologic fractures. *Clin Orthop* 1989;249:256–264.
83. Damron TA. Critical evaluation of the Mirels rating system for impending pathologic femur fractures. Presented at the Second North American Symposium on Skeletal Complications of Malignancy. Montreal, Quebec, Canada, 1999.
84. Hipp JA, Springfield DS, Hayes WC. Predicting pathologic fracture risk in the management of metastatic bone defects. *Clin Orthop* 1995;312:120–135.
85. Snyder BD, Hecht AC, Tedrow JR, et al. Structural rigidity measured by CT accurately predicts fracture in children with benign tumors of the appendicular skeleton. *Transactions of the 46th Orthopaedic Research Society* 2000;25:243.
86. Rodriguez R, Carter HB. The current management of carcinoma of the prostate. *Adv Surg* 1999;33:181–196.
87. Lu-Yao GL, Potosky AL, Albertsen PC, et al. Follow-up prostate cancer treatments after radical prostatectomy: a

population based study. *J Natl Cancer Inst* 1996;88:166–172.

88. Huggins C, Hodges CV. Studies on prostate cancer. I. The effect of estrogen and of androgen injection on serum phosphatases in metastatic carcinoma of the prostate. *Cancer Res* 1941;1:293–297.
89. Daniell HW. Osteoporosis after orchiectomy for prostate cancer. *J Urol* 1997;157:439–444.
90. Brage ME, Simon MA. Evaluation, prognosis, and medical treatment considerations of metastatic bone tumors. *Orthopedics* 1992;15:589–596.
91. Berges RB, Vukanovic J, Epstein JI, et al. Implication of cell kinetic changes during the progression of human prostatic cancer. *Clin Cancer Res* 1995;1:1473–1480.
92. Lin JH. Bisphosphonates: a review of their pharmacokinetic properties. *Bone* 1996;18:75–85.
93. Coleman RE. Bisphosphonate treatment of bone metastases and hypercalcemia of malignancy. *Oncology* 1991;5:55–62.
94. Adami S, Mian M. Clodronate therapy of metastatic bone disease in patients with prostate cancer. *Recent Results Cancer Res* 1989;116:567–572.
95. Boissier S, Magnetto S, Frappart L, et al. Bisphosphonates inhibit prostate and breast carcinoma cell adhesion to unmineralized and mineralized bone extracellular matrices. *Cancer Res* 1997;57:3890–3894.
96. Diel IJ, Solomayer EF, Bastert G. Bisphosphonates and the prevention of metastasis. *Cancer Supp* 2000;88:3080–3087.
97. Charhon SA, Chapuy MC, Delvin EE, et al. Histomorphometric analysis of sclerotic bone metastases from prostatic carcinoma with special reference to osteomalacia. *Cancer* 1983;51:918–924.
98. Schocker JD, Brady LW. Radiation therapy for bone metastasis. *Clin Orthop Rel Res* 1982;169:38–43.
99. Fitzpatrick PJ. Wide-field irradiation of bone metastases. In: Weiss R, Gilbert W, eds. *Bone metastasis*. Boston: GK Hall, 1981:399–428.
100. Bessler W. *Breast cancer*. New York: Alan R. Liss, 1977.
101. Mertens WC. Radionuclide therapy of bone metastases: prospects for enhancement of therapeutic efficacy. *Semin Oncol* 1993;20:49–55.
102. Nielsen OS, Munro AJ, Tannock IF. Bone metastases: pathophysiology and management policy. *J Clin Oncol* 1991;9: 509–524.
103. Scher HI, Chung LW. Bone metastases: improving the therapeutic index. *Semin Oncol* 1994;21:630–656.
104. Serafini AN. Samarium Sm-153 lexidronam for the palliation of bone pain associated with metastases. *Cancer Supp* 2000;88:2934–2939.
105. Harrington KD. Anterior decompression and stabilization of the spine as a treatment for vertebral collapse and spinal cord compression from metastatic malignancy. *Clin Orthop* 1988;233:177–197.
106. Parrish FF, Murray JA. Surgical treatment for secondary neoplastic fractures: a retrospective study of ninety-six patients. *J Bone Joint Surg Am* 1970;52:665–686.
107. Sim FH. Instructional course lectures: metastatic bone disease. In: *Instructional course lectures*, vol. 49. Anaheim, CA: American Academy of Orthopaedic Surgeons, 1999.
108. Frankel VH, Burstein AH. The application of engineering to the musculoskeletal system. In: Frankel VH, Bursteain AH, eds. *Orthopaedic biomechanics*. Philadelphia: Lea & Febiger, 1970:24–28.
109. Bonarigo BC, Rubin P. Nonunion of pathologic fracture after radiation therapy. *Radiology* 1967;88:889–898.
110. Murray JA, Bruels MC, Lindberg RD. Irradiation of polymethylmethacrylate. In vitro gamma radiation effect. *J Bone Joint Surg* 1974;56A:311–312.
111. Dijstra S, Wiggers T, van Geel BN, et al. Impending and actual pathological fractures in patients with bone metastases of the long bones: a retrospective study of 233 surgically treated fractures. *Eur J Surg* 1994;160:535–542.
112. Gilbert RW, Kim JH, Posner JB. Epidural spinal cord compression from metastatic tumor: diagnosis and treatment. *Ann Neurol* 1978;3:40–51.
113. Harrington KD. The management of acetabular insufficiency secondary to metastatic malignant disease. *J Bone Joint Surg* 1981;63:653–664.
114. Francis KC, Higinbotham NL, Carroll RF, et al. The treatment of pathological fractures of the femoral neck by resection. *J Trauma* 1962;2:465–473.
115. Damron TA, Sim FH. Operative treatment for metastatic disease of the pelvis and the proximal end of the femur. *J Bone Joint Surg* 2000;82A:114–125.
116. Dube MA, Pollack AN, Price N, et al. A comparison of fixation devices for the treatment of unstable subtrochanteric femur fractures. Presented at the Meeting of the Orthopaedic Trauma Association. Louisville, Kentucky, 1997.
117. Kraemer WJ, Hearn TC, Powell JN, et al. Fixation of segmental subtrochanteric fractures. A biomechanical study. *Clin Orthop* 1996;332:71–79.
118. DiPuccio G, Lunati P, Franceschi G, et al. The long gamma nail: indications and results. *Chir Org Mov* 1997;82:49–52.
119. Lefevre C, Yaacoub C, Dubrana F, et al. Long gamma locking nails: results of a prospective European multicentric study of 120 cases. *J Bone Joint Surg* 1997;79B:28.
120. Hecht A, Wright RJ, Ready J. Surgical treatment of pathologic subtrochanteric femur fractures in patients with metastatic disease with unreamed spiral interlocking nail. Read at the Annual Meeting of the Musculoskeletal Tumor Society, Washington, DC, 1998.
121. Sim FH, Frassica FJ, Chao EYS. Orthopaedic management using new devices and prostheses. *Clin Orthop* 1995;312: 160–172.
122. Healey JH, Brown HK. Complications of bone metastases. *Cancer* 2000;88:2940–2951.
123. Healey JH, Lane JM. Treatment of pathologic fractures of the distal femur with the Zickel supracondylar nail. *Clin Orthop* 1990;250:216–220.
124. Douglas HO, Shukla SK, Mindell I. Treatment of pathological fractures of long bones excluding those due to breast cancer. *J Bone Joint Surg* 1976;58A:1055–1061.
125. Flemming JE, Beals RK. Pathologic fracture of the humerus. *Clin Orthop* 1986;203:258–260.
126. Townsend PW, Smalley SR, Cozad SC, et al. Role of postoperative radiation therapy after stabilization of fractures caused by metastatic disease. *Int J Radiat Oncol Biol Phys* 1995:31:43–49.

49

PSYCHOSOCIAL CONSIDERATIONS IN PROSTATE CANCER

JOHN W. SHARP

Like all cancers, quality of life, psychological, and social concerns have received increasing attention in prostate cancer by oncology professionals. In the early 1980s, the focus of psychosocial interventions in prostate cancer was sexual dysfunction (1). As an old man's disease, prostate cancer received less attention than cancers that affected younger patient groups, such as breast cancer or leukemia. With the onset of new treatments in the late 1980s and improvements in early detection [e.g., prostate-specific antigen (PSA)], the study and treatment of psychosocial problems expanded rapidly (2).

This chapter addresses the complexity of psychosocial issues according to the natural history of the disease. Specifically, it is important to examine the cancer experience from initial diagnosis and treatment, remission or disease- and symptom-free periods, recurrence (after local or distance metastases), and advanced disease. Within each stage, this chapter addresses the impact on the patient and family, treatment decision points, variation in the experience by one's race, and recommended interventions.

SCREENING AND DETECTION

In recent years, a growing body of literature has emerged on the psychosocial aspects of screening for prostate cancer. The general stereotype of men avoiding and delaying screening appears to have some validity. Former Senator Bob Dole, a prostate cancer survivor, observed that many men circled the midway at his state fair with their wives several times before entering the tent offering free PSAs and prostate cancer screening (2a). Studies of heart disease support this avoidant behavior in men. Fears of impotence and misunderstanding of the anatomy of the prostate continue to exacerbate fear and avoidance (3). Three factors are changing this stereotype. First, there was a shift from the digital rectal exam to the PSA (a simple blood test) as the primary screening mechanism. The digital rectal exam was unpopular as an intrusive and embarrassing examination and even abhorrent to some (4). Particularly for African-American men, the digital rectal exam performed by a white male physician echoed the sexual exploitation of the Jim Crow era. Second, the general growth in the awareness of prostate cancer has changed the way screening is perceived. Many hospitals and cancer centers offer free screening during Prostate Cancer Awareness Week, which has now become an annual event (5,6). High-profile celebrities announcing their diagnosis publicly has given prostate cancer equal status with other cancers in terms of public awareness. Third, the availability of new treatments with fewer side effects provides an added incentive. As in other diseases, awareness of such treatments reduces the fear of screening detecting a life-threatening illness. The key concept here is the sense of self-efficacy. With any disease, the patient's belief that their actions can produce an effective result motivates them to seek appropriate care or perform appropriate self-care (7). Whereas a decade or more ago, the diagnosis of prostate cancer meant few treatment options, today the public awareness of effective treatments is growing; men can have the sense that if they go for screening and are diagnosed, effective treatments are available. A study of the chronically ill elderly showed that those with a stronger sense of self-efficacy about their illness were more likely to have a better quality of life and experience fewer symptoms, such as pain (8).

An important study shows the effect of family history and perceived risk on psychological distress. It showed that those presenting for screening experienced greater distress if they had a family history or an elevated perceived risk (6).

The role of family, particularly spouses and adult daughters, is key in promoting health screening in elderly men. The literature on this family interaction is limited; thus, the most effective means for families to encourage screening for prostate cancer remain unclear. Some current research uses the theory of *monitors* versus *blunters*. That is, some men are effective at monitoring for health risks, whereas others blunt their awareness. There is some evidence that prostate cancer screening is more acceptable, particularly in minority communities, when it is presented in the context of community-based health screening. Some cities have health care screening in churches and mosques in underserved neighborhoods. The support of clergy provides an added boost to the acceptability of screening.

The principal barriers to screening for underserved and minority groups continue to be the lack of access to health care and cost. Studies in southern rural and northern urban communities support this hypothesis. Specifically, they show that poor, African-American men see health screening as a low priority as compared to earning enough to live on and personal and family safety. This holds true in spite of their knowledge of being at high risk for the disease (9). Lack of insurance or adequate insurance adds to the barriers to access. Specifically, lower income is related to higher cancer incidence and higher stage of cancer at time of diagnosis. The less insured and educated not only have a poorer understanding of cancer risk and screening but also, once they have a cancer-related symptom, are less likely to have access to quality care or more likely face financial barriers to obtaining quality care (10). Finally, the general distrust of the medical system and clinical trials specifically, largely a result of the Tuskeegee experiment, sustains the cultural barriers between African-Americans and medical care (9).

Programs to bridge these barriers are essential. Early detection and aggressive treatment are now the standard for the white middle-class elderly man who has a primary care physician. For the underserved and minority populations, better access to health care screening and treatment, eliminating or reducing financial disincentives, and improving culturally competent care will be the only ways to improve the lagging survival statistics in these groups. McCoy et al. state that a "lack of preventive care and screening tests in low socioeconomic and disadvantaged populations does not appear to be due entirely to the lack of physician contact. Rather, these data indicate that preventive care is not integrated with the provision of other medical services" (4). They go on to recommend screening for those who attend public health clinics and community-based education with easy access, regardless of ability to pay (4). Three principles must drive innovative screening programs: increasing availability, improving accessibility, and promoting acceptability (11).

DIAGNOSIS AND TREATMENT: EARLY-STAGE DISEASE

The diagnosis of prostate cancer presents as a major stress event for any man. McDaniel summarizes the initial shock in this way: "Receiving the diagnosis of cancer may result in a cascade of emotional responses. Feelings of sadness are an expected response to painful life experiences. . . . These feelings may be coupled with reactions of shock, disbelief, anxiety. . ." (12). The level of distress can vary greatly based on exacerbating and buffering factors. One factor that may worsen the shock, depression, and anxiety associated with the statement, "You have cancer" includes the patient's ability to cope with prior stressful life events. Specifically, Does he have the emotional resources to cope, such as a problem-solving approach? Does he tend to become fatalistic, hopeless, or angry, and unable to moderate these emotions? Does he have a history of mental illness, especially depression, even if not previously diagnosed? Is this associated with suicidal thoughts or a history of suicidal attempts? A history of substance abuse, physical abuse, or self-injury are additional risk factors for depression in early disease (13). A family history of cancer and especially prostate cancer may increase the risk of poor coping if the patient recalls only that his relative experienced a slow painful death and assumes this will be his fate. Living alone or without family support in near proximity is another potential risk factor. Widowers with unresolved grief may be at additional risk (14).

Factors that buffer this shock of diagnosis balance out the risk factors for most men. Family support is the best studied of these buffering forces (13). In addition to general emotional support, families provide an additional communication link with the medical team to absorb important diagnosis and treatment specifics and report on symptoms. In some cases, because male urologists treat much of early-stage prostate cancer, spouses can believe they are excluded from the exam room in which men are discussing a male problem. For men in any stage of treatment, spouses and adult children should be invited and encouraged to attend discussions of treatment plans.

Other buffering factors include a knowledge of others who have been successfully treated. This awareness could be of public figures, family members, or neighbors, such as in retirement communities. Many support groups for prostate cancer can provide key information and support for the man who has been newly diagnosed and is attempting to choose the best treatment among several options. These support groups often include men who have had prostatectomies, external beam radiation therapy, or brachytherapy and can discuss their experience. However, outreach from these groups is needed to reach those who are newly diagnosed and are in the throws of making a decision on initial treatment. In addition, these groups fail to reach into minority communities. Reaching the African-American who has been newly diagnosed may be more effective on a one-to-one basis, but more study is needed in this area (15).

ADULT DEVELOPMENT AND THE EXPERIENCE OF PROSTATE CANCER

Some have compared the experience of women with breast cancer to men's experience with prostate cancer. Both are solid tumors with hormonal correlates. Both potentially have consequences for sexuality. The major difference is the age of onset, which on average is two decades later for prostate cancer. Men in their 50s, 60s, or 70s may be retired or more established in their careers. They are more likely to have grown children. There are more similarities in older women with breast cancer (16). Studies of distress for those newly diagnosed with cancer show that distress varies inversely with age; the older the cancer patient, the lower the level of distress, on average (17). A number of theories have been advanced to explain this phenomenon, including relative stability due to life stage, a longer history of coping with life crises, and broader acceptance of death.

At the same time, increasing age has its own risks that necessitate psychosocial screening in prostate cancer patients. Older men are at higher risk for depression, suicide, and alcohol abuse. Those living alone have an increased risk of these psychological problems and higher cancer mortality in general. Several authors note the underdiagnosis of depression in cancer patients in general. Reasons cited include the "belief that depression is a normal reaction to a serious disease and partly because of the belief that . . . weight loss, sleep disturbance, or emotional/cognitive signs of depression often are attributable to the medical illness" (18). In addition, responding to a depressed person is perceived as time consuming; a patient's lack of cooperation may be labeled as noncompliance or another negative attribute, or depression leading to suicidal thoughts is accepted as suicide becomes a socially accepted alternative for cancer patients (13). It should be noted that many elderly men have healthy, active lifestyles and may have high expectations of quality of life after initial treatment. Stereotypes of elderly men living with chronic, disabling illness are largely a myth. Some centers are reporting successful results of radical prostatectomies in 80-year-olds.

REACTIONS TO NERVE-SPARING RADICAL PROSTATECTOMY

The nerve-sparing radical prostatectomy, the standard of care for many men with stage B prostate cancer, has become an increasingly common treatment choice. Nerve-sparing has given men hope of avoiding or limiting the two most dreaded side effects of prostate cancer treatment: impotence and incontinence (18). Men may have unrealistic expectations of the surgery, assuming that, in spite of statistics, they will be successful in avoiding complications. Clear education before surgery is essential (19). This should fully inform surgical candidates of the following:

1. The cancer may have spread locally and the prostate may not be removed.
2. The cancer may be too close to the nerve bundles to allow the nerve-sparing procedure.
3. Even if nerve sparing is accomplished and the prostate is removed, it may take months to recover potency and continence.

If fully informed of these risks and even percentages for the cancer center or surgeon, the patient is less likely to become angry and disappointed by the surgical results (20).

SEXUAL DYSFUNCTION IN EARLY-STAGE DISEASE

The incidence of sexual dysfunction for surgery or radiation treatments in early-stage disease is decreasing but still occurs. Although men undergoing nerve-sparing radical prostatectomy may find the rates of recovery of potency at 75% or higher for younger men and 50% for men older than 70 years, there are still some patients for whom the nerve bundle must be sacrificed to achieve adequate margins (21). The typical scenario for men with successful nerve sparing is to gradually achieve successful erections after weeks or months of recovery. For external beam radiation of the prostate, the more typical experience is to gradually lose potency over a period of months posttreatment, whereas up to 30% or more of patients may never lose potency (22). The treatment of sexual dysfunction has traditionally included

1. Vacuum pumps
2. Prosthesis
3. Injections
4. Counseling (23)

More recently, sildenafil (Viagra) has been prescribed for men with impotence related to prostate cancer with some success. In the absence of hormonal treatment, sexual desire remains intact. Treatments for sexual dysfunction in prostate cancer are a strong interest area in support groups. Openness among these men to ask questions about sexual problems and treatments is common (24).

Male identity and sexual dysfunction produce strong emotional reactions to this treatment side effect. The sense of needing to have an erection to maintain one's identity persists. In a study by Singer, 50 men were willing to trade off survival to preserve sexual potency (25). The results were independent of age, interest in sex, frequency of intercourse, or ability to achieve erections (25). Although this study has not been replicated, it does illustrate the kinds of trade-offs that go into decision making in prostate cancer treatment.

In counseling patients regarding the potential for treatment-related sexual dysfunction, there are three important considerations: premorbid sexual function, age, and the sexual partner. Because prostate cancer is more common in older men, the potential for sexual dysfunction from other causes is higher. For example, men on hypertensive medication for diabetes or pain problems, such as rheumatoid arthritis, may have limited sexual function or impotence before surgery (26). Chronic disease in the sexual partner may also mean a curtailment or end to the couple's sex life before the diagnosis of prostate cancer.

Regarding age issues, there are still misconceptions about sexual activity in the elderly. Some studies show that more than 50% of men are sexually active in their 60s and 30% in their 70s. Even for couples who are not practicing coitus, they may participate in other sexual activity that is satisfying to them. Ofman notes, "Even patients who are not sexually active are likely to be invested in their ability to perform sexually if they wanted to" (26). The physician treating the patient may need to rephrase the question from "Are you and your wife having sex?" to "Is your ability to have an erection important to you so that you would like to have it preserved if possible?"

Besides being life threatening, prostate cancer has many consequences for the partner. The sexual consequences may not all be related to the ability to have an erection or an active libido. For example, role changes as a result of treatment and recovery may impact the man's self-concept, giving him a broader sense of impotence about his ability to perform tasks around the house or work that was important to his identity as a man. This can lead to resentment for both the patient and his spouse and interfere with open communication. Communication can be inhibited by feelings of shame (3). For some older couples, open discussion of sexual function and anatomy may be uncomfortable. Both may believe in the need to put up a strong front to the other, not revealing fears or uncertainties or discussing death (27). Incontinence can be another block to intimacy. For men with even mild incontinence from treatment, shame and fear of spillage may inhibit moves toward intercourse. Finally, unspoken fears of contamination create a barrier to intimacy. In addition to not talking with each other about this, the couple who has these beliefs rarely discusses them with the medical team (26). Breaking through these barriers is a major challenge for the treatment team. Questions about the couple's beliefs about sexual dysfunction can be presented sensitively by the physician, nurse, or social worker. Literature is available that can help the couple learn about sexual issues and how to discuss them (28). In some cases, referral to a sex therapist is indicated, such as when couples need help in learning how to be intimate again in the presence or absence of anatomic dysfunction (20).

Long-term dysfunction that is unsuccessfully treated may lead to depression or even suicidal thoughts (20). Successful treatment requires the inclusion of the sexual partner; having partner consensus on the mode of treatment increases the cooperation and comfort of the spouse with the potential for renewed intercourse (26).

OBSERVATION IN LOCAL DISEASE MANAGEMENT

Among the complex choices facing the patient with localized prostate cancer and his family is whether to accept observation only or pursue active treatment. The conservative management of localized prostate cancer was proposed by Whitmore as an alternative to early endocrine therapy (29). With older men, particularly those with coexisting diseases, the morbidity from treatment could have a greater impact on quality of life than would no treatment. Because prostate cancer is a slow-growing tumor in some men and can be safely monitored with PSA levels and other techniques, observation is an option chosen by some men to avoid the potential complications of treatment. One study involving 140 men whose average age was 66 years that examined the preference of men for observation versus treatment found that 53% preferred surgery and 42% preferred observation. The main factor in those preferring surgery was their desire to have the tumor completely removed. In those preferring observation, a large majority were strongly influenced by the potential for surgical complications. Older men were more likely to choose expectant management (30).

In expectant management, discussion with the family is particularly essential. Adult children or spouses of men offered observation might be as split about the decision as the group of men in the previously mentioned study. By providing the same information to the family and patient, some conflicts can be avoided. However, because cancer has traditionally been approached more aggressively, the idea of "doing nothing" and allowing the cancer to remain in the body under observation is a concept that may be difficult for some to accept (31).

ENHANCING COPING IN EARLY-STAGE DISEASE

By understanding the diagnosis of cancer as a traumatic event, the provision of psychosocial services to enhance coping is essential. A recent study of patients receiving radiation therapy for local prostate cancer noted that intrusive thoughts about their cancer were common; *intrusive thoughts* are defined as unwanted negative ideas that present persistently, even when one tries to drive them out of their mind. The study also found that fatigue was a common complaint that had an impact on quality of life (32). In a study from Canada, men with prostate cancer reported being well informed about their disease and treatment but were dissatisfied with the lack of information about emotional reactions, how to meet other prostate cancer survivors, where counseling was available, and how to find a support group (33). Clearly, men with prostate cancer are eager for help in coping with their disease.

The key aids to enhance coping in the early phases of prostate cancer are best illustrated by the *Cancer Survivor's Toolbox*, a set of audiotapes developed for cancer survivors (34). The Toolbox covers six topics: (a) communicating what you think and feel to family and the medical team, (b) finding information by using the resources that are available, (c) making decisions about treatment by weighing the pros and cons, (d) solving problems that affect daily activities, (e) negotiating with those involved in patient care to maximize quality of life, and (f) standing up for your rights or self-advocacy (34). Because cancer challenges even the strongest of families with fears of the unknown, a set of basic tools like this provide needed skills to meet these challenges.

A number of cognitive and behavioral interventions have been demonstrated as effective in reducing distress and uncertainty and improving confidence in cancer patients' ability to manage their illness. These interventions include individual counseling, group interventions, biofeedback and relaxation, and imagery, to mention a few (35). One example of an intensive individual intervention was conducted in Canada, randomizing 60 prostate cancer patients into two groups—one receiving information and counseling about a self-efficacy approach to managing their illness and the other receiving only written information. The experimental group had a more active approach to treatment decisions and lower anxiety at 6 weeks after the intervention (36). Interventions that promote self-care have also been demonstrated to positively affect mood among pessimistic prostate cancer patients in a study of those receiving radiation therapy (37,38).

Support groups have become a widely available resource at all stages of prostate cancer. Many, such as the American Cancer Society program Man-to-Man, also provide one-to-one contact with long-term prostate cancer survivors, especially during the critical stage of deciding on initial treatment. Support groups for prostate cancer tend to emphasize problem solving over affective expression, with new treatments being a common topic, along with practical ways to deal with symptoms and even encouraging political action (39,40).

Several books are now available to enhance coping with prostate cancer. Some are personal stories about how men coped with their diagnosis and treatment; others written by physicians describe current treatment alternatives; others view prostate cancer as an illness that requires family involvement. These books can be effective tools in the early stages of uncertainty and shock (Table 49-1). The Internet is emerging as a universal resource for finding information and support for prostate cancer. Several high-quality web sites and e-mail discussion groups (listservs) provide information on standard treatment, alternative treatment, and personal stories (Table 49-1). As noted earlier, if, during psychosocial screening, severe distress is identified, then referral to one of several mental health professionals with oncology experience is indicated. This may involve individual or family psychotherapy; psychotropic medication; and, in rare cases, psychiatric hospitalization. The Distress Management Guidelines developed by the National Comprehensive Cancer Network are the most comprehensive guides to evaluating distress in cancer (41) (Fig. 49-1).

TABLE 49-1. RECOMMENDED BOOKS AND WEBSITES FOR PROSTATE CANCER

Books
- Kantoff P, McConnell M. *Prostate cancer: a family consultation*. New York: Houghton-Mifflin, 1996.
- Bostwick D, MacLennan GT, Larson TR. *Prostate cancer: what every man—and his family—needs to know*. New York: Villard Books, 1996.
- Salowe, AE. *Prostate cancer: overcoming denial with action. A guide to screening, treatment, and planning*. New York: St. Martin's Griffin, 1997.

Websites
- Man-to-Man (American Cancer Society), http://www.cancer.org/m2m/m2m.html
- US TOO! International, Inc., http://www.ustoo.com
- Phoenix5, http://www.phoenix5.org
- Prostate Pointers, http://www.prostatepointers.org

IMPACT OF RECURRENCE AND TREATMENT FAILURE

The impact of recurrence in cancer is well known to exacerbate anxiety and depression. Every cancer patient lives with the possibility of recurrence and worries that this fear will become a reality. A few studies have shown lower anxiety after recurrence in those that anticipated its probability and developed strong coping skills after their initial diagnosis. In a study by Cella et al., recurrence is characterized as a traumatic event; the subjects who were completely surprised by recurrence or who were undergoing their first recurrence experienced a higher rate of intrusive thoughts and exhibited more avoidant behavior (42). Again, psychosocial screening is helpful in differentiating the level of distress and coping abilities in the face of this second threat. Patients and families are not only faced with the news of the recurrent cancer but also another set of complex treatment decisions.

As PSA has become the principal tumor marker for prostate cancer, some anxiety and obsession with PSA levels can occur in men fearing recurrence. This hypervigilance can interfere with daily functioning. A similar phenomenon has been observed in other diseases, such as T-cell counts in patients with human immunodeficiency virus (43). Education and reassurance are adequate to reduce this anxiety for most men, but those who truly become obsessed should be referred to a social worker, psychologist, or psychiatrist.

Treatment side effects can create additional coping problems. For instance, antiandrogen treatment can result in demasculinization, such as loss of libido, hot flashes, and breast enlargement or pain (26). These symptoms may be subtle and go unnoticed by family; owing to the embarrassing nature of the symptoms, the patient may be reluctant to tell his family or physician. These symptoms can lead to a triple insult to the male ego: having cancer, being impotent, and developing female characteristics (44). Men who find this triple insult unbearable are certainly candidates for depression and suicidal thoughts. Evaluation of the

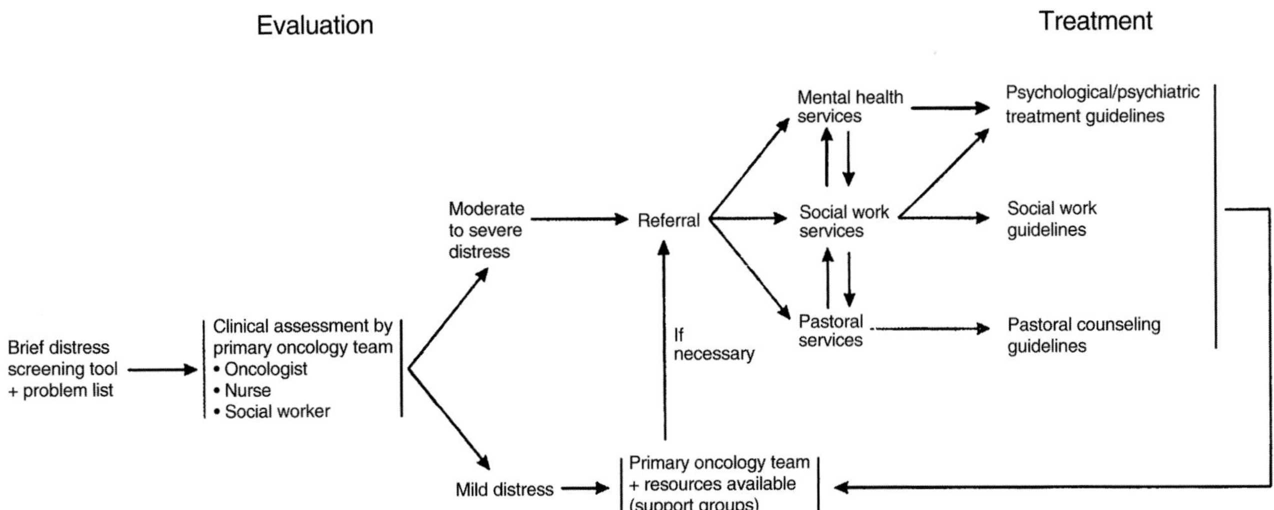

FIGURE 49-1. Distress management. (From the National Comprehensive Cancer Network, Inc., with permission.)

impact of new symptoms is essential, whether done by the physician or another member of the medical team. Monitoring quality of life can help identify changes in the patients' activities of daily living and the effects of treatment. Clark et al. developed a scale identifying nine areas of concern in men with metastatic prostate cancer: body image, sexual problems, spouse affection, spouse worry, masculinity, cancer-related self-image, cancer distress, cancer acceptance, and regret of treatment decision (44).

These middle stages of prostate cancer are characterized by periods of active symptoms and remission from symptoms. Typically, antiandrogen treatment produces a successful decrease in physical symptoms that may produce a parallel sense of emotional relief and hopefulness. With the onset of side effects from these treatments, men may become discouraged and question the treatment's benefit and regret their decision to pursue their chosen course of treatment. In cases of severe toxicity, some may prefer withdrawal from treatment (45,46).

Often during periods of uncertainty and disappointment at traditional treatment, cancer survivors will seek out complementary and alternative treatments. These may be as straightforward as prayer or relaxation tapes or may be more extreme, nontraditional treatments such as shark cartilage (47). The physician should encourage the patient to discuss in a nonjudgmental way the types of treatments he is experimenting with to avoid further alienating the patient. Once the patient believes he has been heard on his reasons for trying these treatments, the physician and the medical team can lay out their recommendations and opinions on these treatments. Often, a compromise can be reached in finding ways to have alternative treatments complement rather than conflict with standard treatment (48). Some ethnic differences in distress and uncertainty have been found, such as spiritual factors and the quality of the home environment being more important for African-American men; however, there are more similarities than differences in coping with uncertainty (45).

One treatment with special implications is the bilateral orchiectomy or surgical castration as opposed to medical castration with antiandrogens. Although castration makes sense for a select group of men with advanced disease, the impact on their self-concept must be considered. In a study by Montgomery et al., no differences in self-concept were seen in comparison to men who underwent transurethral resection of the prostate (49). However, subscales, measuring physical self and identity, did show significant changes. Ofman notes, "Because of its symbolic nature, bilateral orchiectomy has potential body image repercussions that far exceed . . . the changes from testosterone ablation" (22).

Advanced Disease

Advanced disease is more frequently being referred to as hormonal-resistant prostate cancer and is an active area of treatment investigation. As with an initial recurrence, failure of hormonal therapy can signal the return of depression and a loss of hope. In addition, symptoms may be more debilitating. Pain, especially related to bone metastases, becomes a major symptom but can be successfully controlled. Fatigue related to pain, tumor, or treatment can worsen. Fortunately, cancer-related fatigue is now a better-identified symptom with several successful nursing and medical interventions. The psychosocial aspects of fatigue need to be attended to, because men especially can perceive it as laziness or a loss of manhood. Depression can be intermingled with fatigue, clouding a clear diagnosis and treatment of either (50). Spinal metastases bring the threat of paralysis.

In this context, it is important to provide home care and aggressive symptom relief. Men should be encouraged to shed a macho image and report symptoms of pain and fatigue early and specifically. There may be communication problems within the family or between the patient and physician that interfere with cancer pain relief. A team approach to pain, which provides continual reassessment and open communication, is essential (51). Hope in clinical trials can give patients the will to go on. Even the promise of basic research for future prostate cancer treatments provides hope and encouragement. During this time of greater uncertainty and symptoms, many men report an increased desire for intimacy (45). This provides needed comfort and reassurance that they will not be abandoned in death.

Caregivers

As the disease advances and symptoms increase, the family must mobilize to assist the patient at home. From a review of the literature, Northouse et al. note the three major concerns of caregivers: "dealing with the fear and threat associated with a cancer diagnosis, helping partners to deal with the emotional repercussions of cancer, and managing the changes and disruptions of daily life brought on by the disease" (52). Studies are inconclusive about the effect of recurrence on the spouse. Given and colleagues' results showed an increase in depression of caregivers during the 6 months after recurrence, with a more symptomatic patient producing a more pronounced effect in caregivers (53). Caregivers and patients can benefit from problem-solving interventions. In a study by Blanchard et al., cancer patients became less depressed than those patients whose family caregivers did not receive the intervention (54). The Prepared Family Caregiver Course and the accompanying book, *Home Care Guide for Cancer* (55), provide excellent tools to improve the problem-solving skills in a symptom-focused format (56).

Referral to palliative care, hospice, or a pain service is an anticipated step in the natural history of prostate cancer. The timing of this step depends on the severity of symptoms, availability of treatments, and the patient and family's perception of end-of-life care. Some may resist the idea of hospice care because of its association with their perception of dying and death. Most often, acceptance of hospice and palliative care comes with a compassionate explanation of the inevitable transition from treatment for cure to comfort care. This is most effectively accomplished through a family conference (57). Again, a sense of nonabandonment is important, as is a reassurance that effective treatments were tried and failed. This will help reduce the sense of regret about prior treatment decisions (44).

LONG-TERM SURVIVORS

With the advent of improved and new treatments for prostate cancer since 1990, a large population of long-term survivors has emerged. Many of these men may return to work or proceed with a relatively normal retirement. Each year, more are becoming cancer activists (58). These men become support-group leaders and friendly visitors. Others volunteer in hospitals and cancer centers. Still others have become active in political advocacy for prostate cancer research and public speaking or fund raising. The future of prostate cancer research and treatment can only benefit from this kind of activism.

CONCLUSION

The psychosocial aspects of prostate cancer are beginning to gain broader scientific study beyond the issue of sexual dysfunction. It is clear that screening patients for depression and other quality of life problems is key to effective treatment. With the availability of effective psychosocial interventions, patients and caregivers can benefit from individual counseling and education, support groups, books, and the Internet. Sexual dysfunction continues to be of concern for many men approaching surgical and hormonal treatment; however, these concerns are complex and include one's sense of self-concept and self-worth. Support groups for prostate cancer are now broadly available and provide an effective intervention for men at all stages of the disease. The specific effects of these groups require further study. In general, psychosocial research in prostate cancer is in its infancy. More research is needed on how men make treatment decisions and what tools can most effectively help them make decisions, balancing the trade-offs of various treatment modalities. Research is needed to explore whether the incidence of depression or anxiety is higher or lower in prostate cancer than other cancers. Caregiver research needs to explore the specific relationship of the spouse and adult children in dealing with issues of pain, depression, incontinence, and fatigue in the context of prostate cancer.

REFERENCES

1. Schover LR, Von Eschenbach AC, Smith DB, et al. Sexual rehabilitation of urologic cancer patients: a practical approach. *CA Cancer J Clin* 1984;34:66–74.
2. Sharp JW, Blum D, Aviv L. Elderly men with cancer: social work interventions in prostate cancer. *Soc Work Health Care* 1993;19:91–107.

2a. Dole R. Speech delivered at The March: Coming Together to Conquer Cancer. Washington, DC. 25–26 September 1998.

3. Heyman EN, Rosner TT. Prostate cancer: an intimate view from patients and wives. *Urol Nurs* 1996;16:37–44.

4. McCoy CB, Anwyl RS, Metsch LR, et al. Prostate cancer in Florida: knowledge, attitudes, practices, and beliefs. *Cancer Pract* 1995;3:88–93.
5. Mettlin C, Murphy GP, Ray P, et al. American Cancer Society—National Prostate Cancer Detection Project. *Cancer* 1993;71:891–898.
6. Taylor KL, DiPlacido J, Redd WH, et al. Demographics, family histories, and psychological characteristics of prostate carcinoma screening participants. *Cancer* 1999;85:1305–1312.
7. Adderley-Kelly B, Green PM. Breast cancer education, self-efficacy, and screening in older African-American women. *J Natl Black Nurs Assoc* 1997;9:45–57.
8. Kempen GI, Jelicic M, Ormel J. Personality, chronic medical morbidity and health-related quality of life among older persons. *Health Psychol* 1997;16:539–546.
9. Underwood SM. African-American men: perceptual determinants of early cancer detection and cancer risk reduction. *Cancer Nurs* 1991;14:281–288.
10. Freeman HP. Cancer and the economically disadvantaged. *Cancer* 1989;64(Suppl):324–334.
11. McCoy CB, Nielsen BB, Chitwood DD, et al. Increasing the cancer screening of the medically underserved in South Florida. *Cancer* 1991;67(Suppl):1808–1813.
12. McDaniel S, Musselman DL, Porter MR, et al. Depression in patients with cancer: diagnosis, biology, and treatment. *Arch Gen Psychiat* 1995;52:89–99.
13. Valente SM, Saunders JM, Cohen MZ. Evaluating depression among patients with cancer. *Cancer Pract* 1994;2:65–71.
14. Godding PR, McAnulty RD, Wittrock DA, et al. Predictors of depression among male cancer patients. *J Nerv Ment Dis* 1995;183:95–98.
15. Coreil J, Bebal R. Man to man prostate cancer support groups. *Cancer Pract* 1999;7:122–129.
16. Steward DE, Cheung AM, et al. Informational needs and decisional preferences of women with breast cancer compared to men with prostate cancer. Academy of Psychosomatic Medicine Proceedings, 45th annual meeting, 1997.
17. Zabora JR, Blanchard CG, Smith ED, et al. Psychological distress among cancer patients across the disease continuum. *J Psychosoc Oncol* 1997;15:73–87.
18. Catalona WJ, Bigg SW. Nerve-sparing radical prostatectomy: evaluation of results after 250 patients. *J Urol* 1990;143:538–544.
19. Montie JE. Counseling the patient with regional metastasis of prostate cancer. *Cancer* 1993;71:1019–1023.
20. Schover LR. Sexual rehabilitation after treatment for prostate cancer. *Cancer* 1993;71:1024–1030.
21. Catalona WJ. Surgical management of prostate cancer: contemporary results with anatomic radical prostatectomy. *Cancer* 1995;75:1903–1908.
22. Ofman US. Preservation of function in genitourinary cancers: psychosexual and psychosocial issues. *Cancer Invest* 1995;13:125–131.
23. Sprouse DO. Sexual rehabilitation of the prostate cancer patient. *Cancer* 1995;75:1957–1962.
24. Calabrese DA. Prostate cancer groups. *Cancer* 1995;75: 1897–1899.
25. Singer PA, Tasch ES, Stocking C, et al. Sex or survival? Trade-offs between quality and quantity of life. *J Clin Oncol* 1991;9:328–334.
26. Ofman US. Sexual quality of life in men with prostate cancer. *Cancer* 1995;75:1949–1953.
27. Ofman US. Psychosocial and sexual implications of genitourinary cancers. *Semin Oncol Nurs* 1993;9:286–292.
28. Schover LR. *Sexuality and fertility after cancer.* New York: John Wiley & Sons, 1997.
29. Whitmore WF. Conservative approaches to the management of localized prostatic cancer. *Cancer* 1993;71:970–975.
30. Mazur DJ, Hickam DH. Patient preferences for management of localized prostate cancer. *West J Med* 1996;165:26–30.
31. Gray RE, Fitch MI, Phillips C, et al. Presurgery experiences of prostate cancer patients and their spouses. *Cancer Pract* 1999;7:130–135.
32. Walker BL, Nail LM, Larsen L, et al. Concerns, affect, and cognitive disruption following completion of radiation treatment for localized breast or prostate cancer. *Oncol Nurs Forum* 1996;23:1181–1187.
33. Fitch MI, Johnson B, Gray R, et al. Survivor's perspectives on the impact of prostate cancer: implications for oncology nurses. *Can Oncol Nurs J* 1999;9:23–34.
34. *Cancer survivor's toolbox.* Washington, DC: National Coalition of Cancer Survivors, 1998.
35. Lovejoy NC, Matteis M. Cognitive-behavioral interventions to manage depression in patients with cancer: research and theoretical initiatives. *Cancer Nurs* 1997;20:155–167.
36. Davison BJ, Degner LF. Empowerment of men newly diagnosed with prostate cancer. *Cancer Nurs* 1997;20:187–196.
37. Johnson JE. Coping with radiation therapy: optimism and the effect of preparatory interventions. *Res Nurs Health* 1996;19:3–12.
38. Johnson JE, Fieler VK, Wlasowicz GS, et al. The effects of nursing care guided by self-regulation theory on coping with radiation therapy. *Oncol Nurs Forum* 1997;24:1041–1050.
39. Krizek C, Roberts C, Ragan R, et al. Gender and cancer support group participation. *Cancer Pract* 1999;7:86–92.
40. Gray RE, Fitch M, Davis C, et al. Interviews with men with prostate cancer about their self-help group experience. *J Pall Care* 1997;13:15–21.
41. National Comprehensive Cancer Network. *Distress management practice guidelines.* Washington, DC: National Coalition of Cancer Survivors, 1999.
42. Cella DF, Mahon SM, Donovan MI. Cancer as a traumatic event. *Behav Med* 1990;16:15–22.
43. Griffin KW, Rabkin JG. Psychological distress in people with HIV/AIDS: prevalence rates and methodological issues. *AIDS Behav* 1997;1:29–42.
44. Clark JA, Wray N, Brody B, et al. Dimensions of quality of life expressed by men treated for metastatic prostate cancer. *Soc Sci Med* 1997;45:1299–1309.
45. Germino BB, Mishel MH, Belyea M, et al. Uncertainty in prostate cancer: ethnic and family patterns. *Cancer Pract* 1998;6:107–113.
46. Cassileth BR, Seidmon EJ, Soloway MS, et al. Patient's choice of treatment in stage D prostate cancer. *Urology* 1989;33:57–62.
47. Jenkins RA, Paargament KI. Religion and spirituality as resources for coping with cancer. *J Psychosoc Oncol* 1995; 13:51–74.
48. Wyatt GK, Friedman LL, Given CW, et al. Complementary therapy use among older cancer patients. *Cancer Pract* 1999; 7:136–144.

49. Montgomery P, Shanti G. The influence of bilateral orchiectomy on self-concept: a pilot study. *J Adv Nurs* 1996;24: 1249–1256.
50. Hann DM, Jacobsen PB, Azzerello LM. Measurement of fatigue in cancer patients: development and validation of the Fatigue Symptom Inventory. *Qual Life Res* 1998;7:301–310.
51. Glajchen M, Fitzmartin RD, Blum D, et al. Psychosocial barriers to cancer pain relief. *Cancer Pract* 1995;3:76–87.
52. Northouse LL, Peters-Golden H. Cancer and the family: strategies to assist spouses. *Semin Oncol Nurs* 1993;9:75.
53. Given BA, Given CW, Helms E, et al. Determinants of family caregiver reaction: new and recurrent cancer. *Cancer Pract* 1997;5:17–24.
54. Blanchard CG, Toseland RW, McCallion P. The effects of a problem-solving intervention with spouses of cancer patients. *J Psychosoc Oncol* 1996;14:1–21.
55. Houts P, Nezu AM, Nezu CM, et al. *Home care guide for cancer.* Philadelphia: American College of Physicians, 1996.
56. Bucher JA, Houts PS, Nezu CM, et al. Improving problem-solving skills of family caregivers through group education. *J Psychosoc Oncol* 1999;16:73–84.
57. Miller R, Krech R, Walsh TD. The role of the palliative care service family conference in the management of the patient with advanced cancer. *Pall Med* 1991;5:34–39.
58. Zakarian B. *The activist cancer patient: how to take charge of your treatment.* New York: John Wiley & Sons, 1996.

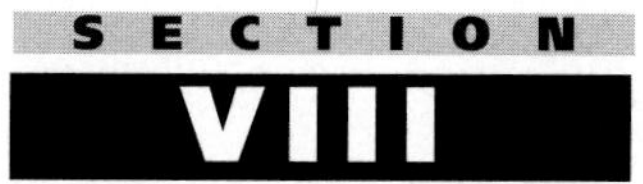

HORMONE REFRACTORY DISEASE—CURRENT STANDARDS AND FUTURE DIRECTIONS

50

CLINICAL TRIAL DESIGN FOR PROSTATE CANCER

MICHAEL J. MORRIS
HOWARD I. SCHER

Clinical trial design for prostate cancer has historically been a difficult and controversial endeavor, as several unique features of the disease complicate, if not impede, the testing of new agents. For example, the majority of patients with metastases lacks disease in the soft tissues, and objective changes in measurable lesions are rarely applicable. Changes in the radionuclide bone scan can occur months after a drug's antitumor effect and are reader dependent. As a result, greater emphasis is placed on biochemical response criteria, namely that of the prostate-specific antigen (PSA). Whether a treatment-induced PSA decline confers a clinical benefit to a patient, however, is debatable. Furthermore, novel biologic agents may modulate the PSA in ways traditionally not associated with an antitumor effect.

Patient selection is complicated by the fact that a patient diagnosed with prostate cancer may not develop symptoms of the disease or die of it, recurrent disease may not require immediate treatment, and slowing the rate of disease progression may be sufficient to reduce prostate cancer–specific mortality.

In the past, the selection of agents available for trials was limited primarily to hormones or cytotoxic agents, both of which have significant side effects. The appropriate clinical setting in which investigational agents were tested was limited as well, as the balance between morbidity from therapy versus morbidity from disease favored the treatment of patients with advanced disease. Newer therapies have altered this balance. As a result, clinical scenarios that were previously inappropriate for trials now exist: the treatment of patients without evidence of disease, of those who have biochemically relapsed, and of patients who have metastatic disease but are androgen-dependent. As these new agents and new treatment opportunities emerge, a reassessment of the purpose of clinical trials and their appropriate design is in order.

This chapter addresses each of these factors independently. First, disease states are discussed as a model for describing not only tumor progression but trial design as well. Second, the elements of trials are discussed (i.e., entry criteria, interventions, and end points). Third, the integration of the disease state with individual elements of the clinical trial is reviewed state by state to highlight state-specific design considerations.

CLINICAL TRIAL DESIGN AS A FUNCTION OF NATURAL HISTORY

A clinical trial is composed of a defined aim, an intervention, a treatment population, end points relevant to the intervention and population, and a decision rule on whether evaluation should continue. In this context, a universal set of "rules" cannot be applied to all states of the disease.

In an effort to clarify trial design, we have proposed a model of disease progression, shown in Figure 50-1 (1). This model segregates patients on the basis of their place in the continuum of the disease from diagnosis to death. It focuses on how the therapeutic approach being evaluated relates to the patient's point in the natural history, as shown in Table 50-1. A unique aspect of the model is that it highlights the objectives of the treatment and not the treatment itself. In addition, unlike traditional staging schema based on the characteristics of the primary tumor, nodal status, and metastatic involvement at diagnosis, the model is not fixed at a static point but is descriptive of the entire disease course throughout time. Illustrated are the competing causes of death for a patient with prostate cancer—disease or other causes—and the shift in the relative significance of these causes to the individual depending on the point in the illness. An additional consideration is the distinction between *cure*, elimination of all cancer cells, and *control*, modulation of growth rates so that the patient dies a non-cancer–related death.

The states in the model identify points in the history of the disease where an intervention might be considered or a

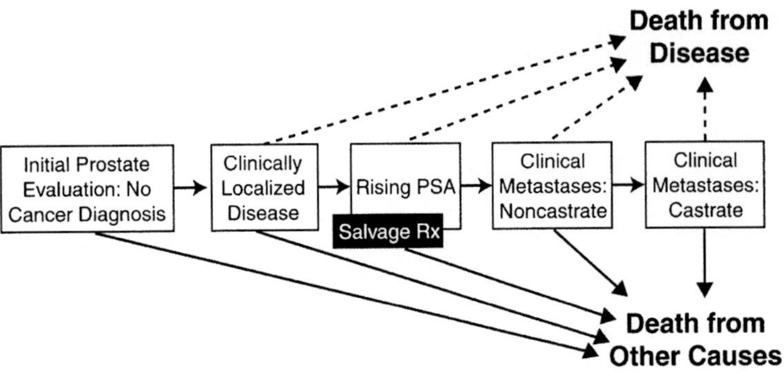

FIGURE 50-1. Clinical disease states in prostate cancer: clinical states model. PSA, prostate-specific antigen; Rx, therapy.

clinical trial question addressed. By implication, progression from one state to another represents a treatment failure, although this does not imply that the patient will require another intervention. Patients who do not progress remain in a given state, allowing the determination of "time within a state" to be calculated reliably.

The ultimate goal of all cancer therapies is to prolong quality-adjusted life expectancy. There are, however, other short-term measures of benefit that may be clinically relevant to a patient. These include the elimination of a specific manifestation of the disease that is identified at a particular point in time (e.g., pain) and the prevention of disease-related events in the future, underscoring the fact that end points are often state specific and therapy specific. The decision to continue development of a strategy ultimately rests on a combination of how many patients benefited (however that is defined) from the treatment and how long that benefit was maintained.

INTERVENTIONS

Hormonal therapy was the past focus of drug development for prostate cancer. Later, traditional cytotoxic approaches were applied, primarily in late-stage disease. Because the molecular lesions underlying the tumorigenesis, growth, and resistance of prostate cancer are better understood, mechanism-based approaches are now undergoing investigation. Potential strategies include targeting cell signaling through the Her2 gene product (2–5), epidermal growth factor receptor (6), and farnesyl transferase (7–9); tumor suppressor genes, such as p53 (10,11); apoptotic pathways, such as bcl-2 (12); histone acetylation; and cellular differentiation through the vitamin D receptor (13,14), retinoic acid receptor (15,16), and peroxisome proliferator-induced receptor gamma (17). In addition, strategies that are directed against tumor invasion and angiogenesis are undergoing clinical testing, as are *in vivo* and *ex vivo* immune strategies using active and passive immunity (18–20).

TABLE 50-1. THERAPEUTIC OBJECTIVES AS A FUNCTION OF DISEASE STATE

Disease state	Therapeutic objective
No prostate cancer diagnosis	Prevent a prostate cancer diagnosis
Localized disease	Elimination of all cancer
Rising prostate-specific antigen: local or systemic	Elimination of all cancer
Clinical metastatic disease: noncastrate	Prevent hormone independence
Clinical metastatic disease: castrate	Prolong life

Many of these agents are cytostatic in their effects, whereas others are designed to slow progression. Each of these interventions may alter the natural history by delaying death; however, their short-term effects on a specific disease-related manifestation, such as changes in a gene's expression or on a biochemical marker such as PSA, are unclear.

In the states model, the application of a specific therapeutic strategy is determined by the characteristics of the patients in that state and the end points of the trial, as shown in Table 50-2. The therapeutic targets vary. Some, such as prostate-specific membrane antigen, PSA, or prostate stem-cell antigen, are relatively prostate specific. Others are oncogenic proteins, altered tumor suppressor gene products, and differentiation antigens that are not cancer- or organ-site specific. Some targets are therapeutically appropriate only within specific disease states, whereas others are valid across various phases of the disease. For example, targets associated with metastatic disease such as bcl-2 may be effective in narrowly defined clinical scenarios, whereas targets such as prostate-specific membrane antigen may be exploited across clinical states.

ELIGIBILITY

The purpose of eligibility criteria is to assure that the aims or goals of a trial are precisely defined and the diversity of factors impacting an outcome are as restricted as possible. An unfortunate historical reality is that eligibility criteria have varied across trials. For example, disease progression may be defined on the basis of changes in soft-tissue involvement, bony disease, symptoms, or PSA, as shown in Table 50-3.

TABLE 50-2. RELATIONSHIP BETWEEN DISEASE STATE, INTERVENTION, AND END POINT

Disease state	Therapeutic objective	Interventions	End point
No prostate cancer diagnosis	Prevent a prostate cancer diagnosis	Chemopreventive drugs, intraprostatic injections, dietary modulation, differentiating agents	No cancer
Localized disease			No cancer
Probability of local control	Complete elimination of all cancer	Local therapies	
Probability of local failure		Adjuvant local therapy	
Probability of systemic failure	Prevention of rising PSA	Combined modality approaches, systemic adjuvant therapy	
Postprostatectomy			
High-risk local failure	Prevent local recurrence	Local radiation therapy	No detectable PSA, no local recurrence
High-risk systemic failure	Prevent systemic relapse	Vaccination approaches	No detectable PSA, no systemic recurrence
Rising PSA			
Local	Complete elimination of all cancer	Salvage therapies: Surgery postradiation Radiation postsurgery	No detectable PSA No further rise in PSA
Systemic	Preventing clinically detectable metastases	Experimental systemic therapies	No detectable PSA, change in PSA rate of rise, negative imaging studies
Clinical metastatic disease			
Noncastrate	Prevent emergence of androgen independence, increase response rates (complete elimination of all cancer)	Secondary therapy to prevent emergence of androgen independence, chemohormonal therapy	No detectable PSA, no progression after initial response, no detectable PSA
Castrate	Prolong life	Secondary hormones Nonhormonal therapies: Vaccination strategies Gene therapy Biologic agents Differentiating agents Antimetastatic drugs Angiogenesis inhibitors Proapoptotic drugs Chemotherapy	Prolongation of life

PSA, prostate-specific antigen.
From Morris MJ, Scher HI. Novel strategies and therapeutics for the treatment of prostate carcinoma. *Cancer* 2000;89:1329–1348.

Specific criteria exist for progression in measurable soft-tissue disease, including a defined increase (greater than 25%) in the area of an existing lesion or the development of a new lesion. Progression in bone includes the development of new sites of metastases, although the significance of an increase in the area of an existing lesion in the absence of new lesions is more controversial (21). The definition of biochemical progression is even more confusing, although a minimum of three sequential rising values is generally an accepted convention. There is no concensus, however, on the proportional increase and the time interval between determinations, although many investigators follow a rule of thumb that a 50% increase from a baseline represents a significant rise. The minimum value will vary. For example, progression after radical prostatectomy is any detectable PSA (greater than 0.4 ng per mL), whereas progression after radiation therapy can be greater than 0.5 ng per mL or 1.0 ng per mL.

Disease progression defined by virtue of worsening symptoms is established with the onset of new symptoms or an increase in intensity of preexisting symptoms. There is disagreement on the quantification of symptomatology, which will differ from trial to trial and state to state.

Another challenge to consistent eligibility criteria is that the availability and use of technology and expertise vary from center to center. For example, trials assessing salvage radiation therapy in relapsed patients after radical prostatectomy can enroll patients on the basis of biochemical parameters, biopsy samples, ProstaScint scans, or any combination of these. However, the results of the trial will likely vary as a function of which criteria are used. Biologic assays, such as assessments of Her2, bcl-2, p53, or others, are also increasingly used in many centers to select patients for studies. In these situations, the site from which the tissue was obtained (prostate vs. bone vs. soft tissue), the

TABLE 50-3. DEFINITIONS OF PROGRESSIVE DISEASE

Prostate-specific antigen
- Three sequential rising values
- Proportional increase not defined; suggest a >50% increase from a baseline value
- Time interval between determinations not defined; suggest a minimum of 2 wk apart
- Minimum value not defined but will vary by disease state

Measurable disease
- A >25% increase in bidimensionally measurable soft tissue disease or the appearance of new sites of disease

Bone scan
- New lesions: a minimum of one
- Controversial: an increase in area or intensity of an existing lesion with or without new symptoms in the area

androgen dependence of the tumor, the techniques used to obtain and prepare the tissue, and the definition of a positive result will all affect whether a result is "positive" or "negative." For example, differences in Her2 expression have been reported on the basis of whether immunohistochemistry or fluorescence *in situ* hybridization was used (22). Details of the methods used are critical parts of the eligibility criteria in trials that use these assays.

Elibigility criteria will also vary according to disease state, as shown in Table 50-4. For example, treatments intended to reduce symptoms must be tested on (a) patients with active disease and (b) those who experience symptoms that directly relate to the disease burden. By contrast, a patient who has no detectable PSA after radical prostatectomy typically has no cancer-related symptoms requiring control and would undergo treatment based on a predicted risk of relapse; thus, such patients are inappropriate for studying palliative therapies. The disease state dictates the rationale of the study; the rationale dictates the treatment population and, by implication, the eligibility criteria.

Finally, prior treatments and outcomes must, at least in part, be a part of decisions regarding eligibility. Prior exposure to hormonal agents, chemotherapy, and biologic drugs is relevant to present outcomes. Patients who are currently taking an antiandrogen or steroid hormone should be observed for a response to withdrawal of these drugs, with documentation of progression after withdrawal. Failure to do so may lead to the false attribution of response to an intervention and overestimation of the level of benefit of the drug. Relevant manifestations of the disease, such as a rising PSA or symptoms, medications taken (including alternative medications), dietary habits, and a record of each involved site and the method of assessment, must be documented.

DEFINING END POINTS

Perhaps the most difficult element to plan in prostate cancer clinical trials is the selection of appropriate end points. The reasons for this are multifold. First, most patients do not have measurable disease. Second, bone scans have interreader variability and lag relative to the clinical effect. Third, changes in PSA can vary as a function of the mechanism of treatment, and there is no agreement on the degree to which the PSA must change to be "significant." Fourth, outcomes that merely demonstrate that a drug is targeting its intended pathway are often confused with those that translate into a clinical benefit in later trials. As a result of these ongoing ambiguities, it is often difficult to tell whether a drug has "made a difference" and, therefore, when a strategy should be abandoned rather than pursued.

The outcome measures used to assess treatment effects in the course of routine clinical practice or in the context of a clinical trial are ultimately developed to address a single question: Do the results justify continued use or further clinical evaluation? A rational developmental strategy for any new agent is the sequential determination of the dose and toxicity (phase I), efficacy (phase II), and overall level of benefit relative to other treatments (phase III).

This sequence, particularly as drugs enter phase III trials, is costly in dollars and time. Such trials generally involve large numbers of patients and many different treatment centers. The decision to design and conduct these trials must therefore be based on reproducible and objective data to insure that such an endeavor is appropriate. An accurate estimation of the expected level of difference in outcome is necessary so that a cohort of appropriate size can be enrolled and followed for a sufficient time. Any error in these factors can have disastrous results on a drug's development: Underestimation of the level of benefit can lead to the abandonment of a strategy, whereas overestimation can lead to underpowered and inconclusive results.

To avoid such errors, establishing valid and informative response criteria is critical. Such criteria allow investigators to standardize the reporting of results and determine whether a treatment or intervention performs well enough to continue use and further clinical development is justified. They must be reproducible and quantitative, qualities that have heretofore been elusive.

The specific outcome measures of a trial are derived from the hypothesis under study, the intervention used, and the manifestations of the disease at the stage or disease state targeted. Therefore, they vary according to who is being treated, what they are being treated with, and why they are being treated. The anticipated measures of response must each be defined independently, *a priori*, based on all of the preclinical data available (Table 50-5).

Measurable Disease

Only 15% to 20% of patients with metastases will have soft tissue disease. Even in those patients with soft tissue and bone involvement, it is unclear that disease in the soft tis-

TABLE 50-4. RELATIONSHIP BETWEEN ELIGIBILITY CRITERIA, STATE, AND END POINT

Disease state	Eligibility	Interventions	End point
No cancer diagnosis	High-risk profile: Age Race Family history Elevated PSA	Chemopreventive drugs Intraprostatic injections Dietary modulation Differentiating agents	Decrease in frequency of PIN in radical prostatectomy specimens
Localized disease			
Probability of local control high with surgery	Multiplex staging: T stage, grade, Gleason Number of cores	Local treatment to the prostate: Radical surgery	No detectable PSA
	Pathologic markers (MVD, ploidy, p53, e-cadherin, vascular invasion)	Radiation therapy: External or implantation Evaluation in good prognosis localized disease before prostatectomy (window of opportunity designs)	PSA <0.5 No rise in PSA Negative prostate biopsy
	Prevention of a rising PSA	Experimental: Cryosurgery Hyperthermia Intraprostatic gene therapy Differentiating agents	PSA nadir not established Negative prostate biopsy Removal of the prostate shows no cancer PSA change not defined Negative prostate biopsy Removal of the prostate shows no cancer
Rising PSA			
Local	Complete elimination of all cancer	Salvage therapies: Surgery postradiation	Complete removal of the prostate with negative margins of resection No detectable PSA
Systemic	Preventing clinically detectable metastases	Experimental systemic therapies	No detectable PSA, change in rate of PSA rise, negative imaging studies
Clinical metastatic disease			
Noncastrate	Prevention of hormone independence	Secondary therapy to prevent emergence of androgen independence	Assess individual manifestations of disease independently
Good prognosis (minimal metastatic disease)	Toxicity reduction	Intermittent therapy, noncastrating hormones, window of opportunity, castration	Assess individual manifestations of disease independently: PSA Soft tissue Bone Symptoms
Poor prognosis (advanced metastatic disease, high grade, visceral spread, symptoms)	Increase complete response proportions	Chemohormonal therapy	Assess individual manifestations of disease independently: PSA Soft tissue Bone Symptoms
Castrate	Prolong life	Secondary hormones Nonhormonal therapies: Vaccination strategies Gene therapy Biologic agents Differentiating agents Antimetastatic drugs Angiogenesis inhibitors Proapoptotic drugs Chemotherapy	Assess individual manifestations of disease independently: PSA Soft tissue Bone Symptoms

MVD, microvessel density; PIN, prostatic intraepithelial neoplasia; PSA, prostate-specific antigen.

sues mirrors that in the bone in response to treatment. The limited data that exist suggest that disease in bone is more resistant to treatment and more likely to relapse after treatment than soft-tissue disease, suggesting that the latter is a poor surrogate for the former (23).

Osseous Disease

The radionuclide bone scan is an imperfect tool for assessing osseous disease. First, it is an indirect measure of tumor activity, because there is no direct visualization of the

TABLE 50-5. ANTICIPATED CHANGES IN RESPONSE INDICATORS WILL VARY AS A FUNCTION OF THE MECHANISM OF THE INTERVENTION

Therapeutic intervention	Measurable disease	Bone scan	Posttherapy changes in PSA	Symptoms	Time to progression/ survival
Hormones	↓	Improved	↓	Improved	↑
Cytotoxic chemotherapy	↓	Improved	↓	Improved	↑
Differentiation	↔	↔	↑ then ↓	Improved	↑
Antiangiogenesis	↑	↔	↑	Improved	↑
Antimetastatic	↑	↔	↑	Improved	↑
Cytostatic	↔	↔	↔	Improved	↑
Proapoptotic	↑ then ↓	↑ then ↓	↑ then ↓	Improved	↑

↑, increase; ↓, decrease; ↔, (either or no change); PSA, prostate-specific antigen.
From Morris MJ, Scher HI. Novel strategies and therapeutics for the treatment of prostate carcinoma. *Cancer* 2000;89:1329–1348.

tumor, but, rather, the reactive changes in the bone induced by tumor. Radionuclide bone scans may take several months to reflect a change, even in the setting of receiving effective therapy, and can take years to fully resolve after an otherwise complete remission. Confounding the picture is the existence of the "flare phenomenon." This apparent worsening of the bone scan occurs as osteoblastic activity increases due to healing when the tumor regresses. Therefore, a worsened bone scan may not reflect true progression but pseudoprogression, a sign that a drug is indeed working (24). The distinction is further obfuscated when scans are obtained at short intervals, and in practice, 12-week intervals are probably the minimum necessary to show appropriate correlations with clinical outcomes.

The criteria by which bone scans are interpreted also vary. For example, one group may consider only the appearance of new lesions to establish progressive disease; another might consider new lesions and increased intensity of existing lesions; a third might consider increased intensity of existing lesions in combination with a rising PSA or increased pain at the involved site. Investigators must use care when using methods of assessing outcomes that have not been validated (25).

New approaches have focused on quantifying and standardizing radionuclide bone scan data. For example, at Memorial Sloan-Kettering Cancer Center, a bone scan index (BSI) has been developed to quantify the extent of skeletal involvement by tumor (26). The BSI is based on the known proportional weights of each of the 158 bones that were derived from the reference man, a standardized skeleton in which autopsy-based individual bone weights were reported for the average adult. A preliminary analysis showed that changes in the BSI paralleled changes in PSA, with minimal interobserver variability.

Tumor Metabolism

Positron emission tomography (PET) scans offer the promise of assessing disease in the soft tissues and bones using one modality and, unlike bone scans, can directly assess the activity of the tumor. PET scanning is therefore undergoing study as a complement to, if not a substitution for, radionuclide bone scans (27). However, PET scanning has traditionally been used to distinguish benign from metastatic disease and not as a means of sequentially following a tumor response to a novel agent. This application continues to be explored (28). Various labeled compounds are being investigated, including 2-[F-18] fluoro-D-glucose, C-11 methionine, and, most recently, fluorine-18–labeled androgen receptor ligands, such as dihydrotestosterone (29). The latter promises to be a highly specific method of imaging the prostate cells and other tissue with high androgen receptor content.

Biochemical

Having a biochemical marker to assess outcomes is not unique to prostate cancer, as tumor markers exist for germ-cell tumors, breast cancer, colon cancer, and others. However, the role that the marker plays in prostate cancer clinical trials is uniquely important. The rarity of measurable disease, ambiguities of radionuclide bone scans, and lack of alternative measures of response confer singular importance to the use of the posttherapy decline in PSA as an outcome measure in clinical trials. Drugs that might otherwise have been discarded for lack of an observable response are now advanced on the basis of the biochemical response. This use of the marker is grounded in the observation that a post-treatment decline in PSA correlates with survival (30), which has been demonstrated in multivariate analyses validated against an independent data set (31). This correlation has also been observed in models that examine PSA velocities as opposed to absolute change over time, although these have not been validated (32–34).

This use for the PSA is rife with potential pitfalls, however. There is still no consensus on how much of a decline is "significant," on the accepted time interval over which that decline should be observed, and on the significance of the starting baseline (35,36). As a result, there is no consensus regarding the validity and use of this end point (37–43) as an indication that the natural history of the disease

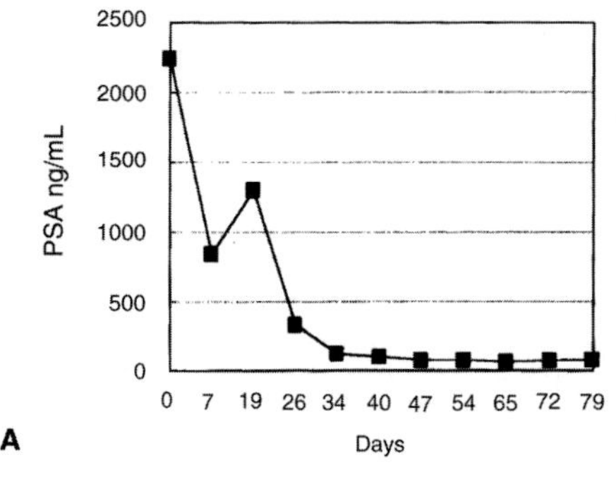

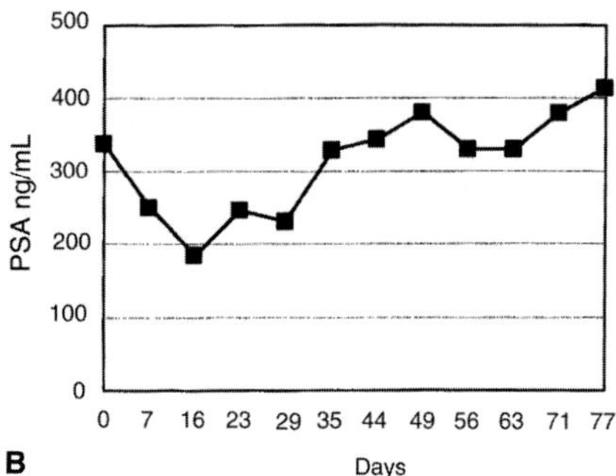

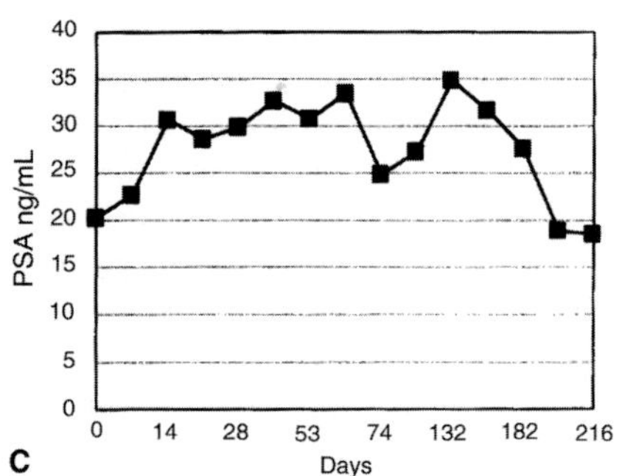

FIGURE 50-2. Changes in prostate-specific antigen (PSA) vary as a function of the mechanism of therapy. **A:** Taxane-based chemotherapy. **B:** Suramin. **C:** Differentiating agent (interferon and *cis*-retinoic acid).

has been altered or that a clinically significant event has been prevented.

With the introduction of mechanism-based therapy, the interpretation of a PSA change as a measure of response is made more complex. The variability of the PSA in response to treatment is seen in Figure 50-2. Figure 50-2A illustrates the PSA change in a patient successfully treated with a cytotoxic combination. The PSA declines markedly with treatment and remains suppressed throughout the treatment period. Figure 50-2B shows an initial PSA decline after treatment with suramin (44), given over 5 days every 21 days. Despite an initial decline, each 21-day cycle is characterized by an increase in PSA consistent with an ineffective drug or schedule. Figure 50-2C shows a projection based on preclinical data of the expected change in PSA after treatment with a differentiating agent. After an initial rise due to tumor cell maturation, the PSA then declines as the cells undergo apoptosis.

The PSA change in response to new drugs that act through novel mechanisms, such as angiogenesis inhibitors and matrix metalloproteinase inhibitors, is at present unknown. These drugs and others may inhibit growth but may not substantially reduce existing tumor burden. A slowing of the rate of rise may be all that is seen, even if these drugs ultimately prove to be active.

It is essential to remember that the "PSA definition" must be considered in the context of other pretreatment prognostic and posttherapy treatment predictive factors using multivariable analytic techniques. Some proposed models fail to analyze other factors that may be impacting survival, such as performance status, hemoglobin, Gleason score, or lactic dehydrogenase. Furthermore, models based on a single center's experience or on a single trial's treatment population should be validated against an independent data set. Only when the association is retained using multivariate techniques and validated using independent data sets of patients is it considered significant (31,45).

Symptoms

Treatments can effectively alleviate pain but may not have a significant antitumor effect. Studies of the radioisotopes samarium-153-ethylene diamine tetramethylene phosphonate and rhenium-186-hydroxyethylidene diphosphonate demonstrated that outcome measures of palliation, such as changes in narcotic use, were seen in excess relative to indicators of tumor response, such as changes in PSA (46,47). This was also found in trials of chemotherapeutics. In a trial of mitoxantrone and prednisone versus prednisone alone, patients on the chemotherapy arm enjoyed a greater palliative benefit than those who received steroids alone (48). This was seen despite the fact that, as an antitumor agent, mitoxantrone has only modest activity as a single agent (49), and, even in combination with prednisone, the palliative benefit exceeded the proportion of patients who had a decline in PSA. The lesson drawn from these experiences is that symptomatic effects should be considered independently of other measures of antitumor activity. If not, a drug that can significantly impact a patient's quality of life might be underestimated because of a disappointing impact on the PSA or bone scan in the face of an improvement in the patient's symptoms. Drugs without direct actions on the disease can still impact the bony microenvironment, osteoclasts, neurohumoral pain mediators, and psychological elements, all of which will modulate a patient's level of suffering.

Reporting End Points

Although preclinical data may suggest the pattern that end points may manifest in response to treatment, the actual clinical experience frequently differs considerably from the predictive model. As a result, end points must be clearly defined, reproducible from trial to trial, assessed at identical time points for each patient, and independently assessed and reported.

In addition, factors that might affect the interpretation of outcomes should also be accounted for and reported, as these can confound the results of a trial. This is especially true of trials using PSA end points. Over-the-counter drugs, diet, vitamins, and supplements (e.g., soy, vitamin D, and nonsteroidal antiinflammatory agents that impact the cyclooxygenase pathway) may all have effects on the PSA, that have yet to be fully established. Unless these agents are recorded and assessed, potential associations of a therapy with outcome (favorable or unfavorable) cannot be explored.

DISTINGUISHING "RESPONSE" FROM "CLINICAL BENEFIT": THE PHASE II TO PHASE III TRANSITION

Despite the extensive search for valid end points for phase I and II trials, the majority of the phase III trials that have been conducted in prostate cancer has been negative. There are many factors in the phase II study design that contribute to the failure of a drug in phase III. These include the use of a surrogate end point in the phase II trial that does not accurately reflect the end point of interest in the phase III study, differences in the patient populations enrolled in the respective studies, an overestimation of the level of benefit of the new therapy through misinterpretation of the reported outcomes observed in prior studies, and a failure to identify clinically beneficial approaches through underpowered trials. Furthermore, drugs that induce a response in earlier trials are often found to have no durable benefit, particularly in terms of survival, in the phase III setting.

The other side of this coin is that drugs that may show no response in early trials may indeed have the potential to confer a durable benefit to the patient. This is particularly true of cytostatic drugs in which a short-term response may be difficult to assess. Hence, differentiating agents, antimetastatic compounds or angiogenesis inhibitors, vaccination studies, or dietary manipulations may be difficult to assess in the short term, but they may offer long-term benefits if they can be shown to slow or arrest the process of disease progression. Although these agents might be abandoned in early-phase trials because they fail to show a response, they might also be brought prematurely to the phase III setting using a survival end point. The inability to detect this error before the level of the phase III investigation is particularly harmful, because these trials are resource intensive, require hundreds of patients, vast sums of money, and often take many years to complete.

Because of the difficulties in transitioning from the questions addressed in the phase I or II trial to those of the phase III trial, we have proposed that an intermediate trial design, phase IIb, be incorporated into the sequence of drug development (50). In this model, the phase IIb follows preliminary screening trials for efficacy but precedes large multicenter comparative phase III trials. The phase IIb study population is larger and more heterogenous that those in phase IIa trials, which typically contain small groups of highly selected patients treated in single centers and that consequently overestimate the treatment effect. Furthermore, the end points of the phase IIb trial replicate those of phase III trials in measuring clinically relevant end points, such as survival, rather than biologic, biochemical, or radiographic surrogates. The proposed phase IIb design has the potential to identify effective and ineffective treatments earlier in the clinical trial process. It allows ineffective treatments to be weeded out earlier in the process and effective ones to proceed. A larger number of patients than is typically applied to phase II studies is required. Nevertheless, in the long run, by reducing the number of approaches that is tested in the phase III setting, more patients will be spared ineffective treatments, and fewer patients will need to be enrolled in trials to identify those that are indeed active.

INTEGRATION OF DISEASE STATE WITH CLINICAL TRIAL DESIGN

No Cancer Diagnosis

Increasingly, medical oncologists are managing patients without disease but who are at high risk of developing cancer. Prophylactic interventions have been shown to be beneficial in preventing a number of cancers: Women at high risk for breast cancer can reduce that risk by prophylactic mastectomy (51) and patients at risk for developing second primary head and neck cancers have been shown to benefit using chemopreventive strategies (52). In the past, preventive strategies were not an option for patients at high risk for prostate cancer, as the toxicities of radical surgery, radiation, or hormonal therapy precluded treatment in the documented absence of disease.

As mechanism-based treatments are introduced into the clinic, patients at risk of developing prostate cancer can be treated with agents sufficiently low in toxicity to warrant

TABLE 50-6. ELEMENTS OF CLINICAL TRIALS FOR PATIENTS WITHOUT DISEASE

Cancer prevention	Entry	End point
Demographics	General population	—
	Age	
	High risk	
	Ethnicity	
	Family history	
	Diet	
PSA	Normal	
	Elevated	Age specific
	Defined rate of rise	>0.75 ng/mL/yr
	% Free	
Pathology	Prior negative biopsy	No cancer
	Documentation of PIN	No invasive cancer
Measurable	NA	NA
Bone	NA	NA

NA, not applicable; PIN, prostatic intraepithelial neoplasia; PSA, prostate-specific antigen.

TABLE 50-7. CLINICAL TRIAL DESIGN FOR PATIENTS WITH LOCALIZED DISEASE

Clinically localized disease	Entry	End point
Demographics	Local disease extent	NA
Tumor	DRE	No tumor
	Imaging (sonography, MRI, ± ProstaScint)	
PSA	Multiplex models	Radical prostatectomy—NMA
	DRE, Gleason score, PSA	Radiation therapy—<0.5–1.0 ng/mL
Pathology	Gleason score	No cancer
	Number of cores	
	Percentage of cores	
Measurable	NA	NA
Bone	NA	NA

DRE, digital rectal examination; MRI, magnetic resonance imaging; NA, not applicable; NMA, no measurable amount; PSA, prostate-specific antigen.

study, the design of which is outlined in Table 50-6. The treatment population ideally would represent patients at high risk of developing prostate cancer and who are young enough to derive a significant benefit from a preventive strategy. These patients might be identified on the basis of family history, diet, the presence of prostatic intraepithelial neoplasia (PIN), or an abnormal PSA.

Patients in this category can have normal, elevated, or rising PSA values. Whether a decline in PSA in patients without cancer is beneficial has yet to be established. Conversely, a rise in PSA is not necessarily an indicator of treatment failure in this population, as patients may develop elevated PSA concentrations secondary to benign conditions unrelated to treatment success or failure. Pathologic criteria, which can be used to assess changes in atypia in patients with PIN or establish a diagnosis in patients without cancer, are singularly appropriate in this population, as few other response criteria such as cancer-related symptoms, measurable soft-tissue disease, or assessable bony disease are available. Ultimately, the clinically relevant end point for these patients is lengthening the time in which they remain within their defined state (i.e., remain disease free). An alteration in the time to diagnosis suggests that the drug should be advanced in development.

Localized Disease

A truly localized prostate cancer is one that can be cured if the prostate were completely removed (surgically) or eliminated (by radiation or a medical therapy). The methodology to assess localized disease continues to evolve. In the past, it was based solely on the results of a digital rectal examination; more recently, it has involved using multiplex models based on the findings of digital rectal examination, Gleason score, and PSA (53), with or without imaging studies (54). Equally important in the assessment of a localized prostate cancer is the determination of the probability of spread to distant sites (55). Although patients with documented local disease are potentially curable, some will relapse locally while others will already have micrometastatic disease at the time of treatment. Patients with advanced local lesions, high PSAs, and high Gleason scores are at risk of failing single-modality local treatments (56,57). The ultimate aim of these trials is to render a patient who is at risk of relapse as curable, as shown in Table 50-7. For the medical oncologist, this implies an intervention before or after surgery or radiation.

The advantage of testing novel agents as neoadjuvant therapy is that many patients will undergo definitive surgery after treatment; tissue can be easily obtained to assess indicators of biologic activity, such as histologic appearance, genetic or protein assays, or measures of apoptosis. Changes in PSA, tumor size, or surgical margins can be used to assess whether these biologic phenomena correlate with clinical effects and local or systemic drug levels. Furthermore, these trials can be conducted using patients with tumors unexposed to prior treatments and with an intact and virgin androgen receptor axis.

Neoadjuvant therapy is ultimately intended as an adjunct to achieving cure. A reduction in tumor burden is inconsequential unless it is associated with an increase in the cure rate after definitive local therapy. This is the essence of the challenge of the phase II to phase III transition—that is, to show that changes in biology are reflected in a reduction in the rate of relapse or an increase in survival.

Outcome measures for adjuvant treatments are more difficult to define than for equivalent treatments used as neoadjuvants. In this disease state, the PSA may be normal or undetectable, there is no identifiable tumor volume, and tissue is unavailable to assess biologic activity. The clinically relevant end point for such trials, therefore, is the length of time patients remain in the disease state. Adjuvant therapies warrant further study if they delay the time to the detection of local or systemic relapse.

Rising Prostate-Specific Antigen Postprimary Therapy

Patients with a rising PSA after primary therapy, be it radical prostatectomy, radiation therapy, a combined modality approach, or deferred therapy, represent an increasing proportion of the prostate cancer population. For these patients, therapy is directed toward preventing progression to the point in which the disease becomes clinically detectable or symptomatic, at which point the probability of death from disease increases significantly and the patient is faced with disease-related morbidity and mortality (64). Nevertheless, an important distinction is that a rise in PSA does not universally lead to death from prostate cancer nor does it signify the need for immediate intervention (65).

Patients who relapse biochemically in the absence of symptomatic or radiographic disease represent a unique treatment opportunity. The tumor burden is low and the disease has been exposed only to limited prior therapy. However, care should be taken to distinguish those factors that contributed to the failure of local therapy, as shown in Table 50-8. These elements include demographic data such as the patient's family history and race, the original stage of the tumor, the pretreatment likelihood of relapse, the nature of the surgery (if performed) and the pathologic findings, and the dose and type of radiation (pelvic vs. three-dimensional conformal with or without beam modulation).

Outcome measures are limited in this clinical scenario. The only evidence that these patients have cancer is by virtue of an abnormal marker, and, therefore, the efficacy of a new agent is defined by the modulation of that marker. As discussed earlier, some agents may, in the face of an antitumor effect, stimulate PSA expression. However, in a population with no disease-related symptoms and no assessable disease other than the PSA, it is difficult to know whether a drug that appears to promote PSA expression should be abandoned. Knowledge of the mechanism of the drug, the biologic role of the targeted pathway, and preclinical data should be applied, but all effects obviously cannot be predicted *a priori*. This again underscores having a clinically significant end point, such as progression-free survival or overall survival, early in the sequence of trials.

Metastatic Disease (Detectable Tumor on Imaging Studies)

There are multiple routes to clinically detectable disease. Some patients have extensive involvement at diagnosis and others develop it after a rising PSA. In some cases, metastases arise without a change in PSA. Regardless of the path or the time to clinically detectable metastases, once they are identified, the disease has progressed to the point in which the overwhelming cause of death is cancer and not co-morbid conditions (64).

Patients with metastatic disease can be divided into two groups: those who are newly diagnosed and have noncastrate levels of testosterone and those who are androgen independent and have castrate testosterone serum concen-

TABLE 50-8. CLINICAL TRIAL DESIGN FOR PATIENTS WITH A RISING PROSTATE-SPECIFIC ANTIGEN (PSA) ONLY

Rising PSA	Entry	End point
Demographics	Prior treatment history Probability of relapse	NA
Tumor	Initial tumor stage ProstaScint scanning	NA
PSA	Rate of rise (doubling time) Time to relapse	Salvage prostatectomy—NMA Salvage radiation therapy—undetectable (no further rise) Change in slope, decline, disappearance
Pathology	Initial tumor characteristics Gleason score Number and % of cores (radiation therapy) EOD at prostatectomy Extent Vascular/lymphatic invasion Margin status Molecular/biologic determinants, e.g., Ploidy, p27, e-cadherin, and others Biopsy of prostate/prostatic bed	Negative biopsy
Measurable	NA	No detectable disease
Bone	NA	No detectable disease

EOD, extent of disease; NA, not applicable; NMA, no measurable amount.

TABLE 50-9. CLINICAL TRIAL DESIGN FOR PATIENTS WITH METASTATIC DISEASE (NONCASTRATE LEVELS OF TESTOSTERONE)

Clinical metastatic disease: noncastrate	Entry	End point
Demographics	Prior treatment Duration of benefit	NA
Tumor	Initial disease extent Grade	NA
PSA	Rate of rise	Undetectable Change in pattern (degree of rise, decline in rate of rise, stabilization, decline from baseline) Time to progression
Pathology	Molecular/biologic determinants Her2 Bcl-2	Modulation of determinant (to assess biologic effect) Differentiation
Measurable	If present	Table 50-3
Bone	If present	Table 50-3
Symptoms	If present	Quality of life end points

NA, not applicable; PSA, prostate-specific antigen.

trations. It is the latter that has classically served as the testing ground for new drug development, as these patients have the fewest treatment options. No therapeutic strategy for this group has significantly improved survival. However, even patients who have noncastrate levels of testosterone should be candidates for new treatments as (a) responses to hormonal treatments are generally short-lived, (b) hormonal treatments are associated with significant morbidity, and (c) it is unclear whether deferral of hormonal treatments is of disadvantage to the patient.

Therapy for patients who have noncastrate levels of testosterone has the potential to delay the emergence of androgen independence and to enhance the response rates of existing hormonal treatments. The advantages of treating patients who are androgen dependent are (a) the androgen receptor axis is naïve, (b) tumor exposure to prior treatments is minimal, as may be resistance, and (c) PSA and radiographic evidence of disease may be used to assess response. Treatment in this setting is directed at delaying the need for hormonal therapy by using drugs that act via mechanisms other than mediation through the androgen receptor or, if hormonal therapy has already been instituted, prolonging the period of responsiveness to hormonal treatments. As shown in Table 50-9, assessments of the success or failure of these strategies can be measured by changes in the PSA, pathologic assays of targeted pathways, radiographic and scintigraphic manifestations of disease, and symptoms.

The median survival after the documentation of androgen-independent metastatic disease is 9 to 12 months. For these patients, the overwhelming considerations are to control disease-related symptoms, prevent their occurrence or recurrence, and prolong life. As such, outcome measures in early trials can include changes in clinical symptoms; measurable disease, if present; improvements on bone scans; biochemical markers; and targeted biologic pathways, depending on the therapy, as shown in Table 50-10. End points for later trials assess disease-free survival, overall survival, and quality of life. These patients have few treatment alternatives and a limited expected survival after the establishment of androgen independence. They are also the most difficult patients to treat, as they often have a substantial burden of disease, may have

TABLE 50-10. CLINICAL TRIAL DESIGN FOR PATIENTS WITH CLINICAL METASTATIC DISEASE (CASTRATE LEVELS OF TESTOSTERONE)

Clinical metastatic disease: castrate	Entry	End point
Demographics	NA	NA
Tumor	Grade Initial disease extent (BSI, sites of disease, symptoms)	NA
PSA	Value	Undetectable Percentage decline Time to progression
Pathology	Molecular/biologic determinants Ploidy, p27, e-cadherin, and others	Negative biopsy
Measurable	If present	Regression No progression
Bone	If present	Disappearance Regression No progression
Symptoms	If present	Improvement Regression No progression

BSI, bone scan index; NA, not applicable; PSA, prostate-specific antigen.

been extensively pretreated, and may have a significantly impaired performance status.

An essential component of the therapeutic approaches currently under evaluation is an understanding of the molecular and phenotypic differences that exist between a tumor that is proliferating in the primary, as opposed to the metastatic, site. These changes involve multiple genetic events and occur in parallel with the evolution of androgen independence. Pathways or mutations that are not significant in the growth of an androgen-dependent primary tumor may indeed be critical to androgen-independent metastatic growth, and vice versa. For example, p53 alterations have a higher frequency in androgen-independent metastases compared to hormone-naïve primary tumors (66). Similarly, progression to androgen independence is associated with an increase in the proportion of cells that express bcl-2 (67). Preliminary data show that the frequency of mutations increases as prostate cancers become resistant to androgen ablation (68–72). The results suggest that functionally significant mutations can be identified in human material (73), whereas recent results show that the specific alterations influence sensitivity to treatment (74). Most reports have evaluated cell lines, primary tumors, or regional lymph nodes removed during the performance of a radical prostatectomy; few studies evaluate distant metastases before or after androgen deprivation.

Recent work has shown that among the mechanisms associated with the development of androgen independence are continued signaling through a functional but altered androgen receptor, ligand-independent activation of the receptor by receptor tyrosine kinase–signaling molecules, inhibition of apoptosis, and the increased expression of markers of drug resistance.

Therefore, to understand the role of biologic therapies in the treatment of metastatic disease, it is important to (a) characterize the status of the pathway being targeted (e.g., mutations, overexpression, and others), (b) define the sensitivity and specificity of the technique used, and (c) establish the impact of that drug on the pathway. As many of these agents may be dosed according to optimal biologic dose and not maximum tolerated dose, validating biologic activity is critical to advancing a drug through development. Although biologic end points have yet to be shown to predict for clinical outcome (and in particular, survival), they are indicators that an approach is at least capable of inducing an *in vivo* biologic change, a necessary initial step before conducting trials with end points of time-to-progression, disease-free survival, or overall survival.

CONCLUSION

Clinical trial design in prostate cancer is at a crossroads. A greater understanding of the molecular basis of prostate cancer has led to the introduction of a variety of new biologic agents in the clinic. New treatment opportunities, which were previously inappropriate given the limited efficacy and significant morbidity associated with available treatments, are now being considered. Now more than ever, investigators are faced with the challenge to rationally apply these strategies.

Trial design requires an *a priori* defined rationale and aim, eligibility criteria that ensure that the treatment population reflects the goals of the trial, an intervention, and end points that provide an assessment of whether the intervention is inducing a response. These elements are complicated by the unique manner in which prostate cancer is manifest and the variability in the need to treat the disease at various junctures in the natural history. Furthermore, phase II end points may have no bearing on appropriate designs for phase III trials, which has led us to propose that phase III questions be asked earlier in the drug development process through a modified phase II design. The elements of the clinical trial are variables defined by disease state and clinical context, as each state represents a discreet treatment opportunity. Finally, the basic understanding of the molecular pathways that distinguish one disease state from another must be advanced.

REFERENCES

1. Scher HI, Heller G. Clinical states in prostate cancer: towards a dynamic model of disease progression. *Urology* 2000;55:323–327.
2. Carter P, Presta L, Gorman CM, et al. Humanization of an anti-p185HER2 antibody for human cancer treatment. *Proc Natl Acad Sci U S A* 1992;89:4285–4289.
3. Lyne JC, Melhem MF, Finley GG, et al. Tissue expression of neu differentiation factor/heregulin and its receptor complex in prostate cancer and its biologic effects on prostate cancer cells in vitro. *Cancer J Sci Am* 1997;3:21–30.
4. Ross JS, Sheehan C, Hayner-Buchan AM, et al. HER-2/neu gene amplification status in prostate cancer by fluorescence in situ hybridization. *Human Pathol* 1998;28:827–833.
5. Shepard HM, Lewis GD, Sarup JC, et al. Monoclonal antibody therapy of human cancer: taking the her2 protooncogene to the clinic. *J Clin Immunol* 1991;11:117–127.
6. Slovin SF, Kelly WK, Cohen R, et al. Epidermal growth factor receptor (EGFr) monoclonal antibody (MoAb) C225 and doxorubicin (DOC) in androgen-independent (AI) prostate cancer (PC): results of a phase Ib/IIa study. *Proc Am Soc Clin Oncol* 1997;16:311.
7. Reference deleted by author.
8. Scher H, Sepp-Lorenzino L, Bos M, et al. Farnesyltransferase inhibition reverses the transformed phenotype of malignant prostate epithelial cells. Breast and prostate cancer: basic mechanisms. *Keystone Symposium*, 1996:46.
9. Sepp-Lorenzino L, Ma Z, Rands E, et al. A peptidomimetic inhibitor of farnesyl:protein transferase blocks the anchorage-dependent and -independent growth of human tumor cell lines. *Cancer Res* 1995;55:5302–5309.

10. Eastham JA, Hall SJ, Sehgal I, et al. In vivo gene therapy with p53 or p21 adenovirus for prostate cancer. *Cancer Res* 1995;55:5151–5155.
11. Logothetis CJ, Hossan E, Evans R, et al. Ad5CMV-p53 intraprostatic gene therapy preceding radical prostatectomy (RP): an in vivo model for targeted therapy development. *Proc Am Soc Clin Oncol* 1999;18:313a.
12. Morris MJ, Tong W, Osman I, et al. A phase I/IIa dose-escalating trial of BCL-2 antisense (G3139) treatment by 14-day continuous intravenous infusion (CI) for patients with androgen-independent prostate cancer or other advanced solid tumor malignancies. *Proc Am Soc Clin Oncol* 1999;18: 323a.
13. Peehl DM, Skowronski RJ, Leung GK, et al. Antiproliferative effects of 1,25-dihydroxyvitamin D3 on primary cultures of human prostatic cells. *Cancer Res* 1994;54:805–810.
14. Smith DC, Johnson CS, Osborn J, et al. Phase I trial of subcutaneous calcitriol (1,25-(OH)2D3) with and without prednisone in advanced solid tumors. *Proc Annu Meet Am Assoc Cancer Res* 1996;37:A1137.
15. DiPaola RS, Weiss R, Goodin S, et al. The clinical and biological effects of 13 cis-retinoic acid (CRA) and alpha interferon (IFN-A) in patients with prostate-specific antigen (PSA) progression after initial local therapy for prostate cancer. *Proc Am Soc Clin Oncol* 1997;16:A1185.
16. Kelly WK, Curley T, Liebertz C, et al. Phase II trial of 13-cis-retinoic acid and interferon-alpha 2α in patients with adenocarcinoma of the prostate. *Proc Am Soc Clin Oncol* 1996;15:250.
17. Smith M, Mueller E, Demetri G, et al. Preliminary results: phase II trial of troglitazone for androgen-dependent (AD) and androgen-independent (AI) prostate cancer. *Proc Am Soc Clin Oncol* 1999;18:328a.
18. Slovin SF, Livingston PO, Rosen N, et al. Targeted therapy for prostate cancer: the MSKCC approach. *Semin Oncol* 1996;23:41–48.
19. Slovin SF, Livingston P, Zhang S, et al. Targeted therapy in prostate cancer (PC): vaccination with a glycoprotein, MUC-1-KLH-QS-21 peptide conjugate. *Proc Am Soc Clin Oncol* 1997;16:311.
20. Slovin SF, Scher HI. Peptide and carbohydrate vaccines in relapsed prostate cancer: immunogenicity of synthetic vaccines in man-clinical trials at Memorial Sloan-Kettering Cancer Center. *Semin Oncol* 1999;26:1–8.
21. Smith PH, Bono A, Calais da Silva F, et al. Some limitations of the radioisotope bone scan in patients with metastatic prostatic cancer. *Cancer* 1990;66:1009–1016.
22. Ross JS, Sheehan C, Hayner-Buchan AM, et al. HER-2/neu gene amplification status in prostate cancer by fluorescence in situ hybridization. *Hum Pathol* 1998;28:827–833.
23. Goldenberg SL, Bruchovsky N, Rennie PS, et al. The combination of cyproterone acetate and low dose diethylstilbestrol in the treatment of advanced prostatic carcinoma. *J Urol* 1988;138:1460–1465.
24. Johns WD, Garnick MB, Kaplan WD. Leuprolide therapy for prostate cancer. An association with scintigraphic "flare" on bone scan. *Clin Nucl Med* 1990;15:485–487.
25. Kelly WK, Scher HI, Mazumdar M, et al. Suramin and hydrocortisone: determining drug efficacy in androgen-independent prostate cancer. *J Clin Oncol* 1995;13:2214–2222.
26. Imbriaco M, Larson SM, Yeung HW, et al. A new parameter for measuring metastatic bone involvement by prostate cancer: the bone scan index. *Clin Cancer Res* 1998;4:1765–1772.
27. Larson SM. Positron emission tomography in oncology and allied diseases. In: DeVita VT, Hellman S, Rosenberg SA, eds. *Cancer: principles and practice of oncology*, 2nd ed. Philadelphia: JB Lippincott Co, 1989:1–12.
28. Osman I, Akhurst T, Macapinlac H, et al. C-11 methionine and F-18 PET imaging: use in the evaluation of progressive prostate cancer. *Proc Am Soc Clin Oncol* 1998;18:1203(abst).
29. Bonasera TA, O'Neil JP, Xu M, et al. Preclinical evaluation of fluorine-18-labeled androgen receptor ligands in baboons. *J Nucl Med* 1996;37:1009–1015.
30. Kelly WK, Curley T, Leibertz C, et al. Prospective evaluation of hydrocortisone and suramin. *J Clin Oncol* 1995;13:2208–2213.
31. Scher HI, Kelly WK, Zhang Z-F, et al. Post-therapy serum prostate specific antigen level and survival in patients with androgen-independent prostate cancer. *J Natl Cancer Inst* 1999;91:244–251.
32. Carter H, Pearson J. PSA velocity for the diagnosis of early prostate cancer. A new concept. *Urol Clin North Am* 1993; 20:665–670.
33. Vollmer RT, Dawson NA, Vogelzang NJ. The dynamics of prostate specific antigen in hormone refractory prostate carcinoma: an analysis of cancer and leukemia group B study 9181 of megestrol acetate. *Cancer* 1998;83:1989–1994.
34. Vollmer RT, Kantoff PW, Dawson NA, et al. A prognostic score for hormone-refractory prostate cancer: analysis of two Cancer and Leukemia Group B studies. *Clin Cancer Res* 1999;5:831–837.
35. Dawson N. Apples and oranges: building a consensus for standardized eligibility criteria and end points in prostate cancer clinical trials. *J Clin Oncol* 1998;16:3398–3405.
36. Scher HI, Mazumdar M, Kelly WK. Clinical trials in relapsed prostate cancer: defining the target [Review] [90 refs]. *J Natl Cancer Inst* 1996;88:1623–1634.
37. Chackal-Roy M, Niemeyer C, Moore M, et al. Stimulation of human prostatic carcinoma cell growth by factors present in human bone marrow. *J Clin Invest* 1989;84:43–50.
38. Sella A, Kilbourn R, Amato R, et al. A phase II study of ketoconazole (KC) combined with weekly doxorubicin (DOX) in patients (PTS) with hormone refractory prostate cancer (PC). *Proc Am Soc Clin Oncol* 1992;11:219.
39. Pienta KJ, Redman B, Hussain M, et al. Phase II evaluation of oral estramustine and oral etoposide in hormone-refractory adenocarcinoma of the prostate. *J Clin Oncol* 1994;12: 2005–2012.
40. Dimopoulos MA, Panopoulos C, Bamia C, et al. Oral estramustine and oral etoposide for hormone-refractory prostate cancer. *Urology* 1997;50:754–758.
41. Kobayashi K, Vokes EE, Janisch L, et al. Suramin (SUR) is safe and active in prostate cancer without adaptive control: evidence for a dose-response. *Proc Am Soc Clin Oncol* 1994; 13:140.
42. Sridhara R, Eisenberger MA, Sinibaldi VJ, et al. Evaluation of prostate-specific antigen as a surrogate marker for response of hormone-refractory prostate cancer to suramin therapy. *J Clin Oncol* 1995;13:2944–2953.

43. Eisenberger MA, Nelson WG. How much can we rely on the level of prostate-specific antigen as an end point for evaluation of clinical trials? A word of caution! *J Natl Cancer Inst* 1996;88:779–781.
44. Reference deleted by author.
45. Kelly WK, Scher HI, Mazumdar M, et al. Prostate specific antigen as a measure of disease outcome in hormone-refractory prostatic cancer. *J Clin Oncol* 1993;11:607–615.
46. Scher H, Curley T, Graham M, et al. Phase I trial of escalated dose of rhenium-186-hydroxyethylidene diphosphonate [RE-186-HEDP] in patients with metastatic prostate cancer to bone. *Proc Am Soc Clin Oncol* 1994;13:242.
47. Turner JH, Claringbold PG, Hetherington EL, et al. A phase I study of samarium-153 ethylenediaminetetramethylene phosphonate therapy for disseminated skeletal metastases. *J Clin Oncol* 1989;7:1926–1931.
48. Tannock IF, Osoba D, Stockler MR, et al. Chemotherapy with mitoxantrone plus prednisone or prednisone alone for symptomatic hormone-resistant prostate cancer: a Canadian randomized trial with palliative end points. *J Clin Oncol* 1996;14:1756–1764.
49. Osborne CK, Drelichman A, Von Hoff DD, et al. Mitoxantrone: modest activity in a phase II trial in advanced prostate cancer. *Cancer Treat Rep* 1983;67:1133–1135.
50. Fazzari M, Heller G, Scher HI. The phase II/III transition: towards the proof of efficacy in cancer clinical trials. *Control Clin Trials* 2000;21:360–368.
51. Hartmann LC, Schaid DJ, Woods JE, et al. Efficacy of bilateral prophylactic mastectomy in women with a family history of breast cancer. *N Engl J Med* 1999;340:77–84.
52. Hong WK, Lippman SM, Itri LM, et al. Prevention of second primary tumors with isotretinoin in squamous-cell carcinoma of the head and neck. *N Engl J Med* 1990;323:795–801.
53. Partin AW, Subong EN, Walsh PC, et al. Combination of prostate-specific antigen, clinical stage, and Gleason score to predict pathological stage of localized prostate cancer: a multi-institutional update. *JAMA* 1997;277:1445–1451.
54. Montie JE. Current prognostic factors for prostate carcinoma. *Cancer* 1996;78:341–344.
55. Kattan MW, Eastham JA, Stapleton AMF, et al. A preoperative nomogram for disease recurrence following radical prostatectomy for prostate cancer. *J Natl Cancer Inst* 1998;90:766–771.
56. Partin A, Yoo J, Carter HB, et al. The use of prostate specific antigen, clinical stage and Gleason score to predict pathological stage in men with localized prostate cancer. *J Urol* 1993;150:110–114.
57. Huland H, Hammerer P, Henke R-P, et al. Preoperative prediction of tumor heterogeneity and recurrence after radical prostatectomy for localized prostate carcinoma with digital rectal examination, prostate specific antigen and the results of 6 systematic biopsies. *J Urol* 1996;155:1344–1347.
58. Reference deleted by author.
59. Reference deleted by author.
60. Reference deleted by author.
61. Reference deleted by author.
62. Reference deleted by author.
63. Reference deleted by author.
64. Pound CR, Partin AW, Eisenberger MA, et al. Natural history of progression after PSA elevation following radical prostatectomy. *JAMA* 1999;281:1591–1597.
65. Scher HI. Management of prostate cancer after prostatectomy: treating the patient, not the PSA. *JAMA* 1999;281: 1642–1645.
66. Bookstein R, MacGrogan D, Hilsenbck SG, et al. p53 is mutated in a subset of advanced-stage prostate cancers. *Cancer Res* 1993;53:3369–3373.
67. Furuya Y, Krajewski S, Epstein JI, et al. Expression of bcl-2 and the progression of human and rodent prostatic cancers. *Clin Cancer Res* 1998;2:389–398.
68. Culig Z, Hobisch A, Cronauer MV, et al. Mutant androgen receptor detected in an advanced-stage prostatic carcinoma is activated by adrenal androgens and progesterone. *Mol Endocrinol* 1993;7:1541–1550.
69. Veldscholte J, Ris-Stalpers C, Kuiper GG, et al. A mutation in the ligand binding domain of the androgen receptor of human LNCaP cells affects steroid binding characteristics and response to anti-androgens. *Biochem Biophys Res Commun* 1990;173:534–543.
70. Gaddipati JP, McLeod DG, Heidenberg HB, et al. Frequent detection of codon 877 mutation in the androgen receptor gene in advanced prostate cancers. *Cancer Res* 1994;54: 2861–2864.
71. Tilley WD, Lim-Tio SS, Horsfall DJ, et al. Detection of discrete androgen receptor epitopes in prostate cancer by immunostaining: measurement by color video image analysis. *Cancer Res* 1994;54:4096–4102.
72. Tilley WD, Buchanan G, Hickey TE, et al. Mutations in the androgen receptor gene are associated with progression of human prostate cancer to androgen-independence. *Clin Cancer Res* 1996;2:274.
73. Scher HI, Bentel JM, Buchanan G, et al. Androgen receptor expression in androgen-independent prostate cancer: relation to flutamide withdrawal. *Proc Am Soc Clin Oncol* 1996;37.
74. Scher HI, Liebertz C, Kelly WK, et al. Bicalutamide for advanced prostate cancer: the natural vs. treated history of disease. *J Clin Oncol* 1997;15:2928–2938.

51

CHEMOTHERAPY FOR ANDROGEN-INDEPENDENT PROSTATE CANCER

DAVID B. SOLIT
WILLIAM K. KELLY

For more than 50 years, androgen ablation has been standard treatment for patients with metastatic prostate cancer. Despite an initial response to medical or surgical castration, disease progression to an androgen-independent state occurs in the majority of patients. Secondary and tertiary hormonal manipulations provide a brief palliative response in 30% to 40% of patients, followed by progression to a truly hormone-refractory state. Studies have not been able to fully elucidate the sequence of events leading to androgen independence, but the surviving cells are thought to be resistant to standard cytotoxic chemotherapies. This premise is supported by the lack of activity seen in clinical trials of patients with androgen-independent prostate cancer (AIPC). In one review of 26 trials reported between 1987 and 1991, only 8% of 1,683 patients with AIPC treated with chemotherapy achieved a complete or partial remission (1). Based on these data, many physicians have questioned the role of systemic therapy in the treatment of androgen-independent disease and have recommended palliative care as the patient's best and only treatment option.

Before 1990, the majority of the patients entered on clinical trials for advanced prostate cancer was symptomatic, had large tumor burdens and overall had a poor performance status (Table 51-1). Given the strong correlation between advancing age and prostate cancer, it is not surprising that many patients with prostate cancer have significant comorbid diseases. Dramatic improvements in medical care over the past decade have increased the number of elderly patients with prostate cancer eligible to receive chemotherapeutic treatment. This, coupled with the widespread use of prostate-specific antigen (PSA) and further improvements in imaging in the past decade, has significantly changed the profile of patients with advanced metastatic prostate cancer. The majority of patients who present today has minimal disease with few symptoms attributable to their prostate cancer. They now often have a good performance status and few, if any, comorbid conditions that would limit their treatment options. To date, no randomized trial of chemotherapy in patients with AIPC has demonstrated a survival benefit, although recent trials have demonstrated clinical benefit using a range of end points, including measures of tumor regression and improvements in quality of life (QOL). Furthermore, the antitumor activity of contemporary combination regimens suggests that AIPC is not as resistant to chemotherapy as previously believed. This chapter reviews the improvements in prostate cancer clinical trial methodology adopted since 1990 and the results of contemporary systemic therapy for patients with progressive AIPC.

PROGRESS IN PROSTATE CANCER CLINICAL TRIAL METHODOLOGY

Data obtained from prospective randomized trials remain the gold standard in the evaluation of promising new therapies (2). Given the time and expense required to complete such trials, only a limited number of those treatments with activity in the phase II setting will ultimately be evaluated in definitive randomized studies. Therefore, to efficiently select those regimens with the greatest promise, rigid entry criteria and reproducible measures of outcome are required for screening phase II studies.

The development of effective systemic therapy for AIPC has long been hindered by an osseous pattern of disease progression that precludes the use of traditional phase II end points. In contrast to many solid tumors, fewer than 30% of patients with AIPC develop bidimensionally measurable disease that can be quantitated on computed tomography or magnetic resonance imaging scans (3). In response, many early investigators restricted clinical trial entry to patients with measurable soft-tissue disease, despite the realization that objective responses in this small subset of patients did not necessarily predict for activity in patients with bone-only disease (4,5).

Pain and fatigue are the two most common disease-associated symptoms in patients with AIPC who are candi-

TABLE 51-1. ADVANCED PROSTATE CANCER: CHANGING LANDSCAPE

Pre-1990s	1990s
Clinical metastatic disease	Clinical metastatic disease
Symptomatic	Asymptomatic
Large tumor burdens	Rising prostate-specific antigen only
Poor Karnofsky performance status	Locally advanced disease with minimal local symptoms
Multiple co-morbidities	Co-morbidities controlled

TABLE 51-2. GUIDELINES FOR PHASE II CLINICAL TRIALS IN ANDROGEN-INDEPENDENT PROSTATE CANCER

General:
- Consensus guidelines on the use of PSA decline to guide the selection of agents for further testing and randomized evaluation.

Eligibility criteria:
- Patients must demonstrate progressive disease in bone, measurable disease, or a rising PSA.
- Patients need to show progression of disease after withdrawal of the antiandrogen.
- Patients should have castrate levels of testosterone (serum testosterone <50 ng/mL).
- Patients who are not surgically castrated should be maintained on medical castration.

Reporting trial outcomes:
- Posttherapy changes in PSA (minimum criteria): a posttherapy decline of ≥50% confirmed by a second PSA at a minimum of 4 wk apart without clinical or radiographic evidence of disease progression.
- Objective response: use traditional response criteria or Response Evaluation Criteria in Solid Tumors (RECISTS).
- Osseous disease: response parameters not addressed.
- Disease progression:
  - PSA: 25% increase over baseline or nadir value.
  - Osseous disease: one or more new lesions on the bone scan not associated with bone "flare".
  - Objective disease: standard criteria.
- Time to PSA progression: time from initiation of treatment to time of a 50% increase from the nadir or a 25% increase from baseline PSA if no PSA decline achieved.

PSA, prostate-specific antigen.

dates for systemic therapy. With the goal of identifying therapies that provide palliative benefit, pain and QOL measures were developed and incorporated into phase II trial designs (6). The impact of these instruments is evident in their selection as the primary study end point in several large prospective randomized trials (7,8). With the widespread adoption of PSA, these measures of outcome have become less applicable, as the majority of patients now presents without disease-associated symptoms or minimal radiographic disease.

PSA is elevated in more than 90% of patients with AIPC, and posttherapy decline in PSA has been proposed as a mechanism to screen novel cytotoxic agents. In a multivariate analysis of 254 AIPC patients treated at Memorial Sloan-Kettering Cancer Center, a posttherapy decline in PSA levels of 50% or greater achieved at 8 or 12 weeks was a statistically significant factor associated with survival (9). Several groups have shown similar findings and have refined our understanding of the dynamics of posttherapy PSA change in this population (10–12). For example, Vollmer et al. demonstrated that the log and average velocity of PSA change significantly correlated with survival, further supporting the use of PSA as a marker of clinical benefit (12).

To better define the minimal criteria for eligibility and response parameters for phase II clinical trials in androgen-independent disease, a consensus conference sponsored by the National Cancer Institute was convened to formulate guidelines (13). The purpose of this meeting was to develop a common approach to analyzing and reporting the outcomes of clinical trials by agreeing on definitions and values for a minimum set of parameters for eligibility and posttherapy changes in PSA (Table 51-2). Before trial enrollment, it was recommend that all patients demonstrate disease progression after the withdrawal of an antiandrogen. In reporting outcomes, no overall response categories were recommended, but the posttherapy changes in PSA, objective measurable disease, and osseous disease were to be evaluated individually. A PSA decline of at least 50% from baseline confirmed by a second PSA determination at a minimum of 4 weeks apart without other evidence of clinical or radiographic progression was defined as the minimum accepted PSA response criteria (13). A 25% increase in the PSA from baseline or nadir value was acceptable criteria for establishing disease progression. For patients who had measurable disease on computed tomography scan or magnetic resonance imaging scan, the traditional phase II criteria for evaluating objective disease response was recommended. The panel also recognized that some agents might produce changes in serum PSA independent of changes in tumor burden (14). One such example was the differentiating agent all-*trans*-retinoic acid (15). This agent often produces an initial rise in serum PSA that may be misinterpreted as "treatment failure." Given the large number of novel biologic agents entering early clinical trials, novel methods of assessing treatment response, such as positron emission tomography, may be required.

The appearance of a new lesion on bone scan is universally accepted as evidence of disease progression. In contrast, serial bone scans are limited in their ability in assess treatment-associated improvements in preexisting bone lesions. Reproducible methods to quantify changes on serial radionuclide scans have not been established and were not part of the response criteria in this consensus conference (13). Imbriaco et al. have developed a reproducible parameter for quantitative assessment of bone involvement in patients with AIPC (16). The system assigns a bone scan index (a distinct value) that quantitates the amount of

TABLE 51-3. CONTEMPORARY CLINICAL TRIALS WITH SINGLE AGENTS

Therapy	Reference	Year	Treatment schedule	Objective response (%)	PSA decline >50%
Carboplatin	21	1993	150 mg/m^2 q wk	16	—
Carboplatin	107	1998	400 mg/m^2 q4wk	4	—
Coumarin	108	1992	3 g daily	8	—
Cyclophosphamide (oral)	23	1993	100 mg/m^2 × 14 d q2wk	20	—
Dexamethasone	109	1995	0.75 mg b.i.d. daily	—	61%
Docetaxel	20	1999	75 mg/m^2 q3wk	28	46%
Epidoxorubicin	110	1997	35 mg/m^2 weekly	28	—
Epirubicin	111	1992	90 mg/m^2 q4wk	55	—
Epirubicin	112	1993	75 mg/m^2 q3wk	12	—
Etoposide	41	1994	50 mg/m^2 × 21 d q4wk	9	—
10-ethyl-10-deaza-aminopterin	113	1994	80 mg/m^2 q wk	0	0%
Gallium nitrate	114	1987	200 mg/m^2 CI × 7 d q4wk	10	—
Gemcitabine	115	1997	1,000 mg/m^2 days 1, 8, 15 q4wk	5	—
Ifosfamide	116	1990	2 g/m^2 × 2 d q3wk	0	—
Interferon-alpha	117	1992	10 × 10^6 U/m^2 3 × wk	5	—
Interferon-beta	118	1986	6 × 10^6 U 3 × wk	0	—
Irinotecan	119	1998	125 mg/m^2 q wk × 4 followed by a 2-wk break	0	0%
Mitomycin C	22	1997	12 mg/m^2 q4wk	27	—
Mitoxantrone	120	1993	1.0–1.5 mg/m^2 i.v. CI × 14 days q2wk	14	—
Paclitaxel	48	1993	135–170 mg/m^2 × 24 h q3wk	4	—
Paclitaxel	121	2000	150 mg/m^2 weekly, 6 wk q8wk	22	39%
Topotecan	122	1995	1.1–1.5 mg/m^2 × 5 d q3wk	8	18%
Trimetrexate	3	1990	8 mg/m^2 daily × 5 q3wk	17	—
Vinblastine	123	1985	1.5 mg/m^2 q.d. × 5 d q3–4wk	21	—
Vinorelbine	124	1997	25 mg/m^2 q wk	6	—

CI, continuous infusion; PSA, prostate-specific antigen.

osseous disease. The bone scan index has been demonstrated to be an independent prognostic factor in AIPC and can be used to monitor serial changes in osseous metastatic disease (17). Widespread adoption of this technique has been limited by the time necessary to perform the analysis. Computer automation will be needed before the widespread application and incorporation of this technique into clinical trials.

The recommendations of the Prostate-Specific Antigen Working Group were general, but the conference has given investigators a common platform to standardize clinical trial design and the reporting of response data. These guidelines are still evolving and will need further refinements as novel agents are developed for this disease.

MONOTHERAPY TRIALS IN PATIENTS WITH ANDROGEN-INDEPENDENT PROSTATE CANCER

Table 51-3 reports the objective and, when applicable, PSA response data from selected single-agent studies of patients with AIPC reported over the past decade. The majority of the agents demonstrated modest activity with objective responses in fewer than 15% of patients. However, few used currently accepted criteria for assessing PSA response, making comparisons between trials difficult. The greatest activity has been noted with anthracyclines and cytoskeletal targeting agents, such as estramustine, the vinca alkaloids, and taxanes (18–20). Limited activity has also been reported with the platinum compounds, mitomycin C, and cyclophosphamide (21–23).

Despite these historically disappointing results, the recently reported trial of single-agent docetaxel allows for cautious optimism (20). Using an every 3-week schedule, objective responses were noted in 28% of patients and posttherapy PSA declines of 50% or greater were noted in 46% of patients. Therapy was generally well tolerated and toxicity acceptable. These results have prompted further study of this agent alone and in combination.

COMBINATION CHEMOTHERAPY FOR ANDROGEN-INDEPENDENT PROSTATE CANCER

In contrast to the limited activity of single-agent chemotherapy in AIPC, several combination regimens have demonstrated significant palliative benefit and antitumor effects in patients (Table 51-4). Most of these combination regimens are based on the anthracycline derivatives and cytoskeletal-targeting agents.

TABLE 51-4. CONTEMPORARY COMBINATION CHEMOTHERAPY TRIALS IN ANDROGEN-INDEPENDENT PROSTATE CANCER

Author (ref)	Regimen	Year	n	Objective response	PSA decline >50%	Median survival (mo)
Non-estramustine-containing regimens						
Small et al. (25)	Doxorubicin (40 mg/m^2) + cyclophosphamide (800–2,000 mg/m^2) + G-CSF q3wk	1996	35	5/15 (33%)	16/35 (46%)	11
Wozniak et al. (125)	Cyclophosphamide (100 mg/m^2) P.O. daily + methotrexate (15 mg/m^2) q wk + 5-fluorouracil (300 mg/m^2) q wk	1993	57	0/19 (0%)	—	12
Blumenstein et al. (26)	Doxorubicin (35–50 mg/m^2) days 1 and 29 + mitomycin C (7.5–10.0 mg/m^2) day 1 + 5-fluorouracil (500–750 mg/m^2) days 1, 2, 29, and 30	1993	68	16/68 (24%), NPCP criteria	—	10
Dik et al. (126)	Mitomycin C (15 mg/m^2) q6wk + aminoglutethimide (250 mg) P.O. b.i.d. + cortisone 37.5 mg P.O. daily	1992	24	4/24 (17%)	—	—
Osborne et al. (127)	Cisplatin (60 mg/m^2) + mitoxantrone (8–10 mg/m^2) q4wk	1992	43	2/17 (12%)	—	—
Sella et al. (28)	Ketoconazole (1,200 mg) daily + doxorubicin (20 mg/m^2) CI × 24 h weekly	1994	39	7/12 (58%)	21/38 (55%)	15.5
Berlin et al. (128)	5-Fluorouracil (450 mg/m^2) + leucovorin (20 mg/m^2) daily × 5 d q4wk	1998	38	3/38 (7.9%)	2/38 (5%)	11.6
Chao et al. (129)	5-Fluorouracil (200 mg/m^2) CI + cisplatin (60 mg/m^2) + epirubicin (40 mg/m^2) q3wk	1997	24	3/8 (38%)	8/20 (40%)	—
Maulard-Durdux (129a)	Cyclophosphamide (100 mg/day) + etoposide P.O. (50 mg/day) × 14 d q4wk	1996	20	7/20 (35%)	2/8 (25%)	11
Estramustine-containing regimens						
Seidman et al. (37)	EMP (10 mg/kg/d) + vinblastine (4 mg/m^2) i.v. q wk	1992	25	2/5 (40%)	13/24 (54%)	—
Hudes et al. (38)	EMP (600 mg/m^2) daily + vinblastine (4 mg/m^2) i.v. q wk	1992	36	1/7 (14%)	22/36 (61%)	—
Ellerhorst et al. (47)	Doxorubicin (20 mg/m^2) CI × 24 h + ketoconazole (400 mg) P.O. t.i.d., wk 1, 3, 5 alternating with vinblastine (5 mg/m^2) + EMP (140 mg) P.O. t.i.d., wk 2, 4, 5	1997	46	31/46 (67%)	12/16 (75%)	19
Pienta et al. (130)	EMP (10 mg/kg/d) + etoposide (50 mg/m^2) × 21 d q4wk	1997	62	8/15 (53%)	24/62 (39%)	12.9
Hudes et al. (49)	EMP (600 mg/m^2) daily + paclitaxel (120 mg/m^2) CI × 96 h	1997	34	4/9 (44%)	17/32 (53%)	15.9
Smith et al. (50)	EMP (10 mg/kg/d) × 14 d + etoposide (50 mg/m^2/d) × 14 d + paclitaxel (135 mg/m^2) i.v. day 2 q3wk	1999	40	10/22 (45%)	26/40 (65%)	12.8
Kelly et al. (51)	EMP (240 mg) t.i.d. + Paclitaxel (100 mg/m^2) q wk + carboplatin (AUC = 6 d1) q4wk	2000	56	15/33 (45%)	36/54 (67%)	19.9
Petrylak et al. (52)	EMP (280 mg) t.i.d., days 1–5 + docetaxel (70–80 mg/m^2) day 1 q3wk	1999	34	5/18 (28%)	20/32 (63%)	22.8
Savarese et al. (54)	EMP (10 mg/kg/d) day 1–5 + docetaxel (70 mg/m^2) day 1, q3wk + hydrocortisone (40 mg) daily	1999	40	4/21 (19%)	27/39 (69%)	—
Kreis et al. (53)	EMP (14 mg/kg) daily + docetaxel (40–80 mg/m^2) day 1, q3wk	1999	17	1/6 (17%)	14/17 (82%)	—
Sinibaldi et al. (131)	EMP (280 mg) q6h × 5 doses + docetaxel (70 mg/m^2) q3wk	1999	18	2/8 (25%)	7/18 (39%)	—
Hernes et al. (45)	EMP (10 mg/kg) daily + epirubicin (100 mg/m^2) i.v. q3wk	1997	24	0/9 (0)	13/24 (54%)	—
Culine et al. (46)	EMP (600 mg) P.O. daily + doxorubicin (20 mg/m^2) i.v. q wk	1998	31	5/11 (45%)	18/31 (58%)	12
Colleoni et al. (44)	EMP (400 mg/m^2) P.O. daily + etoposide (50 mg/m^2) day 1–14, day 28–42 + vinorelbine (20 mg/m^2) day 1, 8, 28, and 35 q8wk	1997	25	2/3 (67%)	14/25 (56%)	11.7

AUC, area under the curve; CI, continuous infusion; EMP, estramustine phosphate; G-CSF, granulocyte colony-stimulating factor; NPCP, National Prostate Cancer Project; PSA, prostate-specific antigen.

Anthracycline-Based Regimens

Doxorubicin Combinations

Trials of single agent doxorubicin performed in the pre–PSA era demonstrated only modest palliative benefit. One trial reported by Rangel et al. randomized patients to weekly doxorubicin in combination with prednisone or prednisone alone (18). Toxicity was minimal, and significantly more subjective responders were noted in the doxorubicin arm, but overall survival was not prolonged.

Doxorubicin and cyclophosphamide combinations have been evaluated by a number of investigators. The Hoosier Oncology Group compared cyclophosphamide to the combination of cyclophosphamide, doxorubicin, and methotrexate in a randomized phase III trial (24) (Table 51-5). Toxicity was tolerable and primarily hematologic. Overall results were disappointing, with only four patients demonstrating a response [three partial responses (PRs) in the combination arm, one PR in the cyclophosphamide arm]. No differences in overall survival or time to disease progression were noted between the single-agent cyclophosphamide and combination arms.

More recently, Small et al. studied doxorubicin in combination with dose-escalated cyclophosphamide (25). Patients

TABLE 51-5. CONTEMPORARY RANDOMIZED TRIALS IN PATIENTS WITH ANDROGEN-INDEPENDENT PROSTATE CANCER

Reference	Year	Treatment arms	N	Time to progression (mo)	Overall survival (mo)
Cervellino et al. (132)	1990	DES-DP	20	3	11.8
		vs.			
		DES + vindesine	31	4	10.2
Patel et al. (133)	1990	Megestrol acetate	29	—	9.1
		vs.			
		Dexamethasone	29	—	8.4 (p = .2)
Rangel et al. (18)	1992	Doxorubicin + prednisone	59	5	8.8
		vs.			
		Prednisone	51	3.8 (p = .07)	8.2 (p = .26)
Laurie et al. (27)	1992	5-Fluorouracil + doxorubicin + mitomycin C	70	—	8.65
		vs.			
		Mitomycin C → doxorubicin → 5-fluorouracil (sequential)	72	—	7.07 (p = .025)
Saxman et al. (24)	1992	Cyclophosphamide	53	4.4[a]	9.0[b]
		vs.			
		Cyclophosphamide + doxorubicin + methotrexate	50	6.2[a]	9.5[b] (p = .93)
Newling et al. (134)	1993	Mitomycin C	86	5	10
		vs.			
		Estramustine	85	5 (p = .46)	10 (p = .60)
Tannock et al. (7)	1996	Mitoxantrone + prednisone	80	10[c]	~10
		vs.			
		Prednisone	81	4.5[c] (p <.0001)	~10 (p = .27)
Iversen et al. (19)	1997	Estramustine	61	4.6	9.4
		vs.			
		Placebo	68	5	6.1 (p = .90)
Kantoff et al. (30)	1999	Mitoxantrone + hydrocortisone	119	3.7	12.3
		vs.			
		Hydrocortisone	123	2.3 (p = .025)	12.6 (p = .77)
Hudes et al. (40)	1999	Estramustine + vinblastine	95	3.7	11.9
		vs.			
		Vinblastine	98	2.2 (p <.001)	9.2 (p = .08)
Small (8)	2000	Suramin + hydrocortisone	229	—	9.4
		vs.			
		Hydrocortisone	231	—	9.2 (p = NS)
Halabi et al. (61)	2000	Suramin: low	NA	NA	14.7
		vs.			
		Intermediate	NA	NA	13.2
		vs.			
		High dose	NA	NA	12.9

DES-DP, diethylstilbestrol diphosphate; NA, not available, NS, not specified.
[a]Responders only.
[b]Good performance patients only.
[c]Palliative response duration.

were treated with doxorubicin at a dose of 40 mg per m^2 every 21 days while the dose of cyclophosphamide was escalated from 800 to 2,000 mg per m^2. All patients were supported with granulocyte colony-stimulating factor. Five of 15 (33%) patients with bidimensionally measurable disease had an objective response, and three patients with bone-only disease had an improvement on bone scan. A posttherapy PSA decline of 50% or greater was seen in 46% of the patients. Toxicity with this regimen was primarily hematologic, with 33% of all cycles resulting in grade 4 neutropenia. This study established that cyclophosphamide could be escalated safely in this population; however, higher doses of cyclophosphamide did not clearly translate into greater clinical activity.

Several investigators have evaluated doxorubicin in combination with 5-fluoruracil and mitomycin C (26,27). Laurie et al. reported on a randomized comparison of 5-fluoruracil, doxorubicin, and mitomycin C and the same three agents administered sequentially at the time of disease progression (27). A minimal improvement in median survival of questionable clinical significance (1.1 months, p = .025) was noted in the combination arm; however, toxicity with the 5-fluoruracil, doxorubicin, and mitomycin C arm was significant, with 91% of the patients developing severe leukopenia and 21% developing severe thrombocytopenia. The excessive toxicity and minimal improvement in survival limited the used of this regimen to the clinical trial setting.

Based on the demonstration of preclinical synergy between doxorubicin and the antifungal agent ketoconazole, Sella et al. studied this combination in patients with AIPC (28). Daily, continuous ketoconazole was combined with doxorubicin administered on a weekly 24-hour infusion schedule. A posttherapy decline in PSA of 50% or greater was noted in 21 of 38 (55%) assessable patients. Seven out of 12 (58%) patients with bidimensionally measurable disease had a PR. Despite limiting the total dose of doxorubicin to 400 mg per m^2, significant adverse events were seen with two patients dying of sudden cardiac death and an additional 45% requiring hospitalization for treatment-associated complications. Clinically apparent adrenal insufficiency resulting from the high-dose ketoconazole occurred in 63% of patients. Eleven patients (29%) developed a syndrome of grade III or IV acral erythema of the palms and soles accompanied by stomatitis and often anal and urethral mucositis.

Mitoxantrone Combinations

Many consider the combination of mitoxantrone plus a corticosteroid as a treatment standard for patients with symptomatic AIPC. This conclusion is based on a prospective randomized trial demonstrating a palliative benefit of mitoxantrone and prednisone when compared to prednisone alone (7). Although no survival benefit was noted, this study represented a milestone in this disease, as it was the first to demonstrate a clear role for chemotherapy in the treatment of patients with symptomatic androgen-independent disease.

In this Canadian multiinstitutional randomized trial, entry was restricted to patients with symptomatic AIPC, and the primary study end point was a palliative response as indicated by a reduction in pain (7). A response was defined as a 2-point reduction in pain as assessed by the 6-point McGill-Melzack Pain Questionnaire (or complete loss of pain if initially 1+) maintained for a minimum of 3 weeks (7,29). Secondary end points included a 50% or greater reduction in analgesic use without an increase in pain, duration of response, and survival. QOL measures were also evaluated. Although no survival difference was found, an increased proportion of patients treated with the combination reported a decrease in pain (29% vs. 12%, p = .01). Duration of palliation was also longer in the chemotherapy arm (median 43 vs. 18 weeks, p <.0001). Toxicity was primarily hematologic, and nausea and alopecia were minimal with this regimen. Five patients treated with cumulative doses of 116 to 214 mg per m^2 developed possible cardiac toxicity. In two of these five cases, symptomatic congestive heart failure developed.

A second randomized trial of mitoxantrone plus hydrocortisone or hydrocortisone alone was recently reported by the Cancer and Leukemia Group B (CALGB) (30). In this study, survival was the primary end point, and entry was not restricted to symptomatic patients only. Secondary end points included time to disease progression, time to treatment failure, response rate, and QOL. No statistically significant difference in overall survival between the two treatment arms was reported. Median survival was 12.3 months and 12.6 months for the hydrocortisone plus mitoxantrone and hydrocortisone only arms, respectively. Time to disease progression and the time to treatment failure favored the combination of mitoxantrone and hydrocortisone (3.7 months vs. 2.3 months, p = .25), but there was no difference in response based on improvements in objective disease or posttherapy decline in PSA 4 to 8 weeks after the initiation of therapy. The time to PSA nadir was longer than initially predicted and, in a post hoc analysis, a greater percentage of patients in the mitoxantrone arm had a 50% or greater maximum reduction in PSA (38% vs. 22%, p = .008). Furthermore, patients who achieved a 50% or greater or an 80% or greater decline from baseline had a longer median survival duration than those that did not (20.5 months vs. 10.2 months). In the QOL analysis, a trend for improved pain control for mitoxantrone plus hydrocortisone, compared to hydrocortisone, also did not reach statistical significance.

Although the CALGB study did not confirm the findings of the Canadian investigators, this may have been the result of differences in the primary study objectives and patient selection. In the Canadian study, pain was the primary end point and a prerequisite for entry into the study (7). In contrast, only one-third of the patients enrolled in the CALGB trial required analgesics at the time of study entry (30). In addition, there were differences in the QOL instruments used, and many patients in the CALGB study were not compliant in completing the QOL questionnaires. Overall, these trials suggest that mitoxantrone plus prednisone has clinical benefit in selected symptomatic patients with AIPC, and further studies of mitoxantrone-based combinations are warranted.

Cytoskeleton Agents: Estramustine-Based Regimens

Estramustine phosphate (EMP) consists of estradiol with a phosphate group at the C17 position covalently linked to nitrogen mustard by a carbamate ester bond (31). EMP was initially developed with the expectation that the estrogen moiety would target the molecule to tumor cells, and the nitrogen mustard would be cleaved inside the cell, resulting in the activation of this alkylating agent. Only later was it demonstrated that the carbamate ester bond is resistant to cleavage *in vivo*. An antimitotic mechanism of action has since been demonstrated *in vitro* and *in vivo* (32). EMP binds to microtubule assembly proteins, causing microtubule disassembly, mitotic block, and eventual cell death (33,34). This mechanism is distinct from other microtubule-targeted agents, such as the vinca alkaloids and taxanes, which both bind to tubulin (35). The taxanes bind directly to polymerized tubulin to promote microtubule assembly and stabilize microtubules from depolymerization. These stabilized microtubules lose their normal dynamic reorganization properties, resulting in a loss of function and cell death (35).

Nontaxane Estramustine Phosphate Combinations

Based on observed synergy *in vitro*, several groups investigated the combination of estramustine and vinblastine in patients with AIPC (36). The combined results of three phase II trials demonstrated that a significant decline in PSA can be achieved in more than half of patients (56%, 46 of 82), and approximately one-third of the patients will have measurable disease regression (complete response or PR) (37–39). Peripheral edema and nausea are the most common adverse effects.

These studies were followed by a randomized comparison of EMP plus vinblastine and vinblastine in 193 patients with hormone-refractory disease (40). The primary study end point was survival. Although no statistically significant overall survival benefit for the combination was reported, a trend in favor of the EMP plus vinblastine arm was detected (11.9 months vs. 9.2 months, $p = .08$). For patients treated with the combination, there was a significant improvement in the time to progression (3.7 Months vs. 2.2 months, $p < .001$); a greater proportion of patients achieved measurable disease regression (18% vs. 6%); and more patients had a 50% or greater posttherapy decline in PSA (25% vs. 3.2%, $p < .0001$). Patients treated with estramustine and vinblastine experienced significantly less granulocytopenia, suggesting that EMP may have a marrow-protecting effect. Nausea and peripheral edema, as expected, were more common in the estramustine arm.

Etoposide, a topoisomerase II inhibitor that acts at the level of the nuclear matrix, has been combined with EMP with promising results. Although single-agent oral etoposide demonstrated only minimal palliative benefit in a study by Hussain et al., a preclinical laboratory study suggested synergistic antitumor effects when etoposide was combined with estramustine (41,42). Pienta and Lehr demonstrated binding of estramustine to the nuclear matrix, the RNA-protein network of the nucleus hypothesized to play an important role in DNA replication and gene expression (42). Furthermore, EMP and etoposide appeared to act synergistically to inhibit tumor growth in the Dunning rat prostate cancer model (42).

In a study of 42 patients with AIPC reported by Pienta et al., the combination of daily oral EMP and etoposide demonstrated significant activity (43). Nine of 18 patients (50%) with measurable soft-tissue disease demonstrated a complete (three) or partial (six) response. Of 24 patients with bone-only disease, six (25%) demonstrated an improvement on bone scan. Twenty-two of 42 (53%) had posttherapy declines in PSA of 50% or greater, and 21% had declines of 75% or greater. Nausea and hematologic toxicity, however, were significant. In total, 25% of the patients required a reduction in etoposide dose as a result of grades 3 or 4 leukopenia, and two patients withdrew from the study within 2 weeks of registration due to persistent nausea and vomiting. Five patients developed neutropenic fever and one died of complete bone marrow failure 12 weeks after beginning therapy. Four patients also developed deep venous thrombosis. In summary, although this active and easily administered oral regimen has gained some popularity, toxicity has limited its widespread adoption.

Based on the promising activity of estramustine and vinblastine and estramustine etoposide combinations, Colleoni et al. studied the three-drug combination of estramustine, etoposide, and the newer semisynthetic vinca alkaloid vinorelbine (44). Fourteen of 25 (56%) treated patients had a 50% or greater decline in PSA. PRs were also noted in two patients with measurable soft-tissue disease, and six patients demonstrated an improvement in osseous disease on serial bone scans. In contrast to the report by Pienta et al., toxicity was mild with this regimen, with only 12% developing grade III or IV neutropenia. This difference in toxicity profile may have been attributable to the reduced duration of etoposide treatment (14 of 56 days per cycle vs. 21 of 28 days) (43,44).

Combinations of EMP and the anthracyclines doxorubicin and epirubicin have also been reported (45,46). Combining daily oral estramustine and epirubicin administered on an every 3-week schedule, Hernes et al. reported a 50% or greater reduction in PSA in 13 of 24 (54%) patients and subjective improvement in 7 of 24 patients (45). No objective responses were seen. Of note, no correlation between PSA decline and subjective improvement was detected in this study. Adverse effects included nausea, gynecomastia (50%), and hematologic toxicity (42% with grade 3 or 4). One patient developed deep venous thrombosis, one developed cardiomyopathy, and two developed grade 2 arrhythmia. Culine et al. reported on the combination of daily oral estramustine and weekly doxorubicin (46). In this phase II study, 18 of 31 patients with AIPC had a 50% or greater decline in PSA and 5 of 11 (45%) patients with bidimensionally measurable disease achieved a PR in liver or retroperitoneal lymph nodes (46). Twelve (38%) patients who received at minimum 4 weeks of therapy experienced grade 3 or 4 neutropenia. Two developed febrile neutropenia, and one died of septic shock. Two patients had deep venous thrombosis requiring anticoagulant therapy, and one patient had grade 3 hepatic toxicity. No patients developed congestive heart failure.

A unique approach to combining estramustine with an anthracycline was pursued by investigators from the M. D. Anderson Cancer Center (47). Two active regimens, estramustine plus vinblastine and doxorubicin plus ketoconazole, were alternated weekly (47). Patients were treated with doxorubicin and ketoconazole weeks 1, 3, and 5 and estramustine plus vinblastine weeks 2, 4, and 6. Thirty-one of 46 (67%) patients had a 50% or greater posttherapy decline in PSA, and 12 of 16 (75%) had measurable disease regression. The median duration of response was 8.4 months (range, 1.8 months to 14.9 months), with a median duration of response after discontinuation of chemotherapy of 4.2 months. Therapy was well tolerated, but, as with most estramustine-based combinations, peripheral edema (49%), deep venous thrombosis (18%), and cardiac events (4%) were prominent and dose limiting in some cases.

Estramustine Phosphate–Taxane Combinations

The activity of the taxanes in several diverse solid tumors prompted the preclinical and clinical evaluation of these agents in AIPC. Paclitaxel binds to tubulin and interferes with the depolymerization of microtubules necessary to complete cell division. Cells treated with paclitaxel are arrested in the M-phase of the cell cycle and ultimately undergo apoptosis. The initial phase II study of paclitaxel in AIPC was performed by the Eastern Cooperative Oncology Group using a 24-hour continuous infusion schedule every 21 days (48). In this trial, only 1 of 23 patients (4.3%) experienced a PR lasting 9 months. Four other patients had radiographically stable disease and declines in PSA of 16% to 24%. Marrow toxicity was dose limiting, with 74% of patients developing grades III or IV leukopenia and 26% developing neutropenic fever. Of further concern, three patients developed sudden cardiovascular events during or shortly after completing therapy. One was a nonfatal myocardial infarction during paclitaxel infusion in a patient who died of progressive prostate cancer 4 months later. The other two were sudden deaths occurring within 1 month of the last paclitaxel treatment.

These results may have limited further evaluation of this agent in AIPC, had preclinical laboratory data not suggested synergy with estramustine (35). Speicher et al. studied the combination of paclitaxel and estramustine using estramustine-resistant and wild-type androgen-independent DU145 human prostatic carcinoma cell lines (35). In the estramustine-resistant and wild-type cells, synergistic antitumor effects were noted with the combination of estramustine and paclitaxel. In contrast, evidence of synergy was not found with the combination of paclitaxel and vinblastine, another microtubule-targeting drug. Furthermore, taxanes and EMP have nonoverlapping toxicities, suggesting that the combination of these agents may be clinically useful.

Hudes et al. studied the combination of estramustine and paclitaxel using a 96-hour continuous infusion paclitaxel schedule in combination with daily oral estramustine (49). Significant activity was noted with this combination as measured by posttherapy decline in PSA and reductions in measurable disease. In total, 53% (9 of 32) and 28% of patients with an elevated PSA before treatment had 50% or greater and 80% or greater declines in PSA, respectively. Four of nine patients with measurable disease had a complete response or PR. Nausea, leukopenia, fluid retention, and fatigue were the major adverse effects. Thrombotic complications occurred in three patients. All three developed subclavian thromboses associated with a central venous catheter. One patient also developed a cerebrovascular thrombosis during therapy.

In an effort to improve the efficacy and toxicity profile of this combination, three drug combinations and shorter infusion schedules of paclitaxel have been investigated. A study combining oral estramustine and etoposide for 7 days with a 1-hour infusion of paclitaxel every 21 days was reported by Smith et al. (50). In this study, 26 of 40 patients demonstrated a 50% or greater posttherapy decline in PSA, and 45% of assessable patients with bidimensionally measurable disease had disease regression. The primary toxicity was hematologic. The study also assessed the Functional Assessment of Cancer Therapy–Prostate, which showed there was no significant change in QOL as a result of the therapy.

In a multiinstitutional study, weekly paclitaxel was evaluated in combination with estramustine and monthly carboplatin (51). This regimen was active and well tolerated, with 67% of patients demonstrating a 50% or greater posttherapy decline in PSA. Forty-five percent of the patients showed regression in measurable disease and four patients had resolution of bone lesions on serial radionuclide scans that were accompanied by an improvement in the bone scan index. The overall median time to progression was 21 weeks, with a median survival of 19.9 months. The regimen was well tolerated, with the most common toxicities being low-grade nausea (77%) and deep vein thrombosis (21%). Significant leukopenia, thrombocytopenia, and peripheral neuropathy were not observed.

Docetaxel is a semisynthetic taxane that has significant single-agent activity in AIPC (20). Consistent with the results reported for paclitaxel, docetaxel has been studied in combination with estramustine with promising early results. Petrylak et al. reported the results of a phase I study of docetaxel and estramustine (52). Docetaxel was administered every 21 days and estramustine was administered on days 1 through 5 of each cycle. Patients were stratified into minimally pretreated and extensively pretreated groups. The recommended dose of docetaxel was 70 mg per m^2 in the minimally pretreated group and 60 mg per m^2 in the extensively pretreated group. Overall, 63% of the patients had a 50% or greater posttherapy decline in PSA, and 40% of the patients had an 80% or greater decline. Five of 18 (28%) patients with bidimensionally measurable disease achieved a PR. More than half of the patients who were on narcotic analgesics before treatment were able to discontinue their pain medications. Fluid retention, grade 3 or 4 neutropenia without neutropenic fever, and nausea were the major toxicities. In contrast to other estramustine-based combinations, the incidence of deep venous thrombosis was only 8.8% in this trial. This may have been the result of the reduced duration of estramustine treatment during this regimen. Although survival data from phase I studies need to be interpreted with caution, the median survival of 22.8 months reported with this regimen was far in excess of the 10- to 12-month median survival reported in contemporary randomized studies of AIPC. Further evaluation of this regimen will be required to confirm these findings.

Kreis et al. reported the results of a phase I study of continuous oral estramustine and docetaxel administered every 3 weeks (53). Of 17 treated patients, 14 (82%) had significant posttherapy declines in PSA. Leukopenia and fatigue were the dose-limiting toxicities in this study. Preliminary results from a multiinstitutional CALGB phase II study of estramustine, docetaxel, and low-dose hydrocortisone are consistent with the results reported by Petrylak et al. and Kreis et al., suggesting significant antitumor activity with this combination (54).

The data available do not allow for a direct comparison between the two taxanes, paclitaxel and docetaxel, in the treatment of AIPC. Laboratory studies have detected differences in nontubulin binding between paclitaxel and docetaxel, suggesting that clinically significant differences may exist (55). As an example, docetaxel treatment of prostate cancer cell lines results in increased phosphorylation and inactivation of the antiapoptotic protein bcl-2 in comparison to paclitaxel treatment (55). Whether these nonmicrotubule targets of paclitaxel and docetaxel are relevant *in vivo* will require further study. Given the high level of activity reported by Picus et al. for single-agent docetaxel, further study is also needed to determine the added benefit of EMP when combined with this agent and whether the additional benefit outweighs the added toxicity of EMP (20).

In summary, EMP-based combination regimens have significant antitumor activity in patients with AIPC. Despite these early results, randomized phase III trials will be required to confirm these promising results and to establish the role of estramustine and taxane-based therapies in the treatment of patients with advanced prostate cancer.

THE SURAMIN EXPERIENCE

Suramin is a polysulfonated naphthylurea with a diverse range of proposed antitumor effects, including the modulation of soluble polypeptide growth factors (56). The development of suramin as a treatment for AIPC illustrates many of the pitfalls that may arise in the development of effective agents for the treatment of this disease. Interest in suramin as a treatment for AIPC began more than a decade ago with a report by Myers et al. of major antitumor responses in four of eight patients with measurable disease and significant PSA declines in 7 of 11 patients treated with continuous infusion suramin (57). Of particular interest was the durability of several of the reported responses. These findings sparked several additional studies of suramin in AIPC using a variety of intermittent and continuous dosing schedules. One study by Eisenberger et al. using an intermittent infusion schedule reported measurable disease regressions in 6 of 12 cases and a more than 50% decline in PSA in 24 of 31 patients (77%) (58). Several other studies noted much lower response proportions (56). A direct comparison between the various phase II studies was confounded by significant differences in patient selection and the wide diversity of treatment schedules used.

In retrospect, although suramin has clinically meaningful activity in a subset of patients with AIPC, patient selection and differences in the criteria used to assess PSA response likely accounted for the wide range of response rates reported in several of the early phase I and II studies. In addition to differences in disease burden and the extent of previous treatment, confounding variables common to all solid tumors, several characteristics unique to AIPC merit further discussion. At the time of the initial suramin studies, the flutamide withdrawal syndrome had not been characterized (59). It is now well established that meaningful disease regression can occur on the withdrawal of antiandrogen therapy (59). A significant proportion of patients enrolled on the initial phase I and II trials of suramin had previously received an antiandrogen, and androgen withdrawal may have accounted for a percentage of the responses noted. Furthermore, the need for glucocorticoid

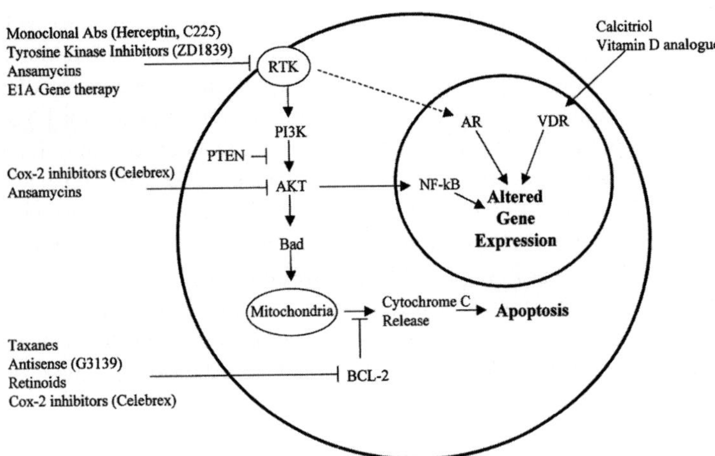

FIGURE 51-1. Novel targets for prostate cancer therapy. Numbers represent the four targets with drugs pointing to them 1: Receptor tyrosine kinases (RTKs), including epidermal growth factor receptor and Her2. 2: The PTEN/Akt pathway. 3: The anti-apoptotic protein Bcl-2. 4: The vitamin D receptor (VDR). Therapies targeting tumor-stromal interactions, including angiogenesis inhibitors, matrix metalloproteases, and bisphosphonates, are also in clinical development. AR, androgen receptor; PI3K, phosphatidylinositol 3'-kinase.

supplementation to address the adrenal inhibitory effects of suramin represents a further potentially confounding variable. As a significant number of patients with AIPC will have a response to second-line hormonal manipulations, a proportion of the benefit derived by patients treated with the combination may have been attributable to the hydrocortisone.

To account for the confounding effects of androgen withdrawal and corticosteroid therapy, a perspective trial of suramin was performed at Memorial Sloan-Kettering Cancer Center in which patients did not receive suramin until disease progression after withdrawal of flutamide and, later, hydrocortisone alone (60). In this trial of 30 patients, suramin had only limited clinical activity in patients who had progressed on hydrocortisone (60). No objective responses were noted, and only 18% of patients demonstrated a greater than 50% decline in PSA.

Recently, the results of two large randomized trials of suramin in AIPC were reported (8,61). Small et al. published the results of a double-blind placebo-controlled randomized comparison of suramin plus hydrocortisone versus placebo plus hydrocortisone in patients with painful bone metastases necessitating opioid analgesics (8). Posttherapy changes in pain and opioid use were the primary end points. For this trial, a 5-day loading schedule of suramin was followed by twice weekly infusions for 2 weeks and then weekly infusions during weeks 4 through 12. The study demonstrated moderate palliative benefit, with a greater proportion of patients in the suramin arm reporting a pain response. A modest delay in disease progression without survival benefit was also noted. A higher proportion of patients (33% vs. 16%, $p = .01$) in the suramin arm had a greater than 50% decline in PSA. Crossover to open-label suramin at the time of disease progression was allowed and occurred in 71.3% of the patients randomized to the placebo arm.

The Intergroup led by the CALGB recently reported preliminary results of a three-arm randomized phase III trial designed to assess suramin dose escalation (61). Patients were randomized to receive low- (3.19 g per m^2), intermediate- (5.32 g per m^2), or high-dose (7.66 g per m^2) suramin administered on days 1, 2, 8, and 9 of a 28-day cycle for three cycles (61). Although dose escalation resulted in an increase in the proportion of patients with an objective response or a PSA decline of 50% or greater, these trends did not reach statistical significance, and no improvement in overall survival was detected. Furthermore, a statistically significant increase in grade III and IV toxicities were seen with the higher-dose schedules.

In summary, suramin has limited activity in AIPC and is not currently in use outside of the clinical trial setting. The experience with suramin emphasizes the importance of prospectively validated standardized enrollment and outcome criteria. Given the large number of novel targeted therapies now in preclinical development, further improvements in clinical trial design and outcome assessment will be required to effectively select those agents with greatest promise for prospective randomized evaluation.

NOVEL TARGET

Since 1990, dramatic advances have been achieved in understanding the molecular pathways responsible for tumorigenesis and treatment failure. These discoveries have led to the identification of novel targets for systemic therapy. Novel agents designed to target pathways required for prostate cancer growth and survival are in early clinical and preclinical development (Fig. 51-1). These therapies hold the promise of increased antitumor activity with less toxicity by targeting pathways critical to malignant but not normal cell survival.

Differentiating Agents

Retinoids

Enthusiasm for using retinoids as therapeutic agents for AIPC is based on epidemiologic studies suggesting that consumption of vitamin A is correlated with reduced prostate cancer incidence. Preclinical study further established that retinoids have growth-inhibitory and differentiating activity in prostate cancer and are effective in preventing the emergence of primary prostate cancer in animal models (62,63). Based on this data, Trump et al. studied all-*trans*-retinoic acid in 17 patients with AIPC (64). No clinical activity was seen.

Kelly et al. reported on the treatment of 14 AIPC patients with all-*trans*-retinoic acid and 16 AIPC and 4 androgen-dependent patients with 13-*cis*-retinoic acid and interferon-2a (CRA/IFN) (15). No responses in bone, measurable disease, or PSA were noted with all-*trans*-retinoic acid. CRA/IFN had minimal clinical activity, with the majority of patients developing symptomatic disease progression within 2 to 3 months. One patient with measurable disease treated with CRA/IFN had a PR and one patient had a 50% or greater decline in PSA. Prolonged stabilization of disease was noted in several patients, including all four patients with androgen-dependent disease. One patient had an initial steady rise in PSA without evidence of progression in measurable soft-tissue or osseous disease followed by a decline in PSA to below his pretherapy value at 4 months. This patient continued on therapy for 9 months until measurable disease regression was documented. On discontinuation of therapy, a greater than 50% decline in PSA and stable measurable disease was documented and maintained for 4 months without additional therapy. This case illustrates that retinoids may modulate the level of serum PSA independent of changes in overall disease burden, complicating the use of PSA as a clinical trial end point. In summary, the experience with retinoids to date suggests that these agents have minimal activity in advanced AIPC. Although the study by Kelly et al. suggests that these agents may have activity in androgen-dependent patients earlier in the course of their disease, further study will be necessary to confirm this finding.

Vitamin D

Vitamin D is a steroid hormone with a well-characterized role in the regulation of calcium and bone homeostasis. An epidemiologic link between vitamin D metabolism and prostate cancer has been proposed on the basis of an increased incidence of this disease in African-American men and men living in northern latitudes (65). Some studies of serum calcitriol, the active form of vitamin D, also support a link between vitamin D metabolism and prostate cancer, and vitamin D–receptor expression has been documented in human prostate cancer. Calcitriol has antiproliferative and proapoptotic activity in prostate cancer models and has entered human clinical trials (66). The major toxicity, as predicted, has been hypercalcemia. To address this limitation, analogs that retain the antitumor effects of vitamin D but produce less hypercalcemia have been developed with promising preclinical activity. Other approaches have combined calcitriol with steroids and bisphosphonates, agents that attenuate the hypercalcemic response. Because each of these agents may have antitumor effects in prostate cancer, well-designed clinical trials will be necessary to separate out the contribution of calcitriol (67).

Growth Factor Pathways

The epidermal growth factor receptor (EGFR) and Her2/neu are related transmembrane tyrosine kinase receptors implicated in prostate cancer progression and the development of androgen-independent disease (68,69). In one survey of primary and metastatic lesions reported by Scher et al., a change in transforming growth factor alpha (TGF-alpha) expression pattern was noted with progression from primary carcinoma to the androgen-independent metastatic state (68). In the primary samples, TGF-alpha expression was present predominantly within the stromal cells. In contrast, 14 of 18 evaluable androgen-independent lesions demonstrated coexpression of TGF-alpha and EGFR, suggesting a shift from paracrine to autocrine receptor stimulation. C225, a monoclonal antibody that binds to the EGFR, has antitumor activity in xenograft models of prostate cancer and has been studied in combination with doxorubicin in patients with AIPC (70,71). Modest activity was noted with this combination, as measured by soft tissue regression in one patient and stable measurable disease in three patients (71).

Her2/neu-kinase activity may also contribute to prostate cancer progression, and the development of androgen-independent disease and Her2/neu expression may serve as a marker for poor clinical outcome (69,72). Herceptin, a monoclonal antibody approved for use in patients with breast cancer whose tumors overexpress Her2/neu, has demonstrated activity in preclinical models of prostate cancer and is now under investigation in patients with advanced prostate cancer (73,74). Small molecules that selectively inhibit the tyrosine kinase activity of EGFR and Her2/neu are areas of intense investigation. Preclinical studies demonstrate activity in prostate cancer and one such agent, ZD1839, an inhibitor of EGFR, has clinical activity in the phase I setting (75,76).

Geldanamycin and 17-allyl-amino-geldanamycin are ansamycin antibiotics that bind to Hsp90 and cause the proteasomal degradation of a subset of proteins, including steroid receptors, Raf, and certain transmembrane tyrosine kinases (77). Treatment of breast cancer cells lines with ansamycins results in a rapid reduction in Her2/neu protein expression, and cell lines that overexpress Her2/neu are particularly sensitive to these agents (77). 17-Allyl-amino-geldanamycin has been chosen as the lead agent for this class by the NCI and has now entered phase I testing at several institutions. Antisense and gene therapy approaches targeting the Her-kinase axis are also in preclinical development (78,79).

Modulators of Apoptosis

Bcl-2

Pathways that regulate apoptosis (or programmed cell death) contribute to tumorigenesis and resistance to therapy. Bcl-2 and its homologues are structurally similar family members that regulate apoptosis in prostate cancer cells (80). The bcl-2 protein was initially identified in lymphomas in which a t(14;18) results in the placement of the bcl-2 protooncogene under the control of the immunoglobulin heavy chain locus (81). Bcl-2 family members segregate into proapoptotic members, such as Bad, BAX, and Bid, and antiapoptotic proteins, such as bcl-2 and bcl-x_L, and evidence suggests that the cellular balance between pro- and antiapoptotic family members determines cell survival or death (82).

Strong evidence exists that overexpression of bcl-2 confers resistance to chemotherapy and radiation therapy by preventing treatment-associated apoptosis, and a reduction in bcl-2 levels may enhance cytotoxic cell kill (83). The incidence of bcl-2 expression has been studied by immunohistochemistry in early and advanced prostate cancers (84). Studies in prostate cancer suggest that bcl-2 overexpression increases with progression to metastatic and androgen-independent states. Furthermore, bcl-2 expression has been correlated with recurrence-free survival after radical prostatectomy and recurrence after radiation therapy (85,86). Taken together, these data suggest that agents that target the bcl-2 apoptotic pathway may be potential therapeutic targets.

Several agents with preclinical activity in prostate cancer have now been demonstrated to modulate bcl-2. The taxanes paclitaxel and docetaxel inhibit bcl-2 activity by inducing bcl-2 phosphorylation (55). Modulation of the bcl-2 pathway may also contribute to the antitumor effects noted with the nonsteroidal antiinflammatory drugs and cyclooxygenase-2–specific inhibitors (87). Antisense oligonucleotides that down-regulate bcl-2 have antitumor activity in preclinical models of prostate cancer and are now in early clinical trial (88). Retinoids have also been demonstrated to reduce bcl-2 expression and to act synergistically with interferon-alpha to inhibit growth (89). DiPaola et al. combined paclitaxel with CRA/IFN based on the hypothesis that the CRA/IFN, by decreasing bcl-2 expression, would sensitize tumor cells to the antitumor effects of paclitaxel (89). In this report, CRA/IFN decreased bcl-2 expression in prostate cancer cell lines and in peripheral blood mononuclear cells drawn from CRA/IFN-treated patients (89).

PTEN/Akt

The search for novel targets has also identified the PTEN-phosphatidylinositol 3'-kinase-Akt pathway as a contributor to prostate cancer development and progression (90). PTEN, also referred to as MMAC1 (*P*utative *P*rotein *T*yrosine *P*hosphatase/*M*utated in *M*ultiple *A*dvanced *C*ancers), is a candidate tumor suppressor gene that maps to human chromosome 10q23 (91,92). This gene encodes a protein and lipid phosphatase that negatively regulates the Akt/protein kinase B kinase. The Akt-signaling pathway serves as a dominant regulator of growth factor–mediated apoptosis through its regulation of NFκB, Forkhead transcription factors, and the bcl-2 family member Bad (93).

PTEN is frequently mutated in prostate cancer cell lines, and loss of heterozygosity has been demonstrated at the 10q23 locus (94,95). Furthermore, loss of PTEN protein expression has been detected as a frequent event in prostate cancer xenograft models in the absence of gene deletion or mutation (96). McMenamin et al. examined 109 prostatectomy specimens for PTEN protein expression by immunohistochemistry (97). Loss of PTEN expression was common and correlated with higher Gleason scores and advanced pathologic stages (97). Efforts are under way to identify agents that selectively inactivate the PTEN-Akt pathway. One such agent may be the COX-2 inhibitor celecoxib (Celebrex) (98). Treatment of the LNCaP and PC3 prostate cancer cell lines with this agent results in the induction of apoptosis through a bcl-2–independent pathway (98). Apoptosis was preceded by a reduction in Akt activity as measured by protein phosphorylation, and apoptosis could be prevented by the transfection of a constitutively active form of Akt (98).

Stromal Targets

Angiogenesis

An accumulating body of evidence suggests a central role for angiogenesis in tumor growth and metastasis. Soluble pro- and antiangiogenic factors have been identified, and agents that target angiogenic pathways are in development. One soluble growth factor with a well-established role in angiogenesis is the vascular endothelial growth factor (VEGF) (99). VEGF is overexpressed in many human cancers, including prostate cancer (100). Antibodies that bind to the VEGF ligand and VEGF-receptor tyrosine kinase inhibitors demonstrate preclinical activity in prostate cancer and have entered clinical trial (99).

Matrix Metalloproteinase

The matrix metalloproteinases (MMPs) are a family of proteases that degrade extracellular matrix and basement membrane components. By allowing for tumor invasion and spread to distant sites, MMPs facilitate metastatic tumor progression. High levels of MMPs have been detected in prostate cancer, and an inhibitor of MMPs (A-177430) has been demonstrated to prevent tumor growth and metastasis in a prostate cancer–animal model (101). Selective MMP inhibitors are now in early human clinical trial.

Bisphosphonates

Bisphosphonates are powerful inhibitors of osteoclastic bone resorption that have established clinical benefit in breast cancer and multiple myeloma (102). These malignancies are frequently characterized by the development of painful osteolytic bone metastases that result in significant morbidity and mortality. In contrast, prostate cancer bone disease is almost always osteoblastic in nature. Despite these differences in biology, a role for bisphosphonates in prostate cancer is supported by several observations. In a study of adjuvant clodronate treatment, patients with primary breast cancer and tumor cells in the bone marrow were randomized to receive 2 years of clodronate therapy or standard care (103). A statistically significant reduction in the incidence and number of distant metastases and an improvement in overall survival were observed in the clodronate-treated patients (103). Surprisingly, the reduction in distant metastases was not confined to bone but was also seen in visceral sites, suggesting additional nonosteoclastic antitumor effects. In preclinical models of prostate cancer, bisphosphonates inhibit prostate cancer cell adhesion and invasion, providing a mechanistic basis for their use as prophylactic therapy in preventing or delaying the establishment of osteoblastic metastatic lesions (104,105). Although this body of data suggests a rationale for bisphosphonate therapy in prostate cancer, definitive clinical trials of bisphosphonates in this disease will be necessary.

To date, the success of targeted therapies for prostate cancer has been hindered by limited direct evidence that particular pathways are important for prostate cancer tumorigenesis and progression. Prostate cancer likely represents a heterogenous collection of genetically and molecularly distinct diseases, and the success of current and future approaches will depend on our ability to predict through preclinical study patients likely to benefit from specific targeted approaches. Despite these obstacles, the promise of a curative therapy with low toxicity will continue to encourage the development of novel targeted approaches.

CONCLUSION

No randomized trial of chemotherapy in patients with AIPC has demonstrated a survival benefit when compared to a control population. Contemporary taxane-based combinations consistently demonstrate significant antitumor activity as measured by posttherapy decline in PSA, a reduction in measurable soft-tissue disease, and palliation of disease related symptoms. The level of activity reported in these trials compares favorably with that of other solid tumors in which chemotherapy confers a meaningful survival benefit. This suggests that a large phase III trial of taxane-based combination therapy with survival as the primary end point is now justified. This hypothesis is now being tested in a randomized comparison of estramustine and docetaxel or mitoxantrone and prednisone being led by the Southwest Oncology Group (106). This study of 620 patients will be the largest AIPC trial to date and will likely establish further benefits of chemotherapy in the treatment of this disease.

REFERENCES

1. Yagoda A, Petrylak D. Cytotoxic chemotherapy for advanced hormone-resistant prostate cancer. *Cancer* 1993;71:1098–1109.
2. Fazzari M, Heller G, Scher HI. The phase II/III transition. Toward the proof of efficacy in cancer clinical trials. *Control Clin Trials* 2000;21:360–368.
3. Scher HI, Curley T, Geller N, et al. Trimetrexate in prostatic cancer: preliminary observations on the use of prostate-specific antigen and acid phosphatase as a marker in measurable hormone-refractory disease. *J Clin Oncol* 1990;8: 1830–1838.
4. Yagoda A, Watson RC, Natale RB, et al. A critical analysis of response criteria in patients with prostatic cancer treated with *cis*-diamminedichloride platinum II. *Cancer* 1979;44: 1553–1562.
5. Schroeder FH. Treatment response criteria for prostatic cancer. *Prostate* 1984;5:181–191.
6. Moore MJ, Osoba D, Murphy K, et al. Use of palliative end points to evaluate the effects of mitoxantrone and low-dose prednisone in patients with hormonally resistant prostate cancer. *J Clin Oncol* 1994;12:689–694.
7. Tannock IF, Osoba D, Stockler MR, et al. Chemotherapy with mitoxantrone plus prednisone or prednisone alone for symptomatic hormone-resistant prostate cancer: a Canadian randomized trial with palliative end points [see comments]. *J Clin Oncol* 1996;14:1756–1764.
8. Small EJ, Meyer M, Marshall ME, et al. Suramin therapy for patients with symptomatic hormone-refractory prostate cancer: results of a randomized phase III trial comparing suramin plus hydrocortisone to placebo plus hydrocortisone. *J Clin Oncol* 2000;18:1440–1450.
9. Scher HI, Kelly WM, Zhang ZF, et al. Post-therapy serum prostate-specific antigen level and survival in patients with androgen-independent prostate cancer. *J Natl Cancer Inst* 1999;91:244–251.
10. Sridhara R, Eisenberger MA, Sinibaldi VJ, et al. Evaluation of prostate-specific antigen as a surrogate marker for response of hormone-refractory prostate cancer to suramin therapy. *J Clin Oncol* 1995;13:2944–2953.
11. Smith DC, Dunn RL, Strawderman MS, et al. Change in serum prostate-specific antigen as a marker of response to cytotoxic therapy for hormone-refractory prostate cancer. *J Clin Oncol* 1998;16:1835–1843.
12. Vollmer RT, Dawson NA, Vogelzang NJ. The dynamics of prostate specific antigen in hormone refractory prostate carcinoma: an analysis of cancer and leukemia group B study 9181 of megestrol acetate. *Cancer* 1998;83:1989–1994.
13. Bubley GJ, Carducci M, Dahut W, et al. Eligibility and response guidelines for phase II clinical trials in androgen-independent prostate cancer: recommendations from the Prostate-Specific Antigen Working Group [published erra-

tum appears in *J Clin Oncol* 2000;18:2644]. *J Clin Oncol* 1999;17:3461–3467.
14. Scher HI, Mazumdar M, Kelly WK. Clinical trials in relapsed prostate cancer: defining the target. *J Natl Cancer Inst* 1996;88:1623–1634.
15. Kelly WK, Osman I, Reuter VE, et al. The development of biologic end points in patients treated with differentiation agents: an experience of retinoids in prostate cancer. *Clin Cancer Res* 2000;6:838–846.
16. Imbriaco M, Larson SM, Yeung HW, et al. A new parameter for measuring metastatic bone involvement by prostate cancer: the bone scan index. *Clin Cancer Res* 1998;4:1765–1772.
17. Sabbatini P, Larson SM, Kremer A, et al. Prognostic significance of extent of disease in bone in patients with androgen-independent prostate cancer. *J Clin Oncol* 1999;17:948–957.
18. Rangel C, Matzkin H, Soloway MS. Experience with weekly doxorubicin (adriamycin) in hormone-refractory stage D2 prostate cancer. *Urology* 1992;39:577–582.
19. Iversen P, Rasmussen F, Asmussen C, et al. Estramustine phosphate versus placebo as second line treatment after orchiectomy in patients with metastatic prostate cancer: DAPROCA study 9002. Danish Prostatic Cancer Group. *J Urol* 1997;157:929–934.
20. Picus J, Schultz M. Docetaxel (taxotere) as monotherapy in the treatment of hormone-refractory prostate cancer: preliminary results. *Semin Oncol* 1999;26:14–18.
21. Canobbio L, Guarneri D, Miglietta L, et al. Carboplatin in advanced hormone refractory prostatic cancer patients. *Eur J Cancer* 1993;15:2094–2096.
22. Coppin C, Murray N, Bryce C, et al. Mitomycin C revisited for androgen-independent prostate cancer (AIPC). *Proc ASCO* 1997;16:331a.
23. Raghavan D, Cox K, Pearson BS, et al. Oral cyclophosphamide for the management of hormone-refractory prostate cancer. *Br J Urol* 1993;72:625–628.
24. Saxman S, Ansari R, Drasga R, et al. Phase III trial of cyclophosphamide versus cyclophosphamide, doxorubicin, and methotrexate in hormone-refractory prostatic cancer. A Hoosier Oncology Group study. *Cancer* 1992;70:2488–2492.
25. Small EJ, Srinivas S, Egan B, et al. Doxorubicin and dose-escalated cyclophosphamide with granulocyte colony-stimulating factor for the treatment of hormone-resistant prostate cancer. *J Clin Oncol* 1996;14:1617–1625.
26. Blumenstein B, Crawford ED, Saiers JH, et al. Doxorubicin, mitomycin C, and 5-fluorouracil in the treatment of hormone refractory adenocarcinoma of the prostate: a Southwest Oncology Group study. *J Urol* 1993;150:411–413.
27. Laurie JA, Hahn RG, Therneau TM, et al. Chemotherapy for hormonally refractory advanced prostate carcinoma. A comparison of combined versus sequential treatment with mitomycin C, doxorubicin, and 5-fluorouracil. *Cancer* 1992;69:1440–1444.
28. Sella A, Kilbourn R, Amato R, et al. Phase II study of ketoconazole combined with weekly doxorubicin in patients with androgen-independent prostate cancer. *J Clin Oncol* 1994;12:683–688.
29. Melzack R. The McGill Pain Questionnaire: major properties and scoring methods. *Pain* 1975;1:277–299.
30. Kantoff PW, Halabi S, Conaway M, et al. Hydrocortisone with or without mitoxantrone in men with hormone-refractory prostate cancer: results of the cancer and leukemia group B 9182 study [see comments]. *J Clin Oncol* 1999;17:2506–2513.
31. Perry CM, McTavish D. Estramustine phosphate sodium: a review of its pharmacodynamic and pharmacokinetic properties, and therapeutic efficacy in prostate cancer. *Drugs Aging* 1995;7:49–74.
32. Eklov S, Nilsson S, Larson A, et al. Evidence for a non-estrogenic cytostatic effect of estramustine on human prostatic carcinoma cells in vivo. *Prostate* 1992;20:43–50.
33. Stearns ME, Tew KD. Estramustine binds MAP-2 to inhibit microtubule assembly in vitro. *J Cell Sci* 1988;89:331–342.
34. Hartley-Asp B. Estramustine-induced mitotic arrest in two human prostate carcinoma cell lines DU 145 and PC-3. *Prostate* 1984;5:93–100.
35. Speicher LA, Barone L, Tew KD. Combined antimicrotubule activity of estramustine and Taxol in human prostatic carcinoma cell lines. *Cancer Res* 1992;52:4433–4440.
36. Mareel MM, Storme GA, Dragonetti CH, et al. Antiinvasive activity of estramustine on malignant MO4 mouse cells and on DU-145 human prostate carcinoma cells in vitro. *Cancer Res* 1988;48:1842–1849.
37. Seidman AD, Scher HI, Petrylak D, et al. Estramustine and vinblastine: use of prostate specific antigen as a clinical trial end point for hormone refractory prostatic cancer. *J Urol* 1992;147:931–934.
38. Hudes GR, Greenberg R, Krigel RL, et al. Phase II study of estramustine and vinblastine, two microtubule inhibitors, in hormone-refractory prostate cancer. *J Clin Oncol* 1992;10: 1754–1761.
39. Amato R, Logothetis C, Sella A, et al. Preliminary results of a phase II trial of estramustine (EMCYT), vinblastine (VLB), and mitomycin-C (MMC) for patients (pts) with progressive androgen independent prostate cancer (AIPCa). *Proc AACR* 1993;34.
40. Hudes G, Einhorn L, Ross E, et al. Vinblastine versus vinblastine plus oral estramustine phosphate for patients with hormone-refractory prostate cancer: a Hoosier Oncology Group and Fox Chase Network phase III trial. *J Clin Oncol* 1999;17:3160–3166.
41. Hussain MH, Pienta KJ, Redman BG, et al. Oral etoposide in the treatment of hormone-refractory prostate cancer. *Cancer* 1994;74:100–103.
42. Pienta KJ, Lehr JE. Inhibition of prostate cancer growth by estramustine and etoposide: evidence for interaction at the nuclear matrix. *J Urol* 1993;149:1622–1625.
43. Pienta KJ, Redman B, Hussain M, et al. Phase II evaluation of oral estramustine and oral etoposide in hormone-refractory adenocarcinoma of the prostate [see comments]. *J Clin Oncol* 1994;12:2005–2012.
44. Colleoni M, Graiff C, Vicario G, et al. Phase II study of estramustine, oral etoposide, and vinorelbine in hormone-refractory prostate cancer. *Am J Clin Oncol* 1997;20:383–386.
45. Hernes EH, Fossa SD, Vaage S, et al. Epirubicin combined with estramustine phosphate in hormone-resistant prostate cancer: a phase II study. *Br J Cancer* 1997;76:93–99.
46. Culine S, Kattan J, Zanetta S, et al. Evaluation of estramustine phosphate combined with weekly doxorubicin in patients with androgen-independent prostate cancer. *Am J Clin Oncol* 1998;21:470–474.

47. Ellerhorst JA, Tu SM, Amato RJ, et al. Phase II trial of alternating weekly chemohormonal therapy for patients with androgen-independent prostate cancer. *Clin Cancer Res* 1997;3:2371–2376.
48. Roth BJ, Yeap BY, Wilding G, et al. Taxol in advanced hormone-refractory carcinoma of the prostate. A phase II trial of the Eastern Cooperative Oncology Group. *Cancer* 1993; 72:2457–2460.
49. Hudes GR, Nathan F, Khater C, et al. Phase II trial of 96-hour paclitaxel plus oral estramustine phosphate in metastatic hormone-refractory prostate cancer. *J Clin Oncol* 1997; 15:3156–3163.
50. Smith DC, Esper P, Strawderman M, et al. Phase II trial of oral estramustine, oral etoposide, and intravenous paclitaxel in hormone-refractory prostate cancer. *J Clin Oncol* 1999; 17:1664–1671.
51. Kelly WK, Curley T, Slovin S, et al. Paclitaxel, estramustine, and carboplatin (TEC) in patients with advanced prostate cancer. *J Clin Oncol* 2001;19:44–53.
52. Petrylak DP, Macarthur RB, O'Connor J, et al. Phase I trial of docetaxel with estramustine in androgen-independent prostate cancer. *J Clin Oncol* 1999;17:958–967.
53. Kreis W, Budman DR, Fetten J, et al. Phase I trial of the combination of daily estramustine phosphate and intermittent docetaxel in patients with metastatic hormone refractory prostate carcinoma. *Ann Oncol* 1999;10:33–38.
54. Savarese DM, Taplin M-E, Marchesani B, et al. A phase II study of docetaxel, estramustine, and low dose hydrocortisone in hormone refractory prostate cancer: CALGB 9780. *Proc ASCO* 1999:321a.
55. Haldar S, Basu A, Croce CM. Bcl2 is the guardian of microtubule integrity. *Cancer Res* 1997;57:229–233.
56. Scher HI, Kelly WK. Suramin: defining the role in the clinic. *PPO Updates* 1993;7:1–15.
57. Myers CE, Stein C, LaRocca R, et al. Suramin: an antagonist of heparin binding tumor growth factors with activity against a broad spectrum of human tumors. *Proc ASCO* 1989;8:66.
58. Eisenberger MA, Reyno LM, Jodrell DI, et al. Suramin, an active drug for prostate cancer: interim observations in a phase I trial [see comments] [published erratum appears in *J Natl Cancer Inst* 1994;86:639–640]. *J Natl Cancer Inst* 1993;85:611–621.
59. Scher HI, Kelly WK. Flutamide withdrawal syndrome: its impact on clinical trials in hormone-refractory prostate cancer. *J Clin Oncol* 1993;11:1566–1572.
60. Kelly WK, Curley T, Leibretz C, et al. Prospective evaluation of hydrocortisone and suramin in patients with androgen-independent prostate cancer. *J Clin Oncol* 1995;13:2208–2213.
61. Halabi S, Small EJ, Ansari RH, et al. Results of CALGB 9480, a phase III trial of 3 different doses of suramin for the treatment of hormone refractory prostate cancer (HRPC). *Proc ASCO* 2000;19.
62. Greco KE, Kulawiak L. Prostate cancer prevention: risk reduction through life-style, diet, and chemoprevention. *Oncol Nurs Forum* 1994;21:1504–1511.
63. Pollard M, Luckert PH, Sporn MB. Prevention of primary prostate cancer in Lobund-Wistar rats by N-(4-hydroxyphenyl)retinamide. *Cancer Res* 1991;51:3610–3611.
64. Trump DL, Smith DC, Stiff D, et al. A phase II trial of all-*trans*-retinoic acid in hormone-refractory prostate cancer: a clinical trial with detailed pharmacokinetic analysis. *Cancer Chemother Pharmacol* 1997;39:349–356.
65. Schwartz GG, Hulka BS. Is vitamin D deficiency a risk factor for prostate cancer? (Hypothesis.) *Anticancer Res* 1990; 10:1307–1311.
66. Smith DC, Johnson CS, Freeman CC, et al. A Phase I trial of calcitriol (1,25-dihydroxycholecalciferol) in patients with advanced malignancy. *Clin Cancer Res* 1999;5:1339–1345.
67. Carlin BI, Andriole GL. The natural history, skeletal complications, and management of bone metastases in patients with prostate carcinoma. *Cancer* 2000;88:2989–2994.
68. Scher HI, Sarkis A, Reuter V, et al. Changing pattern of expression of the epidermal growth factor receptor and transforming growth factor alpha in the progression of prostatic neoplasms. *Clin Cancer Res* 1995;1:545–550.
69. Craft N, Shostak Y, Carey M, et al. A mechanism for hormone-independent prostate cancer through modulation of androgen receptor signaling by the HER-2/neu tyrosine kinase [see comments]. *Nat Med* 1999;5:280–285.
70. Prewett M, Rockwell P, Rockwell RF, et al. The biologic effects of C225, a chimeric monoclonal antibody to the EGFR, on human prostate carcinoma. *J Immunother Emphasis Tumor Immunol* 1996;19:419–427.
71. Slovin SF, Kelly WF, Cohen R, et al. Epidermal growth factor receptor (EGFr) monoclonal antibody (MoAb) C225 and doxorubicin (DOC) in androgen-independent prostate cancer (PC): results of a phase Ib/IIa study. *Proc ACSO* 1997;16:311a.
72. Ross JS, Sheehan CE, Hayner-Buchan AM, et al. Prognostic significance of HER-2/neu gene amplification status by fluorescence in situ hybridization of prostate carcinoma. *Cancer* 1997;79:2162–2170.
73. Agus DB, Scher HI, Higgins B, et al. Response of prostate cancer to anti-Her-2/neu antibody in androgen-dependent and -independent human xenograft models. *Cancer Res* 1999;59:4761–4764.
74. Morris MJ, Reuter VE, Kelly WK, et al. A phase II trial of Herceptin alone and with Taxol for the treatment of prostate cancer. *Proc ASCO* 2000;19:330a.
75. Sirotnak FM, Miller VA, Scher HI, et al. Efficacy of cytotoxic agents against human tumor xenografts is markedly enhanced by co-administration of ZD1839 (IressaTM), an inhibitor of EGF receptor tyrosine kinase. *Proc AACR-NCI-EORTC Intl Conf* 1999;5.
76. Baselga J, Ranson M, Ferry D, et al. A pharmacokinetic/pharmacodynamic trial of ZD1839 (IRESSATM), a novel oral epidermal growth factor receptor tyrosine kinase (EGFR-TK) inhibitor, in patients with 5 selected tumor types (a phase I/II trial of continuous once-daily treatment). *Proc AACR-NCI-EORTC Intl Conf* 1999;5:3735s.
77. Munster PN, Zheng FF, Srethapakdi M, et al. Induction of differentiation and apoptosis in human breast cancer cell lines by modified geldanamycin derivative (17-AAG). *Proc AACR-NCI-EORTC Intl Conf* 1999;5:3802s.
78. Roh H, Hirose CB, Boswell CB, et al. Synergistic antitumor effects of HER2/neu antisense oligodeoxynucleotides and conventional chemotherapeutic agents. *Surgery* 1999;126:413–421.
79. Hortobagyi GN, Hung MC, Lopez-Berestein G. A phase I multicenter study of E1A gene therapy for patients with metastatic breast cancer and epithelial ovarian cancer that

overexpresses HER-2/neu or epithelial ovarian cancer. *Hum Gene Ther* 1998;9:1775–1798.
80. Liu QY, Stein CA. Taxol and estramustine-induced modulation of human prostate cancer cell apoptosis via alteration in bcl-xL and bak expression. *Clin Cancer Res* 1997;3:2039–2046.
81. Weiss LM, Warnke RA, Sklar J, et al. Molecular analysis of the t(14;18) chromosomal translocation in malignant lymphomas. *N Engl J Med* 1987;317:1185–1189.
82. Gross A, McDonnell JM, Korsmeyer SJ. BCL-2 family members and the mitochondria in apoptosis. *Genes Dev* 1999;13:1899–1911.
83. Tu SM, McConnell K, Marin MC, et al. Combination adriamycin and suramin induces apoptosis in bcl-2 expressing prostate carcinoma cells [published erratum appears in *Cancer Lett* 1996;99:247]. *Cancer Lett* 1995;93:147–155.
84. Sullivan GF, Amenta PS, Villanueva JD, et al. The expression of drug resistance gene products during the progression of human prostate cancer. *Clin Cancer Res* 1998;4:1393–1403.
85. Keshgegian AA, Johnston E, Cnaan A. Bcl-2 oncoprotein positivity and high MIB-1 (Ki-67) proliferative rate are independent predictive markers for recurrence in prostate carcinoma. *Am J Clin Pathol* 1998;110:443–449.
86. Huang A, Gandour-Edwards R, Rosenthal SA, et al. p53 and bcl-2 immunohistochemical alterations in prostate cancer treated with radiation therapy. *Urology* 1998;51:346–351.
87. Liu XH, Yao S, Kirschenbaum A, et al. NS398, a selective cyclooxygenase-2 inhibitor, induces apoptosis and down-regulates bcl-2 expression in LNCaP cells. *Cancer Res* 1998; 58:4245–4259.
88. Scher HI, Morris MJ, Tong WP, et al. A phase I trial of G3139 (Genta, Inc.), a BCL2 antisense drug, by continuous infusion (CI) as a single agent and with weekly Taxol (T). *Proc ASCO* 2000;19.
89. DiPaola RS, Rafi MM, Vyas V, et al. Phase I clinical and pharmacologic study of 13-cis-retinoic acid, interferon alfa, and paclitaxel in patients with prostate cancer and other advanced malignancies. *J Clin Oncol* 1999;17:2213–2218.
90. Graff JR, Konicek BW, McNulty AM, et al. Increased AKT activity contributes to prostate cancer progression by dramatically accelerating prostate tumor growth and diminishing p27Kip1 expression. *J Biol Chem* 2000;275:24500–24505.
91. Li J, Yen C, Liaw D, et al. PTEN, a putative protein tyrosine phosphatase gene mutated in human brain, breast, and prostate cancer [see comments]. *Science* 1997;275:1943–1947.
92. Steck PA, Pershouse MA, Jasser SA, et al. Identification of a candidate tumour suppressor gene, MMAC1, at chromosome 10q23.3 that is mutated in multiple advanced cancers. *Nat Genet* 1997;15:356–362.
93. Datta SR, Brunet A, Greenberg ME. Cellular survival: a play in three Akts. *Genes Dev* 1999;13:2905–2927.
94. Vlietstra RJ, van Alewijk DC, Hermans KG, et al. Frequent inactivation of PTEN in prostate cancer cell lines and xenografts. *Cancer Res* 1998;58:2720–2723.
95. Pesche S, Latil A, Muzeau F, et al. PTEN/MMAC1/TEP1 involvement in primary prostate cancers. *Oncogene* 1998; 16:2879–2883.
96. Whang YE, Wu X, Suzuki H, et al. Inactivation of the tumor suppressor PTEN/MMAC1 in advanced human prostate cancer through loss of expression. *Proc Natl Acad Sci U S A* 1998;95:5246–5250.
97. McMenamin ME, Soung P, Perera S, et al. Loss of PTEN expression in paraffin-embedded primary prostate cancer correlates with high Gleason score and advanced stage. *Cancer Res* 1999;59:4291–4296.
98. Hsu AL, Ching TT, Wang DS, et al. The cyclooxygenase-2 inhibitor celecoxib induces apoptosis by blocking Akt activation in human prostate cancer cells independently of Bcl-2. *J Biol Chem* 2000;275:11397–11403.
99. Schlaeppi JM, Wood JM. Targeting vascular endothelial growth factor (VEGF) for anti-tumor therapy by anti-VEGF neutralizing monoclonal antibodies or by VEGF receptor tyrosine-kinase inhibitors. *Cancer Metastasis Rev* 1999;18:473–481.
100. Duque JL, Loughlin KR, Adam RM, et al. Plasma levels of vascular endothelial growth factor are increased in patients with metastatic prostate cancer. *Urology* 1999;54:523–527.
101. Rabbani SA, Harakidas P, Guo Y, et al. Synthetic inhibitor of matrix metalloproteases decreases tumor growth and metastases in a syngeneic model of rat prostate cancer in vivo. *Int J Cancer* 2000;87:276–282.
102. Bloomfield DJ. Should bisphosphonates be part of the standard therapy of patients with multiple myeloma or bone metastases from other cancers? An evidence-based review [see comments]. *J Clin Oncol* 1998;16:1218–1225.
103. Diel IJ, Solomayer EF, Costa SD, et al. Reduction in new metastases in breast cancer with adjuvant clodronate treatment [see comments]. *N Engl J Med* 1998;339:357–363.
104. Boissier S, Magnetto S, Frappart L, et al. Bisphosphonates inhibit prostate and breast carcinoma cell adhesion to unmineralized and mineralized bone extracellular matrices. *Cancer Res* 1997;57:3890–3894.
105. Boissier S, Ferreras M, Peyruchaud O, et al. Bisphosphonates inhibit breast and prostate carcinoma cell invasion, an early event in the formation of bone metastases. *Cancer Res* 2000;60:2949–2954.
106. Hussain M, Petrylak D, Fisher E, et al. Docetaxel (Taxotere) and estramustine versus mitoxantrone and prednisone for hormone-refractory prostate cancer: scientific basis and design of Southwest Oncology Group Study 9916. *Semin Oncol* 1999;26:55–60.
107. Jungi WF, Bernhard J, Hurny C, et al. Effect of carboplatin on response and palliation in hormone-refractory prostate cancer. Swiss Group for Clinical Cancer Research (SAKK). *Supp Care Cancer* 1998;6:462–468.
108. Mohler JL, Gomella LG, Crawford ED, et al. Phase II evaluation of coumarin (1,2-benzopyrone) in metastatic prostatic carcinoma. *Prostate* 1992;20:123–131.
109. Storlie JA, Buckner JC, Wiseman GA, et al. Prostate specific antigen levels and clinical response to low dose dexamethasone for hormone-refractory metastatic prostate carcinoma. *Cancer* 1995;76:96–100.
110. Neri B, Barbagli G, Bellesi P, et al. Weekly epidoxorubicin therapy in hormone-refractory metastatic prostate cancer. *Anticancer Res* 1997;17:3817–3820.
111. Delaere KP, Leliefeld H, Peulen F, et al. Phase II study of epirubicin in advanced hormone-resistant prostatic carcinoma. *Br J Urol* 1992;70:641–642.
112. Tannock IF, Erwin TJ, Stewart DJ, et al. Phase II multicenter study of epirubicin for hormone-resistant prostatic

cancer with measurable soft tissue disease. *Am J Clin Oncol* 1993;16:156–158.

113. Schultz PK, Kelly WK, Begg C, et al. Post-therapy change in prostate-specific antigen levels as a clinical trial endpoint in hormone-refractory prostatic cancer: a trial with 10-ethyl-deaza-aminopterin. *Urology* 1994;44:237–242.
114. Scher HI, Curley T, Geller N, et al. Gallium nitrate in prostatic cancer: evaluation of antitumor activity and effects on bone turnover. *Cancer Treat Rep* 1987;71:887–893.
115. Morant R, Ackermann D, Trinkler F, et al. Gemcitabine in hormone refractory metastatic prostate carcinoma—a phase II study of the SAKK. *Proc ASCO* 1997;16:311a.
116. Mahjoubi M, Azab M, Ghosn M, et al. Phase II trial of ifosfamide in the treatment of metastatic hormone-refractory patients with prostatic cancer. *Cancer Invest* 1990;8:477–481.
117. van Haelst-Pisani CM, Richardson RL, Su J, et al. A phase II study of recombinant human alpha-interferon in advanced hormone-refractory prostate cancer. *Cancer* 1992;70:2310–2312.
118. Bulbul MA, Huben RP, Murphy GP. Interferon-beta treatment of metastatic prostate cancer. *J Surg Oncol* 1986;33: 231–233.
119. Reese DM, Tchekmedyian S, Chapman Y, et al. A phase II trial of irinotecan in hormone-refractory prostate cancer. *Invest New Drugs* 1998;16:353–359.
120. Kantoff PW, Block C, Letvak L, et al. 14-Day continuous infusion of mitoxantrone in hormone-refractory metastatic adenocarcinoma of the prostate. *Am J Clin Oncol* 1993;16: 489–491.
121. Trivedi C, Redman B, Flaherty LE, et al. Weekly 1-hour infusion of paclitaxel. Clinical feasibility and efficacy in patients with hormone-refractory prostate carcinoma. *Cancer* 2000;89:431–436.
122. Hudes GR, Kosierowski R, Greenberg R, et al. Phase II study of topotecan in metastatic hormone-refractory prostate cancer. *Invest New Drugs* 1995;13:235–240.
123. Dexeus F, Logothetis CJ, Samuels ML, et al. Continuous infusion of vinblastine for advanced hormone-refractory prostate cancer. *Cancer Treat Rep* 1985;69:885–886.
124. Caty A, Oudard S, Humblet Y, et al. Phase II study of vinorelbine in patients with hormone refractory prostate cancer. *Proc ASCO* 1997;16:311a.
125. Wozniak AJ, Blumenstein BA, Crawford ED, et al. Cyclophosphamide, methotrexate, and 5-fluorouracil in the treatment of metastatic prostate cancer. A Southwest Oncology Group study. *Cancer* 1993;71:3975–3978.
126. Dik P, Blom JH, Schroder FH. Mitomycin C and aminoglutethimide in the treatment of metastatic prostatic cancer: a phase II study. *Br J Urol* 1992;70:542–545.
127. Osborne CK, Blumenstein BA, Crawford ED, et al. Phase II study of platinum and mitoxantrone in metastatic prostate cancer: a Southwest Oncology Group study. *Eur J Cancer* 1992;28:477–468.
128. Berlin JD, Propert KJ, Trump D, et al. 5-Fluorouracil and leucovorin in patients with hormone refractory prostate cancer. *Am J Clin Oncol* 1998;21:171–176.
129. Chao D, von Schlippe M, Harland SJ. A phase II study of continuous infusion 5-fluorouracil (5-FU) with epirubicin and cisplatin in metastatic, hormone-resistant prostate cancer: an active new regimen. *Eur J Cancer* 1997;33:1230–1233.

129a. Moulard-Durdux C, Dufour B, Hennequin C, et al. Phase II study of oral cyclophosphamide and oral etoposide combination in hormone-refractory prostate carcinoma patients. *Cancer* 1996;77:1144–1148

130. Pienta KJ, Redman BG, Bandekar R, et al. A phase II trial of oral estramustine and oral etoposide in hormone refractory prostate cancer. *Urology* 1997;50:401–406.
131. Sinibaldi VJ, Carducci M, Laufer M, et al. Preliminary evaluation of a short course of estramustine phosphate and docetaxel (Taxotere) in the treatment of hormone-refractory prostate cancer. *Semin Oncol* 1999;26:45–48.
132. Cervellino JC, Araujo CE, Pirisi C, et al. Combined hormonal therapy with high-dose diethylstilbestrol diphosphate (DES-DP) intravenous infusion plus vindesine (VND) for the treatment of advanced prostatic carcinoma: a controlled study. *J Surg Oncol* 1990;43:250–253.
133. Patel SR, Kvols LK, Hahn RG, et al. A phase II randomized trial of megestrol acetate or dexamethasone in the treatment of hormonally refractory advanced carcinoma of the prostate. *Cancer* 1990;66:655–658.
134. Newling DW, Fossa SD, Tunn UW, et al. Mitomycin C versus estramustine in the treatment of hormone resistant metastatic prostate cancer: the final analysis of the European Organization for Research and Treatment of Cancer genitourinary group prospective randomized phase III study (30865). *J Urol* 1993;150:1840–1844.

52

NOVEL TUMOR-DIRECTED THERAPEUTIC STRATEGIES FOR HORMONE-REFRACTORY PROSTATE CANCER

DANIEL J. GEORGE
GEORGE WILDING

Despite nearly 60 years of androgen ablative therapy for advanced prostate cancer, no treatment has been demonstrated to prolong survival of patients with hormone-refractory disease. Many of these patients progress with systemic symptoms (including weight loss and fatigue) and local complications (e.g., bone pain, cord compression, and urinary obstruction). For these reasons, new treatment strategies are needed to target prostate cancer cells in an androgen-independent manner. Unfortunately, novel treatments for hormone-refractory prostate cancer (HRPC) are limited by our understanding of the biology of this disease, identification of functional targets for therapy, response assessment, and new drug development. Clinical trials of novel therapeutics currently reflect these limitations. However, as new functional targets, surrogate end points, and drugs emerge, improvements in patient selection, trial design, and response assessment may increase our success. Ultimately, prolonged survival and improved quality of life are the clinical end points by which all new treatments must be judged, but given the difficulty in performing phase III studies in HRPC patients, few novel agents have undergone such testing. The focus of this chapter is to outline the preclinical and clinical data regarding some tumor-directed treatment strategies currently in development, including those that target differentiation and growth factor signaling.

DIFFERENTIATION THERAPY

Differentiation is the process whereby immature cells develop into a characteristic phenotype of a mature cell. In cancer, differentiation is often characterized by a cell-cycle arrest (sometimes referred to as terminal differentiation); expression of cellular functions similar to nonmalignant cells; and, in some cases, results in programmed cell death or apoptosis. The concept of promoting differentiation of cancer cells as a means of stopping their growth has been well established in preclinical models for years (1); however, not until French and Chinese investigators showed that patients with promyelocytic leukemia could achieve complete remission by taking high doses of retinoic acid (RA) did differentiation therapy demonstrate a clinical benefit (2,3). Since then, a number of agents have been tested in various malignancies, including prostate cancer. Using *in vitro* and *in vivo* tumor models of HRPC, a number of research groups have demonstrated data supporting the hypothesis that inducing the differentiation of these cancer cells can slow the progression of disease. Below is a summary of preclinical and clinical data on several classes of differentiation agents that have been tested in HRPC, including RA, peroxisome proliferator–activated receptor (PPAR) agonists, short-chain fatty acids, and vitamin D analogs.

Retinoic Acid

Vitamin A (retinol) and its derivative RA are endogenous compounds that have been implicated in the growth and differentiation of epithelial cells (4). RA and its derivatives, collectively known as the retinoids, bind to two classes of nuclear receptors: RA receptors (RARs) and retinoid X receptors (RXRs). The RXR ligand-receptor complexes occur as homodimers or heterodimers, whereas the RAR ligand-receptor complexes always form heterodimers with RXRs. Once formed, these receptor dimers interact with retinoid response elements on the regulatory sequences of genes to modulate gene expression directly or indirectly by inhibiting transcription factors, such as AP-1.

In prostate cancer cells, retinoids and their cognate receptors are present but appear to be less abundant than in normal prostate tissue or benign prostatic hyperplasia (5). Early studies showed that an RA analog, N-4-(hydroxyphenyl) retinamide, could diminish the incidence of primary and metastatic prostate carcinoma in rats and inhibit the growth of human PC3 cells through a G1/S cell-cycle arrest and suppression of *c-myc* gene expression (6–8). More recently, synthetic retinoids were shown to induce marked growth inhibition of androgen-sensitive and androgen-independent prostate cell lines through a cell-cycle arrest at S phase, followed by an increase in reactive oxygen species and rate of apoptosis (9,10). Furthermore, use of synthetic retinoids selective for RXR or RAR receptors has shown that both can inhibit prostate cancer cell growth (11). However, RA itself has shown mixed results, resulting in growth promotion of some cell lines and growth inhibition of others, with no association to RAR subtype expression (12).

Based on the preclinical evidence mentioned earlier, as well as other reports, and an anecdotal clinical effect of all-*trans*-RA in an HRPC patient, a phase II study using all-*trans*-RA in HRPC was completed at the University of Pittsburgh Cancer Institute. Seventeen patients received 50 mg per m^2 of all-*trans*-RA orally three times a day for 2 weeks, followed by a 1-week hiatus repeated every 22 days (13). Unfortunately, in 13 evaluable patients, there were no responses, due in part to an increased clearance that occurred with a few days of beginning treatment. One possible solution is to inhibit the metabolism of RA. Liarozole (R75251) is an imidazole derivative that has been shown to inhibit RA metabolism and to result in RA-mimetic effects *in vivo* (14). In prostate cancer tumor models, liarozole inhibited androgen-dependent (Dunning G and H) and androgen-independent (PIF1 and AT-6) tumors (15,16). Based on these and other preclinical data, researchers from the Netherlands began clinical trials of liarozole in HRPC patients.

A phase II study using two dosing schemes of oral liarozole (150 mg and 300 mg twice a day) was completed in HRPC patients who had failed at least first-line androgen-ablative therapy (17). Of 42 patients who were evaluated, 23 experienced at least one point improvement in their pain score. Furthermore, 11 patients improved their World Health Organization performance status by one point. With regard to prostate-specific antigen (PSA) response, 17 out of 42 patients exhibited a 50% or greater decline in serum PSA levels, compared to baseline. Based on these results, a European multicenter randomized phase III trial comparing liarozole to a secondary hormonal treatment was undertaken.

Using cyproterone acetate, a synthetic steroid with progestational and antiandrogenic properties, as the standard second line hormonal therapy, patients were randomized to receive liarozole or cyproterone acetate (18). In this study of 321 patients, those that received liarozole demonstrated a 20% PSA response rate compared to 4% with cyproterone acetate ($p < .001$) and had an adjusted hazards ratio for survival of 0.74 (18). Although these results suggest patients benefited from liarozole, other secondary hormonal manipulations have shown similar or greater response rates in the United States. Therefore, liarozole has not been adopted as standard therapy in this country. More randomized studies are needed to further define the efficacy of liarozole and retinoid pathway, in general, as a target for therapy.

Peroxisome Proliferator–Activated Receptor Agonists

Similar to other nuclear receptors, PPAR-gamma functions as a regulator of numerous genes, some of which appear to induce differentiation in specific tissues. For example, PPAR-gamma is highly expressed in adipocytes and induces differentiation of several preadipocyte cell lines (19), whereas overexpression of PPAR-gamma in fibroblasts and myoblast cells induces adipocyte differentiation (20). PPAR-gamma forms a heterodimer complex with the RXR, which binds to specific recognition sites on DNA. On binding of ligand for either receptor, the complex activates transcription of specific genes that promote adipocyte differentiation. Several natural and synthetic ligands for PPAR-gamma have been identified, such as prostaglandins and arachidonic acid metabolites (21,22). Also included in this group of agonists is troglitazone, a member of the thiazolidinedione class of drugs, which is also a new class of antidiabetic drugs developed since 1990 (23).

Recent studies have demonstrated that troglitazone induces differentiation of liposarcoma, breast cancer, and prostate cancer cell lines *in vitro* (24–26). In prostate cancer studies, troglitazone was shown to decrease proliferation, induce morphologic changes, and, in PSA-producing LNCaP cells, decrease PSA production by 50%, independent of growth inhibition (26). In liposarcoma patients, a "proof of principle" open-label phase II trial was recently published demonstrating evidence that *in vivo* troglitazone induced differentiation. In this study, patients were treated with daily oral troglitazone and underwent serial tumor biopsies, revealing evidence of differentiation, including histologic changes, decreases in the mitotic index, altered gene expression, and altered triglyceride metabolites by proton nuclear magnetic resonance spectroscopy (27). These results led to the first study of troglitazone in prostate cancer patients.

Using the U.S. Food and Drug Administration–approved daily dose of 800 mg orally, we tested 40 prostate cancer patients with evidence of a rising serum PSA level after local therapy (hormone-naïve) or androgen-ablative therapy (hormone-refractory). The initial results showed no response by the criteria established for the study—specifically, a 50% drop in two consecutive serum PSA levels, compared to the pretreatment level; however, approximately one-fourth of the men demonstrated a sustained stabilization or a decrease in their serum PSA levels (28). Toxicity was noted in only one patient who experienced grade 2 transaminitis that completely reversed with discontinuation of the drug. These results suggest that, as is the case preclinically, PPAR-gamma agonists may result in some growth-inhibitory effect, perhaps through differentiation, with minimal toxicity, but further investigation is needed to determine the significance of these findings.

Phenylacetate and Phenylbutyrate

The phenyl fatty acids phenylacetate (PA) and phenylbutyrate (PB) represent a class of agents that has been shown to induce differentiation of HRPC cells. Originally developed as a treatment for children with urea cycle disorders (29), PA has also been used safely in children with sickle cell anemia and thalassemia to induce fetal hemoglobin production (30,31) and to treat adults with chemotherapy-induced hyperammonemia syndrome (32). In these settings, PA appears to be safe and well tolerated. Samid et al. first demonstrated that PA induced differentiation of various human leukemic cell lines *in vitro* (33). Against prostate cancer cell lines, treatment with PA resulted in dose-dependent growth arrest *in vitro* while inducing markers of differentiation, including morphologic changes (e.g., lipid deposition) and altered gene expression patterns consistent with phenotypic differentiation (34). Although the mechanism of action of PA remains unresolved, effects on gene expression by modifications of lipid metabolism and DNA methylation, inhibition of isoprenylation, and glutamine depletion have been proposed (35,36). Recently, several phase I studies have been conducted with this agent in patients with various solid tumors, including HRPC (37,38). Although neurotoxicity appears to be dose limiting, high concentrations of PA were achieved at well-tolerated doses. Unfortunately, *in vitro* data suggest that with differentiation, PA may actually induce PSA expression (39), making assessment of tumor response in many HRPC patients difficult in future studies.

Similar in structure, PB is β oxidized *in vivo* to PA in mitochondria of the liver and kidney, yet PB seems to exhibit distinct cellular and molecular effects from PA. Because this metabolism does not occur *in vitro*, parallel studies have shown that PB may have more potent cytotoxic effects than PA, independent of p53 mutational status or *mdr-1* expression (40). PB also induced multiple acetylated forms of histone H4 and inhibited telomerase activity in prostate cancer cells (41). Although the exact mechanism of action of PB is not known, at least two effects (i.e., inhibition of histone deacetylation and activation of PPAR-gamma) are likely involved. PB has also undergone initial phase I testing, showing excellent tolerance and safety; however, the effects on serum PSA are of unclear significance. In a comparison between intravenous and oral formulations, 5 of 19 (intravenous-formulated) and 4 of 11 (oral) HRPC patients demonstrated stable disease for 6 months or greater (42). Serum PSA levels typically rose during the dosing of PB and later returned to baseline. Further studies of both agents, perhaps in combination with other putative differentiating drugs, are anticipated.

Vitamin D

Over the past decade, mounting molecular, genetic, epidemiologic, and preclinical data suggest that 1,25-dihydroxyvitamin D [1,25$(OH)_2$ vitamin D] plays an important role in the carcinogenesis and progression of prostate cancer. Molecular studies have revealed that vitamin D receptors are present on prostate epithelial cells and in a number of prostate cancer cell lines (43,44). These prostate cell lines also express 24-hydroxylase activity, which is necessary to convert 25(OH) vitamin D to its active 1,25$(OH)_2$ form (45). Several groups have demonstrated that 1,25$(OH)_2$ vitamin D increases expression of the androgen receptor (AR), as well as androgen-regulated genes, including PSA (46–48). In addition, genetic studies have demonstrated that a polymorphic variant resulting in an elongated poly-A microsatellite in the 3'-untranslated region is associated with an increased risk of developing prostate cancer and is more likely associated with advanced disease (49).

Epidemiologic studies have further supported the significance of serum vitamin D levels in the development of prostate cancer. In 1990, Schwartz et al. showed a relationship with known risk factors for prostate cancer, including age, race, and living in northern latitudes, was associated with low serum levels of vitamin D (50). Later, Corder et al. showed that low serum 1,25$(OH)_2$ vitamin D levels correlated with an increased risk of palpable and high-grade tumors (51). Since then, Chan et al. and Giovannucci have shown a link between high dietary calcium intake and prostate cancer risk, hypothesizing that chronically high calcium intake might confer this risk by resulting in lower endogenous 1,25$(OH)_2$ vitamin D levels (52,53).

As a treatment, 1,25$(OH)_2$ vitamin D appears to have therapeutic efficacy in preclinical models. *In vitro* studies have demonstrated that various concentrations of 1,25$(OH)_2$ vitamin D can induce differentiation while reducing proliferation and metastasis (54–56). In animal models, treatment with 1,25$(OH)_2$ vitamin D has demonstrated therapeutic efficacy. Early studies demonstrated that 1,25$(OH)_2$ vitamin D inhibited growth of prostate xenografts (57). Because of concerns of dose-limiting hypercalcemia, a number of synthetic derivatives have been developed. Several of the compounds inhibit not only proliferation but also metastasis and invasion (58–60). Finally, there may be synergistic effects combining vitamin D or synthetic analogs with other targeted therapies. Most notably, synergistic effects have been demonstrated with vitamin D and RA, as well as with cisplatin (55,61).

Based on these and other data, a phase I study of 1,25$(OH)_2$ vitamin D was completed at the University of Pittsburgh. Doses ranged from 2 to 10 μg by mouth every other day (62). Unfortunately, hypercalcemia was seen at all dose levels and was the dose-limiting toxicity at the 10-µg dose. For this reason, vitamin D analogs with less hypercalcemic effects are currently under clinical development. These compounds should offer a larger therapeutic index and greater possibilities in combination with other differentiating agents or traditional cytotoxic agents.

Other Agents

In addition to the classes of agents mentioned earlier, a number of other targets have been identified for their potential differentiating properties. Cyclooxygenase inhibitors, for example, have been shown to inhibit the metabolism of arachidonic acid and thus decrease the production of a number of eicosanoids, some of which have been implicated in prostate carcinogenesis. Likewise, isoflavones and polyphenols, which may be prevalent in many eastern diets, are also thought to impact on the aggressiveness of prostate cancer. Finally, hybrid polar compounds, including hexamethylene bisacetamide, suberolanilide hydroxamic acid, and m-carboxycinamic acid bis-hydoxamide, may inhibit histone deacetylation similar to PA and PB, representing another class of agents to target differentiation (63). In the future, as the mechanisms of differentiation are further defined, more of these agents may be used in conjunction with other therapies.

SIGNAL TRANSDUCTION INHIBITORS

Androgen stimulation of prostate epithelial cells and cancer cells results in transcriptional activation of numerous genes affecting various cellular functions. Many of these androgen-regulated genes are small peptide growth factors that can alter cell growth, survival, and differentiation in an autocrine or paracrine loop. Because ARs are present in prostate cancer cells and the surrounding stromal elements, it is possible that androgen produces altered gene expression within the cancer cell itself or in the stromal cells, or both. Growth factors released by the cancer cells could bind to cognate receptors on the surface of the cancer cell and thus create an autocrine loop, whereas those secreted by the stromal cells might bind to receptors on nearby prostate cancer cells, resulting in paracrine activation. Much of the work leading to the therapeutic development of signal transduction inhibitors is based on molecular studies demonstrating the functional significance of these pathways. Table 52-1 represents some of the many signal transduction receptor pathways implicated in the growth and development of prostate cancer. Below is an overview of some of the growth factor signaling pathways that have been implicated in prostate cancer growth and survival and specific inhibitors under development.

Growth factor signal transduction is a multistep process (Fig. 52-1). Ligands bind with high affinity to extracellular sites on transmembrane receptor tyrosine kinases (RTKs), resulting in homodimerization of the receptors and cross-phosphorylation of specific tyrosine residues. Several different intracellular pathways can be activated through phosphorylation of these specific sites. For Ras activation, this process continues through binding and activation of docking molecules (e.g., Shc) and adaptor proteins (e.g., Grb2), which then bind to deoxyguanosine triphosphate-exchange factors that result in the phosphorylation of Ras. Ras activation propagates

TABLE 52-1. GROWTH FACTOR PATHWAYS IMPLICATED IN PROSTATE CANCER

Transforming growth factor (TGF)-beta family
Fibroblast growth factors (FGFs) (basic FGF, acidic FGF)
Epidermal growth factors (TGF-alpha, amphiregulin)
Her2/neu
Insulinlike growth factors (I and II)
Platelet-derived growth factor (A and B)
Neurotrophins (nerve growth factor)
Vascular endothelial growth factors
Neurotensin
Endothelins
Keratinocyte family
Colony-stimulating factors (CSFs) (granulocyte macrophage-CSF, macrophage-CSF, SCF)

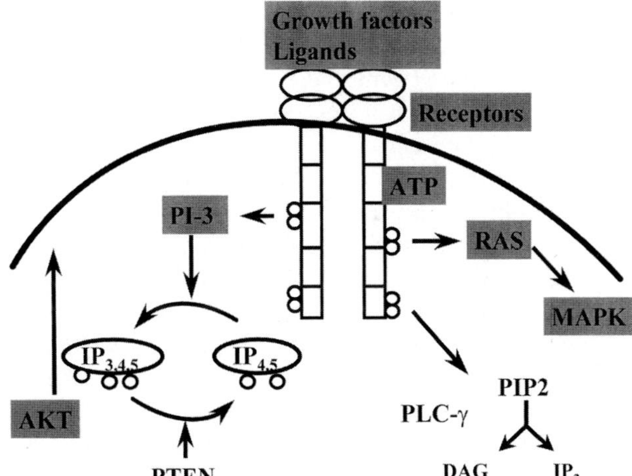

FIGURE 52-1. Drug targets for signal transduction inhibition. Growth factor signal transduction is thought to offer a promising array of targets for therapeutic intervention in cancer. Neutralizing antibodies can sequester growth factor ligands and/or competitively inhibit their binding to cell surface tyrosine kinase receptors. Small molecules can bind to the adenosine triphosphate–binding sites of these receptors and selectively inhibit specific receptor types. Farnesyl transferase inhibitors can block the activation of RAS, a critical molecule in many of these pathways, while selective kinase inhibitors of phosphatidylinositol-3 kinase and various mitogen-activated protein kinases are in development. Akt activation, regulated by the tumor suppressor gene PTEN, may also represent an important future target. Antisense strategies may be useful at decreasing the expression of any one of these targets. Other pathways, including phospholipase C signaling, appear less critical. ATP, adenosine triphosphate; DAG, diacylglycerol; IP_3, inositol 3-phosphate; MAPK, mitogen-activated protein kinase; PI-3, phosphatidylinositol 3; PIP2, phosphatidylinositol-4,5-bisphosphate; PLCγ, phospholipase Cγ.

its signal through a series of serine-threonine kinases [known collectively as mitogen-activated protein kinases (MAPKs)], which amplify the signal with each successive step. Ultimately, this cascade leads to transcriptional activation of genes that function in a number of cellular processes, including proliferation, survival, and differentiation. Other intracellular signaling pathways activated by RTK include phosphatidylinositol-3 (PI-3) kinase/Akt, phospholipase C, and Janus tyrosine kinase/signal transducers and activators of transcription (STAT).

Inhibition of these signal transduction pathways can occur at several sites (Fig. 52-1). Specific ligands can be inhibited competitively (by antibodies or other molecules blocking the binding site on cell surface receptors) or noncompetitively by sequestering or otherwise altering ligand presentation. Alternatively, these pathways can be semispecifically inhibited by small molecules that penetrate the cell membrane and bind to ATP-binding sites on the cytosolic portion of RTK. In addition, inhibiting downstream intermediate proteins such as MAPK, PI-3 kinase, Akt, or other common targets can potentially block multiple RTK pathways. Other nonspecific methods of signal transduction inhibition include targeting immunophilins or chaperone proteins, which can alter the half-life of critical proteins in these pathways. Finally, gene therapy and antisense nucleotides can affect expression of one or more specific proteins that may alter the kinetics of these intracellular signals.

There have been numerous specific growth factors implicated in the growth and survival of prostate cancer. Although the mechanisms of androgen-independent growth of prostate cancer are poorly understood, many of these growth factor genes can be amplified in this setting. Although initially regulated by androgen, it is possible that through genetic changes, genes encoding one or more of these growth factors could be deregulated from androgen control. Furthermore, in the androgen-independent state, there may be cross-talk between the signal transduction pathways of peptide growth factors and the AR pathway. One example of this phenomenon has recently been demonstrated to involve the oncogene Her2/neu (64).

Her2/neu

The Her2/neu oncogene encodes a transmembrane glycoprotein with a tyrosine kinase domain that is structurally related to the epidermal growth factor (EGF) receptor superfamily (65). Gene amplification of Her2/neu has been detected in various solid tumors and correlates with a poor prognosis. In prostate cancer, amplification of Her2/neu varies, ranging from 8% to 44% in several series using fluorescence *in situ* hybridization analysis (66–68). Recently, Craft et al. demonstrated that overexpression of Her2/neu in an otherwise androgen-dependent prostate cancer cell line stimulated androgen-independent growth (64). Interestingly, androgen-regulated genes (including PSA) were expressed in the absence of androgen but only if AR was present, indicating that overexpression of Her2/neu could activate the AR pathway independent of androgen (64). This model suggests a novel mechanism for androgen- (ligand-) independent growth of prostate cancer and further points to peptide growth factor pathways as targets for new therapeutics.

Driven by these findings and the successful development of a humanized monoclonal anti-Her2/neu antibody (Herceptin) in combination with chemotherapy as first line treatment for women with Her2/neu–positive metastatic breast cancer (69), investigators are beginning to study combinations of chemotherapeutic agents (with activity in HRPC) and Herceptin. Most notably, a multicenter phase II study with paclitaxel and Herceptin is ongoing in HRPC patients. Although therapeutic antibodies such as Herceptin have demonstrated efficacy in solid tumors, they are limited by the development of antiidiotype antibodies and increased clearance. Alternatively, many growth factor pathways can be semispecifically blocked using small peptides that competitively inhibit the ATP-binding site of RTK. Because these growth factor pathways require energy-dependent phosphorylation for signal transduction, small peptide inhibitors can effectively block propagation of signaling at low nanomolar concentrations. Using such inhibitors, several other growth factor pathways have been targeted.

Epidermal Growth Factor

Like Her2/neu, other members of the EGF superfamily of growth factors and their cognate receptors may represent additional targets of future treatments of prostate cancer. As one of the first growth factors recognized to signal through a transmembrane tyrosine kinase receptor, EGF was soon found to be abundantly present in human prostatic fluid and prostate cancer cells (70,71). Receptors for EGF, which are also expressed by normal and malignant prostate epithelium under androgen control, can be activated by EGF or transforming growth factor (TGF)-α, both of which are mitogenic to human prostatic carcinoma *in vitro* (72–74). Since 1990, interactions between EGF, TGF-α, and other mitogens with growth inhibitory factors (TGF-β and the like) have been further characterized, suggesting a delicate biologic balance (75–78). This balance is clearly under androgen control in the normal prostate and many prostate cancer cell lines; androgen deprivation results in down-regulation of EGF receptor, whereas androgen and EGF down-regulate p27 and stimulate proliferation (79,80). EGF stimulation also activates androgen receptors while enhancing prekallikrein activator activity through MAPK signaling (81,82). Finally, EGF activity may be even more significant in androgen-independent prostate cancer, because these cell lines exhibit greater EGF receptor expression (83,84). For these reasons, inhibitors of the EGF pathway have been tested preclinically in prostate cancer animal models.

Using small peptide inhibitors semispecific for the EGF receptor, investigators have shown *in vitro* growth inhibition of a wide range of EGF-producing tumor cell lines, including prostate cancers (85,86). These results were enhanced when coupled with C225, a human EGF receptor monoclonal antibody (85). Both compounds have gone on to phase I testing, and C225 is currently being developed in conjunction with conventional chemotherapeutic regimens (87).

Platelet-Derived Growth Factor

Although data linking platelet-derived growth factor (PDGF) to prostate cancer growth and survival is less convincing than EGF, PDGF may also represent a functional target for therapy. Two closely related genes (PDGF A and B) comprise the PDGF family and bind to two receptors, PDGFα and -β, respectively. PDGF A is closely related to v-sis, the simian oncogene originally shown to transform cells by an autocrine loop (88). Like many polypeptide growth factors, the effects of PDGF are largely localized within the tissues in which it is produced; however, unlike its oncogenic relative, PDGF A and B appear to function to regulate epithelial and stromal interactions more through a paracrine model. For example, PDGF blocks the differentiation of prostatic stromal cells by TGF-beta (89). PDGF A may also function in prostatic carcinogenesis, because its expression is not seen in normal prostate and benign prostatic hyperplasia tissue, whereas in high-grade prostatic intraepithelial neoplasia and adenocarcinoma, PDGF A and PDGFα are overexpressed (90,91). PDGF has many possible functions in proliferation and transformation. In prostate cancer, however, it may also help to regulate apoptosis. In p53-deficient prostate cancer, overexpression of PDGF-mediated, radiation-induced apoptosis; however, the clinical significance of this finding remains unknown (92). Nonetheless, inhibition of PDGF receptors using small peptide inhibitors has also been successfully shown in prostate cancer models to effectively inhibit tumor growth (93). Unfortunately, results of these agents in clinical trials have not yet been reported.

Nerve Growth Factor

More than 20 years ago, the nerve growth factor (NGF) was found to be highly concentrated in the prostate of mammals, yet its clinical significance remains unclear (94). Although some researchers still contend that NGF and the family of related peptides collectively known as *neurotrophins* are neuron-specific growth factors, a body of evidence is growing to suggest that these growth factors may also influence the proliferation, differentiation, and survival of several epithelial cells and malignant cell types. The neurotrophins bind to specific transmembrane tyrosine kinase receptors known as *trk* receptors, which are expressed in nonneuronal tumors, including Wilms' tumor and prostate cancer (95,96). An oncogenic form of the trkA receptor has also been found in colon and papillary thyroid carcinomas (97,98). In prostate cancer, no mutated forms of trkA have been found (99); however, by immunocytochemistry, more than 90% of primary and metastatic human tumors express one of the trk receptors (100).

In the normal prostate, NGF appears to function as a paracrine growth factor. First, prostatic stroma–conditioned medium is rich in a number of growth factors, including NGF. Djakiew et al. showed that treating this conditioned medium with an anti-NGF antibody completely abrogated the growth stimulation, whereas antibodies of other growth factors did not (101). In addition, NGF appears to increase epithelial cell motility and prostate cancer invasiveness (102,103). For these reasons, specific inhibitors of the trk receptors have been developed for possible applications in prostate cancer treatment.

A lead compound known as CEP-751 (Cephalon, Inc.) is an indolocarbazole with potent inhibitory effects on all trk receptors (104). *In vitro* studies showed concentration that inhibits 50% of value for the trkA receptor in the low nanomolar concentrations, whereas *in vivo* studies using trkA-transformed cell lines showed antitumor activity (104). CEP-751 was also growth inhibitory in various prostate cancer cell lines and tumor models (100). Finally, using the Dunning H androgen-dependent tumor model, combinations of CEP-751 with androgen ablative therapy was additive (105). To date, two trk inhibitors, CEP-2563 and an oral form known as CEP-701, have been tested in phase I clinical trials, and definitive efficacy trials in HRPC are planned for CEP-701 in the near future.

Insulinlike Growth Factors

Insulinlike growth factors (IGFs) are thought to play an important role in the development of the prostate. The IGF family is composed of two genes (IGF-I and -II) and two distinct receptors: type I, which is a tyrosine kinase receptor that binds IGF-I and -II with equal affinity, and type II, which binds IGF-II exclusively. IGF-I and -II can be detected in the serum of humans and are largely bound to proteins called IGF-binding proteins (IGFBP). Like the previously mentioned growth factors, IGF-I and -II levels are elevated in prostatic tissues. In transgenic knockout mice deficient in IGF-I (–/–), prostate glands were significantly smaller with fewer duct tips than those seen in wild-type mice (106). Furthermore, this size difference could be partially reversed by administering exogenous IGF-1 to the IGF-I–null mice.

In prostate cancer, several different lines of evidence suggest that IGF-II may be important in prostate cancer growth. First, several prostate xenograft models express IGF-I and -II as well as receptors for each (107). In serum-free media PC3 cells, an androgen-independent prostate cancer cell line secretes IGF-II as well as IGFBP (-2, -3, -4, and -6) (108). *In vitro* cell growth of PC3 was inhibited by the addition of monoclonal antibodies to type 1 receptor or a serine protease inhibitor (blocking the proteolysis of IGFBP-3), suggesting an autocrine loop involving IGF-II and IGFBP-3 (108). Finally, *in situ* hybridization and immunohistochemistry of type 1 IGF receptor (IGFR) and IGF-II of prostatectomy samples revealed a decrease of type 1 IGFR in high-grade prostatic intraepithelial neoplasia and adenocarcinoma compared to normal epithelium, whereas IGF-II was increased in the same adenocarcinoma lesions, suggesting a role in prostate carcinogenesis (109).

IGF-I is also present in prostate cancer tumor models and is likely to play an important role in prostate cancer progression. In a large T antigen transgenic adenocarcinoma of a mouse prostate model, IGF-I expression increased with the progression of prostate cancer in the androgen-dependent but remained at nontransgenic levels in the androgen-independent stage, whereas IGF-II expression remained low throughout (110). IGF-I has also been shown to have growth stimulatory effects on DU-145, another androgen-independent prostate cancer cell line, and PC3 cells (107) that are blocked by type 1 IGFR antisense or small peptide competitive inhibitors of IGF-I binding (111).

Adding to the complexity of the IGF axis is IGFBP, which may control the function of IGF-I and -II. Castration of mice bearing the androgen-dependent Shionogi carcinomas results in increased expression of IGFBP-5 and a decrease in IGFBP-3 and -4, coinciding with 90% tumor reduction (112). In contrast, the androgen-dependent CWR22 prostate cancer cell line decreased IGFBP-5 expression with castration (113). IGFBP-3 has been demonstrated to stimulate prostate cancer proliferation through proteolysis or release of IGF-II at concentrations from 20 to 50 ng per mL but inhibited growth at concentrations greater than 150 ng per mL (114,115). Meanwhile, IGFBP-1 was found to block the mitogenic effects of IGF-II in DU-145 (116). Finally, PSA, a serine protease, has been shown to cleave IGFBP-3; however, the functional significance of this finding remains unknown (117).

Perhaps the most compelling evidence indicating the functional importance of IGF-I comes from population studies. In 1998, Chan et al. reported on the relationship between plasma IGF-1 levels and prostate cancer, citing a relative risk of 4.3 for men in the highest quartile compared to men in the lowest quartile (118). This association was independent of PSA levels. Furthermore, IGF levels increased the detection rate of prostate cancer over PSA alone (119).

Based on the previously mentioned data, specific inhibitors of the IGF axis are actively being developed. Unfortunately, to date no agents have completed clinical testing. One intriguing possibility is the use of somatostatin to lower IGF levels in patients with tumors, such as prostate cancer. Two small studies have been reported showing the feasibility of lowering serum IGF levels in patients; however, no clinical efficacy has been described (120,121).

Endothelin 1

Endothelin 1 (ET-1) is a potent vasoconstrictor that has been identified as a mitogen for several cancer cell types and may represent a unique target for therapy in HRPC. Originally isolated from endothelial cells, ET-1 is the prototype of the ET family, which includes ET-2 and ET-3. These ligands bind to the cell surface, G-coupled receptors ET_A and ET_B. ET_A has a high affinity for ET-1, whereas ET_B is nonselective for ET-1, -2, and -3. Although ET-1 is produced by a number of cell types, it is concentrated in seminal fluid and overexpressed by the epithelial cells of the prostate (122). ET_A receptors are expressed largely on the prostatic stroma, whereas ET_B predominates on the epithelium (123).

In prostate cancer, ET-1 may play an important role in the progression and morbidity of advanced disease. Nelson et al. demonstrated an elevated median plasma level of ET-1 in HRPC patients, compared to those with localized prostate cancer or normal controls (124). In contrast to benign prostate epithelium, prostate adenocarcinoma expresses very little of the ET_B receptor, at least in some cases, because of methylation, whereas ET_A expression is unchanged (125). In prostate cancer cell lines, ET-1 appears to be up-regulated by interleukin-1, tumor necrosis factor-alpha, and TGF-beta (126). Although ET-1 appears to demonstrate weak mitogenic activity by itself, *in vitro* it appears to act synergistically with several other polypeptide growth factors (127). Recently, ET-1 has been shown to cooperate with nitric oxide in promoting endothelial cell migration and increased vascularity in gliomas, suggesting a role in angiogenesis (128,129). In addition, ET-1 has been shown to promote new bone formation (124,130). Finally, because of its homology to the snake venom sarafotoxins, it may possess nociceptive properties as well (131). For these reasons, selective ET_A inhibitors have been developed for clinical study in prostate cancer.

Recently, an orally bioavailable, racemic version of a highly potent and selective ET_A-receptor antagonist called ABT-627 was tested in two phase I studies, including HRPC patients. Overall, the drug was well tolerated and resulted in reduced subjective pain or narcotic use in 70% of the patients treated (132). Moreover, serum PSA levels stabilized or declined in 68% of patients treated. Although no measurable responses were noted, these results warranted further investigation. Currently, randomized phase II trials are ongoing.

Downstream Targets

As stated earlier, many of the cell surface growth factor receptor pathways activate common downstream proteins that may represent appropriate targets for therapy. For example, the MAPK cascade is a series of serine/threonine and tyrosine kinases that propagate cell surface signals when activated by phosphorylation. Many of these signals result in transcriptional activation and, ultimately, growth and differentiation. The kinetics of this pathway may in turn control the end result of this signal, and various cell surface receptors may differ in this manner. Nonetheless, because many pathways important to prostate cancer growth, including EGF, NGF, PDGF, and Her2/neu, activate MAPKs, these proteins may represent important targets for therapy. Currently, MAPK inhibitors are early in development, but several are likely to reach clinical trials in the near future.

Parallel to the MAPK signal transduction cascade, many receptor tyrosine kinase pathways result in the phosphorylation and activation of PI-3 kinase and Akt. Recent studies have demonstrated that these proteins are regulated by an important tumor suppressor gene in prostate cancer and therefore may represent another important and common downstream target in prostate cancer. PTEN is a known dual-specificity phosphatase with protein and phospholipid substrates (133). Recently, PTEN was shown to dephosphorylate lipid substrates for PI-3 kinase, including those that function in the activation of Akt (134,135). Like MAPK, PI-3 kinase/Akt is a common downstream pathway activated by many cell surface growth factor receptors. Furthermore, in androgen-independent prostate cancer cell lines with loss of PTEN expression, Akt appears to be constitutively active, suggesting that PTEN may function in part as a negative regulator of this survival pathway. Therefore, inhibition of Akt, especially in prostate cancer in which PTEN function is impaired, represents another promising target. Although development of such inhibitors is active, no drugs are yet available for clinical testing.

As illustrated in Figure 52-1, a third downstream pathway involves the activation of phospholipase C and downstream signaling through protein kinase C isoforms. Perturbations of this pathway with agonists and antagonists have demonstrated significant antitumor effects. Currently, bryostatin-1 is a partial agonist/antagonist of the protein kinase C family that is in clinical trials as a single agent and in combination with chemotherapy against several solid tumors, including HRPC.

REFERENCES

1. Sacks L. Control of normal cell differentiation and the phenotypic reversion of malignancy in myeloid leukemia. *Nature* 1978;274:535–539.
2. Castaigne S, Chomienne C, Daniel MT, et al. All-*trans* retinoic acid as a differentiation therapy for acute promyelocytic leukemia. I. Clinical results. *Blood* 1990;76(9):1704–1709.
3. Chen ZX, Xue YQ, Zhang R, et al. A clinical and experimental study on all-*trans* retinoic acid-treated acute promyelocytic leukemia patients. *Blood* 1991;78(6):1413–1419.
4. Lotan R. Mechanisms of action of retinoids. *Cancer* 1986;38:13–26.
5. Pasquali D, Thaller C, Eichele G. Abnormal level of retinoic acid in prostate cancer tissues. *J Clin Endocrinol Metab* 1996;81:2186–2191.
6. Pollard M, Luckert PH, Sporn MB. Prevention of primary prostate cancer in Lobund-Wistar rats by N-(4-hydroxyphenyl) retinamide. *Cancer Res* 1991;51:3610–3611.
7. Slawin K, Kadmon D, Park SH, et al. Dietary fenretinide, a synthetic retinoid, decreases the tumor incidence and the tumor mass of ras+myc–induced carcinomas in the mouse prostate reconstitution model system. *Cancer Res* 1993;53: 4461–4465.
8. Igawa M, Tanabe T, Chodak GW, et al. N-(4-hydroxyphenyl) retinamide induces cell cycle specific growth inhibition in PC-3 cells. *Prostate* 1994;24:299–305.
9. Liang JY, Fontana JA, Rao JN, et al. Synthetic retinoid CD437 induces S phase arrest and apoptosis in human prostate cancer cells LNCaP and PC-3. *Prostate* 1999;38: 228–236.
10. Sun SY, Yue P, Lotan R. Induction of apoptosis by N-(4-hydroxyphenyl) retinamide and its association with reactive oxygen species, nuclear retinoic acid receptors, and apoptosis-related genes in human prostate carcinoma cells. *Mol Pharmacol* 1999;55:403–410.
11. De Vos S, Dawson MI, Holden S, et al. Effects of retinoid X receptor-selective ligands on proliferation of prostate cancer cells. *Prostate* 1997;32:115–121.
12. Jones HE, Eaton CL, Barrow D, et al. Response of cell growth and retinoic acid receptor expression to retinoic acid in neoplastic and non-neoplastic prostate cell lines. *Prostate* 1997;30:174–182.
13. Trump DL, Smith DC, Stiff D, et al. A Phase II trial of all-*trans*-retinoic acid in hormone-refractory prostate cancer: a clinical trial with detailed pharmacokinetic analysis. *Cancer Chemother Pharmacol* 1997;39:349–356.
14. Van Wauwe J, Van Nyen G, Coene MC, et al. Liarozole, an inhibitor of retinoic acid metabolism, exerts retinoid-mimetic effects in vivo. *J Pharmacol Exp Ther* 1992;261:773–779.
15. Van Ginckel R, De Coster R, Wouters W, et al. Antitumoral effects of R75251 on the growth of transplantable R3327 prostate adenocarcinomas in rats. *Prostate* 1990;16:313–323.
16. Dijkman GA, Van Moorselaar RJ, Van Ginckel R, et al. Antitumoral effects of liarozole in androgen-dependent and independent R3327 Dunning prostate adenocarcinomas. *J Urol* 1994;151:217–222.
17. Dijkman GA, Fernandez del Moral P, Bruynseels J, et al. Liarozole (R75251) in hormone-resistant prostate cancer patients. *Prostate* 1997;33:26–31.
18. Debruyne FM, Murray R, Fradet Y, et al. Liarozole—a novel treatment approach for advanced prostate cancer: results of a large randomized trial versus cyproterone acetate. *Urology* 1998;52:72–81.
19. Chawla A, Schwarz EJ, Dimaculangan DD, et al. Peroxisome proliferator-activated receptor (PPAR)γ: adipose-predominant expression and induction early in adipocyte differentiation. *Endocrinology* 1994;135:798–800.
20. Tontonoz P, Hu E, Spiegelman BM. Stimulation of adipogenesis in fibroblasts by PPAR γ 2, a lipid-activated transcription factor. *Cell* 1994;79:1147–1156.
21. Kliewer SA, Forman BM, Blumberg B, et al. Differential expression and activation of a family of murine peroxisome proliferator-activated receptors. *Proc Natl Acad Sci U S A* 1994;91:7355–7359.
22. Yu K, Bayona W, Kallen W, et al. Differential activation of the peroxisome proliferator-activated receptors by eicosanoids. *J Biol Chem* 1995;270:23975–23983.

23. Nolan JJ, Ludvik B, Beerdsen P, et al. Improvement in glucose tolerance and insulin resistance in obese subjects treated with troglitazone. *N Engl J Med* 1994;331:1188–1193.
24. Tontonoz P, Singer S, Forman BM, et al. Terminal differentiation of human liposarcoma cells induced by ligands for peroxisome proliferator-activated receptor γ and the retinoid X receptor. *Proc Natl Acad Sci U S A* 1997;94:237–241.
25. Mueller E, Sarraf P, Tontonoz P, et al. Terminal differentiation of human breast cancer through PPARγ. *Mol Cell* 1998;1:465–470.
26. Kubota T, Koshizuka K, Williamson EA, et al. Ligand for peroxisome proliferator-activated receptor γ (Troglitazone) has potent antitumor effect against human prostate cancer both in vitro and in vivo. *Cancer Res* 1998;58:3344–3352.
27. Demetri GD, Fletcher CD, Mueller E, et al. Induction of solid tumor differentiation by the peroxisome proliferator-activated receptor-γ ligand troglitazone in patients with liposarcoma. *Proc Natl Acad Sci U S A* 1999;90:3951–3956.
28. Mueller E, Smith M, Sarraf P, et al. Effects of ligand activation of peroxisome proliferator-activated receptor gamma in human prostate cancer. *Proc Natl Acad Sci U S A* 2000;97:10990–10995.
29. Brusilow SW, Danney M, Waber LJ, et al. Treatment of episodic hyperammonemia in children with inborn errors of urea synthesis. *N Engl J Med* 1984;310:1630–1634.
30. Fibach E, Prasanna P, Rodgers GP, et al. Enhanced fetal hemoglobin production by phenylacetate and 4-phenylbutyrate in erythroid precursors derived from normal donors and patients with sickle cell anemia and beta-thalassemia. *Blood* 1993;82:2203–2209.
31. Dover GJ, Brusilow S, Charache S. Induction of fetal hemoglobin production in subjects with sickle cell anemia by oral sodium phenylbutyrate. *Blood* 1994;84:339–343.
32. Mitchell RB, Wagner JE, Karp JE, et al. Syndrome of idiopathic hyperammonemia after high-dose chemotherapy: review of nine cases. *Am J Med* 1988;85:662–667.
33. Samid D, Yeh A, Prasanna P. Induction of erythroid differentiation and fetal hemoglobin production in human leukemic cells treated with phenylacetate. *Blood* 1992;80:1576–1581.
34. Samid D, Shack S, Myers CE. Selective growth arrest and phenotypic reversion of prostate cancer cells in vitro by nontoxic pharmacological concentrations of phenylacetate. *J Clin Invest* 1993;91:2288–2295.
35. Hudgins WR, Pineau T, Sher T, et al. Anticancer activity of phenylacetate and related aromatic fatty acids: correlation with lipophilicity and capacity to activate nuclear receptor. *Proc Am Assoc Cancer Res* 1994;35:391–395.
36. Samid D, Hudgins WR, Shack S, et al. Phenylacetate and derivatives: simple compounds with complex antitumor activities. *Proc Am Assoc Cancer Res* 1994;35:408–413.
37. Thibault A, Cooper MR, Figg WD, et al. A phase I and pharmacokinetic study of intravenous phenylacetate in patients with cancer. *Cancer Res* 1994;54:1690–1694.
38. Thibault A, Samid D, Cooper MR, et al. Phase I study of phenylacetate administered twice daily to patients with cancer. *Cancer* 1995;75:2932–2938.
39. Wood CG, Lee C, Grayhack JT, et al. Phenylacetate and phenylbutyrate promote cellular differentiation in human prostate cancer systems. *Proc Am Assoc Cancer Res* 1994;35: 403–407.
40. Carducci MA, Nelson JB, Chan-Tack KM, et al. Phenylbutyrate induces apoptosis in human prostate cancer and is more potent than phenylacetate. *Clin Cancer Res* 1996;2: 379–387.
41. Tong KP, David-Beabes G, Meeker A, et al. Phenylbutyrate (PB) has pleiotropic effects on gene transcription and inhibits telomerase activity in human prostate cancer. *Anticancer Res* 1997;17:3953–3958.
42. Carducci MA, Bowling MK, Eisenberger MA, et al. Phenylbutyrate (PB) for refractory solid tumors: a phase I clinical and pharmacologic evaluation of intravenous versus oral PB. *Anticancer Res* 1997;17:3972–3978.
43. Miller GJ, Stapleton GE, Ferrara JA, et al. The human prostatic carcinoma cell line LNCaP expresses biologically active, specific receptors of 1α,25-dihydroxyvitamin D_3. *Cancer Res* 1992;52:515–520.
44. Miller GJ, Stapleton GE, Houmiel KL, et al. Specific receptors for vitamin D3 in human prostatic carcinoma cells. In: Karr JP, Coffey DS, Smith RB, et al., eds. *Molecular and cellular biology of prostate cancer.* New York: Plenum Publishing, 1991:253–259.
45. Miller GJ, Stapleton GE, Hedlund TE, et al. Vitamin D receptor expression, 24-hydroxylase activity, and inhibition of growth by 1α,25-dihydroxyvitamin D_3 in seven human prostatic carcinoma cell lines. *Clin Cancer Res* 1995;1:997–1003.
46. Hsieh TY, Ng CY, Mallouh C, et al. Regulation of growth, PSA/PAP, and androgen receptor expression by 1 alpha,25-dihydroxyvitamin D3 in the androgen-dependent LNCaP cells. *Biochem Biophys Res Commun* 1996;223:141–146.
47. Blutt SE, Allegretto EA, Pike JW, et al. 1,25-dihydroxyvitamin D3 and 9-cis-retinoic acid act synergistically to inhibit the growth of LNCaP prostate cells and cause accumulation of cells in G1. *Endocrinology* 1997;138:1491–1497.
48. Zhao XY, Ly LH, Peehl DM, et al. Induction of androgen receptor by 1alpha,25-dihydroxyvitamin D3 and 9-cis retinoic acid in LNCaP human prostate cancer cells. *Endocrinology* 1999;140:1205–1212.
49. Ingles SA, Ross RK, Yu MC, et al. Association of prostate cancer risk with genetic polymorphisms in vitamin D receptor and androgen receptor. *J Natl Cancer Inst* 1997;89:166–170.
50. Schwartz GG, Hulka BS. Is vitamin D deficiency a risk factor for prostate cancer? (Hypothesis). *Anticancer Res* 1990;10: 1307–1311.
51. Corder EH, Guess HA, Hulka BS, et al. Vitamin D and prostate cancer: a prediagnostic study with stored sera. *Cancer Epidemiol Biomarkers Prev* 1993;2:467–472.
52. Chan JM, Giovannucci E, Andersson SO, et al. Dairy products, calcium, phosphorous, vitamin D, and risk of prostate cancer. *Cancer Causes Control* 1998;9:559–566.
53. Giovannucci E. Dietary influences of 1,25$(OH)_2$ vitamin D in relation to prostate cancer: a hypothesis. *Cancer Causes Control* 1998;9:567–582.
54. Peehl DM, Skowronski RJ, Leung GK, et al. Antiproliferative effects of 1,25-dihydroxyvitamin D3 on primary cultures of human prostatic cells. *Cancer Res* 1994;54:805–810.
55. Skowronski RJ, Peehl DM, Feldman D. Vitamin D and prostate cancer: 1,25 dihydroxyvitamin D3 receptors and actions in human prostate cancer cell lines. *Endocrinology* 1993;132:1952–1960.

56. Esquenet M, Swinnen JV, Heyns W, et al. Control of LNCaP proliferation and differentiation: actions and interactions of androgens, 1alpha,25-dihydroxycholecalciferol, all-trans retinoic acid, 9-cis retinoic acid, and phenylacetate. *Prostate* 1996;28:182–194.
57. Schwartz GG, Hill CC, Oeler TA, et al. 1,25-Dihydroxy-16-ene-23-yne-vitamin D3 and prostate cancer cell proliferation in vivo. *Urology* 1995;46:365–369.
58. Schwartz GG, Wang MH, Zang M, et al. 1 alpha,25-Dihydroxyvitamin D (calcitriol) inhibits the invasiveness of human prostate cancer cells. *Cancer Epidemiol Biomarkers Prev* 1997;6:727–732.
59. Getzenberg RH, Light BW, Lapco PE, et al. Vitamin D inhibition of prostate adenocarcinoma growth and metastasis in the Dunning rat prostate model system. *Urology* 1997;50:999–1006.
60. Lokeshwar BL, Schwartz GG, Selzer MG, et al. Inhibition of prostate cancer metastasis in vivo: a comparison of 1,23-dihydroxyvitamin D (calcitriol) and EB1089. *Cancer Epidemiol Biomarkers Prev* 1999;8:241–248.
61. Moffatt KA, Johannes WU, Miller GJ. 1Alpha,25dihydroxyvitamin D3 and platinum drugs act synergistically to inhibit the growth of prostate cancer cell lines. *Clin Cancer Res* 1999;5:695–703.
62. Smith DC, Johnson CS, Freeman CC, et al. A Phase I trial of calcitriol (1,25-dihydroxycholecalciferol) in patients with advanced malignancy. *Clin Cancer Res* 1999;5:1339–1345.
63. Wood HM, Carducci MA. Differentiation therapy for prostate cancer. *Prostate* 1999 (In press).
64. Craft N, Shostak Y, Carey M, et al. A mechanism for hormone-independent prostate cancer through modulation of androgen signaling by the Her-2/neu tyrosine kinase. *Nat Med* 1999;5:280–285.
65. Coussens L, Yang-Feng TL, Liao YC, et al. Tyrosine kinase receptor with extensive homology to EGF receptor shares chromosomal location with neu oncogene. *Science* 1985;230:1132–1139.
66. Ross JS, Sheehan C, Hayner-Buchan AM, et al. HER-2/neu gene amplification status in prostate cancer by fluorescence in situ hybridization. *Hum Pathol* 1997;28:827–833.
67. Kallakury BV, Sheehan CE, Ambros RA, et al. Correlation of p34cdc2 cyclin-dependent kinase overexpression, CD44s downregulation, and HER-2/neu oncogene amplification with recurrence in prostatic adenocarcinomas. *J Clin Oncol* 1998;16:1302–1309.
68. Mark HF, Feldman D, Das S, et al. Fluorescence in situ hybridization study of HER-2/neu oncogene amplification in prostate cancer. *Exp Mol Pathol* 1999;66:170–178.
69. Pegram MD, Lipton A, Hayes DF, et al. Phase II study of receptor-enhanced chemosensitivity using recombinant humanized anti-p185HER2/neu monoclonal antibody plus cisplatin in patients with HER2/neu-overexpressing metastatic breast cancer refractory to chemotherapy treatment. *J Clin Oncol* 1998;16:2659–2671.
70. Elson SD, Browne CA, Thorburn GD. Identification of epidermal growth factor-like activity in human male reproductive tissue and fluids. *J Clin Endocrinol Metab* 1984;58:589–595.
71. Fowler JE, Lau JL, Ghosh L, et al. Epidermal growth factor and prostatic carcinoma: an immunohistochemical study. *J Urol* 1988;139:857–865.
72. Maddy SQ, Chisholm GD, Hawkins RA, et al. Localization of epidermal growth factor receptors in the human prostate by biochemical and immunocytochemical methods. *J Endocrinol* 1987;113:147–153.
73. Schuurmans AL, Bolt J, Mulder E. Androgens stimulate both growth rate and epidermal growth factor receptor activity of the human prostate tumor cell LNCaP. *Prostate* 1988;12:55–63.
74. Wilding G, Valverius E, Knabbe C, et al. Role of transforming growth factor-alpha in human prostate cell growth. *Prostate* 1989;15:1–9.
75. Sutkowski DM, Fong CJ, Sensibar JA, et al. Interaction of epidermal growth factor and transforming growth factor beta in human prostatic epithelial cells in culture. *Prostate* 1992;21:133–143.
76. Steiner MS. Role of peptide growth factors in the prostate: a review. *Urology* 1993;42:99–110.
77. Byrne RL, Leung H, Neal DE. Peptide growth factors in the prostate as mediators of stromal epithelial interactions. *Br J Urol* 1996;77:627–633.
78. Culig Z, Hobisch A, Cronauer MV, et al. Regulation of prostatic growth and function by peptide growth factors. *Prostate* 1996;28:392–405.
79. Myers RB, Oelschlager D, Manne U, et al. Androgenic regulation of growth factor and growth factor receptor expression in the CWR22 model of prostatic adenocarcinoma. *Int J Cancer* 1999;82:424–429.
80. Ye D, Mendelsohn J, Fan Z. Androgen and epidermal growth factor down-regulate cyclin-dependent kinase inhibitor p27Kip1 and costimulate proliferation of MDA PCa 2a and MDA PCa 2b prostate cancer cells. *Clin Cancer Res* 1999;5:2171–2177.
81. Culig Z, Hobisch A, Cronauer MV, et al. Androgen receptor activation in prostatic tumor cell lines by insulin-like growth factor-I, keratinocyte growth factor, and epidermal growth factor. *Cancer Res* 1994;54:5474–5478.
82. Putz T, Culig Z, Eder IE, et al. Epidermal growth factor (EGF) receptor blockade inhibits the action of EGF, insulin-like growth factor I, and a protein kinase A activator on the mitogen-activated protein kinase pathway in prostate cancer cell lines. *Cancer Res* 1999;59:227–233.
83. Sherwood ER, Van Dongen JL, Wood CG, et al. Epidermal growth factor receptor activation in androgen-independent but not androgen-stimulated growth of human prostatic carcinoma cells. *Br J Cancer* 1998;77:855–861.
84. MacDonald A, Habib FK. Divergent responses to epidermal growth factor in hormone sensitive and insensitive human prostate cancer cell lines. *Br J Cancer* 1992;65:177–182.
85. Bos M, Mendelsohn J, Kim YM, et al. PD153035, a tyrosine kinase inhibitor, prevents epidermal growth factor receptor activation and inhibits growth of cancer cells in a receptor number-dependent manner. *Clin Cancer Res* 1997;3:2099–2106.
86. Jones HE, Dutkowski CM, Barrow D, et al. New EGF-R selective tyrosine kinase inhibitor reveals variable growth responses in prostate carcinoma cell lines PC-3 and DU-145. *Int J Cancer* 1997;71:1010–1018.
87. Mendelsohn J. Epidermal growth factor inhibition by a monoclonal antibody as anticancer therapy. *Clin Cancer Res* 1997;3:2703–2707.

88. Bejeck B, Li D, Deuel TF. Transformation by v-sis occurs by an internal autoactivation mechanism. *Science* 1989;245: 1496–1499.
89. Peehl DM, Sellers RG. Basic FGF, EGF, and PDGF modify TGFbeta-induction of smooth muscle cell phenotype in human prostatic stromal cells. *Prostate* 1998;35:125–134.
90. Fudge K, Wang CY, Stearns ME. Immunohistochemistry analysis of platelet-derived growth factor A and B chains and platelet-derived growth factor alpha and beta receptor expression in benign prostatic hyperplasias and Gleason-graded human prostate adenocarcinomas. *Mod Pathol* 1994;7:549–556.
91. Fudge K, Bostwick DG, Stearns ME. Platelet-derived growth factor A and B chains and the alpha and beta receptors in prostatic intraepithelial neoplasia. *Prostate* 1996;29: 282–286.
92. Kim HE, Han SJ, Kasza T, et al. Platelet-derived growth factor (PDGF)-signaling mediates radiation-induced apoptosis in human prostate cancer cells with loss of p53 function. *Int J Radiat Oncol Biol Phys* 1997;39:731–736.
93. Shawver LK, Schwartz DP, Mann E, et al. Inhibition of platelet-derived growth factor-mediated signal transduction and tumor growth by N-[4-(trifluoromethyl)-phenyl]5-methylisoxazole-4-carboxamide. *Clin Cancer Res* 1997;3:1167–1177.
94. Harper GP, Barde YA, Burnstock YA, et al. Guinea pig prostate is a rich source of nerve growth factor. *Nature* 1979;350:678–682.
95. Donovan MJ, Hempstead B, Huber LJ, et al. Identification of the neurotrophin receptors p75 and trk in a series of Wilms' tumors. *Am J Pathol* 1994;145:792–801.
96. Pflug BR, Dionne C, Kaplan DR, et al. Expression of a trk high affinity nerve growth factor receptor in human prostate. *Endocrinology* 1995;136:262–268.
97. Martin-Zanca D, Hughes SH, Barbacid M, et al. A human oncogene formed by the fusion of truncated tropomyosin and protein tyrosine kinase sequences. *Nature* 1986;319:743–748.
98. Pierotti MA, Bongarzone I, Borrello MG, et al. Cytogenetics and molecular genetics of carcinomas arising from thyroid epithelial follicular cells. *Genes Chromosomes Cancer* 1996;16:1–14.
99. George DJ, Susuki H, Bova GS, et al. Mutational analysis of the trk A gene in prostate cancer. *Prostate* 1998;36:172–180.
100. Dionne CA, Jani J, Camoratto AM, et al. Cell cycle independent death of prostate adenocarcinoma is induced by the trk tyrosine kinase inhibitor, CEP-751. *Clin Cancer Res* 1998;4:1887–1898.
101. Djakiew D, Delsite R, Pflug BR, et al. Regulation of growth by a nerve growth factor-like protein which modulates paracrine interactions between a neoplastic epithelial cell line and stromal cells of the human prostate. *Cancer Res* 1991;51:3304–3310.
102. Djakiew D, Pflug BR, Delsite R, et al. Chemotaxis and chemokinesis of human prostate cancer cell lines in response to human prostate stromal cell secretory proteins containing a nerve growth factor-like protein. *Cancer Res* 1993;53:1416–1420.
103. Geldof AA, DeKleijn MAT, Roa BR, et al. Nerve growth factor stimulates in vivo invasive capacity of DU-145 human prostate cancer cells. *J Cancer Res Clin Oncol* 1997;123:107–112.
104. Camoratto AM, Jani J, Angeles TS, et al. CEP-751 inhibits trk receptor tyrosine kinase activity in vitro and exhibits anti-tumor activity. *Int J Cancer* 1997;72:673–679.
105. George DJ, Dionne CA, Jani J, et al. Sustained in vivo regression of Dunning H rat prostate cancers treated with combinations of androgen ablation and trk tyrosine kinase inhibitors, CEP-751(KT-6587) or CEP-701(KT-5555). *Cancer Res* 1999;59:2395–2401.
106. Ruan W, Powell-Braxton L, Kopchick JJ, et al. Evidence that insulin-like growth factor I and growth hormone are required for prostate gland development. *Endocrinology* 1999;140:1984–1989.
107. Iwamura M, Sluss PM, Casamento JB, et al. Insulin-like growth factor I: action and receptor characterization in human prostate cancer cell lines. *Prostate* 1993;22:243–252.
108. Angelloz-Nicoud P, Binoux M. Autocrine regulation of cell proliferation by the insulin-like growth factor (IGF) and IGF binding protein-3 protease system in a human prostate carcinoma cell line (PC-3). *Endocrinology* 1995;136:5485–5492.
109. Tennant MK, Thrasher JB, Twomey PA, et al. Protein and messenger ribonucleic acid (mRNA) for the type 1 insulin-like growth factor (IGF) receptor is decreased and IGF-II mRNA is increased in human prostate carcinoma compared to benign prostate epithelium. *J Clin Endocrinol Metab* 1996;81:3774–3782.
110. Kaplan PJ, Mohan S, Cohen P, et al. The insulin-like growth factor axis and prostate cancer: lessons from the transgenic adenocarcinoma of mouse prostate (TRAMP) model. *Cancer Res* 1999;59:2203–2209.
111. Pietrzkowski Z, Mulholland G, Gomella L, et al. Inhibition of growth of prostatic cancer cell lines by peptide analogues of insulin-like growth factor 1. *Cancer Res* 1993;53:1102–1106.
112. Nickerson T, Miyake H, Gleave ME, et al. Castration-induced apoptosis of androgen-dependent Shionogi carcinoma is associated with increased expression of genes encoding insulin-like growth factor-binding proteins. *Cancer Res* 1999;59:3392–3395.
113. Gregory CW, Kim D, Ye P, et al. Androgen receptor up-regulates insulin-like growth factor binding protein-5 (IGFBP-5) expression in a human prostate cancer xenograft. *Endocrinology* 1999;140:2372–2381.
114. Kaicer E, Blat C, Imbenotte J, et al. IGF binding protein-3 secreted by the prostate adenocarcinoma cells (PC-3): differential effect on PC-3 and normal prostate cell growth. *Growth Regul* 1993;3:180–189.
115. Angelloz-Nicoud P, Harel L, Binoux M. Recombinant human insulin-like growth factor (IGF) binding protein-3 stimulates prostate carcinoma cell proliferation via an IGF-dependent mechanism. Role of serine proteases. *Growth Regul* 1996;6:130–136.
116. Figueroa JA, Lee AV, Jackson JG, et al. Proliferation of cultured human prostate cancer cells is inhibited by insulin-like growth factor (IGF) binding protein-1: evidence for an IGF-II autocrine growth loop. *J Clin Endocrinol Metab* 1995;80:3476–3482.
117. Cohen P, Graves HC, Peehl DM, et al. Prostate-specific antigen (PSA) is an insulin-like growth factor binding protein-3 protease found in seminal plasma. *J Clin Endocrinol Metab* 1992;75:1046–1053.

118. Chan JM, Stampfer MJ, Giovannucci E, et al. Plasma insulin-like growth factor-I and prostate cancer risk: a prospective study. *Science* 1998;279:563–566.
119. Djavan B, Bursa B, Seitz C, et al. Insulin-like growth factor 1 (IGF-1), IGF-1 density, and IGF-1/PSA ratio for prostate cancer detection. *Urology* 1999;54:603–606.
120. Pollak MN, Polychronakos C, Guyda H. Somatostatin analogue SMS 201-995 reduces serum IGF-1 levels in patients with neoplasms dependent on IGF-1. *Anticancer Res* 1989; 9:889–892.
121. Figg WD, Thibault A, Cooper MR, et al. A phase I study of somatostatin analogue Somuatuline in patients with metastatic hormone-refractory prostate cancer. *Cancer* 1995;75: 2159–2164.
122. Casey ML, Byrd W, MacDonald PC. Massive amounts of immunoreactive endothelin in human seminal fluid. *J Clin Endoc Metabol* 1992;74:223–225.
123. Kobayashi S, Tang R, Wang B, et al. Localization of endothelin receptors in the human prostate. *J Urol* 1994;151: 763–766.
124. Nelson JB, Hedican SP, George DJ, et al. Identification of endothelin-1 in the pathophysiology of metastatic adenocarcinoma of the prostate. *Nat Med* 1995;1:944–949.
125. Nelson JB, Lee WH, Nguyen SH, et al. Methylation of the 5' CpG island of the endothelin B receptor gene is common in human prostate cancer. *Cancer Res* 1997;57:35–37.
126. Le Brun G, Aubin P, Soliman H, et al. Upregulation of endothelin 1 and its precursor by IL-1beta, TNF-alpha, and TGF-beta in the PC3 human prostate cancer cell line. *Cytokine* 1999;11:157–162.
127. Nelson JB, Chan-Tack K, Hedican SP, et al. Endothelin-1 production and decreased endothelin B receptor expression in advanced prostate cancer. *Cancer Res* 1996;56:663–668.
128. Stiles JD, Ostrow PT, Balos LL, et al. Correlation of endothelin-1 and transforming growth factor beta 1 with malignancy and vascularity in human gliomas. *J Neuropathol Exp Neurol* 1997;56:435–439.
129. Goligorsky MS, Budzikowski AS, Tsukahara H, et al. Cooperation between endothelin and nitric oxide in promoting endothelial cell migration and angiogenesis. *Clin Exp Pharmacol Physiol* 1999;26:269–271.
130. Nelson JB, Nguyen SH, Wu-Wong JR, et al. New bone formation in an osteoblastic tumor model is increased by endothelin-1 overexpression and decreased by endothelin A receptor blockade. *Urology* 1999;53:1063–1069.
131. Dahlof B, Gustafsson D, Hedner T, et al. Regional haemodynamic effects of endothelin-1 in rat and man: unexpected adverse reaction. *J Hypertens* 1990;8:811–817.
132. Nelson JB, Carducci MA. The role of the endothelin axis in prostate cancer. *Prostate J* 1999;1:126–130.
133. Myers MP, Pass I, Batty IH, et al. The lipid phosphatase activity of PTEN is critical for its tumor suppressor function. *Proc Natl Acad Sci U S A* 1998;95:13513–13517.
134. Maehama T, Dixon JE. The tumor suppressor, PTEN/MMAC1, dephosphorylates the lipid second messenger, phosphatidylinositol 3,4,5-trisphosphate. *J Bio Chem* 1998; 273:13375–13381.
135. Stambolic V, Suzuki A, de la Pompa JL, et al. Negative regulation of PKB/Akt-dependent cell survival by the tumor suppressor PTEN. *Cell* 1998;95:29–36.

53

TUMOR ENVIRONMENT AS THE TARGET: NOVEL THERAPEUTICS, INCLUDING ANTIANGIOGENESIS AND ANTIMETASTATICS

ROBERTO PILI
MICHAEL A. CARDUCCI
SAMUEL R. DENMEADE

In this chapter, a thorough overview of angiogenesis as it pertains to prostate cancer (CaP) is explored, with a clear understanding that many of the data are extrapolated from other tumor types. Although the process of angiogenesis and targeting it as an antitumor strategy is not new, the clinical development remains in its earliest stages. We review many of the targets for antiangiogenesis, including specific growth factors and degradative enzymes responsible for continued growth and proliferation based on providing adequate tumor blood supply. A limited review of agents in or about to enter clinical trial closes the chapter.

ANGIOGENESIS: AN OVERVIEW

Angiogenesis is an essential component of tumor growth and metastasis. In the earliest stages of tumor growth before angiogenesis, tumor size does not exceed more than 2 mm (1). Within this avascular tumor, tumor cell proliferation is balanced by an equal rate of cell death (2), and human tumors can persist in this *in situ* state for months to years without neovascularization. Further growth occurs when a subgroup of cells in the tumor "switch on" to an angiogenic phenotype (1). This switch involves a change in the local levels of positive and negative regulators of microvessel growth (3,4). The tumor overrides the normally tightly controlled process of angiogenesis by directly secreting angiogenic substances or by activating or releasing angiogenic substances within the extracellular matrix (ECM) (5). In addition, tumors can recruit host cells, such as lymphocytes and macrophages, that produce their own angiogenic substances (4). The net result is the activation of endothelial cells to undergo a stereotypic process that culminates in new blood vessel formation.

The complex angiogenic process can be broken down into a series of discrete steps (5). It begins with local degradation of the capillary basement membrane to create an area of vascular deformity in an established blood vessel. Under the direction of an angiogenic stimulus, endothelial cells migrate into the surrounding stroma. This endothelial cell migration is followed by proliferation of endothelial cells at the leading edge of the migrating column. The endothelial cells then undergo a structural reorganization and form new capillary tubes with subsequent remodeling to form anastomosis and blood flow (5).

Once the growing tumor has established a vascular supply, the metastatic process can continue. Tumor cells invade the thin-walled venules and enter the circulation (5). Those cells that are not destroyed in the circulation must arrest in capillary beds of organs and extravasate into the tissue parenchyma. If these cells can evade the host immune system, they will begin to proliferate in the new microenvironment. These newly established tumors must then activate angiogenesis to produce a clinically detectable metastasis and potentially reinitiate the metastatic process. What is clear is that to produce a metastasis, tumor cells must complete every step in the process; failure to complete one or more steps results in cell elimination (6–8). Each step of the process is essential and represents a potential site of therapeutic manipulation.

REGULATION OF ANGIOGENESIS

Angiogenesis is fundamental to many normal processes, including reproduction, development, and wound healing (9). Nevertheless, other than these processes, angiogenesis rarely occurs in mature tissue (9). It has been estimated that under normal conditions only 0.01% of endothelial cells in the body are actively proliferating at any one time (10). Normal cells have been demonstrated to secrete high levels of angiogenesis inhibitors that maintain endothelial cells in a proliferatively quiescent state. The balance of inducers and inhibitors of angiogenesis in the tissue microenvironment determines the angiogenic response (11). In tumors, this balance favors neovascularization due to an increase in positive regulators and a decreased production of inhibitory molecules (11).

A large number of angiogenic substances have now been described. Those most commonly found in tumors include basic fibroblast growth factor (bFGF) (12,13) and vascular endothelial growth factor (VEGF) (14–16). Other important angiogenic substances are listed in Table 53-1 (9,17). Some of these substances, such as VEGF and scatter factor, bind to specific receptors on endothelial cells. In addition, degradative enzymes can be produced by tumors that lead to release of substances such as bFGF that are stored in a bound form within the ECM (12). Angiogenic peptides can also be derived from proteolysis of basement membrane components. Many of these angiogenesis inducers are growth factors or cytokines that have multiple physiologic functions.

A variety of potential angiogenesis inducers have been identified in CaP (17). Increased expression of VEGF, bFGF, transforming growth factor alpha and beta, platelet-derived growth factor (PDGF), and interleukin (IL)-8 has been demonstrated in CaPs, compared to normal controls (18–32). Serine proteases [i.e., urokinase, prostate-specific antigen (PSA), and human glandular kallikrein 2], matrix metalloproteinases (MMPs), and hyaluronidase have also been detected at high levels in CaP cells and these degradative enzymes may also promote angiogenesis (17,31).

Growth of the prostate in rodents has been shown to be regulated by vascular endothelial cells that are responding to angiogenic/trophic factors produced by the normal prostate epithelium under testosterone stimulation (21,22,33). VEGF, in particular, is produced by normal, hyperplastic, and malignant prostate epithelial cells (20,21,34). Several recent studies have demonstrated that VEGF expression is regulated by androgen (20,21,35,36). Using the androgen-dependent CaP xenograft, Joseph et al. (21) demonstrated an 85% decrease in VEGF levels after castration. In further studies, castration resulted in an 80% decrease in VEGF levels in the ventral prostates of castrated rats, whereas androgen replacement resulted in an eightfold rise in VEGF levels (21). Moon et al. (35) have also recently demonstrated that after androgen ablative therapy, there is a profound decrease in endothelial cell proliferative index in human CaPs that is associated with a significant reduction in VEGF expression in the cancer tissue. The vascular regression induced by castration has been shown to precede the cell death of malignant prostate epithelial cells (37). These results suggest that VEGF contributes to the establishment and progression of malignant prostate disease and that androgen ablation can curtail the process of the disease by inhibiting angiogenesis via decreasing VEGF levels within these cancers and inducing apoptosis of androgen-dependent CaP cells.

TABLE 53-1. ENDOGENOUS ANGIOGENIC SUBSTANCES

Angiogenin	Placental growth factor
Acidic fibroblast growth factor	Platelet-derived endothelial cell growth factor
Basic fibroblast growth factor	Proliferin
Epidermal growth factor	Scatter factor
Granulocyte colony-stimulating factor	Transforming growth factor alpha
Hepatocyte growth factor	Transforming growth factor beta
Interleukin-8	Tumor necrosis factor α
	Vascular endothelial growth factor

Androgen-dependent cells eventually progress to become androgen independent. These androgen-independent CaP cells can be of two distinct subtypes. One subtype retains expression of the androgen receptor and a degree of growth stimulation by androgen, although the cells are able to grow progressively after androgen ablation. These androgen-sensitive cells do not undergo apoptosis after androgen withdrawal. Using androgen-sensitive cell lines such as LNCaP, Joseph et al. demonstrated that VEGF levels continue to be regulated by androgen (20). This finding provides an explanation as to how such cancer cells can retain sensitivity to androgen stimulation without being androgen dependent. The second cell type is completely insensitive to androgen-induced growth stimulation and does not express the androgen receptor. Using such androgen-independent cell lines, Joseph et al. (21) determined that VEGF is constitutively expressed and is up-regulated not by androgens but by cellular hypoxia. Other growth factors, such as bFGF or PDGF, are not induced by hypoxia, suggesting that VEGF may be the central mediator of hypoxia-induced angiogenesis (21).

During the final steps of angiogenesis, the forming vasculature needs to become a stable mature blood vessel bed (38). This process involves investment of vessels with mural cells (pericytes or smooth muscle cells), production of basement membrane, and induction of vessel bed specialization (38). Selective vascular regression can also occur during this process. Recent studies have suggested that the association between the vascular tube and mural cells regulates these maturational changes (38). The incorporation of pericytes within the basement membrane of proliferating capillaries appears to inhibit capillary proliferation (39).

It has previously been demonstrated that newly formed vessels are dependent on exogenous survival factors such as VEGF for a critical period of time during their development (40). The association of forming vessels with mural cells marks the end of this period of growth factor dependence (41). In a recent study, Benjamin et al. (41) have demonstrated that in the absence of associated pericytes or smooth muscle cells, the vascular tube is unstable and prone to regression. In addition, the vascular tube requires VEGF for survival (41).

Benjamin et al. (41) further demonstrated that in the normal prostate and CaPs, a large percentage of the blood vessels are immature and have few pericytes. These immature vessels are dependent on VEGF for survival. After androgen ablation, VEGF levels decline and immature vessels are selectively obliterated (41). This finding may, in part, explain the reduction in tumor and normal prostate mass seen in the prostate after castration (37). These studies provide a mechanistic framework for VEGF regulation of CaP growth and suggest that CaPs may be particularly susceptible to anti-VEGF therapies. In support of these findings, several groups have demonstrated that treatment of CaPs with neutralizing anti-VEGF antibodies can inhibit angiogenesis and growth and metastasis of CaP xenografts *in vivo* (42,43). Other strategies using agents that directly block the VEGF receptor or block the kinase activity of the receptor may prove particularly effective and are actively under development.

ENDOGENOUS ANGIOGENESIS INHIBITORS

Angiogenesis does not typically occur in normal tissue due to the presence of an excess of angiogenesis inhibitors (2). When endothelial cells do proliferate during physiologic angiogenesis, the resulting neovascularization is turned off abruptly (44). Local administration of angiogenic factors results in neovascularization, but, with discontinuation of the stimulus, rapid involution occurs and the capillary vessel is not sustained (44). In contrast, pathologic angiogenesis induced by malignancies is not easily reversible, suggesting that in addition to increased production of angiogenesis inducers, local endogenous inhibitors of blood vessel growth may also be down-regulated in tumors (44). Genetic changes resulting in decreased expression of angiogenesis inhibitors can occur that lead to the development of the angiogenic phenotype. For example, loss of normal p53 function in human fibroblasts is associated with a sharp decline in the expression of thrombospondin-1, an endogenous angiogenesis inhibitor (3).

Recently, a variety of endogenous inhibitors of angiogenesis have been described (44,45). In most cases, the endothelial inhibitor has proven to be a fragment of a larger protein that itself lacks inhibitory activity (44). Examples of such inhibitors include angiostatin (a 38-kd fragment of plasminogen) (46), endostatin (a 20-kd fragment of collagen XVIII) (47), the 16-kd fragment of prolactin (48), and thrombospondin-1 (fragments of matrix thrombospondin-1) (49,50). Many malignant tumors can generate these inhibitory fragments, including angiostatin, endostatin, and thrombospondin-1 (47). Inhibitors can also be generated by other nontumor cell types such as tumor macrophages that, under certain conditions, can secrete an elastase capable of cleaving plasminogen to produce angiostatin (51).

Angiostatin and endostatin are examples of endogenous protein fragments that directly inhibit endothelial cell proliferation (47). Recently, it has been demonstrated that a serine protease from human CaP cell lines can proteolytically cleave plasminogen to produce angiostatin (52). In addition, tumors derived from the human CaP cell line PC3 can be maintained in a dormant state *in vivo* by systemic administration of angiostatin (53). Preclinical trials with angiostatin and endostatin have demonstrated that these agents can induce nearly complete suppression of tumor-induced angiogenesis in a variety of cancer cell types (46,47). In addition, chronic administration of these agents does not induce acquired drug resistance (54). This last finding is particularly critical due to the fact that these types of agents may require long-term administration to maintain tumor dormancy.

A variety of other endogenous angiogenesis inhibitors have also been described. Unlike angiostatin and endostatin, these proteins do not directly inhibit endothelial cell proliferation. Inhibitors such as interferon-alpha and interferon-beta may prevent tumor cells from secreting certain angiogenic inducers such as bFGF (55). Recently Dong et al. (56) demonstrated that overexpression of interferon-beta in the human CaP cell line PC3 was able to suppress angiogenesis and metastasis, possibly by activation of host effector cells such as macrophages.

Levels of circulating angiogenic factors secreted by tumors may be regulated by soluble receptors such as the FLT-1 receptor that binds VEGF with high affinity (57). Binding proteins for acidic and bFGF have also been demonstrated in human plasma (58). Other potential endogenous angiogenesis inhibitors include MMP inhibitors such as tissue inhibitor of metalloproteinase (TIMP)-1 and other inhibitors of matrix-degradative proteases (59,60). Finally, a series of other angiogenesis inhibitors have been described whose mechanism of inhibition is unknown. These include platelet factor 4 (61), human interferon–inducible protein 10 (62,63), the 16-kd N-terminal fragment of prolactin (48), and a variety of ILs, such as IL-10 and -12 (64,65). Recently, it has been demonstrated that IL-10 can reduce secretion of MMPs 2 and 9 while inducing production of the endogenous MMP inhibitor TIMP-1 in immortalized primary human CaP cells (65).

The role many of these proteins play in regulating angiogenesis in CaPs is not yet known. These studies, however, have identified proteins and protein fragments that could be tested in clinical trials. Endostatin, for example, is currently entering clinical trials as treatment for a variety of cancers, including CaP. In addition, protein targets have been discovered whose inhibition by small molecules may prove to be effective antiangiogenic therapy for CaP. Examples of such targets include the VEGF receptor and MMPs, and clinical trials are under way to test the activity of agents that inhibit these angiogenic proteins.

VASCULARIZATION AND PROSTATE CANCER PROGRESSION

More than 50% of men with clinically localized CaP treated with radical prostatectomy (RP) and pelvic lymph-node dissection are understaged, using established preoperative clinical, biochemical, and pathologic results (66). Additional prognostic indicators that can more accurately predict outcome are needed to identify those patients who would benefit from more aggressive therapy. An increasing number of studies have attempted to quantify microvessel density (MVD) in RP specimens to determine correlation with pathologic stage and usefulness as an indicator of progression (67). These studies have produced mixed results, with some studies demonstrating a correlation between vascular density and pathologic stage or risk of progression, or both, whereas others have found no correlation. Although it is beyond the scope of this chapter to review in detail each individual study, key points from several of the larger studies are addressed.

In the earliest study, Weidner et al. counted microvessels in the most active area of neovascularization (i.e., "hot spot") within the initial invasive CaP from 74 patients (68). Endothelial cells were detected by immunostaining, using an antibody to factor VIII-related antigen. In this study, the primary tumors of cases with metastatic disease had increased vascular density, compared to those without metastatic disease. In a multivariate analysis, vascular density was a better predictor of higher stage than Gleason score but was only predictive for metastases in high-grade carcinomas (Gleason scores 8 to 10) and not for low- and intermediate-grade tumors (68).

Silberman et al. (69) examined the relationship between MVD in intermediate-grade CaP and stage at RP and progression after RP. In this study, specimens were stained using the endothelial-specific antibody CD31, and "hot spot" microvessels were quantitated. In patients with Gleason grade 6 to 7 cancers, there was no observed relationship between MVD and stage at the time of RP (69). The mean vascular density in tumors that progressed was significantly higher than in nonprogressors (69). Most importantly, vascular density was found to be an independent significant predictor of progression after RP for tumors with Gleason scores 5 to 7 (69). In another study using CD31, Rubin et al. (70) looked at the MVD in RP specimens from 87 patients and found no correlation with stage, nor was MVD predictive of subsequent progression. In two other large studies (71,72), MVD was not useful in predicting progression; however, one of the studies did demonstrate a correlation with pathologic stage (71).

MVD quantification may prove useful in stratifying patients into groups to better evaluate adjuvant therapies after resection. A more important potential role is to identify, before RP, those patients likely to have insignificant tumor. Preoperative identification may allow these patients to be managed expectantly. Few studies to date have looked at MVD in diagnostic specimens. In a large retrospective analysis, Borre et al. (73) examined transurethral resection of the prostate specimens in patients subjected to watchful waiting and found that MVD correlated with clinical stage and histopathologic grade. Although a retrospective analysis, this study found that MVD was a significant predictor of disease-free survival in the entire cancer population and, more importantly, in the clinically localized cancer population (73). In a similar study, Lissbrant et al. (74) also retrospectively examined diagnostic transurethral resection of the prostate specimens and found that MVD was an independent predictor of cancer-free survival.

One study by Bostwick et al. (75) measured MVD in needle biopsy specimens and found a statistically significant contribution of MVD (along with serum PSA and Gleason score) in the prediction of organ-confined disease. Although these results are promising, it remains to be determined whether analysis of MVD will be as predictive of tumor biology in needle biopsy specimens as assessment in larger tissue specimens.

In summary, several studies have defined MVD as a potential prognostic factor in clinically localized CaP. In other studies, however, MVD does not appear to be an independent prognostic factor when subjected to multivariate analysis. Such disparate findings may be due to the use of different endothelial-specific antibodies and immunohistochemical techniques. It may also be due to the subjective nature of analyzing only the "hot spots" in the specimen. Standardization and validation in prospective studies will be required before analysis of MVD is of widespread clinical usefulness.

Aside from MVD, investigators have looked at circulating levels of cell adhesion molecules bFGF and VEGF as potential markers of progression or response to therapy. Circulating levels of these molecules have poorly correlated with tissue activity and ongoing angiogenic properties. It is known that alterations in cell adhesion are an important step in the metastatic cascade. Decreases [E-cadherin (76), C-cell adhesion molecule (C-CAM) (77)] and increases in cell adhesion molecules (E-CAM, N-CAM) are associated with CaP progression (78). Soluble and membrane-shed CAMs exist and can be assayed in circulation. A study of serum levels of I-CAM-1, V-CAM-1, N-CAM, and E-selectin in men with benign prostatic hyperplasia (n = 50) and CaP (n = 26) found no clinical use for these adhesion molecules as biomarkers of malignancy for predicting progression, for identifying metastatic potential, or for monitoring therapy (79).

bFGF is mitogenic to prostatic stromal cells, epithelial cells, and endothelial cells (80–82). Androgen-independent CaP cell lines and primary and metastatic CaPs produce bFGF (83). Mean serum levels of bFGF were significantly elevated (6.64 ± 1 pg per mL) in a group of 36 men with CaP, when compared with a group of healthy controls (1.28 ± 0.3 pg per mL) (83). There was no correlation between bFGF levels and age, PSA, tumor grade, and stage. There was also significant overlap of bFGF levels between normal controls, men with benign prostatic hyperplasia, and men with CaP. bFGF concentrations increased in four of five men with disease progression. Another study found a direct relationship between log bFGF and the odds of cancer in

11 men with PSA levels less than 4.0 ng per mL. Using an arbitrary cut off of 1.0 pg per mL, the sensitivity was 83% and the specificity 44% in this group of men. Whether bFGF concentrations correlate with angiogenesis and MVD is unknown, but the lack of correlation between bFGF and pathologic stage makes such a correlation *a priori* unlikely. To date, little information is available about VEGF in circulation in men with CaP.

MATRIX METALLOPROTEINASES AND PROSTATE CANCER

A step-wise hypothesis of tumor progression postulates that tumor cells are required to degrade the ECM to locally invade and systemically metastasize (4). During this dynamic process, tumor cells exert their ability to degrade proteins in the ECM, adhere and detach from the ECM, and, finally, migrate through it. These steps appear to occur simultaneously and continuously through the long and complex process of the tumor development. Tumor cells need to break their basement membrane first to invade the local tissue, reach the lymphatics and capillaries, and establish new metastatic sites through the "intravasation" and "extravasation" processes (84). Invasion and remodeling of the basement membrane are necessary steps for endothelial cells before they proliferate, migrate, and differentiate in the formation of new blood vessels (85).

Among various proteolytic enzymes, Zn^{2+}-dependent MMPs are a representative endopeptidase family of at least 17 structurally related proteases possessing broad spectrum proteolytic activity for a variety of ECM components, including collagen I through IV, laminin, fibronectin, gelatin, elastin, and proteoglycans (86). The MMP family can be divided into different subclasses according to substrate specificity and structural similarity (Table 53-2). These are the gelatinases (MMP-2 and MMP-9), collagenases (MMP-1 and MMP-8), stromelysins (MMP-3, MMP-10, and the related matrilysin MMP-7 and metalloelastase MMP-12), membrane-type MMPs [membrane-type (MT)1-4MMPs)], and a subgroup including stromelysin-3 (MMP-11, MMP-19, and MMP-20).

MMP gene expression is primarily regulated at the transcriptional level by growth factors, cytokines, and contact to ECM (87,88). Several studies demonstrate the role of mitogen-activated protein kinase pathways in the regulation of MMP transcription in response to different signals, including hypoxia and hyperthermia (86). MMPs are expressed by several cells, including fibroblasts, keratinocytes, chondrocytes, monocytes and macrophages, hepatocytes, and a variety of tumor cells.

These proteases were originally cloned from human tumors, such as breast carcinoma tissue (MMP-3 and MMP-11) and invasive lung cancer cells (MT1-MMP). Each enzyme has a highly conserved active site containing a zinc atom held within a metal-binding domain. The secreted inactive form of these enzymes undergoes activation through conformational modification and proteolytic cleavage of the pro-domain (89). Once activated, the MMPs are subject to control by endogenous inhibitors such as TIMPs that bind to the highly conserved zinc-binding site of active MMPs at molar equivalence.

TABLE 53-2. HUMAN MATRIX METALLOPROTEINASE (MMP) FAMILY

Enzyme	MMP number	Substrates
Collagenases		
Fibroblast collagenase	MMP-1	Fibrillar collagens types I, II, III
Neutrophil collagenase	MMP-8	Fibrillar collagens types I, II, III
Collagenase-3	MMP-13	Type I collagen
Gelatinases		
Gelatinase-A (72 kd)	MMP-2	Non-fibrillar collagens, fibronectin, laminin
Gelatinase-B (92 kd)	MMP-9	Non-fibrillar collagens, types IV and V
Stromelysins		
Stromelysin-1	MMP-3	Non-fibrillar collagens, proteoglycan, laminin
Stromelysin-2	MMP-10	Non-fibrillar collagens, proteoglycan, laminin
Stromelysin-3	MMP-11	Serine protease inhibitor (serpins)
Metalloelastase	MMP-12	Elastin, non-fibrillar collagen
Matrilysin	MMP-7	Non-fibrillar collagens, proteoglycan, laminin
Membrane-type MMPs		
MT1-MMP	MMP-14	Progelatinase A
MT2-MMP	MMP-15	?
MT3-MMP	MMP-16	Progelatinase A
MT4-MMP	MMP-17	?
Novel MMPs		
MMP-19	RASI-1	?
Enamelysin	MMP-20	Amelogenins

?, unknown.

The TIMP gene family consists of four structurally related members (90,91), three of which are soluble (TIMP-1, -2, and -4), and one is associated with ECM (TIMP-4). The proteolytic degradation of the ECM by MMPs not only removes a physical barrier but also interferes with the mechanisms controlling cell proliferation. Overexpression of TIMP-2 in melanoma cells inhibits tumor growth secondary to G_1/S arrest induced by fibrillar type I collagen (91). Modulation of MMP-7 in colon cancer cells has been shown to affect cell proliferation and tumorigenicity (92). Overexpression of TIMP-1 and TIMP-2 not only inhibits local invasion but also affects the growth of primary tumor and established metastasis in mice (93,94).

Several mechanisms can be envisioned to explain the inhibitory effect of TIMPs and synthetic inhibitors of MMPs on tumor growth (91). Inhibition of angiogenesis is likely to play an important role, because TIMPs and synthetic inhibitors of MMPs have been shown to affect the proliferation and invasion of endothelial cells *in vitro* and neovascularization *in vivo* (60,61,95,96). Some of the growth factors are also bound to the ECM and are released as the ECM is degraded or proteolytically activated from a latent form by MMPs (i.e., transforming growth factor-beta and insulinlike growth factor-2) (97,98). Furthermore, the preservation of the contact between the cells and an intact ECM exerts a restrictive growth signal generated by the contact (99). Thus, the role of TIMPs and synthetic inhibitors of MMPs has been recently expanded to include important regulatory functions of the cell-ECM and cell-cell interactions on essential cellular functions such as proliferation.

The proposed role of MMPs in tumor invasion is based on the observation of high-level expression of distinct MMPs in invasive malignant tumors (100,101). Direct evidence that MMPs play an important role in tumor invasion and progression comes from several *in vivo* studies in which overexpression of TIMPs results in reduced invasion and metastatic potential of transformed cells (102,103). Furthermore, MMP knockout mice lacking MMP-2 and MMP-7 showed reduced angiogenesis and tumor progression and inhibition of intestinal tumorigenesis, respectively (104,105).

The expression of MMPs in the tumor is regulated in a paracrine manner by growth factors and cytokines secreted by tumor-infiltrating inflammatory cells as well as by tumor or stromal cells (86). A continuous interplay between tumor cells and the stroma has been envisioned during tumor progression, suggesting that a specific tumor stroma undergoing extensive remodeling is present at the primary and metastatic sites (106). *In vivo* expression of MMPs is localized in tumor, stromal, and endothelial cells. Increased expression of MMP-1, MMP-2, and MMP-9 has been shown in different malignancy, including lung carcinoma, breast carcinoma, head and neck and colorectal tumors, and CaP (107–111).

In particular, there are several reports that show high expression of MMPs in CaP and a significant correlation with the disease grade or stage. A significant correlation between the expression of MMP-7 and the pathologic state or lymph-node metastasis was found in patients with CaP (112), and a direct correlation was observed between the intensity of MMP-2 expression and Gleason score (113). Condition media of fresh tissue from normal and neoplastic prostate showed that normal and neoplastic tissue secrete latent and active forms of MMP-2 and MMP-9. However, samples from malignant prostate explants contained a higher proportion of the active form of MMP-2, with markedly reduced or not detectable free TIMPs. These findings suggest that there is an imbalance of secretion between MMPs and TIMPs in CaP (114). Another report showed that TIMP-1 and TIMP-2 were expressed at elevated levels in the stroma of Gleason sum 5 tissue, whereas MMP-2 and MMP-9 were expressed at relatively low levels (115). In higher Gleason sum tissue (Gleason sum 8 to 10), TIMP-1 and TIMP-2 were not expressed, whereas MMP-2 and MMP-9 were intensely expressed. Furthermore, TIMP-1/TIMP-2 and MMP-2/MMP-9 expression was, respectively, higher and lower in organ-confined specimens in comparison with specimens with capsular penetration and samples with surgical margin; seminal vesicle, and/or lymph node involvement. A positive correlation of TIMP and MMP expression with GS and pathologic stage versus cure rate was also found, suggesting a possible role for TIMP1/TIMP-2 and MMP-2/MMP-9 as independent predictors of outcome.

Overproduction of MMPs by a prostate tumor might result in increased MMP levels found in body fluid, such as blood or urine. Elevated levels of MMPs have been found in serum and plasma of animals bearing experimental tumors and human patients. Serum MMP-2 and MMP-2 density (serum level divided by the prostate volume) correlates with the presence of organ-confined and metastatic disease in CaP patients (116). A recent study showed that the presence of biologically active MMP-2 or MMP-9 in the urine of cancer patients (40% with CaP and a Gleason grade 5 to 7) was an independent predictor of organ-confined cancer, and the high molecular weight species was an independent predictor of metastatic cancer (117).

One of the first reports of blood measurements in CaP patients showed increased TIMP-1 and MMP-1, unchanged MMP-3, and decreased TIMP-2 serum concentrations (118). In contrast, a different study reported that only plasma concentrations of TIMP-1 and MMP-3 were elevated in CaP patients with metastasis, compared with controls, patients with BPH, and patients with organ-confined disease. These differences were attributed to the different blood components analyzed (119). In the same report, the author also found a correlation between TIMP-1 and PSA. The interesting finding of elevated TIMP-1 in patients with metastatic CaP correlates with increased amounts of TIMP-1, as found in advanced colon cancer and hepatocellular carcinoma tissues (120,121). Apparently, TIMP-1 is a potent inhibitor of tumor progression as an antagonist of metalloproteinases and a growth promoting agent. These two different and paradoxical properties are apparently exerted at different concentrations.

Finally, neuropeptides, including calcitonin, serotonin, bombesin, neurotensin, and others, have been reported to be expressed in several malignancies, including CaP (122). Interestingly, neuropeptide hormones stimulate secreted activity of MMP-9 in human CaP lines, suggesting a role for these molecules in the CaP progression (123). Although there are several studies investigating the role of MMPs in tumor progression, the scenario depicted to date may be more complex. Several MMPs—for example, MMP-3, MMP-7, MMP-9, and MMP-12—have been recently shown to degrade plasminogen to angiostatin, a potent endogenous angiogenesis inhibitor, suggesting the possibility that the expression of MMPs in the peritumoral area may in fact be a reactive inhibitory response (124,125). Further *in vivo* studies are necessary to elucidate the complex role of MMPs in tumor development.

In summary, the multiple steps of tumor development (initiation, migration/invasion), angiogenesis, and metastasis-associated events (intravasation/extravasation) have been shown to be controlled by MMPs and their physiologic inhibitors, TIMPs. It was on the basis of this hypothesis that several investigators began the development of MMP inhibitors in the mid-1980s (126).

Clinical Testing of Metalloproteinases

The first MMP inhibitors were designed to mimic part of the peptide sequence, surrounding the point in the collagen molecule first cleaved by interstitial collagenase so that the inhibitor binds the MMP-active site in a stereospecific manner. The problem of this approach using peptide-based MMP inhibitors was the poor oral availability (with the exception of marimastat). Marimastat is a low-molecular weight broad-spectrum inhibitor not active against MMP-3 only. More recently, based on x-ray crystallographic information, nonpeptidic inhibitors have been designed, such as the compounds CGS 27023A, AG3340, and Bay 12-9566. Using the x-ray crystallographic data, it is possible to make these compounds more selective by maintaining the inhibitory activity against one or more MMPs, such as the gelatinase "selective" inhibitor AG3340 and Bay 12-9566.

Several preclinical studies have shown the efficacy of different MMP inhibitors in animal models (126). The broad spectrum MMP inhibitor batimastat has shown the ability to suppress micrometastatic disease in a rat mammary carcinoma model (127). Animals treated with a long course of the drug developed silent lymphatic micrometastases. Additional studies with batimastat showed inhibition of local growth and dissemination of orthotopic human colorectal carcinoma (128) and local regrowth of MBA-MD-435 breast carcinoma (129). The selective MMP inhibitors AG3340 and Bay 12-9566 have also been shown to inhibit tumor growth in several models, including Lewis lung carcinoma, B16 melanoma, and human glioma (130,131). Furthermore, direct angiogenesis inhibition has been demonstrated with batimastat and the more selective Bay 12-9566 (132,133). Interestingly, further studies with AG3340 in combination with cisplatin or cyclophosphamide in the Lewis lung carcinoma model and batimastat in combination with cisplatin in a human ovarian cancer model have shown additive antitumor effects without additional toxicities (134,135). These preclinical studies evaluating the possibility of combined MMP inhibitors with standard chemotherapy have been particularly encouraging for a feasible clinical application in the adjuvant settings in which micrometastatic disease is more likely to respond to cytostatic agents.

However, the synthetic MMP inhibitors have followed the traditional safety and efficacy study approach in patients with advanced disease despite the preclinical indication.

Batimastat was the first compound to enter clinical trials but, because of its poor bioavailability, was rapidly dismissed. Chemical modification of this compound resulted in the synthesis of marimastat (BB-2516), which retains the same biologic activity but has good oral availability. Marimastat is a broad spectrum MMP inhibitor currently in clinical trials (136). Phase I evaluation was performed in 31 healthy volunteers in two placebo-controlled escalating-dose studies (137). The drug showed a good pharmacokinetic profile with peak plasma concentration at 1.5 to 3.0 hours, with a terminal elimination half-life of 8 to 10 hours and no toxicity detected. The main side effect associated with marimastat was detected only in later studies in which cancer patients had prolonged administration of the drug with evidence of different pharmacokinesis between healthy volunteers and cancer patients.

A phase II study was designed with a different strategy from the one used with standard cytoreductive chemotherapy. Although the preclinical data showed not only tumor stabilization but also volume reduction secondary probably to angiogenesis inhibition, a classical response in terms of tumor mass shrinkage was not expected, and change in tumor antigen levels was used as a surrogate marker to monitor the biologic effect of marimastat. Six parallel phase II studies conducted in North America and Europe assessed the biologic activity of marimastat in patients with advanced serologically progressive ovarian, prostatic, pancreatic, and colorectal cancer by serial measurements of the serum markers CA125, PSA, CA19-9, and CEA, respectively (138). Patients received marimastat at doses of 25 mg b.i.d., escalating in cohorts to 75 mg twice a day over a 4-week period, with measurements of the tumor markers at the beginning and the end.

Partial biologic effect (PBE) was a less than 25% rise in markers over the 4-week period and a BE was a decrease in markers. Four hundred and fifteen patients were recruited with only 54% of patients completing the treatment. A pooled analysis across the six studies showed a dose-dependent increase in the number of patients with a BE or PBE with no apparent difference among the different tumor types. Although changes in tumor markers have never been validated as surrogate markers for anticancer activity, interestingly, survival curves showed a greater median survival time for patients who achieved a BE or PBE.

A more encouraging phase II study was performed in 14 patients with inoperable gastric carcinoma (139), with stable disease in seven patients and histological evidence of biologic activity suggested by increased stromal tissue. Interestingly, combination studies of marimastat (10 or 20 mg twice a day) coadministered with carboplatin in patients with advanced ovarian cancer (140), gemcitabine in pancreatic cancer (141), and carboplatin/paclitaxel in metastatic or locally advanced non–small cell lung cancer have recently shown good tolerability and no additional toxicities (142). These clinical results confirmed preclinical data, which indicate that if used early in combination with chemotherapy, MMP inhibitors may reach their best efficacy (134,135).

Based on these clinical data, several phase III studies assessing the efficacy of marimastat in several tumor types, including lung, gastric, ovarian, pancreatic, breast, and prostate cancers, have been started. The preliminary safety profile from ongoing phase III studies with more than 4,000 patients enrolled indicates single agent marimastat (10 mg by mouth, twice a day) to be well tolerated and suitable for long-term dosing. Approximately one-fifth of patients develop musculoskeletal toxicity that is clinically manageable in three-quarters of patients (143).

Other synthetic nonpeptide MMP inhibitors have been testing in phase I/II, among them AG3340 and Bay 12-9566. AG3340 is a selective inhibitor associated with growing tumors (e.g., MMP-2, MMP-3, MMP-9, and MMP-14, and Ki 30 to 330 pm) and is less potent against enzymes responsible for collagen maintenance in joints (MMP-1, Ki 8,300 pm). A recent preclinical report showed an inhibition of membrane-type MMP-1 in human CaP (144). Phase I with AG3340 as a single agent orally administered twice a day showed no dose-limiting toxicities, with only reversible joint-related toxicities at higher doses. The phase III development of AG330 is ongoing with randomized double-blind trials in combination with standard front-line chemotherapy in patients with unresectable non–small cell lung cancer or metastatic hormone-refractory prostate cancer (HRPC). In men with HRPC, treatment consists of mitoxantrone/carboplatin plus AG3340 or placebo. Other than standard toxicities due to chemotherapy, toxicities attributable to the AG3340 have been minimal (145).

Bay 12-9566 is a selective nonpeptidic inhibitor of MMP-2 and -9. Expression of these MMPs is associated with a poor prognosis in ovarian, lung, and colorectal carcinomas. A phase I trial was recently performed to determine the tolerability and pharmacokinetics of Bay 12-9566 when administered with standard doses of paclitaxel, carboplatin, and combination (146). Coadministration of Bay 12-9566 did not significantly alter paclitaxel clearance and was shown to be safe. Phase III trials are under way in patients with ovarian and pancreatic cancer.

In conclusion, the trial design for MMP inhibitors has been complex but extremely challenging. The hypothesis to achieve a significant tumor volume reduction equivalent to partial or complete responses to cytotoxic chemotherapy has been disregarded since the beginning. The original tumor marker measurements envisioned as surrogate markers to assess biologic activity lately have been substituted with other end points. In view of the cytostatic properties of this new class of drugs, direct measures of clinical outcomes have been established. The focus of the current phase III trials is the time to progression, quality of life, and most importantly (but harder to achieve), survival in patients with advanced disease in combination with chemotherapy. If these ongoing trials enrolling patients with advanced malignancies, including CaP, confirm the preclinical data and provide additional safety data, then the adjuvant setting will be the natural development for the MMP inhibitors, and some of the future trials already envision this possibility.

ANTIANGIOGENIC AGENTS FOR PROSTATE CANCER

Preclinical data, such as those described earlier, have led to clinical testing of antiangiogenic agents. To date, the agents available for clinical testing have been relatively few in number. The MMPs are in clinical testing. Agents such as thalidomide and TNP-470 (a synthetic fumagillin analog that inhibits endothelial cell growth) have been tested with a suggestion of mild clinical activity that requires further exploration (147,148). The mechanism behind thalidomide's antiangiogenic properties has not been elucidated. Thalidomide, like many other agents, including cytotoxic agents such as docetaxel or paclitaxel or cytostatic agents such as retinoic acid or vitamin D, has been shown to have antiangiogenic properties in preclinical testing involving simple matrigel or chick chorioallantoic membrane assays (149–151).

Antiangiogenic agents have been broadly grouped into drugs that block activators of angiogenesis, inhibit endothelial cells directly, block matrix breakdown (already reviewed), inhibit endothelial-specific integrin and survival signaling, and drugs with nonspecific mechanisms of action. The drugs that block activators of angiogenesis primarily target VEGF directly or through inhibition of VEGF receptor signaling. Genetech and Sugen have multiple agents in this category undergoing clinical investigation (152,153). Sugen's SU101 has completed phase II testing in hormone-refractory CaP. SU101 inhibits PDGF-mediated signaling. In a multicenter study, 44 patients with rising PSAs in the hormone-refractory state received this compound after a 4-day induction followed by ten weekly infusions. One patient had his PSA return to normal, two had a greater than 50% decline in PSA, and ten had PSA stabilization over the course of therapy. An improvement in pain was noted in 26%. Asthenia, nausea, anorexia, and anemia were the most frequent side effects (152). SU101 has entered phase III testing in combination with mitoxantrone and prednisone (154).

Agents that inhibit endothelial cells directly include TNP-470, thalidomide, squalamine, and endostatin. TNP-470 and thalidomide have completed phase II testing, but the reports of these studies are pending. Squalamine and endostatin are undergoing phase I testing.

Agents that inhibit endothelial-specific integrin/survival signaling are antibodies or small molecules that block integrins present on endothelial cell surfaces. Vitaxin, developed by Ixsys, is in phase II testing (155). Other compounds that exhibit nonspecific mechanisms of action include carboxyamidotriazole (an inhibitor of calcium influx), phenylbutyrate (activator of peroxisome proliferator–activated receptor gamma and inhibitor of histone deacetylase), IL-12 (up-regulator of interferon gamma and interferon-inducible protein 10) (156–159). Not all of these agents are specifically designed for CaP and many will not be tested in CaP unless activity is seen in more vascular tumor types, such as renal cell cancer or mesothelioma.

In a recent summary of antiangiogenesis and its role in targeting cancer, the ideal characteristics that inhibitors of angiogenesis should possess were outlined: They should be specific for a particular step or component of the neovascularization process, have a broad spectrum of antitumor activity across tumor types, lack documented resistance, be relatively nontoxic, and be easy to combine with other anticancer therapies (160).

Clinical trials of antiangiogenic agents have proven difficult so far, as the end point is not clear. Direct antitumor effects with subsequent shrinkage of tumor mass have not been seen except in a few select cases. Disease stabilization or tumor marker stabilization has been a consistent finding, yet the significance of this is of unclear importance. Clearly, patients are happy with agents that maintain disease and a good quality of life. Scientifically, it has been challenging to attribute disease stabilization to these agents and not to the heterogeneity of cancer. Numerous markers of antiangiogenesis are being explored in biopsied or surgical material after therapy. These markers include assays of apoptosis rate, proliferative rate, overall effect on MVD, and alterations in endothelial cell–specific receptors and their ligands. Not all tumor types, especially CaP, lend themselves well to frequent procurement of tissue while on therapy. Current radiographic studies are limited in their assessment of antitumor effects through antiangiogenic mechanisms. Ultrasound of flow in and out of tumors may be a surrogate to assess activity associated with tumor blood flow into a tumor bed. Once again, the ability to ultrasound tumor deposits is fairly limited. Nuclear magnetic resonance imaging is rapidly becoming the imaging technique of choice to follow antiangiogenic effects directly by assessing global blood flow and using spectroscopy of metabolites of a hypoxic or hyperoxic environment. Positron emission tomography scanning remains reserved to specialized centers that can follow tumor blood flow.

Trial designs and end points have also hindered development of these agents. As each agent may have a potentially different target and outcome, drug-specific trials are often set up, rather than consistent trial designs, to attempt to understand the role of these agents in cancer therapy and halting cancer progression. Single-arm studies need to be controlled to historical controls and often need to be repeated in the randomized setting with a no-therapy arm or with different doses or schedules of the agent. Combination with other agents is also a common design. Treating a tumor to best response or to give a therapy with a known response rate and add the investigational agent to explore any enhanced efficacy is a common trial design. Trials of this nature can seek hard end points such as prolongation of survival or soft end points such as delay in time to progression or improvement in progression-free survival.

At this time, antiangiogenic therapy remains uncharted territory in the frontier of cancer therapies. It has the potential for great promise. New agents are leading to bolder trial designs and the validation of new end points once not thought feasible or of clinical significance. The timing of agents and targeting of therapy remain unclear. Certainly, angiogenesis is an early event in cancer progression and the role of these therapies in prevention needs exploration. It is likely that in subsequent editions of this text there will be significantly more information regarding antiangiogenesis as an antitumor strategy than that which is currently available.

REFERENCES

1. Folkman J. Tumor angiogenesis. In: Mendelsohn J, Howley PM, Israel MA, et al., eds. *The molecular basis of cancer.* Philadelphia: WB Saunders, 1995:206–232.
2. Holmgren L, O'Reilly MS, Folkman J. Dormancy of micrometastases: balanced proliferation and apoptosis in the presence of angiogenesis suppression. *Nat Med* 1995;1:149–153.
3. Dameron KM, Volpert OV, Tainsky MA, et al. Control of angiogenesis in fibroblasts by p53 regulation of thrombospondin-1. *Science* 1994;265:1582–1584.
4. Liotta LA, Stetler-Stevenson WG. Tumor invasion and metastasis: an imbalance of positive and negative regulation (review). *Cancer Res* 1991;51:5054s–5059s.
5. Fidler IJ. Molecular determinants of angiogenesis in cancer metastases. *Cancer J Sci Am* 1998;(Suppl 1):S58–S66.
6. Poste G, Fidler IJ. The pathogenesis of cancer metastasis. *Nature* 1980;283:139–146.
7. Hart IR, Goode NT, Wilson RE. Molecular aspects of the metastatic cascade. *Biochim Biophys Acta* 1989;989:65–87.
8. Price JE, Aukerman SL, Fidler IJ. Evidence that the process of murine melanoma metastasis is sequential and selective and contains stochastic elements. *Cancer Res* 1986;46:5172–5178.
9. Folkman J. Clinical applications of research on angiogenesis. *N Engl J Med* 1995;333:1757–1763.
10. Denekamp J. Angiogenesis, neovascular proliferation, and vascular pathophysiology as targets for cancer therapy. *Br J Radiol* 1993;66:181–196.
11. Hanahan D, Folkman J. Patterns and emerging mechanisms of the angiogenic switch during tumorigenesis. *Cell* 1996;86:353–364.

12. Folkman J, Klagburn M. Angiogenic factors. *Science* 1987;235:444–447.
13. Shing Y, Folkman J, Haudenschild C, et al. Angiogenesis is stimulated by a tumor-derived endothelial cell growth factor. *J Cell Biochem* 1985;29:275–287.
14. Leung DW, Cachianes G, Kuang WJ, et al. Vascular endothelial growth factor is a secreted angiogenic mitogen. *Science* 1989;246:1306–1309.
15. Connolly DT, Heuvelman DM, Nelson R, et al. Tumor vascular permeability factor stimulates endothelial cell growth and angiogenesis. *J Clin Invest* 1989;84:1470–1478.
16. Plate KH, Breier G, Weich HA, et al. Vascular endothelial growth factor is a potential tumor angiogenesis factor in human gliomas in vivo. *Nature* 1992;359:845–848.
17. Campbell SC. Advances in angiogenesis research: relevance to urologic oncology. *J Urology* 1997;158:1663–1674.
18. Ferrer FA, McKenna PH, Bauer B, et al. Angiogenesis and prostate cancer: in vivo and in vitro expression of angiogenesis factors by prostate cancer cells. *Urology* 1998;51:161–167.
19. Jackson MW, Bentel JM, Tilley WD. Vascular endothelial growth factor (VEGF) expression in prostate cancer and benign prostatic hyperplasia. *J Urol* 1997;157:2323–2328.
20. Joseph IB, Isaacs JT. Potentiation of the antiangiogenic ability of linomide by androgen ablation involves down-regulation of vascular endothelial growth factor in human androgen-responsive prostatic cancers. *Cancer Res* 1997;57:1054–1057.
21. Joseph IB, Nelson JB, Denmeade SR, et al. Androgens regulate vascular endothelial growth factor content in normal and malignant prostatic tissue. *Clin Cancer Res* 1997;3:2507–2511.
22. Mansson E, Adams P, Kan M, et al. Heparin-binding growth factor gene expression and receptor characteristics in normal rat prostate and two transplantable rat prostate tumors. *Cancer Res* 1989;49:2485.
23. Nakamoto T, Chang C, Li A, et al. Basic fibroblast growth factor in human prostate cancer cells. *Cancer Res* 1992;52:571–577.
24. Ikeda T, Lioubin MN, Marquardt H. Human transforming growth factor type beta 2: production by a prostate adenocarcinoma cell line, purification, and initial characterization. *Biochemistry* 1987;26:2406–2410.
25. Truong LD, Kadmon D, McCune BK, et al. Association of transforming growth factor-beta 1 with prostate cancer: an immunohistochemical study. *Hum Path* 1993;24:4–9.
26. Steiner MS, Zhou ZZ, Tonb DC, et al. Expression of transforming growth factor-beta 1 in prostate cancer. *Endocrinology* 1994;135:2240–2247.
27. Hofer DR, Sherwood ER, Bromberg WD, et al. Autonomous growth of androgen-independent human prostatic carcinoma cells: role of transforming growth factor alpha. *Cancer Res* 1991;51:2780–2785.
28. Harper ME, Goddard L, Glynne-Jones E, et al. An immunocytochemical analysis of TGF alpha expression in benign and malignant prostatic tumors. *Prostate* 1993;23:9–23.
29. Sitaras NM, Sariban E, Bravo M, et al. Constitutive production of platelet derived growth factor-like proteins by human prostate carcinoma cell lines. *Cancer Res* 1988;48: 1930–1935.
30. Fudge K, Wang CY, Stearns ME. Immunohistochemistry analysis of platelet-derived growth factor A and B chains and platelet-derived growth factor alpha and beta receptor expression in benign prostatic hyperplasias and Gleason-graded human prostate adenocarcinomas. *Mol Path* 1994;7: 549–554.
31. Koch AE, Polverini PJ, Kunkel SL, et al. Interleukin-8 as a macrophage-derived mediator of angiogenesis. *Science* 1992; 258:1798–1801.
32. Lokeshwar VB, Lokeshwar BL, Pham HT, et al. Association of elevated levels of hyaluronidase matrix-degrading enzyme, with prostate cancer progression. *Cancer Res* 1996;56:651–657.
33. Franck-Lissbrant I, Haggstrom S, Damber J-E, et al. Testosterone stimulates angiogenesis and vascular regrowth in the ventral prostate in castrated rats. *Endocrinology* 1988;139: 451–456.
34. Brown LF, Yeo K-T, Berse B, et al. Vascular permeability factor (vascular endothelial growth factor) is strongly expressed in the normal male genital tract and is present in substantial quantities in semen. *J Urol* 1995;154:576–579.
35. Moon W-C, Choi IR, Moon SY. Endocrine therapy inhibits expression of vascular endothelial growth factor and angiogenesis in prostate cancer. *J Urol* 1997;157(Suppl):223.
36. Sordello S, Bertrand N, Plouet J. Vascular endothelial growth factor is up-regulated in vitro and in vivo by androgens. *Biochem Biophys Res Commun* 1998;251:287–290.
37. Jain RK, Safabakhsh N, Sckell A, et al. Endothelial cell death, angiogenesis and microvascular function following castration in an androgen-dependent tumor: role of VEGF. *Proc Natl Acad Sci U S A* 1998;181:10820–10825.
38. Darland DC, D'Amore PA. Blood vessel maturation: vascular development comes of age. *J Clin Invest* 1999;103:157–165.
39. Crocker DJ, Murad TM, Greer JC. Role of the pericyte in wound healing. An ultrastructural study. *Exp Mol Pathol* 1970;13:51–65.
40. Alon T, Hemo I, Itin A, et al. Vascular endothelial growth factor acts as a survival factor for newly formed retinal vessels and has implications for retinopathy of prematurity. *Nat Med* 1995;1:1024–1028.
41. Benjamin LE, Golijanin D, Itin A, et al. Selective ablation of immature blood vessels in established human tumors follows vascular endothelial growth factor withdrawal. *J Clin Invest* 1999;103:159–165.
42. Borgstrom P, Bourdon MA, Hillan KJ, et al. Neutralizing anti-vascular endothelial growth factor antibody completely inhibits angiogenesis and growth of human prostate carcinoma micro tumors in vivo. *Prostate* 1998;35:1–10.
43. Melnyk O, Zimmerman M, Kim KJ, et al. Neutralizing anti-vascular endothelial growth factor antibody inhibits further growth of established prostate cancer and metastases in a pre-clinical model. *J Urology* 1999;161:960–963.
44. Folkman J. Angiogenesis and angiogenesis inhibition: an overview. In: Goldberg ID, Rosen EM, eds. *Regulation of angiogenesis.* Basel, Switzerland: Birkhauser Verlag, 1997:1–7.
45. Chen C, Parangi S, Tolentino MJ, et al. A strategy to discover circulating angiogenesis inhibitors generated by human tumors. *Cancer Res* 1995;55:4230–4233.
46. O'Reilly MS, Holmgren L, Shing Y, et al. Angiostatin: a novel angiogenesis inhibitor that mediates the suppression of metastases by Lewis lung carcinoma. *Cell* 1994;79:315–328.

47. O'Reilly MS, Boehm T, Shing Y, et al. Endostatin: an endogenous inhibitor of angiogenesis and tumor growth. *Cell* 1997;88:277–285.
48. Clapp C, Martial JA, Guzman RC, et al. The 16-kilo-dalton N-terminal fragment of human prolactin is a potent inhibitor of angiogenesis. *Endocrinology* 1993;133:1292–1299.
49. Good DJ, Polverini PJ, Rastinejad F, et al. A tumor suppressor-dependent inhibitor of angiogenesis is immunologically and functionally indistinguishable from a fragment of thrombospondin. *Proc Natl Acad Sci U S A* 1990;87:6624–6628.
50. Tolsma SS, Volpert OV, Good DJ, et al. Peptides derived from two separate domains of the matrix protein thrombospondin-1 have antiangiogenic activity. *J Cell Biol* 1993;122:497–511.
51. Dong Z, Kumar R, Fidler IJ. Generation of the angiogenesis inhibitor, angiostatin, by Lewis lung carcinoma is mediated by macrophage elastase. *Proc Am Assoc Cancer Res* 1996;37:58.
52. Gately S, Twardowski P, Stack MS, et al. Human prostate carcinoma cells express enzymatic activity that converts human plasminogen to the angiogenesis inhibitor, angiostatin. *Cancer Res* 1996;56:4887–4990.
53. O'Reilly MS, Holmgren L, Chen CC, et al. Angiostatin induces and sustains dormancy of human primary tumors in mice. *Nature Med* 1996;2:689–692.
54. Boehm T, Folkman J, Browder T, et al. Antiangiogenic therapy of experimental cancers does not induce acquired drug resistance. *Nature* 1997;390:404–407.
55. Singh R, Gutman M, Bucana CD, et al. Interferons alpha and beta down-regulate the expression of basic fibroblast growth factor in human carcinomas. *Proc Natl Acad Sci U S A* 1995;92:4562–4566.
56. Dong Z, Greene G, Pettaway C, et al. Suppression of angiogenesis, tumorigenicity, and metastasis by human prostate cancer cells engineered to produce interferon-beta. *Cancer Res* 1999;59:872–879.
57. Kendall RL, Thomas KA. Inhibition of vascular endothelial growth factor activity by an endogenously encoded soluble receptor. *Proc Natl Acad Sci U S A* 1993;90:10705–10709.
58. Hanneken A, Ying W, Ling N, et al. Identification of soluble forms of the fibroblast growth factor receptor in blood. *Proc Natl Acad Sci U S A* 1994;91:9170–9174.
59. Takigawa M, Nishida Y, Suzuki F, et al. Induction of angiogenesis in chick-yolk-sac membrane by polyamines and its inhibition by tissue inhibitors of metalloproteinases (TIMP and TIMP-2). *Biochem Biophys Res Commun* 1990;171:1264–1272.
60. Johnson MD, Kim HR, Chesler L, et al. Inhibition of angiogenesis by tissue inhibitor of metalloproteinase. *J Cell Physiol* 1994;160:194–202.
61. Maione TE, Gray GS, Petro J, et al. Inhibition of angiogenesis by recombinant human platelet factor-4 and related peptides. *Science* 1990;247:77–79.
62. Strieter RM, Kunkel SL, Arenberg DA, et al. Human interferon-inducible protein 10 (IP-10), a member of the C-X-C chemokine family, is an inhibitor of angiogenesis. *Biochem Biophys Res Commun* 1995;219:51–57.
63. Angiollo AL, Sgadari C, Taub DD, et al. Human interferon-inducible protein 10 is a potent inhibitor of angiogenesis in vivo. *J Exp Med* 1995;182:155–162.
64. Voest EE, Kenyon BM, O'Reilly MS, et al. Inhibition of angiogenesis in vivo by interleukin-12. *J Natl Cancer Inst* 1995;87:581–586.
65. Stearns ME, Rhim J, Wang M. Interleukin 10 (IL-10) inhibition of primary human prostate cell-induced angiogenesis: IL-10 stimulation of tissue inhibitor of metalloproteinase-1 and inhibition of matrix metalloproteinase (MMP)-2/MMP-9 secretion. *Clin Cancer Res* 1999;5:189–196.
66. Partin AW, Kattan MW, Subong EN, et al. Combination of prostate-specific antigen, clinical stage, and Gleason score to predict pathological stage of localized prostate cancer. A multi-institutional update. *JAMA* 1997;277:1445–1451.
67. Weidner N. Intratumoral vascularity as a prognostic factor in cancers of the urogenital tract. *Eur J Cancer* 1996;32:2506–2512.
68. Weidner N, Carroll P, Flax J, et al. Tumor angiogenesis correlates with metastasis in invasive prostate carcinoma. *Am J Pathol* 1993;143:401–409.
69. Silberman M, Partin A, Veltri R, et al. Tumor angiogenesis correlates with progression after radical prostatectomy but not with pathologic stage in Gleason sum 5 to 7 adenocarcinoma. *Cancer* 1997;79:772–779.
70. Rubin MA, Buyyounouski M, Bagiella S, et al. Microvessel density in prostate cancer: lack of correlation with tumor grade, pathologic stage, and clinical outcome. *Urology* 1999; 53:542–547.
71. Bettencourt MC, Bauer JJ, Sesterhenn IA, et al. CD34 immunohistochemical assessment of angiogenesis as a prognostic marker for prostate cancer recurrence after radical prostatectomy. *J Urol* 1998;160:459–465.
72. Gettman M, Bergstralh E, Blute M, et al. Prediction of patient outcome in pathologic stage T2 adenocarcinoma of the prostate: lack of significance of microvessel density analysis. *Urology* 1998;51:79–85.
73. Borre M, Offersen BV, Nerstrom B, et al. Microvessel density predicts survival in prostate cancer patients subjected to watchful waiting. *Br J Cancer* 1998;78:940–944.
74. Lissbrant IF, Stattin P, Damber JE, et al. Vascular density is a predictor of cancer-specific survival in prostatic carcinoma. *Prostate* 1997;33:38–45.
75. Bostwick DG, Wheeler TM, Blute M, et al. Optimized microvessel density analysis improves prediction of cancer stage from prostate needle biopsies. *Urology* 1996;48:47–57.
76. Umbas R, Isaacs WB, Bringuier PP, et al. Decreased E-cadherin expression is associated with poor prognosis in patients with prostate cancer. *Cancer Res* 1994;54:3929–3933.
77. Kleinerman DI, Troncoso P, Lin S-H, et al. Consistent expression of an epithelial cell adhesion molecule (C-CAM) during human prostate development and loss of expression in prostate cancer: Implications as a tumor suppressor. *Cancer Res* 1995;55:1215–1220.
78. Banks RE, Gearing AJ, Hemingway IK, et al. Circulating intracellular adhesion molecule-1 (ICAM-1), E-selectin, and vascular cell adhesion molecule-1 (V-CAM-1) in human malignancies. *Br J Cancer* 1993;68:122–126.
79. Lynch DF, Hassen W, Clements MA, et al. Serum levels of endothelial and neural cell adhesion molecules in prostate cancer. *Prostate* 1997;32:214–220.
80. Sherwood ER, Fong CJ, Lee C, et al. Basic fibroblast growth factor: a potential mediator of stromal growth in the human prostate. *Endocrinology* 1992;130:2955–2963.
81. Marengo SR, Chung LW. An orthotopic model for the study of growth factors in the ventral prostate of the rat:

effects of epidermal growth factor and basic fibroblast growth factor. *J Androl* 1994;15:277–286.

82. Folkman J, Klagsbrun M. Angiogenic factors. *Science* 1987;235:442–447.
83. Cronauer MV, Hittmair A, Eder IE, et al. Basic fibroblast growth factor levels in cancer cells and in sera of patients suffering from proliferative disorders of the prostate. *Prostate* 1997;31:223–233.
84. Folkman J. What is the evidence that tumors are angiogenesis dependent? *J Natl Cancer Inst* 1990;82:4–6.
85. Liotta LA, Steeg PS, Stetler-Stevenson WG. Angiogenesis: an imbalance of positive and negative regulation. *Cell* 1991;64:327–336.
86. Westermarck J, Kahari VM. Regulations of matrix metalloproteinase expression in tumor invasion. *FASEB J* 1999;13: 781–792.
87. Woessner JF. The matrix metalloproteinase family. In: Parks WC, Mecham RP, eds. *Matrix metalloproteinases.* San Diego: Academic Press 1998:1–14.
88. Vincenti MP, White LA, Schroen DJ, et al. Regulating expression of the gene for matrix metalloproteinase-1 (collagenase): mechanisms that control enzyme activity, transcription, and mRNA stability. *Crit Rev Eukaryot Gene Exp* 1996;6:391–411.
89. Kleiner DJ, Stetler-Stevenson WG. Structural biochemistry and activation of matrix metalloproteinases. *Curr Opin Cell Biol* 1993;5:891–897.
90. Gomez DE, Alonso DF, Yoshiji H, et al. Tissue inhibitors of metalloproteinases—structure, regulation and biological functions. *Eur J Cell Biol* 1997;74:111–122.
91. Henriet P, Blavier L, Declerck YA. Tissue inhibitors of metalloproteinases (TIMP) in invasion and proliferation. *APMIS* 1999;107:111–119.
92. Witty JP, McDonnell S, Newell KJ, et al. Modulation of matrylisin levels in colon carcinoma cell lines affects tumorigenicity in vivo. *Cancer Res* 1994;54:4805–4812.
93. Declerk YA, Perez N, Shimada H, et al. Inhibition of invasion and metastasis in cells transfected with an inhibitor of metalloproteinases. *Cancer Res* 1992;52:701–708.
94. Koop S, Khokha R, Schmidt EE, et al. Overexpression of metalloproteinase inhibitor in B16F10 cells does not affect extravasation but reduces tumor growth. *Cancer Res* 1994;54:4791–4797.
95. Murphy AN, Unsworth EJ, Stetler-Stevenson WG. Tissue inhibitor of metalloproteinase-2 inhibits bFGF-induced human microvascular endothelial cell proliferation. *J Cell Physiol* 1993;157:351–358.
96. Schnaper HW, Grant DS, Stetler-Stevenson WG, et al. Type IV collagenase(s) and TIMPs modulate endothelial cell morphogenesis in vitro. *J Cell Physiol* 1993;156:235–246.
97. Vlodavsky I, Korner G, Ishai MR, et al. Extracellular matrix-resident growth factors and enzymes: possible involvement in tumor metastasis and angiogenesis. *Cancer Metastasis Rev* 1990;9:203–226.
98. Fowlkes JL, Enghild JJ, Suzuki K, et al. Matrix metalloproteinases degrade insulin-like growth factor-binding-protein-3 in dermal fibroblast cultures. *J Biol Chem* 1994;269: 25742–25746.
99. Koyama H, Raines EW, Bornfeldt KE, et al. Fibrillar collagen inhibits arterial smooth muscle proliferation through regulation of Cdk2 inhibitors. *Cell* 1996;87:1069–1078.
100. Basset P, Okada A, Chenard MP, et al. Matrix metalloproteinases as stromal effectors of human carcinoma progression: therapeutical implications. *Matrix Biol* 1997;15:535–541.
101. Johnsen M, Lund LR, Romer J, et al. Cancer invasion and tissue remodeling: common themes in proteolytic matrix degradation. *Curr Opin Cell Biol* 1998;10:667–671.
102. Kruger A, Sanchez Sweatman OH, Martin DC, et al. Host TIMP-1 overexpression confers resistance to experimental brain metastasis of a fibrosarcoma cell line. *Oncogene* 1998;16:2419–2423.
103. Ahonen M, Baker A, Kahari VM. Adenovirus mediated gene delivery of tissue inhibitor of metalloproteinases-3 inhibits invasion and induces apoptosis in melanoma cells. *Cancer Res* 1998;58:2310–2315.
104. Itoh T, Tanioka M, Yoshida H, et al. Reduced angiogenesis and tumor progression in gelatinase A-deficient mice. *Cancer Res* 1998;58:1048–1051.
105. Wilson CL, Heppner KJ, Labosky PA, et al. Intestinal tumorigenesis is suppressed in mice lacking the metalloproteinase matrilysin. *Proc Natl Acad Sci U S A* 1997;94:1402–1407.
106. Iozzo R. Tumor stroma as a regulator of neoplastic behavior. Agonist and antagonist elements embedded in the same connective tissue. *Lab Invest* 1995;73:157–160.
107. Heppner KJ, Matrisian LM, Jensen RA, et al. Expression of most matrix metalloproteinase family members in breast cancer represents a tumor-induced host response. *Am J Pathol* 1996;149:273–282.
108. Johanson N, Airola K, Grenman R, et al. Expression of collagenase-3 (MMP-13) in squamous cell carcinoma of the head and neck. *Am J Pathol* 1997;151:499–508.
109. Bolon I, Gouyer V, Devouassoux M, et al. Expression of c-ets-1, collagenase 1, and urokinase–type plasminogen activator genes in lung carcinoma. *Am J Pathol* 1995;147:1298–1310.
110. Brown PD, Bloxidge RE, Stuart NSA, et al. Association between expression of activated 72-kd gelatinase and tumor spread in non–small cell lung carcinoma. *J Natl Cancer Inst* 1993;85:574–578.
111. Hamdy FC, Fadlon EJ, Cottam D, et al. Matrix metalloproteinase 9 expression in primary human prostatic adenocarcinoma and benign prostatic hyperplasia. *Br J Cancer* 1994;69: 177–182.
112. Hashimoto K, Kihira Y, Matuo Y, et al. Expression of matrix metalloproteinase-7 and tissue inhibitor of metalloproteinase-1 in human prostate. *J Urol* 1998;160:1872–1876.
113. Stearns ME, Wang M. Type IV (MW 72000) expression in human prostate: benign and malignant tissue. *Cancer Res* 1993;53:878–883.
114. Lokeshwar BL, Selzer MG, Block NL, et al. Secretion of matrix metalloproteinases and their inhibitors (tissue inhibitor of metalloproteinases) by human prostate in explant cultures: reduced tissue inhibitor of metalloproteinase secretion by malignant tissues. *Cancer Res* 1993;53:4493–4498.
115. Wood M, Fudge K, Mohler JL, et al. In situ hybridization studies of metalloproteinases 2 and 9 and TIMP-1 and TIMP-2 expression in human prostate cancer. *Clin Exp Metastasis* 1997;15:246–258.
116. Gohji H, Fujimoto N, Hara I, et al. Serum matrix metalloproteinase-2 and its density in men with prostate cancer as a

new predictor of disease extension. *Int J Cancer* 1998;79:96–101.
117. Moses MA, Wiederschain D, Loughlin KR, et al. Increased incidence of matrix metalloproteinases in urine of cancer patients. *Cancer Res* 1998;58:1395–1399.
118. Baker T, Tickle S, Wasan H. Serum metalloproteinases and their inhibitors: markers for malignant potential. *Br J Cancer* 1994;70:506–512.
119. Jung K, Nowak L, Lein M, et al. Matrix metalloproteinases 1 and 3, tissue inhibitor of metalloproteinase-1, and the complex of metalloproteinase-1/tissue inhibitor in plasma of patients with prostate cancer. *Int J Cancer* 1997;74:220–223.
120. Zeng ZS, Cohen AM, Zhang ZF, et al. Elevated tissue inhibitor of metalloproteinase 1 RNA in colorectal cancer stroma correlates with lymph node and distant metastases. *Clin Cancer Res* 1995;1:899–906.
121. Nakatsukasa H, Ashida K, Higashi T, et al. Cellular distribution of transcripts for tissue inhibitor of metalloproteinases 1 and 2 in human cellular carcinomas. *Hepatology* 1996;24:82–88.
122. Di Sant'Agnese PA. Neuroendocrine differentiation in carcinoma of the prostate. *Cancer* 1992;70:254–268.
123. Seghal I, Thompson TC. Neuropeptides induce Mr 92,000 type IV collagenase (matrix metalloproteinase-9) activity in human prostate cancer cell lines. *Cancer Res* 1998;58:4288–4291.
124. Patterson BC, Sang QA. Angiostatin-converting enzyme activities of human matrilysin (MMP-7) and gelatinase B/type IV collagenase (MMP-9). *J Biol Chem* 1997;272: 28823–28825.
125. Dong Z, Kumar R, Yang X, et al. Macrophage-derived metalloelastase is responsible for the generation of angiostatin in Lewis lung carcinoma. *Cell* 1997;88:801–810.
126. Brown PD. Clinical studies with matrix metalloproteinase inhibitors. *APMIS* 1999;107:174–180.
127. Eccles SA, Box GM, Court WJ, et al. Control of lymphatic and hematogenous metastases of a rat mammary carcinoma by the matrix metalloproteinase inhibitor batimastat (BB-94). *Cancer Res* 1996;56:2815–2822.
128. Wang X, Fu X, Brown PD, et al. Matrix metalloproteinase inhibitor BB-94 (batimastat) inhibits human colon tumour growth and spread in a patient-like orthotopic model in nude mice. *Cancer Res* 1994;54:4726–4728.
129. Sledge GW, Qulali M, Goulet R, et al. Effect of matrix metalloproteinase inhibitor batimastat on breast cancer regrowth and metastasis in athymic mice. *J Natl Cancer Inst* 1995;87:1546–1550.
130. Price A, Raja JB, Rewcastle NB, et al. Marked inhibition of tumor growth in a malignant glioma tumor model by the novel synthetic matrix metalloproteinase AG3340. *Proc AACR* 1998;39:2058.
131. Bull C, Flynn C, Eberwein D, et al. Activity of the biphenyl matrix metalloproteinase inhibitor BAY 12-9566 in vivo murine models. *Proc AACR* 39:2062.
132. Taraboletti G, Garofalo A, Belotti D, et al. Inhibition of angiogenesis and murine hemangioma growth by batimastat, a synthetic inhibitor of matrix metalloproteinase. *J Natl Cancer Inst* 1995;87:293–298.
133. Hibner B, Card A, Flynn C, et al. BAY-12-9566, a novel biphenyl matrix metalloproteinase inhibitor, demonstrates anti-invasive and anti-angiogenic properties. *Proc AACR* 1998;39:2063.
134. Anderson IC, Shipp MA, Docherty AJP, et al. Combination therapy including a gelatinase inhibitor and cytotoxic agent reduces local invasion and metastasis of murine Lewis lung carcinoma. *Cancer Res* 1996;56:715–718.
135. Giavazzi R, Garofalo A, Lucchini V, et al. Batimastat, a synthetic inhibitor of matrix metalloproteinases, potentiates the anti-tumor activity of cisplatin in ovarian carcinoma xenografts. *Clin Cancer Res* 1998;4:985–992.
136. Steward WP. Marimastat (BB2516): current status of development. *Cancer Chemother Pharmacol* 1999;43:s56–s60.
137. Millar AW, Brown PD, Moore J, et al. Results of single and repeat dose studies of the oral matrix metalloproteinase inhibitor marimastat in healthy male volunteers. *Br J Clin Pharmacol* 1998;45:21.
138. Nemunaitis J, Poole C, Primrose J, et al. Combined analysis of studies of the effects of the matrix metalloproteinase inhibitor marimastat on serum tumor markers in advanced cancer: selection of a biological active and tolerable dose for long-term studies. *Clin Cancer Res* 1998;4:1101–1109.
139. Parson SL, Watson SA, Griffin NR, et al. An open phase I/II study of the oral matrix metalloproteinase inhibitor marimastat in patients with inoperable gastric cancer. *Ann Oncol* 1996;7:47.
140. Adams M, Thomas H. A phase I study of the matrix metalloproteinase inhibitor marimastat administered concurrently with carboplatin to patients with relapsed ovarian cancer. *Proc ASCO* 1998;17:217a.
141. Carmichael J, Ledermann J, Woll PJ, et al. Phase IB study of concurrent administration of marimastat and gemcitabine in non-resectable pancreatic cancer. *Proc ASCO* 1998; 17:232a.
142. Anderson I, Supko J, Eder J, et al. Pilot pharmacokinetic study of marimastat in combination with carboplatin/paclitaxel in patients with metastatic or locally advanced inoperable non–small cell lung cancer. *Proc ASCO* 1999;18:719.
143. Rasmussen H, Rugg T, Brookes C, et al. First placebo controlled safety review of marimastat: a potential new therapeutic class. *Proc ASCO* 1999;18:743.
144. O'Leary J, Young D, Shalinsky D, et al. Identification of membrane type-matrix metalloproteinase-1 (MT-MMP-1) in human prostate cancer and in vivo inhibition of PC3 cell invasion and angiogenesis by AG3340. *Proc ASCO* 1999;18:1198.
145. Collier M, Shepherd F, Ahmann FR, et al. A novel approach to studying the efficacy of AG3340 a selective inhibitor of matrix metalloproteinases (MMPs). *Proc ASCO* 1999;18: 1861.
146. Tolcher A, Rowinsky EK, Rizzo J, et al. A phase I and pharmacokinetic study of the oral matrix metalloproteinase inhibitor Bay 12-9566 in combination with paclitaxel and carboplatin. *Proc ASCO* 1999;18:617.
147. Figg WD, Raje S, Bauer RS, et al. Pharmacokinetics of thalidomide in an elderly prostate cancer population. *J Pharm Sci* 1999;88:121–125.
148. Nonomura MT, Nozawa M, Harada Y, et al. Angiogenesis inhibitor TNP-470 inhibits growth and metastasis of a hormone–independent rat prostatic carcinoma cell line. *J Urol* 1998;160:210–213.

149. Belotti D, Vergani V, Drudis T, et al. The microtube-affecting drug paclitaxel has antiangiogenic activity. *Clin Cancer Res* 1996;2:1843–1849.
150. Bollag W. Experimental basis of cancer combination chemotherapy with retinoids, cytokines, 1,25-dihydroxyvitamin D3, and analogs. *J Cell Biochem* 1994;56:427–435.
151. Majewski S, Shopinska M, Marczak M, et al. Vitamin D3 is a potent inhibitor of tumor-cell induced angiogenesis. *J Invest Dermatol Symp Proc* 1996;1:97–101.
152. Shawyer LK, Schwartz DP, Mann E, et al. Inhibition of platelet-derived growth factor-mediated signal transduction and tumor growth by N-[4-(trifluoromethyl)-phenyl]5-methylisoxazole-4-carboxamide. *Clin Cancer Res* 1997;3: 1167–1177.
153. Reese D, Frolich M, Bok R, et al. A Phase II trial of humanized monoclonal anti-vascular endothelial growth factor antibody (rhuMAb VEGF) in hormone refractory prostate cancer. *Proc Am Soc Clin Oncol* 1999;18:351a.
154. Ko YJ, Chachoua A, Small E, et al. Phase II study of SU-101 in patients with PSA-positive prostate cancer. *Proc Am Soc Clin Oncol* 1999;18:317a.
155. Wu H, Beurelein G, Nie Y, et al. Stepwise in vitro affinity maturation of Vitaxin, an alphav beta3-specific humanized mAB. *Proc Natl Acad Sci U S A* 1998;95:6037–6042.
156. Bauer KS, Figg WD, Hamilton JM, et al. A pharmacokinetically guided phase II study of carboxyamido-triazole in androgen-independent prostate cancer. *Clin Cancer Res* 1999;5:2324–2329.
157. Carducci MA, Nelson JB, Chan-Tack KM, et al. Phenylbutyrate induces apoptosis in human prostate cancer and is more potent than phenylacetate. *Clin Cancer Res* 1996;2: 379–387.
158. Warrell RP, He LZ, Richon V, et al. Therapeutic targeting of transcription in acute promyelocytic leukemia by use of an inhibitor of histone deacetylase. *J Natl Cancer Inst* 1998;90: 1621–1625.
159. Majewski S, Marczak M, Szmurlo A, et al. Interleukin-12 inhibits angiogenesis induced by tumor cell lines in vivo. *J Invest Dermatol* 1996;106:1114–1118.
160. Pluda JM. Tumor-associated angiogenesis: mechanisms, clinical implications, and therapeutic strategies. *Semin Oncol* 1997;24:203–218.

54

CANCER VACCINES AND GENETIC IMMUNOTHERAPY FOR PROSTATE CANCER

JONATHAN W. SIMONS
BEVERLY DRUCKER
JASON REINGOLD

NEW RESEARCH RATIONALE FOR PROSTATE CANCER IMMUNOTHERAPY

New, potent, and specific antineoplastic modalities for prostate cancer (CaP) are imperative (1). Hormonal therapy for CaP is not curative, and a large window of opportunity exists for adjuvant therapy after definitive treatment of the primary. As described in Chapters 21 and 22 of this book, recurrence rates after standard therapy for localized disease, either radiotherapy or surgery, are still more than 20% in the best academic hands. Options for primary treatment failures, such as hormonal therapy, chemotherapy, or radiation, are limited in terms of duration and efficacy. Although hormonal therapies offer significant remissions and palliation of pain from bony metastases, survival has not been significantly improved for the majority of patients who develop the inevitable progression to androgen-refractory disease (2). Furthermore, combinations of cytotoxic drugs active against proliferating cells in S phase (e.g., cisplatinum and etoposide) have currently shown limited therapeutic benefits in providing overall survival improvement in prostate cancer to date since Huggins' first paper in 1941.

Although perhaps ignored by investigators eager to pursue early new drug development, CaPs *in vivo* may in part be "kinetically resistant" to cell-cycle poisons active in breast cancer medical oncology. In patients, many clinical metastatic prostate tumors manifest a very *low* growth fraction and are therefore kinetically resistant to many of these active agents that kill in S phase (2). Osseous metastases from CaP can often have less than 3% of CaP cells in S phase. Thus, nearly one-third of all newly diagnosed CaP patients who have locally advanced or metastatic cancer at diagnosis are ultimately faced with an urgent need for new treatment options in addition to antiproliferative cytotoxic drugs. Thus, modalities that kill independent of cell cycle have become attractive for research. Antibodies, macrophages, natural killer (NK) cells, and T lymphocytes all can kill tumor cells *in vitro*, independent of cell cycle. Given the unmet medical need and measurable explosion in potential new molecular biology applications for cancer immunotherapy, it is logical that clinical and basic research has begun exploration of new directions in CaP immunotherapy since 1993.

Immunotherapy research for solid tumors in the era preceding recombinant DNA has had a venerable past. With some remarkable exceptions, it has also been largely inactive in the clinic. More than a century ago, Coley and colleagues began clinical investigation with cancer immunotherapy using pyogenic bacterial extracts and tumor vaccines (3). In the 1970s, before recombinant DNA biotechnology allowed mechanistic dissection of immune responses, Brannen and colleagues showed it was possible in some patients to detect preexisting systemic immune responses to autologous CaP cell lysates bearing tumor-associated antigens (3). Thus, data suggested that the host immune response can recognize undefined CaP cell–associated antigens. In the clinical development of recombinant interferon-alpha (IFN) and interleukin-2 (IL-2), no significant activity was observed for CaP, and this tumor type was relegated to a class of tumors that was not of priority for immunotherapy development. CaP was viewed by basic scientists as a largely nonimmunogenic tumor type; adjuvants such as bcg with prostate tumor vaccines in pilot trials and animal research with the rat CaP Dunning model had suggested this tumor type was nonimmunogenic—unrecognizable to the B-cell or T-cell arm of the immune system (W.W. Scott, *personal communication*, 1991). As late as 1995, major medical oncology textbooks that dealt comprehensively with CaP clinical trials did not bother to reference negative results of immunotherapy clinical trials for it.

Why has the paradigm shifted to a discussion in this chapter of the vibrant new rationale for research on prostate immunotherapy? At minimum, two major forces are at work. First, the time is right: the science of cancer immunotherapy is readily translatable to clinical research (4). Second, CaP is antigenically attractive for full-scale induction of new therapeutic forms of autoimmunity, a factor considered inconceivable 5 years ago (3).

Fundamentally, there has never been a brighter moment in biomedical research to manipulate therapeutic immune responses against solid tumors previously conceived as immunity resistant. New knowledge exists to do so (Table 54-1). The principal effectors of human immune responses have now been characterized with increasing precision. The understanding of the molecular biology of B- and T-cell activation and regulation has deepened to the point that therapeutic predictions can be made, tested, and interpreted in clinical trials (4). An unanticipated benefit of the human immunodeficiency virus epidemic has been research funding of basic research on human T-cell biology and disclosure of how the T-cell receptor is used to recognize cancer-associated peptides. This essential new knowledge has had a direct leavening influence on new concepts on activating and augmenting T-cell responses to solid tumors, such as CaP. The precise signals and co-stimulatory molecules that activate many immune responses also have been identified (4). More than 40 genes encoding the activation molecules (cytokines and lymphokines) and their ligand-specific receptors have been identified, cloned, and evaluated as molecular therapeutics. This allows each to be considered for use as purified and well-characterized drugs in the form of proteins or DNA. Many of these immunostimulatory molecules have become far more potent therapeutically as adjuvants than bcg or *Cryptosporidium parvum* extracts. This is because they are the human body's own activation molecules for the repertory of immune responses necessary to withstand and survive constant viral, bacterial, and fungal infections. Furthermore, recombinant DNA biotechnology has allowed commercial-scale generation of specific mouse monoclonal antibodies generated against prostate-unique antigens. These can be chimerized so that most of the candidate therapeutic antibody is encoded from the human Fc DNA sequences and thus avoids neutralizing effects of human antimouse monoclonal antibodies (5).

In addition to the new molecular immunology is the scientific realization that CaP is particularly attractive antigenically for novel approaches to immunotherapy. The prostate is an accessory organ that is not needed for potency or fertility; complete eradication of cells bearing prostate-unique antigens using immune responses can be envisioned as a therapeutic goal. Currently, expression sequence–tagged RNA libraries suggest that more than 500 unique genes to the prostate—and no other adult organ—can be considered candidate antigens for defined immunologic attack (6). Current research in T-cell–mediated cancer immunotherapy further suggests that to cure experimental animals with preestablished tumors, it is critical to create T-cells that have autoimmune properties. These T cells are tolerant to normal organs *in situ* but are tumoricidal against tumors expressing these normal antigens at ectopic metastatic sites once these T cells are stimulated by immunotherapeutic manipulations. For example, therapeutic T-cell tumor antigens found in melanoma patients are expressed not only on the melanoma but also on normal melanocytes (MART-1, gp100, tyrosinase, tyrosinase-related protein-1, and tyrosinase-related protein-2). Clinical responses have been identified in human melanoma patients whose activated T cells recognize the MAGE-1 to -3, gp100, and tyrosinase genes. These melanoma-associated antigens are normal "self proteins" that are highly expressed in normal melanocytes, as well as by melanomas at metastatic sites. Furthermore, breast, colon, lung, and even some CaPs can express MAGE antigens. T cells specific for peptides of the self-protein tyrosinase can be isolated from normal individuals and can attack and kill melanoma tumor cells from human leukocyte antigen (HLA)-matched cancer patients (7). These are not necessarily tumor-specific cancer antigens but rather cancer-associated antigens that are immunodominant. Indeed, evidence has grown that the distinction between self antigens and tumor antigens for T cells is vanishing. A class of tumor-associated antigens (MAGE-1, MAGE-3, GAGE-1 and -2, and RAGE) is overexpressed in solid tumors and only elsewhere expressed in the germ cell of the testes. More to the therapeutic point for cancer patients is "breaking immunologic tolerance" to tumor-associated self proteins that can be attacked selectively by autoimmune

TABLE 54-1. NEW RATIONALE FOR PROSTATE CANCER IMMUNOTHERAPY

More than 500 prostate-unique genes in the human genome are also more than 500 potential unique antigens for specific prostate cancer immunotherapy.

Antitumor effector cells have defined activation receptors and co-stimulatory molecules for therapy research and have activity in models of prostate cancer:

- T-cell subsets (CD4 Th1, CD4 Th2, CD8), as well as NK cells, neutrophils, and eosinophils

Potent new tumor peptide antigen presentation pathways have been identified: dendritic cell loading of class I + class II prostate antigens.

Prostate cancer–associated carbohydrate antigens identified.

Prostate-specific peptide antigens recognized by T-cell receptors identified through new antigen discovery technologies.

Humanized murine antiprostate antibodies can be generated by biotechnology to prostate antigens discovered in patients going into remission after treatment with polyvalent vaccine.

Recombinant DNA technology allows clinical trial-based material-grade testing of all of above concepts in a combinatorial fashion.

Th1, T helper cell 1; NK, natural killer.

mechanisms without causing damage to neighboring normal tissues. For example, anti-MAGE–reactive T cells can induce tumor regressions in melanoma without apparent adverse autoimmunity (8). Self antigens of known treatment targets associated with tumors do induce weak autoimmune T- and B-cell responses before diagnosis. For example, women with breast cancer with Her2/neu overexpression have T cells reactive to Her2/neu peptides and immunoglobulins against Her2/neu (10). Because tumors express over more Her2/neu than normal tissues, efforts are focussed on driving autoimmunity against this antigen in breast and ovarian cancer. In summary, interest in driving T cells against similar organ-unique peptide antigens to create autoprostate T-cell immune responses now has a strong basis in the new age of molecular immunology.

HARNESSING IMMUNITY FOR PROSTATE CANCER THERAPEUTICS

Antigens

A basic understanding by the CaP oncologist of the immune system is required to understand emerging research immunotherapy strategies for CaP. An immune response requires two phases: first, a recognition of a pathogen and second, the mounting of a response to eliminate it. The pathogen may be foreign, as in cases of infections, or self antigen, as in cases of cancer or autoimmunity. The distinguishing elements of a pathogen that are recognized by the immune system are antigens. The uniqueness of antigens for recognition is embedded in their coding by amino acid sequence or structure by carbohydrate protein–binding interactions. After recognition of the pathogenic antigen, the effector phase is activated. This consists of the coordinated response of many different cell types that work together to eliminate the source of antigens. These include B lymphocytes, which respond to antigen through production of antibody; T-helper lymphocytes, which direct cell-cell interactions and the release of cytokines; and cytotoxic T cells, which kill cells bearing foreign antigen. Additional cells that are vital to immune process are mixed populations of phagocytic cells whose varied functions include cytokine production, internalization and destruction of pathogens, or presentation of foreign antigens to T or B cells.

Essential properties of the human immune response are specificity and memory. When a particular lymphocyte recognizes antigen, it undergoes a clonal expansion and differentiation to effector and memory cells so that a subsequent encounter with the same antigen will trigger a potentially more effective response. This system is further regulated by the elaboration of cytokines by a host of immune cells that direct the immune response toward the production of antibodies; the production of cytotoxic T-cell responses; antibodies and T cells; or, at times, toward no response, otherwise known as tolerance.

B Cells and Antibodies

B lymphocytes develop in the bone marrow. Each B cell is genetically programmed to encode a unique surface receptor that is specific for a particular antigen. In concept, multiple antibodies might be expanded that recognize tumor-associated antigens. Once the surface receptor binds its specific antigen, it relays a signal that causes the B cell to multiply and differentiate into plasma cells. Plasma cells, in turn, produce large quantities of the receptor molecule in a soluble form known as the antibody. Antibodies are large glycoproteins found in blood and tissue fluids. By maintaining the same molecular-binding specificity as the original B-cell receptor, the antibody can then bind to the same antigen originally recognized by the B cell but now at distant sites. The binding of an antibody to a foreign antigen causes it to be targeted by macrophages and allows it to be more easily internalized by phagocytosis.

T Cells

T lymphocytes are derived from bone marrow cells but mature in the thymus. There are several different types of T cells that are defined by their surface markers and functions. T helper cells (Th) interact with other immune cells to influence their function. Th1 cells interact with mononuclear phagocytes and generally help them to destroy intracellular pathogens such as viruses through the elaboration of various cytokines. Th1 cells are essential in destroying human cells infected with viruses, as they can recognize viral antigens expressed on the cell surface. Th2 cells interact with B cells and help them to divide, differentiate, and make antibodies. Another T-cell population can destroy host cells bearing foreign antigen and are called *cytotoxic T cells*. T cells recognize peptide antigens when they bind to their receptor molecule, the T-cell receptor. Each T cell has a unique antigen-recognition receptor that can bind a specific antigen. T cells are activated to perform their particular function when antigen binds the T-cell receptor together with a major histocompatibility complex (MHC) molecule on the surface of the cell bearing the antigen along with an activator molecule on the same cell surface. Th cells require MHC class II on the target cell surface for activation, whereas cytotoxic T cells require MHC class I on the target cell surface. T cells generate their effects by releasing cytokines, soluble proteins that affect other cells, or direct cell-cell interactions.

T Helper Cells

Th cells are phenotypically defined as those bearing the cell-surface marker protein CD4. Based on murine models, there are two distinct populations of CD4+ cells (Th1 and Th2) that can be distinguished by their functions and cytokine profiles, rather than by surface marker phenotyping. As these cells may each be therapeutically useful, both are under study. Th1 cells secrete cytokines IFN-gamma and tumor necrosis factor α (TNF-α). These cytokines, in turn, mediate responses to viruses, bacteria, and protozoans. Th2 cells secrete cytokines that help B cells proliferate, expand, and differentiate into plasma cells in the face of infection. Th1 responses lead to increased cellular immune responses to tumor, as well as increased secretion of tumoricidal IFN-gamma, and TNF-α T cells have been used for adoptive immunotherapy trials because of their ability to function as cytotoxic effectors, mobile cytokine factories, and antibody production stimulators.

Cytotoxic T Cells

T-killer cells, or cytotoxic T cells, are phenotypically defined as those bearing the CD8 cell surface molecule. Cytotoxic CD8+ T cells require antigen in a complex with MHC class I and beta 2-microglobulin to effect cell killing. Tumor cells that lack class I MHC expressions can therefore escape from class I mediate killing. This is thought to be one of the pathways of resistance of CaP to T-cell killing (12,13). Some preclinical approaches have explored the use of gene therapy to augment or restore class I MHC expression of tumor lines, but clinical applications of this technology have been limited.

Antigen-Presenting Cells: Dendritic Cells and Macrophages

"Professional" antigen-presenting cells (APCs) are essential to the development of tumor-specific responses. Macrophages have the function of presenting antigens to CD4 T cells and B cells. A subtype of APCs, the dendritic cells (DCs) are found in the epidermal layer of the skin, respiratory system, and gastrointestinal system, as well as the interstitial regions of several organs. DCs are the most potent presenters of antigen in the immune system. Only in the past 5 years has their importance for multiple strategies of cancer immunotherapy become evident. On a per cell basis, compared to macrophages, DCs are the most potent APCs in the body (13). DCs can trigger powerful T-cell responses and eradicate experimentally induced infections and tumors (14). DCs capture full-length proteins, proteolytically digest them, and then present the resulting "processed" peptides on their cell membranes bound to MHC antigens (Fig. 54-1). Fully activated, they sprout long dendrites in three dimensions likened to docking arms on space stations. These arms (dendrites) act as docking surfaces for the adherence of T cells on their surface, which attach like small spaceships. In addition to these "docking arms," the cell surface expresses high levels of T-cell co-stimulatory proteins, such as CD80 and CD86, that are needed for full activation of T cells. Protein antigens are presented to cytotoxic lymphocytes as small peptides, eight to ten amino acids in length, bound in a groove of the MHC class I molecule. Antigens presented to Th cells are slightly longer. Activation of the T cells leads to release of cytokines and new surface molecules on the T cells, which further enhances the function of the APCs, causing them to up-regulate expression of MHC molecules, co-stimulatory molecules, and cytokines.

Natural Killer Cells

NK cells are large lymphocytes that can recognize alterations on the surface of host cells. When exposed to high concentrations of IL-2 *in vitro*, NK cells differentiate into lymphokine-activated killer cells that can lyse fresh tumor specimens (15). This leads to a theory that NK cells are partly responsible for tumor surveillance. They do not express antigen receptors and, unlike cytotoxic T cells, they can kill cells that lack MHC molecules. They also can destroy cells that have become coated with antibody. This is known as *antibody-dependent cell-mediated cytotoxicity* or *killer cell activity*. Their primary function is to recognize and kill virus-infected cells and possibly tumor cells. NK

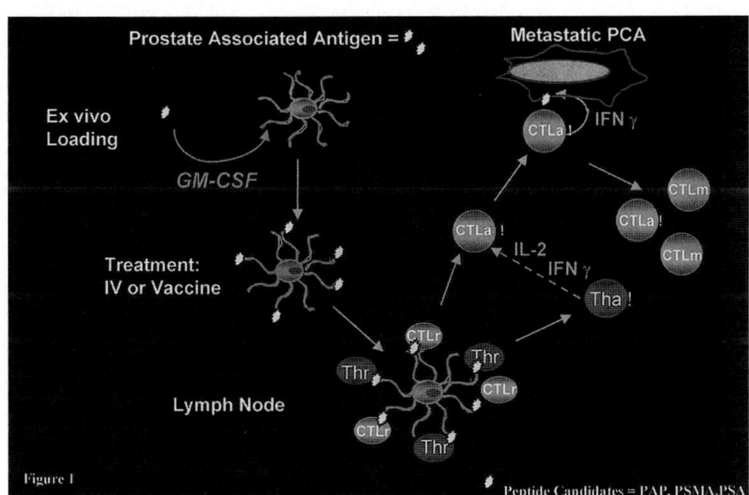

FIGURE 54-1. Prostate peptide loading of dendritic cells. CTLa, cytoxic T lymphocyte–associated antigen; CTLm, CTL memory; GM-CSF, granulocyte-macrophage colony-stimulating factor; IFNγ, interferon-γ; IL-2, interleukin-2; PAP, prostatic acid phosphatase antigen; PCA, prostate cancer; PSA, prostate-specific antigen; PSMA, prostate-specific membrane antigen; Tha, T-cell helper activate; Thr, threonine. (See also color Figure 54-1.)

cells release IFNs, IL-1, and granulocyte-macrophage colony-stimulating factor (GM-CSF) when activated, which may further amplify the immune response. NK cells themselves, by lack of an antigen receptor, are nonspecific. Coordination of their tumoricidal activity requires a cancer antigen–specific antibody or T cell.

Antibodies: Soluble Mediators of Immunity

Antibodies are produced by B cells after stimulation by T cells in the presence of foreign antigen. Each B cell produces a unique antibody with a unique antigen-binding site, termed the *fragment antigen binding* (Fab). All antibodies share a common section, termed the *Fc*, which interacts with other cells of the immune system. Phagocytes can bind the Fc portion of antibodies, which permits easier phagocytosis of the antigen bound by the antibody. The Fc component also binds complement, which consists of a group of proteins that interact in a cascadelike manner to cause the lysis of cells with antibody bound to their surface antigens. Although each antibody has a unique Fab section, it is possible that more than one antibody is capable of binding to the same antigen, as each antibody may recognize a different portion of the antigen. Each segment of the antigen that contains an antibody recognition site is termed an *epitope*. Once antibody is bound to foreign antigen, the complex becomes a target for phagocytic cells to destroy. Antibodies can kill cancer cells by complement-mediated lysis, antibody-dependent cell-mediated cytotoxicity, or by generalized inflammatory reactions (5).

Biotechnology has allowed antibodies to become U.S. Food and Drug Administration (FDA)-approved drugs for cancer. Native, humanized, toxin-conjugated, and radionucleotide-conjugated monoclonal antibodies have all been evaluated in oncology. Anti-CD20 antibodies have been used successfully to cure non-Hodgkin's lymphoma, and treatment with anti-Her2/neu antibodies improves metastatic breast cancer survival in patients whose cancers overexpress Her2/neu (16). Attempts to systemically treat CaP with monoclonal antibodies in clinical trials are discussed in Chapter 52 of this book. Nevertheless, as discussed elsewhere in this volume, radionucleotide-conjugated antibodies directed against prostate-specific membrane antigen (PSMA) (ProstaScint) can bind and allow imaging of CaP metastasis (5). Toxin-linked monoclonal antibodies have been used to treat Hodgkin's disease, but responses were limited by the development of antibodies against the toxins linked to the therapeutic antibody.

Cytokines

Cytokines are the general term for a large group of polypeptide molecules involved in the signaling between cells during immune responses (4). Cytokines are proteins or peptides produced by cells of the immune system. There are distinct families of cytokines, including IFNs, Ils, and colony-stimulating factors. They are small proteins that usually exert their effect in an autocrine (on the cell that produced them) or paracrine (on cells close by) fashion. The production of the molecules is usually transient and tightly regulated. They act by binding to specific transmembrane glycoprotein receptors at the cell surface and set off a cascade of protein interactions that often leads to alterations in gene transcription and translation. Several cytokines have similar actions; there is a redundancy in their roles. They also usually work in concert with other cytokines, although many cytokines like IFN-alpha, IFN-gamma, IL-2, and IL-12 have been tested as drugs and given intravenously in an endocrine fashion. Most work physiologically as *paracrine* signals. Paracrine molecules exert their actions locally at sites of infection or therapeutic vaccination. Cytokines function in a complex network in which the production of one cytokine will influence the production of or response to others. Cytokines such as GM-CSF have emerged in early phase I and phase II trials as potentially critical in making poorly immunogenic CaP cells recognizable to the patient's immune system.

Antigens

The past decade has seen substantial progress in efforts to define the antigens recognized on cancer cells (7). These might include viral antigens in the case of virus-associated tumors or variants of normal tissue antigens that have minor variations that alter their function, leading to oncogenesis. Normal antigens expressed in tumors may be altered by variant glycosylation. Some tumor-associated antigens are common to normal and tumor cells but are overexpressed on tumor cells, such as Her2/neu or MAGE. In these cases, the challenge of the cancer immunotherapist is to exploit these differences to develop a therapy that will destroy tumor cells while sparing normal cells that express similar antigen or lower levels of the identical one. Many groups have begun to ask whether cancer-specific mutant genes such as p53, the most commonly mutated tumor suppressor gene in solid tumors, can be used as antigens. Tumor antigens can also be differentiation antigens, which are expressed by the tumor and the normal differentiated cell from which the tumor originated. Alternatively, they can also be "oncofetal" antigens, which are differentiation antigens expressed strictly during development but not normally on adult tissues. The host's immune system would not recognize any of these antigen types as foreign, because they have been present on normal cells at some time. Immunotherapists for cancer attempt to break this tolerance through nonspecific means via cytokine therapy or through directed approaches to be discussed later. The problem with targeting antigens common to normal and tumor cells is that therapy aimed at destruction of the tumor may also destroy normal cells. For example, some patients receiving immunotherapy for melanoma have developed vitiligo from destruction of normal melanocytes (17). In the case of CaP, the hope is that therapies directed against prostate-specific antigens (PSAs) will have minimal toxicities even if active against normal tissue, as the prostate is not a vital organ (3).

Defining the expression of tumor-associated antigens on primary and metastatic CaP is a key step in selecting appropriate targets for immune attack with vaccines or other strategies. Monoclonal antibodies, directed against tumor cell lines, have helped to identify several tumor antigens. Using immunohistochemistry, Zhang et al. compared the distribution of 18 tumor-associated antigens on primary and metastatic CaP, as well as 16 normal tissue samples (18). They found that granulocyte-macrophage-2, KSA, and MUC2 were strongly expressed on eight of nine metastatic CaP biopsy specimens and that PSMA, transferrin, tension, and sTn were present in 8 of 11 primary CaP specimens. Tn, MUC1, and PSMA were expressed on approximately half of the nine metastatic specimens. Normal tissues were also tested with these antigens. PSMA was the only antigen that was not significantly expressed on any of the normal tissues except prostate epithelium and, weakly, on skeletal muscle cells. MUC7 and Her2/neu, although not frequently expressed by CaPs, were also not found in normal tissues, suggesting they would be excellent targets for other cancer therapies.

Currently, three candidate peptide antigens for CaP vaccines that have undergone clinical investigation are prostatic acid phosphatase (PAP), PSA, and PSMA. PAP is differentially expressed in prostate epithelial and CaP cells. PSA is a serine protease discussed at length in Chapter 15 of this book. More than 90% of CaPs and 100% of epithelial cells lining the ducts and acini of the prostate express the PSA protein. In contrast to PSA, PSMA is an integral membrane glycoprotein. Its expression is highly restricted to prostate epithelial cells, although it is also expressed at very low levels on skeletal muscle as well as small intestine (19). PSMA is expressed on a high proportion of CaPs, with increased expression often correlating with higher-grade cancers, metastatic disease, and hormone-refractory CaPs. It is also intriguing that monoclonal antibodies directed against its extracellular domain react with tumor vascular endothelium of a wide variety of carcinomas (lung, colon, breast) but not normal vascular endothelium, suggesting that effector cells directed against this antigen might attack more than one aspect of the cancer as it is directed against cancer cells and its vascular supply.

In the case of CaP oncology, prostate antigens secreted by the tumor can also be applied as biomarkers for monitoring of therapeutic effects. For example, PSA is detected in sera by enzyme-linked immunoabsorbent assay to monitor CaP development and can be used to monitor response to treatment with cancer vaccines. PSMA has been used diagnostically as part of a CaP imaging method (ProstaScint), which uses a monoclonal antibody specific for PSMA. Levels of PSMA are elevated in the sera of hormone-refractory CaP patients with advanced disease, suggesting that it too, like PSA, could be used to monitor disease progression (20). Enhanced expression of PSMA was detected in hormone-refractory CaP, presenting the possibility that PSMA may be used in the future to predict disease with worse prognosis (21). PSMA has been used as an antigen for loading DC-based vaccines, and PSA has been used to monitor clinical response (22).

Tolerance

Immunologic tolerance is a state of unresponsiveness that is specific for a particular antigen. It is induced by prior exposure to that antigen during a period of immune system development. Tolerance prevents harmful reactivity against the body's own tissues as well as common innocuous antigens that are encountered, such as those in food. Self-tolerance usually occurs during embryonic development but can also occur afterwards, depending on several conditions. Some of these include the nature of the antigen, stage of differentiation when the lymphocytes first encounter the antigen, site of the encounter, nature of the cells presenting the epitope, number of lymphocytes responding to the epitope, and cytokine milieu during the encounter. Some aspects of the antigen influence the type of immune response that occurs. For example, very large doses of antigen can often result in specific T- and sometimes B-cell tolerance. Specific host-antigen interactions may also play a role if there are no epitopes within the antigen that bind the host's MHC subtype. This may help explain certain cancer predispositions occurring with some MHC subtypes. The route of administration of an antigen can also determine whether or not an immune response occurs. Antigens administered subcutaneously or intradermally evoke an immune response, whereas those given intravenously, orally, or as an aerosol may cause tolerance or an immunologic deviation.

The APC presenting the antigen may also influence whether immune responsiveness or tolerance ensues. Effective activation of the T cell requires the expression of co-stimulatory molecules on the surface of the APC. The presentation of antigen by DCs or activated macrophages, both of which express high levels of MHC class II as well as co-stimulatory molecules, results in highly effective T-cell activation. However, if antigen is presented to T cells by a nonprofessional APC incapable of providing co-stimulation, such as the tumor cell itself, then unresponsiveness or tolerance results. The production of different cytokines by different CD4+ helper lymphocyte subpopulations probably influences the development of an immune response versus tolerance. For example, cytokines secreted by Th1 cells such as IFN-gamma can inhibit the responsiveness of Th2 cells. IL-10 made by Th2 cells or by cancer cells themselves can down-regulate B7 and IL-12 by APCs, which in turn inhibit Th1 activation.

Tolerance appears to play a pivotal role in carcinogenesis, as tumor cells have escaped immune recognition at the time of diagnosis. This may be because tumor cells express self-antigens but may also be because they do not express immunogenic co-stimuli or the appropriate adhesion molecules for lymphocytes and macrophages. Many tumors have absent or decreased levels of class I MHC expression on their surface. A preclinical model using transgenic T cells from tumor-bearing mice suggests that antigens expressed on tumor cells still fail to induce immune responses. Some tumors also express immunosuppressive cytokines, which would then give them a selective advantage from blunting antigen recognition. Tumor cells bearing altered MHC proteins that do not bind antigen or the T-cell receptor also have a selective growth advantage. Any of these mechanisms—and others—could result in the induction of immune response protection at the site of tumor cells.

New immunotherapy strategies strive to overcome CaP "tolerance" by manipulating the tumor cells themselves or the conditions under which the immune cells encounter CaP-associated tumor antigens. Some strategies require removing the immune cells to make these modifications, whereas others remove tumor cells, manipulate them, and then reintroduce them to the host in a more immunogenic context. Regardless of the strategy, the objective overall is to "break host tolerance" against CaP in the patient using immunotherapy.

APPROACHES TO PROSTATE CANCER IMMUNOTHERAPY

Two new approaches to cancer immunotherapy are undergoing clinical trial tests: activation immunotherapy with immunization (vaccines) and adoptive immunotherapy (Table 54-2). Both are intended to break tolerance. The development of immunotherapies based on specific stimulation of immune reactions against known characterized tumor antigens is distinctive from previous approaches using cytokines. These earlier approaches used the stimulation of the immune system against uncharacterized antigens with systemic administration of cytokines. Earlier studies used IL-2 to induce broad stimulation of the immune system to obtain FDA approval for use in treating renal cell carcinoma. Systemic use of cytokines to elicit a macroscopic response to attack tumor cells has had limited but clear success in the therapy of melanoma and renal cell carcinoma. IL-2 has no direct cytotoxic effect on cancer cells but rather exerts its immunotherapeutic effect by stimulating T-cell host immune responses that, by being augmented, can now respond to tumor associated antigens.

Newer approaches include the *ex vivo* (out of the body) stimulation of antigen-specific cytotoxic T lymphocytes (CTLs) directed at tumor-specific antigens. DCs can also be cultured from peripheral blood or bone marrow and loaded with peptides or tumor lysates for clinical use (24). The *ex vivo* culture of DCs in the presence of peptides is being used to educate patients' immune systems and stimulate them against specific prostate tumor antigens as described later (Fig. 54-1).

TABLE 54-2. PROSTATE CANCER IMMUNOTHERAPY STRATEGIES

- Activation immunotherapy
  - Prostate cancer immunization: new vaccine formulations
    - Single prostate antigen (full protein or peptide) vaccine
    - Multiple prostate antigens purified (polyvalent)
    - Whole-irradiated prostate cell vaccine unpurified (polyvalent)
    - Recombinant virus vaccine encoding prostate antigen gene
    - Naked DNA vaccine-encoding prostate antigen gene
    - Dendritic cell vaccines:
      - Loaded with prostate antigen peptides
      - Transfected and expressing prostate antigen genes
  - Immunization adjuvants for above vaccines: cytokines
    - Cytokine genes GM-CSF, IL-2, IL-12 encoded in vaccine
    - Recombinant cytokines given systemically with vaccine
- Adoptive immunotherapy
  - Transfer of antiprostate antigen effector cells
    - Intravenous transfer of T cells activated against prostate antigens
    - Intravenous transfer of T cells or B cells transfected with prostate antigen–specific T cell receptors or immunoglobulins
    - Monoclonal antibody to CaP antigen

CaP, prostate cancer; GM-CSF, granulocyte-macrophage colony-stimulating factor; IL-2, interleukin-2; IL-12, interleukin-12.

Other active immunotherapy strategies enhance the immunogenicity of the tumor through gene modification that augments immune recognition by transducing cytokines or co-stimulatory molecules into the tumor cell vaccines (3,24). Gene transfer is accomplished outside of the patient's body, and the approach has been designated *ex vivo gene therapy*. These genetically engineered whole tumor cell vaccines have been a major area of gene therapy research in cancer immunotherapy. These are then used as vaccines to stimulate DCs and T cells to upregulate systemic responses to the immunogens (Fig. 54-2). When compared head to head against many different immunostimulatory genes, one immunostimulatory gene has shown impressive activity in models of poorly immunogenic tumors, including CaP. GM-CSF–secreting cancer cell vaccines, generated from cancer cells by *ex vivo* gene transfer, elicit tumoricidal antitumor immune responses in a variety of animal tumor models, including preclinical models of hormone-refractory CaP and in human clinical trials (3). Irradiated GM-CSF–secreting cancer cell vaccines induce antitumor immune responses by recruiting APCs such as DCs to immunization sites. DCs, the most potent immunostimulatory APCs yet characterized, activate antigen-specific CD4+ and CD8+ T cells by priming them with antigens processed from the dying cancer cells (25). Recent preclinical studies have

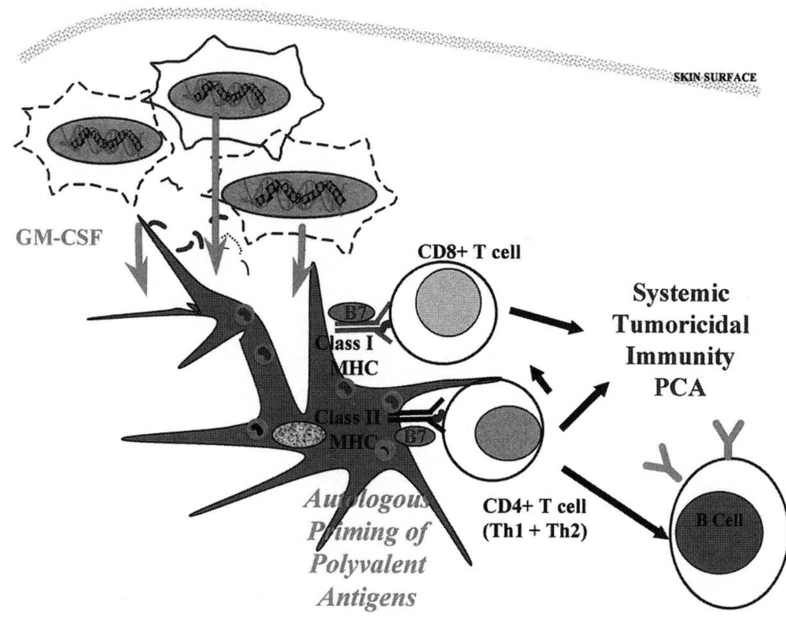

FIGURE 54-2. Granulocyte-macrophage colony-stimulating factor (GM-CSF) cytokine gene–transduced irradiated autologous prostate cancer (PCA) vaccine cells. MHC, major histocompatibility complex; Th1, T helper cell 1.

suggested that CD4+ T cells activated by GM-CSF–secreting cancer cell vaccines do not merely facilitate cancer cell destruction by CD8+ T-cell cells (25). In a phase I clinical trial of this treatment approach for malignant melanoma and advanced CaP, T- and B-cell immune responses against melanoma antigens and prostate antigens were detected (26–28).

NEW CLINICAL TRIALS IN PROSTATE CANCER IMMUNOTHERAPY

With the emergence of a strong molecular rationale for testing new concepts, new concepts of immunotherapy for CaP have entered early clinical investigation. All involve the use of new candidate therapeutic antigens. Although not considered particularly immunogenic, CaP has several unique differentiation antigens that it shares only with the prostate epithelium. In an initial assessment of expressed genes in the human genome project, more than 500 unique-expressed sequence tags, including the PSA gene messenger RNA, were found. Thus, many prostate-unique candidate genes might be potential protein antigens for vaccines that break tolerance to CaP cells. Antigen choices have been the use of glycoproteins, which are immunogenic or prostate-associated antigens in the form of specific proteins or whole tumor cell vaccines. Current clinical trials are directed against portions of defined carbohydrates and glycoproteins specific to CaP. Other strategies use whole tumor cells as vaccines in the hopes that they will provide a wider array of antigens, some of which may not be defined. The strategy behind adoptive immunotherapy is to educate immune cells *ex vivo* to respond to prostate antigens and then reintroduce them to the patient in the hopes of reconstituting a specific immune response against CaP cells. Investigational groups are still evaluating which cell types, immune effector arms, and antigen models are most effective.

Single Peptide Vaccines

Because PSA is an obvious candidate antigen, it has been used as a recombinant peptide as a vaccine. Early clinical development was conducted in phase I/II trials of hormone-refractory CaP, and different adjuvants were tested (25). These vaccines mount T-cell responses in some patients but have not demonstrated significant clinical responses in peer-reviewed literature at this writing. An alternative approach that is still under investigation has been to vaccinate patients with a vaccinia virus vector containing the PSA gene (Sanda, University of Michigan).

Carbohydrate Vaccines for Prostate Cancer

Oncogenesis is often associated with changes in the expression of cell-surface carbohydrates. Globo H is a hexasaccharide, originally isolated by Hakamori and co-workers on a human breast cancer cell line. Although expressed on normal tissues, its expression on cancer cells is more extensive. When synthesized artificially and used as a vaccine in mice, it was found to be highly immunogenic. Immunohistochemical methods detected enhanced expression of this antigen on primary and metastatic CaP (18). It was therefore selected as a rational target for immunotherapy vaccine strategies. Slovin and co-workers at Memorial Sloan-Kettering Cancer Center synthesized globo H hexasaccharide conjugates and used them as a vaccine in patients with relapsed CaP (25). Relapse was defined as three consecutively rising PSA values determined at a minimal interval of 2 weeks or visible metastatic disease. Vaccine was administered as five subcutaneous vaccinations of 36 weeks. No significant side effects were noted, with the major toxicities being local reactions at the injection site, chills, and fever. Patients responded to the vaccine with the expression of significant titers of immunoglobulin M antibody, with maximal response by week 9 and a decline in values by week 19. Despite immunoglobulin M production, all patients continued to have a rise in their PSA during the first 26 weeks of therapy, although in some patients the rate of PSA rise appeared to slow. Several patients who had evidence of disease relapse restricted to a rising PSA had a treatment effect occur within 3 months after completion of the vaccine therapy. The slope of the log of PSA concentration versus time plot after treatment declined, compared with values before treatment. Five patients had stable PSA slope profiles in the absence of any radiographic evidence of disease for 2 years after completing vaccination. The concept of using PSA slope profiles in assessing early treatment effect vaccine trials is not validated but has stimulated further validation in phase II and III trials.

Granulocyte-Macrophage Colony-Stimulating Factor Gene–Transduced Irradiated Whole Cell Tumor Vaccines

The whole cell tumor vaccine was initially proposed with the idea that a tumor cell introduced in a novel manner can provide a platform that expresses whole tumor antigens for antigen processing and, therefore, immune response. This concept has been improved on by combining the basic vaccine platform with cytokine adjuvants. Dranoff and Mulligan screened cytokine complementary DNAlike drugs to establish a rank order of cytokine potency for gene-modified murine melanoma vaccines (30). They used a high-efficiency replication-defective retroviral vector (MFG) to drive expression and secretion of cytokines. GM-CSF was found to be significantly more immunostimulatory in the tumor vaccine setting when compared to other cytokines, with IL-4 and IL-6 also manifesting some activity. Using a rat model, Sanda et al. showed preclinical efficacy and clinical feasibility of using GM-CSF gene-transduced autologous vaccines in the therapy of micrometastatic disease (31).

The first human study of the GM-CSF gene–transduced irradiated tumor was conducted in renal cell carcinoma (32). Patients were treated in a randomized double-blind dose-escalation study with equivalent doses of autologous irradiated renal cell carcinoma vaccine cells with or without *ex vivo* human GM-CSF gene transfer. Patients within a given study arm received escalating doses of cells within that treatment arm until limiting dose toxicities were reached. No dose-limiting toxicities were encountered. Vaccine site pruritus was the major toxicity associated with vaccination and was present in both arms of the study. Biopsies of intradermal sites of injection with GM-CSF–transduced vaccines were positive for macrophage, DC, eosinophil, neutrophil, and T-cell infiltrates. Delayed-type hypersensitivity (DTH) conversion to challenge with irradiated autologous unpassaged renal cell carcinoma after treatment suggested the generation of T-cell responses to antigens expressed on autologous tumor cells.

This same approach to GM-CSF gene–transduced whole tumor vaccines was tested in a phase I trial of CaP patients with advanced CaP discovered at radical prostatectomy (32). Yields from primary culture of tumor cells limited expansion of vaccine cells from primary tumor, but GM-CSF gene transfer was accomplished successfully. Vaccination side effects were limited to pruritus, redness, and swelling, which were all manageable on an outpatient basis. Nevertheless, activation of T-cell responses to autologous prostate tumor cells was observed. Furthermore, associated with the recruitment of DCs and macrophages to the vaccination sites was the induction of oligoclonal antibodies against autologous tumor–associated antigens. Based on these data suggesting that tolerance can be broken to prostate-associated antigens by loading them via vaccination with GM-CSF gene–transduced vaccines, multiinstitutional phase II clinical trials using allogeneic GM-CSF gene–transduced vaccines are under way. The first of these showed clinical responses by National Cancer Institute PSA response criteria and induction of new antibodies associated with clinical response (34). In these trials, a sterile unpassaged autologous tumor is not available from most of the patients, as they often underwent surgery at other institutions as part of standard therapy. Therefore, the tumor cell used in this study is not derived from the patient being treated but instead derived from two preestablished human CaP cell lines. The two cell lines are PC3 (derived from a bone metastasis) and the PSA-expressing LNCaP (derived from a lymph-node metastasis). The two cell lines are used as potential CaP-associated antigen sources in place of the patients' tumors (Fig. 54-3). These vaccines have induced some self-limited toxicity, including pain during administration, low-grade fevers, erythema, and pruritus (Fig. 54-4). This very favorable toxicity profile has allowed several different approaches to clinical development, including combination with hormonal therapy and investigational chemotherapy.

Dendritic Cell–Based Vaccines and Infusions

DCs are considered the most potent APCs of the immune system and are unique in their ability to stimulate naïve T cells. Tumor vaccines that optimally activate DCs are currently receiving the greatest intensity in preclinical and clinical investigation. DCs capture vaccine proteins, proteolytically digest them, and then present the resulting peptides on their cell membranes bound to MHC antigens, making them the cellular mechanism of "adjuvants." DCs

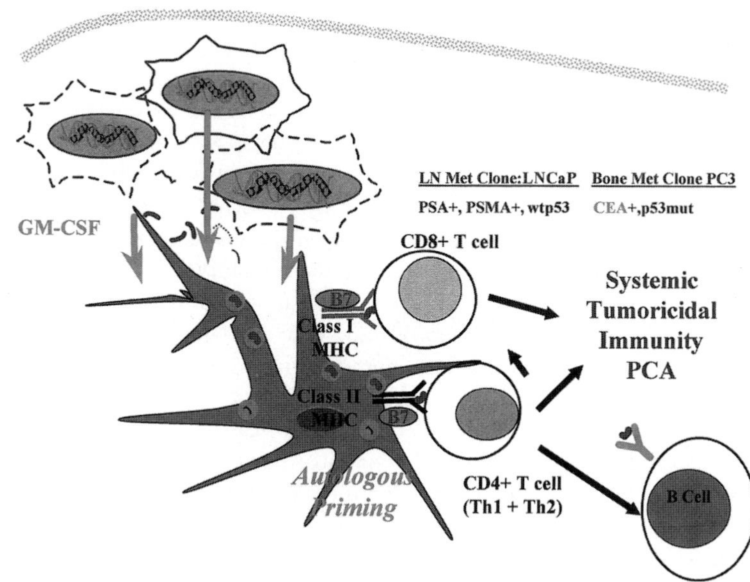

FIGURE 54-3. Granulocyte-macrophage colony-stimulating factor (GM-CSF)–transduced irradiated allogeneic prostate cancer (PCA) vaccine cells LNCaP + PC3. CEA, carcinoembryonic antigen; LN, lymph node; Met, metastasis; MHC, major histocompatibility complex; mut, mutant; PSA, prostate-specific antigen; PSMA, prostate-specific membrane antigen; Th1, T helper cell 1.

also express high levels of the co-stimulatory molecules CD80 and CD86, which are required for T-cell activation. Nevertheless, an alternative to tumor cell vaccination with GM-CSF gene–transduced irradiated vaccine cells is to use *ex vivo* autologous antigen–loaded DCs themselves.

DCs can now be isolated by leukophoresis and cultured with new biotechnology. They are derived from peripheral blood using cytokines, such as GM-CSF, IL-4, and TNF-α, and other growth factors. They then can be loaded with defined antigens. Murphy and colleagues were the first to report on the use of a CaP vaccine that uses patients' DCs and PSMA-derived peptides to induce CaP-specific T cells *in vivo* (22,35). Each participant underwent leukapheresis to harvest DCs from the peripheral blood. DCs are isolated and then cultured in the presence of GM-CSF and IL-4 for 7 days. Cultured DCs were then incubated for 2 hours in the presence of purified peptides derived from PSMA. Peptides (PSM-P1 and -P2) were seven to ten amino acids in length and were selected for their ability to bind the MHC class I-A2 molecule with high affinity. The cells were then washed, resuspended, and infused more than 30 minutes into the patient from which they were isolated. All study participants were followed before, during, and after treatment with periodic PSA levels, free PSA levels, PSMA, complete blood counts, CHEM-22, bone alkaline phosphatase, initial chest x-ray, bone scans, and ProstaScint scans. A DTH test against a panel of common antigens was conducted at the beginning of the phase I study and repeated during the phase II study with each patient to measure their general immune response activity.

The phase I study using this approach was conducted in Seattle in 1995. Its goal was to examine the safety of administering HLA-A2–specific PSMA peptides, autologous DCs, and peptide-pulsed autologous DCs to patients. Fifty-one patients with advanced hormone-refractory CaP were enrolled. The majority of patients (39 of 51) were stage D2 (T4N1-3M1a-c). Fewer than 25% of these patients were considered fully immunocompetent as assessed by DTH skin tests. The initial phase I trial demonstrated that infusions of autologous DCs and HLA-A2–specific PSMA peptides were well tolerated by all 51 study participants. As in the case of prostate tumor vaccines, at the completion of four infusion cycles, the maximum tolerated dose had not been achieved. No significant toxicity, acute or chronic, was observed, except for mild to moderate hypotension associated with the infusion.

Patients were monitored for cellular immune modulation to the appropriate PSMA peptide. An enhanced T-cell response was observed only with HLA-A2 subjects who were infused with PSMA peptide-pulsed DCs but not DCs or peptide alone. Seven patients had partial disease responses as defined by decreases in PSA serum levels (35,36). Average PSA levels increased in the nonresponder group, whereas a

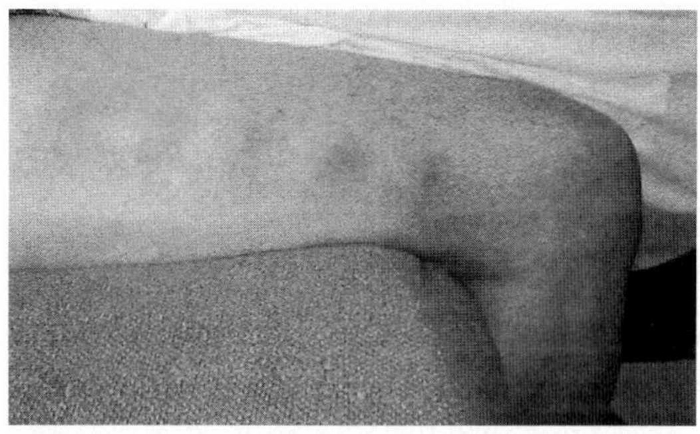

FIGURE 54-4. Outpatient safety of genetically engineered prostate cancer vaccines: activating dendritic cell antigen presentation intradermally 24 hours postvaccination. Allogeneic granulocyte-macrophage colony-stimulating factor gene–transduced irradiated prostate cancer vaccine cells. (See also color Figure 54-4.)

decrease was observed in the seven partial responders. All patients who were on hormone therapy before the trial continued their treatments during the trial. In the locally advanced group (group B), 10 of 41 (27%) were reported as partial responders and one subject had a complete response. Eight patients (22%) showed no significant change in their disease, and 19 patients (49%) showed disease progression. Of note, not all of the responders were HLA-A2 positive. Three of eight (37%) responders were HLA-A2-negative, indicating that although the peptides were selected for their ability to bind HLA-A2, they may also bind other HLA molecules. Further studies will use a recombinant PSMA peptide consisting of the native sequence without the transmembrane domain in the hopes that the processed protein might bind more HLA molecule subtypes.

Using a different antigen and different DC antigen loading technique, Burch and colleagues infused DCs loaded with the PAP (37) (Fig. 54-1). Loading was achieved by preexposing patient-derived DCs to a fusion protein PA2024 consisting of the GM-CSF recombinant protein and human PAP. In this phase I study, 3 of 13 patients with hormone-refractory disease sustained PSA declines associated with T-cell responses and new antibodies generated against CaP. Small and colleagues have extended these findings in hormone-refractory CaP patients (23). After four infusion sessions, three patients with hormone-refractory disease were found to have partial responses by PSA, and time to disease progression in all patients appeared to be correlated with dose of DCs infused and development of immune responses to the PAP antigen. Aside from fever that could be managed with antipyretics, this therapy was well tolerated in outpatients. A pivotal trial evaluating time to progression and overall survival is under way with this GM-CSF–activated DC-based therapy loaded with PAP antigen (E.J. Small, *personal communication*).

Currently, additional approaches are underway to load polyvalent antigens from CaPs into DCs. One strategy is to load the genes encoding CaP-associated antigens into DCs and then have the DCs express the proteins and process them as antigens. Using polymerase chain reaction, a very small amount of the original tumor is required, far less than that needed for creation of tumor vaccine cell lines. Gilboa and colleagues have discovered that by using prostate tumor complementary DNA–loaded DCs, cytotoxic T-cell responses in these patients can be generated against the polypeptide component of telomerase (TERT) (38).

FUTURE DIRECTIONS: COMBINATION THERAPY WITH IMMUNOTHERAPY

Although early in their development, GM-CSF gene–transduced irradiated prostate vaccines, globo H carbohydrate antigen vaccines, and single antigen-loaded DCs have clinical activity in the range of reports for single-agent estramustine. Prolongation of disease-specific survival remains to be demonstrated. Of interest, prolongation of disease-specific survival in animals treated with GM-CSF gene–transduced vaccines was accomplished in a transgenic model of aggressive CaP by combining vaccination with a new therapeutic modality: anti-CTLA4 antibody. CTLA4 normally inactivates expansion of cytolytic T cells to a new antigen and has been studied as a mechanism for suppressing organ transplantation rejection. A monoclonal antibody that selectively blocks CTLA4 actually substantially augments T-cell activation and tumor-cell killing. Subtherapeutic doses of GM-CSF gene–transduced prostate vaccines can be made efficacious in mice with the combinations of CTLA4 antibody and GM-CSF gene–transduced irradiated CaP vaccines (39,40). A major new area of clinical investigation will be the combination of anti-CTLA4 antibodies or small molecule inhibitors with loaded DCs or GM-CSF gene–transduced tumor vaccines to induce longer lasting and more potent T-cell responses to CaPs.

Immunotherapy can be administered to cancer patients alone or in combination with standard chemotherapy. Many chemotherapeutic agents can suppress immune function. Nigam and colleagues screened ten cytotoxic agents representing different classes of conventional antineoplastic drugs combined with GM-CSF gene–transduced tumor cell vaccines in an animal model (41). Included in the screen were cyclophosphamide, doxorubicin, vincristine, vinblastine, etoposide, methotrexate, 5-fluorouracil, cytarabine, cisplatin, levamisole, and dexamethasone. Mice were injected subcutaneously with CT26 murine colon carcinoma cells and then were vaccinated with irradiated CT26 cells expressing GM-CSF or left unvaccinated as a control. Vaccinated mice were then also treated 1 week later with a single intraperitoneal, intravenous, or oral dose of a chemotherapeutic drug. Splenocytes were then harvested 2 weeks after vaccination and assessed for CD8+ T-cell–mediated lysis of CT26 cancer cells. Treatment with the majority of antineoplastic drugs appeared detrimental to tumor-specific CTL generation, with cyclophosphamide having the most pronounced effect. Surprisingly, doxorubicin (Adriamycin) appeared to be immunostimulatory, with increased CTL activity over the baseline. Timing of drug administration was also important, with maximal inhibition occurring when cyclophosphamide was given in conjunction with or after vaccination and maximal immunostimulation occurring when doxorubicin was given before vaccination. As most immunotherapy will require combination with conventional treatments to achieve maximal therapeutic benefit, this study demonstrates the need for a systematic review of new combinations of chemotherapy with genetically engineered immunotherapy. Nonetheless, the fact that topoisomerase II inhibitors can augment the therapeutic activity of GM-CSF gene–transduced vaccines provides strong scientific encouragement of combination therapy in minimal residual disease settings after cytoreduction with surgery, radiotherapy, and cytotoxic drugs.

CONCLUSION

In view of our limited level of understanding of the most therapeutically useful prostate antigens and ignorance of mechanisms of limiting full-blown autoimmunity, the progress made thus far in CaP immunotherapy is impressive. Several concepts are worthy of extensive large-scale clinical investigation. The time from molecular discovery to pivotal phase III trial is shorter than ever with new biotechnologies of therapeutics. Outpatient safety and the absence of a "maximum-tolerated dose" for these approaches have been the rules to date, making them both attractive to the FDA and patients alike. Preclinical models and human trials involving correlative molecular science in patients continues to provide direction for basic science. The most open question is whether a monovalent or polyvalent antigen approach will confer greatest efficacy. Further investigation is needed to rationally define the antigens most useful for sustainable clinical benefits. A critical lesson derived from the accumulation of many individual approaches is that all elements of the immune system may need to be rationally exploited—T-cells, antibodies, effectors such as NK cells, and eosinophils around the vasculature of the tumor—and all must be harnessed to provide an optimal antitumor effect. The question has changed from the early 1990s as to why do immunotherapy research in CaP to how in the twenty-first century can it scientifically realize the greatest benefit to CaP patients?

REFERENCES

1. Landis SH, Murray T, Bolden S, et al. Cancer statistics. *CA Cancer J Clin* 1999;49:8–31.
2. Hseih WS, Simons JW. Systemic therapy of prostate cancer. New concepts from prostate cancer tumor biology. *Cancer Treat Rev* 1992;19:229–260.
3. Simons JW, Mikhak B. Ex vivo gene therapy using cytokine-transduced tumor vaccines: molecular and clinical pharmacology. *Semin Oncol* 1998;25:661–676.
4. Pardoll DM. Cancer vaccines. *Nature Med* 1998;4:525–531.
5. Chang S, Bander NH, Heston WD. Monoclonal antibodies: will they become an integral part of the evaluation and treatment of prostate cancer—focus on prostate-specific membrane antigen? *Curr Opin Urol* 1999;9:391–395.
6. Nelson PS, Ng WL, Schummer M, et al. An expressed-sequence-tag database of the human prostate: sequence analysis of 1168 cDNA clones. *Genomics* 1998;47:12–25.
7. Boon T, van der Bruggen P. Human tumor antigens recognized by T lymphocytes. *J Exp Med* 1996;183:725–729.
8. Rosenberg SA. Identification of cancer antigens: impact on development of cancer immunotherapies. *Cancer J Sci Am* 2000;6(Suppl 3):S200–S207.
9. Reference deleted.
10. Disis M, Schiffman K, Gooley TA, et al. Delayed-type hypersensitivity response is a predictor of peripheral blood T-cell immunity after HER-2/neu peptide immunization. *Clin Cancer Res* 2000;6:1347–1350.
11. Sanda M, Resitfo N, Walsh JC, et al. Molecular characterization of defective antigen presentation in human prostate cancer. *J Natl Cancer Inst* 1995;87:280–285.
12. Blades R, Keating P, McWilliam L, et al. Loss of HLA class I expression in prostate cancer implications for immunotherapy. *Urology* 1995;46:681–687.
13. Steinman RM. The dendritic cell system and its role in immunogenicity. *Annu Rev Immunol* 1991:9:271–296.
14. Mellman I, Turley S, Steinman RM. Antigen processing for amateurs and professionals. *Trends Cell Biol* 1998;8:231–237.
15. Lotze M. The future role of interleukin-2 in cancer therapy. *Cancer J Sci Am* 2000;6(Suppl 1):S58–S60.
16. Pelgram M, Slamon D. Biological rationale for HER2/neu (c-erbB2) as a target for monoclonal antibody therapy. *Semin Oncol* 2000;27(Suppl 9):13–19.
17. Rosenberg S, White T. Vitiligo in patients with melanoma normal tissue antigens as targets for cancer immunotherapy. *J Immunother* 1996;19:81–84.
18. Zhang S, Zhang HS, Reuter VE, et al. Expression of potential target antigens for immunotherapy on primary and metastatic prostate cancers. *Clin Cancer Res* 1998;4:295–302.
19. Gong MC, Chang SS, Sadelain M, et al. Prostate-specific membrane antigen: present and future applications. *Urology* 2000;55:622–629.
20. Murphy GP, Ragde H, Kenny G, et al. Comparison of prostate specific membrane antigen, and prostate specific antigen levels in prostatic cancer patients. *Anticancer Res* 1995; 15:1473–1479.
21. Kawakami M, Nakayama J. Enhanced expression of prostate-specific membrane antigen gene in prostate cancer as revealed by in situ hybridization. *Cancer Res* 1997;15:2321–2324.
22. Murphy GP, Tjoa BA, Simmons SJ, et al. Infusion of dendritic cells pulsed with HLA-A2-specific prostate-specific membrane antigen peptides: a phase II prostate cancer vaccine trial involving patients with hormone-refractory metastatic disease. *Prostate* 1999;38:73–78.
23. Small EJ, Fratesi P, Reese DM, et al. Immunotherapy of hormone-refractory prostate cancer with antigen-loaded dendritic cells. *J Clin Oncol* 2000;18:3894–3903.
24. Gilboa E, Nair SK, Lyerly HK. Immunotherapy of cancer with dendritic-cell-based vaccines. *Cancer Immunol Immunother* 1998;46:82–87.
25. Slovin SF, Ragupathi G, Adluri S, et al. Carbohydrate vaccines in cancer: immunogenicity of a fully synthetic globo H hexasaccharide conjugate in man. *Proc Natl Acad Sci U S A* 1999;96:5710–5715.
26. Dranoff G, Jaffee E, Lazanby A, et al. Vaccination with irradiated tumor cells engineered to secrete murine granulocyte-macrophage colony-stimulating factor stimulates potent, specific, and long-lasting anti-tumor immunity. *Proc Natl Acad Sci U S A* 1993;90:3539–3543.
27. Soiffer R, Lynch T, Mihm M, et al. Vaccination with irradiated autologous melanoma cells engineered to secrete human granulocyte-macrophage colony-stimulating factor generates potent antitumor immunity in patients with metastatic melanoma. *Proc Natl Acad Sci U S A* 1998;95:13141–13146.

28. Simons JW, Mikhak B, Chang JF, et al. Induction of immunity to prostate cancer antigens: results of a clinical trial of vaccination with irradiated autologous prostate tumor cells engineered to secrete granulocyte-macrophage colony-stimulating factor using ex vivo gene transfer. *Cancer Res* 1999;59:5160–5168.
29. Reference deleted.
30. Dranoff G, Mulligan RC. Gene transfer as cancer therapy. *Adv Immunol* 1999;58:417–439.
31. Sanda MG, Ayyagari SR, Jaffee EM, et al. Demonstration of a rational strategy for human prostate cancer gene therapy. *J Urol* 1994;151:622–628.
32. Simons JW, Jaffee EM, Weber C, et al. Bioactivity of human GM-CSF gene transfer in autologous irradiated renal cell carcinoma vaccines. *Cancer Res* 1997;57:1537–1546.
33. Reference deleted.
34. Simons JW, Mikhak B, Chang J, et al. Clinical activity and broken immunologic tolerance from vaccination with ex vivo GM-CSF gene–transduced prostate vaccines. *Proc Am Soc Clin Oncol* 1999;40:1666.
35. Tjoa B, Erickson S, Baren R, et al. In vitro propagated dendritic cells from prostate cancer patients as a component of prostate cancer immunotherapy. *Prostate* 1995;27:63–69.
36. Lodge PA, Jones LA, Bader RA, et al. Dendritic cell-based immunotherapy of prostate cancer: immune monitoring of a phase II clinical trial. *Cancer Res* 2000;60:829–833.
37. Burch PA, Breen JK, Buckner JC, et al. Priming tissue specific cellular immunity in a phase I trial of autologous dendritic cells for prostate cancer. *Clin Cancer Res* 2000;6:2175–2182.
38. Nair SK, Heiser A, Boczkowshi D, et al. Induction of cytotoxic T cell responses and tumor immunity against unrelated tumors using telomerase reverse transcriptase RNA transfected dendritic cells. *Nature Med* 2000;6:1011–1017.
39. Hurwitz AA, Foster BA, Kwon ED, et al. Combination immunotherapy of primary prostate cancer in a transgenic mouse model using CTLA-4 blockade. *Cancer Res* 2000;60: 2444–2448.
40. Kwon ED, Foster BA, Hurwitz AA, et al. Elimination of residual metastatic prostate cancer after surgery and adjunctive cytotoxic T lymphocyte-associated antigen 4 (CTLA-4) blockade immunotherapy. *Proc Natl Acad Sci U S A* 1999;96:15074–15079.
41. Nigam A, Yacavone R, Zahurak M, et al. Immunomodulatory properties of antineoplastic drugs administered in conjunction with GM-CSF secreting cancer cell vaccines. *Int J Oncol* 1998;12:161–170.

55

COMPLEMENTARY AND ALTERNATIVE MEDICINE

BARRIE R. CASSILETH
ANDREW J. VICKERS

Complementary and alternative medicine (CAM) is now a highly visible feature of contemporary health care. No longer restricted to the lay sector, CAM practices are widespread, and use is not uncommon among patients with prostate cancer (CaP). In the United States, as in other countries in the developed world, expenditures for alternative and complementary products and services exceed billions of dollars annually. Despite broad acceptance of CAM by the public, many members of the oncology community remain ambivalent. To some extent, this is attributable to problems of inconsistent terminology and definition, which are discussed later.

This chapter describes the prevalence of CAM use in the general public, among cancer patients overall, and among men with CaP. Specific complementary and alternative therapies are reviewed, and useful and problematic regimens are described.

TERMINOLOGY OF COMPLEMENTARY AND ALTERNATIVE MEDICINE

The terminology associated with unconventional medicine continues to change over time. In a popular European definition, CAM was described as "diagnosis, treatment and/or prevention, which complements mainstream medicine by contributing to a common whole, by satisfying a demand not met by orthodoxy, or by diversifying the conceptual frameworks of medicine" (1). This definition addresses *complementary* medicine, the term commonly applied to CAM in Europe. However, it does not address *alternative* medicine, the umbrella term applied most often to unconventional therapies in the United States.

An advantage to the phrase *alternative and complementary* is that it offers the opportunity to make distinctions between the two terms. *Alternative therapies*, which typically are invasive and biologically active, are promoted as cancer treatments for use instead of mainstream therapy. Conversely, complementary therapies are used as adjuncts to mainstream care for symptom management and to enhance quality of life.

The importance of this useful distinction was validated when the National Institutes of Health changed the name of its Office of Alternative Medicine to the current Center for Complementary and Alternative Medicine and by the results of a recent survey, the largest ever conducted to determine public use of unconventional therapies (2). The study found that only 2% of people who used unconventional remedies did so to replace, rather than complement, mainstream care.

This distinction is especially important in oncology, in which "alternative" methods are promoted as literal alternatives to mainstream care, resulting in some patients' selecting unproved methods instead of surgery or other mainstream therapies after tissue biopsy diagnosis. Alternative therapies by definition are unproved. If data supported their efficacy, then they would be brought in from the fringes of medicine to become part of the standard therapeutic armamentarium.

Patients can be helped to distinguish between these two very different categories by noting proponent claims: Nonmainstream regimens and products that claim to cure cancer or that claim to establish a physiologic environment in which cancer will disappear are unproved alternatives to be avoided. Complementary therapies that address symptoms and improve well-being represent an extension of supportive care, long a needed and valued component of oncology medicine.

COMPLEMENTARY AND ALTERNATIVE MEDICINE USE IN THE GENERAL PUBLIC

Surveys in the U.S. general public show increasing CAM use over time. In 1993, one-third of a representative sample of 1,539 adults was found to use complementary or alternative therapies (3).

Two surveys published in 1997 report prevalence rates of 50% of 113 family practice patients (4) and 42% of 1,500 members of the general public (5). A 1998 publication found 42% CAM use among 2,055 people surveyed (6). Often, these surveys did not define CAM or, more typically, defined it extremely broadly, resulting in the inclusion of lifestyle activities, such as weight loss efforts, exercise, church attendance, and support activities such as group counseling, thus resulting in bloated figures for the use of CAM.

Studies with more restrictive definitions of CAM find lower prevalence rates. The 1999 survey of more than 24,000 individuals reports an 8% use of CAM (2). Prevalence in other surveys ranges from 10% (7) to approximately 30% (8). Similar figures are found for other industrialized countries, such as the United Kingdom (9), Western Europe (10), Australia (11), and Canada (12).

COMPLEMENTARY AND ALTERNATIVE MEDICINE USE AMONG CANCER PATIENTS

A recent systematic review of relevant published data (13) located 26 surveys of cancer patients from 13 countries, including five from the United States. The average prevalence of CAM use across all studies was 31%. Therapies most commonly used around the world included dietary treatments, herbs, homeopathy, hypnotherapy, imagery/visualization, meditation, megavitamins, relaxation, and spiritual healing. Subsequent investigations have reported similar findings (13,15). All but one survey conducted in the United States obtained information about specific therapies used. Patients used Laetrile, metabolic therapies, diets, spiritual healing, megavitamins, imagery, and "immune system stimulants" (13). There is some indication of increased CAM use among cancer patients in recent years (14): A secondary analysis of close to 3,000 cancer patients estimates a 64% increase since 1997 (16).

COMPLEMENTARY AND ALTERNATIVE MEDICINE USE AMONG PATIENTS WITH PROSTATE CANCER

A recent survey focused specifically on the use of CAM therapies by patients with CaP or at high risk for the disease (17). Approximately 25% of patients in outpatient clinics and 40% of those attending a support group used CAM. The most common treatments used included diets, vitamins, garlic, and saw palmetto. It is likely that use of PC-SPES ("PC" for prostate cancer and "SPES" from the Latin for hope) was not reported because this survey was conducted before publication of a major article announcing the merits of PC-SPES (18).

The prevalence of complementary therapy use in the prostate patient survey noted earlier varied significantly by medical status and was highest among men who were disease-free after radical therapy. The authors of this study urged urologists to take account of this pattern of use when assessing patients (17). The fact that approximately three-fourths of patients discussed their use of complementary therapies with their physicians suggests the importance of urologists raising the issue of CAM use.

Although research evidence is scant, the vast majority of cancer patients who use CAM seek complementary, not alternative, medicine. Approximately 8% to 10% of tissue biopsy–diagnosed cancer patients eschew mainstream therapy and seek only alternative care (19).

PHYSICIAN REFERRALS TO COMPLEMENTARY PRACTITIONERS

Data on oncologists' referrals of patients to CAM practitioners are not available and probably are extremely limited. However, generalist physicians are more likely to make such referrals. A survey conducted in Massachusetts, Washington, New Mexico, and Israel, for example, found that more than 60% of physicians had referred patients to alternative providers in the previous year (20). Primary care physicians were more likely than other specialists to use and to refer patients for complementary and alternative therapies, a finding also reported in other studies (20–22).

Referral for and delivery of CAM by doctors are probably more common abroad than in the United States. There are, for example, more than 10,000 doctors practicing homoeopathy in France and Germany and nearly 2,000 doctors practicing acupuncture in the United Kingdom (23). It is likely that application of these therapies to patients with cancer is infrequent and limited to symptom control efforts.

Even if they do not refer patients, many nononcologist physicians hold positive attitudes toward some CAM methods. A survey of 295 family physicians in the Maryland-Virginia region found that 90% view complementary therapies, such as diet and exercise, behavioral medicine, and hypnotherapy, as legitimate medical practices, although many would argue that, in fact, they are legitimate medical or lifestyle practices rather than CAM. Homeopathy, Native American medicine, and traditional Oriental medicine were not generally seen as legitimate (22).

Similar views emerged among 200 Canadian general practitioners, with chiropractic, hypnosis, and acupuncture for chronic pain perceived as effective and reflexology and homoeopathy viewed as ineffective (24). A review of twelve UK-based studies reported that British physicians perceive complementary medicine as moderately effective (25). Younger physicians seem to view CAM more favorably than their older colleagues. Data from oncologists concerning perceptions efficacy of CAM in cancer are not available.

COMPLEMENTARY AND ALTERNATIVE MEDICINE RESEARCH

There is a substantial amount of research in CAM. The registry of the Cochrane Collaboration Field in CAM (26) lists more than 4,000 randomized clinical trials of CAM therapies, a figure that doubles every 5 years (27). Eighty-four percent of trials were published in mainstream medical journals. Slightly more than 200 randomized clinical trials examined the use of CAM with cancer patients, addressing primarily treatment-related symptoms, such as pain and nausea.

Research in CAM is increasingly funded by the National Institutes of Health and conducted at mainstream medical institutions. An Office of Alternative Medicine was established at the National Institutes of Health by Congressional mandate in 1992, with its stated purpose to investigate unconventional medical practices (28). In October 1998, Congress elevated the Office of Alternative Medicine to the National Center for Complementary and Alternative Medicine, appropriating $50 million for its support. Currently, the center supports disease-specific CAM research centers.

COMPLEMENTARY AND ALTERNATIVE MEDICINE ACTIVITY IN MEDICAL SCHOOLS AND MEDICAL CENTERS

Elective courses in CAM and portions of required courses are taught in at least 75 medical schools in the United States (29). This degree of activity displays broad interest, although an academic physician's analysis of the quality of courses found that almost all present material uncritically (30).

Numerous medical centers and cancer centers have developed clinical service programs in CAM. Services range from mind-body sessions only to massage and exercise, the provision of herbs and food supplements, and, rarely, services even more removed from mainstream care, such as colonics and homeopathy. Some clinical "CAM" programs are repackaged support services, previously available to patients as spiritual care, group and individual counseling, art therapy, nutritional guidance, and so on.

INSURANCE COVERAGE OF COMPLEMENTARY AND ALTERNATIVE MEDICINE

Health insurance programs increasingly cover CAM services and providers. More than 30 major insurers, half of them Blue Cross plans, cover more than one alternative method (31,32). Coverage is most likely if the patient has a physician's prescription for that therapy. Acupuncture, massage therapy, and chiropractic services are most likely to be reimbursed.

This expanding coverage reflects not only consumer demand but also the attempt by managed care to control costs. A common as yet undocumented argument is that CAM therapies, which generally do not involve expensive pharmaceuticals or procedures, save money by decreasing drug costs and the use of conventional medicine. However, it is not clear whether CAM represents additional or substituted costs.

A Swiss health insurance company randomized patients to standard coverage or an expanded package including CAM and found no important differences in health costs or quality of life (33). Data from the Blue Cross of Washington and Alaska AlternaPath project have been reported. In 1994 and 1995, 39 cents of each benefit dollar was spent on natural products (34). In 1994, the program took in $170,000 and paid out $650,000 (35). It is believed that some of this cost overrun was due to subscribers stocking up on nutritional supplements (35).

A similar unanticipated cost overrun occurred when Blue Cross of Arizona was obliged legislatively in 1983 to cover chiropractic care. It was assumed that the competition would decrease health care costs. However, the average chiropractic case cost was $576, 8% higher than surgeon's costs and 352% higher than general practice M.D.s (36). The cost-effectiveness of chiropractic services remains a contentious and uncertain issue. These negative experiences, however, may be anomalous. Data on costs and deficits associated with other carriers are not publicly available.

ALTERNATIVE THERAPIES PROMOTED AS CANCER CURES

Many regimens are promoted as exclusive cancer treatments to be used instead of conventional care. Some of the most popular alternative techniques are noted below.

Diet Cures

Advocates and purveyors of alternative dietary cancer cures typically extend mainstream data on the protective effects of fruits, vegetables, soy, fiber, and avoidance of excessive dietary fat in reducing cancer risk to the idea that food or vitamins can cure cancer. Claims about the efficacy of diet cures are found in books with titles such as *The Food Pharmacy: Dramatic New Evidence That Food Is Your Best Medicine*, *Prescription for Nutritional Healing*, and *New Choices in Natural Healing*.

The chapter on cancer in one popular tome, *Alternative Medicine*, criticizes chemotherapy, radiation, and surgery as "highly invasive" interventions that "may shorten the patient's life" and recommends that therapy instead address the entire body and use a "non-toxic approach . . . incorporating treatments that rely on biopharmaceutical, immune enhancement, metabolic, nutritional, and herbal non-toxic methods" (37).

One popular diet promoted for decades as a cancer cure is the macrobiotic diet (38). This approach is based on the ancient Asian concept of yin-yang balance. Although macrobiotics incorporate many features of conventionally recommended diets emphasizing grains, vegetables, and fruits and minimizing fat, the macrobiotic diet is embedded in an idiosyncratic philosophy of living and a fanciful concept of human physiology and disease. This holds, for example, that blood cells are produced in the stomach, where they are birthed by a "mother red blood cell" (39).

There is no evidence that the macrobiotic diet is beneficial for patients who have been diagnosed with cancer. Moreover, versions of this diet are nutritionally deficient (40,41).

Megavitamin and Orthomolecular Therapy

Related to dietary cures is the use of nutritional supplements as primary cancer treatments, an approach that contrasts ironically with alternative medicine's emphasis on "natural" foods and therapies. Some patients and alternative practitioners believe that cancer can be cured with large dosages of vitamins—typically hundreds of pills a day—or with intravenous infusions of high-dose vitamin C.

Nobel Laureate Linus Pauling coined the term *orthomolecular therapy* in 1968 to describe the treatment of disease with large quantities of nutrients (42). Pauling claimed that massive doses of vitamin C could cure cancer, most effectively in patients who had not received chemotherapy. Two randomized trials failed to support vitamin C for cancer (43,44). Despite negative findings, high-dose vitamins and supplements remain popular among cancer patients. Perhaps the simplicity of this approach and the fact that patients can prescribe and provide their own over-the-counter therapies contribute to their appeal.

Metabolic Therapies and Detoxification

Metabolic therapies continue to draw patients from North America to the many clinics in Tijuana, Mexico. One of the best known is the Gerson clinic, which provides treatment based on the belief that toxic products of cancer cells accumulate in the liver, leading to liver failure and death. The Gerson treatment aims to counteract liver damage with a low-salt, high-potassium diet, coffee enemas, and a gallon of fruit and vegetable juice daily. Other Tijuana clinics provide their own versions of metabolic therapy, each applying individualized dietary and detoxification regimens. Additional components of treatment are included according to practitioners' preferences.

Given metabolic practitioners' belief that cancer is a symptom of the accumulation of toxins, *detoxification* is a prime aim of metabolic treatments. This often involves high colonics with infusion into the colon of 20 or more gallons of water containing herbs, coffee, enzymes, or other substances thought to be of benefit.

Neither the toxins thought to be responsible for illness nor the effects of eliminating them have been documented. Serious side effects are not uncommon. These have resulted from colonic irrigation and from other metabolic therapy techniques (45,46). The Gerson clinic's use of liquefied raw calf liver injections, for example, was suspended in 1997 after sepsis occurred in a number of patients.

Metabolic treatments are uncommon in mainstream oncology. Nicholas Gonzalez, M.D., is a rare example of an internist practicing alternative cancer medicine in the United States. He uses a version of metabolic therapy, involving a restrictive diet, pancreatic enzymes, and coffee enemas. After recent documentation of up to a 4-year survival in 11 patients with inoperable pancreatic cancer (47), the National Cancer Institute now supports a phase III clinical trial of Gonzalez regimen at the New York Presbyterian Hospital Cancer Center.

Pharmacologic and Biologic Treatments

One of the best known and most popular alternative pharmacologic therapies today is antineoplastons, developed by Stanislaw Burzynski, M.D., Ph.D., and available in his clinic in Houston, Texas. Although initial laboratory analyses found no evidence that antineoplastons normalized tumor cells (48), a limited clinical trial for pediatric patients with brain tumors was initiated as a joint effort by the National Institutes of Health Office of Alternative Medicine and the National Cancer Institute. However, it failed to accrue patients. Further research received investigational new drug permission, but preliminary data were criticized as uninterpretable and the therapy as useless and toxic (49). Burzynski and his patients continue the antineoplaston therapy and speak out in favor of its efficacy, disclaiming critics (50) and relying on anecdotal reports and some promising preliminary laboratory results (51,52).

Shark Cartilage

Interest in shark cartilage as a cancer therapy was activated by a 1992 book by I. William Lane, Ph.D., entitled *Sharks Don't Get Cancer*, and by a television special, strongly disputed by oncologists in the United States, that displayed apparent remissions in patients treated with shark cartilage in Cuba. Advocates base their therapy on its putative anti-angiogenic properties (53), but the shark cartilage protein molecules are too large to be absorbed by the gut and would be destroyed if they were absorbed. Shark cartilage actually decomposes into inert ingredients and is excreted. A recent phase I/II trial of shark cartilage found no clinical benefit (54).

Cancell

The biologic remedy Cancell appears to be especially popular in Florida and the midwestern United States. Proponents claim that it returns cancer cells to a "primitive state" from which they can be digested and rendered inert. The U.S. Food and Drug Administration laboratory studies, which showed Cancell to be composed of common chemicals, including nitric acid, sodium sulfite, potassium hydroxide, sulfuric acid, and catechol, found no basis for proponent claims of Cancell's effectiveness against cancer (55).

Bioelectromagnetics

Bioelectromagnetics is the study of interactions between living organisms and their electromagnetic fields. According to proponents, magnetic fields penetrate the body and heal damaged tissues, including cancers (37). A newly arrived treatment from Germany, BioResonance Therapy, ". . . indicates a high success rate . . . within tumor cells that allows the cell to naturally self-destruct" (56). No peer-reviewed publications could be located for any cancer-related claims regarding bioelectromagnetics.

Mind-Body Medicine

Mind-body medicine has been used widely for decades to improve quality of life for patients with cancer. However, some proponents argue that mental attributes and mind-body work can prevent or cure cancer. This belief is attractive because it ascribes to patients almost complete control over the course of their illness (57), and because it helps some patients bring meaning to the often senseless nature of their cancer (58).

A well-known proponent link between mental state and cancer is Bernie Siegel, M.D., former surgical oncologist and author of a number of popular books (59). Siegel developed groups of "exceptional cancer patients," based on his belief that mental attitude influences survival time. A study coauthored by Siegel, however, found no difference in length of survival for "exceptional cancer patients" versus controls. Patients in both groups had completed standard mainstream therapy for breast cancer (60). The results of this trial have received scant media attention and have not significantly altered proponent claims. Similarly, the results of a 1986 trial that found increased median survival for women randomized to a support group (61) was widely publicized. That study has been negated (62) but not replicated.

Attending to the psychological health of cancer patients is a fundamental component of good cancer care. Support groups, good doctor-patient relationships, and the emotional and instrumental help of family and friends is vital. However, the idea that patients can influence the course of their disease through mental or emotional work is not substantiated and can evoke feelings of guilt and inadequacy when disease continues to advance despite patients' best spiritual or mental efforts (57,58,63).

Unproved Herbal Remedies for Cancer

Essiac is a popular herbal remedy for cancer in North America. Developed initially by a Native Canadian healer (64), it was popularized by a Canadian nurse, Rene Caisse (Essiac is Caisse spelled backwards). Essiac is comprised of four herbs: burdock, turkey rhubarb, sheep sorrel, and slippery elm. The American and Canadian Cancer Societies deem it without value.

Mistletoe extracts, also known by the trade names Iscador, Helixor, and Eurixor, are popular cancer treatments in Europe and are available in some mainstream European cancer clinics. Mistletoe extracts have been subjected to randomized trials in cancer patients, although not in patients with CaP. Iscador did not increase median survival time in methodologically appropriate studies (65).

Pau d'arco tea is an old Incan Indian remedy applied against many illnesses, including cancer. Made from the bark of an indigenous South American evergreen tree, its active ingredient, lapachol, has been isolated. Although lapachol showed antitumor activity in animal studies conducted in the 1970s, it does not appear to affect human malignancies. The tea induces nausea and vomiting. Despite the absence of efficacy, pau d'arco tea is sold as a cancer remedy in health food stores, by mail, and on the Internet.

Ginkgo biloba is of proven benefit for cerebral insufficiency (66) and peripheral arterial disease (67), suggesting possible efficacy in the treatment of erectile dysfunction. Although a preliminary trial of ginkgo biloba for erectile dysfunction produced encouraging results (68), a subsequent double-blind trial found no difference between groups (69). No trial of ginkgo has examined erectile dysfunction in CaP patients, although many men with CaP self-medicate with this popular herb.

Medical Systems

Herbal, manual, and cleansing therapies drawn from several ancient medical systems, including traditional Chinese medicine, Tibetan medicine, and Ayurvedic (Indian) medicine, are used today to treat illness in developed as well as undeveloped areas of the world. Illness is seen as an imbalance in the body's internal energy (chi in traditional Chinese medicine; prana in the Ayurvedic system), and treatment aims to restore this crucial equilibrium.

Acupuncture, the traditional means manipulating that energy, is probably the most widely practiced component of traditional Chinese medicine. The value of acupuncture in treating cancer pain is not documented, but many patients rely on this technique and find it helpful.

Herbal remedies from the ancient medical systems have been minimally studied. As discussed below, however, some of these time-worn remedies show great promise.

COMPLEMENTARY THERAPIES FOR SYMPTOM CONTROL

Many unproved remedies, some harmful, others worthless, are widely available and heavily adopted by the public. However, many other products and methods are useful and can serve as beneficial adjuncts to mainstream cancer care. Complementary therapies listed in Table 55-1 have been studied and found to provide effective relief during and after cancer treatment. They include a range of adjunctive approaches such as herbal remedies, music and sound therapy, mind-body techniques, and therapeutic massage.

These therapies also offer patients the opportunity to exert control during and after cancer therapy, an important component of cancer care. These well-supported therapies produce measurable physiologic and emotional benefits. Complementary therapies, which are noninvasive, inexpensive, effective means of relieving symptoms and enhancing quality of life, should be available to assist patients through the rigors of cancer treatment and rehabilitation.

NUTRITIONAL REDUCTION OF PROSTATE CANCER RISK

Substantial data support the value of nutrition and dietary elements in preventing CaP. Many investigators observed that the incidence of CaP is substantially lower in Asian men than in Western men (70–80). Evidence suggests that dietary differences probably account for this disparity. The Western diet's dependence on animal fats, which hinder hormone modulation, and the Eastern low-fat diet emphasizing phytoestrogen-rich foods, such as soy products that balance and modify circulating hormones, are cited most frequently in this regard.

Natural estrogenic compounds found in soy, tea, fruits, and vegetables are believed to serve as chemopreventive agents. It is estimated, for example, that the average Japanese male consumes 20 times the amount of isoflavones daily than does his Western counterpart, which translates to a mean genistein plasma level of 180 ng per mL versus less than 10 ng per mL (75).

Case-control human studies, as well as animal research, document the contribution of diet to CaP prevention. A prospective study of 12,395 Seventh-Day Adventist men reported their soy milk intake in 1976. Recent analyses compared 225 men who developed CaP against the majority who did not. Frequent consumption of soy milk was associated with 70% reduction of risk for CaP (81). Data on CaP mortality and food consumption from 59 countries were obtained from the United Nations. Soy products were found to be significantly protective, with an effect four times as large as that for any other dietary factor (78). A similar but less strong relationship between phytoestrogen intake and CaP risk was reported for a smaller study (79).

Research addressing the role of dietary fat is inconsistent. A study of 328 men with CaP and 328 controls conducted in the United Kingdom failed to support the hypothesis that fat increases CaP risk (82). An interview study in Uruguay involving 175 cases and 233 controls found a relationship between total fat intake and CaP risk (83), as did an interview study conducted in 12 cities in China that compared 133 cases of CaP with 265 neighborhood controls. Dietary fat was significantly associated with increased CaP risk (80). Investigations of nutrient intake revealed polyunsaturated fats to be positively associated and vitamin E inversely associated with CaP (84). Vitamin E was associated with lowered risk of CaP in at least one other study (84).

The influence of nutritional supplements in reducing CaP risk has been studied in a number of investigations. Preliminary research suggests a role for vitamin B_6 (82,83) and vitamin C (83). Garlic was associated with reduced risk of CaP in a case-control study (82), and *in vitro* studies showed reduction of CaP cells in culture by garlic thioallyl derivatives (85) and aged garlic extract (86). An ongoing trial in China (87) will produce the first data from a randomized trial to examine the effects of garlic on cancer prevention.

Zinc, which accumulates in highest levels in the prostate (88), also may inhibit prostatic cancer cell growth (89), and lycopene, an antioxidant found in tomato products, reduced CaP risk in a case-control study (90) and in a prospective randomized trial (91).

Perhaps the most substantial body of data linking nutrients to the risk of CaP comes from studies of green tea and selenium. Green tea, made by steaming and then drying standard black tea leaves, has a long history of medicinal use in China and Japan. Epidemiologic studies suggest a preventive effect for green tea against upper gastrointestinal cancers (92).

Cell culture and animal model research documented the value of green tea and its polyphenols against CaP (93–95). Circumstantial evidence comes from China, which has the lowest incidence of CaP in the world and a population that consumes green tea on a regular basis (96). The mechanisms of green tea action appear to be the induction of apoptosis (96–101). Green tea is a component of ongoing trials to explore the preventive and therapeutic effects of diet on cancer.

In a prospective double-blind clinical trial of 1,312 people with a history of basal or squamous cell cancer of the skin, patients were randomly assigned to ingest 200 μg of selenium or a placebo daily for up to 10 years. Although selenium did not affect the incidence of recurring nonmelanoma skin cancer, it was associated with reduced cancers of all kinds and specifically with reduced incidence of CaP (102). Epidemiologic data (103,104) indicate that selenium acts as an effective chemopreventive agent against CaP, and decreased incidence of CaP was found with selenium supplementation (105,106).

TABLE 55-1. COMPLEMENTARY THERAPIES TO HELP SMOOTH THE WAY DURING CANCER TREATMENT AND RECOVERY

Anxiety and stress

Acupressure: Using the fingers of one hand to press the acupoint inside the wrist of the other hand is said to relieve nausea as well as anxiety and stress.

Aroma therapy (127): Those who find fragrance calming add a few drops of "essential oil" of rosemary, lavender, or camomile (available in health food stores and pharmacies) to the bath, or light a scented candle while relaxing.

Meditation and other relaxation techniques (128–132): Patients close their eyes and see themselves in a pleasant, peaceful place while breathing deeply and slowly. Others prefer a slightly different technique, lying down with eyes closed, consciously relaxing each body part from top to bottom. The body and mind relax accordingly.

Music Therapy (133): For many, music has important soothing physiologic as well as emotional benefits.

Therapeutic massage (134–138): Given by a licensed, certified massage therapist experienced with cancer patients or a family member gently massaging neck, shoulders, hands, and feet. Patients with lymphatic cancers should receive only light-touch massage.

Valerian (139,140): In tea or capsules form, valerian is said to reduce anxiety and induce sleep. Should be avoided by those on prescription medication for sleep or anxiety. Long-term use may cause hepatotoxicity.

Yoga (141–143): Instructional videotape and books are available in libraries and bookstores. Yoga involves practicing postures along with deep breathing techniques. Even bedridden patients can benefit.

Kava kava (144,145): A popular herb to relieve anxiety, but new evidence indicates it can cause liver damage. Avoid except under close medical supervision.

Backache or muscle ache

Capsicum cream (146): Hot red peppers contain capsaicin, a pain-relieving chemical that is the active ingredient in many rub-on pharmaceutical products. The homemade version involves adding mashed red pepper to body lotion or cold cream until the lotion turns pink. Keep away from eyes.

Hydrotherapy (147–149): A warm bath or Jacuzzi relaxes muscles.

Massage: A professional massage by a licensed, certified massage therapist or a careful, light touch massage by a friend or relative.

Willow tea: The bark of the willow tree contains salicin, the active ingredient in aspirin. Should be avoided by patients who cannot take aspirin or aspirin substitutes.

Colds and flu

Garlic: Raw or cooked garlic is an old folk remedy for colds and flu.

Echinacea (150): This herb may reduce the duration and relieve the symptoms of colds and flu. Should be avoided by those with allergy to ragweed, daisy, or sunflower.

Eucalyptus or peppermint oil (151): May be beneficial when placed in a steam vaporizer and inhaled.

Ginger: Ginger tea is said to be an effective expectorant and cough suppressant.

Iceland moss and plantain: Tea made with these herbs are old remedies for sore throats and other cold and flu problems.

Watercress tea or fresh watercress: May help treat cough and running nose.

Zinc lozenges (152–154): Studies show they may reduce the duration of colds or flu.

Constipation

Fluid extracts or capsules of cascara or buckthorn bark, a related herb, which are often found in over-the-counter laxatives.

Plantago or psyllium seed should be taken with plenty of water.

Pureed rhubarb flavored with apple juice, lemon, and honey.

Water (6–8 glasses a day) and fiber (fruit, bran cereal, prunes) consumed regularly.

Depression

Hypericum, or St. John's wort, a proven antidepressant for mild or moderate problems (155). Contraindicated for patients on any prescribed medication, especially chemotherapy or antidepressants.

Light therapy: Made specifically to reduce depression, bright-light boxes placed at eye level on a desk or table are especially effective in northern parts of the world where sunlight is rare or during winter months in the Northern Hemisphere. Light boxes are recommended by psychiatrists to treat seasonal affective disorder.

Meditation and yoga (128,129).

Tai Chi (156,157): A gentle exercise program practiced daily by millions of older Chinese. May be learned through books, videos, and classes and practiced to benefit even by bedridden patients.

Diarrhea

Agrimony or peppermint tea.

Applesauce or cooked carrots.

Dried blackberry, blueberry, or raspberry leaves.

Dried blueberry fruit.

Pulverized seeds from the herb fenugreek.

Headache

Acupressure (158): Pressing the acupoint between the eyebrows or in the hollows at the base of the skull on both sides of the spine is said to relieve headache.

Evening primrose tea, sunflower seeds, garlic, and onion are also headache remedies.

Feverfew leaf tea (159) or capsules of fresh or freeze-dried leaf are used against headache. Bay leaves may be added to enhance benefits of feverfew tea.

Progressive relaxation or massage (160): See Anxiety and stress.

Heartburn

Herb teas: especially ginger, camomile, and licorice.

Salad items: including lettuce, onion, garlic, and olives.

Walnuts.

Fennel or anise tea.

Indigestion

Peppermint or chamomile tea.

Nausea

Acupressure (161): Press inside of wrist with fingers of other hand (see Anxiety and stress).

Cinnamon or peppermint tea (162).

Ginger (163,164): Tea, capsules, or candy. Ginger ale or cookies, if made with real ginger and not flavoring.

Hypnosis (165–170).

(*continued*)

TABLE 55-1. (*continued*)

Chronic pain	Sleep problems
Acupuncture (171).	A warm bath scented with lavender oil.
Biofeedback (172,173): This requires equipment and a trained biofeedback therapist. Many pain clinics and pain management experts in hospitals use biofeedback or can make referrals.	Lemon balm herb tea.
Useful herbs: External capsicum (see Backache or muscle ache), mountain mint leaf tea applied to skin, sunflower seeds, willow bark "natural aspirin" tea (avoid by those who cannot take aspirin).	Massage (137,177).
Hypnotherapy (174–176).	Meditation (178).
Massage: See Anxiety and stress.	Tea made from fresh or dried passionflower herbs, valerian root, or chamomile.

Note: All herbs should be discontinued prior to receipt of chemotherapy (herb-drug interactions may occur), radiation therapy (skin may become sensitized), or surgery (potential for herb-anesthesia interactions and interference with coagulation).
Modified from Cassileth BR. The alternative medicine handbook: the complete reference guide to alternative and complementary therapies. New York: WW Norton, 1998.

EVIDENCE FOR NUTRITIONAL REDUCTION OF ESTABLISHED PROSTATE CANCER

Numerous anecdotal reports have led to product claims and books such as *Heal Your Prostate in 90 Days* (80,000 copies sold), but research in support of the therapeutic value of nutrition in patients diagnosed with CaP is beginning to emerge. Dietary soy significantly reduced tumor cell proliferation in mice (107), and CaP tissue in histoculture was inhibited by genistein, a major component of soy (108,109). Similarly, antioxidants such as lycopene, vitamin E, and selenium may play a major role in halting disease progression (110).

HERBAL THERAPIES

PC-SPES is the only herbal remedy for CaP subjected to clinical investigation. The therapy consists of eight herbs, all but two from traditional Chinese medicine: chrysanthemum, *Isatis*, licorice, *Ganoderma lucidum*, *Panax noto ginseng*, *Rabdosia rubescens*, saw palmetto, and *Scutellaria*. Saw palmetto inhibits 5α-reductase, licorice competes with estradiol in estrogen receptor–binding assay, and ginseng induces estrogen-regulated expression of a pS2 in cultured breast cancer cells (18).

In vitro, PC-SPES inhibits proliferation, induces apoptosis, and promotes down-regulation of bcl-6 in Mutu I cells (111). It also inhibits proliferation, reduces secreted prostate-specific antigen (PSA), and promotes down-regulation of proliferating cell nuclear antigen in LNCaP cells (112). PC-SPES has estrogenic activity (18,113) and reduces prostate tumor incidence and rate of growth in rats (114).

In an uncontrolled trial of eight patients with confirmed CaP, PC-SPES caused clinically significant decreases in testosterone and PSA (19). Side effects such as breast tenderness and loss of libido were common and similar to those associated with estrogen therapy. Reduction of PSA and estrogenlike side effects were documented in at least one additional patient on PC-SPES (114).

Research on saw palmetto provides substantial evidence that this herb can decrease the symptoms of benign prostatic hypertrophy. It improves urologic symptoms and urine flow as effectively as finasteride but with less toxicity (115). Although saw palmetto research in CaP is limited to its inclusion in the PC-SPES trial, the use of saw palmetto by CaP patients appears to be fairly common.

REGULATION OF COMPLEMENTARY AND ALTERNATIVE MEDICINE

Practitioners

Major categories of CAM practitioners outside of mainstream medicine include chiropractors, naturopaths, and acupuncturists who often practice a broader range of traditional Chinese medicine involving herbal therapeutics (116). Chiropractic training requires 4 years and prepares students to provide primary clinical services, including wellness maintenance, diagnosis of illness, and primary care, in addition to musculoskeletal care. Fifteen percent of clinical training is devoted to organ systems other than the musculoskeletal system. All 50 states plus the District of Columbia have licensure programs for chiropractors. The accrediting agency for chiropractic medicine was established in 1971, and a standardized national examination was created in 1982 (117).

Training that results in naturopathic doctoral degrees, awarded after 4 years of post-B.A. training, is designed to prepare primary care providers. Training emphasizes health promotion, disease prevention, and the use of natural remedies such as botanicals. All 11 states that license naturopaths permit the designation N.D., doctor of naturopathic medicine (118). The accrediting agency for naturopathy was established in 1978. Standardized tests were first offered in 1986.

TABLE 55-2. HERBAL PRODUCTS WITH SERIOUS TOXIC EFFECTS

Chaparral tea, promoted as an antioxidant, pain reliever, et cetera, has caused liver failure requiring liver transplantation.
Chaste tree berry, used for premenstrual syndrome, can interfere with dopamine-receptor antagonists.
Chomper, an "herbal laxative" and "cleansing" agent to be used as part of a diet regimen. The product is contaminated with digitalis.
Coltsfoot, an expectorant, and other alkaloids have been linked to liver failure.
Comfrey, ingested or used on bruises, can obstruct blood flow to the liver and possibly lead to death.
Feverfew (used for migraines, premenstrual syndrome), garlic (numerous preventive and therapeutic uses), ginger (nausea), and ginkgo (dilates arteries) can interact with anticoagulants and increase bleeding. Anticoagulant effects are possible in unusually high doses or when used in combination.
Jin bu huan, a sedative and analgesic containing morphinelike substances, can cause hepatitis and dangerously slow heart rate.
Kava, used for anxiety, can be hepatoxic.
Laxatives such as senna, cascara, and aloe can cause potassium loss when used repeatedly over time and are particularly dangerous when used with digitalis or prescription diuretics.
Licorice, used to treat peptic ulcers and as an expectorant, is contraindicated with cardiac glycosides.
Lobella, an emetic that may cause coma and death at high doses; lesser effects include rapid heartbeat and breathing problems.
Ma huang, or ephedra, an herbal form of a central nervous system stimulant commonly known as *speed*, sold with names like Herbal Ecstasy, Cloud 9, and Ultimate XPhoria.
Plantain leaves cut or powdered, found in plantain extract, nature cleanse tablets, BotaniCleanse brands, blessed herbs, and others. Contaminated with digitalis glycosides.
"Siberian ginseng" capsules: Some contain a weed comprised of male hormonelike chemicals.
Yohimbe (body builder, "enhances male performance") has caused seizures, kidney failure, and death.

Practitioners of acupuncture and herbal medicine are trained for 3 years. They learn to diagnosis disease using pulse diagnosis and other traditional Chinese medicine techniques and treat common problems with acupuncture and herbal remedies. Acupuncturists are recognized and licensed in 34 states, and three additional jurisdictions permit practice under M.D. supervision (119). Acupuncturists were accredited and their standardized national test was created in 1982.

Products

Botanical remedies are sold in many forms, including capsules, liquids, and tea leaves. They may contain one or a collection of herbs and other ingredients that typically are not described and often are unknown. Adverse events and interactions of herbs have been reported in the literature (120), as summarized in Table 55-2.

No legal standards currently exist for the processing or packaging of herbs in the United States. According to research conducted by Consumer Reports, the content of herbal remedies often differs widely from one bottle to the next, even within the same brand, as well as from claims made on the label (120a). The American Botanical Council even found that some ginseng products contain no ginseng. St. Johns wort, a popular over-the-counter antidepressant, was analyzed recently by an independent laboratory commissioned by the *Los Angeles Times*. This assay revealed that three of ten brands tested contained less than half the potency listed on the label (121).

The California Department of Health conducted an investigation of ingredients in Asian patent medicines. Unsafe levels of mercury and other toxic metals, as well as prescription drug compounds, were discovered in more than one-third of the products tested. Reports of herbal contamination in the literature include steroids in Chinese herbs (122), heart problems resulting from digitalis-contaminated supplements (123), atropine in herbal tea (124), and lead poisoning from Chinese herbs.

Quality-control standards and reviews are needed. Because they are not mandatory, however, few food supplement companies voluntarily self-impose quality evaluation and control. Consumer protection and enforcement agencies cannot provide protection against contaminated or falsely advertised products. Current federal regulations do not permit such oversight, and regulatory capability would prohibit full analysis and ongoing oversight of the estimated 20,000 food supplement items now sold over-the-counter. The lack of data on safety and efficacy and the absence of regulation represent a serious problem that government agencies are now attempting to redress. Given the opposition to regulation of related industries, this is expected to be an uphill battle.

INFORMATION ABOUT COMPLEMENTARY AND ALTERNATIVE MEDICINE

Information available to the public and health professional varies widely in accuracy. Many web sites and publications that appear to be objective are actually sponsored by commercial enterprises that promote and sell the products on which they report.

One apparently common source of information for patients is health food stores (125). A study in which a researcher visited health stores reporting symptoms associated with serious pathology found that the majority of store clerks recommended specific unproven treatments and usually did not suggest consultation with a physician (126).

It is often difficult for patients to distinguish between reputable sources of information and those that present vested interests. Some promotional material and books are

TABLE 55-3. REPUTABLE SOURCES OF COMPLEMENTARY AND ALTERNATIVE MEDICINE (CAM) INFORMATION

Databases
- Medline should be searched using explode "alternative medicine." Herbs can be found by using explode "plants, medicinal" and "drugs, Chinese herbal." The Cochrane Library has many systematic reviews on CAM therapies. It also contains a registry of randomized trials of CAM: use the keyword "COMPMED."

Cancer-specific web sites
- American Association for Cancer Research: http://www.aacr.org
- American Cancer Society: http://www.cancer.org
- Association of Community Cancer Centers: http://www.assoccancer-ctrs.org
- CancerGuide by Steve Dunn: http://cancerguide.org
- CancerNet: a service of the National Cancer Institute: http://www.cancernet.nci.nih.gov/
- Office of Alternative Medicine: http://nccam.nih.gov/
- Oncolink (University of Pennsylvania Cancer Center): http://www.oncolink.org
- St. Jude Children's Research Hospital: http://www.stjude.org
- Tufts University: http://www.altmedicine.com/
- University of Texas Center for Alternative Medicine Research in Cancer: http://sph.uth.tmc.edu/utcam/reslnk.htm

Herb and other food supplement web sites
- American Botanical Council: http://www.herbalgram.org
- Medicinal Herbalism: A Journal for the Clinical Practitioner: http://www.medherb.com
- Pharmaceutical Information Network: http://pharminfo.com
- U.S. Pharmacopoeia Consumer Information (Botanicals): http://www.usp.org/

Regulatory and government agency sites
- U.S. Food and Drug Administration: http://www.fda.gov
- NIH Medline Search: http://www.medscape.com
- National Institutes of Health: http://www.nih.gov

Alternative and unproved methods websites
- National Council Against Health Fraud: http://www.ncahf.org
- Quackwatch: http://www.quackwatch.com

General CAM information
- National Institutes of Health Center for Complementary and Alternative Medicine: http://altmed.od.nih.gov/
- Natural Health Village: http://www.netvillage.com/
- HealthAtoZ: http://www.healthatoz.com
- Bibliographic summary of international CAM information: http://cpmcnet.columbia.edu/dept/rosenthal/databases/AM_databases.html
- HealthTel Corp Links (Medical Matrix): http://www.medmatrix.org/index.asp

Recommended books
- Duke JA. *The green pharmacy*. New York: Rodale Press, 1997.
- Duke JA. *Handbook of medicinal herbs*. Fulton, Maryland: CRC Press, 1987.
- Cassileth BR. *The alternative medicine handbook: the complete reference guide to alternative and complementary therapies*. New York: WW Norton & Company, 1998.
- Tyler VE. *Herbs of choice: the therapeutic use of phytomedicinals*. London: Pharmaceutical Press, 1994.
- Tyler VE. *The honest herbal: a sensible guide to the use of herbs and related remedies*. London: Pharmaceutical Press, 1993.

written by M.D.s and appear to present legitimate information. Reputable sources of information about CAM are listed in Table 55-3.

COMPLEMENTARY AND ALTERNATIVE MEDICINE RESEARCH ISSUES

Many scientists argue against two categories of research—mainstream science and CAM. In fact, research in alternative and complementary medicine requires and deserves standard scientifically accepted research methodologies. Attaining this goal may not be easy. Some practitioners of unproved methods prefer to rely on anecdotal reports and disclaim a need for clinical trials. Simultaneously, some in mainstream science disclaim the relevance of studying complementary therapies, asserting that they are not worthy of study. The challenge for both camps is to mount and accept the results of rigorous inquiry. Recent years have seen major progress toward that goal.

REFERENCES

1. Ernst E, Resch KL, Mills S, et al. Complementary medicine—a definition. *Br J Gen Pract* 1995;45:506.
2. Druss BG, Rosenheck RA. Association between use of unconventional therapies and conventional medical services. *JAMA* 1999;282:651–656.
3. Eisenberg DM, Kessler RC, Foster C, et al. Unconventional medicine in the United States. *N Engl J Med* 1993;328:246–252.
4. Elder NC, Gillcrist A, Minz R. Use of alternative health care by family practice patients. *Arch Fam Med* 1997;6:181–184.
5. The Landmark Report, 1997. http://www.landmarkhealthcare.com.
6. Eisenberg DM, Davis RB, Ettner SL, et al. Trends in alternative medicine use in the United States, 1990–1997: results of a follow-up national survey. *JAMA* 1998;280:1569–1575.
7. Paramore LC. Use of alternative therapies: estimates from the 1994 Robert Wood Johnson Foundation National Access to Care Survey. *J Pain Sympt Manage* 1997;13:83–89.
8. Drivdahl CE, Miser WF. The use of alternative health care by a family practice population. *J Am Board Fam Prac* 1998;11:193–199.
9. Vickers A. Use of complementary therapies. *BMJ* 1994;309:1161.
10. Fisher P, Ward A. Complementary medicine in Europe. *BMJ* 1994;309:107–111.
11. MacLennan AH, Wilson DH, Taylor AW. Prevalence and cost of alternative medicine in Australia. *Lancet* 1996;347:569–573.
12. Millar WJ. Use of alternative health care practitioners by Canadians. *Can J Pub Health* 1997;88:154–158.
13. Ernst E, Cassileth BR. The prevalence of complementary/alternative medicine in cancer: a systematic review. *Cancer* 1998;83:777–782.

14. Crocetti E, Crotti N, Feltrin A, et al. The use of complementary therapies by breast cancer patients attending conventional treatment. *Eur J Cancer* 1998;34:324–328.
15. Miller M, Boyer MJ, Butow PN, et al. The use of unproven methods of treatment by cancer patients. Frequency, expectations and cost. *Support Care Cancer* 1998;6:337–347.
16. Abu-Realh MH, Magwood G, Narayan MC, et al. The use of complementary therapies by cancer patients. *Nursing Connections* 1996;9:3–12.
17. Nam RK, Fleshner N, Rakovitch E, et al. Prevalence and patterns use of complementary therapies among prostate cancer patients: an epidemiological analysis. *J Urol* 1999;161:1521–1524.
18. DiPaola RS, Zhang H, Lambert GH, et al. Clinical and biologic activity of an estrogenic herbal combination (PC-SPES) in prostate cancer. *N Engl J Med* 1998;339:785–791.
19. Cassileth BR, Lusk EJ, Strouse TB, et al. Contemporary unorthodox treatments in cancer Medicine: a study of patients, treatments and practitioners. *Ann Intern Med* 1984;101:105–112.
20. Borkan J, Neher JO, Anson O, et al. Referrals for alternative therapies. *J Fam Pract* 1994;39:545–550.
21. Perkin MR, Pearcy RM, Fraser JS. A comparison attitudes shown by general practitioners, hospital doctors, and medicine students towards alternative medicine. *J Royal Soc Med* 1994;87:523–525.
22. Berman BM, Singh BK, Lao L, et al. Physicians' attitudes toward complementary or alternative medicine: a regional survey. *J Am Board Fam Pract* 1995;8:361–366.
23. Zollman C, Vickers AJ. ABC of complementary medicine: use of complementary medicine and the doctor. *BMJ* 1999;319:1558–1561.
24. Verhoef MJ, Sutherland LR. General practitioners' assessment of and interest in alternative medicine in Canada. *Soc Sci Med* 1995;41:511–515.
25. Ernst E, Resch KL, White AR. Complementary medicine. What physicians think of it: a meta-analysis. *Arch Intern Med* 1995;155:2405–2408.
26. Ezzo J, Berman BM, Vickers AJ, et al. Complementary medicine and the Cochrane Collaboration. *JAMA* 1998;280:1628–1630.
27. Vickers AJ. Bibliometric analysis of randomised controlled trials in complementary medicine. *Complemen Ther Med* 1998;6:185–189.
28. Unconventional medical practices. Senate Appropriations Committee Report, 1992;3:141.
29. Wetzel MS, Eisenberg DM, Kaptchuk TJ. Courses involving complementary and alternative medicine at U.S. medical schools. *JAMA* 1998;280:784–787.
30. Sampson W. The need for educatinal reform in teaching about alternative therapies. *Acad Med* 2001;76:248–250.
31. Cunningham R. Perspectives: expanding coverage signals growing demand, acceptance for alternative care. *Med Health* 1998;52(Suppl):1–4.
32. Moore NG. A review of reimbursement policies for alternative and complementary therapies [news]. *Alt Ther Health Med* 1997;3:26–29.
33. Sommer JH, Burgi M, Theiss R. A randomized experiment effects of including alternative medicine in the mandatory benefit package of health insurance funds in Switzerland. *Complement Ther Med* 1999;7:54–61.
34. Weeks J. The emerging role of alternative medicine in managed care. *Drug Benefit Trends* 1997;9:14–16.
35. Jarvis W. The idea vs. the reality of "alternative" medicine. *NCAHF Newsletter* 1997;20:1–3.
36. Shekelle PG. What role for chiropractic in health care? *N Engl J Med* 1998;339:1074–1075.
37. Burton Goldberg Group. *Alternative medicine: the definitive guide*. Puyallup, WA: Future Publishing, 1993.
38. Newbold V. Complete remission of advanced medicinally incurable cancer in six patients following a macrobiotic approach to healing. *Townsend Lett* 1990;87:638–643.
39. Kushi M. *The macrobiotic approach to cancer*. Wayne, NJ: Avery Publishing Group, 1982.
40. Dagnelie PC, van Staveren WA, van Dusseldorp M. Balancieren zwischen zuviel und zuwenig: Nahrstoffmangel und Aufholwachstum bei vegetarisch ernahrten Kindern. *Erfahrungsheilkunde* 1998;47:477–482.
41. Chitgau R. Beth Ann and macrobioticism. In: Wolfe T, Johnson EW, eds. *The New Journalism*. New York: Harper & Row, 1973.
42. Pauling L, Rath M. An orthomolecular theory of human health and disease. *J Orthomol Med* 1991;6:135–138.
43. Creagan ET, Moertel CG, O'Fallon JR, et al. Failure of high-dose vitamin C (ascorbic acid) therapy to benefit patients with advanced cancer. A controlled trial. *N Engl J Med* 1979;301:687–690.
44. Moertel CG, Fleming TR, Creagan ET, et al. High-dose vitamin C versus placebo in the treatment of patients with advanced cancer who have had no prior chemotherapy. A randomized double-blind comparison. *N Engl J Med* 1985; 312:137–141.
45. Istre GR, Kreiss K, Hopkins RS, et al. An outbreak of amebiasis spread by colonic irrigation at a chiropractic clinic. *N Engl J Med* 1982;307:339–342.
46. Eisele JW, Reay DT. Deaths related to coffee enemas. *JAMA* 1980;244:1608–1609.
47. Gonzalez NJ, Issacs LL. Evaluation of pancreatic proteolytic enzyme treatment of adenocarcinoma pancreas with nutrition and detoxification support. *Nutrition and Cancer* 1999; 33:117–124.
48. Green S. Antineoplastons: an unproved cancer therapy. *JAMA* 1992;267:2924–2928.
49. Anonymous. Experts say interpretable results unlikely in Burzynski's antineoplastons studies. *Cancer Lett* 1998;24:1–16.
50. Burzynski S. Antineoplastons in cancer patients with 5-year follow-up. *Townsend Lett* 1988;56:65–67.
51. Harrison LE, Wojciechowicz DC, Brennan MF, et al. Phenylacetate inhibits isoprenoid biosynthesis and suppresses growth of human pancreatic carcinoma. *Surgery* 1998;124: 541–550.
52. Tsuda H, Sata M, Kumabe T, et al. Quick response of advanced cancer to chemoradiation therapy with antineoplastons. *Oncol Rep* 1998;5:597–600.
53. American Cancer Society. Shark cartilage/angiogenesis. Atlanta: American Cancer Society, report no. 8100, 1992.
54. Miller DR, Anderson GT, Stark JJ, et al. Phase I/II trial safety and efficacy of shark cartilage in the treatment of advanced cancer. *J Clin Oncol* 1998;16:3649–3655.
55. American Cancer Society. Complementary and alternative methods. http://www.cancer.org/alt_therapy/index.html.

56. National Center for Complementary and Alternative Medicine. http://altmed.od.nih.gov/.
57. Cassileth BR. Mental health quackery in cancer treatment. *Int J Ment Health* 1990;19:81–84.
58. Vickers AJ. Against mind-body medicine. *Complementary Ther Med* 1998;6:111–114.
59. Siegel BS. *Love, medicine, and miracles: lessons learned about self-healing from a surgeon's experience.* New York: Harper & Row, 1986.
60. Gellert GA, Maxwell RM, Siegel BS. Survival of breast cancer patients receiving adjunctive psychosocial support therapy: a 10-year follow-up study. *J Clin Oncol* 1993;11:66–69.
61. Spiegel D, Bloom JR, Kraemer HC, et al. Effect of psychosocial treatment on survival of patients with metastatic breast cancer. *Lancet* 1989;2:888–891.
62. Cunningham AJ, Edmonds CV, Lockwood GA. A careful investigation of an important phenomenon. *Psychooncology* 1999;8:364–366.
63. Angell M. Disease as a reflection psyche. *N Engl J Med* 1985;312:1570–1572.
64. LeMoine L. Essiac: an historical perspective. *Can Oncol Nurs J* 1997;7:216–221.
65. Dold U, Edler L, Mäurer HC, et al. *Krebszusatztherapie beim fortgeschrittenen nicht-kleinzelligen Bronchialkarzinom.* Stuttgart: Georg Thieme Verlag, 1991.
66. Hopfenmuller W. Evidence for a therapeutic effect of ginkgo biloba special extract. Meta-analysis of 11 clinical studies in patients with cerebrovascular insufficiency in old age. *Arzneimittel Forschung* 1994;44:1005–1013.
67. Schneider B. Ginkgo biloba extract in peripheral arterial diseases. Meta-analysis of controlled clinical studies. *Arzneimittel Forschung* 1992;42:428–436.
68. Sikora R, Sohn MH, Deutz FJ, et al. Ginkgo biloba extract in the therapy of erectile dysfunction. *J Urol* 1989;141: 188A.
69. Sikora R, Sohn MH, Engelke B, et al. Randomized placebo-controlled study on the effects of oral treatment with ginkgo biloba extract in patients with erectile dysfunction. *J Urol* 1998;159:240A.
70. Stephens FO. The rising incidence of breast cancer in women and prostate cancer in men. Dietary influences: a possible preventive role for nature's sex hormone modifiers—the phytoestrogens [Review]. *Oncol Rep* 1999;6:865–870.
71. Moyad MA. Soy, disease prevention, and prostate cancer. *Semin Urol Oncol* 1999;17:97–102.
72. Kamat AM, Lamm DL. Chemoprevention of urological cancer. *J Urol* 1999;161:1748–1760.
73. Thomas JA. Diet, micronutrients, and the prostate gland. *Nutr Rev* 1999;57:95–103.
74. Fair WR, Fleshner NE, Heston W. Cancer prostate: a nutritional disease? *Urology* 1997;50:840–848.
75. Griffiths K, Morton MS, Denis L. Certain aspects of molecular endocrinology that relate to the influence of dietary factors on the pathogenesis of prostate cancer. *Eur Urol* 1999;35:443–455.
76. Denis L, Morton MS, Griffiths K. Diet and its preventive role in prostatic disease. *Eur Urol* 1999;35:377–387.
77. Yip I, Heber D, Aronson W. Nutrition and prostate cancer. *Urol Clin North Am* 1999;26:403–411.
78. Hebert JR, Hurley TG, Olendzki BC, et al. Nutritional and socioeconomic factors in relation to prostate cancer mortality: a cross-national study. *J Natl Cancer Inst* 1998;90:1637–1647.
79. Strom SS, Yamamura Y, Duphorne CM, et al. Phytoestrogen intake and prostate cancer: a case-control study using a new database. *Nutr Cancer* 1999;33:20–25.
80. Lee MM, Wang RT, Hsing AW, et al. Case-control study of diet and prostate cancer in China. *Cancer Causes Control* 1998;9:545–552.
81. Jacobsen BK, Knutsen SF, Fraser GE. Does high soy milk intake reduce prostate cancer incidence? The Adventist Health Study. *Cancer Causes Control* 1998;9:553–557.
82. Key TJ, Silcocks PB, Davey GK, et al. A case-control study of diet and prostate cancer. *Br J Cancer* 1997;76:678–687.
83. Deneo-Pellegrini H, De Stefani E, Ronco A, et al. Foods, nutrients, and prostate cancer: a case-control study in Uruguay. *Br J Cancer* 1999;80:591–597.
84. Tzonou A, Signorello LB, Lagiou P, et al. Diet and cancer prostate: a case-control study in Greece. *Int J Cancer* 1999;80:704–708.
85. Pinto JT, Qiao C, Xing J, et al. Effects of garlic thioallyl derivatives on growth, glutathione concentration, and polyamine formation of human prostate carcinoma cells in culture. *Am J Clin Nutr* 1997;66:398–405.
86. Sigounas G, Hooker J, Anagnostou A, et al. S-allylmercaptocysteine inhibits cell proliferation and reduces the viability of erythroleukemia, breast, and prostate cancer cell lines. *Nutr Cancer* 1997;27:186–191.
87. Lian Z, Jun Ling M, Wei Dong L. A randomized multi-intervention trial to inhibit gastric cancer in Shandong. *Chinese J Clin Oncol* 1998;25:338–340.
88. Costello LC, Franklin RB. Novel role of zinc in the regulation of prostate citrate metabolism and its implications in prostate cancer. *Prostate* 1998;35:285–296.
89. Liang JY, Liu YY, Zou J, et al. Inhibitory effect of zinc on human prostatic carcinoma cell growth. *Prostate* 1999;40: 200–207.
90. Rao AV, Fleshner N, Agarwal S. Serum and tissue lycopene and biomarkers of oxidation in prostate cancer patients: a case-control study. *Nutr Cancer* 1999;33:159–164.
91. Gann PH, Ma J, Giovannucci E, et al. Lower prostate cancer risk in men with elevated plasma lycopene levels: results of a prospective analysis. *Cancer Res* 1999;59:1225–1230.
92. Gao YT, McLaughlin JK, Blot WJ, et al. Reduced risk of esophageal cancer associated with green tea consumption. *J Natl Cancer Inst* 1994;86:855–858.
93. Huang MT, Ho CT, Wang ZY, et al. Inhibitory effect of topical application of a green tea polyphenol fraction on tumor initiation and promotion in mouse skin. *Carcinogenesis* 1992;13:947–954.
94. Oguni I, Nasu K, Yamamoto S, et al. On the antitumor activity of fresh green tea leaf. *Agric Biol Chem* 1988;52:1879–1880.
95. Gupta S, Ahmad N, Mohan RR, et al. Prostate cancer chemoprevention by green tea. *Cancer Res* 1999;59:2115–2120.
96. Gupta S, Ahmad N, Mukhtar H. Prostate cancer chemoprevention by green tea. *Semin Urol Oncol* 1999;17:70–76.
97. Paschka AG, Butler R, Young CY. Induction of apoptosis in prostate cancer cell lines by the green tea component, (-)-epigallocatechin-3-gallate. *Cancer Lett* 1998;130:1–7.

98. Ahmad N, Feyes DK, Nieminen AL, et al. Green tea constituent epigallocatechin-3-gallate and induction of apoptosis and cell cycle arrest in human carcinoma cells. *J Natl Cancer Inst* 1997;89:1881–1886.
99. Kennedy DO, Matsumoto M, Kojima A, et al. Cellular thiols status and cell death in the effect of green tea polyphenols in Ehrlich ascites tumor cells. *Chem Biol Interact* 1999;122:59–71.
100. Liao S, Umekita Y, Guo J, et al. Growth inhibition and regression of human prostate and breast tumors in athymic mice by tea epigallocatechin gallate. *Cancer Lett* 1995;96: 239–243.
101. Liao S, Hiipakka RA. Selective inhibition of steroid 5 alpha-reductase isozymes by tea epicatechin-3-gallate and epigallocatechin-3-gallate. *Biochem Biophys Res Commun* 1995;214: 833–838.
102. Combs GF Jr., Clark LC, Turnbull BW. Reduction of cancer risk with an oral supplement of selenium. *Biomed Environ Sci* 1997;10:227–234.
103. Nelson MA, Porterfield BW, Jacobs ET, et al. Selenium and prostate cancer prevention. *Semin Urol Oncol* 1999;17:91–96.
104. Kelloff GJ, Lieberman R, Steele VE, et al. Chemoprevention of prostate cancer: concepts and strategies. *Eur Urol* 1999;35:342–350.
105. Yoshizawa K, Willett WC, Morris SJ, et al. Study of prediagnostic selenium level in toenails and the risk of advanced prostate cancer. *J Natl Cancer Inst* 1998;90:1219–1224.
106. Clark LC, Dalkin B, Krongrad A, et al. Decreased incidence of prostate cancer with selenium supplementation: results of a double-blind cancer prevention trial. *Br J Urol* 1998;81: 730–734.
107. Zhou JR, Gugger ET, Tanaka T, et al. Soybean phytochemicals inhibit the growth of transplantable human prostate carcinoma and tumor angiogenesis in mice. *J Nutr* 1999; 129:1628–1635.
108. Geller J, Sionit L, Partido C, et al. Genistein inhibits the growth of human-patient BPH and prostate cancer in histoculture. *Prostate* 1998;34:75–79.
109. Messina M, Bennink M. Soyfoods, isoflavones, and risk of colonic cancer: a review in vitro and in vivo data. *Baillieres Clin Endocrinol Metab* 1998;12:707–728.
110. Fleshner NE, Klotz LH. Diet, androgens, oxidative stress, and prostate cancer susceptibility. *Cancer Metastasis Rev* 1998;17: 325–330.
111. Hsieh TC, Ng C, Chang CC, et al. Induction of apoptosis and down-regulation of bcl-6 in mutu I cells treated with ethanolic extracts Chinese herbal supplement PC-SPES. *Int J Oncol* 1998;13:1199–1202.
112. Hsieh T, Chen SS, Wang X, et al. Regulation of androgen receptor (AR) and prostate specific antigen (PSA) expression in the androgen-responsive human prostate LNCaP cells by ethanolic extracts Chinese herbal preparation PC-SPES. *Biochem Mol Biol Int* 1997;42:535–544.
113. Moyad MA, Pienta KJ, Montie JE. Use of PC-SPES, a commercially available supplement for prostate cancer, in a patient with hormone-naïve disease. *Urology* 1999;54:319–323.
114. Tiwari RK, Geliebter J, Garikapaty VP, et al. Anti-tumour effects of PC-SPES, an herbal formulation in prostate cancer. *Int J Oncol* 1999;14:713–719.
115. Wilt TJ, Ishani A, Stark G, et al. Saw palmetto extracts for treatment of benign prostatic hyperplasia: a systematic review. *JAMA* 1998;280:1604–1609.
116. Cooper RA, Henderson T, Dietrich CL. Roles of nonphysician clinicians as autonomous providers of patient care. *JAMA* 1998;280:795–802.
117. American Chiropractic Association. *Chiropractic: state art.* Arlington, Virginia: American Chiropractic Association, 1994.
118. Weeks J. *Integration strategies for natural healthcare.* http:// www.anma.com 19 July 2001.
119. Ergil KV. Acupuncture licensure, training, and certification in the United States. In: *NIH consensus development conference on acupuncture.* Bethesda, Maryland: National Institutes of Health, 1997.
120. Miller LG. Herbal medicinals: selected clinical considerations focusing on known or potential drug-herb interactions. *Arch Intern Med* 1998;158:2200–2211.

120a. Consumer report: herbal Rx: the promises and pitfalls. *Consumer Reports* 1999;64(3):44–48.

121. Monmaney T. Remedy's sales zoom, but quality control lags; St. John's wort: regulatory vacuum leaves doubt about potency, effects of herb used for depression. *Los Angeles Times* 1998:A1.
122. Graham-Brown RA, Bourke JF, Bumphrey G. Chinese herbal remedies may contain steroids. *BMJ* 1994;308:473.
123. Slifman NR, Obermeyer WR, Aloi BK, et al. Contamination of botanical dietary supplements by *digitalis lanata. N Engl J Med* 1998;339:806–811.
124. Routledge PA, Spriggs TL. Atropine as possible contaminant of comfrey tea. *Lancet* 1989;1:963–964.
125. Worsley A. Perceived reliability of sources of health information. *Health Educ Res* 1989;4:367–376.
126. Vickers AJ, Rees RW, Robin A. Advice given by health food shops: is it clinically safe? *J R Coll Physicians Lond* 1998;32: 426–428.
127. Wilkinson S. Aromatherapy and massage in palliative care. *Int J Pall Nurs* 1995;1:21–30.
128. Bindemann S, Soukop M, Kaye SB. Randomised controlled study of relaxation training. *Eur J Cancer* 1991;27:170–174.
129. Bridge LR, Benson P, Pietroni PC, et al. Relaxation and imagery in the treatment of breast cancer. *BMJ* 1988;297: 1169–1172.
130. Burish TG, Lyles JN. Effectiveness of relaxation training in reducing adverse reactions to cancer chemotherapy. *J Behav Med* 1981;4:65–78.
131. Vasterling J, Jenkins RA, Tope DM, et al. Cognitive distraction and relaxation training for the control of side effects due to cancer chemotherapy. *J Behav Med* 1993;16:65–80.
132. Arakawa S. Use of relaxation to reduce side effects of chemotherapy in Japanese patients. *Cancer Nurs* 1995;18:60–66.
133. Beck SL. The therapeutic use of music for cancer-related pain. *Oncol Nurs Forum* 1991;18:1327–1337.
134. Corner J, Cawley N, Hildebrand S. An evaluation use of massage and essential oils on the well-being of cancer patients. *Int J Pall Nurs* 1995;1:67–73.
135. Weinrich SP, Weinrich MC. The effect of massage on pain in cancer patients. *Applied Nurs Res* 1990;3:140–145.

136. Field T, Morrow C, Valdeon C, et al. Massage reduces anxiety in child and adolescent psychiatric patients. *J Am Acad Child Adolesc Psychiat* 1992;31:125–131.
137. Stevensen C. The psychophysiological effects of aromatherapy massage following cardiac surgery. *Complement Ther Med* 1994;2:27–35.
138. Fraser J, Kerr JR. Psychophysiological effects of back massage on elderly institutionalized patients. *J Advanc Nurs* 1993;18:238–245.
139. Gerhard U, Linnenbrink N, Georghiadou C, et al. Vigilance-decreasing effects of 2 plant-derived sedatives. *Schweizerische Rundschau Medicineizin Praxis* 1996;85:473–481.
140. Lindahl O, Lindwall L. Double blind study of a valerian preparation. *Pharmacol Biochem Behav* 1989;32:1065–1066.
141. Wood C. Mood change and perceptions of vitality: a comparison effects of relaxation, visualization, and yoga. *J R Society Med* 1993;86:254–258.
142. Panjwani U, Gupta HL, Singh SH, et al. Effect of Sahaja yoga practice on stress management in patients of epilepsy. *Indian J Physiol Pharmacol* 1995;39:111–116.
143. Latha D, Kaliappan KV. Efficacy of yoga therapy in the management of headaches. *J Indian Psychol* 1992;10:41–47.
144. Kinzler E, Kromer J, Lehmann E. Effect of a special kava extract in patients with anxiety-, tension-, and excitation states of non-psychotic genesis. Double blind study with placebos over 4 weeks. *Arzneimittel Forschung* 1991;41:584–588.
145. Volz HP, Kieser M. Kava-kava extract WS 1490 versus placebo in anxiety disorders—a randomized placebo-controlled 25-week outpatient trial. *Pharmacopsychiatry* 1997;30:1–5.
146. Puett DW, Griffin MR. Published trials of nonmedicinal and noninvasive therapies for hip and knee osteoarthritis. *Ann Intern Med* 1994;121:133–140.
147. Konrad K, Tatrai T, Hunka A, et al. Controlled trial of balneotherapy in treatment of low back pain. *Ann Rheum Dis* 1992;51:820–822.
148. Guillemin F, Constant F, Collin JF, et al. Short and long-term effect of spa therapy in chronic low back pain. *Br J Rheum* 1994;33:148–151.
149. Constant F, Guillemin F, Collin JF, et al. Use of spa therapy to improve the quality of life of chronic low back pain patients. *Med Care* 1998;36:1309–1314.
150. Melchart D, Linde K, Fischer P. Echinacea for the prevention and treatment of the common cold (Cochrane review). In: *The Cochrane library*, Issue 4, 1998.
151. Zalewski P, Olszewski J, Olszewska Ziaber A, et al. Clinical evaluation of olbas oil effect on nasal mucosa in acute rhinitis patients during common cold. *Otolaryngologia Polska* 1997;51[Suppl 25]:312–314.
152. Godfrey JC, Godfrey NJ, Novick SG. Zinc for treating the common cold: review of all clinical trials since 1984. *Altern Ther Health Med* 1996;2:63–72.
153. Mossad SB, Macknin ML, Medendorp SV, et al. Zinc gluconate lozenges for treating the common cold. A randomized double-blind placebo-controlled study. *Ann Intern Med* 1996;125:81–88.
154. Macknin ML, Piedmonte M, Calendine C, et al. Zinc gluconate lozenges for treating the common cold in children: a randomized controlled trial. *JAMA* 1998;279:1962–1967.
155. Linde K, Ramirez G, Mulrow CD, et al. St John's Wort for depression—an overview and meta-analysis of randomised clinical trials. *BMJ* 1996;313:253–258.
156. Jin P. Efficacy of Tai Chi, brisk walking, meditation, and reading in reducing mental and emotional stress. *J Psychosom Res* 1992;36:361–370.
157. Kutner NG, Barnhart H, Wolf SL, et al. Self-report benefits of Tai Chi practice by older adults. *J Gerontol Psychologic Sci Soc Sci* 1997;52:242–246.
158. Pikoff H. The effects of acupressure on headache pain: a placebo-controlled group outcome study. *Diss Abst Int* 1990;50:5890.
159. Vogler BK, Pittler MH, Ernst E. Feverfew as a preventative treatment for migraine: a systematic review. *Cephalalgia* 1998;18:704–708.
160. Bogaards MC, ter Kuile MM. Treatment of recurrent tension headache: a meta-analytic review. *Clin J Pain* 1994;10:174–190.
161. Vickers AJ. Can acupuncture have specific effects on health? A systematic review of acupuncture antiemesis trials. *J R Soc Med* 1996;89:303–311.
162. Tate S. Peppermint oil: a treatment for postoperative nausea. *J Advanc Nurs* 1997;26:543–549.
163. Bone ME, Wilkinson DJ, Young JR, et al. Ginger root—a new antiemetic. The effect of ginger root on postoperative nausea and vomiting after major gynaecological surgery. *Anaesthesia* 1990;45:669–671.
164. Visalyaputra S, Petchpaisit N, Somcharoen K, et al. The efficacy of ginger root in the prevention of postoperative nausea and vomiting after outpatient gynaecological laparoscopy. *Anaesthesia* 1998;53:506–510.
165. Jacknow DS, Tschann JM, Link MP, et al. Hypnosis in the prevention of chemotherapy-related nausea and vomiting in children: a prospective study. *J Develop Behav Pediatr* 1994;15:258–264.
166. Morrow GR, Morrell C. Behavioral treatment for the anticipatory nausea and vomiting induced by cancer chemotherapy. *N Engl J Med* 1982;307:1476–1480.
167. Troesch LM, Rodehaver CB, Delaney EA, et al. The influence of guided imagery on chemotherapy-related nausea and vomiting. *Oncol Nurs Forum* 1993;20:1179–1185.
168. Cotanch PH, Strom S. Progressive muscle relaxation as antiemetic therapy for cancer patients. *Oncol Nurs Forum* 1987;14:33–37.
169. Holli K. Ineffectiveness of relaxation on vomiting induced by cancer chemotherapy. *Eur J Cancer* 1993;29:1915–1916.
170. Arakawa S. Use of relaxation to reduce side effects of chemotherapy in Japanese patients. *Cancer Nurs* 1995;18:60–66.
171. Melchart D, Linde K, Fischer P, et al. Acupuncture for recurrent headaches: a systematic review of randomized controlled trials. *Cephalalgia* 1999;19:779–786.
172. Newton-John TR, Spence SH, Schotte D. Cognitive-behavioural therapy versus EMG biofeedback in the treatment of chronic low back pain. *Behav Res Ther* 1995;33:691–697.

173. Dalen K, Ellertsen B, Espelid I, et al. EMG feedback in the treatment of myofascial pain dysfunction syndrome. *Acta Odontologica Scandinavica* 1986;44:279–284.
174. Spiegel D, Bloom JR. Group therapy and hypnosis reduce metastatic breast carcinoma pain. *Psychosom Med* 1983; 45:333–339.
175. Sellick SM, Zaza C. Critical review of five nonpharmacologic strategies for managing cancer pain. *Cancer Prevent Control* 1998;2:7–14.
176. NIH Technology Assessment Panel. Integration of behavioral and relaxation approaches into the treatment of chronic pain and insomnia. *JAMA* 1996;276:313–318.
177. Richards KC. Effect of a back massage and relaxation intervention on sleep in critically ill patients. *Am J Crit Care* 1998;7:288–299.
178. McClusky HY, Milby JB, Switzer PK, et al. Efficacy of behavioral versus triazolam treatment in persistent sleep-onset insomnia. *Am J Psychiat* 1991;148:121–126.

INDEX

Note: Page numbers followed by *f* indicate figures, and page numbers followed by *t* indicate tables.

B

S

T